Geriatric Rehabilitation

A Clinical Approach

Jennifer M. Bottomley, PT, MS, PhD
Geriatric Rehabilitation Program Consultant
Wayland, MA

Carole B. Lewis, PT, GCS, MSG, MPA, PhD
President
Physical Therapy Services of Washington

Adjunct Associate Professor
George Washington University
College of Medicine
School of Health Care Sciences
Washington, DC

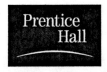

Upper Saddle River, New Jersey 07458

Library of Congress Cataloging-in-Publication Data

Bottomley, Jennifer M.
  Geriatric rehabilitation : a clinical approach / Jennifer M.
Bottomley, Carole B. Lewis.— 2nd ed.
     p.   cm.
  Rev. ed. of: Geriatric physical therapy / Carole B. Lewis,
Jennifer M. Bottomley. c1994.
  Includes bibliographical references and index.
  ISBN 0-8385-2284-X
  1. Physical therapy for the aged. 2. Aged—Rehabilitation.
    [DNLM: 1. Physical Therapy Techniques—Aged. 2. Aging. 3. Geriatric
Assessment. 4. Rehabilitation—Aged. WB 460 B751g 2003] I. Lewis,
Carole Bernstein. II. Lewis, Carole Bernstein. Geriatric physical
therapy. III. Title.
RC953.8.P58 L479 2003
615.8'2'0846—dc21
                                                    2002002685

Publisher: *Julie Levin Alexander*
Executive Assistant: *Regina Bruno*
Senior Acquisitions Editor: *Mark Cohen*
Assistant Editor: *Melissa Kerian*
Editorial Assistant: *Mary Ellen Ruitenberg*
**Director of Production
  and Manufacturing:** *Bruce Johnson*
Managing Editor for Production: *Patrick Walsh*
Production Liaison: *Alexander Ivchenko*
Manufacturing Manager: *Ilene Sanford*
Manufacturing Buyer: *Pat Brown*
Creative Director: *Cheryl Asherman*
Cover Design Coordinator: *Maria Guglielmo-Walsh*
Production Management: *Pine Tree Composition*
Formatting: *Pine Tree Composition*
Marketing Manager: *Nicole Benson*
Product Information Manager: *Rachele Strober*
Printer/Binder: *Courier/Westford*
Copy Editor: *Susan Landry*
Cover Design: *Gary J. Sella*
Cover Printer: *Phoenix Color*

Notice: The authors and the publisher of this volume have taken care to make certain that the doses of drugs and schedules of treatment are correct and compatible with the standards generally accepted at the time of publication. Nevertheless, as new information becomes available, changes in treatment and the use of drugs become necessary. The reader is advised to carefully consult the instruction and information material included in the package insert of each drug or therapeutic agent before administration. This advice is especially important when using new or infrequently used drugs. The publisher disclaims any liability, loss, injury, or damage incurred as a consequence, directly or indirectly, of the use and application of any of the contents of this volume.

Pearson Education LTD.
Pearson Education Australia Pty, Limited
Pearson Education Singapore, Pte. Ltd.
Pearson Education North Asia Ltd
Pearson Education Canada, Ltd
Pearson Educación de Mexico, S.A. de C.V.
Pearson Education—Japan
Pearson Education Malaysia, Pte. Ltd
Pearson Education, Upper Saddle River, New Jersey

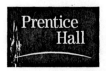

10 9 8 7 6
ISBN 0-8385-2284-X

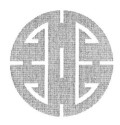

Dedication

To my Mother, who is my continual source of love, inspiration, and strength, who, loving life, continues a valiant fight against cancer . . . and to the loving memory of my Father, the rainbow on the horizon after the rain has passed and the brightest star in my sky, whose influence on my life inspired my desire for knowledge and learning, and my professional growth and direction in geriatric practice.

Jennifer M. Bottomley

With enthusiasm for the new millennium and the changes that this momentous time foreshadows, I dedicate this book to my children, Madison and Gerald, who will live well into this century, and possibly into the next. Your growth has paralleled that of the healthcare industry that has warranted the publication of this revised edition. At the publication of the first edition, Madison, you were but an infant, and you, Gerald, but a thought. Geriatric rehabilitation was also in its infancy, but the eight intervening years have seen remarkable developments. As you both continue to expand your horizons, I wish you a bright future full of promise, joy, and success.

Carole B. Lewis

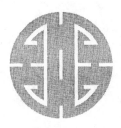

About the Cover

Eastern cultures are known for their respectful treatment of the elderly, who are valued members of their society. A long and healthy life is desirable, as well as attainable. It is with this image and idea that we selected the symbol that appears on the cover as well as throughout the pages of *Geriatric Rehabilitation: A Clinical Approach*. As you read this book, and learn from it, we hope that respect and care will always be a part of the treatment plan for your geriatric patients.

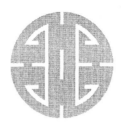

Contents in Brief

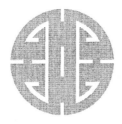

Contents in Detail

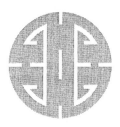

Preface

The second edition of this text adds all of the information that has been requested over the years by readers of the first edition, to enhance their practice of geriatric rehabilitation. The authors have incorporated material from the first edition and expanded each chapter to provide the most up-to-date information possible. As new research and evidence-based practice have evolved in the area of geriatrics over the past few years, much of the information in the first edition has been reviewed, substantiated, and enhanced. This edition provides a comprehensive overview of current science and practice in geriatric rehabilitation. The second edition addresses a wider scope of clinical issues than the first to meet the multiple needs of its readers in managing the geriatric patient. It is the authors' strong belief that the current and future success of geriatric practitioners lies in their ability to ground the practice of geriatric rehabilitation in the foundational sciences and in the concepts and principles of evidence-based geriatric practice.

This book was initially developed to address the need for a geriatric rehabilitation text that transcended the classical clinical and academic texts currently available. The many professions involved in geriatric rehabilitation have evolved rapidly in the past decade, but textbooks have not kept pace with the need for specialized clinical information. With the inauguration of a geriatric specialty examination in rehabilitation therapies, the need became more pressing. This book is designed to provide a single, comprehensive source for the advanced applied science of normal and pathological aging, clinical problems, implications for therapeutic interventions, and considerations specific to the elderly.

The main objective of this textbook is to present therapists with a thorough review of advanced clinical information. The targeted audience for this text is clinicians already exposed to geriatric patients who seek to improve their background and skill level. In addition, advanced master's and doctoral students seeking specific clinical information will find relevant material in the text.

At the time the first edition of this text went into publication, a small group of rehabilitation therapists had successfully passed the first geriatric specialty exam. Many of these therapists, however, had difficulty locating up-to-date information to prepare for the exam, or finding a comprehensive source of information. The authors believe this text addresses both of these criteria.

Both of the authors have worked extensively in the field of geriatrics. They have combined their knowledge to provide clinical information that is grounded in the literature and research-based references.

The text is divided into three parts. Part I provides advanced applied gerontological concepts. These chapters contain the most recent background information available and provide a clinically useful basis for a sound foundation for the following two sections.

Part I covers the important areas of demographic trends in the aging population as well as theories of aging and their impact on clinical strategies. Thorough descriptions of age-related changes in the biology, physiology, anatomy, and functioning of all organ systems of the body are provided, as well as a comprehensive examination of pathological manifestations commonly seen in the aged population.

Descriptions of detailed psychological aspects of aging and a presentation of tools that can be used to evaluate and treat these conditions are provided for the clinician. Background information on assessment tools, particularly functional assessment tools, is presented to provide the reader with objective indices for thorough evaluation in a variety of settings.

Part I also incorporates a clear explanation of some of the common nutritional problems and risk factors seen in the older population, as well as a discussion on the components of good nutritional programs. An emphasis on prevention and health promotion related to dietary considerations is provided. Finally, identification of various drug regimens, adverse drug reactions, and common pathologies seen with inappropriate drug management afford a practical approach to identifying pharmacological aspects of patient intervention. As many of our elderly clients have sought alternative therapies for management of various conditions, a section on herbs, vitamins, and nutraceuticals has been added.

Part II presents a comprehensive consideration of patient care concepts. This section begins with an overview, "Principles and Practices in Geriatric Rehabilitation," which bridges the gap between the background information presented in Part I and advanced clinical concepts. Understanding the importance of immobility and disuse is emphasized. This section provides an introduction to evaluation and presents therapeutic suggestions for common problems, including treatment design and rationale.

Strategies for evaluating and treating orthopedic, neurologic, cardiopulmonary, and integumentary conditions contribute invaluable means for comprehensively addressing problems commonly seen in an elderly population. Practical suggestions guide the rehabilitation therapist in establishing and implementing health maintenance programs, such as the provision of screening programs as a means of preventive health care and early intervention to avoid the pathological consequences of "hypokinetics."

Part III covers administration and management. Effective communication with the aging population is discussed, as well as the evaluation of personal attitudes, cultural biases, ethnic considerations, and other factors relating to the care of the elderly. A discussion of educational services and objectives for the elderly with a differentiation of various learning theories applied to the older population completes this section.

Practical information is also provided on the identification and description of geriatric rehabilitation services, and includes how to address administrative needs, prepare budgets, and develop marketing proposals for nursing homes and outpatient facilities. The role of the consultant and the development of the consultative tasks for geriatric specialists are presented. A thorough discussion of methods for reviewing research includes identifying the various aspects of a research proposal and an examination of research characteristics that make clinical data collection unique for an aging population. Finally, the network of resources available for the older person, including legislative, social, and federal programs, disease-specific organizations, and research grant availability are presented in a user-friendly style. The one-stop information resource provides current contact information and internet sites for the most appropriate services.

The authors hope that this book provides a strong clinical foundation for practicing geriatric therapists, and that it will facilitate the provision of optimum care to their elderly patients.

Jennifer M. Bottomley, PT, MS, PhD

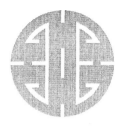

Acknowledgments

I would like to acknowledge, with gratitude, my family and friends for their patience and understanding in allowing me the time to compile materials and spend many hours/days/months in research, reading, and re-scripting this manuscript for the second edition of this text.

Jennifer M. Bottomley

PART I

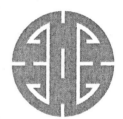

Applied Gerontological Concepts

CHAPTER 1

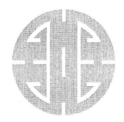

Understanding the Demographics of an Aging Population

Demography is the scientific study of the population. The demography of aging as a subfield of general demography has become increasingly important as it relates to the concerns of social gerontologists.[1] Demography continues to evolve as a fundamental knowledge base for the study of aging. The study of the demography of aging is currently focused on determining: the state of the older population; changes in the numbers, proportionate size, and composition of this subpopulation; the component forces of fertility, mortality, morbidity, migration, and immigration; and the impact of these demographic changes on issues related to the social, economic, and health status of the elderly in an aging society.[1,2]

Distinct subgroups within the older population, somewhat ignored in the past, have also been receiving increased demographic emphasis in the past few years.[3] This development appears to reflect societal concerns about the policy challenges of meeting the welfare and health needs of all components of an aging society.[4]

Gilford[5] has determined that there are serious data gaps in existing demographic information. One such data gap has been identified in the area of the subgroup termed the "oldest-old" (also called the "frail elderly" or the "extremely old"). Because of the special concerns regarding the relatively high rates of illness and disability, and the concomitant implications for health care and social service provisions in this age group, the oldest-old have been presented by demographers as a geriatric imperative for future research.[6] This trend toward specialized demographic studies is also apparent in recent analysis of a broad range of issues specific to the situations of racial and ethnic minorities[3] and older women. These areas will be dealt with more extensively in the latter sections of this chapter.

AN HISTORICAL PERSPECTIVE OF THE STUDY OF POPULATION AGING

The study of population aging has a relatively long history. Attention to population aging emerged in France at the close of the nineteenth century, when the proportion of persons aged 65 years of age and over exceeded 5%. By the 1900s, this had increased to 8%.[7] Sweden also experienced considerable population aging in the nineteenth century.[8] Sundbarg[8] was the first to place emphasis on the relative proportions of aged individuals in a society, and the first demographer to note systematic differences in age composition among countries. By implication, he hypothesized that there would be a demographic shift over time toward an aging population structure in all countries.[9]

For most western countries, the aging of the population has been a distinctly twentieth-century phenomenon. In the United States, concerted demographic attention to the aging process can be found as early as the 1920s,[10] and increasing concern was expressed in the 1930s when the declining fertility of the Depression led demographers to project rapid changes in the age structure of the United States.[11–13] It also led to a growing interest by demographers in capturing the dimensions of this phenomenon. Following World War II, there was a steady increase in the body of literature related to population aging in the United States as well as other western countries.

Today, there is an increasing awareness that population aging will be an important issue in developing countries currently experiencing social and economic growth.[14] Population aging is now recognized as a worldwide phenomenon that commands immediate attention if effective societal responses are to be made to changing demographic realities.[1] As a result, many issues have emerged, such as the degree to which countries are able to make commitments to social welfare and health care policies in light of other priorities they face in the allocation of social and economic resources.[15,16]

DEMOGRAPHIC PROCESSES AND POPULATION AGE STRUCTURE

The demographic view of aging is that it reflects an aggregative process through which the population structure is modified. It is defined in terms of the mean or median age of the population, the size and proportion of various age categories of the population, and ratios between different age categories.[1] Though these are relatively static conceptions, when they are examined over time, demographic patterns and trends begin to develop. In projecting changes in population structure, demographers focus on the rate and timing of events over the entire life course, using chronological age as a reference scale on which to measure important social transitions and identify demographic trends.

Change in the size of a population over time depends on the rate persons join the population through birth or immigration and the rate they leave the population through death or emigration. Persons born in a common year (i.e., classified by common age) are often grouped together as a birth cohort.[17] Such cohorts can be followed to reconstruct population history and to project future population change.

Traditionally, demographers have used the age of 65 for delineating old age. This facilitates standardized analyses and is grounded in social practices (e.g., retirement, Social Security provisions). In addition, because slightly more males than females are born in human populations and the mortality experiences of men and women differ, demographers typically distinguish the sex of persons in constructing models of population change.[3]

The number of persons who survive to any given age depends on the number of persons born into that cohort, the rate at which they survive, and the extent to which their numbers have changed because of cumulative differences between immigrants and emigrants. For example, the number of persons reaching the age of 65 in 1990 depended on the number of persons born in 1925; the cumulative probability that they survived each of the next sixty-five years; and the relative balance between the movement of persons from that age cohort into the United States or out of the United States from 1925 to 1990. The number of persons aged 65 and older in 1990 increased compared to the number of the elderly in 1989 because of the addition of this new cohort to the population of older persons was greater than the subtraction of persons who died in all cohorts aged 65 and older during that year.[3] The population of older persons can thus grow either because the size of the entering birth cohort is much larger than that of previous cohorts or because improvements in survivorship have reduced the number of deaths that might otherwise have occurred among the elderly. Demographers utilize the aging pyramid to graphically depict cohort distribution from year to year. Figure 1–1 shows the age structure of the US population in 1910.[18] Contrast this pyramid with the age structure of the US population in 1980 depicted in Figure 1–2 when the 1900–1910 birth cohort reached the 70 years of age and older category.[18] Figures 1–3, 1–4, and 1–5 demonstrate the significant shift in the aged population that occurred in the year 2000 (Figure 1–3) and the anticipated increase in the elderly population projected for 2025 (Figure 1–4) and 2050 (Figure 1–5). A distinction is drawn between "aging at the apex" (i.e., when the proportion of older persons in a population increases) and "aging from the base" (i.e., when the proportion of younger persons in a population decreases).

In studying the elderly population, the absolute number of older persons, the rate of change in the number of older persons, and the proportion of the total population that is old are each important demo-

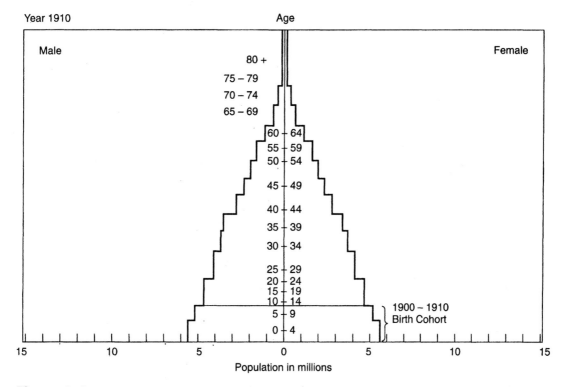

Figure 1-1. Population Pyramid Summary of Age Structure of the US Population: 1910 Census. *(Adapted from the US Bureau of the Census, 1970 Census of Population: United States Summary, General Population Characteristics, PC(1):B1, Washington, DC: US Government Printing Office; 1972. Reproduced with permission from Soldo BJ. America's elderly in 1980's. Pop Bull. 1980; 35(1):1-48.)*

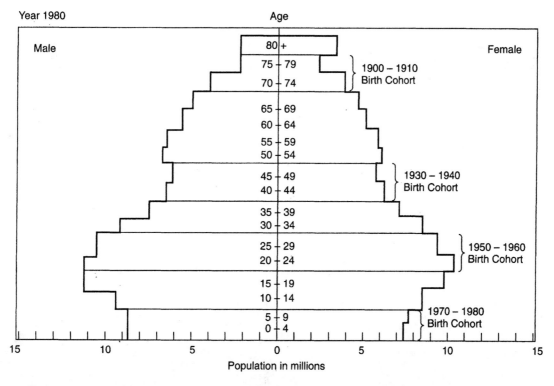

Figure 1-2. Population Pyramid Summary of Age Structure of the US Population: 1980 Census. *(Adapted from Bouvier LF. America's baby boom generation: The fateful bulge. Pop Bull. Vol. 35:1. Washington, DC: Population Reference Bureau; 1980; 35(1):1-48.)*

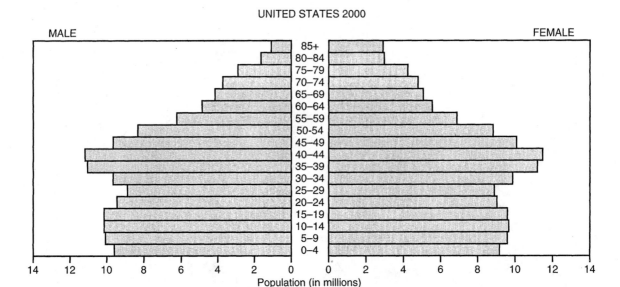

UNITED STATES 2000

Figure 1–3. Population Pyramid US Population in 2000. *(Source: U.S. Census Bureau, International Data Base. US Census Bureau. Accessed online at: http://www.census.gov/population/projections/nation/summary/np-t3-a.txt.)*

graphic components. The aggregate older population is composed of a population that includes persons who range in age over a span of some forty-five years.[1] The relative numbers of men and women at each age and the age characteristics of the elderly are also important compositional factors. Explicit attention to the composition of the aged population leads to the recognition of important changes taking place to modify the population structure, such as the high relative increase in the numbers of extremely old persons, declining sex ratios, shifts in marital status, in living arrangements, and in racial, ethnic, and health status. These aspects of the demography of aging will often be discussed to present a comprehensible global picture of the characteristics of the population aged 65 and over in any given year.

Historically, fertility is the most important determinant of population growth and the age structure of the population. Demographers view fertility as the critical process of renewal. When the fertility rate is high, the cohort born each year has more members than the cohorts that preceded it. At moderate to low levels of mortality, then, the number of newborns added to the population exceeds the number of older

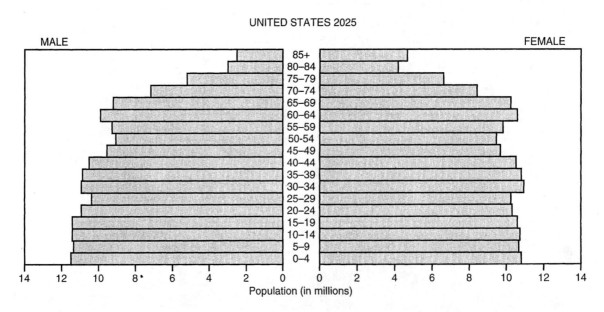

UNITED STATES 2025

Figure 1–4. Population Pyramid Projected US Population: 2025. *(Source: U.S. Census Bureau, International Data Base. US Census Bureau. Accessed online at: http://www.census.gov/population/projections/nation/summary/np-t3-a.txt.)*

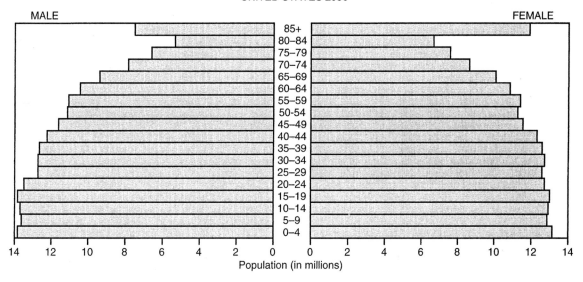

Figure 1–5. Population Pyramid Projected US Population: 2050. *(Source: U.S. Census Bureau, International Data Base. US Census Bureau. Accessed online at: http://www.census.gov/population/projections/nation/summary/np-t3-a.txt.)*

persons who die; the proportion of the population that is young increases, and its median age declines. When the birthrate is low, the proportion of the population that is old increases, and its median age rises.

The effect of a decline in mortality from high to moderate levels, which occurred in the United States in the late nineteenth century and early twentieth century as infectious diseases were brought under control, paradoxically caused the population to become younger.[19] The reason for this relationship between mortality and age structure is that the most important improvements in survivorship during this period occurred in the age groups of infants and children. Recent advances in the prevention and treatment of cardiovascular disease, however, have increased the survivorship of older persons. Since 1940, the major reason for the increase in the number of the oldest-old, those aged 85 years and older, has been the improved survivorship of the old.[20] About two-thirds of the 1980 to 1985 increase in the proportion of older persons in the population was caused by the mortality decline.[21] The tremendous increase in the projected number of elderly during the next fifty years results from the large cohorts born during the post-World War II baby boom reaching old age *and* the improved survivorship at all ages, especially the oldest old.[19]

The growth of the total population is particularly sensitive to declining mortality rates, whereas the growth of the older population, especially in their proportionate size relative to the total population, occurs when the fertility rate declines.[22] In fact, declines in mortality focused at younger ages that are not accompanied by decreases in the fertility rate can lead to an overall younger population. The sustained decrease in mortality that extends into older ages is the main reason for current population aging.[21]

PROJECTED POPULATION TRENDS IN AN AGING SOCIETY

The major demographic forces that alter the size of a population and its age composition are levels of fertility and mortality. Measures used by demographers to estimate these two factors are, respectively, the general fertility rate (i.e., the number of live births per one thousand women annually) and the life expectancy at birth. Demographers, in making their projections, typically utilize low, middle, and high estimates. For the purpose of this chapter, the middle series projections are used unless otherwise indicated.

The projected demographic trends indicate that by the year 2030 there will be over 69 million elderly Americans.[19,23,24] In 1960, Census Bureau statistics indicated that there were 16.7 million persons aged 65 and over. By 1990, an estimated 31.6 million persons were aged 65 and older.[23,24] In 1998, 34.4 million people were aged 65 years or older,[24] reflecting major changes in the population structure of the United States in this century. Figure 1–6 represents the growth of elderly individuals in the United States since 1900 and anticipated growth to the year 2030.

Individuals who had reached their 65th birthday accounted for 4.1% of the total US population in 1900, 6.9% of the population in 1940, and 8.2% of the population in 1950. The number of Americans 65 years of age or older grew at an unprecedented rated between 1950 and 1960 and continues to grow. Proportionally, the elderly made up 9.2% of the American population in 1960 with an increase to 12.6% by 1990. By 1998, one in every eight Americans was over the age of 65, representing 12.7% of the population.[24] The number of older Americans has increased by 3.2 million or 10.1%

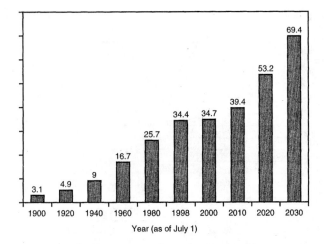

Figure 1–6. Number of Persons 65+, 1900–2030 (numbers in millions). Data for this section compiled primarily from Internet releases of the U.S. Bureau of the Census and the National Center for Health Statistics.

since 1990, compared to an increase of 8.1% for the under-65 population.[25] To put things in perspective, since 1900 the percentage of Americans aged 65 or older has more than tripled (4.1% in 1900 to 12.7% in 1998) and the number has increased eleven times (3.1 million to 34.4 million). If Census Bureau projections are accurate, it is anticipated that these proportions will climb to 17.7% in 2020, to 20% by the year 2030 when the children of the postwar baby boom will be well into old age, and to 22.9% by 2050.[25]

Between the years 1960 and 1990 there was a 2% annual growth in the overall elderly population. This trend is actually expected to decrease to about 1% by the year 2010 as a result of the smaller Depression era and World War II age cohorts that will be reaching the age of 65. However, after 2010, the annual rate of growth will exceed 2% as the baby-boom cohort reaches the age of 65 years. This trend is anticipated to persist until 2030. Between 2030 to 2050, it is projected that the population of elderly Americans will stabilize to a 1% level of growth annually.[19]

Projected demographic trends reflect an assumption that there will be a sharply declining fertility rate accompanied by a decreasing mortality rate until the year 2050.[19] These forecasted changes indicate that there will be a reduction in the growth of the total population to a level of 1% annually.[1] However, even at a level of 1% annual growth, it is anticipated that the total population will double over the next 60 years.[19]

Table 1–1 shows how dramatically life expectancy of the US population has increased from the early 1900s to the projected life expectancy of the year 2050.[18,25] The major part of the current increase in life expectancy occurred because of reduced death rates for children and young adults. Life expectancy at age 65 increased by only 2.4 years between 1900 and 1960, but has increased by 3.3 years since 1960. In fact, life expectancy at birth has increased from 74.3 years in 1982 to 76.7 years in 2000 and is projected to increase to 81 years of age by 2050.[19] In 1997, Americans reaching age 65 had an average life expectancy of an additional 17.6 years (19 years for females and 15.8 years for males).[25] A child born in 1997 can expect to live 76.5 years, about 29 years longer than a child born in 1900.[25] Male life expectancy increased from 70.6 years in 1982 to 72.9 years in the year 2000 and is expected to rise to 76.7 years by the year 2050. Females who could expect to live 78.1 years in 1982, and as projected, attained a life expectancy of 80.5 years in 2000. This life expectancy is anticipated to increase to 85.2 years by 2050 for women. Some researchers feel that it will improve even more than the Census Bureau projections assume.[26–28] Life expectancy is expected to gain an additional 12.8 years if the current demographic trends persist over the next fifty years.

Almost 1.9 million persons celebrated their 65th birthday in 1998 (5,190 per day). In the same year, about 1.75 million persons aged 65 or older died, resulting in a net increase of 145,000 (396 per day).[25]

In 1998, there were 20.2 million older women and 14.2 million older men, or a sex ratio of 143 women for every 100 men. The sex ratio increased with age, ranging from 118 for the 65–69 year old group to a high of 241 for persons aged 85 and over.[25] Female life expectancy has been about 7.5 years

TABLE 1–1. LIFE EXPECTANCY OF US POPULATION AT BIRTH, BY RACE AND GENDER: 1900, 1940, 1950, 1960, 1970, 1980, 1990, 1994, 1997

Race and Gender	Life Expectancy at Birth								
	1900	1940	1950	1960	1970	1980	1990	1994	1997
White									
Men	47	62.1	66.5	67.4	68	70.7	72.7	73.3	73.6
Women	49	66.6	72.2	74.1	75.6	78.1	79.4	79.6	80.5
Nonwhite									
Men	33	51.5	59.1	61.1	61.3	65.3	67	67.6	68.2
Women	34	54.9	62.9	66.3	69.4	73.6	75.2	75.7	76.3

Compiled from data in Singh GK, Kochanek KD, MacDorman MF. Advance report of final mortality statistics, 1994. *Monthly Vital Statistics Report.* 45(3), suppl.:19. Hyattsville, MD: National Center for Health Statistics 1996 AND *Monthly Vital Statistics Report.* 46(12):2. Hyattsville, MD: National Center for Health Statistics 1998.

higher than male life expectancy since 1970.[19] While there is much disagreement as to whether this differential will narrow or widen, several demographers believe it may narrow by several years.[29-31] Others, however, believe it may widen to 10 or 12 years by the turn of the century.[27,28] Spencer[19] predicts that the sex difference in life expectancy will gradually widen to 8.5 years by 2050.

PROJECTED COMPONENTS OF CHANGE IN AN AGING POPULATION

Fertility Patterns

In the middle series for the overall US population, the number of births is expected to remain above the present level of 3.7 million throughout the early 2000s. The peak number of births (3.9 million) may actually have already occurred in the late 1980s.[19] After the early 1990s, the birth rate did not surpass 3.7 million because of a decline in the female population of childbearing age. In the early 2000s the number of births is projected to fluctuate between 3.4 and 3.7 million.

Mortality Patterns

The first year in which 2 million Americans died was 1983, and it is projected that it is not likely that there will ever be a year with fewer than 2 million deaths.[19] Deaths in the next century are expected to steadily increase. Annual death rate reached 2.4 million at the turn of the century and is expected to increase to 3.8 million by the year 2040. After that time, the death rate is predicted to stabilize between 3.8 and 4.0 million deaths a year.

Because we have already established that the population is getting older, it is no surprise that the proportion of all deaths which happen at older ages would increase in the future. Currently, about 70% of deaths occur at age 65 years and older. This proportion is anticipated to increase to 80% by 2030 and remain relatively stable until the end of the twenty-first century. More noteworthy is the likely change in the proportion of deaths that happen at age 85 and over. While 18% of all deaths now occur at such old ages, this percentage is expected to reach 30% by 2010 and increase to more than 43% after 2050.[19]

Immigration and Migration Patterns

A great deal of interest centers on future levels of net immigration and the impact that will have on the size of the US population. This is the only demographic area where projections based on the low, middle, and high estimates from the census data will be covered, because the uncertain immigration rate could have such profound consequences. According to Spencer,[19] if there were no net immigration, the US population would grow to 258 million people in the year 2000 and peak at approximately 275 million people around 2030. However, if the estimate of net migration was relatively low (about 250,000 per year), the population would grow to 264 million in the year 2000. At this rate of growth it would be expected to level off to 294 million in 2040. This population represented 2.1% or 5.5 million people in the year 2000, and is expected to be 6% larger in 2030, and 10% larger by the year 2050. Net immigration at the middle level (450,000 per year) has an interesting effect on the projected population size. Essentially, there would be a zero-growth population after the year 2050. Therefore, if middle fertility and mortality assumptions are correct, net immigration much below 450,000 eventually produces a stable or declining population.[19] The highest net immigration estimates (750,000 per year) show a continuous increase in the population throughout the twenty-first century.

Age Composition of the Aging US Population

It is anticipated that the percentage of the total population aged 65 and over will increase from the current level of approximately 13% in the year 2000 to 21.2% by 2030 (nearly double) utilizing the middle series Census Bureau estimates.[24] The older population will continue to grow significantly in the future (see Figure 1–6). This growth slowed somewhat during the 1990s because of the relatively small number of babies born during the Great Depression of the 1930s. But the older population will burgeon between the years 2010 and 2030 when the baby boomers reach the age of 65.[25] By 2030, there will be about 70 million older persons, twice their numbers in 1998.

The older population itself is getting older. The 85 years of age and over population will grow at a more rapid rate than the entire 65 and over population, assuming that the extremely old will benefit from the improvements in future mortality rates. In 1998, the 65- to 74-year-old age group (18.4 million) was eight times larger than in 1900, but the 75- to 84-year-old group (12.0 million) was sixteen times larger and the over-85 group (4.0 million) was thirty-three times larger.[25] According to population studies, there are currently more than 4 million Americans aged 85 and over. This number is projected to increase during the beginning of the twenty-first century to approximately 4.9 million, and reach 8.6 million persons over the age of 85 by 2030.[19,25] Currently, about 1% of the population is aged 85 years and older. By 2050, 5.2% of the population will be that old. Within the present population of 65 years of age and older, this comprises 9.1% aged 85 and above.[23] Projections indicate that by the year 2050, those 85 years of age and older will make up one-quarter of the entire elderly population.[25,27]

For the population of those aged 100 years and over, a substantial growth in the overall numbers is also anticipated. According to the 1990 Census Bureau report,[23] there were about 32,000 centenarians in the population. By the year 2000, this number grew to 108,000 and is expected to reach an estimated 492,000 persons over the age of 100 by the year 2030. Currently, about ninety elderly persons turn 100 every day, and by the year 2030, two hundred eighty persons each day are expected to be passing their first century of life.[25]

Gender Composition of the Aging US Population

Accompanying the aging of the population is an increasing proportion of females compared to males as age increases. Elderly women outnumbered men by three to two as a result of sex differentials in mortality that favor females at all ages over 65. For those 85 years of age and older, women outnumbered men five to two in 1990,[32] which increased to a ratio of seven to one by 1998.[33,34] In other words, higher proportions of females than males survive to old age. These ratios are expected to sharply increase through the middle of the twenty-first century as large entry cohorts, in which the sex ratios are higher, enter the 65 years of age and older population.[1]

Geographical Distribution of the Aging US Population

Elderly individuals tend to concentrate in specific regions of the country. In 1998, about half (52%) of persons over 65 lived in nine states. California had more than 3.5 million, Florida had 2.7, and New York 2.4 million, Texas and Pennsylvania had almost 2 million, and Ohio, Illinois, Michigan, and New Jersey each had over 1 million individuals 65 years of age and older.[25,34]

Persons over 65 constituted 14% or more of the total population in eleven states in 1998: Florida (18.3%); Pennsylvania (15.9%); Rhode Island (15.6%); West Virginia (15.2%); Iowa (15.1%); North Dakota (14.4%); Connecticut, Arkansas, and South Dakota (14.3%); Maine (14.1%); and Massachusetts (14%).[25]

In sixteen states, the over-65 population increased by 15% or more between 1990 and 1998: Nevada (55%); Alaska (49%); Arizona (29%); Hawaii (27%); Utah (22%); Colorado and New Mexico (21%); Delaware (19%); North Carolina and South Carolina (18%); Wyoming (17%); Texas (16%); and Georgia, California, Florida, and Virginia (15%).[25]

The ten jurisdictions with the highest poverty rates for elderly in the period 1995–1997 were: the District of Columbia (20.6%); Arkansas (17.1%); Mississippi (16.6%); Louisiana (16.3%); Texas (15.8%); New Mexico (15.7%); South Carolina (15.6%); Georgia (14.0%); West Virginia (13.9%); and Tennessee (13.7%).[25]

Persons over 65 were slightly less likely to live in metropolitan areas in 1998 than younger persons (77% of the elderly, 81% of persons under 65). About 28% of older persons lived in central cities and 49% lived in the suburbs.[25]

The elderly are less likely to change residence than other age groups. In 1997, only 5% of persons aged 65 and older had moved since 1996 compared to 18% of persons under 65.[25] A large majority of those elderly (81%) had moved to another home in the same state.[25]

Income Status of the Aging US Population

The median income of older persons in 1998 was $18,166 for males and $10,504 for females. Real median income (after adjusting for inflation) grew more for women (2.8%) than for men (0.7%) since 1997.[25] Households with families headed by persons aged 65 and older reported a median income in 1998 of $31,568 ($32,398 for whites, $22,102 for African Americans, and $21,935 for Hispanics). Approximately one of every seven (13.7%) family households with an elderly head had an income of less than $15,000 and 44.6% had an income of $35,000 or more.[25]

For all older persons reporting income in 1998 (31.7 million), 36% reported less than $10,000. Only 22% reported $25,000 or more. The median income reported was $13,768.[25]

The major sources of income as reported by the Social Security Administration for older persons in 1996 were Social Security (reported by 91% of older persons), income from assets (reported by 63%), public and private pensions (reported by 43%), earnings (reported by 21%), and public assistance (reported by 6%).[25]

In 1996, Social Security benefits accounted for 40% of the aggregate income of the older population. The bulk of the remainder consisted of earnings (20%), pensions (18%), and assets (18%).[25]

The median net worth (assets minus liabilities) of older households ($86,300), including those aged 75 and older ($77,700), was well above the US average ($37,600) in 1993. Net worth was below $10,000 for 16% of older households but was above $250,000 for 17%.[25]

Poverty of the Aging US Population

About 3.4 million elderly persons were below the poverty level in 1998.[25] The poverty rate for persons aged 65 and older was 10.5%, no change from 1997, and the same as the rate for persons aged 18 to 64. Another 2.1 million or 6.3% of the elderly were classified as "near-poor" (income between the poverty level and 125% of this level). In total, one of every six (17%) older persons was poor or near-poor in 1998.[25]

One of every eleven (8.9%) elderly whites was poor in 1998, compared to 16.4% of elderly African Americans and 21% of elderly Hispanics. Higher than average poverty rates for older persons correlated with living in central cities (13.8%), rural areas (12.5%), and in the South (12%).[25]

Older women had a higher poverty rate (12.8%) than older men (7.2%) in 1998.[25] Older persons living alone or with nonrelatives were much more likely to be poor (20.4%) than were older persons living with families (6.4%). The highest poverty rates (49.3%) were experienced by older African American women who lived alone.[25]

Marital Status of the Aging US Population

Another demographic characteristic that warrants examination is the marital status of older persons. The importance of this characteristic is its meaning for the elderly individual and its impact on family status, living arrangements, and available support systems.[35] The composition of the aged population with respect to marital status is influenced by complex patterns of family formation and dissolution that vary cross-culturally as well as by the important constraints imposed by differential mortality rates of males and females.[36] In 1998, older men were much more likely to be married than older women—75% of men and 43% of women (see Figure 1–7). The reduced mortality that distinguishes the demographic transitions reportedly occurring, lengthens the duration of marriage as the joint survival of both men and women is extended. However, with the widening gap in survival between the sexes, widowhood becomes more common for women at older ages. For males over the age of 65 years of age, over 15% were widowed in 1998, but, for females, over 45% are widowed as depicted in Figure 1–7.[24,25] There were four times as many widows (8.4 million) as widowers (2.0 million).[25]

Marital dissolution through divorce or separation, and remarriage in later life, are additional factors that need to be considered. In addition, those never married or those cohabitating certainly confound any clean analysis of living arrangements and support systems for the elderly. The proportion of older persons who were divorced in 1998 was less than 7%, however, their numbers (2.1 million) has increased five times as fast as the older population as a whole since 1990 (2.8 times for men, 7.4 times for women). The proportions of never-married males and females are quite high at approximately 4.0% and 5.0% respectively.[25] Remarriage at older ages plays a relatively small part in modifying the marital status distributions.[37,38]

Projections of marital status in the United States indicate that there will be a slight reduction in the proportions of older males married and widowed as the century progresses, and that there will be proportionately fewer females who are widowed.[37] It is anticipated, however, that cohorts reaching the older ages after 2000 will be more likely to be divorced or separated as a result of the substantially higher proportions of divorced and separated persons in younger cohorts.

Living Arrangements of the Aging US Population

Associated with these marital changes have been pronounced changes in the living arrangements of the elderly. The most notable of these have been the sharp increase in the proportion of women living alone, and the sharp decline in the proportion of women living with other family members.[25,35] There has been relatively little change in the proportion of elderly men living alone or with other family members. The majority (67%) of older noninstitutionalized persons lived in a family setting in 1998. Approximately 10.8 million or 80% of older men, and 10.7 million or 58% of older women, lived in families. The proportion living in a family setting decreased with age.

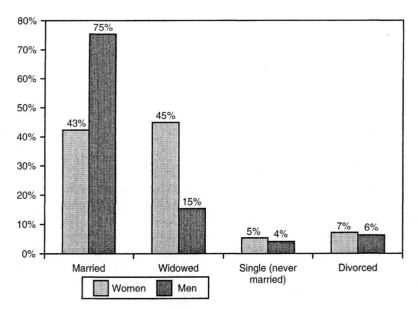

Figure 1–7. Marital Status of Persons 65+, 1998. (Based on data from the U.S. Bureau of the Census. Marital Status and Living Arrangements: March 1998 (Update), Current Population Reports, PPL-100.)

Only 45% of those aged 85 and older lived in family settings in 1998.[25] Elderly men are much more likely to be living with a wife than to be widowed or living with other family members.[25,39] About 13% of older persons over the age of 85 (7% of men, 17% of women) were not living with a spouse but were living with children, siblings, or other relatives in 1998. An additional 3% of men and 2% of women, or 718,000 older persons, lived with nonrelatives.[25]

About 31% (9.9 million) of all noninstitutionalized older persons in 1998 lived alone (7.6 million women, 2.3 million men). They represented 41% of older women and 17% of older men. Living alone correlates with advanced age. Among women aged 85 and over, for example, three of every five lived outside a family setting.[25] The increased tendency of older women, including extremely aged women, to live alone, is likely to continue. It is expected that by 2005, over 70% of women 75 years of age and over will be living alone. The proportion of aged men living alone is not expected to change much.[35] The US Census Bureau indicates that in 1995, about 52% of the households were maintained by persons 75 years and over. Of these households most were maintained by women living alone or with nonrelatives.[24]

The trends towards independent living has come about partly as a result of improvements in the economic and health status of the elderly, partly from a desire not to be dependent on others, and partly, for some, from a simple lack of an alternative.[39]

There is an unfortunate and growing trend for homelessness among the elderly population.[40,41] In the United States, according to the 1990 Population Census *S-Night* (shelter and street count), there were 400,000 homeless elderly people on the streets and in shelters, and 6,000 to 9,000 in temporary accommodations, such as hotels, prisons, and staying with friends.[42] A recent assessment is that anywhere between 60,000 and 400,000 older persons are homeless, and that although the absolute number has recently increased, the proportion of elderly among the total homeless population has declined.[43] Other estimates of the national total are, however, highly variable, as are the reported proportions of homeless aged 50 years and over (2% to 27% in studies of homeless people).[43–45]

While a comparatively small number (1.43 million) and percentage (4.2%) of the over-65 population lived in nursing homes in 1996, the percentage increases dramatically with age, ranging from 1.1% for persons from 65 to 74 years old to 4.2% for persons aged 75 to 84 and 19.8% for persons over 85.[25,45]

Housing Status of the Aging US Population

Of the 20.9 million households headed by older persons in 1997, 79% were owners and 21% were renters. The median family income of older homeowners was $20,280. The median family income of older renters was $10,867.[25]

About 50% of homes owned by older persons in 1997 were built prior to 1960 (33% for younger owners) and 6% had structural problems.[25]

In 1997, 37% of older homeowners spent more than one-fourth of their income on housing costs, compared to 30% of homeowners under age 65.[25]

In 1997, the median value of homes owned by older persons was $89,294, compared to a median home value of $98,815 for all homeowners. About 77% of older homeowners in 1997 owned their homes free and clear.[25]

Employment Status of the Aging US Population

About 3.7 million older Americans (12%) were in the labor force (working or actively seeking work) in 1998, including 2.2 million men (16%) and 1.6 million women (8%). They constituted 2.8% of the US labor force. About 3.2% were unemployed.[25]

Labor force participation of older men decreased steadily from two of three in 1900 to 15.8% in 1985, and has stayed at 16% to 17% since then. The participation rate for older females rose slightly from one of twelve in 1900 to 10.8% in 1956, fell to 7.3% in 1985, and has been around 8% to 9% since 1988.[25]

Just over half (54%) of the workers over 65 years of age in 1998 were employed part-time: 48% of men and 62% of women.[25]

About 860,000 or 23% of older workers in 1998 were self-employed, compared to 7% for younger workers. Over two-thirds of them (71%) were men.[25]

Educational Status of the Aging US Population

The educational level of the older population is increasing. Between 1970 and 1998, the percentage who had completed high school rose from 28% to 67%. About 15% in 1998 had a bachelor's degree or more.[25] The percentage who had completed high school varied considerably by race and ethnic origin among older persons in 1998: 69% of whites, 43% of African Americans, and 30% of Hispanics.[25]

Health Status of the Aging US Population

Clinical measures clearly indicate the decline of health status with advancing age. The elderly are more likely to have chronic conditions that limit their activities, and they experience about twice as many days of restricted activity because of illness as the general population. However, to be aged in the United States today is not necessarily to be beset with numerous and complex disabilities. Life after age 65 years is not a period inexorably marked with massive physical deterioration.[46] Nevertheless, increasing life expectancy of those reaching age 65 years has had an important impact on the prevalence of disease and functional disability in the elderly population.

Life expectancy is a summary measure of the overall health of a population. It represents the average number of years of life remaining to a person at a given age if death rates were to remain constant. In the United States, improvements in health have resulted in increased life expectancy and contributed to the growth of the older population over the past century. In 1900, life expectancy at birth was about 49 years. By 1960, life expectancy had increased to 70 years, and in 1997, life expectancy at birth was 79 years for women and 74 years for men.[34] Life expectancies at age 65 and 85 have also increased. Under current mortality conditions, people who survive to age 65 can expect to live an average of nearly 18 more years, more than five years longer than persons aged 65 in 1900. The life expectancy of persons who survive to age 85 today is about seven years for women and six years for men.[25] Other variables come into play with health and well-being. Educational attainment is associated with higher life expectancy. The life expectancy of high school graduates at age 65 is approximately one year longer than the life expectancy at that age for persons who did not graduate from high school.[47] Life expectancy also varies by race, but the difference decreases with age. In 1997, life expectancy at birth was six years higher for white persons than for African American persons. At age 65, white persons can expect to live an average of two years longer than their African American counterparts. The declining race differences in life expectancy at older ages are subject to debate. Some research shows that age misreporting may have artificially increased life expectancy for African American persons, particularly when birth certificates were not available.[48] Other research suggests that black persons who survive to the oldest ages may be healthier than white persons and have lower mortality rates.[49]

Overall, death rates in the US population have declined during the past century. For some diseases, however, death rates among older Americans have increased in recent years.[50,51] Between 1980 and 1997, age-adjusted death rates for heart disease and stroke declined by approximately one-third. Death rates for cancer, pneumonia, and influenza increased slightly over the same period. Age-adjusted death rates for diabetes increased by 32% since 1980, and death rates for chronic obstructive pulmonary diseases increased by 57%.[51,52]

In 1997, the leading cause of death among persons aged 65 or older was heart disease (1,832 deaths per 100,000 persons), followed by cancer (1,133 per 100,000), stroke (426 per 100,000), chronic obstructive pulmonary diseases (281 per 100,000), pneumonia and influenza (237 per 1000,000), and diabetes (141 per 100,000). Among persons aged 85 or older, heart disease was responsible for 40% of all deaths.[50]

Death rates in 1997 were higher for older men than for older women at every age except the very oldest, persons aged 95 or older, for whom men's and women's rates were nearly equal.[51]

The relative importance of certain causes of death varied according to sex and race and ethnic group. For instance, in 1997, diabetes was the third leading cause of death among American Indian and Alaska Native men and women aged 65 or older, the fourth leading cause of death among older Hispanic men and women, and ranked sixth among older white men and women and older Asian and Pacific Islander men. Alzheimer's disease was the sixth leading cause of death among white women aged 85 or older, however, it was less common among African American women in the same age group or men of either race.[50,51]

Chronic diseases and long-term illnesses can become significant health and financial burdens, not only to those persons who have them, but also to their families and the nation's health care system. Chronic conditions such as arthritis, diabetes, and heart disease negatively affect quality of life, contributing to declines in functioning and the inability to remain in the community.[52] Five of the six leading causes of death, discussed above, among older Americans are chronic diseases.

Between 1984 and 1998, the prevalence of stroke increased by 1%, diabetes by 2%, arthritis by 3%, heart disease by 5%, and cancer by 7%.[52] The prevalence of hypertension remained fairly constant over this same period. These trends are generally evident among older persons regardless of age, sex, or race.[52]

In 1998, about 58% of persons aged 70 or older reported having arthritis, 45% reported having hypertension, and 21% reported having heart disease. Other chronic diseases included cancer (19%), diabetes (12%), and stroke (9%). About 64% of older women reported having arthritis, 48% reported having hypertension, and 19% reported having heart disease. Older men were less likely to report having arthritis (50%) and hypertension (41%), but were more likely to report having heart disease (25%). Men were also more likely to have had cancer (23%), compared with women (17%).[52]

The prevalence of chronic conditions also varies by race and ethnicity in the older population. In 1998, arthritis was reported by 67% of non-Hispanic black persons, 58% of non-Hispanic white persons, and 50% of Hispanic persons. Non-Hispanic African Americans were also more likely to report having diabetes, stroke, and hypertension than either non-Hispanic white persons or Hispanic persons. Cancer was reported by 21% of non-Hispanic white persons, compared with 9% of non-Hispanic black persons and 11% of Hispanic persons.[52]

Memory skills are important to general cognitive function, and declining scores on tests of memory are indicators of general cognitive loss for older adults. Low cognitive functioning (e.g., memory impairment) is a major risk factor for entering a nursing home.[53] The prevalence of moderate or severe memory impairment was 35% of women aged 85 or older, compared with 37% of men in the same age group.[52] In 1998, the percentage of older adults with moderate or severe memory impairment ranged from about 4% among persons aged 65 to 69 to about 36% among persons aged 85 or older.[52]

Depressive symptoms are an important indicator of general well-being and mental health among older Americans. Higher levels of depressive symptoms are associated with higher rates of physical illness, greater functional disability, and higher health care resource utilization.[54] Women between the ages of 65 and 84 are more likely than men to have severe depressive symptoms. Among persons age 85 or older, men and women have a similar prevalence of severe depressive symptoms. In 1998, about 15% of persons ages 65 to 69, 70 to 74, and 75 to 79 had severe symptoms of depression, compared with 21% of persons aged 80 to 84, and 23% of persons aged 85 or older.[52]

Asking people to rate their own health as excellent, very good, good, fair, or poor provides a common indicator of health easily measured in surveys. It represents physical, emotional, and social aspects of health and well-being. Good to excellent self-reported health correlates with lower risk of mortality.[55] During the period 1994 to 1996, 72% of older Americans reported their health as good, very good, or excellent. Women and men reported comparable levels of health status. Positive health evaluations decline with age. Among non-Hispanic white men aged 65 to 74, 76% reported good to excellent health, compared with 67% among non-Hispanic white men aged 85 or older. A similar decline with age was reported by non-Hispanic black and Hispanic older men, and by women, with the exception of non-Hispanic black women. Among older men and women in every age group, non-Hispanic black and Hispanic persons were less likely to report good health than non-Hispanic white persons.[52]

In 1996, 27% of older persons assessed their health as fair or poor (compared to 9.2% for all persons). There was little difference between sexes on this measure, but older African Americans (41.6%) and older Hispanics (35.1%) were much more likely to rate their health as fair or poor than were older whites (26%).[25]

Functioning in later years may be diminished if illness, chronic disease, or injury limits physical and/or mental abilities. Changes in disability rates

have important implications for work and retirement policies, health and long-term care needs, and the social well-being of the older population. By monitoring and understanding these trends, policymakers are better able to make informed decisions.

The National Health Interview Survey conducted in 1981 by the National Center for Health Statistics provided national estimates of the level of functioning of the noninstitutionalized aged in the United States.[56] Table 1–2 provides a summary of the data collected in that survey. In 1981, about 20% of those community-dwelling elders aged 65 years of age or older reported some restrictions in their mobility. A similar trend is seen with respect to restrictions in elders' major daily activities. Forty-three percent reported some limitation in their amount or kind of functional activity.[56.]

Looking at trends in disability, the proportion of Americans aged 65 or older with a chronic disability declined from 24% in 1982 to 21% in 1994. Figure 1–5 presents the percentage of Medicare beneficiaries aged 65 or older who were chronically disabled, by level and category of disability in repeat surveys by researchers, using the National Long Term Care Survey, between 1982 and 1994. Despite the decline in rates of disability noted in Figure 1–5, the number of older adults with chronic disabilities increased by about 600,000 from 6.4 million in 1982 to 7.0 million in 1994.[25] This is because the overall population of older persons was growing fast enough to outweigh the decline in disability rates. However, if disability rates had not declined from 1982 to 1994, then the disabled population would have increased by almost 1.5 million bringing the total number of older Americans with chronic disabilities close to 7.9 million, a strong policy argument for screening and preventive interventions on the part of rehabilitation professionals.

Different indicators can be used to monitor disability including limitations of Activities of Daily Living (ADLs) and Instrumental Activities of Daily Living (IADLs), and measures of physical, cognitive, and social functioning. Aspects of physical functioning such as the ability to climb stairs, walk a quarter mile, or reach up over one's head are more closely linked to physiological capabilities than are ADLs and IADLs, which may be influenced by social and cultural role expectations and by changes in technology.

TABLE 1–2.   PREVALENCE OF DISABILITY IN SELF-REPORTED LIMITATIONS IN FUNCTIONAL ACTIVITIES, BASIC ADL AND INSTRUMENTAL ADL IN ADULTS 65 AND OVER: UNITED STATES 1994

	Age		
Disability	65–74 (%)	75–84 (%)	85+ (%)
Self-reported functional limitations	27.8	42.6	60.8
Needs help in one or more Basic ADL	5.2	12.4	26.6
Needs help in one or more Instrumental ADL	15.6	28.2	53.0

Source: Compiled from National Center for Health Statistics (1996). Data File Documentation, National Health Interview Survey of Disability, Phase I, 1994. Hyattsville, MD: National Center for Health Statistics. 1996.

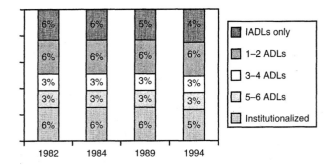

Figure 1–8. Percentage of Medicare beneficiaries aged 65 or older who are chronically disabled by level and category of disability. 1982 to 1994. *(Source: National Long Term Care Survey 1982, 1984, 1989, 1994.)*

Between 1984 and 1995, older adults reported improvements in physical functioning in the ability to walk a quarter mile, climb stairs, reach up over one's head, and stoop, crouch, or kneel.[57] The percentage unable to perform at least one of nine physical activities without assistance or special equipment was higher among women than men but declined for both groups. In 1995, older African Americans were more likely than older white persons to be unable to perform at least one of nine physical activities (33% and 25%, respectively).[57]

Viewed as a homogeneous group, the majority of elders are free from disability. For most, the later years of life are characterized by substantial physical ability.[58]

DEMOGRAPHIC TRENDS AND PROJECTIONS IN THE MINORITY ELDERLY

The aging of the US population will affect every institution and every individual in our society. Projections of the proportion of the population 65 years of age and over anticipate dramatic increases over the next 50 years.[3] This phenomenon of population aging is of particular importance in minority groups in America.

In 1998, 15.7% of persons aged 65 and older were minorities: 8% were African Americans, 2.1% were Asians or Pacific Islanders, and fewer than 1% were American Indians or Native Alaskans. Persons of Hispanic origin (who may be of any race) represented 5.1% of the older population.[25,59] Only 7.2% of minority race and Hispanic populations were aged 65 and older in 1998 compared with 14.8% of whites.

Minority populations are projected to represent 25% of the elderly population in the United States by 2030, up from almost 16% in 1998.[25] Between 1998 and 2030, the older white population is projected to increase by 79% compared with 226% of older minorities, including Hispanics (341%), African Americans (130%), American Indians, Eskimos, and Aleuts (150%), and Asians and Pacific Islanders (323%).[25,59] There is a marked differential between majority and minority aging with respect to fertility, mortality, and

migration and it is expected that the racial and ethnic diversity of the aged in the United States will increase rapidly as we proceed through the twenty-first century. In other words, as the elderly population becomes a larger percentage of the overall population, a greater proportion of the elderly will be minority group members. This shift in the composition of the elderly population will have great impact on public policy development in the arenas of social welfare and the health care system. This section of the chapter examines the projected demographic trends and the compositional changes in the United States of the minority group elderly.

Age is sometimes called the great equalizer,[3] however, today's elderly are a highly diverse group, and this makes simple analysis difficult. Age, gender, race, and ethnicity determine an individual's status in American society, and as a result, influence life-course experiences. Differences in income, health, and social supports significantly affect the elderly person's quality of life. Each of these demographic variables is important to understanding the intergenerational family relations, the social and economic status, and the health status and longevity of the elderly. The status and resources of many minority elderly reflect social and economic discrimination experienced earlier in life. Many, especially those who migrated to the United States, face cultural and language differences as well. Demographic data provides a sound foundation upon which to examine health status, life expectancy, economic status, family patterns, household structure, and support systems of minority elderly.

Projected Population Trends in the Minority Elderly

Projected demographic trends indicate that by the year 2050 there will be 69 million elderly Americans. Within that group 54 million will be white, 10 million will be black, and 5 million will be comprised of other ethnic and racial groups.[60] Eight million of these elderly (of any race) will be of Hispanic origin.[61] If life expectancy improves more rapidly than presently anticipated, these numbers could increase even more dramatically.[60]

Projections of minority elderly population growth are based on the "middle series," intermediate assumptions by the Census Bureau.[19,59] The growing statistical significance of the elderly population as a whole, and of the minority aged population in particular, is clearly illustrated in the recent rapid growth rates reported by the Census Bureau over the past three decades and the trends extrapolated from that data into the middle of the twenty-first century.[59]

In 1990, 89.9% of America's elderly were white; in fact, the total number of elderly white persons nearly doubled between 1960 and 1990, from 15.4 million to 28.3 million, however, demographic shifts reveal that this situation is changing rapidly. Though it is projected that the white elderly population will double again by the year 2030, it is estimated that the number of minority elderly will grow at a more rapid rate compared with white elderly over the next 50 years.[3] As a consequence, the percentage of America's elderly that comprise blacks and other races other than white would increase from 10.2% in 1990 to 18.3% in 2020, and to 25.3% in 2030. The number of black elderly doubles as well from 1960 to 1990 (1.2 million to 2.6 million) and will nearly triple by 2050.[59] In fact, it is anticipated that the number of black minority elderly will escalate to 9.6 million by the year 2050. Races other than white or black will increase from 600,000 to 5.0 million. Hispanic elderly of any race, the fastest-growing population group in America, will increase from 1.1 million in 1990 more than doubling to 2.5 million by 2010, reaching 5.6 million by 2030, and escalating to 7.9 million in 2050. All non-white and non-black elderly populations have shown a considerable increase from 81,000 in 1960 to 603,000 in 1990. Based on the middle series projections, this number would increase to 1.5 million persons in 2010, doubling aging by 2030.[19] From these statistics it appears that although non-Hispanic white elderly will remain the majority group, blacks, Hispanics, and other racial and ethnic groups will grow at a faster rate and become a large and important component of the aging American populace.

It is also expected that there will be a projected increase in the proportion of elders in each ethnic group. In 1960, 6% of the black population was 65 years of age or older. This percentage is anticipated to increase to 10% by 2010 and go beyond 17% in 2030. The other races, including Asian, Native American, Eskimo, and Aleut, could more than double between now and the middle of this century from 7% elderly to 16.1% in 2030. The Hispanic population would also age considerably. Currently 6% of the Hispanic population is 65 years of age or older. By 2030 this is expected to increase to 13%.[59]

Between the years 1960 and 1990 there was a 2% annual growth in the white elderly population. This is expected to decrease to about 1% from 1990 to the year 2010. This drop is anticipated as the small Depression era and World War II cohorts reach old age. When the baby boom cohort reaches 65 years of age, the rate of growth of elderly whites will exceed 2% per year until 2030.[19] Between 2030 to 2050, projections indicate that there will be no increase in the population of white elderly Americans. Similar growth patterns for the black elderly will also occur, however, it is expected that their rate of increase will be substantially greater than that of the white elderly. On average, the black elderly population will increase at a rate of 1 to 1.5% higher than the white elderly each year.[59] For elderly of other races, there was a 7% annual increase from 1960 to 1990. It is projected that this group will grow at a rate of 5% per year between 1990 and 2020; between 2020 and 2050 growth will remain relatively constant at 2% annually. Hispanic elderly are expected to continue at a steady increase of 4% per year from 1990 to 2030.[62]

Projected Components of Change in the Minority Elderly

The demographic processes of minority populations in the United States typically vary from the majority population on the demographic dimensions of fertility, mortality, immigration, and migration.[3] For instance, African Americans, Native Americans, and Mexican Americans have a higher mortality rate when compared to whites. Conversely, Japanese Americans tend to show a lower mortality rate than whites.[21] In addition, age and gender characteristics seem to influence mortality within a minority group. For example, infants and young men in the black minority have a substantially higher mortality rate when compared to other age groups and young women.[3]

Fertility Patterns The number of births is projected to fluctuate between 3.4 and 3.7 million from 1990 into the middle of the twenty-first century.[19,59] The minority population birth statistics are grouped in the census data as "Black-and-Other Races." The number of black-and-other races births is already at an all-time high of 725,000.[19] If the middle series proves correct, the number of black-and-other races births would increase to almost 900,000 in 2030 and then stabilize. There was not much of a decline in black-and-other races births during the 1990s because the number of women of childbearing age in the minority populations continued to increase.

Mortality Patterns The pattern of mortality rates in minority elders varies substantially from that seen in the white population as a result of differences in life expectancy and health status.[52] Since declines in the mortality rates for blacks have historically lagged behind white mortality declines, the life expectancy of blacks is not projected to reach white levels until 2080 under all assumptions.[19] Overall life expectancy is projected to decline substantially in the future, and it is not deemed likely that blacks could attain white mortality levels any sooner than 2080. Even with this postponement of convergence, black life expectancy at birth is expected to improve two to four times more rapidly than white life expectancy.[59] There is a good deal of evidence that black and white differences in life expectancy for women are narrowing more quickly than those of men, and this trend is expected to continue.[19,59] Other than the black population, other ethnic subgroups have not been isolated for specific demographic analysis.

Immigration and Migration Patterns of Minority Elders As a result of high fertility rates and high levels of immigration, Hispanics are a relatively young population. Between 1970 and 1980, the Hispanic population as a whole grew 61%,[61] a surge that makes Hispanics the fastest-growing population in the United States. During the first half of the twenty-first century an overall growth and proportion of the aged among Hispanics is expected to occur. Though the separate Hispanic national origin groups (Mexican Americans, Puerto Ricans, Cuban Americans, and Central and South Americans) have not been isolated in demographic projections, examination of the national origins of current older Hispanics reveals the diversity of the elderly Hispanic population.[59,62] The importance of immigration patterns in the history of this ethnic group is clear.

Fewer than 5% of Hispanic of Mexicans, Puerto Rican, South and Central American origin were 65 years of age or older in 1989.[3] On the other hand, Hispanics from Cuba aged 65 and over made up approximately 20% of the entire Cuban American population, making them a relatively "old" proportion of Hispanics. Mexican Americans (also known as Chicanos) constitute 48%, Puerto Ricans 11%, Cuban Americans represent 18%, and Central and South Americans 8% of the total elderly Hispanic population. One reason for this heterogeneity within the older Hispanic population of the United States is their varied immigration histories.[62] Some Mexican Americans immigrated to the southwestern United States during colonial times. Others arrived during the "bracero" period, when the use of temporary Mexican agricultural labor was encouraged in the United States. Recent documented and undocumented immigrants to the United States from Mexico have further increased the size of the Mexican American population.[59] While the early immigrants of the colonial and "bracero" times are now reaching or have reached the age of 65, the more recent immigrants are relatively young.[62] It is the aging of this latter group that will play a major role in the growth of the Hispanic elderly in this next century.

The current aging of the Cuban subgroup is a result of their immigration to the United States as political refugees of the Castro regime during the 1960s. They came to America as young and middle-aged families, and now they are turning 65 years of age. That is why the Cuban Americans constitute a much larger proportion of the Hispanic elderly compared to the overall Hispanic population.

There is much diversity within the Asian elderly population as well. This population is also growing at a relatively rapid rate and will become an increasingly significant proportion of the United States population in the first half of the twenty-first century. In 1980, 6% of the Asian origin population was 65 and older.[63] The Asian population is made up of Chinese, Filipino, Japanese, and most recently, a subgroup of Vietnamese and Cambodians. Each of these Asian origin groups comprise about one-quarter of Asian elderly.[59,63]

The immigration history of each of these Asian subgroups varies considerably and constitutes three primary immigration waves. The oldest group are those Asians who came to the United States as young persons in the eary 1900s; a second wave is primarily made up of the children, born in the United States to the earliest immigrants from Asia, and the last group are middle-aged and elderly persons who emigrated after changes in the US immigration laws in the mid-1960s.[63] In contrast, the Vietnamese and Cambodians came to the United States as political refugees after immigration quotas were lifted in 1965 and will comprise the future wave of Asian elderly.[63]

The elderly Native American population are the "statistically invisible" subgroup of the Native American population. Approximately 80,000 Native Americans 65 years of age and over were counted in the 1999 census.[59] Elderly persons make up approximately 5% of the total Native American population. It is suggested that due to the low proportions of the Native American population who are aged, and due to changing patterns of self-identification as Native Americans, that this group of minority elderly are virtually imperceptible within the census.[3] Overall, less than 1% of the minority aged are Native Americans.[59] Between 1970 and 1980 the older Native American population grew at nearly twice the rate of the population of elderly whites or blacks.[60] This apparent increase is credited to a renewed sense of ethnic awareness that developed among Native Americans following the Wounded Knee uprising in 1970.

Geographic Distribution of Minority Elders The population distribution of minority elders is affected by patterns of international immigration and migration within the United States. Approximately one-fifth of black elderly live in rural areas, and more than 59% are concentrated in the Southeastern states. Of the remainder, most live either in the North Central or Northeast regions of the United States.[25,64,65] The vast majority of Hispanic elderly live in four states, each with a different concentration of Hispanic groups. The majority of the Hispanic population in California and Texas are from Mexico and Central America; Florida attracts the Cuban population, while New York receives a large number of immigrants from Puerto Rico and the Caribbean Islands.[62]

The proportion of Hispanic elderly living in rural areas is approximately 11%, less than half that of the rural white elderly population, which is estimated to be 26%.[25,65] The 1999 census shows that approximately 10% of Asian Pacific Islander elderly live in rural areas, and that over 55% are concentrated in California, Hawaii, and the state of Washington. Of the remainder, most live in New York and New Jersey metropolitan areas, or in Illinois and Texas.[59] About one-quarter of Native American elderly live on American Indian reservations or in Alaskan Native villages. Over half are concentrated in the Southwestern states of Oklahoma, California, Arizona, New Mexico, and Texas. Of the remainder, most live along the Canadian border. A far greater proportion (52%) of Native American elderly live in rural areas than any other subgroup of the population.[65] It becomes apparent that the population distribution and migration within the United States creates substantial variations in the age structure of populations in the various states and regions of the nation. Demographic studies indicate that racial and ethnic minorities are more geographically concentrated than the majority population.[60]

Race Distribution Trends The black-and-other races population grew from 33.6 million in 1990 to 45.3 million in the year 2000, and is expected to increase to 63.2 million in 2030, and 79.1 million by 2080.[59] About two-thirds of the growth is predicted to occur during the next half century, and the rate of growth thereafter will slow relative to any previous time.[19] In contrast, the white population is projected to increase from 198.5 million in 1990, reaching 222.7 million by the year 2000. Continued growth is expected, peaking at almost 242 million shortly after 2030, and then declining slowly to 231.6 million in 2080.[19,59]

Future projections indicate that the white population will never increase more than about 40% as rapidly as does the black-and-other races population.[59] The effect of this is that the proportion of the population that is comprised of black-and-other races will continue to rise. In 1950 this proportion was 10.7%, increasing in 1970 to 12.4% and 14.5% in 1982.[64] This proportion reached 16.9% in the year 2000. It is expected that this proportion will increase about 1.3 percentage points a decade with the black-and-other races reaching over 25% in 2030, and 29.5% by 2080.[59]

Conversely, the fraction of the black-and-other races population that is black will continue to decline. Blacks constituted 89.7% of the black-and-other races population in 1970 and 82.5% of the black-and-other races population in 1982.[64] That proportion decreased to 78.9% in 2000, and is expected to continue to decrease to 75.4% in 2030, and 70.4% in 2080.[59] This occurs despite the fact that black fertility is assumed to be considerably above the other races. In large part, the black proportion declines because of the relatively high net immigration of races other than white or black.[19]

Even if there were no growth resulting from net immigration, the proportion of black-and-other races is projected to increase because of higher future black fertility and the younger age structure of the black-and-other races population as compared to the white population. In fact, it is expected that the black-and-other races population will eventually exceed 25%.[25,60]

Age Composition of Minority Elderly The age composition of the minority aged is another important demographic feature, because the elderly population is aging within itself. People of all races are living longer. Blacks aged 85 and older increased from 67,000 in 1960 to 251,000 in 1990, and it is expected that the number of "old-old" Blacks will increase to 500,000 by 2010 and 1.8 million by the year 2050.[19,59] Between 1980 and 1990, the oldest-old Hispanics nearly doubled, increasing from 49,000 to 95,000. It is anticipated that this minority subgroup will number more than 1.5

million by 2050.[59,62] The very old for all other races increased from 4,000 in 1960 to 41,000 in 1990, a remarkable ten-fold growth rate.[63]

Projected estimates of minority population growth indicate that the most significant and dramatic changes will occur between 2020 and 2050.[19,59] Currently, around 62% of the aged in all minority groups fall within the 65 to 74 years of age range. By 2050, the numbers in this age group will decrease to about 50% for Hispanics and other races, and to about 55% of the blacks.[59] Growth is projected to occur in the percent of the aged who are 85 and older. Currently, fewer than one in ten of the minority elderly are in the oldest-old age range, but it is anticipated that this ratio will increase to one in five by the year 2050.[19,59]

Gender Composition of the Minority Elderly The gender composition of the minority aged varies considerably from gender differences in the US elderly population as a whole. In the entire population, elderly women outnumber men by three to two as a result of differences in the life expectancy between males and females. For those 85 years of age and older, women outnumber men five to two.[60,64] In the minority elderly, both because of the gender imbalances in previous migration patterns and variations in the extent to which females have better survival rates than males, these ratios become more equalized.[47] If sex ratio is defined as the number of males per 100 females, the following ratios for elderly minority groups were calculated for 2000.[59] In the young-old group (65 to 74 years old), the sex ratio for non-Hispanic whites was 81:100, for blacks it was 71:100, among Mexican American and Puerto Rican Hispanics the ratio was 100:100, for Hispanics of Cuban and Central and South American origin the ratio was 91:100, and 95:100 among Asian Americans. The sex ratio of the young elderly was more balanced among those ethnic groups that had a substantial history of immigration.[59] The less balanced ratio among blacks compared with other minorities is credited to the excess mortality rate of black men at every age.[3]

The sex ratio drops among those minority elders 75 years of age and older in all groups with the exception of Asian elderly.[3] For non-Hispanic whites the ratio becomes 59:100, for blacks it is 63:100, for Hispanics the ratio drops to 72:100, and for Asians the ratio actually increases to 124:100. Asian elderly men outnumber females until they reach the oldest-old age group of 85 years of age and over.[59] It is suggested that the more balanced sex ratio among young-old Asian Americans is the result of differences in male migration history. For example, in the early 1900s, among the Chinese population, there were fourteen males for every one female. It is expected that in the future, the relative number of Asian men to women will evolve to resemble more closely the ratios of other Asian cohorts, which had more sex-balanced immigration patterns (e.g., Asian immigrants since 1965), and the increased proportion of the Asian American elderly who were born in America.[63]

Marital Status of the Minority Elderly   Among both whites and blacks aged 65 or older, the majority of men are married and the majority of women are widowed,[65] however, among older males, more than twice as many blacks compared to whites are divorced or separated, and the proportion of widowed black men is also higher.[66] The marital status of older black and white women is generally the same, except that the percentage of older black women divorced or separated is slightly higher.[65,67]

Mirroring the white elderly population, nearly twice as many Hispanic men as women aged 65 and older are married and living with their spouses.[33] Almost twice as many older Hispanic men and women are divorced or separated compared with whites, but the same proportion of Hispanic and white women are widowed.[62,67]

The majority of Asian men aged 65 and over are married, while the majority of women are widowed. Asian women are much more likely to be married than white counterparts with a smaller proportion remaining single in their later years.[67,68]

The marital status of Native Americans is comparable to that of the white elderly population. The majority of elderly men are married, and the majority of women are widowed. Like Asian women, Native American elderly women are more likely to be married in their later years than are white women.[65,67]

Living Arrangements of the Minority Elderly   Household living arrangements of elderly non-Hispanic whites, blacks, Mexican Americans, Puerto Ricans, other Hispanics, and Asians in 1996 reveal some intriguing differences between groups. One-third of whites and blacks live alone, though generally, minority elderly rarely live alone.[67] This is particularly true of Asian elderly who tend to live in multigenerational households.[68] With the exception of black elders, living with a spouse is the most common household situation for most elderly groups.[3] It is interesting that the black elderly are less likely to be married than other minority groups, which reflects their higher rates of marital disruption in the life course.[65] In contrast, Puerto Rican and Asian elderly are three times as likely as non-Hispanic whites to live with others, including family members other than their spouses.[66] One-third of black elderly persons live with others, related or unrelated, as do approximately one-fifth of Mexican Americans and other Hispanics.[21,67]

While about 94% of all elderly live in the community, a slightly higher proportion (96%) of black elderly do.[65,67] Since relatively more older blacks compared to whites are widowed, divorced, or separated, a smaller proportion live with their spouses; sharing a home with a grown child, usually a daughter, is a common living arrangement for older blacks.[66] Only about 3% of all African American elderly are institutionalized, whereas almost 5% of white elderly are. This trend is more apparent among the oldest-old (aged 85 and over) who generally are more likely to be widowed and in need of physical and medical assistance. Among the eldest population, only 12% of blacks live in nursing homes. Twenty-three percent of white elderly over the age of 85 live in nursing homes.[67]

About 97% of Hispanic elderly live in households in the community, either alone, with family members (72% of Hispanic elders live with at least one family member), or with non-relatives. The remaining 3% live in nursing homes.[62] Among elderly Hispanics 85 years of age or older, 10% are in nursing homes compared to 23% of whites.[67]

Among the Asian elderly, 96% live outside of institutions and in the community; only 19% live alone.[67] The proportion of Asian elderly living in nursing home is approximately 2%.[63] Similar to Hispanics, 10% of Asians aged 85 and over reside in nursing homes.[67]

About 96% of Native American elderly live in households in the community with only 4% living in institutions. About the same percentage of Native American elderly compared with white elderly live with family members (66% vs 65%), and for both groups, more men than women live with family members.[65] The proportion of Native American elderly living in nursing homes is low (i.e., less than 0.2%); among the oldest-old, the proportion is similar to the black elderly, 13% of the 85 and above year old population.[59]

Income Status of the Minority Elderly   Blacks as well as other minority elderly typically are less likely to work in professions or jobs with high benefits. Also, less education, fewer skilled jobs, lower salaries, and long periods of unemployment mean that blacks are less likely to accumulate income and other assets, benefits, or pensions.[69,70] As a result, the black elderly, on the average, have less personal postretirement income and are, therefore, more dependent on Social Security benefits for the majority of their retirement.[70] The median income of black elderly Americans is substantially less than that of white elderly. Black elderly men average an annual income of $4,113, and black elderly women average $2,825, compared to $7,408 for white men and $3,894 for elderly white women.[70] The median income of Hispanic men aged 65 years and older is $4,592, or 62% that of white males the same age. Elderly Hispanic women have a median income of $2,873.[70] The income status of Asians is higher than for blacks or Hispanics, with Asian men aged 65 years or older averaging an annual income of $5,551; women have a median income of $3,476 per year. Last, the median income for elderly Native American men is $4,257, and for women 65 years of age or older it is $3,033.[70]

Poverty Status of the Minority Elderly   With the exception of Asians, a higher proportion of minority group elderly compared with non-Hispanic white elderly, live in poverty.[71,72] Living alone makes the situation even worse for the minority group elderly.[65] Over half of black and Puerto Rican elderly persons report household incomes below the poverty level.[3,70] A smaller percentage of Asian and non-Hispanic white elderly who live alone are impoverished compared to other racial and Hispanic groups, and it appears that living with a spouse reduces the fraction of elderly in the poverty groups.[70] Yet, married elderly blacks and Hispanics are three times more likely than non-Hispanic whites and Asians to be poor.[59] This census data indicates that, with the exception of Asians, approximately one in five minority group members who lives with others, lives in poverty.[69]

In urban areas, 32% of black elderly live in poverty (one in three), while 11% older whites are in poverty (one in nine). In rural areas nearly one out of two black elderly live in poverty.[69] In rural areas, almost 40% of white women over the age of 75 are poor but over two-thirds (68%) of rural black women are at or near poverty level.[69]

The percentage of Hispanic elderly with incomes below the poverty level is twice as large (26%) as that among the elderly whites (13%). Hispanic poverty rates are higher in rural than in urban areas, and higher among Hispanic women compared to men. Thus, rural women are the most impoverished Hispanic group of all. For example, among the Hispanic elderly, 38% of rural women have a below-poverty income as compared to 21% of rural white women.[62]

The proportion of Asian elderly living below the poverty level closely compares to the white elderly population. Overall, 14% of Asian elderly and 13% of white elderly live below the poverty level. Twenty-six percent of Asians living in rural areas and 37% in urban areas are poor.[69]

The Native American elderly population is comparable to the black elderly poverty status in that 32% are below the poverty level. In rural areas, the proportion is 39% and in urban areas 25% of the elderly Native Americans are poor.[69]

In light of the demographic trends previously discussed, it appears that we can expect to see a large increase in the number of female-headed households among African Americans and Hispanics, and there seems likely to be an increase in minority elderly who live alone.[73] Both of these trends portend a substantial increase in the number of minority group elderly living in poverty.

PROJECTED TRENDS IN THE WORLD'S AGING POPULATION

Most of us probably are not aware of it, but the population of the world is undergoing an historic change. The older population is growing at a dramatic rate and the balance between the world's young and old is shifting. In many developed countries of Europe, the speed of population growth occurred gradually, taking fifty to one hundred years for the percent of the population aged 65 and over to double from 7% to 14%. However, in most developing countries of the world the same population increase will take place in fewer than thirty years. In approximately thirty years, there will be 850 million elderly worldwide.[74] Here are some pertinent facts:

- In most countries of the world there are declining fertility rates and people are living longer. This means that a country's population age structure will shift towards the older age population.
- Most of the growth in the numbers of elderly is taking place in developing countries.
- In developing countries the speed with which the elderly population is growing is very fast compared with the speed of the same changes in developed/industrialized countries. This contrast is particularly evident if you compare East Asia with Western Europe.
- Europe is the "oldest" world region, with the highest proportion of population aged 65 and older, and Africa is the youngest. Sweden is considered to be the oldest country with 18% of its population aged 65 and older.[75]

Life Expectancy   There are several interesting trends in life expectancy. First, for most countries in the world, more babies are surviving infancy and childhood. Second, during the first half of the twentieth century, developed countries saw the average life expectancy of their population increase by over twenty years. Spain, which had a comparatively low life expectancy in 1900, saw it double by 1995 and equal that of other developed nations.[76]

Beginning in the 1950s, a new trend emerged in developed countries—female life expectancy continued to rise but gains in male life expectancy slowed significantly or leveled off. In most developed countries of the world, women outlive men by five to nine years. By 1995, the life expectancy for females in over fifteen nations was at or exceeded eighty years.[77] The fourth trend is that the oldest-old (aged 80 and older) are the fastest growing segment of many nations' populations. In most developed countries the oldest-old already account for more than 20% of the overall elderly population. For the Scandinavian countries, France, and Switzerland, the oldest-old are approximately 4% of the total population.[77] The final trend is that increases in life expectancy are not uniform for all people living within a country. Indigenous populations living in developed countries have population pyramids that are more typical of developing countries within the African continent (e.g., they have high fertility and mortality levels across all age groups) than they are of the developed country in which they live. For example, American Indian, Eskimo, and Aleut populations have an age structure more like Morocco than that of the United States; and the Aborigines and Torres Strait Islanders of Australia have a population pattern that is roughly the same as in Ethiopia.[74]

A new study[77] finds that the life expectancy of people in the industrialized nations—Canada, France, Germany, Italy, Japan, the United Kingdom, and the United States (Group of 7, or G-7)—may be greater than official estimates now predict. By 2050, populations in these countries may be living from 1.3 years (UK) to 8 years (Japan) longer than formerly projected. In the United States, the current government estimate is 80.45 years; the new study estimate is 82.91 years.[77] The study is based on newer demographic models that incorporate mortality data for the past fifty years. The differences in forecasted life expectancy influence the ratio of the population over age 65 to the population aged 20 through 64. This so-called dependency ratio has important implications for planning retirement systems and health care programs. It is projected that by 2050 these ratios will be higher by between 6% (UK) and 40% (Japan), suggesting that programs for old-age support need to be reexamined worldwide.[77]

The Dependency/Support Ratio   How do we measure the impact of world aging? As mentioned above, dependency or support ratios are used. The dependency or support ratio is the ratio of the number of older people in the population to the population in the age categories most closely associated with employment (generally 20 to 64 years of age).[76] This ratio is intended to give an estimation of the size of the elderly population in comparison to the size of the population that can be expected to pay taxes to support benefits for the older group. This is a less than perfect measure since there are many people over the age of 64 still working and many younger people who are unemployed. It also does not take into consideration that many retired older people provide child care, which allows adult parents to enter or remain in the workforce. However, the ratio is a frequently cited statistic used by policy makers. The apparently favorable economic effect of slowing population growth in terms of total dependency/support ratio, actually increases the old-age dependency ratio.[78] Because older dependents lay claim to more public resources than do young dependents, the weight of the "old" component has great economic significance. For example, it is estimated that by the year 2025, in East Asia there will be about thirty-two older people for every one hundred working age people.[74] With change in the age structure of the population consumption patterns of the people will change. The needs of older people are very different from the needs of middle-aged and younger people. Thus, businesses will have to reorient their policies. Entirely new products and marketing strategies will need to be developed.

Health and Disability   The number of disabled persons is likely to increase rapidly as populations grow older. Emerging morbidity patterns in developing countries may require a reevaluation of health services and service provision.

Given the nonmedical factors that can affect health status, the World Health Organization (WHO) takes a broad view of health, involving the health sector in the larger context of improving the quality of life. This is in accord with the organization's definition of health as complete physical, mental, and social well-being. In regard to the elderly segment of the world population, specific health goals that have been articulated include: promotion of maximum independence and productivity; prevention of debilitating conditions in old age through healthier lifestyles, early diagnosis, environmental safety, and health education.

As might be anticipated, chronic conditions are more prevalent than acute disorders and infection among the world's elderly. However, on an international level there are substantial short falls in the provision of primary health care services to the aging, and in the provision of health aids, particularly in underdeveloped countries and rural areas.[75] There is a high prevalence of physical disability, particularly as regards sight, hearing, ambulation, and nutrition.

Among the world's elderly, arthritis, high blood pressure, foot problems, heart disease, lung disease, and stomach ulcers are the most common problems.[79] As an example of the prevalence of arthritis, for instance, cross-national surveys regarding morbidity indicate that 35.8% of all elderly persons in Myanmar reported suffering from arthritis, 11.9% in Korea, 49.1% in Indonesia, 31.3% in Sri Lanka, and 59.5% in Thailand. Quite substantial proportions of the elderly suffer from hypertension and heart disease, lung problems, foot ulcers, and stomach ulcers. These diseases, along with impaired vision and hearing, greatly affect their ability to carry out daily activities, self-care functions, and employment. Chronic illnesses also impose a huge burden on the national health expenditure in each country.[75,79]

Accessibility and availability of health services are limited in many countries. Of eleven countries surveyed by the United Nations,[75] only a few countries (Korea, Sri Lanka, India) reported that more than 90% of their citizens have access to a health facility within one hour's travel time. The geriatric services, if they exist, are mostly located in urban settings. Although services and programs of nongovernmental organizations and charitable agencies are gradually emerging, the number, scale, and scope of their activities are woefully inadequate to accommodate the health care needs of the vast number of the elderly population of the world. Technological advances in the field of medicine have created a parallel demand for their utilization. However, this potential comes at a huge cost that many older people are unable to afford.[79] Compared to a developed country, reported illness among elderly in developing countries is much higher, but actual utilization of health services is considerably lower.[80]

Social and Cultural Aspects of Our Aging Societies
In recent decades, older persons have begun to concentrate more in urban areas of each country and this trend is projected to continue. In developing countries, estimates of elderly people currently living in urban areas ranges from 25 to 30%. This is likely to increase to 40% by the year 2005.[75]

For able older persons, continued employment can serve simultaneously to maintain personal earnings, to promote participation in the social and economic life of the community, and to ease the burden placed on national resources for support of the economically inactive elderly. Yet, the frequency of unemployment among older workers is generally increasing, and provisions for early retirement in most industrialized nations are becoming more prevalent. At the same time, however, pressure for adaptation of work places to suit the needs of older employees, the introduction of part-time work schedules, and inclusion of older workers in vocational training programs is gaining strength in many countries.[81]

A question of concern is this: If the trend toward urbanization of countries continues, will it create conflicts among generations in both rural and urban areas? Still, the process of urbanization in developing countries seems to have a negative effect on opportunities for employment in rural areas, particularly in traditional trades. For example, if self-employed craftsmen lose their source of income, they tend to experience great difficulty in obtaining another job. Within cities, the employment problems of older persons are particularly severe, often jeopardizing their sole means of subsistence. When older, for the most part untrained, workers find themselves without jobs late in life, they often have no way to sustain themselves and no recourse to other sources of support—neither through the traditional extended family nor state-based social welfare systems. The concept of retirement has little meaning in self-employed farming and other small-scale economic activities; older persons in the rural sector of developing countries tend to continue working far longer than in any other sector of the economy. In this context, the problem is not one of opportunities to work, but rather access to sufficient resources to permit withdrawal from the labor force as physical capabilities decline.

The basic needs in old age are essentially the same as for an individual of any age: secure housing, financial security, good health, availability of essential commodities and services, harmonious relationships with family and neighbors, and activities that can provide a sense of self-worth. The quantity of these basic needs is variable and how they will be met differs from culture to culture. In some societies, aged individuals have minimal demands and expectations and these can frequently be met within the family. In other societies, older individuals have much higher expectations and demands and these can be met only with the assistance of the broader society. Significant social, demographic, and cultural changes, as well as scientific and technical advances, are occurring around the world that will substantially affect the elderly of today and will affect the elderly of tomorrow even more so.

How an aged individual lives today and will live tomorrow depends very much on the local culture, traditions, and policies of their society. Not only are there substantial nation-to-nation differences, there are also significant differences in urban and rural areas within regions and between different groups within any area.

How countries decide to use their resources for assuring health care and material security for the elderly is important. Among developed countries for example, cultural expectations can lead to different actions. Traditionally, Sweden and Japan have had very different social goals regarding the elderly when it comes to living arrangements. In Sweden, approximately 6% of the elderly, compared to 65% in Japan, live with their children. Sweden's social policy emphasizes that an independent life is desirable and that older people should live in their own homes. There are many ways in which the Swedish government supports the elderly living on their own, such as having various types of specialized housing and social services. In Japan, prewar tradition supports the elderly living within their family—preferably with the eldest son—and Japanese culture and government has generally stressed that older parents are a family responsibility. However, there has been a gradual shift in Japanese opinion. Based on a 1997 Japanese national attitude survey, researchers found that only half the people they surveyed believed that parents should live with their adult children. However, in times of need, such as when a parent is widowed or sick, 80% of Japanese surveyed felt that parents should reside with their adult children.[82]

The proportion of elderly people living with their children in developed countries in western Europe and North America changed between the 1950s and the 1990s. A five-nation study found a dramatic decline in intergenerational coresidence. Sweden, which has always had the smallest proportion of elderly living with their children as noted previously, declined from a high coresidence of approximately 28% in the 1950s to 6% in the 1990s.[83] The United States, France, and Britian also showed declines, with Britian experiencing a particularly sharp drop (42% to 18%). Coresidence is the standard throughout the rest of the world. In Asia, about three-quarters of the elderly live with their adult offspring. However, demographers report that in a number of east Asian countries, most notably Japan (a developed country) coresidence is declining. The proportion of elderly Japanese living with their adult children shifted from 77% in 1970 to approximately 65% in 1985.[83]

While the overall picture still shows that in developing countries the elderly reside with their families and in developed countries the elderly reside on their own in the community, there are changes occurring that may alter these patterns. Urban migration in many developing countries is depleting the number of young people living in rural areas. This has led, or is leading, to large increases in the number of elderly who must shift for themselves. For example, in some areas of India, older people already have no children living with them to provide support.[84] Due to economic pressures in urban areas, their children are not able to send money back home to the village to support their parents. Until recently, the practice of apartheid frequently separated elderly blacks living in South African townships from their children.[85] Urban-dwelling blacks, who had lived and worked in townships for their entire adult lives, were not allowed to remain in those townships after retirement and were forced to return to their villages of origin. This separated them from their adult children who, for economic reasons, had to remain in the township.[84]

Living arrangements appear to be related to gender as well. Very old widowed women are more likely than older men to reside alone. This appears to be the case in both developed and developing nations due to the longer life span of women relative to men and to the tendency for women to marry men who are older than them.[84] According to global study findings,[79] in most of the developing countries, almost half of the male elderly reside with their spouses, around a quarter with spouse and children, another 23% with only their children and only 2 to 3% of elderly males live alone. This is not the case for elderly females. About 18% are living with their spouses, 75 to 78% live with children or nonrelatives, and 5 to 6% or more are living alone. In developed countries, the number and proportion of older women living alone is much greater. In the United States, while only 16% of older men lived alone in 1987, 41% of older women did so. For women over the age of 75 in the United States, approximately half are living alone. In Western Europe, the number is even higher. For example, in Great Britain approximately 80% of women aged 75 and older lived alone in 1985.[84] Similarly in Japan while only 4.3% of elderly men live alone, about 11% of elderly women reside alone.

Institutionalization in nursing homes is low in most countries. In Japan, the proportion of the elderly aged 65 and older living in institutions is about 1.6%; in the United States, it is about 5%; in Germany, 4%; in Australia, 6%; and in Sweden, 9%.[84]

In some countries, fewer than one in ten older persons can read and write.[81] Secondary school completion rates of 2% or less are not uncommon among older populations, especially females. Literacy rates among the elderly, reflecting limited opportunities for education, were shown to be low in developing countries,

primarily in the rural areas. This means that the elderly, particularly elderly women, tend to be disadvantaged in areas where education and adaptation to new roles may be an important factor such as, in reemployment, knowledge of health and social issues, and in managing daily affairs without assistance.

CONCLUSION

Over the next 30 years, the number of Americans who are 65 years of age or older will increase to nearly 20% of the population, an increase from the present level of just under 12%. As the population ages, increasing levels of functional disability will impact the need for rehabilitative services for home and nursing home care. Within this older age group, there will be a growing number who will reach extreme old age (100 and beyond) within the proportion of the population that is the 85 years and older. It is this latter group who will have a significant impact on the nation's health care needs and costs.

At present, 20% of those 85 years of age and older are institutionalized and this statistic is not likely to change. The 85 years and older group in the United States is anticipated to increase eightfold, creating an increased demand for home care, nursing home care, and services from all health care providers. Health care providers must begin to plan now for this increase to ensure that as the demand for home care and nursing home care grows, the necessary rehabilitative and restorative services, provisions for nursing care, and financing mechanisms will be available.

Census information and research data are scarce for minority elderly populations. In fact, some researchers have alluded to the statistical invisibility of the minority aged.[3] Census data often underrepresents ethnic minorities and does not provide information on health and disability, which are essential indicators of well-being for the elderly.[86] Most of the research surveys available provide data for blacks and whites and for those of Hispanic origin. Very little information is available on other subgroups of the American culture.

Clearly, in the field of gerontology we need to become more conscious of the increasing ethnic diversity of America's aged and to attend seriously to that diversity in the design and execution of research on the elderly. All too often the elderly are seen as a homogeneous group. The elderly in the United States are a melange of different social classes, national origins, and family types, and this diversity will lead to a set of conflicting demands on our social institutions and will require creative policy solutions.

The status of minority elderly is not likely to improve greatly in the immediate future; however, the importance of projections of the minority aged population—not only in terms of total size but in terms of social characteristics of the older minority populations—should assist in directly effective policy development and implementation. An expanded database will permit interactive projections that will enable analyses to be made of the social and economic implications of demographic developments implicit in the process of majority and minority aging in the United States. This will have an important bearing on the public policy decision making needed for a constructive response to an aging population.

We can expect that a society in which a huge proportion of the population is over 65 years old will function quite differently than a society where there are few elderly. Just think about how the baby boom generation influenced social trends during the 1960s, primarily because of sheer numbers. The new demographic change will likely have a strong impact as well. For example, we can foresee a heavy demand on pension plans and the health care system. Advertising will emphasize goods and services for an aging market. Music and fashion will be aimed at older tastes. Relationships too, will change. For example, in 1800, by the time a woman was 37, she could expect both her parents to be dead. Today, about half of all 60-year-old women have living mothers. In the future, as this trend persists, more and more of the middle-aged will have elderly parents, many of whom will need care and suport.

From a demographic prospective, the patterns that surface in the changing size and composition of the aged population modify consumer demands, political constituencies, economic conditions, and social structures. A focus on the aged as a subpopulation emphasizes the needs that arise from the absolute number and differing types of older persons, as well as from their relative proportion in the total population. This is particularly important for public policy development and program implementation. It calls attention to the need to recognize the differential demands on public and private services and resources that arise from the growth and changing composition of the aged population.

PEARLS

- Consideration of population aging began in Europe in the 1800s but is now a recognized worldwide, twentieth and twenty-first century phenomenon.
- Change in population size depends on the rates of birth, immigration, death, and emigration. Growth in the total population is most sensitive to a decline in mortality rates, whereas growth in the older population is due to a decline in fertility rates.
- The elderly made up 12.6% of the US population in 1990, and this figure is expected to climb to 20% by 2030.
- The US birthrate will stay below 3.7 million per year or decline, and the death rate will steadily decrease.

- The current ratio of elderly women to elderly men is three to two, and it is five to two for those over age 85. These ratios are expected gradually to increase through the twenty-first century.
- Viewed as a homogeneous group, the majority of elderly are free of disability until extreme old age.
- It is estimated that the number of minority elderly will grow at a more rapid rate than the number of white elderly over the next 60 years.
- In approximately 30 years, there will be 850 million elderly worldwide.

REFERENCES

1. Myers GC. Demography of aging. In: Binstock RH, George LK, eds. *Handbook of Aging and the Social Sciences*. 3rd ed. San Diego: Academic Press, Inc.; 1990.
2. Zofp FE, Jr. *America's Older Population*. Houston: Cap & Gown Press; 1986.
3. Angel JL, Hogan DP. The demography of minority aging populations. In: *Minority Elders: Longevity, Economics and Health: Building Public Policy Base*. Washington, DC: Gerontological Society of America; 1991.
4. Committee on an Aging Society, Institute of Medicine/National Research Council. In: *Health in an Older Society*. Washington, DC: National Academy Press; 1985.
5. Gilford DM, ed. *The Aging Population in the Twenty-First Century*. Washington, DC: National Academy Press; 1988.
6. Rosenwaike I, Logue B. *The Extreme Aged in America: A Portrait of an Expanding Population*. Westport, CT: Greenwood Press; 1985.
7. United Nations. *The Aging of Populations and Its Economic and Social Implications*. New York: United Nations; 1956. (ST/SOA/SER.A/26).
8. Sundbarg G. *Grunddragen of befolkningslaren*. Stockholm. 1894.
9. Sundbarg G. Sur la repartition de la population par age et sur les taux de mortalite [On the separation of the population by age and the rates of mortality]. *Bul Internat Institute Statistics*. 1900; 12 (99):89–94.
10. Dublin LI. *Health and Wealth: A Survey of the Economics of World Health: The Problem of Age*. New York: Harper; 1928; 149–168.
11. Pearl R. The aging of populations. *J Am Statistical Assoc Am*. 1940; 209:277–297.
12. Dublin LI, Lotka AJ. *Length of Life: A Study of the Life Table*. New York: Ronald Press; 1937.
13. Thompson WS, Whelpton PK. *Population Trends in the United States*. New York: McGraw-Hill; 1933.
14. Kinsella K. *Aging in the Third World*. Washington, DC: US Government Printing Office; 1988. US Bureau of the Census, International Population Reports, Series P-95, No. 79.
15. United Nations. *Economic and Social Implications of Population Aging*. New York: United Nations; 1988. (ST/ESA/SER.R/85).

16. Treas J, Logue B. Economic development and the older population. *Pop Dev Rev.* 1987; 12:645–673.

17. Winsborough HH. A demographic approach to the life cycle. In: Back KW, ed. *Life Course Integrative Theories and Exemplary Populations.* Boulder, CO: Westview; 1980. (AAAS Selected Symposium 41).

18. Soldo BJ. America's elderly in the 1980's. *Population Bull.* 1980; 35(4):1–48.

19. Spencer G. *Projections of the Population of the United States by Age, Sex, and Race: 1982 to 2050.* Washington, DC: US Bureau of the Census. Current Population Reports, Series P-25, No. 1007; 1989.

20. Rosenwaike I. A demographic portrait of the oldest-old. *Milbank Memorial Fund Quarterly Health and Society.* 1985; 63:187–205.

21. Preston SH, Himes C, Eggers M. Demographic conditions responsible for population aging. *Demography.* 1989; 26:691–704.

22. Grigsby JS. *The Demographic Components of Population Aging.* University of Michigan and Pomona College; 1988. Working paper.

23. US Bureau of the Census. *Population Estimates by Age, Sex, Race, and Hispanic Origin: 1980 to 1988.* Washington, DC: US Government Printing Office; 1990. Current Population Reports, series P-25, no. 1045.

24. US Bureau of the Census. *Statistical Abstract of the United States. Profiles of Older Americans: 1999.* Washington DC: US Government Printing Office; 2000.

25. Administration on Aging. Older Americans 2000: Key Indicators of Well-Being. Federal Interagency. Forum on Aging-Related Statistics. Washington DC: Bureau of the Census. 2000.

26. Bourgeois-Pichat J. *Future Outlook for Mortality Decline in the World.* United Nations, Population Bulletin of the United Nations, 1978. No. 11; 12–41.

27. Crimmins EM. Implications of recent mortality trends for the size and composition of the population over 65. *Rev Public Data Use.* 1983; 11(l): 37–48.

28. Rice DP. Long life to you. *American Demographics.* 1979; 1(9):9–15.

29. Siegel JS, Envidson M. *Demographic and Socioeconomic Aspects of Aging in the United States.* Washington, DC: US Bureau of the Census. Current Population Reports, series P-23, 1991.

30. Verbrugge LM. Recent trends in sex mortality differentials in the United States. *Women and Health.* 1980; 5(3):17–37.

31. Waldon I. Sex differences in longevity. In: Haynes SG, Feinleib M, eds. *Second Conference on the Epidemiology of Aging.* 1980; 163–186. Washington, DC: NIH Publication No. SO-969.

32. Taeuber C. Diversity: the dramatic reality. In: Bass SA, Kutza EA, Torres-Gil FM, eds. *Diversity in Aging.* Glenview, Ill: Scott, Foresman & Co.; 1990.

33. US Bureau of the Census. *Current Population Reports: Poverty in the United States: 1998.* P60-207, September 1999 Report; Washington DC: US Bureau of the Census. 1999.

34. Kalache A, Keller I. The greying world: a challenge for the twenty-first century. *Sci Prog.* 2000; 83(Pt 1):33–54.

35. Soldo BJ, Agree EM. America's elderly. *Population Bull.* 1988; 43(3):1–51.

36. Myers G, Nathanson C. Aging and the family. *World Health Stat Quart.* 1982; 35:225–238.

37. Myers GC, Manton KG, Bacellar H. Sociodemographic aspects of future unpaid productive roles. *Productive Roles in an Older Society.* Washington, DC: National Academy Press. Committee on an Aging Society, Institute of Medicine and National Research Council; 1986; 110–147.

38. US Bureau of the Census. *Projections of the Number of Households and Families: 1979 to 1995.* Washington, DC: US Government Printing Office; 1989. Current Population Reports, series P-25, no. 805.

39. Riley AG. *Aging and Society: Notes on the Development of New Understandings.* Ann Arbor: University of Michigan Press; 1983.

40. Gore T, Bottomley JM. Legislative and public policy issues related to elder homelessness. *Topics Geriatr Rehab.* 2001; 7(1):14–22.

41. Crane M, Warnes AM. Older people and homelessness: prevalence and causes. *Topics Geriatr Rehab.* 2001; 6(4)1–14.

42. Wright J, Rubin B, Devine J. *Beside the Golden Door: Policy, Politics and the Homeless.* New York: Aldine de Gruyter; 1998.

43. Cohen C. Aging and homelessness. *Gerontologist.* 1999; 39(1):5–14.

44. Burt M. Homelessness: definitions and counts. In: Baumohl J, ed. *Homelessness in America.* Phoenix, AZ: Oryx Pubs; 1996; 15–23.

45. US Bureau of the Census. *Population Projections of the United States by Age, Sex, Race and Hispanic Origin: 1995–2050.* Current Population Reports. 1999; series P-25, no. 1130.

46. Jette AM, Branch LG. The Framingham disability study: II: Physical disability among the aging. *Am J Public Health.* 1981; 71:1211–1216.

47. Richards H, Berry R. U.S. life tables for 1990 by sex, race, and education. *J Forensic Economics.* 1998; 11:9–26.

48. Preston SH, Elo IT, Rosenwaike I, Hill M. African-American mortality at older ages: Results of a matching study. *Demography.* 1996; 33(2):193–209.

49. Manton KC, Stallard E, Wing S. Analyses of black and white differentials in the age trajectory of mortality in two closed cohort studies. *Stat Med.* 1991; 10:1043–1059.

50. National Center for Health Statistics. *Health, United States, 1999, with Health and Aging Chartbook.* Hyattsville, MD: National Center for Health Statistics, 1999; 36–37.

51. National Center for Health Statistics. *Health, United States, 1999, with Health and Aging Chartbook.* Hyattsville, MD: National Center for Health Statistics, 1999; 34–35.

52. Centers for Disease Control and Prevention. *Unrealized Prevention Opportunities: Reducing the Health and Economic Burden of Chronic Disease.* Atlanta,

GA: Centers for Disease Control and Prevention, National Center for Chronic Disease Prevention and Health Promotion. 1997.

53. Wygaard HA, Albreksten G. Risk factors for admission to a nursing home. A study of elderly people receiving home nursing. *Scand J Primary Health Care.* 1992; 10:128–133.

54. Wells KB, Stewart A, Hays RD, et al. The functioning and well-being of depressed patients. Results from the Medical Outcomes Study. *JAMA.* 1989; 262:914–919.

55. Idler IL, Benyamini Y. Self-reported health and mortality: a review of twenty-seven community studies. *J Health & Social Behavior.* 1997; 38:21–37.

56. National Center for Health Statistics. *Current Estimates from the National Health Interview Survey: United States, 1981.* Washington, DC: US Government Printing Office; 1982. US Department of Health and Human Services Publication No. 10-141.

57. US Department of Health and Human Services. *Physical Activity and Health: A Report of the Surgeon General.* Atlanta, GA: Centers for Disease Control and Prevention, National Center for Chronic Disease Prevention and Health Promotion. 1996.

58. Butler RN, Davis R, Lewis CB, Nelson ME, Strauss E. Physical fitness: benefits of exercise for the older patient. *Geriatrics.* 1998; 53(10):46–62.

59. US Census Bureau. *Projections of Population Trends.* Available from: *http://www.census.gov/population/projections/nation/summary/np-t3-a.txt.*

60. Taeuber C, Smith D. Minority elderly: an overview of demographic characteristics and 1990 census plans. Presented to the National Council on Aging Symposium; 1988; Washington, DC.

61. Torres-Gil. Hispanics: a special challenge. In: Pifer A, Bronte L, eds. *Our Aging Society: Paradox and Promise,* New York: Norton & Co. 1986; 219–242.

62. Cubillos HL, Prieto MM. *The Hispanic Elderly: A Demographic Profile.* Washington, DC: Policy Analysis Center, National Council of La Raza; 1987.

63. Agree E. *Portrait of Asian Elderly.* Washington, DC: American Association of Retired Persons, Minority Affairs Initiative. Georgetown University Population Research Center; 1985.

64. US Bureau of the Census. *Preliminary Estimates of the Population of the United States by Age, Sex, and Race: 1970 to 1981.* Washington, DC: US Government Printing Office; 1982. Current Population Reports, series P-25, no. 917.

65. Agree E. *A Portrait of Older Minorities.* Washington, DC: American Association of Retired Persons, Minority Affairs Initiative. Georgetown University Population Research Center; 1985.

66. Siegel JS, Taeuber CM. Demographic perspectives on the long-live society. *Daedalus.* 1986; 115: 77–117.

67. Saluter AF, Lugaila TA. *Marital Status and Living Arrangements: March 1996.* US Census Bureau, Current Population Reports. P60–207. Washington, DC: US Government Printing Office. 1998.

68. Kim PK. Demography of Asian-Pacific elderly: Selected problems and implications. In: McNeely RL, Colen JL, eds. *Aging in Minority Groups.* Beverly Hills: Sage Publications; 1983; 29–41.

69. Dalaker J. *Poverty in the United States: 1998.* Table 2. US Census Bureau, Current Population Reports. P60–207. Washington, DC: US Government Printing Office. September 1999.

70. Social Security Administration. *Income of the Population 55 or Older, 1998.* Tables VIII.4 and VIII.11. Washington DC: US Government Printing Office. 2000.

71. Smith JP. Wealth inequality among older Americans. *J Gerontol.* 1997; 52B (Special Issue):74–81.

72. Crystal S. Economic status of the elderly. In: Binstock RH, George LK, eds. *Handbook of Aging and the Social Sciences.* 4th Ed. San Diego, CA: Academic Press, 1996.

73. Worobey JL, Angel RJ. Functional capacity and living arrangements of unmarried elderly persons. *J Gerontol.* 1990; 45(3):95–101.

74. Diczfalusy E. The third age, the Third World and the third millennium. *Contraception.* 1996; 53(1):1–7.

75. United Nations. *World Population Prospects: The 1998 Revision.* Vol. 1. Comprehensive Tables. New York: United Nations; 1999.

76. Wilmoth JR, Horiuchi S. Demography 1999. *Demograph.* 1999; 36:475–495.

77. Tuljapurkar SD, Li N, Boe C. Life expectancy in G-7 nations may exceed past predictions. *Nature.* June 15, 2000; 405:789–792.

78. Horiuchi S. Demography: Greater lifetime expectations. *Nature.* June 15, 2000; 405:744–745.

79. Butler RN. Global Ageing: Challenges and opportunities of the next century. *Aging International.* Summer 1996.

80. Gilford DM. *The Aging Population in the Twenty-First Century: Statistics for Health Policy.* Washington DC: National Academy Press. 1998.

81. Restrepo HE, Rozental R. The social impact of aging populations: Some major issues. *Soc Sci Med.* 39(9):1323–1338, 1994.

82. Andrews GR. Ageing in Asia and the Pacific: A multidimensional cross-national study in four countries. *Comparative Gerontology.* 1997; 1:24–32.

83. Hafez G. The "greying" of the nations. *World Health.* 1994; July–Aug 47(4).

84. Myers GC, Agree EM. The world ages, the family changes: A demographic perspective. *Aging International.* March 1994.

85. Allain TJ, Wilson AO, Gomo ZA, Mushangi E, Senanje B, Adamchak DJ, Matenga JA. Morbidity and disability in elderly Zimbabweans. *Age and Ageing.* 26:115–121, 1997.

86. Jette AM, Bottomley JM. The graying of America. *Am J Phys Ther.* 1987; 67(10):1527–1542.

Additional Recommended Reading

Berkman CS, Gurland GJ. The relationship among income, other socioeconomic indicators, and functional level in older persons. *J Aging Health.* 1998; 10:81–98.

Bureau of the Census. *Statistical Abstract of the United States. Profiles of Older Americans: 1998.* Washington DC: Bureau of the Census. 1999.

Current Population Reports. In: *Developments of Aging: 1997.* Vol. 25. Washington DC: US Senate Special Committee on Aging. 1998.

Dey AN. Characteristics of elderly nursing home residents: Data from the 1995 National Nursing Home Survey. *Advance Data From Vital and Health Statistics,* No. 289. Hyattsville, MD: Public Health Service, DHHS Publication No (PHS) 97-1250, 1997.

Elo IT, Preston SH. Racial and ethnic differences in mortality at older ages. In: Martin LG, Soldo BJ, eds. *Racial and Ethnic Differences in the Health of Older Americans.* Washington DC: National Academy Press, 1997.

Jette AM, Branch LG. Inpairment and disability in the aged. *Chronic Dis.* 1985; 38:59–66.

Kalache A, Keller I. The greying world: a challenge for the twenty-first century. *Sci Prog.* 2000; 83(Pt 1):33–54.

Kingston RS, Smith JP. Socioeconomic status and racial and ethnic differences in functional status associated with chronic diseases. *Amer J Publ Health.* 1997; 87: 805–810.

Krauss NA, Altman BM. Characteristics of nursing home residents—1996. *MEPS Research Findings.* No. 5. Rockville, MD: Agency for Health Care Policy and Research, 1998; Pub No 99-0006.

Miller B. Minority use of community long-term care services: A comparative analysis. *J Gerontol.* 1996; 51B:S70–S81.

Norgard TM, Rodgers WL. Patterns of in-home care among elderly black and white Americans. *J Gerontol.* 1997; 52B (Special Issue):93–101.

Peck CW. Differences by race in the decline of health over time. *J Gerontol.* 1997; 52B:S336–S344.

Smith JP. Wealth inequality among older Americans. *J Gerontol.* 1997; 52B (Special Issue):74–81.

Tennstedt S, Chang B. The relative contribution of ethnicity versus socioeconomic status in explaining differences in disability and receipt of informal care. *J Gerontol.* 1998; 53B:S61–S70.

CHAPTER 2

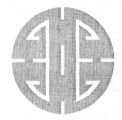

Comparing and Contrasting
the Theories of Aging

The search for the arcana of that nemesis called old age has enticed many scientists to theorize and experiment with explanations for the mechanisms involved in the aging process. What determines how we age? Are there some biological prognosticators that determine how quickly and/or how well we age? How do external factors affect our predisposed genetic makeup? The study of gerontology is a relatively young discipline, and the excitement of exploring new territory has seduced many scientific minds to delve into potential explications of how the human species ages. Several theories of aging have been proposed and the most prominent of these will be reviewed and compared in this chapter. With the decoding of the human genomes, new theories are evolving related to the potential of correcting gene coding that potentiates disease in old age and also to the possibility of extending the length of life. This critical look at current theories will provide a basic framework for understanding and evaluating the subsequent chapters on normal and pathological aging as well as clinical observations and strategies for managing the care of elderly individuals.

HISTORICAL PERSPECTIVE

The study of aging has a long history. Much of the research in the biology of aging has focused on prolongation studies rather than on the actual mechanisms of aging.[1,2] In a comprehensive monograph written in 1979 by Freeman[3] presents research on aging over the last 250 years. From the 1990s, reviews of theories of aging are reported by Rose,[1] Austad,[2] and Harman.[4] The reader is referred to these sources for a more in-depth look at the history and progress of research on aging.

Research on aging began around the turn of the twentieth century.[3] Metchnikoff introduced the concept that aging was caused by the continuous absorption of toxins from intestinal bacteria; he received the Nobel Prize in 1908 for his contributions to biology and the study of aging. Systematic studies that described the aging phenomenon in terms of cell morphology, physiology, and biochemistry began to flourish around 1950.[5] There were improvements in experimental designs in gerontological research which led to more accurate definitions of valid and reliable hypotheses. Two primary groups of aging theories evolved from the studies in the 1950s. Comfort[5] describes the first group of theories about aging as "fundamentalist" or *development-genetic theories*. These theories are based on the premise of "wear and tear,"[6] and aging is attributed to pathological decrements that are tissue-specific (e.g., connective, nervous, vascular, endocrine tissue). The second group of theories conceive of aging as an epiphenomenon in which environmental insults such as gravity, toxins, and cosmic rays impact the aging process. These theories are termed "nongenetic," environmental, or *stochastic theories* of aging. Many additional theories not contained in these two theoretical groups (though could be arguably forced into one of the categories) view aging as a continuum with development and morphogenesis,[7] while others relate aging to a cessation of somatic cell growth[8] and energy depletion.[9]

Current modified versions of these theories have incorporated research on the immune system, the neuroendocrine system, failures in deoxyribonucleic acid (DNA) repair, random mutation in somatic cells, errors in protein synthesis, and random damage from free radicals.[10] Specific theories related to sleep and the rate of aging, growth hormone, dehydroepiandrosterone (DHEA), telomeres, and cell culture models of aging involving specific proteins have evolved. The most recent theories identify genetic characteristics (genotypes) and their effects on survival and the "rate-of-change."[11]

These theories, though often presented as separate from each other, are not mutually exclusive. Clearly, there has not been any one theory that fully identifies all of the causes, mechanisms, or basis of aging. The processes regulating the rate of aging may be different in different cell types and in different tissues, and the combined effects of environmental damage and intrinsic pathologies may further obscure a fundamental mechanism for aging. Clear mechanisms of aging may depend on interdependent sets of variables and causes and affected by an individuals genetic makeup, life style, and environmental influences.

From a historical perspective, the concept of aging as a cell-based phenomenon versus organismic aging is comparatively new. Weissman[8] was the first to emphasize the distinction between somatic cells which age and germ cells which do not age. He suggested that the inability of somatic cells to replicate indefinitely was the reason for limited life span in the human. This theory was subjected to serious questioning because of a flawed series of experiments by Carrel,[12–14] and the study of cellular aging was set back by this historic event in biologic science. In 1912, Carrel and Ebeling[13] began a series of experiments using normal chick embryo fibroblasts cultured in vitro. Based on Carrel's experiments, it was thought that fibroblasts could replicate indefinitely and were immortal. The findings were considered to be compelling evidence that individual cells could live forever. This hypothesis dominated gerontology until 1950, and it was an accepted fact that cells did not characteristically age. It was thought that cells were immortal in isolation and that it was the tissues that were involved in aging. Scientists later discovered that the method Carrel used to prepare the chick embryo extract was contaminated with the continual addition of fresh embryonic cells. The result was erratic mitotic activity coinciding with the periodic addition of chick embryo extract.[15] In summary, these cells lived forever because young embryo cells were mixed with the older prepared culture.

In 1961, a landmark study by two then unknown cell biologists, Hayflick and Moorehead,[16] turned the study of senescence of cultured cells completely around. They concluded from their in vitro studies of fetal fibroblast cells (lung, skin, muscle, heart) that human fibroblasts have a limited life span in culture. Hayflick and Moorhead reported that there was a period of rapid and vigorous cellular proliferation consistently followed by a decline in proliferative activity and characteristic senescent changes (e.g., decreased replication and wasting). They proposed that aging was a cellular as well as an organismic phenomenon. The loss in functional capacity of the aging person reflected the summation of the loss of critical functional capabilities within individual cells. For instance, the loss of type II fibers in the muscle with aging results in atrophy and a decrease in the muscle force production, thereby decreasing functional capacity. The Hayflick and Moorehead experiment altered the direction and interpretation of aging research and cellular biology. In essence, they were among the first scientists to set the course of the philosophy of modern biology and gerontology. From this basis, the subsequent theories evolved.

ANIMAL MODELS OF AGING

The tortoise and the lobster exhibit remarkably few features of aging, albeit for reasons not yet known. In fruit flies, the activation of the methuselah gene confers approximately a 30% extension of longevity. In the laboratory, neuronal sprouting can be stimulated by either apolipoprotein Apo E-3 or Apo E-4, whose production is increased by estrogen.[17] Apo-E transgenic knockout mice (mice without these apolipoproteins) do not exhibit neurite outgrowth in response to estrogen. This finding may be pertinent to the presumed role of estrogen in the prevention of neuronal aging and Alzheimer's disease. Estrogen also induces glial fibrillary acidic protein in astrocytes and their abutment and retraction from regulatory gamma-aminobutyric acid (GABA)-producing terminals that synapse on gonadotropin-releasing hormone (GnRH) neurons in the young female rat, but not in older animals that have lost the capacity to generate a luteinizing hormone (LH) surge.[17] The important new concept of defective hormone-sensitive neuronal plasticity with aging will require further experimental appraisal.

Dietary restriction (DR) has also been found to increase life span in many types of animals.[18] It has been suggested that the response to chronic dietary restriction may be an adaptation to environments with variable food levels. The ability to slow aging when food levels are low purportedly postpones reproductive senescence and therefore allows reproduction when food levels are high.[19] Harrison and Archer[19] predicted that the response to DR should be strongest in species with short reproductive life spans, because these species would be more likely to encounter periods of low food that are longer than their normal reproductive life spans. In contrast, Phelan and Austad[20] noted that reproductive senescence may be uncommon in nature and suggested that the increase in life span in response to DR is not an adaptation to variable food levels, but is instead a "secondary consequence of its effect in delaying age at maturity and decreasing the subsequent rate of reproduction." They predicted that the response to DR should be strongest in those species with early maturity and high reproductive rates. Recent investigations into animal models of aging with DR found that most species, but not all, responded by increasing mean life span, maximum life span, reproductive life span, mortality rate doubling time, and initial mortality rate.[18] Interspecific comparisons did not show the predicted correlations between the strength of the response to DR and either reproductive life span, age of first reproduction, or total reproduction. There was support for the idea that the response to chronic DR is associated with changes in reproductive allocation during short-term periods of starvation. In other words, species that reduced reproduction when starved increased their life spans under DR, whereas species that continued to reproduce when starved decreased their life spans under DR.[18]

Gene studies provide a foundation of convincing proof for age- and genotype-specific effects on gene expression and longevity. These studies reveal key similarities in genetic makeup among the growing number of animal models of decelerated aging.[21] Animal models of aging have been extrapolated and tested in attempts to explain aging and longevity in the human species.

FUNDAMENTAL CONSIDERATIONS

A discussion of the theories of aging must include a review of the observations and correlations associated with the aging process. A great deal remains unknown about the nature of the mechanisms involved in aging; therefore, the study of aging is intrinsically difficult. The myriad of aging scenarios and trajectories that occur in nature, the different combinations of environmental and intrinsic changes, the lack of measurable transition points or biomarkers to define the kinetics of the process of aging, and the lack of a measurable means for aging other than death all serve to obscure any unifying principles.

It is even difficult to define "aging," although it is characterized by an increasing vulnerability to environmental changes, and it is known that increasing chronological age results in functional losses and increases the probability of death.[22] There are several underlying assumptions related to theoretic gerontology. The following fundamental considerations are an important basis upon which to build further knowledge in the studying of aging.

Aging is developmental. This concept is very simple: we do not suddenly age. Our aging time capsules do not ignite at the age of 65. We evolve into mature adults and grow older developmentally, not chronologically. Aging is unique among all developmental stages. A 70-year-old person in chronological age may have the physiologic makeup of a 50-year-old person. Yet a 50-year-old person with chronic diseases may parallel the physiologic decline of a 90-year-old person.

Old age is a gift of twentieth-century technology and scientific advancement. The gerontologist, James Birren, has penned the notion that the extended life expectancy that we now have is really a gift of modern medicine and technology. Some biologists argue that the "survivorship kinetics" of biological aging may be an artifact of civilization and domestication. In nature, populations of species (including humans) only recently began to live long enough to show the characteristic kinetics of biological aging. Since the discovery of insulin, vaccination for diseases, improved sanitation, a decline in infant mortality, and the development of modern surgical techniques and advanced treatment modes for formerly fatal diseases, humans now experience longer lives. We are also staying older longer (not younger longer) throughout the twentieth century. The whole phenomenon of aging is new. Now that we've entered the twenty-first century, it is likely that longevity will significantly increase to the point where humans can expect to live well into their ninth and tenth decades.[1]

The effects of normal aging versus pathologic aging must be differentiated if possible. A confounding problem in understanding aging is the fact that there is a vast spectrum of aging changes. The process of aging is probably multifactorial in its regulation; however, it is virtually impossible to tell which changes are primary to a senescence-regulated event and which are secondary. Often we assume that a functional decline is due to aging. However, disease may often cause functional decline, which is not a normal aging process. For example, if one has adult-onset diabetes, then the probability of cardiovascular disease increases as a result of the effect of the diabetes. It is not "normal" to get diabetes; it is a function of lifestyle and heredity. The relationship between aging, disease, and dying is confusing. Aging characteristically brings a loss in homeostasis and with it increased vulnerability to diseases, some of which result in death. Death has been used as the end point measurement of aging; however, death can occur from many causes, some of which are related to the aging process only secondarily, and in some cases totally unrelated to the process, as is true of accidents.

There is no universally accepted theory of aging. Aging does not occur in all species or in all organisms of the same species in exactly the same way. While one tissue may be losing functional capacity rapidly, others may be comparatively quite "young" functionally. (A more comprehensive discussion of this is in Chapter 3: Comparing and Contrasting Age-Related Changes in Biology, Physiology, Anatomy, and Function.) Although aging is a universal phenomenon, no one really knows what causes it or why we age at different rates. Chronological age is a much less useful and definitive measure of functional capacity than scientists would like.

Amid all these confusing assumptions of aging, a set of consistent aging characteristics has been identified. First, there is increased mortality with age.[23] Second, consistent changes in the biochemical composition of the body with age have been well documented,[24] including a decrease in lean body mass and an increase in fat. There are also characteristic increases in lipofuscin in certain tissues and an increase of cross-linkage in matrix molecules such as collagen.[23] Third, cross-sectional and longitudinal studies have provided evidence of a broad spectrum of progressive deteriorative changes.[25] (These changes will be discussed in detail in Chapter 3, Comparing and Contrasting Age-Related Changes in Biology, Physiology, Anatomy, and Function.) Fourth, there is a reduced ability to respond adaptively to environmental change—perhaps the hallmark of aging. This can be demonstrated at all levels from an individual molecule to the complete organism.[26] Thus, the changes of age are not so much the resting pulse rate nor the fasting serum glucose, but the ability to return these parameters to normal after a physiological stress. Last, there is an increased vulnerability to many diseases with age,[25] which occurs even at the cellular level. Aging is a process that is distinct from disease. The fundamental changes of aging provide the substratum in which age-associated diseases can flourish.

Aging theories can be divided into two major categories: genetic (fundamentalist) and nongenetic (environmental). Genetic theories focus on the mechanisms for aging located within the nucleus of the cell, while nongenetic theories focus on areas located elsewhere, such as in organs, tissues, systems in the body, or extrinsic environmental causes. In order to understand both of the theories of aging, a basic understanding of three somatic cell types is necessary.

Not all somatic cells age at the same rate, nor do they have similar aging characteristics. Somatic cells are divided into three categories: (1) continuously proliferating or mitotic cells, (2) reverting postmitotic cells, and (3) fixed postmitotic cells.[27] Continuously proliferating mitotic cells never cease to replicate themselves, and injury done to these cells is healed through regeneration. Such cells can be found as superficial skin cells, red blood cells, cells of the lining of the intestine, and bone marrow cells. Reverting postmitotic cells have a slower rate of division than the continuously proliferating cells; but when there is injury, the rate of division is speeded up and regeneration is possible. An example of these are kidney and liver cells. The final type of somatic cells, fixed postmitotic cells, never replicate once the cells reach maturity.[15,27] Muscle cells and nerve cells are primary examples of fixed postmitotic cells. Humans have all fixed postmitotic cells they will ever get once they have reached biological maturity (for females at the time of menses; for males at the time they stop growing).

In our adult life, nerve and muscle cells replicate and repair themselves only if the nucleus is intact. Because the postmitotic cell will not replicate itself, no new vital cells are produced. Therefore, the need for residual fixed somatic cells to remain vital is crucial to the well-being and life expectancy of the individual.

THEORIES OF AGING

Historically, one of the major problems in gerontology has been the ease and frequency with which new theories have appeared.[28] There is still not one theory that fully explains the process of aging. Researchers have viewed aging as an event that happens, rather than as a period in the life of an organism that begins at maturity (or conception?) and lasts for the rest of the life span. It seems that aging should be considered a developmental process. Numerous primary and secondary changes occur during development and aging. Some changes are programmed and directed within the body, while some changes are caused by the environment. Understanding aging and formulating coherent, testable hypotheses requires that various aspects of aging be dissected from each other and examined critically. Different authors use different classification systems for the theories of aging. All are useful, and all have inherent difficulties. One effective way to present this information is to group the multiplicity of theories into two classes based on their fundamental conceptual basis, as defined previously, and then describe prominent examples of each of these categories. The reader is reminded that this classification is operational only and that neither the categories of theories nor the theories themselves are mutually exclusive.

Developmental-Genetic Theories

The developmental-genetic theorists consider the process of aging to be part of a continuum with development genetically controlled and programmed. Opposition to this idea comes from two sources. Some researchers believe that there is a selection for aging mechanisms through evolution. In other words, aging processes are controlled extrinsically by environmental influences. The second source is the result of an intuitive sense that the diverse scenarios and trajectories of aging are not likely to be controlled by one process whose mechanisms regulate the precise sequence of development.[24] That is, that aging is not dependent on a single developmental process, but rather influenced by multifactoral ascendants.

There is no question that environmental factors can regulate or modify mortality, and in some cases influence the rate of aging (e.g., the aging of the skin is accelerated by exposure to the sun); however, the dimension of aging controlled by genetic processes clearly has some solid foundations. Gerontologists agree that the maximum life span and the rate of aging are regulated intrinsically. The primary evidence of this is the species-specific maximum life span. Variation in life span is far greater among species than within species. Because maximum life span is a species characteristic, it would seem evident that this is genetically determined. Further supporting evidence for the genetic basis of aging and maximal life span comes from the recognition of genetic disease of precocious aging, such as in genetic progeroid syndromes.[29] The classic progeria—Werner syndrome, Hutchinson-Guilford syndrome, and Down syndrome—are among these diseases. The precise mechanism of human aging is not replicated at an accelerated rate in these individuals, however, many of the commonly recognized aging changes occur more rapidly. These diseases are important probes in the study of aging.

Studies that compare the longevity of monozygotic and dizygotic twins and nontwin siblings are relevant to this discussion. It has been shown that there is a remarkable similarity in longevity between human fibroblast cell cultures in monozygotic twins that is not demonstrated in the other two groups.[29,30] A greater similarity of cell behavior and replicative life span is observed in these twins when compared to nontwin, age-matched controls.[31] One could argue that genetics governs susceptibility to certain diseases but not to aging per se. Alternatively, a certain vigor could be inherited that protects against the developmental susceptibility to a wide variety of diseases. It is difficult to distinguish between the two mechanisms; nonetheless, there is circumstantial evidence for genetically controlled mechanisms of aging that potentially operate in a similar way to developmental processes.

Hayflick Limit Theory Hayflick and Moorhead[16] were able to show that a deterioration in cells (e.g., mitotic and mitochondrial activity) was not dependent on environmental influences, but rather, that cell aging was intrinsic to the cells. They found that there was a limited number of cell population doublings or replications ranging from forty to sixty, the average doubling being fifty per life cycle of the cell. The developmental senescence process of cultured cells includes three phases. Phase I is the beginning stage of cell life, phase II involves a rapid cell proliferation, and the final cessation of cell division occurs in phase III. Hayflick and others have repeatedly shown that phase III is nearly always between forty and sixty population doublings for embryo cells. Hayflick noted alterations and degeneration occurred within the cells before their growth limit,[32] evident in the cell organelles, membranes, and genetic material. Hayflick demonstrated that functional changes within cells are responsible for aging and that the cumulative effect of improper functioning of cells and eventual loss of cells in organs and tissues is probably responsible for the aging phenomenon. Transformation can occur at any point in the life of the cell. Cells acquire a constellation of abnormal characteristics, including chromosomal abnormalities and an in-

definite life span (e.g., properties of tumor cells). The generality of the Hayflick phenomenon is that, in the absence of transformations in the cells, senescence always occurs.

Hayflick's limit of cellular life has served as a model to other investigators who have shown that cell replication potential is a function of donor age.[33,34] In other words, an inverse correlation exists between donor age and the population doubling potential[34] and this correlation is directly related to the maximum life span of the species.[35] Evidence of the Hayflick limit has also been seen in cultures taken from individuals with progeria (Hutchinson-Guilford syndrome and Werner's syndrome). Inasmuch as progeria is a premature aging syndrome, the decreased life span of the donor cells shows a lower Hayflick limit, as expected.[27] The length of the longest life span for different species and the number of cell replications are correlated. For example, the Galápagos tortoise has a maximum life span of 175 years, with a maximum doubling of 125, whereas the human maximum life span is 110 years, with a maximum doubling of 60.[36]

The relationship between the cellular aging phenomenon in culture and aging of the individual is not specific to fibroblasts. It has been demonstrated in smooth-muscle cells, endothelial cells, glial cells, and lymphocytes. Several changes that occur during in vitro senescence are parallel to those that occur in vivo with advancing age. It is not clear that the observed cellular aging in culture, however, actually contributes to what we recognize as the in vivo aging phenomenon of the organism. There is no evidence to support that the in vitro replication life span of mesenchymal cells is important in determining the life span of the organism. Contrary to this, living cells maintain their functional capacity through processes of replacement and repair over long periods of time. So proliferative homeostasis needs to be evaluated with regards to the ability of the organism to respond to environmental stresses. It is also important to keep in mind the aging of proliferating or mitotic cells may be quite different from that of fixed postmitotic or reverting postmitotic cells. The results of the studies cited suggest that, underlying the effects of various proposed "master timekeeping" systems, cells have individual "clocks" that ultimately limit their life span.

Evolutionary Theory of Aging The evolutionary theory of aging is an expansion of the concept of natural selection as Darwin proposed decades ago.[37] This theory predicts that the frequency for deleterious mutations of genes will reach equilibrium from one generation to the next. In other words, there will be an increase in age of onset of mutation of a gene because of postponed selection. This makes each successive generation more resistant to mutations, and when mutations do occur, they occur at a later age.[38] According to the mutation hypothesis, one would expect the genetic variability for survival to increase with age. This has been observed in human aging as discussed in Chapter 1. The life expectancy of the human species has clearly increased since the 1900s. However, the importance of confounding variables (e.g., better sanitation, immunization, and technological advances) must be considered. Often the theory of evolution and a concurrent hypothesis may apply to the aging of the same individual.[39,40] A delay in the onset of mutations may also be dictated by the health of the organism, or as Darwin hypothesized, survival of the fittest.

One theory under the evolutionary model, the network theory of aging, extends the argument that a global reduction in the capacity to cope with a variety of stressors and a concomitant progressive increase in proinflammatory status are major characteristics of the aging process.[41] This phenomenon, which Franceschi and associates[41] refer to as "inflamm-aging," is hypothetically provoked by a continuous antigenic load and stress. On the basis of evolutionary studies, these researchers argue that the immune and the stress responses are equivalent and that antigens are nothing other than particular types of stressors. This theory proposes that the persistence of inflammatory stimuli over time represents the biologic background (first hit) favoring the susceptibility to age-related diseases/ disabilities. A second hit (absence of robust gene variants or the presence of frail gene variants) is likely necessary to develop overt organ-specific age-related diseases having an inflammatory pathogenesis, such as atherosclerosis, Alzheimer's disease, osteoporosis, and diabetes.[41,42] Following this perspective, these researchers found several paradoxes in healthy centenarians, such as an increase of plasma levels of inflammatory cytokines, acute phase proteins, and coagulation factors. Therefore, they conclude that the beneficial effects of inflammation devoted to the neutralization of dangerous and harmful agents early in life and adulthood become detrimental late in life.[41,42]

Stress Theory of Aging Along this same line of thought the stress theory of aging is also an evolutionary model. According to this theory, aging is considered in the context of the abiotic stresses to which free-living organisms are normally exposed.[43] Stress is defined in terms of adequate nutrition and degree of exposure to environmental strains and stressors. Assuming that the primary target of selection of stress is at the level of energy carriers, trade-offs under the rate-of-living theory of aging predict increased longevity from selection for stress resistance. Changes in longevity then become incidental to selection for resistance. Parsons[43] suggests that the primary trait inherited is resistance to stress. Consequently, at extreme ages those with inherited resistance to abiotic stress should dominate, and the reduction in homeostasis manifested by deteriorating ability to adapt to abiotic stress as aging proceeds should be slowest in those surviving the longest.[43] In other words, survival to old age is enhanced by high vitality and resilience associated with substantial physiological and morphological homeostasis. This is underlaid by genes for stress resistance, which confer high metabolic efficiency and hence adaptation to the energy costs of physiological and environmental stress.[44]

Neuroendocrine and Hormonal Theory The endocrine system regulates body composition, fat deposition, skeletal mass, muscle strength, metabolism, body weight, and physical well-being. Multiple endocrine changes evolve with aging in all species and, not surprisingly, some of the physiologic manifestations of aging are related to the effects of declining hormone levels.

One of the earliest investigations into the possible role of the endocrine system in the aging process was conducted by Charles Edward Brown-Séquard (1817–1894),[45] a French-educated physician and professor of physiology and neuropathology at Harvard in the late nineteenth century. At the age of 72 years, Brown-Séquard injected himself intramuscularly with the aqueous extracts of testicular tissue from young dogs and guinea pigs. In 1889, he proclaimed that this treatment produced an increase in grip strength and in sexual vigor, and he subsequently advocated the medical use of testicular extracts as a means to prolong life.[2,3]

The ensemble view of the neuroendocrine axis in systems as the core in aging highlights the role of the hypothalamic-pituitary axis. The central nervous system (CNS) regulates the pituitary gland, which secretes hormones to target tissues that, in turn, produce substances that feed back on the hypothalamic-pituitary axis. This feedback-control network can be assessed via novel entropy statistics, which assess the ensemble synchrony of a feedback axis. Entropy calculations quantify the progressive age-related loss of orderliness of single-hormone secretion of growth hormone (GH), adrenocorticotropic hormone (ACTH), luteinizing hormone (LH), and insulin, as well as the erosion of coordinate 2-hormone section for ACTH-cortisol, LH-testosterone, LH-follicle-stimulating hormone (FSH), and LH-prolactin.[46] LH secretion, sleep-stage transitions, and nocturnal penile tumescence (NPT) oscillations also exhibit marked loss of synchrony with aging.[46]

In humans, aging is associated with a decrease in the gonadal production of estrogen in females (menopause) and testosterone in males (andropause); a decrease in the adrenal production of dehydroepiandrosterone (DHEA) and DHEA sulfate (DHEA-S) (adrenopause); and a decrease in the activity of GH/insulin-like growth factor (IGF)/insulin (I) axis (somatopause).[47] (See Chapter 3 for further discussion of these "pauses.") As a result, hormone replacement regimens are being developed as a strategy to delay or prevent some of the consequences of aging. In some cases, however, the use of hormone replacement therapy for this purpose is controversial.

Unknown mechanisms link aging-related parallel declines in the GH-IGF-I axis (somatopause), gonadal axis (gonadopause), and adrenal androgen secretion (adrenopause). Epidemiological studies reveal consistent decrements in DHEA and DHEA-S secretion in aging men and women.[48–50] However, neither the basis for nor the medical implications of this attrition in the adrenal zona-fasciculata function are known.

The group of theories purporting the neuroendocrine basis of aging regard functional decrements in neurons and their associated hormones as central to the aging process. Given the major interactive role of the neuroendocrine system in physiology, this is an attractive approach. D. Donner Denckla, an endocrinologist turned gerontologist, believes that the center of aging is located in the brain.[45] He bases his theory on past studies of hypothyroidism, a disease that mimics mature aging (e.g., a depressed immune system, wrinkling of the skin, gray hair, and a slowed metabolic rate). Hypothyroidism can be fatal if untreated with thyroxine, inasmuch as all the manifestations of aging are evidenced.

Another aspect of the neuroendocrine basis of aging depends on the role of the pituitary hormones.[51,52] The anterior pituitary gland controls the thyroid gland by the thyroid stimulating hormone, and thus the secretion of thyroxine. Thyroxine is the master rate-controlling hormone within the body for metabolism and protein synthesis. The focus of this theory is the proposed ability of the anterior pituitary to release a blocking hormone labeled DECO (decreasing oxygen consumption) that blocks the cell membrane from taking up thyroxine as a check-balance in the human system. Denckla has not isolated the anti-aging serum, but what Denckla has given us is an alternative philosophic point of view in theoretic gerontology: the in vivo versus the in vitro controversy. Denckla believes that the aging process in vitro is an artifact and unrelated in any meaningful way to true aging. Denckla says, "I don't care what happens to cells in tissue culture. What is important is what people die of." He believes that for good evolutionary reasons—to ensure the turnover of generations so that mutations can take place that enable a species to adapt to a changing environment—nature cannot trust to chance (wear and tear). There must, therefore, exist "an absolutely failsafe killing mechanism without which the species would not survive."[45]

Denckla[53] has shown that elderly rats have a lower O_2 consumption and a reduced increase in O_2 consumption in response to the thyroid hormone T_4. This effect is abolished with hypophysectomy and hormone replacement. Denckla concluded that this finding provided evidence for the presence of a previously undescribed pituitary hormone called "decreasing oxygen consumption hormone" (DECO), which probably begins to be produced at puberty

under stimulation by the thyroid hormone. DECO is proposed to be responsible for the decreasing oxygen consumption and the reduced effect of thyroid hormone observed in aging.[53]

There have been other theories proposed with regard to functional decline of various aging organs and aging systems. As Hayflick[54] notes, aging changes may simply be the result of more fundamental causes, or the organ system in question may not be universally present in all aging animals.

An important version of Denckla's theory proposes that the hypothalamic-pituitary-adrenal (HPA) axis is the master timekeeper for the organism and the primary regulator of the aging process. Functional changes in this system are accompanied by or regulated by decrements throughout the organism. The cascade effect of functional decrements in the hypothalamus, for example, and their potential sequelae have been documented in humans.[55] The neuroendocrine system regulates early development, growth, puberty, the control of the reproductive system, metabolism, and in part, the activities of all the major organ systems. Support of the neuroendocrine and hormonal theories of aging is evidenced by the decline in reproductive capacity due to a decrease in the release of gonadotropin releasing hormone by the hypothalamus, which appears to be the result of diminished activity of hypothalamic catecholamines.[55] Similarly, it has been shown that the release of pulsatile growth hormone declines with age.[56] These changes would have profound effects on estrogen and progesterone release and subsequently on functional capacity. Wise[56] has suggested that there is a loss of neurons in discrete areas of the brain and a loss of neurotransmitter responsiveness by the remaining neurons.

Satisfactory evidence to relate endocrine function to aging is not present to substantiate a significant contribution of endocrine gland function to the process of aging.[57] In response to stress and trophic hormones, the adrenal cortex and thyroid gland remain intact. For women, menopause is a hormone-mediated event that chronicles but does not regulate aging.[57] The ovary is the sole endocrine gland whose functional capacity predictably declines with normal aging. On the other hand, androgen production by the testes is not as predictable because there are individual differences.

The importance of neuroendocrine research cannot be overemphasized. Critics of these theories, however, point out that the master timekeeper of aging, the neuroendocrine system, lacks universality. Many organisms that age (e.g., higher vertebrates) have no complex neuroendocrine system. It can also be argued that the changes that occur in the neuroendocrine system are fundamental changes and occur in all tissues. Aging of the brain, however, produces secondary effects that, although not fundamental to aging, contribute to the development of the overall aging process. What the neuroendocrine system contributes to the aging process is evidenced by the effect of the lack of estrogen on bone density and vascularity. Its contribution to other aging processes remains to be determined.

The Theory of Intrinsic Mutagenesis Another development-genetic theory is referred to as the theory of intrinsic mutagenesis. This idea was first proposed by Burnett[58] and is an attempt to reconcile stochastic theories of aging with the genetic regulation of maximum life span. Burnett suggests that each species is endowed with a specific genetic constitution that "regulates the fidelity of the genetic material and its replication." The degree of fidelity regulates the rate of appearance of mutations or errors, thereby affecting the life span. Alternatively, we can envision a case in which new "fidelity regulators" appear at different stages in an animal's life. Each successive evolutionary set of regulators could have a decreased capacity allowing an increase in mutational events. Another aspect of intrinsic mutagenesis is concerned with the increase in DNA excision repair associated with maximal life span.[59] There is evidence that the accuracy of DNA polymerase may decrease with age,[60–62] but the research in support of both of these hypotheses is rather controversial.

It has been found that the role of DNA methylation as a regulatory factor may have some implications in light of the intrinsic mutagenesis theory. For example, diploid fibroblasts in culture are unable to maintain a constant level of 5-methylcytosine,[63–65] and in other systems DNA methylation patterns have been linked to X chromosome inactivation-reactivation.[66] These hypotheses are potentially important but need further testing before a reliable and valid body of evidence can emerge.

Immunological Theory The immunological theory of aging is another theory categorized as a developmental-genetic theory. This theory was proposed by Walford[67] and has two major observations: (1) that the functional capacity of the immune system declines with age as a result of reduced T-cell function[68] and a reduced resistance to infectious diseases, and (2) that the fidelity of the immune system declines with age as evidenced by the striking age-associated increase in autoimmune diseases. Walford[69] has related these immune system changes to the genes of the major histocompatibility complex genes in rats and mice. Congenic animals that differ only at the major histocompatibility locus appear to have different maximal life spans, suggesting that life span is regulated, at least in part, by this locus. Interestingly, this locus also regulates superoxide dismutase and mixed-function oxidase levels, a finding that relates the immunological theory of aging to the free radical theory of aging, which will be discussed subsequently.

As was the neuroendocrine theory, the immunological theory is attractive in several respects. The immune system has a primary integrative role and is of major importance in health maintenance. Conversely, life span differences could simply be due to the prevention of diseases. The same argument can be leveled at the immunological theory as at the neuroendocrine theory. It lacks universality and it is difficult to defend the immune system's role as the primary timekeeper in the biology of all organisms. The inability to distinguish between primary and secondary effects on aging and the possibility that changes in the immune system are no different from changes in other cell types makes interpretation of this theory difficult.

Free Radical Theory There are more than 300 theories to explain the aging phenomenon. Many of them originate from the study of changes that accumulate with time. Among all the theories, the free radical theory of aging, postulated by Harman,[70] is the most popular and widely tested.[71] It is based on the chemical nature and ubiquitous presence of free radicals. This review aims to recapitulate various studies on the role of free radicals in DNA damage, both nuclear as well as mitochondrial, the oxidative stress they impose on cells, the role of antioxidants, the presence of autoantibodies, and their overall impact on the aging process.

What is a free radical reaction? Biochemical insults arise within aging cells, in part from the action of reactive oxygen species generated and scavenged incompletely throughout the cell cycle. Aging-associated changes occur between and among cells via alterations in the intercellular matrix, the intercellular exchange of trophic factors, the release of inflammatory cytokine mediators, and the degree of infiltration by other cell types (e.g., glial interactions with neurons). It is not known why free radical damage does not adversely affect certain types of cells (e.g., gonadal germ cells).[72]

The free radical theory is another example of development-genetic theory. This theory is attributed to Harman,[73–75] who proposed that aging changes are due to damage caused by radicals. Basically, free radicals are highly charged ions whose outer orbits contain an unpaired electron. Chemically, they are highly reactive species that are generated commonly in single-electron transfer reactions of metabolism. Free radicals have been shown to damage cell membranes, lysosomes, mitochondria, and nuclear membranes through a chemical reaction called lipid peroxidation. Both membrane damage and cross-linking of biomolecules result from free radical chain reactions.[76] The net result of free radical reactions, as summarized by Leibovitz and Siegel,[77] is a decline in cellular integrity caused by reduced enzyme activities, error-prone nucleic acid metabolism, damaged membrane functions, and the accumulation of aging pigments (lipofuscin) in lysosomes.

Free radicals are rapidly destroyed by protective enzyme systems, such as superoxide dismutase. According to this theory, however, some free radicals escape destruction and cause damage that accumulates in important biological structures. This accumulation of damage eventually interferes with function and ultimately causes death. The accumulation of age pigments is an example, and does not refer to the dark brown spots on one's hands. Age pigments (lipofuscin) are seen at microscopic levels in self-selected tissues of the body, such as nerve and muscle tissue. Lipofuscin is the oxidation product of free radical action on polyunsaturated fatty acids. The rate of accumulation of age pigments is a good index of chronologic age and perhaps one of the few aging phenomena universally demonstrated in mammals. Age pigments as an entity are examples of degenerative change. When accumulated in tissue, they cut off oxygen and nutrient supplies to surrounding areas, causing further degeneration and eventual death of tissue.

There is much support for the theory of free radical reactions and their implications in the aging process, as well as their probable pathologic effects as cancer-causing and atherosclerosis-causing agents. This is an appealing theory because it provides a mechanism for aging that does not depend on tissue-specific action but is fundamental to all aerobic tissues. Although this theory has an aspect of random damage, it is not included in the nongenetic stochastic theories because some observations about free radicals are more suggestive of the developmental-genetic theory. For example, Rubner[9] found that the larger the mammal, the lower its metabolic rate. The adaptive significance of this is that as animals get bigger, their surface-to-volume ratio changes. This results in a reduction in the animal's ability to dissipate the heat produced in metabolic reactions. Therefore, a high metabolic rate could cause a hyperthermic effect in a large mammal. Another observation is that life span is a function of body size.[78] Larger animals live longer. This suggests an inverse relationship between metabolic rate and life span. Researchers have speculated that each species is capable of burning a given number of calories in its lifetime.

Metabolic rate is related directly to free radical generation and inversely to life span. It is reasonable to hypothesize that the rate of free radical production is in some way related to life span determination or to senescence. Proponents of this theory suggest that caloric restriction can increase the mean and maximal life span of a species. The notion is that caloric restriction lowers the metabolic rate and therefore decreases the free radical production.

The Caloric Restriction Theory Walford[79] is a staunch proponent of caloric restriction, also known as energy restriction (ER) or DR, as previously described. Dr. Walford himself serves as living evidence of the in vivo experiment and that a life-style committed to the high-nutrient/ low-calorie diet, moderate vitamin and mineral supplementation, and a regular exercise regimen is beneficial. Caloric restriction and its effect on life span extension is perhaps one of the most promising probes of the mechanisms of aging. Caloric restriction may exert its effectiveness through the neuroendocrine system. Everitt[80] has shown a striking similarity between dietary restriction and hypophysectomy demonstrated in Denkla's neuroendocrine studies previously cited.[51,52]

This high-nutrient/low-calorie diet is a result of years of animal in vivo experimentation, exploring longevity and maximum life span potential. Dr. Walford's experiments have been well received and respected, and other noted theorists, such as Leonard Hayflick, have acknowledged Walford's work.[81]

Walford's caloric restriction program prescribes that an individual gradually lose weight over several years until a point of maximum metabolic efficiency is reached for optimum health and life span.[81] Despite some recent reports associating being a little overweight as "healthier" than being underweight, most recent results from the National Institutes of Health Nutrition Committee and the Centers for Disease Control have concluded that "the weights associated with the greatest longevity are below average weights of the population," as long as such weights are not associated with diseases. The result of the high-quality but low-caloric diet serves to retard aging in the sense that one would be chronologically old but functionally younger.

The calorie restricted diet influences both aging rate and disease susceptibility. It has been said that the immune system is the pacemaker of aging,[57] and caloric restriction has been shown to affect the immune system. For example, it slows down the immune system's decline and inhibits the increased autoimmune reaction.[68] Further, pilot studies in mice provide supportive evidence that caloric restriction may also slow the decline in DNA repair capacity,[82] as well as affect the generation or persistence of free radicals.[83] Recent studies regarding the free radical theory show that lipid peroxidation is lower and that catalase reactions are higher in calorie-restricted mice compared with noncalorie restricted controls.[84]

Reducing food intake to well below that of ad libitum fed animals increased life span in a study by Masoro.[85] This action, which gerontologists often refer to as the antiaging action of dietary restriction (DR), maintains physiological processes in a youthful state and delays the occurrence, or slows the progression, of age-related disease processes.[85] It is hypothesized that the DR effect results from the reduced intake of calories, which in turn reduces body fat, alters the characteristics of carbohydrate metabolism and of oxidative metabolism, and slows the aging process down. One theory proported to support this claim is that DR protects against the damaging actions of acute stressors.[85]

What is the relationship of energy restriction to other aging theories? Caloric restriction influences widely diverse phenomena, particularly those whose mechanistic possibilities include effects on the immune system, cell basal state and proliferation potential, metabolic rate, DNA repair, levels of free radical scavengers, chromatin structure, and protein synthesis and turnover.[18]

As can be seen by other theories discussed in this chapter, aging may be caused by a single factor or by many. Thus, the energy restriction model might be useful in analyzing single-factor theories of aging; it might also clarify the significance of physiologic aging markers that correlate with differences in maximum life spans between species.[18,79]

A simple extrapolation of the free radical theory of aging leads to the conclusion that active persons would have a shorter life span than nonactive ones. There is no evidence to support this view. Intuitively, the beneficial effects of exercise preclude this logical extrapolation. Paffenberger[86] has shown that greater caloric expenditure is positively correlated with increasing life span and health in humans. A caveat here, as with other statements, is that exercise could have beneficial effects in preventing disease while at the same time accelerating aging through increased free radical generation. On the other hand, disease prevention through exercise could completely obscure the effects of free radicals.

Extensive research has been done regarding the use of antioxidants with free radicals. Vitamin E, vitamin C, selenium, gluthathione peroxidase, and superoxide dismultase have been used as free radical and lipid peroxidase inhibitors.[77] The implication is that there appear to be effective free radical inhibitors that may prevent further cellular degeneration, such as reduced accumulation of lipofusion.

Stochastic Theories of Aging

The second category of theories is described as stochastic theories. These theories purport that aging at the molecular level is caused by an accumulation of insults from the environment. The result of these insults is that the organism eventually reaches a level incompatible with life.[87]

There is limited evidence (this is evolving via the genome studies discussed subsequently) that genetics plays a role in the aging process *per se,* although the genomic complement regulates longevity. Aging at the molecular level can be viewed as a stochastic process resulting from increased disorderliness of intra- and intercellular regulatory mechanisms. This results in reduced robustness of the organism to intercurrent stress and disease. The notion of greater disorderliness in aging is also evident at the whole organismic level, as illustrated by the erosion of the orderly neuroendocrine feedback regulation of the secretion of GH, LH, FSH, and ACTH.[46]

Error Theory The error theory, also known as the error catastrophe theory, was first presented by Orgel in 1963.[88] It states that, although random errors in

protein synthesis may occur, the error-containing protein molecule will be turned over, and the next copy will be error free. If the error-containing protein is one that is involved in synthesis of the genetic material or in the protein synthesizing machinery, however, then this molecule could cause further errors. If this is the case, the number of error-containing proteins expands to result in an "error crisis" that would be incompatible with proper function and life. The theory specifies that "any accident or error in either the machinery or the process of making proteins would cascade into mutliple effects."[89] A decrease in the fidelity or accuracy of protein synthesis was specifically hypothesized to be caused by errors in proper initiation of the pairing of messenger RNA codon with an anticodon of tranfer RNA. However, "it may not be possible to distinguish between contributions to cellular aging caused by errors in protein synthesis from those due to accumulation of somatic mutations."[54] It is questionable whether accurate protein synthesis is distinguishable from inaccurate DNA synthesis and whether the accuracy of both processes are dependent on the fidelity of the other. The interdependence and cumulative effects of errors remain deeply intertwined and somewhat indistinguishable.[90]

Recent experiments contradict Orgel and undermine support for the error theory. In human cell cultures fed two amino acids (*p*-fluorophenylalanine and ethionine) early in their life spans, both the short-term, high-dose cultures and the long-term, low-dose cultures had essentially the same replicative life spans.[91] This result seems irreconcilable with the error theory. It is an appealing theory because of its apparently straightforward testability through the detection of missynthesized proteins. Experiments have shown that not all aged cells accumulate missynthesized protein molecules and that aging is not necessarily accelerated when missynthesized protein molecules are purposely introduced.[54] Despite numerous reports of altered proteins in aging,[92] no direct evidence of age-dependent malsynthesis has yet been obtained. Altered proteins do occur in aging cells and tissues, however, at present it seems that the accuracy of the protein synthesizing mechanism does not decrease with age.[93] Rather, the capacity of the protein removal machinery in old cells is compromised.[93,94] It may follow that old cells that contain many modified copies of functionally important proteins could have impaired functional capacity. From a historical viewpoint, the error theory was important to test these hypotheses in order to move toward a more plausible theory.

Redundant DNA Theory Another dimension of the error theory is the premise that the ability to repair damage to the genetic material is somehow associated with aging or the rate of aging.[95] Medvedev[95] suggests that biologic age changes are a result of errors accumulating in functioning genes. As these errors accumulate, reserve genetic sequences with identical information take over until the system's redundancy is exhausted. This theory is known as the redundant message theory. Medvedev[95] writes that different species' life spans may be a function of the degree of repeated genetic sequences. If error occurred in a nonrepeated gene sequence, the chance of preserving a final intact gene product during evolution or a long life span would be diminished. Hart and Setlow[59] obtained evidence that the ability to repair DNA cells after ultraviolet damage in cell cultures derived from various species of different maximum life spans and was directly correlated to maximum life span potential.

Redundancy seems to protect mammals from losing vital genetic information during the life span.[95] The major criticism of Medvedev's theory is that it fails to explain other possible aging factors, such as radiation-induced aging and quantitative aspects of normal aging. Although the idea that differences in DNA repair provide the basis for the life span differences in species, current experimental support for this theory remains inconclusive.[94] It is probable that if DNA repair is involved in the determination of maximum life span, it is more likely to be site-specific than generalized.[24]

The mitochondrial theory of aging, based on the redundant DNA theory, states that the slow accumulation of impaired mitochondria is the driving force of the aging process.[96] The discovery of age-related mitochondrial DNA deletions have shown that damaged mitochondria have a decreased degradation rate, and tend to accumulate as a result. The underlying mechanism of the accumulation of defective mitochondria remains unclear, however, this hypothesis solves inconsistencies of the current model of redundancy.[96]

Somatic Mutation Theory   One of the most prominent theories in the stochastic theories category is the somatic mutation theory of aging.[97,98] This theory emerged following World War II as a result of increased research in the area of radiation biology. The theory hypothesizes that mutations or genetic damage result from radiation and that radiomimetic agents accumulate and eventually create functional failure and the death of the organism. The somatic mutation theory is based on the scientific observation that exposure to ionizing radiation shortens the life span. Szilard[98] showed that exposure to radiation was recessive. It requires two or more "hits" from radiation to inactivate a given locus and the exposure must occur in a sufficient number of cells for the damage to be manifested. Comparison of chromosomal aberrations in dividing liver cells in mice support this view.[99] Curtis and Miller[99] found a higher frequency of these chromosomal abnormalities in short-lived compared to long-lived strains of mice, which supports the somatic mutation theory. There are at least two arguments against the somatic mutation theory.

(1) Shortening life span by radiation does not define whether the life span mechanism bears any relationship to the normal mechanism of aging.[24] Numerous treatments that would shorten life span are not related to normal aging (e.g., radiation treatment). (2) Inbred animals would have a longer life span than outbred animals because inbred animals would be homologous at most genetic loci and, therefore, more resistant to random damage. In fact the opposite is true as exemplified in the well-known phenomenon of hybrid vigor. Maynard-Smith[100] showed that inbreeding actually shortened the life span in mice. Some of the most compelling experiments addressing somatic mutation were done on the effects of radiation and life span comparing haploid and diploid animals.[101] Although the haploid animals were much more sensitive to ionizing radiation, both haploids and diploids had the same life span when radiation was withheld. This finding is difficult to reconcile in light of the somatic mutation theory.

Cell senescence, or somatic mutation of cells, limits cell divisions in normal somatic cells and may play a central role in age-related diseases. In other words, cell senescence underlies and is a pivotal event in human aging and disease.[102] There is in vitro and ex vivo data to support the theory that this cell senescence leads to pathologies such as artherosclerosis, osteoarthritis, immune senescence, skin aging, Alzheimer's, and cancer.[102] Such data, if confirmed, has stunning therapeutic (as well as commercial) consequences.

Interestingly, the caloric restriction theory supports the theory of somatic mutation. A key prediction of the somatic mutation theory of aging is that there is an invariant relationship between life span and the number of random mutations. A number of studies have shown that somatic mutations of a variety of types accumulate with age, and that dietary restriction prolongs life span by slowing the accumulation of mutant genes.[103]

Transcription Theory   Other scientists have developed theories focused specifically on stages of genetic processing. One of these processes, transcription, is the first stage in the transfer of information from DNA to protein synthesis. It entails the formation of messenger RNA so that it contains, in the linear sequence of its nucleotides, the genetic information located in the DNA gene from which messenger RNA is transcribed. Hayflick's[54] theory maintains that with increasing age, deleterious changes occur in the metabolism of differentiated postmitotic cells. He also suggests that the alterations are the results of primary events occurring within the nuclear chromatin. A control mechanism responsible for the appearance and the sequence of the primary aging events exists in the nuclear chromatin complex.

Insufficient experimentation to test this hypothesis exists, though Hayflick[54] suggests this should not imply that the hypothesis is wrong. When contemplating these theories thus far, one must ask, why is it that some cells, such as germ cells and some cancer cells never age or die? Hayflick[54] suggests that "in order to maintain immortality, genetic information is exchanged between these cells in the same way that the genetic cards are reshuffled when egg and sperm fuse." The reshuffling of a fused sperm and egg cell may lead to a fixed life span. In all species, there appears to be a specific time for decrement and eventual death. Hayflick[54] and others refer to this as "mean time to failure." Perhaps species-specific genetic apparatus runs out of correctly programmed material, and some species-related repair systems are better than others because they have a longer life span.

Cross-Linkage Theory   A theory related to the redundant DNA theory is based on cross-linking in macromolecules. In 1942, Johan Bjorksten first related the concept of cross-linkage to developmental aging.[104,105] Prior to the 1940s, cross-linking was used as a method to stabilize macromolecules for individual purposes, such as vulcanizing rubber. Although cross-linking is not restricted to proteins, most experimental research has been on collagen and elastin because these molecules are accessible, do not readily turn over, and show increased cross-linking with age. Bjorksten[104] looked at large reactive protein molecules within the body, such as collagen, elastin, and DNA molecules, and surmised that their cross-linkage was responsible for secondary and tertiary causes of aging. According to Bjorksten[105]

> Cross-linking reactions result in the union of at least two large molecules. A bridge or link between these is usually formed by a cross-linking agent: a small, motile molecule or free radical with a reactive hook or some other mechanism at both ends, capable of reacting with at least two large molecules. It is also possible for two large molecules to become cross-linked by the action of their own side chains or reactive groups present on one or both of them, or pathologically formed by ionizing radiation.

Matrix molecules constitute more than 20% of mammalian body weight. The vital physiological processes that occur in a bed of matrix molecules will not be able to proceed effectively because cross-linking increases with age. The concepts underlying this theory are probably overly simplistic. Though collagen shows increasing cross-linking with age, is there more to matrix molecule metabolism than simply cross-linking? Some collagen types are replaced by other collagen types in development and aging. Cross-linking is a process of maturation for which increased cross-linking at some sites leads to improved function, but at other sites impairs function.[106] Further investigation needs to be done to learn more about the matrix molecules.

Bjorksten[104] implies that cross-linking is the primary cause of sclerosis, failure of the immune system, and loss of elasticity. Aging of the skin is perhaps the most obvious example of cross-linking and exposure to solar radiation promotes cross-linkage. Loss of flexibility of the aging body was thought due to the cross-linking of tendon, ligament, and muscle tissue. We now see active aging individuals remain more flexible despite constant exposure to cross-linking agents (e.g., unsaturated fats, polyvalent metal ions such as aluminum, magnesium, zinc, radiation), and few if any researchers view collagen cross-linking as a major underlying cause of aging.

The glycosylation theory suggests that the health of the collagen fibers is affected by the creation of modified forms of proteins and macromolecules as a result of the presence of nonenzymatic glycosylation molecules.[4] In this reaction (termed glycation), glucose combines with certain amino acids in protein resulting in an altered amino acid and ultimately a dysfunctional protein, which accumulates in the collagen fibers. Glycated forms of human collagen accumulate in tendons, muscles, and skin causing losses in flexibility and overall mobility. This process can affect any of the connective tissues of the body and, therefore, results in changes to the eye, blood vessels, blood viscosity, and intestinal tract—anywhere there is collagen (which is everywhere). It is hypothesized that the presence of glycation has been associated with an increased likelihood of developing Alzheimer's disease and increasing the deleterious effects of diabetes.[1–4]

New Theories on Aging

Sleep and Aging   Sleep, or the lack thereof, has been implicated as a factor in exacerbating the aging process. The importance of sleep is often overlooked. Sleep curtailment constitutes an increasingly common condition in industrialized societies and is thought to afftect mood and performance, as well as physiological functions.[107,108] It is during the deepest levels of sleep (Stages III and IV) that the human species repairs tissues and synthesizes the neuroendocrines that comprise a homeostatic hormonal system.

There is evidence that prolonged sleep loss affects the homeostasis of the important hypothalamo-pituitary-adrenal (HPA) axis and increases the secretion of the so-called stress hormone, cortisol. Leproult and associates[107] evaluated the effects of acute partial or total sleep deprivation on the nighttime and daytime profiles of cortisol levels. Alterations in cortisol levels were demonstrated during the evening following the night of sleep deprivation. After normal sleep, plasma cortisol levels were found to be within normal limits. After partial and total sleep deprivation, plasma cortisol levels were found to be higher, and the onset of the quiescent period of cortisol secretion was delayed. Even partial acute sleep loss was found to delay the recovery of the HPA axis from early morning circadian stimulation and is likely to involve an alteration in negative glucocorticoid feedback regulation.[107] In other words, sleep loss could affect the resiliency of the stress response and accelerate the development of immunologic, metabolic, and cognitive consequences of glucocorticoid excess, thereby accelerating the breakdown of tissues.

The production of growth hormone (GH) is one of the most important neuroendocrine processes involved in the regulation and repair of tissues at the cellular level. The major daily peak in plasma growth hormone level normally occurs during the early part of nocturnal sleep.[108] Mullington and colleagues[108] investigated possible factors associated with nocturnal peaks of GH in the absence of sleep, including subjectively defined sleepiness; electroencephalographically defined drowsiness during short lapses into sleep (napping); measures of cortisol levels; and body temperature. In studying subjects aged 16 to 84 years old, the researchers found age to be a significant negative predictor of nocturnal GH peak levels in sleep-deprived subjects compared to subjects experiencing normal sleep. These results suggest that the well-known suppressive effect of sleep deprivation on GH secretion is an age-dependent phenomenon that evolves during early adulthood and increases with age.

Sleep fragmentation, prolonged sleep onset latency, and reduced rapid-eye movement activity are evident in older adults. Some GH-releasing hormones and peptides can trigger sleep in rats, rabbits, and humans.[109] The drugs gamma-hydroxybutyrate and ritanserine can induce both slow-wave sleep and GH secretion, thereby relating sleep and GH release.[110] Conversely, the disordered sleep patterns associated with sleep-apnea syndrome suppress GH secretion. The normal relationship between deep sleep and GH secretion may be eroded in aging. Sleep deprivation in young men elicits some of the same neuroendocrine and metabolic features of aging, such as elevated evening cortisol levels, higher sympathetic tone, and decreased glucose tolerance.[110] These alterations are hypothesized to exacerbate the aging process.

Growth Hormone   The hormonal imbalance-growth factor exposure theory (HI-GFE theory) has been hypothesized as a possible explanation for an exacerbation in the aging process.[111] According to this theory, there is too much growth hormone and not enough insulin. If true, the HI-GFE theory can account for two major aging phenomena: (1) decline in mammalian reserve capacity (the ability to return to physiologic homeostasis following stress) with a consequent increase in diseases of maintenance, and (2) an increase in most age-associated proliferation of diseases, due to an imbalance of both growth hormone and insulin. According to this theory, the decline in the reserve capacity is due to a gradual decline in mitochondrial maximal energy production, which in

turn accounts for the gradual redirection of energy production toward survival functions like ion pumping. This results in the relative detriment of RNA and protein synthesis as seen in lesser synthetic rates and slower turnover with consequent gradual cellular impairment.[111] The hypothetical explanation is that this is triggered by developmental programming and also nutritionally driven. Growth hormone exposure in youth and middle age purportedly promotes events that lead to proliferative diseases that arise coincident to rapidly declining reserve capacity and the cumulative mutational status associated with age. Parr[111] suggests that one possible explanation for this is a lack of available insulin. He proposes that the declining mitochondrial energy production can be reversed, or at least greatly diminished, if there is an improvement in the insulin:growth hormone balance. The result of a lower overall growth factor exposure could potentially lead to a longer, healthier life span than that seen in calorie-restricted models.[111]

In a study of centenarians, it was found that mean levels of insulin-like growth factor-1 (IGF-1) were relatively low, indicating that there is an age-associated decline in this substance even in the extremely old.[112] Interestingly, centenarians with lower IGF-1 levels had a higher prevalence of definitive dementia. This data suggests that serum IGF-1 levels in centenarians appear to reflect their short-term nutritional status of rapid protein turnover and may be involved in the progression of dementia in the oldest-old.[112]

DHEA   The enzymic machinery of the adrenal zona reticularis fails in aging men and women. However, the ability of the zona fasciculata to produce cortisol is preserved.[47] Mineralocorticoid and glucocorticoid receptors in the hippocampus are variably downregulated in aging humans. Excessive lifelong adrenal cortisol feedback on the brain may exacerbate the aging-associated loss in neuronal synapses and plasticity.[48–50]

Extraglandular neuro steroids (typically progestin derivatives) produced by CNS astroglia regulate the activity of neuronal ion-channels (e.g., via GABA-A receptors).[48–50] The mechanisms by which neurosteroids interact with corticosteroids to modulate the cognitive and affective changes of aging have not been described.

Because so much medical and media attention has been drawn to the alleged benefits of dehydroepiandrosterone (DHEA) and its sulfate ester, DHEA-S, it is important to evaluate the effects of replacement therapy on aging parameters. Flynn and associates[113] objectively evaluated DHEA replacement using a double-blind, crossover, randomized research methodology. In their nine-month study of healthy older men, lean body mass, blood hematology, chemistry, and endocrine values, as well as urological and psychological data were measured. Data showed some mild, temporary, but significant positive changes in blood values (blood urea nitrogen, creatinine, uric acid, alanine transaminase, cholesterol, high-density lipoprotein, and potassium) using 100 mg oral DHEA compared with placebo.

Morales and colleagues[114] observed that administration of an oral 100-mg dose of DHEA for six months in elderly men and women resulted in elevation of circulating DHEA and DHEA-S concentrations and the DHEA-S/cortisol ratio. Biotransformation to potent androgens near and slightly above the range of their younger counterparts occurred in women with no detectable change in men. Given this hormonal milieu, an increase in serum (IGF-1) levels was observed in both genders but dimorphic responses were evident in fat body mass and muscle strength in favor of men. The authors of this study suggest that these differences in response of DHEA administration may reflect a gender specific response to DHEA and/or the presence of confounding factors in women, such as estrogen replacement therapy.[114]

Oral DHEA replacement therapy may have a multitude of potential beneficial effects particularly in the presence of DHEA deficiency. Callies[115] hypothesizes that DHEA exerts its action mainly via peripheral bioconversion of DHEA to androgens and estrogens. A daily 50-mg dose of DHEA has been shown to restore low endogenous serum DHEA concentrations to normal youthful levels followed by an increase in circulating androgens and estrogens.[115]

Barnhart and associates[116] studied the effects of DHEA supplementation of 50 mg on perimenopausal symptoms such as altered mood and well-being. Women receiving DHEA did not have any improvements significantly greater than placebo in the severity of perimenopausal symptoms, mood, dysphoria, libido, cognition, memory, or well-being. According to these researchers, DHEA supplementation significantly affects the endocrine and lipid profiles, but does not improve perimenopausal symptoms.[116]

It has been hypothesized that DHEA possibly prevents immunosenescence, and as a neuroactive steroid it may influence processes of cognition and memory.[117] Epidemiological studies revealed an inverse correlation between DHEA-S levels and the incidence of cardiovascular disease in men, but not in women. Arlt and colleagues investigated the effects of 50 mg and 100 mg of DHEA and placebo doses and found that 50 mg was a suitable dose in elderly men, as it leads to serum DHEA-S concentrations usually measured in young healthy adults. The DHEA-induced increase in circulating estrogens was found to have a beneficial effect on immunological measures as well as cognition and memory in men.[117]

Reportedly, DHEA-S levels are negatively influenced by insulin. Additionally, reduced DHEA-S levels have been associated with increased risk for cardiovascular disease, which connotes hyperinsulinemic states, such as obesity. Mazza and associates[118] evaluated serum levels of DHEA-S and insulin as a function of age and body mass index (BMI) in adult women. Interestingly, DHEA-S levels and BMI were positively associated before but not after menopause. The data show that increasing body mass and insulin secretion is not linked with DHEA-S reduction in women. This evidence suggests that DHEA-S is probably not implicated in the pathogenesis of cardiovascular disease in obese women.[118]

Dehydroepiandrosterone sulfate was measured in a randomized, five-year, follow-up study of three age cohorts (age 75, 80, and 85) and determined its associations with clinical diseases and their risk indicators, as well as its prognostic significance in old age.[119] It was found that DHEA-S was higher in men than in women in the 75-year age group. It decreased in men up to 85 years. Compared to healthy men, DHEA-S was lower in men with a history of or manifestation of vascular diseases, presence of dementia, diabetes mellitus, malignancies and musculoskeletal disorders, but was similar in all these disease groups. No differences were found in women. Levels of DHEA-S did not relate to cardioechographic findings, cardiovascular risk factors, or predictors of impaired prognosis. After controlling for age, DHEA-S tended to be lower in the non-surviving than in the surviving men. After controlling for disease, DHEA-S did not predict increased risk of all-cause or cardiovascular mortality during the five-year follow-up. In this study, gender differences in DHEA-S persisted up to the age of 75. The authors concluded that low plasma DHEA-S appears to be a secondary phenomenon rather than a specific risk indicator of common diseases in old age.[119]

Telomeres Telomeres have been implicated in the regulation of cellular senescence. Telomeres consist of tandem repeats of a short nucleotide sequence and are located on the ends of chromosomes. Their length limits the total number of attainable cell generations in a tissue or organ (the so-called "end-replication" problem—the inability of DNA polymerase to completely replicate the end of linear DNA).[120]

In 1971, Olovnikov published a theory in which he first formulated the DNA end-replication problem and explained how it could be solved.[3] The solution to this problem also provided an explanation for the Hayflick Limit, which underpins the discovery in vitro and vivo cell senescence. Olovnikov proposed that the length of the telomeric DNA, located at the ends of chromosomes consists of repeated sequences, which play a buffer role and should diminish in dividing normal somatic cells at each cell doubling.[121] The loss of sequences containing important information could occur after buffer loss (shortening of telomeres) and could cause the onset of cellular senescence. According to this theory it was suggested that for germline cells and for the cells of vegetatively propagated organisms and immortal cell populations like most cancer cell lines, an enzyme might be activated that would prevent the diminution of DNA termini at each cell division, thus protecting the formation containing part of the genome. In recent years, Olovnikov's hypothesis has been authenticated by laboratory evidence. The DNA sequences that shorten in dividing normal cells are telomeres and the enzyme that maintains telomere length constant in immortal cell populations is telomerase.[121] Shortening of the telomere occurs when there is insufficient telomerase. The length of the telomere is predictive of life span for that cell and ultimately predictive of the life span of the organism.

The speculation that the limited proliferative potential of human cells is a result of telomere shortening that occurs during DNA synthesis at each cell division could have some important impact in treating cancer.[72] The extension of telomeres by the enzyme telomerase, which compensates for the loss of a few nucleotides of telomeric DNA during each cell cycle, essentially protects and ensures that the entire linear chromosome is replicated. As a result, telomere length is directly related to the number of cell generations. Transfection of human cells with the gene for telomerase resulted in more than four hundred population doublings.[120] Thus, telomere renewal may be relevant in both cancer pathogenesis and the research of aging.[72,120]

Progress of Cell Culture Aging Models　At the cellular level, several new processes have been proposed as being involved in the physiology of aging and the development of some age-related diseases. Apoptosis, a word coined in 1972, signifies the process of nontraumatic and noninflammatory cell death—and the opposite of cell mitosis—that balances cell proliferation and thus maintains homeostasis. This theme was adumbrated as early as the late 1800s in studies of ovarian follicular atresia. Specific gene products either promote or oppose regulated cell death via mitochondria effects.[122] Dysregulation of apoptosis has been implicated in the development of diseases that are more prevalent in older individuals, such as cancer and the neurodegenerative disorders of Alzheimer's and Parkinson's disease.

Interest in the role of mitochondria in aging has intensified in recent years. This focus on mitochondria originated in part from the free radical theory of aging, which argues that oxidative damage plays a key role in degenerative senescence.[123] Among the numerous mechanisms known to generate oxidants, leakage of the superoxide anion and hydrogen peroxide from the mitochondria electron transport chain are of particular interest, due to the correlation between species-specific metabolic rate ("rate of living") and life span. Phenomenological studies of mitochondrial function long ago noted a decline in mitochondrial function with age,[74,95] and on-going research continues to add to this body of knowledge.[70,96,123] The extranuclear somatic mutation theory of aging proposes that the accumulation of mutations in the mitochondrial genome may be responsible in part for the mitochondrial phenomenol-

ogy of aging. Recent studies of mitochondrial DNA deletions have shown that they increase with age in humans and other mammals.[70,96]

The acceleration of fixed postmitotic cell aging by a high metabolic rate and the age-related loss of mitochondria found in that cell type has led to an oxygen stress-mitochondrial mutation theory of aging.[124] According to this refined theory of mutation, senescence may be linked to mutations of the mitochondrial genome of the irreversibly differentiated cells. This extranuclear somatic gene mutation concept of aging is supported by the fact that mitochondrial DNA synthesis takes place at the inner mitochondrial membrane near the sites of formation of highly reactive oxygen species.[123,124] Mitochondrial DNA may be able to prevent the intrinsic mutagenesis caused by those byproducts of respiration because, in contrast to the nuclear genome, it lacks excision and recombination repair. The resulting mitochondrial impairment and concomitant cell bioenergetic decline may cause the senescent loss of physiological performance and play a key role in the pathogenesis of many age-related degenerative diseases.[124]

These concepts are integrated with classic and contemporary hypotheses in a *unity theory* that reconciles programmed and stochastic concepts of aging.[124] Thus, it is suggested that cells are programmed to differentiate, and then they accumulate mitochondrial-genetic damage because of their high levels of oxyradical stress and the loss of the organelle rejuvenating power of mitosis.[124] This cellular model of aging, which combines previously discussed theories, raises more questions than it answers. Among these are (1) How important are mitochondrial oxidants in determining overall cellular oxidative stress? (2) What are the mechanisms of mitochondrial oxidant generation? (3) How are lesions and mutations in mitochondrial DNA formed? (4) How important are these lesions and mutations in causing mitochondrial dysfunction? (5) How are mitochondria regulated, and how does this regulation change during aging? (6) What are the dynamics of mitochondrial turnover? (7) What is the relationship between mitochondrial damage and lipofuscinogenesis? (8) What are the relationships among mitochondria, apoptosis, and aging, and (9) How can mitochondrial function (ATP generation and the establishment of a membrane potential) and dysfunction (oxidant generation) be modulated and degenerative senescence thereby treated? With the rate of scientific exploration into this area of study, perhaps by the third edition of this text, we'll have answers to some of these questions.

The Genome Project and Implications on Aging
Aging is characterized as a breakdown process and the relevant events occur after reproduction, when the force of natural selection declines. Studies of life histories of species reveal that there is an association between resource allocation and longevity and that

the aging process is retarded when animals are protected from the deleterious consequences of excess metabolic activity. Although the extent to which aging is caused by environmental or genetic factors is unresolved, our understanding of the field has been enriched by the rapid development of the tools of molecular biology.[125] In his pioneering work, Alex Comfort[5] has postulated a hierarchical clock system as a descriptive paradigm of the aging process, and investigations at the molecular level are bringing to light evidence of a genetic link to life span that seems consistent with Comfort's model. With the genome projects now coding the complex structure of genetic material, the appropriate context for these mechanistic observations is just starting to evolve.

Although most studies agree that genetics influence longevity in humans, the magnitude of this effect is debated. A study of children of nonagenarians suggested a strong relation between genetic influences and longevity,[126] as did a study that compared the life span of adopted children with that of their adoptive and biological parents.[127] Studies of twins reared together and twins reared apart suggested, at most, a small genetic influence on longevity.[128,129] There does appear to be, however, a strong relationship between genetics and longevity when centenarians are included in studies. In a recent study by Perls and colleagues, it was demonstrated that the siblings of centenarians are three to four times more likely to survive to the tenth decade of life compared with siblings of noncentenarians.[130] In addition, the immediate ancestors of Jeanne Calment from France, who died at nearly 123 years of age, recently showed that they were ten times more likely to reach age 80 than their general ancestral cohort.[131]

Many genes that determine decreased life expectancy in humans have been identified, cloned, and characterized. These include genes associated with major causes of human (premature) death.[132] For example, the genes associated with breast cancer (e.g., breast cancer genes BRCA1 and BRAC2) and those associated with heart disease and hyperlipidemia (e.g., the low-density lipoprotein receptor, apolipoprotein [apo]B) have been implicated as precursors for these pathologies. Although association studies aimed at identifying longevity association with genes are in their infancy, four candidate genes have been initially implicated in longevity: apoE,[133] angiotensin-converting enzyme (ACE),[134] histocompatibility locus antigen (HLA),[135] and plasminogen activator inhibitor 1 (PAI-1).[136]

The ApoE gene is involved in lipoprotein metabolism and possibly Alzheimer's disease plaque formation. The E2 variant is more frequent in centenarians, although the E4 is half as common compared with younger populations.[133] The ACE gene plays a role in modulating blood pressure, and people with a particular polymorphism have been observed to live longer.[134] The HLA polymorphism has been found with greater frequency in centenarians than in younger populations. This may be attributed to better resistance to infection and inflammatory processes.[135] The PAI-1 protein may modulate blood clotting and, therefore, risk of thromboembolic events (e.g., cerebrovascular and cardiovascular disease).[136]

The four genes have an impact on intermediate traits likely to have effects on longevity, including immune function and levels of plasma homeostatic proteins. Thus, these genes may modulate other efforts on life expectancy by protecting an individual from potentially deadly diseases (e.g., atherosclerosis and infection and/or inflammatory diseases).[132] Furthermore, apoE and PAI-1 are examples of gene variants whose phenotypic expression is likely to be affected by environmental interactions, such as food intake and physical inactivity.[133,136]

Another genetic mechanism for the modulation of life span has been subtested by analysis of the BRCA1 gene. Interestingly, a different polymorphism in or near the BRCA1 gene than that observed in BRCA1 mutations associated with breast cancer is enriched in centenarians compared with control subjects.[137] Thus, different mutations in the same gene may be associated with disease and also protection. Gene variants that decrease free-radical production might be expected to have beneficial effects and to slow aging processes. Recently, certain mitochondrial DNA variants were found significantly more frequently in centenarians,[138] suggesting that oxidative stress may be a relevant mechanism of longevity in humans as well.

Werner syndrome is an interesting disease that is highly relevant to aging. This is a rare autosomal recessive disorder characterized by the premature development of the aging phenotype and a large number of age-related diseases, and is due to a mutation of a helicase gene.[139] This gene is important for the maintenance of cellular function through DNA repair. Potentially, gene variants that slow DNA damage or enhance DNA repair may slow aging and decrease aging-related diseases.

Recent evidence supports a role for important genetic and environmental interactions on longevity in lower organsims.[132] Although less is known in humans, commonality in molecular and biological processes, evolutionary arguments, and epidemiological data would strongly suggest that similar mechanisms also apply. The completion of the Human Genome Project and the rapid innovations in technology will make possible the identification of human longevity-assurance genes.[132] Identification of specific traits relevant to the aging phenotype and genes that promote longevity will provide important mechanistic insights into the molecular basis of aging. Furthermore, these studies will provide insights into how these genes exert their phenotypic influences. The insights may lead to interventions that can be used to promote survival in people who were not fortunate enough to inherit a genome predisposing them to longevity.

Werner Syndrome: Fast-Forwarding Aging Cataracts, osteoporosis, heart disease, and other such ills typically afflict the aged. A disease which mimics and exacerbates the aging process is called Werner syndrome. Though this is not normal aging per se, as it affects individuals early in the life cycle, it is a disease that has been studied in aging studies to determine causal effects of aging. For the unfortunate sufferers of Werner syndrome, the diseases of aging strike, not in the seventh or eighth decade of life, but as early as the third. Such people age abnormally fast and usually die before they reach the age of 50.

This disease is genetic and associated with a dysfunction in the eighth chromosome. It has been found in Werner syndrome that when the DNA sequence of the gene for Werner syndrome is compared with normal genes that it contains a unique class of enzymes called helicases, substances which unwind the double helix of DNA, which is unique to this disease.[1,132] Helicases, of which there are many different types, are crucial enzyme components of all living cells. They help repair DNA and enable messenger RNA molecules to ferry genetic instructions from the nucleus, where DNA resides, throughout the cell, where the instructions are biochemically translated into proteins.[4,7] Although most cellular functions that use DNA or RNA are going to involve a helicase, in order to replicate DNA, the two strands of DNA have to unwind before it can be copied or repaired.[132,139] When chromosomes segregate during cell division, untangling a bunch of chromosomes requires a helicase.[11,132] It is suspected that the enzyme identified in Werner syndrome is not essential to life, but is somehow conducive to a long and healthy one. It is hypothesized that the helicase is not required for DNA replication, but rather it is involved in DNA repair, or in preventing mutation during DNA synthesis. Damaged DNA from people with Werner appears to be capable of repairing itself, however, their DNA seems to accumulate mutations at a higher-than-normal rate. Understanding how the gene works could provide insight into normal aging. It may be that "normal" people carry variants of the gene that influence their life spans or predispose them to an earlier death. Studying Werner could help pinpoint the mechanism that underlies all diseases of aging, which appear in part to be due to the cell slowdown that is such a dramatic feature of this disease.[132,139]

CONCLUSION

Theories of age and aging engage a wide variety of phenomena and levels of explanation. There is a general consensus that aging is a complex process or set of processes, involving many causal inputs and manifold consequences. Two general theoretical orientations that explicitly address complexity have been sketched here. The genetic-based, which is a differential theory of quantitative genetics, and the nongenetic (stochastic) theories, which are based in systems theory.[140] Among the suggestions derived are that it may be advantageous to consider aging to be hierarchically organized, with the corollary that subsystems of an organism can have different functional or biological ages, and that several or many indices will be required to provide an adequate characterization of a single individual. Aging probably proceeds by saltation rather than continuously. Uncertainty associated with bifurcations in complex systems, together with individual differences in timing and magnitude of step changes, may constitute fundamental limitations to the predictability across the full life trajectory. Genetic and environmental influences will differ from heirarchical subsystem to subsystem, and may differ within a subsystem across chronological age.

Gerontology has evolved into a sophisticated scientific realm enabling us to distinguish between logical, plausible explanations and idealistic searches for the fountain of eternal youth. But, the question remains: What causes us to age?

Frolkis, a Soviet gerontologist, was quoted as saying, "the number of hypotheses is generally inversely proportional to the clarity of the problems."[45] This overview of theories should confirm the complicated nature of theoretic gerontology.

It is clear that no one theory adequately explains the entire process of growing old. Aging processes could better be explained if a number of these theories are integrated. For instance, theories on programmed control of aging can readily explain differences in the aging process of different species. The genetic makeup of a species determines the early development of an individual and will determine the rate of growth and metabolism directly affecting aging. Theories that suggest reasons for aging other than genetic makeup are useful in explaining why all members of the same species do not age in an identical manner. It may be that programmed aging directs the similar changes characteristic of all individuals with identical genetic makeup in their earlier years, but eventually bodily changes due to disease, the presence of excessive accumulations of substances in the cells, errors in protein synthesis, and so forth, may alter programmed aging. Because these factors can be expected to vary between individuals, it is expected that individual aging will vary, even among members of the same species.

PEARLS

- Aging research began in the early 1900s, and the two major groups of aging theories that have evolved are the developmental-genetic theories and the environmental stochastic theories.
- Hayflick and Moorehead conducted a landmark study that showed that in culture human fibroblasts have a limited life span.
- Theoretic gerontology uses these fundamental considerations: (1) aging is developmental, (2) old age

is a gift of modern technology, (3) differentiate normal vesus pathological aging, and (4) there is no universally accepted theory of aging.

- The evolutionary theory of aging predicts that the frequency for deleterious mutations of genes will reach equilibrium from one generation to the next (i.e., survival of the fittest).
- Neuroendocrine and hormonal theory regard functional decrements in neurons and their associated hormones as central to the aging process.
- The theory of intrinsic mutagenesis states that successive evolutionary regulations have a decreased capacity allowing an increase in mutations.
- Immunological theory states that the immune system declines with age and exacerbates the aging process.
- According to the free radical theory, free radicals accumulate with age and cause destruction to important biological structures through an oxidative process.
- Caloric restriction theory prescribes that an individual gradually loses weight until a point of maximum metabolic efficiency is reached for maximum health and life span.
- The error theory specifies that any error in the process of making proteins will cascade into multiple effects.
- Redundant DNA theory states that as errors accumulate, reserve genetic sequences with identical information take over until the system's redundancy is exhausted.
- Somatic mutation theory hypothesizes that genetic damage will result from radiation and that radiometric agents accumulate and create functional failure and death of the organism.
- Transcription theory relates to deleterious changes that occur in postmitotic cells in the transcriptive phase of protein synthesis.
- In the cross-linkage theory, cross-linkage of macromolecules is responsible for secondary and tertiary aging.
- Sleep, or the lack thereof, has been implicated as a factor in exacerbating the aging process.
- The hormonal imbalance-growth factor exposure (HI-GFE) theory can account for two major aging phenomena: (1) decline in mammalian reserve capacity with a consequent increase in diseases of maintenance, and (2) an increase in most age-associated proliferation of diseases, due to an imbalance of both growth hormone and insulin.
- The biological role of the adrenal sex steroid precursors dehydroepiandrosterone (DHEA) and DHEA sulphate (DHEA-S) is unclear and why they decline with aging remains incompletely understood.
- Telomeres have been implicated in the regulation of cellular senescence. Telomeres consist of tandem repeats of a short nucleotide sequence and are located on the ends of chromosomes.
- Apoptosis, a word coined in 1972, signifies the process of nontraumatic and noninflammatory cell death—the opposite of cell mitosis—that balances cell proliferation and thus maintains homeostasis.
- Recent compelling evidence supports a role for important genetic and environmental interactions on longevity in lower organsims.
- The completion of the Human Genome Project and the rapid innovations in technology will make possible the identification of human longevity-assurance genes.

REFERENCES

1. Rose MR. Can human aging be postponed? *Sci Am.* 1999; 281(6):106–111.
2. Austad SN. Theories of aging: An overview. *Aging.* 1998; 10(2):146–147.
3. Freeman JT. *Aging, Its History and Literature.* New York: Human Science Press; 1979.
4. Harman D. Aging: Phenomena and theories. *Ann NY Acad Sc.* 1998; 845:1–7.
5. Comfort A. *The Biology of Senescence.* 3rd ed. New York: Elsevier; 1979.
6. Pearl R. *The Rate of Living.* New York: Vropfu; 1928.
7. Warthin AS. *Old Age, the Major Revolution: The Philosophy and Pathology of the Aging Process.* New York: Hoeber; 1929.
8. Weissman A. *Uber die dauer des lebens.* Germany: Jena; 1882.
9. Rubner M. *Das problem der lebensdaver und seine beziebungen zum wachstum und ernabrung.* Munich: Oldenbourg; 1908.
10. Rose MR. *Evolutionary Biology of Aging.* New York: Oxford University Press; 1991.
11. Cauley JA, Dorman JS, Ganguli M. Genetic and aging epidemiology. The merging of two disciplines. *Neurol Clin.* 1996; 14:467–475.
12. Carrel A, Burrows MT. On the physiochemical regulation of the growth of tissues. *J Experimental Med.* 1911; 13:562–569.
13. Carrel A, Ebeling T. On the permanent life of tissues outside the organism. *J Experimental Med.* 1912; 15:516–522.
14. Carrel A. Present condition of a strain of connective tissue twenty-eight months old. *J Experimental Med.* 1914; 20:1–13.
15. Hayflick L. Senescence and cultured cells. In: Shock N, ed. *Perspectives in Experimental Gerontology.* Springfield, Ill: Charles C Thomas; 1966.
16. Hayflick L, Moorehead PS. The serial cultivation of human diploid all strains. *Exp Cell Res.* 1961; 25:585–593.
17. Stone D, Rozovsky I, Morgan T, Anderson C, Finch C. Increases synaptic sprouting in response to estrogen via an apolipoprotein E-dependent mechanism: implications for Alzheimer's disease. *J Neurosci.* 1998; 18:3180–3185.
18. Kirk KL. Dietary restriction and aging: Comparative tests of evolutionary hypotheses. *J Gerontol.* 2001; 56A(3):B123–B129.

19. Harrison DE, Archer JR. Natural selection for extended longevity from food restriction. *Growth Dev Aging.* 1988; 52(2):65.

20. Phelan JP, Austad SN. Natural selection, dietary restriction, and extended longevity. *Growth Dev Aging.* 1989; 53(1):4–6.

21. Dozmorov I, Bartke A, Miller RA. Array-based expression analysis of mouse liver genes: effect of age and longevity. *J Gerontol.* 2001; 56A(2): B72–B80.

22. Gadow S. Aging as death rehearsal: the oppressiveness of reason. *J Clin Ethics.* 1996; 7(1):35–40.

23. Strehler BL. *Time, Cells and Aging.* 2nd ed. New York: Academic Press; 1977.

24. Cristofalo VJ. Overview of biological mechanism of aging. *Annual Review of Gerontology and Geriatrics.* 1991; 6:1–22.

25. Shock NW. Longitudinal studies of aging in human. In: Finch CE, Schneider EL, eds. *Handbook of the Biology of Aging.* New York: Van Nostrand Reinhold; 1985; 721–739.

26. Adelman RC. Hormone interaction during aging. In: Schimke RT, ed. *Biological Mechanisms in Aging.* Washington, DC: US Department of Health and Human Services; 1980.

27. Fries I, Crapo L. *Vitality and Aging.* San Francisco: WH Freeman; 1981.

28. Kirkwood TB. Biological theories of aging: An overview. *Aging.* 1998; 10(2):144–146.

29. Martin GM, Turker M. Genetics of human disease, longevity and aging. In: Hazzard EG, ed. *Textbook of Genetic Medicine.* New York: McGraw-Hill; 1990.

30. Kallman JF, Jarvik LF. Twin data on genetic variations in resistance to tuberculosis. In: Gedda L, ed. *Genetica Della Tuberculosi e dei tumori.* Rome: Gregorio Mendel; 1957; 15–41.

31. Jarvik LF. Survival trends in a senescent twin population. *Am J Human Genetics. 1960;* 12:170–181.

32. Hayflick L. The cellular basis for biological aging. In: Finch C, Hayflick L, eds *The Handbook of the Biology of Aging.* New York: Van Nostrand Reinhold; 1977.

33. Martin GM, Sprague CA, Epstein CJ. Replicative life span of cultivated human cells. *Lab Invest.* 1970; 23:26.

34. Schneider EL, Mitsui Y. The relationship between in vitro cellular aging and in vivo human age. *Proc Natl Acad Sci USA.* 1976; 73:3584–3597.

35. Rohme D. Evidence for a relationship between longevity of mammalian species and life span of normal fibroblasts in vitro and erythrocytes in vivo. *Proc Natl Acad Sci USA.* 1981; 78: 3584–3591.

36. Stanley JF, Pye D, MacGregor A. Comparison of doubling numbers attained by cultural anirnal cells with life span of species. *Nature.* 1975; 255:158.

37. Keller L, Genoud M. Evolutionary theories of aging. 1. The need to understand the process of natural selection. *Gerontology.* 1999; 45(6):336–338.

38. Gavrilova NS, Gavrilov LA, Evdokushkina GN, et.al. Evolution, mutations, and human longevity: European royal and noble families. *Hum Biol.* 1998; 70(4):799–804.

39. LeBourg E. Evolutionary theories of aging: Handle with care. *Gerontology.* 1998; 44(6):345–348.

40. LeBourg E, Beugnon G. Evolutionary theories of aging. 2. The need not to close the debate. *Gerontology.* 1999; 45(6):339–342.

41. Franceschi C, Bonafe M, Valensin S, Olivieri F, De Luca M, Ottaviani E, DeBenedictis G. Inflamm-aging. An evolutionary perspective on immunosenescence. *Ann N Y Acad Sci.* 2000; 908: 244–254.

42. Franceschi C, Ottaviani E. Stress, Inflammation and natural immunity in the aging process: A new theory. *Aging.* 1997; 9(4 Suppl):30–31.

43. Parsons PA. Inherited stress resistance and longevity: A stress theory of aging. *Heredity.* 1995; 75(Pt 2):216–221.

44. Parsons PA. The limit to human longevity: An approach through a stress theory of aging. *Mech Ageing Dev.* 1996; 87(3):211–218.

45. Walford RL. The immunologic theory of aging: Current status. *Fed Proc.* 1974; 33:2020.

46. Pincus S, Mulligan T, Iranmanesh A, Gheorghiu S, Godschalk M, Veldhuis J. Older males secrete luteinizing hormone and testosterone more irregularly, and jointly more asynchronously, than younger males. *Proc Natl Acad Sci USA.* 1996; 93:14100–14105.

47. Veldhuis JD. Conference Report: Endocrinology of Aging. *Diabetes & Endocrinology.* 2000; 10:1–11.

48. Veldhuis JD, Iranmanesh A, Mulligan T. Current insights into hypothalamo-pituitary mechanisms of reproductive aging in men. In: Veldhuis JD. *Toward a Healthier Old Age: Biomedical Advances from Basic Research to Clinical Science.* Barcelona, Spain: Prous Science Publishers; 1999.

49. Veldhuis JD, Iranmanesh A. Pathophysiology of impoverished growth hormone (GH) secretion in aging. In: Veldhuis JD. *Toward a Healthier Old Age: Biomedical Advances from Basic Research to Clinical Science.* Barcelona, Spain: Prous Science Publishers; 1999.

50. Iranmanesh A, Veldhuis J. Functional alterations of the corticotropic axis with advancing aging. In: Veldhuis JD. *Toward a Healthier Old Age: Biomedical Advances from Basic Research to Clinical Science.* Barcelona, Spain: Prous Science Publishers; 1999.

51. Brody H, Jayashankar N. Anatomical changes in the nervous system. In: Finch CE, Hayflick L, eds. *Handbook of the Biology of Aging.* New York: Van Nostrand Reinhold; 1977.

52. Everitt AV. The hypothalamic pituitary control of aging and age-related pathology. *Experimental Gerontol.* 1973; 8:265–269.

53. Denckla WD. Role of the pituitary and thyroid glands in the decline of minimal O_2 consumption with age. *J Clin Investigation.* 1974; 53: 572–577.

54. Hayflick L. Theories of aging. In: Cape R, Coe R, Rodstein M, eds. *Fundamentals of Geriatric Medicine.* New York: Raven Press; 1983.

55. Finch CE, Landfield PW. Neuroendocrine and autonomic functions in aging mammals. In: Finch CE, Schneider EL, eds. *Handbook of the Biology of Aging.* New York: Van Norstrand Reinhold; 1985: 567–579.

56. Wise PA. Aging of the female reproductive system. *Rev Biol Res Aging.* 1983; 1:15–26.

57. Rosenfeld A. Are we programmed to die? *Saturday Rev.* 1976; 10(2):10.

58. Burnett M. *Intrinsic Mutagenesis: A Genetic Approach for Aging.* New York: Wiley; 1974.

59. Hart RW, Setlow RB. Correlation between DNA excision repair and life span in a number of mammalian species. *Pro Natl Acad of Sci USA.* 1974; 71:2169–2183.

60. Krauss SW, Linn S. Studies of DNA polymerases alpha and beta from cultured human cells in various replicative states. *J of Cellular Physiol.* 1986; 126:99–107.

61. Linn S. Decreased fidelity of DNA polymerase activity isolated from aging human fibroblasts. *Proc Natl Acad of Sci USA.* 1976; 13:2818–2826.

62. Murray V, Holliday R. Increased error frequency of DNA polymerases from senescent human fibroblasts. *J of Mol Biology.* 1981; 146:55–82.

63. Fairweather S. The in vitro life span of MRC-5 cells is shortened by 5-azacytidine induced derriethylation. *Experimental Cell Research.* 1987; 168: 153–158.

64. Holliday R. Strong effects of 5-azacytidine on the in vitro life span of human diploid fibroblasts. *Experimental Cell Research.* 1986; 166:543–548.

65. Wilson VL, Jones PA. DNA methylation decreases in aging but not in immortal cells. *Science.* 1983; 220:1054–1071.

66. Wareham VA. Age related reactivation of an X-linked gene. *Nature.* 1987; 327:725–732.

67. Walford RL. Immunopathology of aging. In: Eisdorfer C, ed. *Annual Review of Gerontology and Geriatrics.* 2nd ed., New York: Springer Publishing Co.; 1981:2.

68. Walford RL. *The Immunologic Theory of Aging.* Copenhagen: Munksgaard; 1969.

69. Walford RL. Multigene families, histocompatibility system, transformation, meiosis, stem cells and DNA repair. *Mech Ageing Dev.* 1979; 9:19–28.

70. Ashok BT, Ali R. The aging paradox: free radical theory of aging. *Exp Gerontol.* 1999; 34(3): 293–303.

71. Beckman KB, Ames BN. The free radical theory of aging matures. *Physiol Rev.* 1998; 78(2):547–581.

72. Banks D, Fossel M. Telomeres, cancer, and aging. Altering the human life span. *JAMA.* 1997; 278: 1345–1348.

73. Harmon D. Aging: a theory based on free radical and radiation chemistry. *J Gerontol.* 1956; 11: 298–311.

74. Harmon D. Prolongation of life: roles of free radical reactions in aging. *J Am Geriatr Soc.* 1969; 17:721.

75. Harmon D. The aging process. *Proc Natl Acad Sci USA.* 1981; 78:7124–7141.

76. Tappel AL. Lipid peroxidation damage to cell components. *Fed Proc.* 1973; 32:1870.

77. Leibovitz BE, Siegel B. Aspects of free radical reactions of biological systems: aging. *J Gerontol.* 1980; 35(1):45.

78. Sacher GA, Duffy PH. Genetic relation of life span to metabolic rate for inbred mouse strains and their hybrids. *Fed Proc.* 1979; 38:184–198.

79. Walford RL, Harris S, Weinciruch R. Dietary restriction and aging: historical phases, mechanisms and current directions. *J Nutr.* 1987; 117: 1650–1654.

80. Everitt AV. The effects of hypophysectomy and continuous food restriction, begun at ages 70 and 400 days, on collagen aging, proteinuria, incidence of pathology and longevity in the male rat. *Mech Ageing Dev.* 1980; 12:161–169.

81. Walford RL. *The 120-Year Diet.* New York: Pocket Books; 1986.

82. Weindruch R, Chia D, Barnett EV, Walford RL. Dietary restriction in mice beginning at complex levels. *Age.* 1982; 5:111–112.

83. Harmon D. Free radical theory of aging: Role of free radicals in the origination and evaluation of life, aging, and disease processes. In: Johnson JE, Walford RL, Harinon D, Miguel J, eds. *Free Radicals, Aging, and Degenerative Diseases.* New York: Alan Liss; 1986: 3–50.

84. Koizuini A, Weindruch R, Walford. RL. Influence of dietary restriction and age on live enzyme activities and lipid peroxidation in mice. *J Nutr.* 1987; 11 7:361–367.

85. Masoro EJ. Influence of caloric intake on aging and on the response to stressors. *J Toxicol Environ Health B Crit Rev.* 1998; 1(3):243–257.

86. Paffenberger RS. Physical activity, all-cause mortality, and longevity of college alumni. *N Engl J Med.* 1986; 314:605–609.

87. Pereira-Smith OM. Genetic theories of aging. *Aging.* 1997; 9(6):429–430.

88. Orgel LE. The maintenance of the accuracy of protein synthesis and its relevance to aging. *Proc Natl Acad Sci USA.* 1963; 49:517–531.

89. Sonnebom T. The origin, evolution, nature and causes of aging. In: Behnke J, Fince C, Moment G, eds. *The Biology of Aging.* New York: Plenum Press; 1979; 341.

90. Gallant J, Kurland C, Parker J, Holliday R, Rosenberger R. The error catastrophe theory of aging. *Exp Gerontol.* 1997; 32(3):333–346.

91. Ryan JM, Duda B, Cristofalo VJ. Error accumulation and aging in human diploid cells. *J Gerontol.* 1974; 29:616–627.

92. Holliday R, Tarrant GM. Altered enzymes in aging human fibroblasts. *Nature.* 1972; 238: 26–34.

93. Holliday R. The current status of the protein error theory of aging. *Exp Gerontol.* 1996; 31(4): 449–452.

94. Rothstein M. Age-related changes in enzyme levels and enzyme properties. In: Rothstein M, ed. *Review of Biological Research in Aging.* New York: Alan Liss; 1985; 1:421–444.

95. Medvedev Z. Possible role of repeated nucleotide sequences in DNA in the evolution of life spans of differential cells. *Nature.* 1972; 237–453.

96. Kowald A. The mitochondrial theory of aging: Do damaged mitochondria accumulate by delayed degradations? *Exp Gerontol.* 1999; 34(5):605–612.

97. Failla G. The aging process and carcinogenesis. *Ann NY Acad Sci.* 1958; 71:1124–1130.

98. Szilard L. On the nature of the aging process. *Proc Natl Acad Sci USA.* 1959; 45:30–51.

99. Curtis HF, Miller K. Chromosome aberrations in lower cells of guinea pigs. *J Gerontol.* 1971; 26:292–299.

100. Maynard-Smith J. Review lecturer on senescence: 1. The causes of aging. *Proceedings of the Royal Society of London.* 1962; (B):157:115–124.

101. Clark AM, Rubin NIA. The modification of X-irradiation of the life span of haptoid and diploid hagrogracon. *Radiation Research.* 1961; 14: 244–251.

102. Fossel M. Cell senescence in human aging: A review of the theory. *In Vivo.* 2000; 14(1):29–34.

103. Morley A. Somatic mutation and aging. *Ann NY Acad Sci.* 1998; 854:20–22.

104. Bjorksten J. Cross-linkage and the aging process. In: Rockstein M, ed. *Theoretical Aspects of Aging.* New York: Academic Press; 1974:43.

105. Bjorksten J. The cross-linkage theory of aging: clinical implications. *Compr Ther.* 1976; 11:65.

106. Hall DA. *The Aging of Connective Tissue.* New York: Academic Press; 1976.

107. Leproult R, Copinschi G, Buxton O, Cauter E. Sleep loss results in an elevation of cortisol levels the next evening. *Sleep.* 1997; 20(10): 865–870.

108. Mullington J, Hermann D, Holsboer F, Pollmacher T. Age-dependent suppression of nocturnal growth hormone levels during sleep deprivation. *Neuroendocrinology.* 1996; 64(3):233–241.

109. Giustina A, Veldhuis J. Pathophysiology of neuroregulation of growth hormone secretion in experimental animals and the human. *Endocr Rev.* 1998; 19:717–797.

110. Van Cauter E, Plat L, Leproult R, Copinschi G. Alterations of circadian rhythmicity and sleep in aging: endocrine consequences. *Horm Res.* 1998; 49:147–152.

111. Parr T. Insulin exposure and unifying aging. *Gerontology.* 1999; 45(3):121–135.

112. Yasumichi A, Nobuyoshi H, Yamamura K, Shimizu K, Takayama M, Ebihara Y, Osono Y. Serum insulin-like growth factor-1 in centenarians: implications of IGF-1 as a rapid turnover protein. *J Gerontol.* 2001; 56A(2):M79–M82.

113. Flynn MA, Weaver-Osterholtz D, Sharpe-Timms KL, Allen S, Krause G. Dehydroepiandrosterone replacement in aging humans. *J Clin Endocrinol Metab.* 1999; 84(5):1527–1533.

114. Morales AJ, Haubrich RH, Hwang JY, Asakura H, Yen SS. The effect of six months treatment with a 100 mg daily dose of dehydroepiandrosterone (DHEA) on circulating sex steroids, body composition and muscle strength in age-advanced men and women. *Clin Endocrinol.* 1998; 49(4): 421–432.

115. Callies F. Influence of oral dehydroepiandrosterone (DHEA) on urinary steroid metabolites in males and females. *Steroids.* 2000; 65(2):98–102.

116. Barnhart KT, Freeman E, Grisso JA, Rader DJ, Sammel M, Kapoor S, Nestler JE. The effect of dehydroepiandrosterone supplementation to symptomatic perimenopausal women on serum endocrine profiles, lipid parameters, and health-related quality of life. *Clin Endocrinol.* 1998; 49 (4):433–438.

117. Arlt W, Haas J, Callies F, Reincke M, Hubler D, Oettel M, Ernst M, Schulte HM, Allolio B. Biotransformation of oral dehydroepiandrosterone in elderly men: Significant increase in circulating estrogens. *J Clin Endocrinol Metab.* 1999; 84(6): 2170–2176.

118. Mazza E, Maccario M, Ramunni J, Gauna C, Bertagna A, Barberis AM, Patroncini S, Messina M, Ghigo E. Dehydroepiandrosterone sulfate levels in women. Relationships with age, body mass index and insulin levels. *J Endocrinol Invest.* 1999; 22(9): 681–687.

119. Tilvis RS, Kahonen M, Harkoner M. Dehydroepiandrosterone sulfate, diseases and mortality in a general aged population. *Aging.* 1999; 11(1): 30–34.

120. Hayflick L. How and why we age. *Exp Gerontol.* 1998; 33(6):639–653.

121. Olovnikov AM. Telomeres, telomase, and aging: Origin of the theory. *Exp Gerontol.* 1996; 31(4): 443–448.

122. Perez G, Tilly J. Cumulus cells are required for the increased apoptotic potential in oocytes of aged mice. *Hum Reprod.* 1997; 12:2781–2783.

123. Beckman KB, Ames BN. Mitochondrial aging: Open questions. *Ann NY Acad Sci.* 1998; 854: 118–127.

124. Miquel J. An update on the oxygen stress-mitochondrial mutation theory of aging: genetic and evolutionary implications. *Exp Gerontol.* 1998; 33 (1–2):113–126.

125. Carlson JC, Riley JC. A consideration of some notable aging theories. *Exp Gerontol.* 1998; 33 (1–2):127–134.

126. Abbott M, Abbey H, Bolling D, Murphy E. The familial component in longevity—a study of offspring of nonagenarians: III. Intrafamilial studies. *Am J Med Genetics.* 1978; 2(2):105–120.

127. Sorensen T, Nielsen G, Andersen P, Teasdale T. Genetic and environmental influences on premature death in adult adoptees. *N Engl J Med.* 1988; 318:727–732.

128. Ljungquist B, Berg S, Lanke J, McClearn GE, Pedersen NL. The effect of genetic factors for longevity: a comparison of identidal and fraternal twins in the Swedish Twin Registry. *J Gerontol Med Sci.* 1988; 53A(4):M441–M446.

129. Herskind AM, McGue M, Iachine IA, et al. Untangling genetic influences on smoking, body mass index and longevity: a multivariate study of 2464 Danish twins followed for 28 years. *Hum Genet.* 1996; 98:467–475.

130. Perls TT, Burbrick E, Wager CG, Vijg J, Kruglyak L. Siblings of centenarians live longer. *Lancet.* 1998; 351(3):1560.

131. Robine JM, Allard M. The oldest human. *Science.* 1998; 279:1834.

132. Barzilai N, Shuldiner AR. Searching for human longevity genes: the future history of gerontology in the post-genomic era. *J Gerontol.* 2001; 56A(2): M83–M87.

133. Finch EF, Tanzi RE. Genetics of aging. *Science.* 1997; 279:1834.

134. Schachter F, Faure-Delanef L, Guenot F. Genetic associations with human longevity at the APOE and ACE loci. *Nat Genet.* 1994; 6:29–32.

135. Ivanova R, Henon N Lepage V, Charron D, Vicaut E, Schachter F. HLA-DR alleles display sex-dependent effects on survival and discriminate between individuals and familial longevity. *Hum Mol Genet.* 1998; 7(1):187–194.

136. Mannucci PM, Mari D, Merati G. Gene polymorphisms predicting high plasma levels of coagulation and fibronolysis proteins. A study in centenarians. *Arterioscler Thromb Biol.* 1997; 17: 755–759.

137. Van Orsouw N, Perls TT, Vijg J. Centenarians: defining the "good" polymorphism of longevity enabling genes [abstract]. *The Gerontologist.* 1999; 39(special issue) 1:282. Session 182.

138. De Benedictis G, Rose G, Carrieri G. Mitochondrial DNA inherited variants are associated with successful aging and longevity in humans. *FASEB J.* 1999; 13:1532–1536.

139. Yu C, Oshim J, Wijsman E, et al. Mutations in the consensus helicase domains of the Werner syndrome gene. Werner's Syndrome Collaborative Group. *Am J Hum Genet.* 1997; 60:330–341.

140. McClearn GE. Biogerontologic theories. *Exp Gerontol.* 1997; 32(1–2):3–10.

CHAPTER 3

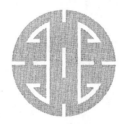

Comparing and Contrasting Age-Related Changes in Biology Physiology, Anatomy, and Function

The aging process occurs along the continuum of life. Beginning at conception and terminating in death, certain biological, anatomical, physiological, and functional changes are recognized as transitional markers in the human aging process. Aging is viewed as characteristically decremental in nature and lacking in defined chronological points of transition, though linear with time.[1]

The notion of a "maximal achievable life span" is inherent in the concepts of aging.[2-4] Identifying and describing changes in function that are common to all individuals and not produced by pathology is a very difficult task. The use of the term eugeric distinguishes changes related to the natural aging process from changes related to pathology.[5] The hypothesis of eugeric death is that the decline of function continues linearly to the point where an internal environment compatible with cell life can no longer be maintained.

The changes that a human experiences with the passage of years can be categorized in several ways. For the purpose of this chapter, these age-related changes will be discussed in terms of the biological, anatomical, physiological, and functional changes that occur eugerically in various systems in the human. While the process of aging is complex and does not uniformly result in decreased functional capacity,[6] this survey of the body's systems will be based on the assumption that the losses associated with the aging process are due to declines in biological cellular functioning. Some changes in function go hand in hand with anatomical or structural changes. In these cases, some functional units are lost, but the remaining units continue to function normally. The kidney is an excellent example of this—function is diminished in proportion to the number of nephrons lost. Skeletal muscle is another example. While muscle mass decreases secondary to the loss of muscle fibers, the remaining muscle mass is capable of oxygenation and consuming metabolic substrates at a constant rate. In some aging processes, there is no anatomical loss but rather reduced physiological efficiency of each unit. The reduced conduction velocity seen in aging nerve fibers is an example of this. The most obvious aging changes are those in which function is totally lost: The capacity of the female to reproduce is an excellent example, while another would be the loss in ability to hear sounds above a certain frequency.

Homeostasis is a concept describing the "constancy of the internal environment." [7] This internal constancy enables humans to survive in many environments and to withstand many biological and physiological challenges, thereby expanding the habitable world of the human. Perhaps the single most salient and age-related difference is the diminishing ability of the body to respond to physical and emotional stress and return to the pre-stress level.[8,9] This decrease in homestatic capacity is seen in all the systems of the body but most marked in neuroendocrine interaction and in the systemic functional alteration in the responsiveness of the nervous and endocrine systems.[7]

The changes associated with aging through adulthood into old age are gradual. During adult life, in the absence of overt pathology, there is a slow decrement in function. Homeostasis can be maintained, albeit at a lower level. Another observation is that the more complex the function, the more decline is seen. There are important differences between the young and old when considering interacting systems. Decrements are greater in the functions involving a number of connections between nerve and nerve, nerve and muscle, nerve and gland. For instance, the decrease in nerve conduction velocity is less than the decrease in maximum breathing capacity. In the former a single system is involved, while in the later the coordination of a number of nerve and muscle activities is required.

Last, it is important to keep in mind that individuals age at different rates. Different tissues and systems within one person demonstrate different aging rates as well. Therefore, while it is useful to discuss the average declines of function, it is important to keep in mind that any one individual may show remarkable variability from his or her peers.

CELLULAR CHANGES IN AGING

General changes in cell growth, division, repair, and regeneration have been found to occur with the aging process. Not all body cells age in the same way or at the same rate; however, in general, the total number of cells in the body decreases with age while remaining cells become less alike in structure and less organized in functions. Within cellular nuclei, nucleoli increase in size and number, loosely coiled fibers of chromatin demonstrate clumping, and the nuclear membrane becomes invaginated. Alterations in the number and shape of mitochondria, distortions of chromosomes, and fragmentation of the Golgi apparatus have been reported to occur. Though also found in younger cells, there is an increased deposition of an autoflourescent chemically inert substance called lipofuscin. The degree of lipofuscin deposition varies among body tissues but is particularly present in critical tissues like the heart and the brain. The possible correlation between lipofuscin accumulation and system pathology is not yet well established. Though general agreement has been reached regarding the existence of these changes, debates continue over their significance as related to cellular function in normal aging.[10]

Cells can be classified in many different ways. For our purposes, cells will be classified as mitotic, those cells that are capable of reproductive division (epithelial cells, hemopoeitic stem cells), and as postmitotic cells (neurons, myocardial cells), which are not capable of division. Mitotic cell life is ultimately ended by cellular division while postmitotic cell life (assuming no trauma) is terminated by senescence or death of the organism.

Mitotic cells were previously, and erroneously, believed to have an infinite capacity for division. Instead, Hayflick and associates[11] demonstrated with human fibroblasts that mitotic cells are capable of approximately fifty cell divisions. As a cell ages, the rate of cellular division decreases and becomes more irregular. Eventually, the cell is incapable of further division, and it dies. Hayflick also found that cellular division could be temporarily interrupted for years via an imposed dormancy with ultracold liquid nitrogen temperatures. Upon thawing, the cells resume their original sequence and rate of division until senescence. This evidence suggests that aging and cell death may be programmed events predetermined by aging genes.[7]

Because enzymes control cellular function, they have been widely studied for age-related changes. Though changes have been observed, the amounts of enzymes available are usually adequate if the system is not challenged. In general, the functional effectiveness of many enzymes does not diminish with age while production under stress may be limited.[12]

CARDIOVASCULAR CHANGES WITH AGE

Cellular Changes

Few cellular changes in the aging heart can be attributed to biological changes alone as evidenced by morphologic studies.[13,14] Age can not be accurately determined by pathologic examination of cardiac muscle cells. The only consistent myofibrillar change documented has been lipofuscin accumulation at the poles of the nuclei of cardiac muscle cells.[14] Baker[15] found that cardiac muscle cell diameter and protein production within the nuclear region of the cell were significantly increased with age. A rise in cellular degeneration was also observed with age, and this included an increase in lipofuscin deposition in the muscle cells, lipid deposition, and tubular dilation in the cardiac muscle cells. A marked decline in the total number of pacemaker cells at the sinoatrial node occurs at the approximate age of sixty and by the age of seventy-five there are less than 10% of pacemaker cells compared to the adult heart.[13-15] It has also been found that there is an increase in interstitial fibrous tissue specifically in the internodal tracts.[14]

Vascular changes with age include a thickening of the supporting membranes of the vessels including capillaries, an elongation of the arteries which become tortuous and calcify, and an increase in amyloidosis (depositing of excess starch-like material in the vessels).[16] The aging process affects each area of the vascular tree differently. Yin[16] reports that changes in the vascular structures are more prominent in the thoracic aorta and less prominent in the renal artery. Changes appear first in the proximal vessels progressing to involve the distal vasculature. It is also noted that the distal vessels undergo the most pronounced changes.[16,17] Changes in the coronary arteries appear first in the left branches, but they do not appear in the right and posterior descending coronary arteries until well into the fifth decade of life.[17]

The endothelial cells of the intima become irregular in size and shape and the cells lose their parallel orientation to the longitudinal axis of the vessel.[16-18] More giant multinucleated cells are present in the intima with age. Thickening of the subendothelial layer is apparent in aging. There is an increase in the connective tissue content, more thinned, frayed, and fragmented elastic laminae and an increase in lipid deposition and calcification around the internal elastic membrane.[16,19]

In the media, the most prominent age-related changes are increased calcification and thickening elastic fragmentation.[16,19,20] The aortic media thickens by approximately 40% (1.21 to 1.67mm) after the fifth decade of life. The thoracic aorta thickens predominantly secondary to an increase in the elastic laminae.[21] In the abdominal aorta, the thickening is due to smooth muscle proliferation.[21] Ninety-eight percent of human aortas demonstrate significant medial calcification by the fourth decade. Calcium binding to decarboxylic acid-containing amino acids demonstrates a parallel increase with age.[21,22]

Anatomic Changes

The heart shows a slight increase in the thickness of the left ventricular wall with age, though there is no significant change in heart chamber sizes.[13] Pomerance also noted that the number of proximal-bundle fascicles connecting the left bundle with the main bundle of the conduction system may be less, and there is a small age-related reduction in the density of the distal conduction fibers.[13] Relatively little change appears in the His' bundle or AV node. The elastic tissue, fat, and collagen content of the myocardium shows only a slight increase in end stage aging, and small areas of fibrosis in the myocardium show an age-related increase. The atrial surface of the atrioventricular and atrial endocardial valves thicken with age. As a result of mechanical stresses induced by repeated contact, nodular thickenings are often noted to form along the line of closure in the atrioventricular valves.

In the vasculature, as previously described, there is an increase in lumen size and thickness in the human aorta.[16] In the renal and carotid arteries there is an increase in the ratio of wall thickness to radius of the vessel. In the aorta and femoral artery there is a decrease in this ratio.[16] The aorta thickness to radius ratio shows a progressive increase in the peripheral vasculature and vascular tortuosity increases significantly with age.[23]

The process of aging results in an increase in collagen in arterial walls, but the blood levels of insulin-like growth factor I (IGF-I) decrease remarkably as adults age.[24] There is an almost simultaneous increase in insulin secretion, particularly in obese individuals. It is not known if, under these hormonal conditions, the enrichment of collagen in the arterial wall is due to insulin. However, Ruiz-Torres and colleagues[24] studied the effect of insulin production of collagen in vascular smooth muscle cells from elderly persons with high levels of insulin secretion after blocking the insulin receptors with a monoclonal antibody. Results were compared to those without insulin receptor blockage and to those with IGF-I. Despite the inhibition of glucose uptake, insulin clearly stimulated the release of procollagen III, and increased the collagen synthesis. The results indicate that under conditions that occur with aging, insulin interacts with nonspecific receptors in vascular smooth muscle cells, especially IGF-I, stimulating these cells to produce collagen.[24]

Physiological Changes

All of these biological and structural changes result in physiologic and functional alterations of the cardiovascular system. Generally there is a decrease in cardiac output at rest, a decline in the cardiovascular system's response to stress, an increase in the systolic blood pressure, and a progressive increase in the peripheral vascular resistance to blood flow.

Heart rate, loading conditions, intrinsic muscle performance, and neurohumoral efficiency all affect cardiac output. The maximum heart rate achievable declines linearly with age at peak exercise levels.[25,26]

Heart rate response is usually not affected at submaximal exercise levels. Heart rate response has been demonstrated to diminish in response to various physiological stimuli, such as coughing, postural changes, or during the Valsalva manuever.[27] The rate with which the heart rate peaks also becomes prolonged with increasing age.[25] Cardiac filling and vascular impedance are loading conditions that influence cardiac output. Diastolic filling rate has been shown to decrease with age,[28] and this is attributed to: prolonged isometric relaxation; thickening and sclerosis of the mitral valve which impedes ventricular filling; and an age-associated decrease in left ventricular compliance.[28] Vascular impedance is affected by the central-aortic stiffness or compliance, peripheral vascular resistance, and the inertial properties of blood.[16] Systolic pressure in the aorta and pulse pressures are increased with age.[14,16] Late systolic pressure exceeds early systolic pressure in the elderly, and the index of elastance (characteristic impedance) and peripheral resistance are increased with age.[29] These changes are indicative of less aortic compliance and a reduced cross-section of the peripheral vasculature, which causes an increase in pulse-wave velocity and an increase in wave reflection. Wei[14,25] hypothesizes that the consequent increase in vascular load could explain the age-associated reductions in stroke volume and cardiac output as well as the development of mild left ventricular hypertrophy and prolonged myocardial relaxation in the elderly.

Intrinsic muscle performance is estimated by the mean velocity of circumferential fiber shortening, and this does not change with age.[28] However, isometric relaxation and early diastolic relaxation are prolonged as age increases.[30] Left ventricular wall thickness may result from prolonged relaxation.[28]

Cardiac output is also affected by neurohumoral regulation. In the myocardium and in the peripheral vessels the end-organ responsiveness is decreased to beta-adrenergic stimulation.[16] The autonomic tone is increased based on plasma catecholamine levels.[31] Reflex activity of the cardiovascular system (e.g., Valsalva maneuver, orthostasis, and cough) are weaker in the aged cardiovascular system, due in part to a decreased baroreceptor sensitivity and associated with changes in the cardiopulmunary system.[25,27,32]

The ability of the body to maintain a homeostatic blood pressure is a function of: the autonomic nervous system; the arterial baroreceptor reflex; circulating neurohumoral factors; local vascular tone; and the extracellular fluid volume. There is an alteration in the homeostatic blood pressure regulatory role as a result of an altered autonomic nervous system with age.[16,32] According to Shimada, an elevation of blood pressure in the elderly can be attributed to an increase in plasma norepinephrine levels, which leads to an increase in the sympathetic responsiveness.[32] The functioning of the arterial baroreceptor reflex is lessened with age.[14,32] Atherosclerosis and the presence of hypertension also decrease the baroreceptor reflex.[32] Catecholamines and circulating neurohumoral factors assist in the maintainance of a homeostatic blood pressure.[33] These factors include renin, aldosterone, vasopressin, atrial natriuretic factor, and angiotensin II. The level of renin in the plasma has been found to remain unchanged or decrease in relation to age. It is hypothesized that this is due to a decrease in the concentration of active renin and not a result of the concentration of renin substrate in the plasma.[33] In proportion to the decreased renin activity in the plasma, there is a related decline in aldosterone and plasma-angiotensin II levels with increasing age.[33] Vasopressin remains unchanged or decreases with age. A decrease in vasopressin activity is most often related to blood loss or dehydration.[34] The level of plasma atrial natriuretic factor does not show a change with age. Vascular tone may show a local increase with age, though the constriction of the vessels is not changed in response to norepinephrine with age.[16]

The effect of these changes on the cardiovascular system is seen in changes in cardiac output, stroke volume, and blood pressure at rest and in response to stress. Resting heart rate does not show a consistent age-related change in humans.[14] Resting cardiac rate and cardiac output remain relatively unchanged, although peripheral resistance (blood pressure) is increased.[35] With age, myocardial weight tends to increase, and myocardial cells show an increase in lipofuscin deposition. Mitochondria decrease in size and myocardial cells are less responsive to catacholamine stimulation. A reduction in baroreceptor response and vascular elasticity combines to result in the tendency for older people to experience postural hypotension.[7,36] When sitting at rest, the cardiac output does not show a change with age; however, when supine there is often an age-related decrease in cardiac output.[14] There is also a similar position-associated change in stroke volume. This is explained by the changes with age in cardiac compliance and preload conditions.[14,16] Resting blood pressures, both diastolic and systolic, tend to show an increase with age.[14] It is not clear whether this increase in blood pressure is a reflection of eugeric aging or the result of heredity, environmental factors, or both.[14]

In response to stress, the cardiovascular system shows a decrease in heart rate acceleration and a decrease in ejection fraction with physical exertion.[14] Postural changes also affect cardiac output and blood pressure as previously discussed. Following a moderately sized meal, the elderly tend to show a decrease in systemic blood pressure.[14] With increasing levels of exercise, there is a concomitant rise in the systemic blood pressure. This rise is credited to the changes in preload conditions during cardiac filling.[14] In the absence of pathology, the cardiovascular responses to increased activity levels are consistently seen with increasing age, however, aerobic conditioning exercises may alter this. The effects of exercise on the cardiovascular system are positive and will be discussed in a subsequent chapter.

PULMONARY CHANGES WITH AGE

In this chapter, aging changes defined by Butler as those changes which are "universal, intrinsic, progressive and irreversible" within the cardiopulmonary system will be discussed.[37] The pathologies of the lung will be further discussed in Chapter 5, Pathological Manifestations of Aging.

In the pulmonary system, age changes can be organized according to mechanical properties, changes in flow, changes in volume, alteration in gas exchange, and impairments of lung defense. Decreases in chest wall compliance and lung elastic recoil tendency are two mechanical properties that are altered with age. Increased calcification of the ribs, a decline in intercostal muscle strength, and changes in the spinal curvature all result in a lower compliance and in increased work of breathing.

At normal lung volume, airway resistance is not increased. However, normal aging results in a reduction of maximum voluntary ventilation, maximum expiratory flow, and forced expiratory volume in one second (alone and in relation to forced vital capacity). Though tidal volume remains fairly constant throughout life, vital capacity decreases while residual volume increases.

Ventilation, diffusion, and pulmonary circulation are the three major components of the respiratory system that lose efficiency with age. There is an increased thickening of the supporting membranes between the alveoli and the capillaries, a decline in total lung capacity, an increase in residual volume, a reduced vital capacity, and a decrease in the resiliency of the lungs. It is difficult to completely separate pulmonary changes resulting with age from those associated with the pathology of emphysema or chronic bronchitis. Throughout a lifetime, exposure to occupational and environmental inhalants as well as cigarette smoke may result in chronic pulmonary changes and lung pathologies. These disease states closely parallel those of the aging process and also increase in incidence with advancing age.[38] "Normal" pulmonary aging includes a loss of elastic tissue leading to expiratory collapse of the larger airways, difficulty with expiration, and dilitation of the terminal air passages.[39]

There are changes in the diffusion efficiency of peripheral vascular system with age. Starting with the pulmonary system, impairment of gas exchange is illustrated by a reduced diffusing capacity of carbon monoxide, a lower resting arterial oxygen tension, and an increased alveolar-arterial oxygen gradient. Alveolar surface area and pulmonary capillary blood volume diminish with age. Small changes in red blood cell metabolism produce a decrease in 2,3 diphosphoglycerate (DPG). As a result, the oxygen dissociation curve shifts to the left, which makes oxygen less available at the tissue level.

The ability to provide oxygen to working tissues is altered as normal aging affects the cardiopulmonary system in a variety of ways. In the absence of pathology, the heart and lungs can generally meet the body's needs; however, reserve capacities are diminished. With any challenge, the body's demand for oxygen and perfusion may exceed available supply.

In an older person, normal changes result in an impairment of pulmonary defenses. Cilia are reduced in number, and those which remain become less strong. The mucous escalator and alveolar macrophages are less effective in removing inhaled particulate matter. In the absence of physiological challenges, the system maintains fairly adequate defenses. However, an older individual who is chronically exposed to air laden with particles will become at risk for pulmonary dysfunction.[7,40]

The recovery period following effort is prolonged in the elderly. Among other factors, this reflects a greater relative work-rate, an increased proportion of anaerobic metabolism, a slower heat elimination, and a lower level of physical fitness. When exercising, elderly individuals need to lengthen the cool down phase of exercise to allow for a more gradual return to the baseline vital signs. Abrupt cessation of exercise without considering an adequate recovery period could have negative effects for a person of any age, but it is particularly important in the elderly to provide adequate recovery time.

MUSCULOSKELETAL CHANGES WITH AGE

Cellular Changes

Extracellular and connective tissue changes with age are related to hydration of the tissues and collagen and elastin extensibility. There are many types of connective tissue in the body (loose, adipose, fibrous, etc.). It is loose connective tissue that binds organs together while holding tissue fluids and permitting cellular-molecular diffusion. Loose connective tissue is located beneath most layers of epithelium and fills spaces between muscles (fascia). The most common type of cells in loose connective tissue are fibroblasts, which work to produce protein fibers called collagen and elastin.[36]

In youth, collagen fibers are strong and flexible, and they are arranged in bundles which crisscross to form structure in the body. As a person ages, there is an increased crisscrossing or cross-linkage of the fibers resulting in more dense extracellular matrices. The collagen structure becomes more stiff as it becomes denser. This increased density also impairs molecular movement of nutrients and wastes at the cellular level.[36]

Structurally, elastin fibers also develop increased cross-linkage with age. Water and elasticity are lost. The elastin fibers become more rigid, may tend to fray, and, in some cases, are replaced by collagen completely.[7]

Connective tissue cells develop from the primitive mesenchymal cell. As a result of this common origin, all connective tissues have similar cellular features. All connective tissue cells secrete collagen, elastin, glycoproteins, hyaluronic acid, and contractile proteins.[41] These substances vary in proportion in different tissue types. For example, the predominant secretion in white fibrous tissue is collagen, elastin is the prevalent secretion in yellow elastic tissue, and glycoprotein is the common secretion in cartilage. The pattern of secretion of these substances by connective tissue is altered under different environmental conditions within the body. In this portion of the chapter, the effects of aging on the production and functional significance of each of these secretions will be considered.

Collagen is the basic protein component in fibrous connective tissue inclusive of bone, tendon, ligament and cartilage.[42,43] Procollagen, a protein material, is secreted by the ribosomes of connective tissue cells. Individual procollagen molecules bind together to form tropocollagen strands. These strands group together in a spiral fashion to form the mature collagen fiber.[44] The diameter of the collagen fiber is increased by the surface aggregation of additional tropocollagen strands with a resulting characteristic of a compressed and increasingly cross-linked central fiber.[45] Further cross-linkages continue to be added even after the fiber has reached maturity. It has been determined that the diameter of collagen fibers is greater in older subjects when compared to younger subjects.[46] Generally, the tensile strength of connective tissue in older persons is greater than that of younger individuals. The increased cross-linkage of collagen fibers is considered a normal change related to aging.

The clinical significance of this increased cross-linking is seen in resultant collagenous contractures. Bonds between adjacent collagen strands can produce shortening and distortion of the collagen fibers. This shortening may result in contractures with a progressive restriction in tissue mobility.[43] Collagen fibers are tough and inelastic, and their bonds can not be broken by mechanical stretching. Of interest clinically, however, has been the determination that some of these chemical bonds are temperature sensitive.[47] Lehmann and associates[47] found that at temperatures of 42.5°C and above, the bonds between collagen fibers become unstable and the tissues can be mobilized. Continuous stretching while heating the tissues followed by thirty minutes of maintained stretch during the cooling period is recommended.[47]

The ribosomes within the connective tissue secrete elastin during the developmental stages.[41] Elastin molecules join together in an end-to-end and branching manner to form a lattice-like network which gives elastin its ability to return to its original length after being stretched.[46] There is a progressive reduction in the amount of elastin in the skin, walls of the arteries, and the bronchial tree with age.[6,7] If the elastin fibers are overstretched to the point of tearing, scarring occurs, which further decreases the elasticity of the tissues.

The glycoproteins form a group of relatively small molecules of soluble protein material. The presence of glycoproteins in the extracellular area produces the osmotic force that is important in maintaining the fluid content of the tissues.[41] The higher the glycoprotein concentration, the greater amount of fluid will be retained in the tissues by osmotic attraction forces. A variety of glycoprotein secretions have been identified and vary among tissue types and locations.[48] The production and release of glycoproteins within the connective tissues is reduced with age and with inactivity. As a result, it becomes increasingly difficult for the tissues to maintain a normal fluid balance. Dehydration is commonly found in the tissues of elderly individuals.[41]

Hyaluronic acid helps to regulate the viscosity of tissues, and is produced by some of the ribosomes in the connective tissue cells, particularly those located in the cartilage. This substance helps to decrease the friction between cellular components during movement. There is a reduction in the amount of hyaluronic acid secreted, which is associated with age and with inactivity, thus reducing the ease of movement (viscosity) of the connective tissues and resulting in tissue degradation.[49] The production of hyaluronic acid is enhanced by activity and weight bearing. Thus, exercise becomes particulary important for maintaining the viscosity of tissues in the elderly. Lack of exercise and activity will negatively affect the production of hyaluronic acid, producing tissue restrictions and further decreasing mobility.

Contractile proteins provide motility within the connective tissues. Their presence provides removal of waste products or debris and enhances mobility within the tissue spaces, as well as facilitates the capacity of cellular proteins to cross a capillary or lymphatic wall.[41] During aging there is a reduction in the secretion and organization of contractile proteins with a resultant decrease in motility.[48] Contractile protein secretion is relatively small in normal fibroblasts. Connective tissue cells that produce abnormally high amounts of contractile protein are called myofibroblasts.[50] Ryan[50] found excessive amounts of contractile protein in chronically restricted tissues, such as the rotator cuff in shoulder-hand syndrome and in Dupuytren's contracture. Again, the importance of activity for the elderly must be stressed to prevent the accumulation of contractile proteins and prevent soft tissue restrictions and contractures.

Fibrinous adhesions have great clinical implications in working with the elderly. Fibrinogen, a soluble plasma protein, is a normal molecular exudate within the capillary, and when this substance passes through the capillary wall into the surrounding tissues, it is converted to strands of insoluble fibrin.[51] Fibrin strands can adhere to tissue structures and restrict movement of these structures. Normally, fibrin is removed as debris by reticuloendothelial cells. With age, as well as with inactivity, the exudation of fibrinogen into the surrounding tissues is increased.[48]

With reduced activity levels, the complete breakdown of fibrin may not occur, which leads to the accumulation of this substance, restricting movement and possibly resulting in adhesions. Following an injury (traumatic or surgically induced), fibrinogen also accumulates at the site of tissue damage. If activity is limited, these strands can consolidate and create an adhesion.[41] Activity enhances the removal of fibrinogen and should be resumed as quickly as possible following an injury to prevent irreversible tissue restriction and contractures. The importance of early intervention and mobilization in the elderly is clear.[50]

Changes in Cartilage

Other connective tissue also affected by aging includes bone, hyaline cartilage, elastic cartilage, and articular cartilage. Changes in bone will be presented separately.

Hyaline cartilage is found in the nose and the rings of the respiratory passages as well as in the joints. Elastic cartilage is found in parts of the larynx and the outer ear. Articular cartilage is found between the intervertebral discs, between the bones of the pelvic girdle, and at most articular joint surfaces.[52] With aging, cartilage tends to dehydrate, becomes stiffer, and thins in weight- bearing areas.

Cartilage is formed when the primitive mesenchymal cells are subjected to compressive forces in an environment of low oxygen concentration. The predominant secretions of the chondroblast are glycoprotein, chondroitin sulfate, and hyaluronic acid. Collagen is produced in lesser amounts than these. Cartilage is a unique connective tissue in that it has no direct blood supply. Blood flow in adjacent bones and synovial fluid provide nutrients to the chondroblasts. A strong osmotic force, created by glycoprotein secretions from the chondroblasts passing from the cells into the surrounding matrix, attracts water with dissolved gases, inorganic salts, and organic materials into the matrix providing materials necessary for normal metabolism. The concentration of glycoproteins in the matrix determines the amount of fluid drawn into the cartilage. Normal aging is accompanied by a reduction in the amount of chondroitin sulfate produced[53] and results in a decrease in osmotic attraction forces and impairment in the ability of the matrix to attract and retain fluids.

Nutrients enter the matrix of the cartilage only when compressive forces are absent.[49,53] In a loaded or compressed state, fluid and nutrient substances are squeezed out. To provide regular movement of substances in and out of the cartilage, it is necessary that alternating application and release of compressive forces occur. Metabolites remain in the matrix in the absence of compression. The presence of metabolites reduces the oxygen content, which results in a decrease in the secretion of glycoproteins and an increase in the amount of procollagen produced. With inactivity, hyaline cartilage is converted to fibrocartilage.[49,53] Therefore, weight-bearing exercises become particularly important in the elderly individual. The movement of nutritional substances in and out of the cartilage with activity could enhance the overall health of the cartilage and preserve the viability of the joints.[53]

In synovial joints the articular surfaces are covered by hyaline cartilage. Secretion of hyaluronic acid by the chondroblasts provides lubrication at the interface of the hyaline cartilage. Hyaluronic acid molecules form a viscous layer covering the hyaline cartilage. Compression facilitates production of hyaluronic acid ensuring continual lubrication of the joint during movement.[49] As previously noted, the secretion of hyaluronic acid decreases with age, thereby reducing the efficiency of the lubrication system of the joint.[53] Degenerative changes of the cartilage are not reversible and rehabilitation efforts need to be directed toward regular compression and release of compression in the aging joint. Normal weight-bearing exercises are recommended to maintain cartilagenous health.

The cartilage that normally covers body joints thins and deteriorates with aging. This especially occurs in the weight-bearing areas. Because cartilage has no blood supply or nerves, erosion within the joint is often advanced before symptoms of pain, crepitation, and limitation of movement are perceived. Decreased hydration, reduced elasticity, and increased fibrous growth around bony prominences contribute to increased stiffness and decreased functioning. Advanced stages of cartilage-joint deterioration are commonly known as osteoarthritis.[7,42,54]

Since some type of connective tissue exists almost everywhere in the body, the effects of aging, especially when superimposed on inactivity, are widespread. The increased rigidity of collagenous and elastin fibers means a greater amount of energy is required to produce a given stretch. Skin becomes less elastic and more wrinkled. Lungs lose some recoil tendency, arteries become more rigid, and the heart becomes less distensible. Joints become stiffer while decreased hydration in the intravertebral discs results in vertebral compaction and shrinkage of height. Cellular repair, nutrition, and waste removal are impaired.[7,55] Other effects of connective tissue changes will be discussed as various systems are reviewed.

Changes in Body Composition

Aging is associated with changes in body composition and weight. The most notable of these changes occurs with the body's fat and water content.[56,57] While extracellular water remains constant, intracellular water decreases, reflecting either a dehydration of the cell or a decrease of cell mass in the presence of adequate hydration.[56–59] Dehydration is a particularly common consequence of aging, especially during exercise. Adequate fluid intake should be encouraged in the elderly and closely monitored in the exercising aged individual.

In general, there is a decrease in lean muscle tissue while there is an increase in fat concentration.[60] It has been estimated that lean body mass declines by as much as 10% to 20% between the ages of 25 and 65.[61] During this period there is an accumulation of adipose tissue, especially in the truncal regions, leading to a net gain in body weight. Accumulation of fat in the central regions of the body has been associated with increased risk for a number of health problems, including hyperinsulinemia, insulin resistance, non-insulin-dependent diabetes, hypercholesterolemia, hypertension, and atherosclerosis. Since the risk of developing diabetes, hypertension, and atherosclerosis is age related, it is important to distinguish the changes in body composition that occur with successful aging from those that are linked to pathology.

Physical inactivitiy with aging contributes to the increased adiposity of older people. Regularly performed exercise protects against the increase in body fat content with aging.[61] Older adults who maintain a high level of activity with advancing age appear to avoid many of the undesirable changes in body composition and fat distribution that typically occur with aging.

Another change in body composition involves the aging of the internal organs. Almost all the organs demonstrate a decrease in weight and mass, with an exception being the prostate, which may actually double in size with age.[59,62]

MUSCLE CHANGES WITH AGE

Cellular Changes

Muscles are composed of postmitotic cells. Intact motor neuron innervation is required for proper functioning and survival. A loss of muscle mass with aging is caused by a reduction in the size and number of muscle fibers.[63] As fewer fibers are lost from the contracting muscles as compared to the opposing muscle mass,[64] the body develops a tendency towards flexion at the joints. Lipofuscin deposition is increased. The density of capillaries per remaining motor unit is decreased, and a reduction in myosin adenosine triphosphate (ATP) activity has been shown.[65] Neuroconduction of muscle impulse is prolonged and coordination is affected. The sum total of these changes includes a decrease in muscle strength and body stability. Deconditioning and malnutrition often compound the effects of normal age-related changes. Though reconditioning will improve muscle function, the speed and degree of potential improvement does decline with age.[66]

Alterations in skeletal muscle with aging resemble those observed with denervation. The classic cross-innervation studies of Buller and associates[67] established the importance of the trophic influence on skeletal muscle function and demonstrated that the metabolic and physiologic profile of a muscle fiber (i.e., the fiber type) was primarily determined by the type of neural innervation (phasic or tonic firing pattern and other trophic factors) received. Adult skeletal muscle is composed of three distinct fiber types: type IIA (fast twitch, high oxidative fiber), type IIB (fast twitch, low oxidative fiber), and type I (slow twitch, high oxidative fiber). Based on the histochemical demonstration of myofibrillar ATPase and the mitochondrial enzyme succinic dehydrogenase, this heterogeneous fiber pattern is lost with aging, and fibers become more homogeneous in respect to their physiological and metabolic profile.[64,65,67]

It is well known that decreases in muscle mass occur with old age, with proximal muscles of the lower extremity particularly affected. This decrease in muscle mass is due to a decrease in both fiber number and diameter. No change in the number of motor neural fibers has been found, but the size of the motor unit decreases due to the loss of muscle fibers. The reported decrease in fiber number primarily affects the red oxidative fiber, the preponderance of evidence based on enzyme histochemistry and physiological properties suggest a greater loss in the fast type II fiber. The decrease occurs in both type IIA and IIB fibers such that the type IIB/IIA fiber ratio is unaltered with increasing age. As a result of this selective loss of type II fibers, the percentage of type I fibers increases from about 40% in 20 to 30 year-olds to 55% in 60 to 65 year-old individuals.[68]

Besides atrophy and decrease in number of fibers, senile skeletal muscle exhibits a number of ultrastructural changes:

1. Thickening and protrusion of the sarcolemma into the extracellular space;
2. An increase in collagenous material in the extracellular space;
3. Disorganized and disrupted myofilaments at the cell perhiphery;
4. Proliferation of the tubular T-system, the sarcoplasmic reticulum, and the terminal cisternae;
5. Enlarged mitochondria with vacuolated matrix, short cristae, and loss of dense granules;
6. Accumulation of ribosomes and polysomes in sub-sarcolemmal region;
7. An increase in lysosomal vesicles and pinocytic activity.

The majority of these age-related changes are located at the fiber surface where considerable cell debris associated with proteolytic activity can be observed.

Cellular changes are found in all organs with aging. Among the most visible signs of aging are alterations in skin and the development of movement dysfunction. As we age, strength and coordination decline and movements tend to become slower. Movement dysfunctions are caused by many factors;

some of these factors are peripheral and central synaptic mechanism changes, motivation, skeletal disorders (such as osteoarthritis or structural imbalances caused by tonal changes in cerebral vascular accidents (CVAs) or other neurological syndromes), and muscle changes. Several factors may be occurring simultaneously. Loss of strength, seen as a decrease in muscle hypertrophy and changes in muscle function, is a result of a complex interaction of factors. For instance, there is a reduced ability of the cardiovascular system to deliver raw materials to working muscles and alterations in the chemical composition of muscle fibers.[69,70] On a quantitative level, all measurements of muscle—physiologic, anatomic, histochemical, or enzymatic—decrease after the age of 40. It is estimated that 20% to 40% of maximal strength is lost by the age of 65 in the nonexercising adult.[71] The general reaction to aging involves a decline in muscular strength accompanied by signs of atrophy. Qualitative measurements of changes in muscle function show loss of lean body mass and primary skeletal muscle. Clinically, it is apparent that aging affects certain muscles more than others. For example, flexor muscles of lower extremities show age-related changes relatively early compared to other muscle groups.

In the aging phenomena there is a decrease in the number of active functional units (motor units or muscle fibers) and a loss in the concentration of specific enzymes or fiber types. The major fiber types show a differential response to aging. Gutmann and Hanzlikova[72] have characterized the essential features of the "senescent motor unit," which indicate that age-related changes are a distinct biological entity. Changes are similar to changes seen in denervated muscle and immobilized muscle, namely:

- Decreased number and size of muscle fibers;
- Proliferation of T tubules and sarcoplasmic reticulum;
- Considerable histochemical evidence of fiber grouping.

Biochemical changes at the cellular level[65] include:

- Loss of activity of glycolytic and oxidative enzymes;
- Decreased concentration of ATP;
- Decreased rate of creatin phosphate resynthesis;
- Changes at the neuromuscular junction altering trophic interactions between muscle and nerve compromising fast synaptic activity (reduced endplate potentials).

Some alterations in aged muscle may be secondary to other age-related changes such as weight loss. Most changes in the senescent motor unit, however, are usually evident before an age-associated loss of body weight. It is unlikely that muscle dysfunction is secondary to weight loss in the elderly unless a true state of malnutrition exists.

Pathologic causes of strength declines are many, and include arthritis, cerebrovascular accidents, cardiovascular disease, and so on, all of which will be covered more extensively in Chapter 5, Pathological Changes with Aging. Functional causes of muscle strength declines can be related to the "use it or lose it" principle. Studies on astronauts in a gravity-eliminated environment as well as research involving immobilization of body parts or the whole body reveal significant parallels to those muscle changes seen as normal aging.[7]

Endurance is another factor of muscle function that appears to be affected by aging. Larsson and his colleagues[68] studied the physiologic, anatomic, and histochemical effects of aging changes in a cross-sectional study of fifty-five healthy men aged 22 to 65 years—all sedentary office workers.

Testing was done using the Cybex[68,73] to determine whether these changes correlated with performance, strength, and endurance. Isometric endurance was measured using the time subjects could maintain 50% of their maximal isometric force, and dynamic endurance was measured by having subjects perform fifty maximal isokinetic contractions at 180 degrees per second. The percent of change was determined by dividing the mean torque of the last three contractions by the mean torque of the first three contractions. It was found that at all velocity settings there was an age-related decline in isometric force and an age-related decrease in the peak isokinetic torque. A decline in maximal knee extension was also noted. There was no age-related difference in muscle mass as measured by thigh circumference. Endurance, both dynamic and isometric, was similar in all age groups. With age, force values linearly declined as did the proportion and area of the type II fibers. However, Larsson[73] postulated, based on multiple regression analysis, that type II fiber atrophy could not account for all of the decline in strength measures. Other factors such as age and activity levels influenced the results. Combining the factors of increased *hydroaldoase dexokinase* (HAD) activity, a shift in lactic dehydrogenase (LDH) isoenzyme patterns, an increased proportion of type I fibers and a decreased area of type II fibers, we see an indication that with aging there is an overall increase in oxidative capacity of the muscle. Another possibly clinically significant finding is the elevated enzyme activities in the older active group compared with the younger sedentary group. The increase in enzyme levels raises the question of how "trainable" the aged motor unit is.[74] Specific measurements of isometric and isokinetic muscle performance all show deterioration. Interestingly, no change in endurance capacity was correlated with age.

Electromyographic patterns indicate an increasing recruitment of motor units for a given task by skeletal muscle with age. In other words, it takes more to do less.[74] This effect is due to the generalized denervation of muscle fibers requiring a larger number of motor units to produce a given force. These physiologic changes in skeletal muscle are associated with the aging process.

Anatomic Changes

Anatomically, a pattern of gross skeletal muscle wasting is seen with aging. On a microscopic level, changes of muscle in aging are similar to those described in myopathy, disuse, and neuropathic atrophy.

The ultrastructure of the sarcoplasm also undergoes some age-related changes. The hypertrophy of the sarcoplasmic reticulum is felt to correlate with an increase in the rate of calcium ion transport or absorption by the reticulum. This effect may in turn cause contractile protein dysfunction due to the paucity of calcium ions available for normal contraction. The thickening of the muscle fibers basement membrane is hypothesized as an explanation of the decreased depolarization sensitivity of aged muscle cell membranes.[75]

Histological Changes

Histopathological changes occur in aging as well as in disuse or denervation. Aging muscles show a general increase in type I muscle fibers. Etiology of this is believed to be twofold: Either there is a selective loss of type II muscle fibers, or there is a reinnervation of denervated type II fiber motor units by type I motor fibers.[76] In the "extremely old" muscle, muscle grouping of fibers of one type occur, a process associated with denervation and subsequent reinnervation. Gutmann[72] found no evidence of disintegration of the terminal axons in senile muscle fibers, but he observed major changes at the neuromuscular junction resulting in muscle atrophy. These changes include an increase in the number and agglutination of presynaptic vesicles, the appearance of neurotubules and neurofilaments in the peripheral axons, the enlargement of primary synaptic clefts, the thickening of the basement membrane, and an increased branching of the junctional folds. These changes produce a slow reduction of synaptic contact in senile muscle and result in a "functional denervation." In addition, the neuromuscular junction in senile muscle shows a reduced frequency of miniature end-plate potentials and a reduced conduction velocity in the presynaptic axons.

It has been proposed that one mechanism for nerve and muscle dysfunction with age involves the mitochondria.[77] Mitochondria contain the only DNA outside the nucleus in mammalian cells. Mitochondrial DNA (mtDNA) has a high mutation rate, and low levels of pathogenic mutations have been found in tissues from elderly subjects. However, the role of these mutations in the aging process is uncertain unless a mechanism can be identified that would lead to a biochemical defect. In muscle tissue from normal elderly subjects, Brierly and associates[77] demonstrated that there are muscle fibers with very low activity of cytochrome c oxidase, suggestive of a mtDNA defect. In these cytochrome c oxidase-deficient fibers, the researchers found very high levels of mutant mtDNA. In addition, different mtDNA mutations are present in different fibers, which explains why there is a low overall incidence of an individual mutation in tissues from elderly subjects. These studies show a direct age-related correlation between a biochemical and genetic defect in normal human tissues and indicate that mtDNA abnormalities are involved in the aging process in human muscle and nerve connection.

The decrease in senile muscle mass is associated with a decrease in total protein and nitrogen concentration and an increase in connective tissue and fat. Intracellular water and potassium are unaltered or decreased, while muscle amino acid concentration increases with aging. Extracellular water, sodium, and chloride are all higher in older adults.

The molecular mechanism of age-related muscle atrophy is not clear, but the process is likely to be linked to the neural and neuromuscular changes already reviewed.

The ability of the muscle to meet energy demands declines linearly with age. It is well known that aging is associated with a progressive decline in physical work capacity. Maximal oxygen uptake (liter/minute VO_2 maximum) shows a steady decline with age and with disuse or in gravity-elimated situations. The decline in maximal VO_2 with age is related to cardiovascular, respiratory, and peripheral skeletal muscle changes.

The effect of age on the oxidative rate of heart and skeletal muscle mitochondria appears to be substrate dependent. The cardiovascular system loses some efficiency with age. The consequence of this is that various proteins are not delivered to the muscle tissue in the same quantity as in the young. Glycoproteins, the small molecules that produce an osmotic force and are important in maintaining fluid content of tissues, decrease in quantity with aging, which makes it increasingly difficult for tissues to retain their normal fluid content.

Chemically, the greatest change is a decrease in the efficiency of the selectively permeable membrane found in muscle cells.[75] Potassium, magnesium, and phosphate ions are normally in high concentration in the sarcoplasm, but, other materials, such as sodium, chloride, and bicarbonate ions, are prevented from entering the cell under resting conditions. A characteristic feature of senescent muscle is a shift from this pattern. In particular, the concentration of potassium is reduced. There is a paucity of potassium ions in aging muscle, which reduces the maximum force of contraction that the muscle is capable of generating. Often, complaints of tiredness and lethargy in the clinic setting are a result of decreased potassium. Exercise in someone with potassium depletion will only fatigue them more, so it is important to check electrolytes.

Functional Changes

The loss of muscle function is not an inevitable consequence of age, but rather a result of an age-related decrease in activity. The mechanisms underlying impaired motor performance in old age are complex and involve the central and peripheral nervous systems and the muscle tissue itself. It is widely accepted that the age-related loss of muscle mass, strength, and quality has a significant detrimental impact on motor performance in old age and on the ability to recover from falls, resulting in an increased risk of fractures and dependency.[78] Therefore, the prevention of falls and gait instability is a very important safety issue, and different intervention strategies have been used to improve motor performance among the aging population. There is general consensus that physical exercise is a powerful intervention to obtain long-term benefits on muscle function, reduce the frequency of falls, and to maintain independence and a high quality of life in older persons.[79,80,81] The results from studies using different types of hormone supplementation therapies, which are discussed in a subsequent section of this chapter, have shown interesting and encouraging effects on skeletal muscle mass and function. However, the potential risks with both growth hormone and androgen treatment are not fully known and long-term clinical trials are needed to address safety concerns and the effects on skeletal muscle. Recent advancement in cellular/molecular, physiological, and molecular biological techniques will significantly facilitate our understanding of age-related impairments of muscle function and contribute to the evaluation of different intervention strategies.[78] From a rehabilitation perspective, there is no medical intervention for maintaining muscle strength and function that can substitute for activity and exercise.

Sarcopenia is the loss of muscle mass and strength that occurs with aging. It is a consequence of normal aging, and not necessarily related to disease, although muscle loss can be accelerated by chronic illness. Muscle wasting occurs in all humans, although it usually goes unnoticed. Sarcopenia results in muscle weakness, reduced activity level, increased prevalence of falls, morbidity, and loss of functional autonomy. It is the major cause of disability and frailty in the elderly.[79] There are many candidate mechanisms leading to sarcopenia, including age-related declines in alpha-motor neurons, growth hormone production, sex steroid levels, and physical activity. Age-related decreases in growth hormone, insulin-like growth factor I and II, estrogen, testosterone, and dehydroepiandrosterone and its sulfates play a major role in sarcopenia.[80,81] In addition, fat gain, increased catabolic cytokines, and inadequate intake of dietary energy and protein are also potentially important causes of sarcopenia. The relative contribution of each of these factors is not yet clear. Sarcopenia can be reversed with high-intensity progressive resistive exercise, which can also slow its development. A major challenge in preventing an epidemic of sarcopenia-induced frailty in the future is developing public health screening and interventions that deliver an anabolic stimulus to the muscle of elderly adults.

SKELETAL CHANGES WITH AGE

The skeletal system functions to support, protect, and shape the body. Additionally, bone has the metabolic functions of blood cell production, the storage of calcium and a role in acid-base balance.

The most commonly known age-related change involving bone is calcium-related loss of mass and density. This loss ultimately causes the pathological condition of osteoporosis, in which bone density is lost from within by a process termed reabsorption. As we grow older, an imbalance occurs between osteoblast activity (bone build up) and osteoclast activity (the breakdown of bone). Osteoclast activity proves to be the stronger. As one ages, a decline in circulating levels of activated vitamin D_3 occurs.[82] This causes less calcium to be absorbed from the gut and more calcium to be absorbed from the bones to meet body needs. In postmenopausal women, decreased estrogren levels influence parathyroid hormone and calcitonin to increase bone reabsorption which in turn decreases bone mass. Certain factors such as immobility, decreased estrogens and progesterones, steroid therapy, and hyperthyroidism, to name a few, are known to accelerate bone erosion to pathological levels. Easily occuring fractures are the most common result.[7,36]

Osteoporosis is a critical disorder in the older adult, because it decreases the bone mineral content and, as a result, bone mass and strength decline with age. It is difficult to draw the line between what is normal and what is pathological in osteoporosis. Bone loss appears to be a normal aging process and has been characterized by a decreased bone mineral composition, an enlarged medullary cavity, a normal mineral composition, and biochemical normalities in plasma and urine. The rate of bone loss is about 1% per year for women starting at age 30 to 35 and for men at age 50 to 55. In elderly subjects, regions of devitalized tissue with osteocyte lacunae and haversian canals containing amorphous mineral deposits have been described.[7] These have been identified as micropetrotic regions and are noted to increase in frequency in the skeleton with age. Thus, it is clear that the mineral content of bone qualitatively changes with age.

Qualitatively, osteoporotic bone exhibits a reduction in bone mass with a resulting decrease in bone strength, and there is some evidence that alterations occur in the composition and structure of bone in the aged. Tensile strength of bone in man is related to the number and size of osteons. It has been found that bone from older humans has smaller osteons and fragments and more cement lines than younger bone, and this would account for some of the reduced bone strength of the older bone specimens. The remaining difference in strength results from the geometric structure of the bone in its distribution per unit area as a response to environmental stress placed upon the bone. A more comprehensive discussion of osteoporosis is in the subsequent Chapter 5, Pathological Manifestations of Aging and in Chapter 11, Orthopedic Treatment Considerations.

Throughout life, red blood cells continue to be replaced after a life span of about 120 days. Some morphological changes do occur with aging. For instance, red cells are slightly smaller and more fragile; however, blood volume is well maintained until approximately 80 years of age. In the absence of pathology, few changes are seen in the white blood cells and in the platelet count. What is lost with aging is the functional reserve to quickly accelerate the production of red blood cells when needed.[7,83]

NEUROMUSCULAR CHANGES WITH AGE

Quantitatively, all muscle measures including biological, anatomical, and physiological, decline after the age of 40.[84] Many of the changes associated with aging indicate a decrease in the number of active functional units (e.g., motor units or muscle fibers) and a loss in concentration of specific enzymes or fiber types.

CENTRAL NEUROLOGICAL CHANGES WITH AGE

After peaking in the early decades of life, brain mass or weight slowly decreases by as much as 6% to 7% by the time a person reaches 80 years old. Though the brain stem appears to be minimally affected by cell loss, widely varied but significant losses occur in the cerebral cortex lobes and cerebellar area. Central nervous system cells are postmitotic. The central neurons that remain continue to decline in numbers and efficiency of function.

Cell number and composition both decrease, and with aging, cells of the hippocampus undergo a degeneration caused by numbers of vacuoles surrounding dense central granules. Amyloid plaques develop, and lipofuscin is deposited within many remaining neuronal cells. After age 60, the number of neuronal microtubular structures may decrease and are often replaced by so-called neurofibrillary tangles. Though plaques and tangles occur with normal aging, they are most commonly associated with the occurrence of senile dementia of the Alzheimer's type (SDAT).

Impulse conduction and cerebral synaptic transmission are both delayed with aging, which affects the transmitter competence of the central nervous system. A particular explanation lies in the general decline of available neurotransmitters. Serotonin, catecholamines, and gamma-aminobutynic acid (GABA) are less prevalent in the older brain. A decrease in the neurotransmitter dopamine is found in normal elderly but is also associated with the pathology of Parkinson's disease.[85]

Conduction velocity of the central nervous system has been shown to decrease with advancing age. A loss of the myelin sheath and a loss of large myelinated fibers decreases axion abilities to transmit impulses, especially in the posterior spinal column tracts. These tracts provide for reflex positive-righting responses. Remembering that balance impairment partially results from cerebellar losses, and now coupled with central nervous system delays, one can begin to see why an older person has a greater tendency to fall and less ability to quickly correct a center of balance before injury occurs.[86]

INTERSYSTEM HOMEOSTASIS

Thermal Regulation

The role of the hypothalamus in homeostatic regulation is a major factor in age-related declines. With increasing age, the hypothalamus becomes less sensitive to the physiological feedback and consequently is less able to maintain the stability of the internal environment of the body. Processes ensue, such as increased body weight, increased serum cholesterol, and decreased glucose tolerance, followed subsequently by diseases.[87] The hypothalamic thermostat is the principle control center for regulating the body's response to ambient, locally applied, and internal temperature gradients. Many investigators have attributed the increased rate of heat stroke, hypothermia, and climate-related deaths among the aged population to faulty thermoregulation.[88]

Not only the hypothalamic thermostat and basal metabolic rate, but also the overall reactivity of the autonomic nervous system, declines with age, altering skin hydration and circulation in turn.[89] The vasomotor system is less responsive to warming and cooling, and the normal transient bursts of vasoconstrictor activity are reduced. It is unclear whether or not thermoreceptors in the skin are altered. Because cold receptors are dependent on a good oxygen supply, it may be reasoned that decreased circulatory supply may decrease perception of cold because of the vulnerability of cold receptors to hypoxia.

Age-related changes in the thermal regulatory response have clinical significance in the elderly individual's ability to maintain homeostasis with increasing exercise levels; the cooling time following exercise is often prolonged. In addition, a decrease in the receptiveness of temperature gradients impacts the application of heat and cold modalities in treatment interventions. Consideration of these changes needs to be employed when treating the elderly patient.

Hormonal Balance

Aging is marked by a deterioration not only in the function of individual cells and organs, but also by a failure of mechanisms for the coordination of function between various parts of the body. A weakening of both neural and hormonal controls reduces the ability to adjust to external and internal stresses. Among other responsibilities, hormones contribute to (1) the regulation of circulating fluid volumes and cardiovascular performance, (2) the mobilization of fuels for exercise (maintenance of blood glucose, liberation of fat, and breakdown of protein), and (3) the repair of body structures with the synthesis of new protein (anabolism). All of the changes in these functions affect exercise tolerance and the healing process in the elderly. The aged are slower to reach homeostasis during exercise, and the return to a balanced homeostatic state following exercise is prolonged. In addition, the healing process is slower due to diminished synthesis of new protein.

Adrenocorticotropic hormone (ACTH) is produced within the cell body of the neuron in a small number of neurons in the central nervous system. Liberation of ACTH from the axon terminals of these neurons produces different effects on different groups of postsynaptic cells. A number of other peptide transmitter substances that have been identified as well as ACTH are produced outside the nervous system by cells of the endocrine system. When produced by endocrine cells, these substances are termed hormones.

At neuron-to-neuron connections, the transmitter molecules are produced in moderate amounts and will be released from the presynaptic cell only through the axon terminals. The small amount of transmitter substance liberated from the terminal is rapidly deactivated at the release site. The effect of release of neurotransmitters is limited to a very localized area for only a short period of time.

Movement of molecules between capillaries and extracellular spaces in the central nervous system is more difficult than in other tissues. Nerve cells have become more sensitive than other types of cells to their immediate chemical environment to facilitate a variety of specific transmitter mechanisms.

The capillary wall thickening is achieved partly by a thickening of the basement membrane of the epithelial cells that form the capillary wall and partly as the result of glial cell activity. The glial cells are tissue cells responsible for producing the connective tissue—packing material for the nerve cells and their fibers. The protein glial membranes that are produced contain finer fibers than those in other connective tissues. The presence of a glial membrane around the small blood vessels and capillaries in the brain produces the so-called blood-brain barrier. While all neuron-to-neuron connections in the brain are protected by the blood-brain barrier, some nerve connections are made with cells outside the nervous system, and these connections form the neuroendocrine system. Connec-

tions from the hypothalamus to the posterior lobe of the pituitary gland belong to this system. Normally, the activity of many endocrine glands is finely balanced and highly coordinated, but in the elderly the coordination is increasingly disrupted.

Much of this disruption is the result of the body's reaction to increasing stress. When a person is exposed to stress, whether physical, emotional, or sociological, changes take place in the body in an attempt to deal with the stress. Many of these changes involve a shift away from the normal endocrine balance. Aging can be a period of chronic and increasing stress, and as a result, the body's defense mechanisms may be unable to cope.

Circulation

A blood flow rate of approximately 40mL/min/ 100 grams of brain tissue is regarded as minimally necessary to maintain adequate cerebral perfusion. As compared to the flow rate of 50–60mL/min/g experienced with youth, an older person may have as much as a 20% reduction in cerebral perfusion by the age of 70. Though cerebral perfusion is adequate if the body is not challenged, in the presence of pathology (e.g., arteriosclerosis, decreased cardiac output), the elderly experience increased risk of cerebral damage.[7]

PERIPHERAL NEUROLOGICAL CHANGES WITH AGE

Aging is often characterized by reduced sensibility, coordination, and cognitive abilities, as well as a reduced ability to react to changing circumstances. A general assumption is made that the loss of nerve tissue (i.e., reduced cell number) is a predominant feature of aging. In reality, although some loss of nerve cells does take place during the aging process, the extent to which this loss occurs is less than usually assumed. The reduced level of nervous system functioning in the elderly is better explained in terms of biochemical changes that take place in neurons during aging and senescence.

Granules of lipofuscin accumulate in the cell bodies of neurons as a function of age, changing the cellular composition. Traditionally, this has been regarded as resulting from wear and tear processes in those cells with high oxidative activity (see the free radical theory of aging in Chapter 2). Lipofuscin appears to be formed from lysosomal material within the cell. There is no evidence to support the notion that the presence of lipofuscin granules within the cytoplasm will have a detrimental influence on the normal functioning of the cell. Indeed, one of the heaviest accumulations of lipofuscin occurs in the inferior olivary nucleus, which appears to function normally and from which no neurons are lost in senescence.

Other changes in cellular composition have been reported. Alterations in the Golgi's complex, the reduction in ribosome concentration in the endoplasmic reticulum, and the lowered fluid content of the cells are not restricted to nerve cells but are generalized characteristics of degenerating and senescent cells of all types.

In the resting state, the interior of the nerve cell and its processes are rich in potassium ions and low in sodium ions, whereas outside the cell the concentration of these ions is reversed. Because of this unequal distribution of ions, together with the fact that the membrane in its resting state is much more permeable to potassium than sodium ions, the nerve has a resting potential of approximately 70mV, the outside being electrically positive with respect to the interior. A nerve impulse is created by the temporary depolarization of the nerve membrane. Channels in the membrane open up to allow the flow of sodium ions into the cell, and a second set of channels allows the outward flow of potassium ions from the cell after a slight delay. A wave of depolarization is conducted over the whole surface of the neuron from the point at which it was initially generated. In myelinated nerve fibers, the nerve impulse jumps quickly from one node of Ranvier to the next. The conduction velocity of nerve impulses along myelinated fibers is up to twenty-five times greater than along unmyelinated fibers of similar diameter. Peripheral nerve conduction velocity shows a progressive decline with aging.

The ionic exchange across the nerve membrane to produce a nerve impulse is a relatively simple mechanism that is altered little during the aging process. In the elderly, there is no significant change in the conduction velocity along a specified portion of a nerve trunk compared to that found in younger adults. In the elderly, as in the younger person, if a reduction in conduction velocity is found, some narrowing of the fiber affecting the integrity of the nerve or some impairment of blood flow to the nerve sheath may be assumed.[75]

SENSORY CHANGES WITH AGE

In the body, information is gathered, interpreted, and transmitted through the integration of the neurosensory system, which includes the nervous system and each of the five senses (touch, smell, taste, vision, and hearing). Each of these systems is highly complex, and structural changes are known to occur with aging. The sum total of these changes results in a decline of neurosensory function.[90]

Touch

Peripheral receptors are responsible for the sense of touch. As with the other senses, touch also declines with age. Specific receptors for touch, pressure, pain, and temperature are found within the dermis and epidermis of the skin. Receptors can be freestanding or arranged in small corpuscular masses. Meissner's cor-

puscles (touch-texture receptors), Pacinian's corpuscles (pressure-vibration receptors), and Krause's corpuscles (temperature receptors), as well as peripheral nerve fibers, are noted to decline; therefore, sensitivity to touch, temperature, and vibration frequently decline with age. Though quantitative studies have produced inconclusive results, since free nerve endings remain relatively unchanged, the ability to sense pain should remain intact; however, the elderly person must take special care to avoid injury from concentrated pressures or temperature on the skin.[42,52] (e.g., pressures from shoes that are too tight, bath water that is too hot, and so forth).

The skin is a very important element in touch. In general, skin wrinkles increase with advancing age, but the directional change of epidermal thickness remains controversial. The dermis becomes thinner, loses elasticity, and has a diminished vascularity.[90] Loss of tissue support for remaining capillaries results in fragility and easy bruising (senile purpura). Though tanning response diminishes, the appearance of flat pigmented lentigos (age spots) increases with exposure to the sun, and such exposure also increases the risk of neoplastic development from actinic keratosis. The previously reviewed decline in cellular division results in a slower rate and efficiency of tissue repair following any trauma.[62]

Changes in the dermal appendages (i.e., hair) also occurs with age. The degree to which hair becomes gray is largely genetically determined, but in general, a reduction in hair follicles produces a reduction of hair. In contrast, after menopause, facial hair tends to increase in women. Nails grow more slowly and develop longitudinal ridges. The number and size of sweat glands is diminished, resulting in a reduction of sweat production.[62]

Health care providers need to be sensitive to the fact that some of the following changes may effect the self-esteem of an older person. If this is the case, sensitive psychological support must be provided in any interactions.

Vision

Though humans are strongly visual creatures, the eye is vulnerable to many age-related changes. Externally, the eyelids show an increase in wrinkling and in ptosis resulting from losses of elastic tissue and orbital fat, and a decrease in muscle tone. Very often the older person will develop an entropion (a turning inward of the eyelid) or an ectropian (an outward relaxation of the eyelid), which is particularly apparent with the lower lids. Aging results in diminished tear production, and ocular inflammation or infection may occur in some elderly people if supplementary artificial tears are not provided.

Arcus Senilis, a deposit of lipids around the outer edge of the cornea, is a well-known, age-related phenomenon which does not interfer with vision. Arcus senilis has been associated with hyperlipidemia in younger people, however, no such association has been shown in the elderly.

In addition to becoming smaller with age, the ocular pupil reacts more slowly to light, and the ability to focus quickly from far-to-near declines. This loss of accommodation is termed presbyopia. The ability to focus is dependent on the ability of the ocular lens to change shape as needed. Presbyopia is partially caused by a decline in ciliary muscle efficiency, however, as a person ages, the ocular lens continues to grow while becoming more dense and inelastic. This change is associated with chronic dehydration of the tissues. Increased stiffness and less flexibility results in a decrease in the ability to change shapes and to focus on desired objects. Far vision is more easily achieved because the ciliary muscles relax and allow the lens to thin. Near vision requires the ciliary muscles to contract, increasing the thickness of the lens. This is why older people may require bifocals, which offer one prescription for far vision and another, stronger one for reading or close vision. Along with reduced accommodation, older people experience a decreased ability to adapt comfortably and quickly to changes of light and dark. Many older people say they had to give up driving at night because of this age-related change.

The older eye demonstrates a tendency toward increased intraocular pressure. As the lens continues to grow into the anterior chamber of the eye, the chamber becomes smaller, and the circulation of aqueous humor is reduced. Though the healthy older eye can tolerate this change, it is possible for a pathologic glaucoma to occur concurrently. The increased density of the lens may lead to a form of cataract which can result in the complete loss of useful vision. On a less serious note, the aqueous humor may also develop a yellowish pigmentation creating difficulty in distinguishing between greens and blues.

An older person may comment to you on the presence of "floaters" in their visual fields. With aging, the vitreous body of the eye loses hydration and tends to demonstrate some clustering of collagen material. This clustering cause shadows or opacities to be projected on the retinal wall. Though the presence of these opacities is normally associated with dehydration, an increase in number and frequency of episodes can be indicative of retinal hemorrhage or detachment.

Age-related changes can ultimately produce a decline in visual acuity. Even when errors of aged refraction are corrected, a loss of visual receptors in the aging retina or macula will result in a decrease of acuity. Although there are some treatments, there is no cure. Fortunately, with modern technology, the majority of older people are able to maintain a high degree of visual function and independence.[91,92]

Hearing

Though a hearing loss may develop at any age, hearing losses do occur more frequently in the later years.

A "sensorineural" hearing loss, called presbycusis, is most common in the elderly. With a sensorineural loss, sound is well conducted through the external and middle ear but age-related impairments of the inner ear or auditory nerve prevent the sound transmission to the brain. Age-related changes that may contribute to a sensorineural hearing loss include sclerotic changes in the tympanic membrane, cochlear otosclerosis, a loss of hair-like receptors in the organ of Corti, and a degeneration of the auditory nerve.

Presbycusis results in a decreased ability to hear and discriminate speech, particularly at higher and lower frequency levels. Because normal speech contains a broad range of frequencies, the older person may realize that he is being spoken to but may not understand all that is being said. The individual loses the ability to hear the "hard" sounds of language (e.g., the beginning and ending of most words). Difficulties increase when the speaker talks too quickly or when the hearing impaired individual is unable to observe the speaker's face.

Contrary to common belief, a sensorineural hearing loss does not always preclude the use of a hearing aid. Vision should be corrected so the skill of visual speech conception can be used as much as possible. When speaking with an elder with sensorineural loss, words should be spoken slowly in a medium pitched voice, and face-to-face communication should always be maintained.

Proprioception/Kinesthesia

Proprioception or kinesthetic sense is provided by sensory nerves which give information concerning movements and position of the body. These receptors are located primarily in the muscles, tendons, and the labyrinth system.[7] Though a greater degree of sensory-perceptual loss results from local system changes (e.g., impaired vision from increased lens density), cerebral cortex cell loss may result in less cellular availability for sensory interpretation.[93] This is of great clinical importance in that, as one ages, there may be a concomitant loss of position and movement sense. Coupled with losses in the other sensory systems, this could significantly affect an elderly individual's awareness of limb or body position, a safety concern during transfers and ambulation (see Chapter 12, Neurological Treatment Considerations).

Vestibular System

The vestibular system changes during the aging process. Degeneration occurs in the sensory receptors in both the otoliths and semicircular canals. The function of the vestibular system is to monitor head position and to detect head movements.[93] When an individual is deprived of visual and lower extremity somatosensory information, the vestibular system is left to provide sensation for control of balance. Healthy young adults are able to balance without meaningful visual or support surface information. Healthy elderly, on the other hand, lose their balance and might even fall when vestibular input is the only spatial orientation information available. All of the major sources of orienting information are compromised during the aging process. Dehydration and diseases further compound this problem. The vestibular system is discussed in more detail in Chapter 12, Neurological Treatment Considerations.

Taste and Smell

The senses of taste and smell become less acute with age.[94] As many as 80% of the taste buds may atrophy and perception of taste sensation (i.e., sweet, salty, bitter, and sour) becomes less sharp. A reduction of saliva flow occurs as a person ages, and this may aggravate an already dulled sense of taste. The olfactory bulb demonstrates age-related cell losses which appear to be associated with decreased perceptions of various smells. It is proposed that the dulling of these sensations contributes to the appetite decline which is observed in and experienced by the majority of elderly people.[62]

Deficits in these chemical senses not only reduce the pleasure and comfort of food, but also represent risk factors for nutritional and immune deficiencies, as well as adherence to specific dietary regimens. Chemosensory decrements can lead to food poisoning or overexposure to environmentally hazardous chemicals that are otherwise detectable by taste and smell.[94]

GASTROINTESTINAL CHANGES WITH AGE

The gastrointestinal tract is subject to many changes throughout life. Though normal aging is not responsible for all gastrointestinal changes, it is sometimes difficult to differentiate the effects of aging from those that result from a lifetime of poor habits involving hygiene, food, and substance abuse. Epidemiological studies are beginning to implicate lifestyle more strongly in relation to some changes in the gut.

It is a fallacy to believe that teeth must be lost with aging. Improved dental hygiene and nutrition can prevent common pathologies of tooth loss such as dental caries and peridontal disease. With age, however, the tooth does lose masticating enameled surface area. Intermaxillary spaces decrease, and tooth pulp may atrophy and regress. If teeth are lost, the older person may experience a migration of the normally opposing teeth, with local oral trauma occurring as a result.[95]

The older esophagus demonstrates a reduction of motility and a hesitance of the lower esophageal sphincter to relax with swallowing. To define these changes, the term presbyesophagus was coined.[96]

When eating, the older person may experience an often uncomfortable substernal sense of fullness as food entry into the stomach is delayed. In contrast, the lower esophageal resting pressure declines with age. This weakening allows gastric contents to more easily reflux into the lower areas of the esophagus causing heartburn to occur. Hiatal hernias frequently develop in the older person who has a reduced resting pressure of the lower esophageal sphincter.[97]

An age-related reduction in motility also affects the stomach, colon, and probably the small intestine. Gastric emptying time often is delayed.[98] Degeneration of gastric mucosa occurs in a small number of elderly and may cause a decrease of intrinsic factor, digestive enzymes, and hydochloric acid. Usually this "atrophic gastritis" is not the sole cause of B_{12} malabsorption and resulting pernicious anemia, but gastrointestinal digestion can be reduced. Medications activated by an acid gastric condition may be less effective in the more alkaline environment of an older stomach. Additionally, an older individual may interpret this gastric discomfort as acid indigestion and further diminish the available acid supply by taking over-the-counter antacids.

A reduced blood supply to the gut and a decrease in the number of absorbing cells can hinder nutrient absorption in the small intestine. Decreased motility in the colon and poor hydration causes the elderly to have a tendency to develop constipation. If the elderly person is particularly immobile or dehydrated, constipation can easily lead into the more serious conditions of fecal impaction and bowel obstruction. Diverticulosis is also common in the elderly. However, its occurrence is probably more related to a diet low in fiber and high in refined, low-residue foods than to aging.[7,97,99]

More on the gastrointestinal changes with aging will be covered in the Chapter 7, Exploring Nutritional Needs.

RENAL, UROGENITAL, AND HEPATIC CHANGES

It is generally accepted that liver mass and blood perfusion both decline with aging. Metabolism of many drugs is decreased and, following injury, regeneration of hepatic cells occurs more slowly. When compared to younger people, no significant differences are found in the serum indicators of liver status of older people. These indicators include measurement of bilirubin clearance, serum glutamic oxaloacetic transaminase (SGOT), serum glutamic pyruvic transaminae (SGPT), and alkaline phosphatase production. Though total serum protein remains relatively stable, reduced albumin to globulin (A/G) ratios result in a decline of colloidal osmotic pressure. Protein binding of medications may also be decreased. Alterations in protein binding and the prolongation of drug effects within the body are two of the more serious results of normal age changes in the liver.[7,12,100]

When discussing these systems, the gallbladder and pancreas should be mentioned, because they also demonstrate functional changes with aging. For example, the incidence of biliary stones increases in the elderly, which is probably related to a reduced efficiency of cholesterol stabilization in the body. Controversy exists over the reduction of pancreatic mass with age. A decline in mass may be hidden by an increase in pancreatic fat deposition. Pancreatic cells become less homogeneous, and studies have generally reported a decline in enzyme volume and concentration, though adequate amounts are available for normal digestive functions.[12,62] Another important endocrine age change is the decreased ability of the peripheral tissues to utilize available insulin produced by the pancreas.[101] The most important pancreatic age change, however, is the decreased ability of the beta cells to increase insulin production in response to a challenge of increased blood glucose.[12,100]

The aged kidney demonstrates both a loss of parenchymal mass and a reduction of total weight. By the time a person is 85 years old, the amount of remaining functioning nephrons may be decreased by as much as 30% to 40% of what was available in youth. Vascular changes, like a reduction in glomerular capillary loops and increased tortuosity of arcuate and interlobar arteries, have been reported. Renal perfusion declines as much as 50% by the later decades of life. The Bowman's capsule basement membrane thickens, glomerular filtration rate declines, and blood urea nitrogen (BUN) tends to show a rise. The renal tubules show a decline in excretory and reabsorptive capacities, and a loss of urine concentrating abilities occurs. Older kidneys can maintain acid-base homeostasis in an unchallenged environment; however, they are unable to handle increased loads of either acid or base. The structural changes observed in the normal aging kidney support the theory that one should expect a decline in renal function as one ages. Reports by renal physiologists, however, suggest that this is not always true.[102] The suggestion is made that vascular adaptations to structural changes may help to preserve glomerular filtration rate by producing a state of hyperperfusion and hyperfiltration in surviving nephrons.[102]

The urinary bladder demonstrates an increased number of uninhibited contractions frequently associated with cerebral arteriosclerotic changes and overconcentration of the urine. Increases in residual urine and reflux into the ureters provide an ideal environment for bacterial growth. Both asymptomatic and symptomatic bacteriuria is common in the elderly.[7,101,103]

ENDOCRINE CHANGES WITH AGE

Most aging individuals die from atherosclerosis, cancer, or dementia; but in the oldest old, loss of muscle strength resulting in frailty is the limiting factor for an individual's chances of living an independent life until death. Three hormonal systems show decreasing circulating hormone concentrations during normal aging: (1) estrogen in *menopause* and testosterone in *andropause*, (2) dehydroepiandrosterone and its suphate in *adrenopause*, and (3) the growth hormone/insulin-like growth factor I axis in *somatopause*. Physical changes during aging have been considered physiologic, but there is evidence that some of these changes are related to this decline in hormonal activity.[104] Hormone replacement strategies have been developed, but many of their aspects remain controversial, and increasing blood hormone levels in aging individuals to the levels of those of mid-adult life has not been uniformly proven safe or beneficial.[104]

Proper functioning of the endocrine system is essential to maintain the majority of the body's regulatory processes. In some cases (e.g., reproductive hormones), age-related changes are well known. In other cases, specific information is nonexistent or unclear. Much available information remains highly controversial.

Although age-related structural changes in the thyroid do occur, in the absence of pathology its function tends to remain adequate for body needs. A decrease in the basal metabolic rate (BMR) is shown in elderly people but seems related to the reduction of lean body mass. The elderly are at risk for both hypo- and hyperthyroid problems. However, these problems are unrelated to changes that occur with normal aging.[7,62,105]

Tests of adrenal function show plasma glucocorticoid levels to be similar in the young and old. The adrenal cortex response to adrenocorticotropic hormone (ACTH) remains intact, as does the pituitary's release of ACTH in response to stress; however, circulating levels of aldosterone do decrease with aging.[7]

The pituitary gland demonstrates a reduction in vascularity and an increase in deposition of connective tissue.[7] A reduction in mass is not well established. With aging, nocturnal elevations in growth hormone (GH) disappear. Serum concentrations of ACTH and GH are unchanged with aging,[12] and in most elderly, thyroid stimulating hormone (TSH) remains normal, although a small percentage develop a slight increase in TSH without obvious symptoms.[106] Postmenopausal women show an increase in the follicle stimulating hormone (FSH) and luteinizing hormone (LH).

Changes in reproductive hormones are most dramatic in the older woman. Following menopause, estrogen and progesterone levels significantly decrease, but serum androgen levels remain relatively unchanged. In the older man, blood levels of testosterone probably decrease, but the controversy over this decline has not yet been resolved.[62]

The uterus, ovaries, and fallopian tubes of the elderly woman become dysfunctional with menopause and decrease in size. A reduction in estrogen causes the vagina to shrink, thin, and lose mucosal protection. The breasts, labia, and clitoris all lose subcutaneous mass, and in advanced years, pubic hair is lost. In contrast, an elderly man will continue to produce sperm throughout his life. However, sperm production and counts are reduced, and spermal abnormalities are increased. The testes may demonstrate very little loss of weight but fibrous tissue deposition increases in the intertubular spaces. With age, the seminiferous tubules basement membrane thickens. Age changes in the prostate begin around age 40 and continue into the elder years. The most disruptive change involves the replacement of smooth prostatic tissue by dense connective tissue. As the connective tissue accumulates, resulting prostatic hypertrophy impinges upon the urethra and interferes with smooth release of urine.[7]

The endocrine system plays a major role in the biologic variability of aging. The remarkable variability in the physical status of the healthy aging population and in the progression of aging-related diseases, such as sarcopenia, osteopenia, and cognitive disorders, may reflect, in part, the natural polymorphisms of key catabolic and/or anabolic gene products. For example, molecular diversity in the glucocorticoid receptor may influence the relative effects of cortisol excess on tissue catabolism. Conversely, polymorphisms of the insulin-like growth factor I (IGF-I) receptor could be relevant in mediating interindividual differences in tissue atrophy in aging.[104]

Neuroendocrine rhythms are altered with aging. For example, although the role of melatonin in human aging is not known, the peak nighttime release of melatonin decreases by approximately 50% with aging. Other CNS timekeeping centers, such as the suprachiasmatic nuclei (SCN), show aging-dependent alterations, as reflected in changing 24-hour rhythms of GH, prolactin, cortisol, TSH, FSH, and LH. For example, over the age range of 18 to 80 years in humans, the secretion of cortisol, which is driven by ACTH, progressively exhibits an earlier maximum (phase advance), a higher late-day nadir, and a smaller variation in secretion over 24 hours.[107] In contrast, the 24-hour periodicity of cortisol secretion remains stable across the life span.[108] With aging, there is a blunting of the presleep peak of TSH. Levels of GH manifest a global (day and night) suppression of amplitude with aging.[107–109]

Neurophysiologic outcomes, such as circadian temperature rhythms, tend to show phase advance and amplitude suppression with aging. Extended daylong and inter-diem monitoring of cardiovascular indices may identify patients at higher risk for arrhythmia or myocardial infarction. Knowledge of circadian rhythms has resulted in the development of chronopharmacotherapy, or timed drug delivery based on the circadian cycle of the older person, in an effort to obviate drug toxicity and enhance medication efficacy.[110]

At least 17% of individuals aged 80 or older will develop type II diabetes mellitus.[111] Adults with low insulin sensitivity (i.e., relative insulin resistance) and reduced glucose effectiveness (i.e., insulin-dependent glucose removal rate) have approximately an 80% risk of developing type II diabetes mellitus over a period of 25 years.[111] In healthy aging individuals, there is a progressive increase in fasting and especially in postprandial plasma glucose levels.[112] As we age, insulin secretion decreases to a variable degree and becomes disorderly.[113] Concomitantly, there is a progressive increase in peripheral resistance to insulin action.[114] In healthy individuals, the aging of the enteroinsular axis shows remarkable between-subject heterogeneity; the underlying basis for this is not completely understood. For example, how the aging-related diabetogenic tendency is related to the age-related increase in visceral obesity is not known. In addition, there are few studies with data to substantiate how well glycosylated hemoglobin levels in healthy aging individuals predict later development of clinical diabetes mellitus.[115]

Biochemically, insulin activates receptor-dependent autophosphorylation as well as phosphorylation of tyrosine residues of multiple insulin-receptor substrates (IRS-1, IRS-2), and multiple isoforms of phosphatidylinositol-3 (PI-3) kinase. Further divergence of these signaling pathways imposes selective control of cellular glucose metabolism, protein and lipid turnover, cell replication and hypertrophy, and gene expression.[115] The use of transgenic mouse signaling gene-knockout models in aging mice have identified a new multiplicity of possible molecular defects associated with aging, in type II diabetes mellitus as well as plausible loci of targeted drug interventions. For example, experimentally disabling the IRS-1 or IRS-2 genes promotes tissue insulin resistance and causes variable intrauterine growth retardation.[116] Although unproven, the pathogenetic sequence that culminates in type II diabetes could be driven by an ensemble of single-allele molecular polymorphisms, which cause progressive insulin resistance in muscle, liver, fat; systemic hyperinsulinemia; and eventual beta-cell failure as the species ages.

Genetic studies discussed in Chapter 2, Theories of Aging further explain this hypothesis. For example, tissue-specific disruption of the muscle insulin receptor promotes visceral fat accumulation and hypertriglyceridemia without producing overt type II diabetes mellitus.[117] Body mass index increases and visceral fat accumulates with age until early senescence, as previously discussed. Levels of the nutritional signaling peptide leptin, mostly produced in white adipose tissue, convey signals to the hypothalamus about fat stores and, in response, hypothalamic efferents regulate food intake and energy expenditure. Leptin inhibits the hypothalamic release of the orexigenic (appetite-inducing) peptide—neuropeptide Y (NPY)—and activates the sympathetic nervous system. In studies of older individuals, fasting suppresses circulating leptin concentrations and stimulates hypothalamic NPY secretion less effectively.

Thus, leptin-receptor signaling may be attenuated in aging causing a higher resistance to insulin.[118]

Menopause

The World Health Organization (WHO) has defined the perimenopausal period as the interval preceding cessation of menses through 1 year after the last bleeding cycle, which according to the findings of the Massachusetts Women's Health Study, is a mean span of about 3½ years. This period of time is termed the *climacteric* period. There is still no known biochemical signal that reliably indicates the onset of menopause. However, serum FSH levels tend to rise in regularly menstruating late-premenopausal women (42 to 50 years of age). The pulsatility and orderliness of LH release also change before menstrual cyclicity falters.[119] Estrogen secretion in the perimenopause is variable, and includes intervals of increased production. A greater stimulation by FSH may increase follicular aromatase activity and induce estrogen excess. Inhibin concentrations fall perimenopausally and contribute to heightened FSH release.[119]

Hot flushes may precede the onset of anovulatory cycles in the perimenopause. Physical complaints, such as breast tenderness, irregular menstrual bleeding, hot flushes, and dyspareunia; and emotional concerns, such as disrupted sleep, fatigue, tension, and irritability, are equally represented among menopausal women.[120] Some of the relevant physiologic effects of estrogen that ameliorate the consequences of menopause may be exerted via the ten or more membrane (nongenomic) binding sites for estradiol, which regulate ion flow and kinase signaling. In addition, the alpha and recently cloned beta isoforms of the estrogen reception mediate classical DNA-dependent interactions within the target cell. New designer estrogens, such as raloxifene (Evista), which act as selective estrogen-receptor modultors, may or may not confer the same neurobiologic effects of estrogen.[121] Increased activity levels (e.g., exercise) has been shown to positively influence circulating levels of estrogen. At a higher metabolic rate, dormant stores of estradiol (which are warehoused in adipose tissue), combine with cholesterol and are converted to an active estrogen (ß-17) compound. Therefore, increasing levels of activity result in a greater supply of available, and natural estrogen sources.[120]

There is a great deal of individual variation in reproductive aging in women. Even in identical (monozygotic) twins, there can be a 12- to 14-year discordance in the age of menopause, albeit 50% of twin pairs are concordant within 2 years. Thus, reproductive aging—even with identical genetic analgen—shows stochastic and/or environmental variability. For the female gonadal axis, this stochastic element could originate from the nonuniformity among individuals in rates of prenatal oocyte and follicle survival. This view highlights the importance of the ovarian oocyte reserve. Clinically, premature menopause holds significant implications for the development of age-associated diseases, such as cardiovascular disease and osteopenia.[120]

Females have a finite nonrenewable complement of oocytes. Hence, control of oocyte depletion is a critical determinant of the human female reproductive life span. A maximal oocyte population of seven million is estimated to exist at twenty weeks gestation. Two million persist until birth, and there are approximately 400,000 at the onset of puberty. Only approximately four-hundred oocytes are actually ovulated during a woman's reproductive years.[104] Understanding the mechanisms that regulate the attrition of oocytes is critical for developing strategies that extend the reproductive life span, intervene in premature ovarian failure, and preserve threatened gonadal function in patients undergoing cancer chemotherapy.

Andropause

Andropause describes the collection of symptoms associated with the age-related decline in gonadal function in men. In contrast to the rapid decline in ovarian function in women at menopause, men experience a gradual decline in testicular function and testosterone production. It is generally accepted that the decline in testosterone production is primarily testicular in origin. There is some evidence to suggest that the central component (i.e., alteration in the hypothalamic-pituitary-gonadal axis) may also have a role.[104] Stress, medications, obesity, malnutrition, and psychiatric conditions, all common in the elderly, tend to reduce testosterone production. However, decreased plasma testosterone levels are also found in healthy elderly individuals.

Reduced testosterone production in men with hypogonadism results in diminished muscular strength, energy, and libido, erectile dysfunction, depression, and osteoporosis and related fractures. Sexual dysfunction in the elderly male is primarily associated with erectile rather than ejaculatory dysfunction. The latter is more often drug-induced or associated with prostate surgery. In the hypogonadal male, reduced libido is often accompanied by diminished well-being and depression that may be relieved by androgen replacement.[122]

Like menopause, andropause is the deficiency in gonadal hormones. A myriad of physiological changes occur with aging, and hormonal levels at andropause may contribute to these. Cognitive decline, visceral obesity, osteopenia, and relative sarcopenia accompany androgen deficiency in aging. Males have a higher prevalence of atherosclerosis and a shorter life span than do women. The effect of testosterone on the serum lipid profile is thought to be one underlying cause of these gender-based differences.[123] Osteoporosis is another significant health problem in men. The rate of hip fracture increases dramatically after the age of 60 years in men and doubles with each decade thereafter. Hypogonadism is a well-established cause of male osteoporosis.[123] These conditions have been found to respond favorably to hormone replacement supplementation, especially in men with very low testosterone levels.[124] Enhanced physical performance has not been established in this context. Few studies have examined whether testosterone or progesterone (or estrogen) supplementation enhances cognitive function in elderly men, as estrogen replacement in women has been found to do.[125] However, in older men, many studies have found that androgen replacement increased the sense of well being, enhanced spatial cognition and had an antidepressent effect. [123] Although it appears that neoplastic transformation of prostate tissue is not elicited by physiologic testosterone repletion, proliferation of existing androgen-responsive carcinomas may be stimulated.

Testosterone supplementation may worsen sleep apnea, induce gynecomastia, elicit erythrocytosis, and elevate blood pressure.[124] Thus, the long-term safety of androgen replacement therapies in healthy adults requires further studies.

Prostate volume increases progressively with age in eugonadal men. Albeit androgen-dependent, this propensity is also modulated by unknown environmental and genetic factors. Estradiol, IGF-I, IGF-II, fibroblast, and keratinocyte growth factors act locally to promote prostate epithelial and stromal growth. The number of cytosine, adenine, and guanine (CAG) repeats in the androgen-receptor gene may also correlate with intense prostate growth.[126]

Adrenopause

Adrenarche is characterized by a prepubertal rise in adrenal secretion of DHEA and DHEA sulfate (DHEA-S) that is independent of the gonads or gonadotropins. Adrenopause is the corresponding diminution in DHEA and DHEA-S concentrations in later life.[127] The mechanisms by which adrenarche and adrenopause are induced and regulated are unknown. Early work focused on identifying hypothetical adrenal androgen regulatory hormones that would induce DHEA in much the same way the adrenocorticotropin induces cortisol, but no such factors have been found.

Replacement therapy with DHEA has been found to have a multitude of potentially beneficial effects, particularly in the presence of DHEA deficiency. Its primary action is to increase the availability of gonadal hormones via peripheral bioconversion of DHEA to androgens and estrogens. A daily dose of 50 mg DHEA has been shown to restore low endogenous serum DHEA concentrations to normal youthful levels followed by an increase in circulating androgens and estrogens.[128] Barnhart and associates[129] found that DHEA supplementation significantly affects the endocrine and lipid profiles, but does not improve perimenopausal symptoms.[129]

It has been hypothesized that DHEA prevents immunosenescence, and as a neuroactive steroid it may influence processes of cognition and memory.[130] Epidemiological studies revealed an inverse correlation between DHEA-S levels and the incidence of cardiovascular disease in men, but not in women. Arlt and colleagues[130] investigated the effects of 50 mg, 100 mg, and placebo doses of DHEA and found that 50 mg was a suitable dose in elderly men, as it leads to serum DHEA-S concentrations usually measured in young healthy adults. The DHEA-induced increase in circulating estrogens was found to have a beneficial effect on immunological measures as well as cognition and memory in men.[130]

Somatopause

The decline in the function of the growth hormone-releasing hormone, growth hormone, insulin-like growth factor (GHRH-GH-IGF) axis has been termed the somatopause. Many of the catabolic sequelae seen in normal aging has been attributed to this decrease in circulating GH and IGF-I.[131,132] Whereas numerous beneficial effects on body composition, strength, and quality of life have been reported in some studies, other studies have reported only marginal functional improvements.[131] Physiological control of GH secretion in adults can be enhanced and the symptoms of somatopause surpressed through exercise.[132,133]

Gender markedly influences GH secretion in young adults. Premenopausal women exhibit a twofold less rapid decline than men in daily GH production with increasing age. Young women also manifest less vulnerability to the suppressive effects of increased total body fat and reduced physical fitness on GH secretion.[134] Withdrawal of estrogen at menopause appears to eliminate much of this gender difference.

An important ongoing clinical issue relates to the uncertain role of sex hormone deficiency in the aging-related impoverishment of GH and IGF-I production in women and men.[135] Preliminary data from clinical studies raise the possibility that combined GH and androgen repletion in older men can have an additive effect on increasing muscle mass.[134] New data indicate that treatment with GH-releasing hormone can restore plasma IGF-I to levels found in young adults and is associated with little evident toxicity.[136–138] Body composition also improves; however, to date this treatment has not enhanced strength and physical aerobic capacity measures. Ongoing investigations are being conducted to evaluate the effects of combining GH, gonadal steroids, and GH secretagogues in older individuals. However, it appears that the relatively brief trials conducted thus far (e.g., six-months duration) may be inadequate to unveil the true spectrum of responses or the possible long-term effects.[139] New prospective interventions corroborate the dose-dependent restoration of plasma IGF-I concentrations by GH injections in older volunteers. Estrogen replacement in older women limits, but does not abolish, the ability of GH to stimulate IGF-I secretion. Treatment with GH consistently reduces visceral adiposity and increases muscle mass in men, though physical performance and maximal aerobic capacity most often do not change.[140]

SLEEP, MEMORY, AND INTELLIGENCE CHANGES

The phenomenon of sleep is not yet totally understood. Four progressively deeper levels of sleep plus an intermediate level associated with rapid eye movements (REM) are known to exist. Once asleep, a younger person seldom awakens, and the deeper sleep levels of three and four are maintained. In the elderly, consecutive sleep time is decreased, awakenings are more frequent, and less sleep time is spent in levels three and four, though total sleep time is normally only slightly reduced. Because of side effects (such as drowsiness and confusion), the use of sedatives should be discouraged in the aged. In most cases, actual sleep loss is minimal. Other therapeutic supports, such as increased daytime activity, exercise, and fewer naps, can be effective in relieving the elderly person's feelings of impaired nocturnal sleep.[12,141]

Aging causes deterioration in various aspects of memory performance in healthy adults.[142] The process of memory is difficult to separate from the total process of learning. After information is perceived, it is stored in either short- or long-term areas of memory. The elderly typically have more difficulty recalling recently experienced information. In order to be properly perceived, information needs to be presented to an older person at a slower rate and with an increased number of repetitions. If the information is presented in a manner that compensates for age-related sensory changes (decreased vision and hearing) and if the information is made to have some personal relevance to the older person, recall of the information is greatly improved.

Different diagnostic classifications have been proposed for use in the characterization of mild cognitive disorders associated with aging. One of the best established of these classifications is age-associated memory impairment (AAMI). Epidemiological data suggest that AAMI is a phenomenon of normal aging rather than a sign of progression from normal aging to a pathological state such as Alzheimer's disease.[142] AAMI appears to occur in a highly heterogeneous group of older individuals, and is of questionable clinical or theoretical significance. The normal aging process is not accompanied by true memory loss as determined by neuropsychological, neuroradiological, and neurophysiological data; however, it is suggested that with sensory losses, as well as poorer oxygen supply from reduced activity levels that cognitive capabilities are slowed, and attentiveness not consistently maintained.[142]

What we characterize as "intelligence" may be affected by pathology, but, even in advanced years it remains unaffected by the physiologic changes of normal aging.[7]

The topics of memory and intelligence will be addressed more thoroughly in Chapter 18, Education and the Older Adult: Learning, Memory, and Intelligence.

CONCLUSION

Aging can be viewed as a stochastic process resulting from a greater disorderliness of regulatory mechanisms, which in turn result in the reduced robustness of the organism to incurrent stress and disease. The notion of greater disorderliness in aging is illustrated by the erosion of the orderly neuroendocrine feedback regulation of the secretion of LH, FSH, ACTH, and GH. These changes are manifested as menopause, andropause, adrenopause, and somatopause. Age-related disruption of metabolic processes is associated with a higher prevalence of diseases such as type II diabetes and other pathologies such as cancer in older individuals.

Although the dysregulation of neurohormone outflow from the CNS constitutes one of the earliest measurable facets of aging, many questions remain to be answered by aging research. What is the exact mechanism of CNS integrative failure? To what degree does peripheral endocrine gland insufficiency (e.g., testis, ovary) contribute to disruption in the aging feedback-axis (e.g., GNRH-LH)? What gender differences underlie the neuroendocrine changes that occur with aging? What is the contribution of the neuroregulatory alterations to the risk of frailty or eventual disability?

Aging as a universal occurrence is regarded as a biological, anatomical, and physiological or "normal" process distinct from pathological processes. As much as aging might be influenced by a predisposition to disease, it is not considered "abnormal." Conceptually, this distinction seems clear enough, but when applied to specific cases, the boundaries become blurred. Some degree of decline is noted in all biological, anatomical, physiological, and functional components of the human body with age, but this is not considered pathological. Aging has been excluded from the domain of disease because it is considered normal. Aging is viewed as the result of the accumulation of unrepaired injuries resulting from mostly unavoidable, universal changes. If one defines disease as a "reaction to injury," then is there a distinct aging process? If a steady accumulation of microinjuries causes a linear decline of function, does the presence of redundancy in any system translate into a linear loss of functional capacity, and, is aging an accelerated age-specific failure of each system? The distinction between aging and disease becomes one of arbitrary degree. A variety of degenerative processes are repeatedly termed normal aging until they proceed far enough to cause clinically significant disability. They then become a "disease." In such cases, the distinction between aging and disease is more semantic than biologically, anatomically, physiologically, or functionally normal. The question remains: Is there a normal aging process?

PEARLS

- Aging is viewed as characteristically decremental in nature and lacking in defined chronological points of transition, though linear with time.
- Not all body cells age in the same way or at the same rate; however, in general, the total number of cells in the body decreases with age while remaining cells become less alike in structure and less organized in function.
- Cardiovascular cellular changes with age are numerous and range from lipofuscin accumulation at the poles of the nuclei of cardiac muscle to increased calcification in the media.
- In the pulmonary system, age changes can be organized according to mechanical properties, changes in flow, gas exchange, and impairment of lung defense.
- The presence of glycoproteins in the extracellular area produces the osmotic force that is important in maintaining the fluid content of the tissues.
- Hyaluronic acid helps to regulate the viscosity of tissues.
- Contractile proteins provide motility within the connective tissues.
- The decrease in aging muscle is associated with a selective loss of type II muscle fibers, a decrease in protein and nitrogen, and an increase in connective tissue and fat.
- Due to change in the thermal regulatory response, the aged have prolonged cooling time following increased activity, as well as a decrease of receptiveness to heat and cold.
- All five senses as well as proprioception/ kinesthesia decline with age.
- The endocrine system plays a major role in the biologic variability of aging.

REFERENCES

1. Eveleth PB, Tanner JM. *Worldwide Variation in Human Growth.* Cambridge, England: Cambridge University Press; 1976.
2. Cutler RG. Evolution of longevity in primates. *J Hum Evol.* 1976; 5:169–202.
3. Fries JF. Aging, natural death and the compression of morbidity. *N Engl J Med.* 1968; 303: 113–123.
4. Kent S. The evolution of longevity. *Geriatrics.* 1980; 35:98–104.
5. Korenchevksy V. *Physiological and Pathological Aging.* New York: Hafner; 1961.
6. Andres R. Normal aging versus disease in the elderly. In: Andres EL, Bierman EL, Hazard WR, eds. *Principles in Geriatric Medicine.* New York: McGraw-Hill; 1985:38–41.
7. Kenney RA. *Physiology of Aging.* Symposium of the Aging Process Clinics in Geriatric Medicine. Feb 1985; 1(1).
8. Shock NW. Physiological theories of aging. In: Rothstein JL, et al, eds. *Theoretical Aspects of Aging.* New York: Academic Press; 1974:119–136.
9. Seyle HA. Stress and aging. *J Am Geriatrics Society.* 1970; 18(9):669–690.
10. Rowlatt C, Franks LM. Aging in tissues and cells. In: Brocklehurst JC. *Textbook of Geriatric Medicine and Gerontology.* New York: Longman Group Ltd.; 1978.
11. Hayflick L. The cellular basis for biological aging. In: Finch C, Hayflick L, eds. *The Handbook of the Biology of Aging.* New York: Van Nostrand Reinhold; 1977.
12. Goldman R. Decline in organ function with age. In: Rossman I, ed. *Clinical Geriatrics.* 2nd ed. Philadelphia: Lippincott, 1979.
13. Pomerance A. Pathology of the myocardium and valves. In: Caird FI, Dalle JLC, Kennedy RD, eds. *Cardiology in Old Age.* New York: Plenum Press; 1976:11–53.
14. Wei JY. Heart disease in the elderly. *Cardiovasc Med.* 1984; 9:971–982.
15. Baker PB, Arn AR, Unverferth DV. Hypertrophic and degenerative changes in human hearts with aging. *J Coll Cardiol.* 1985; 5:536A.
16. Yin FCP. The aging vasculature and its effects on the heart. In: Weisfeldt ML, ed. *The Aging Heart.* New York: Raven Press; 1980:2.
17. Cotton R, Wartman WB. Endothelial patterns in human arteries, their relation to age, vessel site and atherosclerosis. *Arch Pathol.* 1961; 2:15–24.
18. Movat HZ, More RH, Haust MD. The diffuse intimal thickening of the human aorta with aging. *Am J Pathol.* 1958; 34:1023–1030.
19. Milch RA. Matrix properties of the aging arterial wall. *Monogr Surg Sci.* 1965; 2:261–341.
20. Auerbach O, Hammond EC, Garfinkel L. Thickening of wall of arterioles and small arteries in relation to age and smoking habits. *N Engl J Med.* 1968; 278:980–984.
21. Wolinsky H, Glagov S. Structural basis for the static mechanical properties of the aorta media. *Circ Res.* 1964; 14:301–309.
22. Schlatman TJM, Becker AE. Histologic changes in the normal aging aorta: Implications for aortic aneurysm. *Am J Cardiol.* 1977; 39:13–20.
23. Hutchins GM. Structure of the aging heart. In: Weisfeldt ML, ed. *The Aging Heart.* New York; Raven Press; 1980: 269–295.
24. Ruiz-Torres A, Melon J, Munoz FJ. Insulin stimulates collagen synthesis in vascular smooth muscle cells from elderly patients. *Gerontology.* 1998; 44 (3):144–148.
25. Wei JY. Cardiovascular anatomic and physiologic changes with age. *Topics in Ger Rehab.* 1986; 2(1): 10–16.

26. Rodeheffer RJ, Gerstenblith G, Becker LC, et al. Exercise cardiac output is maintained with advancing age in health human subjects: Cardiac dilatation and increased stroke volume compensates for diminished heart rate. *Circulation.* 1984; 69: 203–213.
27. Shannon RP, Wei JY, Rosa RM, et al. The effect of age and sodium depletion on cardiovascular response to orthostasis. *Hypertension.* 1986; 4: 229–242.
28. Gerstenblith G, Frederikson J, Yin FCP, et al. Echocardiographic assessment of a normal adult aging population. *Circulation.* 1977; 56:273–278.
29. Nichols WW, O'Rourke MF, Avolio AP, et al. Effects of age on ventricular-vascular coupling. *Am J Cardiol.* 1985; 55:1179–1184.
30. Miyatake K, Okamoto M, Kinoshita N, et al. Augmentation of atrial contribution to left ventricular inflow with aging as assessed by intracardiac Doppler flowmetry. *Am J Cardiol.* 1984; 53:586–589.
31. Ziegler MG, Lake CR, Kopin IJ. Plasma noradrenalin increase with age. *Nature.* 1976; 261:333–334.
32. Shimada K, Kitazumi T, Sadakne N, et al. Age related changes of baroreflex function, plasma norepinephrine, and blood pressure. *Hypertension.* 1985; 7:113–117.
33. Tsunoda K, Abe K, Goto T, et al. Effect of age on the renin-angiotensin-aldosterone system in normal subjects: simultaneous measurement of active and inactive renin, renin substrate, and aldosterone in plasma. *J Clin Endocrinol Metab.* 1986; 62:384–389.
34. Shannon RP, Minaker KL, Rowe JW. Aging and water balance in humans. *Semin Nephrol.* 1984; 4:346–353.
35. Weisfeldt ML, Gerstenblith G, Lakatta EG. Alterations in circulatory function. In: Andres R, ed. *Principles of Geriatric Medicine.* New York: McGraw-Hill Co.; 1985.
36. Ham RS, Marcy ML. *Normal Aging: A Review of Systems/The Maintenance of Health in Primary Care Geriatrics.* Boston: John Wright, PSG, Inc.; 1983.
37. Butler RN. Current definitions of aging. In: *Epidemiology of Aging.* Bethesda, Md: National Institutes of Health Publication No. 80-969; 1980:7–8.
38. Zadai CC. Cardiopulmonary issues in the geriatric population: Implications for rehabilitation. *Topics in Ger Rehab.* 1986:2(1):1–9.
39. Cummings G, Semple SG. *Disorders of the Respiratory System.* Oxford, England: Blackwell; 1973.
40. Wynne JW. Pulmonary disease in the elderly. In: Rossman I, ed. *Clinical Geriatrics.* 2nd ed. Philadelphia: Lippincott, 1979.
41. Pickles LW. Effects of aging on connective tissues. *Geriatrics.* 1983; 38(1):71–78.
42. Goldberg AL, Goodman HM. Effects of disuse and denervation on amino acid transport by skeletal muscle. *Am J Physiol.* 1975; 216: 1116–1119.
43. Hamlin CR, Luschin JH, Kohn RR. Aging of collagen: Comparative rates in four mammalian species. *Exp Gerontol.* 1980; 15:393–398.
44. Chapman EA, DeVries HA, Swezey R. joint stiffness: Effects of exercise on young and old men. *J Gerontol.* 1972; 27:218–221.
45. Viidik A. Function properties of collagenous tissue. *Int Rev Conn Tissue Res.* 1982; 6:127–215.
46. Klein FA, Rajan RK. Normal aging: effects on connective tissue metabolism and structure. *J Gerontol.* 1985; 40(5):579–585.
47. Lehman J, Warren C, Scham S. Therapeutic heat and cold. *Clin Orthop.* 1974; 99:207–209.
48. Meyer K. Mucopolysacchrides of costal cartilage. *Science.* 1958; 128:896.
49. Donatelli R, Owens-Burkart H. Effects of immobilization on the extensibility of periarticular connective tissue. *JOSPT.* 1981; 3(2):67–71.
50. Ryan AJ. The role of tissue viscosity in injury prevention. In: Ryan AJ, Allman FL., eds. *Sports Medicine.* New York: Academic Press; 1974.
51. Astrand PO, Rodahl K. *Textbook of Work Physiology.* San Francisco, London: McGraw-Hill; 1970.
52. Hole JW. *Human Anatomy and Physiology.* Boston: Wm. C. Brown Co.; 1988.
53. Walker J. Connective tissue plasticity: issues in histological and light microscopy studies of exercise and aging in articular cartilage. *JOSPT.* 1991; 14(5):189–197.
54. Gardner DL. Aging of articular cartilage. In: Brocklehurst JC, ed. *Textbook of Geriatric Medicine and Gerontology.* New York: Longman Group Ltd.; 1978.
55. Akeson WH, Amiel D, Abel MF, et al. Effects of immobilization on joints. *Clin Ortho & Rel Res.* 1987; 219:28–36.
56. Steen B. Body composition and aging. *Nutr Rev.* 1988; 46:45–51.
57. Going S, Williams D, Lohman T. Aging and body composition: Biological changes and methodological issues. *Exercise Sports Science Review.* 1995; 23:411–458.
58. Borkan GA, Norris AH. Assessment of biological age using a profile of physical pararneters. *J Gerontol.* 1980; 35:177–184.
59. Borkan GA, Hults DE, Gerzof SG, et al. Age changes in body composition revealed by computed tomography. *J Gerontol.* 1983; 38:673–677.
60. Gallagher D. Appendicular skeletal muscle mass: Effect of age, gender and ethnicity. *J Applied Physiol.* 1999; 83:229–239.
61. Kohrt WM, Malley MT, Dalsky GP, Holloszy JO. Body composition of healthy sedentary and trained, young and older men and women. *Med Sci Sports Exerc.* 1992; 24(7):832–837.
62. Jacobs R. Physical changes in the aged. In: O'Hara-Devereaux M, Andrus LH, Scott CD, eds. *Eldercare.* New York: Grune & Stratton; 1981.
63. Brown MB, Rose SJ. The effects of aging and exercise on skeletal muscle-clinical considerations. *Top Ger Rehabil.* 1985; 1:20–30.
64. Brown MB. Resistance exercise effects on aging skeletal muscle in rats. *Phys Ther.* 1989; 69(1): 46–53.
65. Albert NR, Gale HH, Taylor N. The effect of age on contractile protein ATPase activity and the veloc-

ity for shortening. In: Tanz RD, Kavaler F, Roberts J. eds. *Factors Influencing Myocardial Contractility.* New York: Academic Press; 1967.

66. Cress ME, Schultz E. Aging muscle: functional, morphologic, biochemical and regenerative capacity. In: Smith EL, ed. *Top Geriatr Rehabil.* 1985; l(l):11–19.

67. Buller AJ, Eccles JC, Eccles RM. Interaction between motoneurons and muscles in respect of the characteristic speeds of their responses. *J Physiol.* 1960; 150:417–439.

68. Larsson L. Physical training effects on muscle morphology in sedentary males at different ages. *Med Sci Sports Exerc.* 1982; 14:203–206.

69. Aniansson A, Grimby G, Hedberg M, Krotkiewske M. Muscle morphology, enzyme activity and muscle strength in elderly men and women. *Clin Physiol.* 1981; 1:73–86.

70. Aniansson A, Hedberg M, Henning GB, et al. Muscle morphology, enzyme activity, and muscle strength in elderly men: A follow-up study. *Muscle Nerve.* 1986; 9:585–591.

71. Aniansson A, Sperling L, Rundgren A, et al. Muscle function in 75-year-old men and women: A longitudinal study. *Scand J Rehabil Med.* 1983; 9(suppl):92–102.

72. Gutmann E, Hanzlikova V. Basic mechanisms of aging in the neuromuscular system. *Mech Ageing Dev.* 1972; 1:327–349.

73. Larsson L, Grimby G, Karlsson J. Muscle strength and speed of movement in relation to age and muscle morphology. *J Appl Physiol.* 1979; 46: 451–456.

74. Gollnick PD, Armstrong RB, Saltin B, et al. Effect of training on enzyme activity and fiber composition of human skeletal muscle. *J Appl Physiol.* 1973; 34:107–111.

75. Grimby G. Physical activity and muscle training in the elderly. *Acta Med Scand.* 1986; 711(suppl): 233–237.

76. Monemi M, Eriksson PO, Eriksson A, Thomell LE. Adverse changes in fibre type composition of the human masseter versus biceps brachii muscle during aging. *J Neurol Sci.* 1998; 154(1):35:48.

77. Brierly EJ, Johnson MA, Lightowlers RN, James OF, Turnbull DM. Role of mitochondrial DNA mutations in human aging: implications for the central nervous system and muscle. *Ann Neurol.* 1998; 43(2):217–223.

78. Larsson L, Ramamurthy B. Aging-related changes in skeletal muscle. Mechanisms and interventions. *Drugs Aging.* 2000; 17(4):303–316.

79. Roubenoff R. Sarcopenia: a major modifiable cause of frailty in the elderly. *J Nutr Health Aging.* 2000; 4(3):140–142.

80. Tseng BS, Marsh DR, Hamilton MT, Booth FW. Strength and aerobic training attenuate muscle wasting and improve resistance to the development of disability with aging. *J Gerontol.* 1995; 50:113–119.

81. Booth FW, Weeden SH, Tseng BS. Effect of aging on human skeletal muscle and motor function. *Med Sci Sports Exerc.* 1994; 26(5):556–560.

82. Bidlack WR, Kirsh A, Meskin MS. Nutritional requirements of the elderly. *Food Technology.* 1988; 40:61–70.

83. Batata M, Spray GH, Bolton FG, Higgins G, Wollner L. Blood and bone marrow changes in elderly patients, with particular reference to folic acid, vitamin B12, iron and ascorbic acid. *Br Med J.* 1967; 2:667–669.

84. Jokl E. *Physiology of Exercise.* Springfield, III: Charles C Thomas Publishers; 1984; 108–112.

85. Burchinsky SC. Neurotransmitter receptors in the central nervous system and aging: pharmacological aspects (review). *Experimental Aging.* 1984; 19: 227–239.

86. Bohannon RW, Larkin PA, Cook AC, et al. Decrease in timed balance test scores with aging. *Phys Ther.* 1984; 64:1067–1070.

87. Besdine RW, Harris TB. Alterations in body temperature (hypothermia and hyperthermia). In: Andres R, Bierman EL, and Hazzard WR, eds. *Principles in Geriatric Medicine.* New York: McGraw-Hill; 1985:209–217.

88. Asmussen E. Aging and exercise. In: Horvath SM, Yousef MK, eds. *Environmental Physiology, Aging, Heat and Altitude.* New York: Elsevier/ North Holland; 1981.

89. Ajiduah AO, Paolone AM, Wailgum TD, Irion G, Kendrick ZV. The effect of age on tolerance of thermal stress during exercise. *Med Sci Spts Exerc.* 1983; 15:168. Abstract.

90. Corso JE. sensory processes and age effects of normal adults. *J Gerontol.* 1971; 26:90–105.

91. Kasper RL. Eye problems of the aged. In: Reichel PE, ed. *Clinical Aspects of Aging.* Baltimore: Williams and Wilkins Co.; 1988.

92. Boyer GG. Vision problems. In: Camevali P, Patrick B, eds. *Nursing Management for the Elderly.* Philadelphia: Lippincott; 1989.

93. Woollacott MH, Shumway-Cook A, Nasner LM. Aging and posture control: changes in sensory organization and muscular coordination. *Int J Aging Hum Dev.* 1986; 23:97–114.

94. Schiffman SS. Taste and smell losses in normal aging and disease. *JAMA.* 1997; 278(16): 1357–1362.

95. Bennet J, Creamer H, Fontana-Smith DJ. Dentistry. In: O'Hara-Devereaux M, Andrus LH, Scott CD, eds. *Eldercare.* New York: Grune & Stratton; 1981.

96. Khan TA, Shragge BW, Crippen JS, et al. Esophageal mobility in the elderly. *Am J Digestive Dis.* 1977; 22:1049–1054.

97. Bartol MA, Heitkemper M. Gastrointestinal problems. In: Carnevali P, Patrick B, eds. *Nursing Management for the Elderly.* Philadelphia: Lippincott, 1989.

98. Horowitz M, Maddern GT, Chateron BE, et al. Changes in gastric emptying rates with age. *Clin Sci.* 1984; 67:213–218.

99. Morgan W, Thomas C, Schuster M. Gastrointestinal system. In: O'Hara-Devereaux M, Andrus LH, Scott CD, eds. *Eldercare.* New York: Grune & Stratton; 1981.

100. Hyans DE. The liver and biliary system. In: Brocklehurst JC, ed. *Textbook of Geriatric Medicine and Gerontology.* New York: Longman Group Ltd.; 1978.

101. Fink RL. Mechanisms of insulin resistance in aging. *J Clin Invest.* 1983; 71:1523–1535.

102. Lindeman RD. Is the decline in renal function with normal aging inevitable? *Geriatr Nephrol Urol.* 1998; 8(1):7–9.

103. Sourander LB. The aging kidney. In: Brocklehurst JC, ed. *Textbook of Geriatric Medicine and Gerontology.* New York: Longman Group Ltd.; 1978.

104. Lamberts S, van den Beld A, van der Lely A. The endocrinology of aging. *Science.* 1997; 278(5337): 419–424.

105. Sundwall DN, Ralond J, Thorn GW. Endocrine and metabolic. In: O'Hara-Devereaux M, Andrus LH, Scott CD, eds. *Eldercare.* New York: Grune & Stratton; 1981.

106. Savin CT, Deepak C. The aging thyroid: increased prevalence of elevated serum thyrotrophin levels in the elderly. *JAMA.* 1989; 242(3):247–250.

107. Van Cauter E, Plat L, Leproult R, Copinschi G. Alterations of circadian rhythmicity and sleep in aging: endocrine consequences. *Horm Res.* 1998; 49:147–152.

108. Czeisler C, Duffy J, Shanahan T. Stability, precision, and near-24-hour period of the human circadian pacemaker. *Science.* 1999; 284: 2177–2181.

109. Veldhuis J, Iranmanesh A, Weltman A. Elements in the pathophysiology of diminished growth hormone (GH) secretion in aging humans. *Endocrine.* 1997; 7:41–48.

110. Halberg F, Cornelissen G. Commentary: Chromosomes: time structures within the physiological range identify early disease risk aiming at primary prevention. *J Gerontol A Biol Sci Med Sci.* 1999; 54:M309–M311.

111. Martin B, Warram J, Krolewski A, Bergman R, Soeldner J, Kahn C. Role of glucose and insulin resistance in development of type 2 diabetes mellitus: results of a 25-year follow-up study. *Lancet.* 1992; 340:925–929.

112. Iozzo P, Beck-Nielsen H, Laakso M, Smith U, Yki-Jarvinen H, Ferrannini E. Independent influence of age on basal insulin secretion in nondiabetic humans. European Group for the Study of Insulin Resistance. *J Clin Endocrinol Metab.* 1999; 84: 863–868.

113. Meneilly G, Veldhuis J, Elahi D. Disruption of the pulsatile and entropic modes of insulin release during an unvarying glucose stimulus in elderly individuals. *J Clin Endocrinol Metab.* 1999; 84: 1938–1943.

114. Shimokata H, Muller D, Fleg J, Sorkin J, Ziemba A, Andres R. Age as independent determinant of glucose tolerance. *Diabetes.* 1991; 40:44–51.

115. Edelstein S, Knowler W, Bain R. Predictors of progression from impaired glucose tolerance to NIDDM: an analysis of six prospective studies. *Diabetes.* 1997; 46:701–710.

116. Accili D, Drago J, Lee E. Early neonatal death in mice homozygous for a null allele of the insulin receptor gene. *Nat Genet.* 1996; 12(1):106–109.

117. Rowe J, Kahn R. Successful aging. *Gerontologist.* 1997; 37:433–440.

118. Li H, Matheny M, Turner N, Scarpace P. Aging and fasting regulation of leptin and hypothalamic neuropeptide Y gene expression. *Am J Physiol.* 1998; 275:E405–E411.

119. Pincus S, Mulligan T, Iranmanesh A, Gheorghiu S, Godschalk M, Veldhuis J. Older males secrete luteinizing hormone and testosterone more irregularly, and jointly more asynchronously, than younger males. *Proc Natl Acad Sci USA.* 1996; 93:14100–14105.

120. Scheiber M, Rebar R. Isoflavones and postmenopausal bone health: a viable alternative to estrogen therapy? *Menopause.* 1999; 6(2): 233–241.

121. Stone D, Rozovsky I, Morgan T, Anderson C, Finch C. Increased synaptic sprouting in response to estrogen via an apolipoprotein E-dependent mechanism: implications for Alzheimer's disease. *J Neurosci.* 1998; 18:3180–3185.

122. Wang C, Iranmanesh A, Berman N. Comparative pharmacokinetics of three doses of percutaneous dihydrotestosterone gel in healthy elderly men—a clinical research center study. *J Clin Endocrinol Metab.* 1998; 83:2749–2757.

123. Bassaria S, Dobs AS. Risks versus benefits of testosterone therapy in elderly men. *Drugs Aging.* 1999; 15(2):131–142.

124. Synder P, Peachey H, Hannoush P. Effect of testosterone treatment on body composition and muscle strength in men over 65 years of age. *J Clin Endocrinol Metab.* 1999; 84:2647–2653.

125. Bhasin S, Bagatell C, Bremner W. Issues in testosterone replacement in older men. *J Clin Endocrinol Metab.* 1998; 83:3435–3448.

126. Morley J, Perry HR. Androgen deficiency in aging men. *Med Clin North Am.* 1999; 83:1279–1289.

127. Miller WL. Mechanisms of adrenarche and adrenopause. *Acta Paediatr Suppl.* 1999; 88(433): 60–66.

128. Callies F. Influence of oral dehydroepiandrosterone (DHEA) on urinary steroid metabolites in males and females. *Steroids.* 2000; 65(2):98–102.

129. Barnhart KT, Freeman E, Grisso JA, Rader DJ, Sammel M, Kapoor S, Nestler JE. The effect of dehydroepiandrosterone supplementation to symptomatic perimenopausal women on serum endocrine profiles, lipid parameters, and health- related quality of life. *Clin Endocrinol.* 1998; 49(4):433–438.

130. Arlt W, Haas J, Callies F, Reincke M, Hubler D, Oettel M, Ernst M, Schulte HM, Allolio B. Biotransformation of oral dehydroepiandrosterone in elderly men: Significant increase in circulating estrogens. *J Clin Endocrinol Metab.* 1999; 84(6): 2170–2176.

131. Hoffman AR, Lieberman SA, Butterfield G, Thompson J, Hintz RL, Ceda GP, Marcus R. Somatopause and the effects of replacement therapy in the elderly. *Endocrine.* 1997; 7(1):73–76.

132. Martin FC, Yeo AL, Sonksen PH. Growth hormone secretion in the elderly: ageing and the somatopause. *Baillieres Clin Endocrinol Metab.* 1997; 11(2):223–250.

133. Lamberts SW. The somatopause: To treat or not to treat? *Horm Res.* 2000; 53 Suppl 3:42–43.

134. Wideman L, Weltman J, Shah N, Story S, Veldhuis J, Weltman A. Effects of gender on exercise-induced growth hormone release. *J Appl Physiol.* 1999; 87:1154–1162.

135. Veldhuis J, Evans W, Shah N, Storey S, Bray M, Anderson S. Proposed mechanisms of sex-steroid hormone neuromodulation of the human GH-IGF-I axis. In: Veldhuis J, Giustina A, eds. *Sex, Steroid Interactions With Growth Hormone.* New York, NY: Springler-Verlag Inc; 1999; 93–121.

136. Vittone J, Blackman M, Busby-Whitehead J. Effects of single nightly injections of growth hormone-releasing hormone (GHRH- 1–29) in healthy elderly men. *Metabolism.* 1997; 46:89–96.

137. Thorner M, Chapman I, Gaylinn B, Pezzoli S, Hartman M. Growth hormone-releasing hormone and growth hormone releasing peptide as therapeutic agents to enhance growth hormone secretion in disease and aging. *Recent Prog Horm Res.* 1997; 52:215–244; discussion 244–246.

138. Cress M, Buchner D, Questad K, Esselman P, deLateur B, Schwartz R. Exercise: effects on physical functional performance in independent older adults. *J Gerontol A Biol Sci Med Sci.* 1999; 54: M242–248.

139. Merriam G, Buchner D, Prinz P, Schwartz R, Vitiello M. Potential applications of GH secretagogs in the evaluation and treatment of the age-related decline in growth hormone secretion. *Endocrine.* 1997; 7:49–52.

140. Giustina A, Veldhuis J. Pathophysiology of the neuroregulation of growth hormone secretion in experimental animals and the human. *Endocr Rev.* 1998; 19:717–797.

141. Guilleminault C. Sleep and sleep disorders. In: Cassel S, Walsh B, eds. *Geriatric Medicine.* New York: Springer-Verlag; 1984:11.

142. Hanninen T. Soininen H. Age-associated memory impairment. Normal aging or warning of dementia? *Drugs Aging.* 1997; 11(6):480–489.

CHAPTER 4

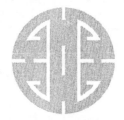

Describing Psychosocial Aspects of Aging

The aging process of human life is not one dimensional. Besides the obvious physical component, there exist the psychological, emotional, and spiritual components of aging. This chapter will address the psychosocial components. Even though physical health is extremely important, studies and life experience illustrate the effects of cognitive perception on life satisfaction and physical health.[1,2] One study on hip fracture outcomes for older persons showed that the most important variable in successful rehabilitation was the presence or absence of depression.[1] This study alone has tremendous implications for physical and occupational therapists, because it illustrates that unless the older person's emotional and mental abilities are addressed, the physical efforts may have minimal effect.

How does a physical or occupational therapist work in the psychosocial realm? Rehabilitation therapists are not psychologists and do not receive extensive training in the social and psychological sciences. Nevertheless, they can use specific information as an adjunct to daily treatment. For example, examining one's attitudes with respect to the various psychosocial theories of aging may provide information about a patient's satisfaction or motivation and enhance a therapist's ability to communicate with an older per-

son. In addition, since the goal of therapy is to achieve optimal functioning, it is imperative that the therapist be able to recognize situations that require coping mechanisms and provide some assistance in these situations.

This chapter will explore the theories of aging and the cognitive changes in late life. Situations, both normal and pathological, that require coping mechanisms will be described in detail as well as society's view of aging and the lifestyle adaptations of older persons.

PSYCHOSOCIAL THEORIES OF AGING

Aging is another developmental period within the circle of life. In the early 1900s, life expectancy (for both sexes) was 47 years of age.[3] Now an individual has a mean life expectancy of approximately 82 years of age (for both sexes), another lifetime beyond retirement at the age of 65 years. It is a period in which adjustments to changes in social roles, employment status, financial stability, loss of family and friends through relocation and death—as well as one's own perceptions of aging, "the golden years," and mortality—will be powerful elements in one's psychosocial response to the process of aging.

In the last 30 years, many psychological theories of aging have been proposed. Prior to this time, however, few theories existed. The mainstream of thought centered around the theories of Freud and Piaget, which placed all the emphasis on the psychological development on the child while essentially ignoring the adult. The theories to be discussed in this section are either full life development theories or late life psychological development theories.

Full Life Development Theories

Erikson Eric Erikson was one of the first psychological theorists to develop a personality theory that extended into old age. Erikson viewed the process of human development as a series of stages that one goes through in order to fully develop one's ego.[4] Erikson describes eight stages in this process. These stages are listed in Table 4–1. Each of these stages represents a choice in the development of the expanding ego. The last two stages are of particular interest to the practitioner working with the older person.

A successful life choice of generativity, as Erikson calls it, consists of guiding, parenting, and monitoring the next generation. If an adult person does not experience generativity then stagnation will predominate. Stagnation is characterized by anger, hurt, and self-absorption. The final stage of Erikson's theory suggests that the older person must accept his or her life with the sense that "If I had to do it all over again, I'd do it pretty much the same."[5] At this stage the person experiences an active concern with life, even in the face of death, and learns to experience his or her own wisdom.

Jung Carl Jung was also a pioneer, and designated adult stages on the basis of his own experience in clinical theory and practice.[6] His theory of development describes youth, from puberty to middle age, as a stage in which the person is concerned with sexual instincts, broadening horizons, and conquering feelings of inferiority. The adult period, between the ages of 35 to 40, involve the transport of the youthful self into the middle years. During this stage, Jung theorized that the person's convictions strengthen until

TABLE 4–1. ERIKSON'S STAGES OF PERSONALITY AND EGO DEVELOPMENT

Period in Life	Erikson's Stage
0–12 months	Trust vs. mistrust
2–4 years	Autonomy vs. shame
4–5 years	Initiative vs. guilt
6–11 years	Industry vs. inferiority
12–18 years	Identity vs. identity confusion
Young adulthood	Intimacy vs. isolation
Adulthood	Generativity vs. stagnation
Late life	Integrity vs. despair

Reprinted with permission from Erikson EH. *Identity, Youth and Crisis.* New York: Norton; 1968.

they become somewhat more rigid at the age of 50. In later years, Jung suggests that activity levels decrease, that men become more expressive and nurturing, and women become more "instrumental," providing care and continuation of the generations they have nurtured in their lives.[6,7] Jung also suggests that the later years are years in which the older person confronts his or her own death. Success in this involves the acceptance of death as a part of the cycle of life, not something to be feared.

Maslow Abraham Maslow's hierarchy of human needs is not a theory singular to aging, but it is an excellent framework for exploring growth, development, and motivation.[8] Maslow's hierarchy is a pyramid of needs, each of which builds upon the other. In the lowest level, "biological and physiological integrity," the critical needs for an individual are food and clothing. At the second level, "safety and security," the primary need is protection against the elements and against other people. This cannot be achieved unless the person is first fed and clothed. In the third level, "belonging or love needs," the person begins to seek love from others, such as a parent or a significant other. When the person satisfies the need for love, he or she then progresses to the next level, "self-esteem," where the person in turn learns to cherish him- or herself, respects his or her own values and ideas, and feels good about who he or she is. Finally, at the level of "self-actualization," the person no longer worries about the lower needs, but is now able to give to others and has reached a higher level transcending the lower self-esteem needs. At the pinnacle of the pyramid of need, individuals can nurture and feed others, develop their own ideas, and actually live their own values and ideas in the community. According to Maslow, very few people in society are self-actualized. Some of our great leaders such as Martin Luther King, Winston Churchill, and Golda Meir were self-actualized people.

One must successfully fill each lower need before ascending to the next higher need. When one is at a given level, one's energies are consumed at that level.[9] One rarely stays at a higher level, but rather the person reverts to lower levels during periods when the lower needs are no longer being met. For example, a recently widowed woman may feel isolated or lonely and be unable to experience the higher levels of self-esteem or self-actualization until her grief has subsided.

This theory is particularly useful in the area of motivation. Since older persons are more likely to have physical decline, their needs will descend to the lower levels of the hierarchy. Therefore, motivation strategies should be aimed at the level of the person's needs. For example, if the person is unstable when walking, then strategies to encourage exercises in this area should appeal to their sense of safety if the person is at that level. If, however, the same person is more concerned about hunger during a treatment session, they will be unable to focus on the exercises.

Maslow believes, though, that it is the older person who truly has the knowledge and experience of life to be able to experience self-actualization, the highest level of the paradigm.[9]

Late Life Theories

Peck Robert C. Peck's theory describes tasks that must be accomplished to achieve integrity in old age. In this theory, the burden is placed on the older person to redefine the self, dismiss occupational identity, and go beyond self-centeredness. Peck's proposed tasks, in order to accomplish this, follow.

1. *Ego differentiation versus work role preoccupation.* In this instance, a retired person must look for new meaning and values beyond their previous work roles.
2. *Body transcendence versus body preoccupation.* Since old age may carry with it ill health, the older person must learn new ways to gain mental, physical, social, and spiritual pleasure that transcend physical discomfort.
3. *Ego transcendence versus ego preoccupation.* This last stage is a way of minimizing the prospect of death by giving to children and making charitable contributions to leave an enduring legacy.[10]

Buehler's Biophysical Model of Later Life Cheryl Buehler adopts a biophysical model of a living open system in which both maintenance and change of the organism are equally important.[7] She purports two kinds of maintenance: satisfying need and maintaining internal order. Two types of change are also proposed: adaptation and creativity. According to Buehler's theory, maturity is the age of fulfillment and in order to proceed successfully, these four basic elements (the two kinds of maintenance and the two types of change) must be met to ensure acceptance of old age. Successful passage through each of these stages requires integrating and balancing conflicting and competing trends from earlier stages. In middle age, self-assessment evolves and whatever order existed previously is questioned. Self-assessment succeeds when the self and others are accepted for what they are; when the individual attains a fresh appreciation of people and the world; and when he or she can be autonomous and serene. The final result is self-actualization. This introspection and re-evaluation of maintenance and change determine how one faces old age: optimistically or pessimistically.

Neugarten Bernice Neugarten also describes the tasks that must be accomplished in order to be a successfully aging older person. The following are a few of her tasks that directly impact the rehabilitation milieu.

1. Accepting the increasing reality and imminence of death,
2. Coping with physical illness,
3. Coordinating the necessary dependence on support and accurately assessing the independent choices that can still be made to achieve maximum life satisfaction,
4. Giving and obtaining emotional gratification.[11]

Disengagement Theory The controversial disengagement theory credited to Cummings and Henry in the 1950s postulated that older people and society mutually withdraw. This withdrawal is characterized by a positive change in psychological well-being for the older person.[12] This theory, though not widely accepted at present, spawned much debate on the subject of late life adaptation. This theory is based on the sociologic perspective of functionalism, it is assumed that society has certain needs that must be met if stability and equilibrium are to be maintained. A structure is said to have a function if it contributes to the fulfillment of one or more of the social needs of the system.[13]

The disengagement theory depicts aging as a process of gradual physical, psychological, and social withdrawal. Disengagement is considered as functional during the aging process, purportedly preparing the person and society to face the inevitability of death. Changes in the personality of the individual are viewed as either the cause or the effect of decreased involvement with others. The authors of this theory claim that once this process starts it is irreversible, and that morale may remain high or improve as part of the process of disengagement.

Within this process, Cummings and Henry described three types of changes resulting in an older person's becoming less tied to the social system.[12] There are changes in the amount of interaction, the purposes of interaction, and the style of interaction with others. In outlining their theory, Cummings and Henry indicate that the process is both intrinsic and inevitable, and that the process is not only a correlate of successful aging but may also be a condition of it, since those who accept this inevitable reduction in social and personal interactions in old age are usually satified with their lives.[12]

Today, however, this theory has been largely discredited. Lipman and Smith,[14] while agreeing that a person's death may be dysfunctional for the social system if it is not prepared for, found that those who reduce their activities as they age tend to suffer a reduction in overall life satisfaction. This revised view is substantiated by recent studies of centenarians where successful aging includes, as the second most important factor, attitude, outlook, and social relationships.[15]

Functionalism-versus-Conflict Theory The challenge to functionalism and the disengagement theory came from several sources one of which is called The Conflict Theory. It was believed that functionalism was too consensus oriented, with a built-in conservative bias, and that it treated both change and conflict in society negatively. Whereas the functionalists emphasized order, stability, and equilibrium, and therefore can devise an orientation that assumes that the person and the society mutually acquiesce to the withdrawal of the older adult, the conflict perspective is radically different. From the conflict perspective, consent and acquiescence take place through oppression, coercion, domination, and exploitation of one group by another. The conflict perspective stresses that there are always competing interests as groups struggle over claims to scarce resources, including status, power, and social class. While functionalists also assume that stratification is based on scarcity, the problem is often defined by functionalists as how to integrate the different sectors, groups, or classes. Conflict theorists, however, see the solution to this scarcity as occurring through the reduction of structural inequalities. These structural changes, they argue, will occur only in the presence of intense struggle.[16] This perspective is also shared by de Beauvoir,[17] who views aging as a class struggle. Estes, in her landmark analysis of the Older Americans Act, states that her research attempts to "make explicit how certain ways of thinking about the aged as a social problem . . . are rooted in the structure of social and power relations."[18(p2)]

Exchange Theory Another theoretical orientation that emerged as a reaction to functionalism is the exchange theory. Based on the belief that functionalism is too abstract and structural, and cannot explain actual human behavior, exchange theory is firmly rooted in rationalism. That is, human beings tend to choose courses of action on the basis of anticipated outcomes from among a known range of alternatives. Underlying this rational view of human behavior is the principle of hedonism, expressed in the contention that people tend to chose alternatives that will provide the most beneficial outcome. Everyone attempts to optimize gratification; that is, people continually try to satisfy needs and wants and to attain certain goals, and most of this occurs through interaction with other persons or groups. People attempt to maximize rewards, while reducing costs. Voluntary social behavior is motivated by the expectation of the return or reward this behavior will bring from others. One gives things in the hope of getting something in exchange.[19]

Another proposition essential to the exchange theory is the principle of reciprocity. In its simplest form it can be stated that a person should help (and not hurt) those who have helped her or him. The principle of reciprocity further assumes that a person chooses between alternative modes of behaving by comparing the anticipated rewards, the possible costs that may be incurred, and the magnitude of investment required to achieve those rewarding outcomes. Accordingly, rewards in human social interaction should be proportional to investment, and costs should not exceed re-

wards, or else the person will avoid that activity. Homans[20] has extended the principle of reciprocity to include another concept, which he calls distributive justice. When rewards are not proportional to investments over the long term, Homan asserts, people tend to feel angry with social relations, instability is created, and the propensities for conflict increase.

People exchange not only tangible, material objects, but also intangibles, such as the expression of love, admiration, respect, power, or influence. A good example of this theory might be that in the social exchange between the elderly and society, the elderly lose availability of resources. By losing power, the elderly are increasingly unable to enter into equal exchange relationships with significant others and all that remains for them is the capacity to comply.[21] Just as the conflict theorists focus on inequities and class struggle, the exchange theorists believe that to understand the situation of the aged, we must examine the role of society's stratification system in the aging process.[21]

Continuity and Activity Theories Two well-known theories that developed in response to the disengagement theory are the continuity and activity theories. The continuity theory proposes that activities in old age reflect a continuation of earlier life patterns,[22] while, in contrast, the activity theory states that successful adaption in late life is associated with maintaining as high a level of activity as possible. The older person should find substitutes when a meaningful activity, such as work, must be terminated. The person should develop an active rather than passive role toward their daily life as well as toward biological and social changes that are taking place.[23]

The continuity theory assumes that in the process of becoming adults, persons develop habits and preferences that become part of their personalities throughout their life experience, and which are carried into old age. The continuity theory claims that neither activity nor inactivity assumes happiness. It posits that most older people want to remain engaged with their social environment and that the magnitude of this engagement varies with the person according to life-long established patterns and self-concepts.[22] It further recognizes the interrelationships of biologic and environmental factors with psychological preferences. Positive aging becomes an adaptive process with interaction among all elements.

The activity theory, which is related to social role concepts, was advanced as an alternative interpretation to disengagement. It affirms that the continued maintenance of a high degree of involvement in social life is an important basis for deriving and sustaining satisfaction. It claims that those who maintain extensive social contacts, who engage in regular activities, similar to their engagement level in midlife, age most successfully. Declines in activity and role loss are thus associated with lower levels of satisfaction.[23]

In sum, continuity and activity theories assume the need for continued involvement throughout life; disengagement assumes mutuality in decline of involvement. Exchange theory assumes neither. It posits that the degree of engagement is the outcome of a specific change relationship between the person and society in which the more powerful exchange partner dictates the terms of relationship.

Havighurst Robert J. Havighurst's theory on aging relates successful aging to social competence and flexibility in adaption to new roles. He believes in the importance of finding new and meaningful roles in old age, while maintaining comfort with the customs of the time.[24,25] Later, Neugarten and Havighurst noted that successful adaptation to age was related to personality and not age per se. They noted the following four personality types.

1. *Integrated.* Shows a high degree of competence in daily activities and a complex inner life. This type is generally the best adapter.
2. *Passive dependent.* Seeks others to satisfy his or her emotional needs.
3. *Armored.* Attempts to control his or her environment and impulses and tends to be a high achiever.
4. *Unintegrated.* Shows poor emotional control and intellectual competency. This type tends to have the poorest adaptation in late life.[24]

Levinson While Erikson focuses on ego and personality development, Havighurst, Neugarten,[22] and Levinson[27] are concerned with the social tasks and roles that must be managed at each developmental stage of the person's life. Daniel Levinson[27] approaches the stages or "seasons" of adulthood as a developmental process involving occupation, love relationships, marriage and family, relation to self, use of solitude, and roles in various social contexts (e.g., relationships with individuals, groups, and institutions that have significance for their lives). According to Levinson, these components make up the underlying structure or pattern of a person's life. He refers to this pattern as the person's "life structure." Two basic types of developmental periods are hypothesized as determining life structure: structure building and structure change.

Levinson identifies a "novice" phase of adult development, which consists of three seasons: early adult transition (a structure-changing phase); entering the adult world (structure building); and transition (during which structure changing again takes place). The most important developmental tasks of early adulthood, according to Levinson are: entering an occupation; developing mentor relationships; and forming a love or marriage relationship. During the transition phase, the primary task is reappraisal of the first part of adulthood and redirection and change as determined by this examination of earlier life choices. The transition may be relatively easy or diffi-

cult, but it is characteristic of this phase to either make new life choices or reaffirm old choices.

The next phase is the settling-down phase. Here the individuals establish their niche in society (e.g., occupation, family, community) and work toward advancement. This is followed by the mid-life transition phase. Reappraisal of the settling-down period, and dealing with and resolving polarities between the individual's sense of her- or himself and the world. Levinson offers some examples of polarities such as: young/old, destructive/creative, masculine/feminine, and attachment/separateness. The most important task is coming to terms with real or impending biologic decline, accompanied by the recognition of mortality, as well as the societal attitudes that denigrate or devalue the status of middle age in favor of youth.

The next phase is another structure-building period. Having faced the polarities of the mid-life transition, the person now makes new choices or reaffirms old ones. As an individual moves to the end of this period, yet another structure-changing phase is entered as the person once again reevaluates upon entry into "old age."

Positive aging is out of the hands of rehabilitation therapists. However, the more therapists understand stages that men and women are likely to undergo as they age, the more responsive they can be to persons in their care. Developing a meaningful context within which the transformations of aging can be understood will be aided by information offered by all who work with the elderly, especially those involved in their day-to-day rehabilitation.

COGNITIVE CHANGES IN LATE LIFE

Are cognitive declines an inevitable consequence of aging? Is there a continuum from normal aging to pathological states such as Alzheimer's dementia. According to the Seattle Longitudinal Study only 20% of adults exhibited reliable age-related decline from 60 to 67 years of age; 36% experienced decline between 67 to 74 years; and more than 60% of elderly adults showed a decline between the ages of 74 to 81 years.[28] Community surveys indicate that more than 50% of people over age 60 report memory problems,[29] and Crook and associates found the incidence is even higher in people referred *to a geriatric screening program.*[30] However, normative studies are difficult to accomplish without contaminating the data to a certain degree. Normative studies of the elderly, without longitudinal follow-up, typically have included individuals with preclinical dementia who have begun to decline cognitively but still perform within normal limits on neuropsychological testing.[31,32] This results in an underestimation of true level of normal cognitive performance. Estimates of variability are inflated due to the mix of individuals with and without preclinical dementia and it is difficult to identify healthy elderly individuals who have unrecognized preclinical dementia.[32]

There is a significant variability in the pattern and rate of change in cognitive abilities. Verbal abilities reach peak performance in the sixth and seventh decades of life and reliable age-related decline does not occur until the middle of the eighth decade.[28]

Table 4–2 summarizes the changes in cognition generally associated with normal aging.[33]

Memory

Several important components of cognition are thought to be affected by age. These are memory, learning, affect, and reasoning. Each of these components of cognition will be discussed in terms of normal aging and pathological mechanisms.

Memory has been extensively studied for many years, and yet no definitive conclusions have been obtained.[34,35] Some studies show a decrease in memory with age, while others show no change.[34,35] Studies agree that older persons do have poorer techniques for organizing new information into a usable form that will impact information retrieval.[36] In addition, older persons perform better on more familiar memory tasks.[37] Older adults perform at a lower level on most memory tasks and tend to use more external (physical) rather than internal (mental) memory strategies.[38]

Some problems are inherent in research of aging memory. The population may have an undiagnosed pathology affecting memory. In addition, older persons do not perform as well in unfamiliar laboratories or in paper-and-pencil situations as younger subjects do.[37] Therefore, in the area of normal aging, there is no definitive conclusions as to decline or improvement in memory.

A recently defined clinical state, called age-associated memory impairment (AAMI), describes the loss of memory function in healthy persons aged 50 and over, and it is very modest. Nevertheless AAMI is common enough to be considered a feature of aging. In AAMI, memory complaints are reflected in everyday memory problems with gradually increasing memory loss. Inclusion criteria for this diagnosis include a score of 24 or greater on the Mini-Mental State Examination (MMSE) and a score of 9 or greater on the vocabulary subtest of the WAIS (see Chapter 6 for details on administration and scoring of these tools). The diagnosis of AAMI is excluded in the presence of any cognitive deterioration, confusion or delirium, brain disease, cerebral vascular pathology or head injury, any major psychiatric disorders (including depression), alcoholism, or drug dependency. The present use of any psychotropic drug that may affect cognitive functioning or any medical disorder that could produce cognitive deterioration are exclusion criteria for the diagnosis of AAMI.

The estimates of prevalence of AAMI vary widely from 18% to 85%.[30] The diagnosis of AAMI is a disputed entity. Some argue that it is really the preclinical phase of dementia,[31] while it has been found that most subjects with AAMI do not progress to Alzheimer's disease (AD).[32] Self-report of memory performance is congruent with actual memory ability.[39] AAMI is associated with impairments in executive functions and linked to self-efficacy, one's sense of competence and confidence related to a specific performance in a given domain. The differences between AAMI and Alzheimer's dementia are quite specific. Alzheimer's is the decline in cognitive functioning, particularly memory, that is unaccounted for by normal changes with aging and that cannot be explained by other medical or psychological conditions.[40] The *Diagnostic and Statistical Manual of Mental Disorder, Fourth Edition* (DSM-IV) definition of AD requires both a memory impairment and one or more of the following cognitive disturbances: aphasia, apraxia, agnosia, executive dysfunction. These impairments must significantly limit social or occupational functioning and represent a decline from a previous level of functioning. Studies suggest that cognitive deficits can be detected a minimum

TABLE 4–2. CHANGES IN COGNITION WITH NORMAL AGING

Cognitive Abilities	Changes
Intelligence	Performance scale of the WAIS shows more decline than the verbal scale
Problem solving	Declined delayed until late 6th decade
	Older adults may be less proficient on laboratory tests
Memory	
Sensory memory	Little if any decline
Short term memory	No decline
Long term (secondary)	Some decline; deficits in encoding processes; deficits more pronounced in free recall than recognition
Long term (remote)	Little decline
Psychomotor skills	Decline may begin in the early 50s
Information processing	Decline may begin in the early 50s
Verbal skills	Declines do not occur until after age of 80 if at all
Abstract reasoning	Mental flexibility or set shifting in reasoning task have been shown to decline

Compiled from: Riley KP. Cognitive Development. In Bonder BR, Wagner MB, eds. *Functional Performance in Older Adults*. Philadelphia, PA: FA Davis Company; 1994.

of one to seven years before clinical diagnosis of AD. This has been called the preclinical phase by some researchers.[31,32] One of the primary differences between AAMI and AD is that patients with pathological cognitive decline typically have MMSE scores of 23 and below and the cutoff score on the Global Deterioration Scale is 4.

Deterioration in any major cognitive domain, memory and learning, attention and concentration, thinking (e.g., problem solving, abstraction), language (e.g., comprehension, word finding), and visuospatial function, is termed age-associated cognitive disorder (AACD).[40] This diagnosis is based upon a comprehensive evaluation of cognition in which the person scores 1 SD below age- and education-specific standards in neuropsychological tests. In more involved symptomatology, memory performance is paired with learning.

Benign senescent forgetfulness is a term used to describe otherwise healthy elderly individuals who experience fleeting periods of cognitive decline relative to their age peers.[41] It is attributed more to inattentiveness and distractions than to the aging process per se. Most of us, regardless of age, experience lapses in memory primarily because we are not paying attention, are uninterested in the information, or in typical "work ethic" fashion—because we are multitasking! With sensory deficits, older adults may be unable to absorb and integrate information accurately, therefore giving the appearance of forgetfulness.

Pathologically, there are several implications of memory loss. First, complaints of memory loss (not actual memory loss) are related to depressive symptomatology.[42,43] Therefore, patient complaints about memory loss should alert the practitioner to check for depression. Actual memory loss is a classic characteristic of dementia or brain syndrome. (See the section on dementia later in this chapter for specifics on brain syndrome and memory loss.) Character features of depression can closely parallel those displayed by patients with subcortical dementia.[44] With depression, there is a tendency to significantly underestimate performance both before and after the task. A depressed individual is unlikely to make errors of intrusion or patently incorrect errors (false negatives). The tendency to give up easily saying "I don't know," or to make errors of omission is a more common feature with the depressed elder. Though there is a decrease in immediate recall, a depressed older adult retains information repeated over a period of time. Recognition performance is frequently normal in comparison to significantly impaired free recall scores on both immediate and delayed recall. This could be the result of weak or incomplete encoding strategies and with intervention for the depression, these scores can be reversed.[44] Depressed individuals have intact incidental learning, such as knowing places, recent events, and knowing names. They do better on retrieval of information if they are given more time and encouragement.[44]

In a study by King and associates,[45] verbal learning and memory performance of a group of elderly individuals with unipolar major depression were compared to that of nondepressed controls. The effect of age within this elderly sample was also examined, controlling for sex, educational attainment, and estimated level of intelligence. Except for verbal retention, the depressive individuals had deficits in most aspects of performance, including cued and uncued recall and delayed recognition memory. There were also interactions between depression effects and age effects on some measures. Performance for depressives declined more rapidly with age than did the performance of controls. This study shows that there is consistent evidence that elderly depressed persons have significant deficits in a range of explicit verbal learning functions.[45]

The neurochemical basis of cognitive dysfunction and memory loss is currently being explored.[45–51] This is more thoroughly discussed in relationship to Alzheimer's disease in Chapter 5, Pathological Manifestations of Aging.

One's sense of competence and confidence related to a specific performance in a given domain has also been found to affect memory. Some studies have found a lack of correlation between self-reports and cognitive performance.[52] This is likely due to expectations about aging and memory loss rather than declining abilities. A self-perceived negative assessment of memory functioning was found to be associated with greater concern about developing disease.[52] If memory loss is not viewed as a problem by the elderly themselves, it does not interfere with their level of functioning and the achievement of everyday goals and cognitive performance scores remain within normal ranges. There is also evidence that learning occurs into advanced age.[52]

Treatment techniques for memory loss include the use of classes and educational strategies to assist memory. Classes in self-esteem, accurate record keeping, and the use of mnemonic devices can be helpful. Two additional hints in helping memory are to keep techniques as familiar as possible and to develop some type of reward system. (Refer to Chapter 18, Education and the Older Adult: Learning, Memory, and Intelligence, for learning strategies.)

Intelligence and Learning

The actual measurement of intelligence is not possible; what can be measured is the performance of the person's intelligence. Performance can easily be influenced by health, motivation, and sensory acuity. Even though the word "intelligence" is used, it is not singular. Intelligence can be subdivided into fluid intelligence and crystallized intelligence.[53]

Crystallized intelligence depends on sociocultural influence and involves the ability to perceive relations, engage in formal reasoning, and understand intellectual and cultural heritage.[54] The growth of crystallized intelligence, even after age 60, can be obtained through self-directed learning and education.[55]

Fluid intelligence depends primarily on the genetic endowment of the individual and the individual's ability to use short-term memory, create concepts, perceive complex relationships, and undertake abstract reasoning. This involves items that are mostly neuropsychologic in nature, which may decline after 60.[56]

The implications of this information for the therapist hoping to capitalize on intellectual performance and learning follow.

1. Expect the intellectual ranges in older persons to be varied.
2. Poor performance may not mean poor learning.
3. Emphasize new knowledge that will be consistent with previous learning.[57]
4. Concentrate on one task at a time and be sure that the item is successfully learned before proceeding to the next.[56]
5. Reduce potential for distraction.
6. Space learning experiences sufficiently.
7. Allow for as much self-pacing as possible.
8. Assist older persons in organizing the information to be learned.
9. Present the information in the mode in which it will be used.[58]
10. Make the learning experience as concrete as possible.
11. Use supportive versus neutral instruction.
12. Use as many of the senses as possible to facilitate learning.
13. Provide as much feedback as possible.[59]

These suggestions have come from various studies[53–59] on changes in intelligence and performance and are presented as techniques to improve performance.

Affect and reasoning appear to remain unchanged as one ages.[55,56] Again, dementia and drug complications are the major causes of decline in these areas.[55,56] (See section later in this chapter for specific changes associated with dementia. Also see Chapter 8, Pharmacology, for changes associated with drug interventions.)

SITUATIONS REQUIRING COPING MECHANISMS

Depression

The statistics on the prevalence of depression are varied. Nevertheless, the following quote aptly describes what many medical professionals may see in the health care setting, "Depression has been termed the common cold of the elderly."[60] Many older people cope with the depressive symptoms, and the statistics are quite significant. Depending on the source, cited depressive illness can be found in 5% to 65% of the older population.[61,62] Nevertheless, studies show that

it is not aging per se that causes depression but the added variables of cognitive impairment, incontinence, chronic conditions, and disabilities, as well as significant personal and emotional losses.[63]

The DSM-IV[40] describes five categories of depression, all of which have relevance to geriatric patients. They are (1) major depression, (2) organic mood syndrome, (3) adjustment disorder with depression, (4) dysthymic disorder, and (5) dementia with depression.

A listing of symptoms of these disorders is found in Table 4–3. Major depression is characterized by having at least five of the symptoms listed for a period of at least two weeks. This type of disorder usually appears suddenly, and the symptoms are severe and are likely to end in a suicide attempt.[31] This disorder may occur in one single episode, or it may be recurrent with partial or full remissions between episodes. Mania, or euphoria, can occur between the episodes, but this is more characteristic of bipolar disease, which is much more severe.

Organic mood syndrome is related to a specific organic cause. For example, a patient with a cerebrovascular accident (particularly patients with hemisphere lesions) may suffer from this type of depression. Endocrinopathies; hypo- or hyperthyroidism, and excessive psychotropic medication are also typical organic factors associated with an organic mood syndrome.[64]

An adjustment disorder with depression is usually the result of a depressive reaction to a psychosocial stressor, such as a physical disability. It is only considered a depressive disorder when the symptoms last longer than six months. The major symptom is a depressed mood that impairs physical and social functioning in excess of what one would expect from the physical stressor.

TABLE 4–3. DEPRESSIVE SYMPTOMS

Cognitive Symptoms:	Poor concentration
	Low self-esteem
	Indecisiveness
	Guilt
	Hopelessness
	Inability to concentrate
	Suicidal ideations
Somatic Symptoms:	Fatigue
	Altered sleep patterns
	Weight gain or loss
	Tearfulness
	Agitation
	Heart palpitations
	Overall weakness
Affective Symptoms:	Sadness
	Anxiety
	Irritability
	Fear
	Anger
	Depersonalization
	Feelings of isolation (loneliness)

Dysthymic disorders represent the most difficult treatment challenge of all the diagnostic categories. Patients with this type of disorder display at least two of the depressive symptoms listed in Table 4–3 over a period of two years. In addition, these patients do not maintain a normal mood for longer than two months. This disorder may be a consequence of a pre-existing disorder, such as rheumatoid arthritis.

Dementia with depression is seen in the early stages of the dementia process as the person realizes that he or she is losing cognitive function. This early manifestation of depression may successfully hide the beginning stages of the dementia.

From the description of the different types of depressions, it becomes obvious how important the clinical interview can be. This interview is the first and most important aspect of the evaluation of depression. During the interview, the clinician asks about the history of this and previous episodes, the patient's responses to any interventions used in previous episodes, the history of drug or alcohol use, and the patient's social and physical functioning. The next stage is a complete clinical examination including routine laboratory studies. The clinician may also choose to do a mental status examination. (See Chapter 6, Assessment Instruments, for a complete explanation of use and implications of mental status examinations and depression scales.)

The clinician can also choose to conduct biological marker studies for dexamethasone suppression or titrated imipramine binding, as well as optional tests, such as magnetic resonance imaging (MRI). However, it should be noted that these tests are still somewhat controversial as to their usefulness in a differential diagnosis,[63] because they are not definitive for diagnosing other psychological problems. Paper-and-pencil tests and psychological interviews prove just as useful in detecting various dementia and depressions as the more expensive tests. Therefore, physicians should be skeptical when using biological markers to prove a differential diagnosis between dementia and depression.

The treatment of depression consists of a four-pronged approach involving psychotherapy, pharmacotherapy, electroconvulsive therapy (ECT), and family therapy. The benefits of insight-oriented psychotherapy have been questioned, in contrast to the benefits of behavioral and educationally oriented therapy, which appears to be quite helpful in older depressed patients.[65]

Anyone who talks to the patient in essence is providing psychotherapy. Therefore, the physical and occupational therapist should be aware of the treatment plans and goals for the individual patient. In addition, the therapist should be aware of some of the themes that emerge when working with the depressed older person. Older depressed patients must learn to adjust to new family roles, body image, and a measure of dependency, and they must learn to accept these changes without shame and continue to maintain intimacy with loved ones. In addition, patients must learn

healthier coping mechanisms. For example, anticipating future discomfort, rather than denying future difficulties, is a healthier choice. Using humor, sublimation, and altruism helps the patient focus less on the illness and depression and more on other situations.

Pharmacotherapy primarily involves the use of antidepressants. (For specific information on the use of antidepressants, see Chapter 8.) A general rule on the use of antidepressants is to start the dose at one-third to one-half the adult dose; the clinician and patient must realize, therefore, that it may take three to four weeks before a significant response occurs. The clinician also needs to remember that the therapeutic-to-toxic dose range is narrow with these kind of drugs. If any side effects are noted, the therapist, patient, or both should consult a pharmacist or physician immediately.

Electroconvulsive shock therapy (ECT) is regaining popularity, and it can be very useful in the treatment of severe depressions that are resistant to pharmacological management. It may be especially useful in older patients because of the absence of cardiovascular side effects. The major side effects of ECT are memory loss and confusion, however, these can be decreased with unilateral nondominant application.[66]

Family therapy has proven to be a double-edged sword. The family must be helped to cope with the patient's depression, and the family must learn how to be effective with the older patient. Family therapy involves several strategies, such as conflict resolution, problem solving, and family role assessment. The family can err in several ways, especially by being too helpful, thereby inhibiting the patient's autonomy. They can also deny the problem and display an overly optimistic attitude that overwhelms the older patient.

Social Isolation

Social isolation can be divided into four types.[67,68] One is geographic isolation, and it is a result of territorial restriction. The second, presentation isolation, results from an unacceptable appearance, while the third, behavioral isolation, results from unacceptable actions. Finally, attitudinal isolation arises from cultural or personal bound values. Any one of these types or any combination of them, bars the older person from full acceptance by others. This will cause the person to feel alienated and out of step, and it will affect his or her self-esteem.

Geographic Isolation Geographic isolation is usually a result of widowhood, urban crowding, rural life-style, or institutionalization. In all of these situations the older person may be alienated. For example, in the urban situation older people may be faced with a fast-paced, depersonalized lifestyle that gives them little opportunity to come in contact with close friends. (Institutionalization will be discussed in the next section.) The intervention techniques for geographic isolation include building upon formal and informal support systems.

TABLE 4–4. SUPPORT SYSTEMS FOR GEOGRAPHICAL ISOLATION

TABLE 4–4. SUPPORT SYSTEMS FOR GEOGRAPHICAL ISOLATION

Formal Support Systems:	Involvement in social issues for seniors Senior centers Volunteer activities Friends of the library National Retired Teachers Association Retired Senior Volunteer Program Foster grandparenting programs Grandparenting (child care)
Information Support Systems:	Neighbors/Friends/Family Social groups Home or nursing home therapists Medical visits (office or home) Pets Fictional kin (books-on-tape, soap operas) Beauty salons, restaurants, shops, etc. Housekeepers Retirement communities Churches

Table 4–4 lists formal and informal support systems.[68] In addition, the older person must examine the ramifications of any move they plan for an extended period of time in terms of the significance and size of the social support system they will be leaving behind versus the one they will be gaining.

Presentation Isolation Unfortunately, in our society many judgments are made on superficial appearance, and as the body ages, its appearance no longer conforms to the Madison Avenue stereotype. On top of this is the disfigurement that accompanies many physical disabilities associated with aging. The physical therapist can help older patients to deal with presentation isolation in several ways:

1. By teaching them to avoid overexposure to individuals with similar image deficiencies, because the older person may capitalize on their weaknesses rather than their strengths.
2. By helping them to establish new relationships with people that can accept them as they are now.
3. By giving lots of positive feedback on present strengths.
4. By asking questions to see what the person really thinks about themselves, and what experience they have had with similar conditions.
5. By teaching them to develop reasonable expectations.[67]

Behavioral Isolation Behavioral isolation occurs when an older person displays behaviors that are unacceptable. The behaviors most likely to fall into this category are eccentricity, confusion, incontinence, and deviant behavior. The physical or occupational therapist can play a role by helping the person to identify the behavior and seek appropriate intervention for alleviating the problem.

Attitudinal Isolation Attitudinal isolation is strongly entrenched in society's response to the older person. (Society's response will be discussed later in this chapter.) Ageism and the belief that it is acceptable and expected for older persons to be lonely are held by both the older person and the health professional. The intervention for this type of isolation is for both groups to evaluate their prejudices and misconceptions. In addition, the therapist must explore whether or not it is, in fact, desirable for the older person to be alone. To do this, the therapist should understand the difference between loneliness and being alone. Loneliness is a state of longing and emptiness, whereas being alone is being apart, solitary, and undisturbed. Figure 4–1 shows Maslow's factors of loneliness and isolation,[68] which may help the rehabilitation therapist in this assessment.

Institutionalization

Institutionalization appears to be a bizarre subheading under "situations requiring coping mechanisms." Nevertheless, organizational structure can have a profound impact on an individual's behavior. The classic text on the behavioral effects of institutionalization is *Asylums* by Goffman.[69] He identifies five aspects of a total institution (any institution where an individual spends 24 hours a day in residence), and they are

1. A hierarchical authority exists with residents on the lowest rung. This type of authority results in situations where the staff is always right, and the residents are punished or reprimanded.
2. Total institutions take control of personal habits. For example, mealtimes are regulated, as well as urination and defecation. This makes it difficult for the resident to satisfy personal needs in an efficient way.
3. Residents of institutions are often made to feel humiliated, and an example of this is that many residents of institutions are not allowed to close their doors.
4. The setting often makes it impossible for the person to engage in face-saving behaviors. Any defensive behavior a resident may take after being rebuked may then become the focus of a new attack. For example, if a resident becomes angry because the doors must remain open, the staff may then begin to rebuke the resident for inappropriate anger.
5. The person's status within the institution is solely defined by his or her status within the institution and any outside roles are rarely counted. For example, a physical therapist who has worked hard for years to help people in an outside role will be treated the same as a criminal in an institution.

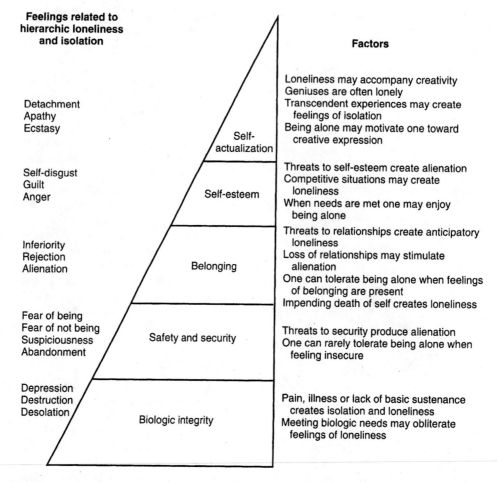

Figure 4–1.   Factors of loneliness and isolation. *(Adapted from Ebersol P., Hess P.* Towards health aging: human needs and nursing response. *St. Louis, Mosby Co.; 1981, with permission.)*

Interventions for helping the older person cope with institutionalization, short of changing the entire system, begin with the individual. The following list gives ways to help personalize the institutional setting for the clinician working with an older patient population.

1. Develop meaningful relationships.
2. Give accurate information.
3. Involve the family.
4. Recognize accomplishments with plaques, posters, and so forth.
5. Recognize and address people by their preferred name.
6. Recognize birthdays on the appropriate day.
7. Provide memorials for residents that have died.
8. Conduct life reviews.
9. Establish contacts with plants, pets, and children.
10. Every person must have some personal items with them.
11. Room sharing should only be done with a compatible resident.
12. Provide legal aid to protect the resident's rights.
13. Provide choices in all matters.

Anxiety Disorders

Anxiety disorders in the older person are frequently underreported and missed.[70] The incidence of anxiety disorders increases with age and is more frequent in women than in men.[71,72] Anxiety disorders either present with symptoms of fear, worry, or nervousness, or as a somatic problem without any physical cause. The DSM-IV of the American Psychiatric Association identifies three classes of disorders that share the characteristic of anxiety.[40] These three classes are (1) adjustment disorders with anxious mood, (2) anxiety states, and (3) phobic states. Table 4–5 shows the most common anxiety disorders and their central features.

In the assessment of anxiety disorders, the clinician should be aware of the descriptions listed in Table 4–5, as well as some of the frequent symptoms associated with anxiety in the elderly. While the list is quite extensive, several symptoms are seen more frequently by occupational and physical therapists,[73] and these include tremor, headaches, chest pain, weakness and fatigue, neck and back pain, dry mouth, dizziness, paresthesia, and a nonproductive

TABLE 4-5. THE ANXIETY DISORDERS AND THEIR CENTRAL FEATURES

Disorder	Central Features
Adjustment disorder with anxious mood	Nervousness/anxiety in reaction to identifiable psychosocial stressor
Anxiety states	Persistent or recurrent anxiety not provoked by identifiable stimulus, generally non-situational
Obsessive-compulsive disorder	Intrusive thoughts and/or repetitive behaviors performed under a sense of pressure Attempts to resist increased anxiety
Posttraumatic stress disorder	Acute and delayed reactions to a traumatic event Involves "reliving" the experience, emotional numbing, and development of somatic symptoms
Panic disorder	Sudden, unpredictable panic attacks involving intense apprehension and physical symptoms
Generalized anxiety disorder	Generalized, persistent anxiety for more than one month Includes three of the following: motor tension, autonomic hyperactivity, apprehension, and hypervigilance
Phobic disorders	Persistent, irrational fear or anxiety provoked by stimulus object, activity, or situation Avoidance of stimulus Fear recognized by patient as irrational or excessive
Agoraphobia	Feared stimulus: being alone or in a public place where escape would be difficult or help hard to find Occurs with or without panic attacks
Social phobia	Fear stimulus: social situations involving possible embarrassment or humiliation
Simple phobia	Fear stimulus: situations similar to a previous terrifying experience

Adapted and reprinted with permission from *Geriatrics*. August 1985; 40(8):80.

cough.[73] The presence of these symptoms does not mean that the older person has an anxiety disorder, because there may be physical causes as well as organic causes, such as caffeine, hypoglycemia, or thyroid disease. In addition, therapists should screen for the symptoms of depression already described, as depression may cause some of the symptoms of anxiety disorders.

Finally, physical and occupational therapists should seek additional information. For example, a patient may not tell you that she has a simple phobia; however, when you visit her at home, she may tell you that people are spying on her, listening to her through the walls, and tapping the phone. In further conversations, you discover that this patient had a terrifying experience as a child when she was left alone or when she was harassed and abused by Nazi soldiers. In this instance, the patient has developed a "simple phobic" reaction to always having people around—seen in terms of spying on her—to avoid her deep-seated fear of being alone.

The treatment for anxiety disorders is condensed in Table 4-6. In treating anxiety disorders, the therapist can act in several ways. First, the physical or occupational therapist can alert the physician to the problem. Second, the therapist may be able to share additional information collected from the frequent rehabilitation therapy sessions. Third, the therapist can play an integral role in any of the behavioral therapies. Finally, the therapist can teach the patient stress management techniques, stress reduction interventions, and assertiveness ideas. These will be discussed in detail at the end of this chapter.

Chronic Illness

As mentioned earlier in this chapter, the importance of coping with chronic illness is imperative for successful aging. In the older population, the percentage of persons with physical illness is staggering. According to Weg, 70% of people over the age of 65 have some type of chronic illness.[74] The three major illnesses for older persons are (1) heart conditions, (2) visual impairments, and (3) arthritis.[74] These types of chronic illnesses can be mild, thereby causing only minimal adaptations or lifestyle changes, or they can be devastating and cause major lifestyle modification. Serious illness or a devastating life event can cause profound changes in a person's appreciation of life,[75] and often this will result in a shift in goals, relationships, and values.

Physical and occupational therapists can recognize their roles in this area by enhancing the older patient's new realizations and thought processes. The following list offers some suggestions to enhance this process.

1. Realize that patients may have a heightened sense of beauty and of caring relationships.
2. Provide opportunities for the patient to talk about these new changes in values.
3. Encourage the patient in these new realizations, and let them know that these types of thoughts are part of the growth process.
4. Foster communication between the patient and their family, especially in light of the patient's new values.

TABLE 4–6. ANXIETY DISORDERS AND THEIR MANAGEMENT

Disorders	Management
Adjustment disorder with anxious mood	Supportive "brief psychotherapies" Stress management techniques Assertiveness training Interventions to eliminate or reduce stressors
Anxiety states Obsessive-compulsive disorder	Tricyclic antidepressants Avoid use of benzodiazepines Psychotherapy
Posttraumatic stress disorder	Crisis intervention techniques Supportive brief psychotherapies
Panic disorder	Short-acting benzodiazepines Frequent evaluations of medication effects; avoid abrupt withdrawal Shield eyes from fluorescent lights Stress management techniques
Generalized anxiety disorder	Short-acting benzodiazepines, with frequent evaluations; avoid abrupt withdrawal Supportive "brief psychotherapies" Stress management techniques
Phobic disorders Agoraphobia	Avoid use of most benzodiazepines Daily tricyclic antidepressants or MAO inhibitors With panic attacks, shield eyes from fluorescent lighting
Social phobia	Behavior therapies
Simple phobia	Behavior therapies

Adapted and reprinted with permission from *Geriatrics.* August 1985; 40(8):80

5. Suggest participating in discussion groups for patients recovering from similar conditions.

Death, Dying, Grief, and Multiple Losses

These final situations that require coping mechanisms fit together well because the insights, manifestations, and mechanisms of coping for each are similar. The legal and ethical aspects of death and dying will be discussed in Chapter 17.

Many people think of aging as a time of loss. In reality, aging represents not just one loss, rather it is a time of multiple losses. Some of the most common losses include the loss of the patient's mobility, productivity, usefulness, body image, time left to live, health, income, and status. These and other losses occur throughout life, however, their frequency increases with old age, and their cumulative effect increases the emotional impact as a person ages. Another very important variable affecting loss is the person's general personality and their ability to tolerate loss. Some people view loss as giving up what one had, while others focus happily on what they have.

The physical or occupational therapist constantly works with people who have lost something, whether it is health, mobility, body image, or independence. The therapist's role is extremely important. To evaluate the loss, the therapist must consider if the loss is simple, compound, or symbolic. Losing $10.00 might be simple—if the person is financially healthy. However, if that $10.00 was borrowed with high interest to pay a long-standing debt, then it becomes compound and more emotional. In another situation, the

$10.00 may be the first money ever received in a business and, therefore, may be symbolic. When evaluating a loss, first check for its type by assessing its significance and by discussing it with the patient and family.

To assist the person, be sure to review the loss with the person and any supportive family and friends. Remember to constantly reorient the person to the reality of the situation. The therapist should not make false promises and set unrealistic goals (see Chapter 14 for treatment suggestions to assist patients with limb loss). Be realistic and set short-term, attainable goals. Watch for signs of chronic grief.

Symptoms of a single loss should subside in six weeks, however, it may take longer in old age to resolve grief.[76] The symptoms are weakness, tiredness, sighing, and digestive symptoms. The patient may exhibit feelings of anger, deprivation, and guilt, but chronic grief in the older person may be much more subtle. For example, they may not cry, but they may sigh frequently when talking or complain of constant tiredness. The most useful treatment suggestion for the physical or occupational therapist working with a grief-stricken patient is to listen and care. This can help bridge the isolation. A recommendation for psychological counseling is also imperative.

To some, the death of an older person is viewed as a blessing or the final chapter in a full and rich life. This, unfortunately, does not hold for all older people, because many older people feel they are not ready to die and that they have not fulfilled their lives. According to Kalish, though, the fear of death diminishes as one ages.[77] This may be due to the increased exposure to dying with the aging of family and friends.

Dying has a special significance for the older patient. The following list gives six areas that are different for the older versus the younger patient.

1. Older persons tend to reminisce as a way of integrating their life prior to dying.
2. Older people are less likely to have an advocate. This is especially true for older women, because they tend to outlive their husbands.
3. Older persons are less able to be communicative than younger patients when dying because of brain syndromes or confusion. This lack of communicative ability makes it more difficult for the health team to provide caring without a reciprocal response.
4. Older people may get less than optimum care because of the belief that they will die soon anyway.
5. The social value of an older person's life is thought to be less than that of younger person's.[77]

Much has been written about the process of dying. The most well-known author in this area is Kübler-Ross. She is most well known for her stages of dying, which are (1) denial, (2) anger, (3) bargaining, (4) depression, and (5) acceptance.[78] Even though her stages have not been proven to be consistent, they have received great acceptance. In interpreting her stages, it is important to note that not all people go through all the stages. For example, someone may not experience anger and go straight from denial to bargaining. In addition, there are no time limits on these various stages. Other studies have postulated stages of the dying or grief process. Bowlby[79] and Engel,[80] for example, have similar stages but end their stages with the process of reorganization.

The interventions for therapists working with the dying patient are to enhance the older person's ability to die with dignity and achieve final growth, and this can be done by recognizing impediments to growth. (These impediments are described in the sections on isolation and institutionalization.)

In addition, the physical or occupational therapist can help to fulfill the unmet needs of the dying person. The most common unmet needs are freedom from pain and loneliness, conservation of energy, and maintenance of self-esteem. Physical therapists are well versed in pain management, and a full discussion of loneliness can be found in the isolation section.

Physical and occupational therapists can also provide environmental and ergonometric assessment by evaluating an older patient's daily program and provide helpful suggestions to the patient and caregiver to reduce excessive energy expenditure. Finally, there are a few helpful hints for bolstering the self-esteem of an older person who is dying. Be sure that their physical comfort is assured (e.g., cleanliness, personal appearance, and lack of odor). Therapists should use as much sensory feedback as possible in the visual, auditory, and tactile realms. Also, therapists should focus on the immediate future and present opportunities; they should not confuse their values with those of the dying person's. Dying is very individual, and everyone perceives it differently.

The final topic under death, dying, grief, and loss focuses on the health care provider. It is imperative that the provider working with dying patients realizes the extreme amount of stress in this situation. Harper has developed stages that health care providers may experience when working with dying patients for a one- to two-year period.[81] They are

1. *Intellectualization* usually occurs in the beginning of employment. The health professional is quite accurate about their job, however, they avoid discussions about death.
2. *Emotional Survival* is characterized by an understanding of the pain and suffering. Here the provider may be unable to face—and may question—his or her own mortality.
3. Depression is a stage where the provider accepts the reality of death or quits. Feelings of grief are classic here.
4. *Emotional Arrival* is characterized by a deeper awareness and sensitivity of the dying person.
5. *Deep Compassion* is characterized by full maturity. Here the provider is extremely constructive and has clear emotions on his or her own and others' issues of death.[81]

DELIRIUM

The syndrome of delirium is a common, serious, and often life-threatening condition in the elderly patient. Often unrecognized, it is the second most common syndrome involving cognitive failure in the geriatric population.[82] It may be the most common adverse outcome of hospitalization and surgery in older patients.[83,84]

Though there are many synonyms used to describe this clinical state (e.g., acute brain syndrome, acute confusional state, metabolic encephalopathy, toxic or exogenous psychosis[85]), the DSM-IV[40] defines delirium as an abrupt change in mental status and behavior, with global, fluctuating impairment in cognitive processes and alterations in attention. There is disturbed psychomotor activity, disorientation, disordered thinking, and inability to correctly process information from the environment. As a result, memory is impaired and the patient is easily distracted and has difficulty concentrating and following commands. Behavioral changes may range from withdrawal to agitation, with or without psychotic symptoms. Illusions and paranoid ideation frequently occur due to misinterpretation of visual or auditory stimuli. Sleep-wake disturbances and sundowning (increased agitation in late afternoon and early evening) are common.[82,84]

Delirium can be a sign of multiple diseases and medical syndromes. When it is acute it is usually caused by drugs or medical illnesses and is often reversible. In the elderly, it may be the first clinical sign of an acute medical or surgical emergency.[82] The syndrome of delirium in the hospitalized patient is associated with increased morbidity, mortality and rate of institutionalization, as well as increased length of stay and cost of hospitalization.[86]

Etiologies of delirium, dominated by drug causes and medical conditions, can be divided into several categories, including vascular causes, infections, nutritional causes, drugs, injury, cardiac causes, autoimmune causes, tumors, and endocrinologic causes, as well as psychiatric and environmental problems. Drugs are the most common cause of delirium and can be accounted for by multiple factors that place the geriatric patient at risk for adverse drug reactions, intoxication, or withdrawal.[83] The elderly tend to have multiple medical problems requiring polypharmacy, which increases the chance of drug-drug interactions. Both prescription and nonprescription drugs may be involved.

Dementia is another strong risk factor for delirium.[87,88] Individuals with dementia are more sensitive to anticholinergic drugs and may be more sensitive to other insults as well. Many have baseline confusion, visuospatial and verbal dysfunction, and impaired responses to the environment.[89] Delirium in an individual with dementia is significantly more difficult to diagnose.

There are multiple other risk factors for the syndrome of delirium including depression, hypotension, azotemia, fever, fracture, infection, previous delirium, illicit substance abuse, and sensory deficits.[82] Malnutrition and hypoalbuminemia affect levels of protein-bound drugs and lead to greater toxic potential in those with CNS toxicity.[83] Vitamin B_{12} and thiamine deficiency can produce cognitive dysfunction.[90] Factors shown to increase risk in surgical patients include dementia, low cardiac output, perioperative hypotension, postoperative hypoxia, and use of anticholinergic drugs.[82] Other conditions associated with delirium include sleep deprivation, incontinence, fecal impaction, and changes in environment.[82]

It is important for the physical or occupational therapist to remember that each patient has a unique presentation that can change over the course of a few minutes. Symptoms and signs generally wax and wane.[84] The decreased awareness associated with the state is characteristically termed "clouding of consciousness"; this fluctuates between extremes of alertness to lethargy. Decreased awareness and inability to concentrate affect memory and cause misinterpretations and agitation, with changes in normal psychomotor activity, personality, and affect.[83] Generally, hyperactive states are typical of drug withdrawal delirium, and stuporous or hypervigilant states are more likely associated with altered metabolic states.[82]

Signs of increased motor activity include picking, pacing, and general restlessness. In the elderly, other major nonspecific presentations of disease such as new onset of falls or incontinence can also coexist. It might be prudent, then, to consider delirium as a possible reason for those elderly with new onset of falls or acute increase in falls.[83]

Immediate recall, short-term, and long-term memory may be impaired by the syndrome of delirium. Anterograde memory formation is impaired by inability to focus attention. Retrograde memory is affected by changes in cerebral neurotransmittors.[83] Disorders of speech are frequent in delirium and reflect disorganized thinking. Speech can be chaotic and disorganized, slurred or rapid, with use of neologisms and aphasic errors. Eating and sleeping patterns can be grossly abnormal. Disturbances in the sleep cycle can lead to "sundowning," which is frequently the first sign of the onset of delirium.[82,83]

Autonomic changes often occur in delirious patients, especially in those who have hyperactivity. Hypertension and tachycardia are the most common signs. Individuals with autonomic symptoms and signs frequently have increased irritability and startle responses, and are acutely sensitive to light and sound.[82]

General principles of managing patients with delirium include the first element, which is to provide enough fluids and nutrition to keep the patient from becoming dehydrated. A calm and quiet environment that enhances cognitive function, maximizes comfort, and minimizes environmental stress should be provided. A low level of lighting without shadows that can induce perceptual disturbances is optimal. Exposure to natural lighting through a window may be beneficial. Reorienting the individual frequently with simple, clear explanations for activities taking place is important. Having familiar objects, clocks, and calendars present will help with orientation. Eyeglasses and hearing aids should be in place to correct sensory deficits. Presence of familiar individuals, such as family members and friends is usually reassuring, and they can often help provide one-to-one observation when staffing is inadequate.

It is preferable to avoid restraining the agitated patient with delirium. Attempts to "escape" restraints often place the delirious patient at great risk for injury and falls.

Dementia

Millions of older Americans are victims of dementias. Because of this, dementia or cognitive impairment is the major cause of disability in older persons. The statistics are staggering: In the United States the estimated number of people suffering moderate to severe dementia ranges from 1.5 million to 2.3 million.[91,92] One study equates these figures to, "One family in every three will see one of their parents succumb to this disease."[91] The prevalence of dementia also increases with age. The estimate for people over 65 is 5%, but for those over 75, it is estimated that 20% will have some degree of cognitive impairment.[91] In addition, in the nursing home setting it is estimated that the prevalence reaches 50%.[93] Besides the amazing emotional burdens, the economic burdens are immense. The care for persons with Alzheimer's disease alone in 1983 was $31 billion.[94]

The categorization of Alzheimer's disease as a cognitive impairment emphasizes the need for precision when describing and categorizing pathologies. The categorization and description of the cognitive impairments of older persons is probably the most important aspect of its assessment and treatment, and yet descriptions and classifications are not always in perfect agreement. This chapter will generally follow a classification scheme derived from the works of Rossman, Eisdorfer, and Cohen.[95,96]

1. *Acute disorders.* These are potentially reversible. Under this subheading is delirium, depression, multiple causes, and accidents.
2. *Chronic disorders.* These are the irreversible cognitive impairments, including Alzheimer's disease, vascular disease, and subcortical disorders.
3. *Presenile dementias.* These diseases tend to be rarer and to occur in younger populations. They are also not reversible.

Acute cognitive disorders have been romanticized in American society. While acute disorders are reversible, their prevalence is not as great as was once reported.[97] In an article entitled "The Reversible Dementias: Do They Reverse?" the results showed only a 3% full resolution and an 8% partial resolution of the dementias.[98]

Despite the less than impressive response rates to treatment, it is still important to understand this aspect of dementia, because it can be reversed. Acute disorders often have multiple causes. Among these causes are drugs, translocation, infection, neoplasm, trauma, malnutrition, toxic states, metabolic imbalances, and depression. According to Clarfield, the most common reversible causes were drugs (28.2%), depression (26.2%), and metabolic changes (15.5%).[98]

The symptoms of this type of cognitive impairment (except for the acute delirium caused by depression) are characterized by a rapidly developing confusion state. The person will often display clouded, fluctuating consciousness accompanied by agitation. In addition the patient will have alterations in the following processes:

1. *Perception.* The person may be hypersensitive to light or sound and suffer from visual, auditory, or tactile hallucinations.
2. *Memory.* This can be significantly impaired—more so in the short term than in the long term. New information may be difficult to learn, possibly because of the delirious patient's decreased attention span.
3. *Thinking.* Delirious patients tend to have illogical and disjointed thoughts. They may have difficulty with problem solving and word finding. Finally, these patients may also have persecution delusions, which they may forget when they recover.
4. *Orientation.* The delirious patient classically is disoriented to time. They may lose orientation to place as the disease progresses, however they rarely lose orientation to person.
5. *Alertness.* The delirious patient may be either hypo- or hyperalert. They may display increased pulse or pressure or decreased alertness.

The manifestation of delirium due to depression differs in several major aspects. The depressed patient will have a slower onset of these symptoms, a longer history of somatic complaints, and a lower self-esteem. The depressed patient will tend to be on the hypo side of alertness. The greatest cognitive decline in the depressed patient will be the ability to process information, and this will be blunted. (For more information on depression in general see the previous section.)

The chronic causes of dementia or cognitive impairment are numerous, with Alzheimer's disease accounting for an estimated 50% of the chronic disorders.[94] Alzheimer's disease results from neuronal degeneration, and it is characterized by neurofibrillary tangles and plaques. However, neuritic plaques and neurofibrillary tangles—the hallmarks of Alzheimer's disease, have recently undergone intense study as scientists search for ways to delay, treat, and prevent the disease.[48,50] (See Chapter 5, Pathological Manifestations of Aging.) While the exact cause is unknown, some researchers theorize that Alzheimer's is genetically linked, metabolic,[49,51] or related to a slow virus.[48,50] The cognitive decline is very slow and gradual, and affects three times as many women as men. The findings from the Nun Study are of interest to the topic of cognition in the elderly.[99] Snowdon and associates[99] investigated the relationship of linguistic ability (as measured by hand-written autobiographies—diaries—completed between the ages of 19 and 37) in early life to the neuropathology of Alzheimer's disease and cerebrovascular disease. Findings from this component of the Nun Study indicate that low linguistic ability in early life has a strong association with dementia and premature death in late life. These researchers suggest that low linguistic ability in early life may reflect suboptimal neurological and cognitive development, which might increase susceptibility to the development of Alzheimer's disease pathology.[99] Further discussion of Alzheimer's disease can be found in Chapter 5, Pathological Manifestations of Aging, and Chapter 12, Neurological Treatment Considerations.

A second category of chronic dementia is vascular disease or multi-infarct dementia. This type of dementia affects twice as many men as women. The cognitive decline may be due to small cerebral infarcts, arteriosclerotic disease, major cerebrovascular accidents, vertebrobasilar insufficiency, diabetic deterioration of blood vessels, carotid atherosclerosis, and diffuse cerebrovascular ischemia. This type is characterized by a stepwise decline. An example of this type of dementia was varified in a study by Gregg and colleagues.[100] These researchers found that elderly diabetics scored significantly lower on three tests of cognitive function compared to non-diabetics. It is suggested that an understanding of the neurobiologic mechanisms underlying the association of dementias with vascular diseases could provide insight into both prevention and treatment of cognitive decline.

The third type of chronic dementias are the subcortical disorders. Korsakoff's psychosis is one cause of subcortical disorders, caused by prolonged vitamin B_1 deficiency, which is usually a result of alcoholism. In a study by Oscar-Berman and Pulaski,[47] association learning and recognition memory in elderly alcoholic men was compared to age-matched nonalcoholic men.[47] Wernicke's encephalopathy is a more advanced stage of this vitamin B_1 deficiency. Parkinson's disease can also cause irreversible dementia due to the dopamine deficiency. Finally, Huntington's chorea, which is genetically transmitted, can cause profound dementia.

The fourth type of chronic dementias are the presenile dementias. Creutzfeldt-Jakob disease is of particular interest to the geriatrician. Even though this disease can occur as early as the second decade of life, it generally occurs in the fifth to sixth decade. It is a rapidly dementing disease thought to be activated by a slow virus of genetic predisposition. Pick's disease is an extremely rare form of dementia involving the frontal and temporal regions that has symptoms similar to Alzheimer's disease and is often confused with Alzheimer's. It can only be definitively diagnosed at autopsy.

What separates the chronic dementias already noted from the acute dementias is their onset and permanence. All chronic dementias will show signs of cognitive impairment over a course of several months. The family may describe a slow loss of short-term memory with accompanying anxiety or depression. Unlike the acute dementias, the level of consciousness does not fluctuate.

The general characteristics of chronic brain syndrome can be summarized by the following mnemonic device, JAMCO.[5]

J— *Judgment*. The person may show inappropriate behavior as a result of improper information processing. For example, the patient walks out of his or her room undressed.

A— *Affect*. The person's affect is more labile, causing them to laugh or cry easily or uncontrollably. An example might be the patient who constantly giggles or weeps.

M— *Memory*. The person will lose their memory, first short-term and then long-term. An example might be the patient who evades current questions by relating anecdotes from the past, however, when forced to answer the current questions the patient is unable to do so.

C— *Cognition*. Cognition will be disjointed and illogical, as well as delusional and hallucinatory. The therapist may be talking to the patient about the patient's exercises and the patient may relate a story about the FBI watching the nursing home.

O— *Orientation*. The person may, in general, have a flat level of awareness. The therapist may find that if the patient is left alone to do exercises, they fall asleep or into a daydreaming state.[5]

Alzheimer's disease deserves additional description in terms of manifestations. Typically, three stages of AD are recognized. Occasionally a fourth stage is identified.[101] Hayter has described various stages of Alzheimer's disease.[102] The first stage lasts two to four years and is characterized by moodiness, hypochondriasis, time disorientation, lack of spontaneity, poor judgment, blaming others, and a sense of helplessness and worthlessness. Generally, the person has difficulty with social adaptation and may display catastrophic reactions to stressful events.

The second stage may last several years, and it is characterized by an increase in symptoms. At this point the person is usually in the health care system (e.g., hospital or nursing home) due to unsafe behaviors, such as constant movement, paranoia and hallucinations, and physical abusiveness. The person may display sleep pattern disturbances, as well as incontinence. The third or final stage has no time limit and is characterized by irritability, seizures, disorientation on all spheres, illogical communication, severe anorexia, rigid postures, and explosive sounds and behaviors.

With all the various types and manifestations of dementia, assessment can be very difficult. Assessing orientation (patient is oriented times three) is not enough because frequently cognitive impairment is missed or dementia and depression are confused. For example, a well-known study found that 64% of the residents of a rehabilitation unit had significant cognitive impairment, yet physicians were unaware of the deficit in 15% of the cases.[103] In addition, Lazarus and associates noted a significant coexistence of depression and dementia in older patients and described methods of differentiating such complications.[104]

What should be in a mental status evaluation and what should be the goals of such an examination? Some suggested goals are to establish a baseline, screen for dementia or depression, determine the patient's ability to follow a rehabilitation program, identify cognitive impairment, and evaluate motor and language skills.[105] The suggested components of a mental status evaluation that can be used by the rehabilitation professional in daily practice are:

Cortical functioning. Including orientation, attention, concentration, memory, judgment, reasoning, and calculation. Ask questions about the patient's current situation.

Perceptual functioning. Assess the deficits of the sensory system. Present information with varying intensities of sensory input (e.g., talk loudly and then softly and check the patient's response).

Speech and thought functioning. Examine appropriateness of questions and statements. Ask questions and note carefully the context appropriateness and complexity of the answer.

Emotional functioning. Assess affect, mood, and flexibility. Discuss emotionally charged issues, and note the resident's response.

General appearance. Note posture, dress, hygiene, expressions, motor responses, and general behavior.[105]

The simple and brief tests that meet these goals range from the Blessed Dementia Scale[106] to Pfeiffer's Short Portable Mental Status Questionnaire.[107] Nevertheless, one of the most widely used tools for assessing cognitive impairment in the clinical setting is the Mini-Mental State Exam.[108] This can be easily administered in less than half an hour, and it meets the criteria already given. (See Chapter 6 for details on administration and scoring of this test.)

Unfortunately, cognitive impairment cannot be assessed by simply administering a simple paper and pencil test. The administration of mental status tests may be very difficult with a demented patient. Often these patients are resentful or suspicious. In addition, they may have developed evasive skills that may fool the novice evaluator. To minimize these complications, the evaluator should explain clearly and honestly why the test is being administered, and that although some of the items may seem silly, it is important that the individual try to answer them. The therapist should also let the patient know that they will have plenty of time to answer. If the patient appears to avoid questions or to be guessing, the evaluator should repeat the question at a later time, possibly in a different form.

The final aspect of the cognitive impairment evaluation is the recognition of its physiological manifestations. Since the rehabilitation professional is most likely to see the patient on a frequent basis, he or she may notice these abnormalities, which include altered vital signs, such as an increase or a decrease in heart rate, blood pressure, or respiration. The skin may change in color, wetness, and temperature. Finally, the person could also display changes in neurological, cardiorespiratory, gastrointestinal, or urinary functions. It should be noted that all of these manifestations may be a result of an infection, drug complications, or an undetected pathology that can be corrected and may result in a decrease or amelioration of cognitive impaired status.[104]

What is the physical or occupational therapist's role in working with the patient with cognitive impairment? A diagnosis of Alzheimer's is often a cause for denial of payment for physical and occupational therapy. Many intermediaries cite the inability of Alzheimer's patients to learn as a reason for denial, because rehabilitation is structured around learning, the benefits derived would be minimal. While this argument has its merits, Alzheimer's patients can learn. In addition, therapy is more than learning. A large part of rehabilitation is environmental and physical modification. For example, if a patient with Alzheimer's disease is sent to physical therapy because of muscle weakness in the legs and an increased incidence of falls, then the physical therapist would be judicious in administering a strengthening program on a daily basis to the weakened muscles. Also, an environmental assessment for potential falls might be indicated. Occupational therapy may often be involved in activities that assist the demented patient in reorienting to their surroundings. Therefore, it is appropriate to design and execute programs for the cognitively impaired elderly with treatable functional decline. In addition, the training and education of the family is crucial to any in-home rehabilitation program.

Some general guidelines for working with the cognitively impaired elderly follow.[109]

1. *Simplify.* That includes simplifying the instructions, programs, and environment.
2. *Explain.* This should be done thoroughly, frequently, constantly, and repetitively, if necessary.
3. *Reorient.* In normal conversation, if possible, remind the patient of the time, place, and activity. Have clocks, calendars, and orienting pictures in view.
4. *Slow down.* Take your time in all aspects. Have a slow, low voice.
5. *Avoid change.* Change should be avoided in the environment, with the personnel, and in all aspects of programming, if possible.
6. *Encourage familiarity.* The environment should have as many familiar objects as possible, exercises should mimic familiar activities, and familiar people should be encouraged to visit.
7. *Touch.* Encourage as much touching as possible. This conveys caring and support to a patient who is going through an uncontrollable change and may desperately need support.
8. *Encourage independence.* This may necessitate simplifying commands and labeling items for ease of recognition.
9. *Respect individual dignity.* Encourage the patient to discuss and demonstrate previous successes and accomplishments. Display pictures of the patient in memorable moments. Respect modesty and dignity.
10. *Educate and support the family.* Be prepared to confront denial in the family and patient. Provide information on additional support services for cognitively impaired patients (see Chapter 22, Aging Network Resources, for listing). Frequently bring up the topic of additional support. (Families

frequently refuse initial offerings of help.) Reinforce that the patient's behavior is not volitional. Offer helpful suggestions for ways to tell others about the disease when the family is ready.

11. *Listen to the patient.* Even if the patient is not making sense try to listen. Every once in awhile a lucid statement will be verbalized.

12. *Take care of yourself.* Working with cognitively impaired patients can be emotionally exhausting. If a patient is combative or abusive, tell the patient that this type of behavior upsets you and take time out from the patient.

BELIEF SYSTEMS REGARDING THE AGING PROCESS

Ageism is the term Butler coined to denote a prejudice against a person or group of persons due to their age.[110] A myth is a belief that a person holds with or without the appropriate facts to gain control of an ambiguous situation. Society holds many of these beliefs. The current belief that is biased toward youth sprung out of the post-depression era. The focus for hope shifted from the older generation to the new, bright-futured baby boomers. The parents who had nothing growing up in The Depression could now give it all to their children with the hope that they would make a better world. The focus unfortunately shifted from the older population. This shift has combined with the birth of high technology and self-absorption and has led to low self-esteem and negative attitudes for older people.

The Facts on Aging Quiz, by Erdman Palmore (Fig. 4–2) is an important tool for assessing bias against older persons.[111] To score this quiz, all the odd-numbered questions are false, and all the even-numbered questions are true. This quiz can be used to test a person's myths, biases, and knowledge.

The problem of ageism or negative attitudes toward older people are particularly pronounced in the health arena. Older patients may be seen as complaining, somatasizing, uninteresting, or helpless. In addition they may not receive the same services as younger persons. In the United States, for example, physicians are often overaggressive with diagnostic tests for older persons but less aggressive in providing rehabilitation services,[112] and physical therapists have been shown to be less aggressive in goal setting for older patients.[113]

The evaluation and treatment of the social misinterpretation of aging is not an easy task. Both the evaluation and the treatment must begin on a personal level. Self-evaluation of myths, belief systems, and the personal evaluation of individual patients must be done daily.

A simple treatment is to show others (by example) healthy and positive ways of working with older persons. The ultimate goal is not to display negative prejudices to other groups in hopes of valuing the older population, but to develop a society with a healthy mixture and respect for all groups. A society to strive for would be one of bright youths, secure middle-aged adults, and wise older persons.

LIFESTYLE ADAPTATION, STRESS

Retirement, illness, and changes in living conditions are all possible lifestyle adaptations in late life. Are these good or bad situations? Do they cause growth or decline? A simple way of viewing some of these lifestyle adaptations is through the stress mechanism. Stress, as defined by Hans Selye, is the response of the body to any demand made on it.[114] Stress has both a physical and psychological component.

On the physical level, stress has been shown to increase the secretion of adrenalin and cortisol, as well as lower the body's sensitivity to insulin and its tolerance to carbohydrates.[115] These physiological changes can cause an increase in blood pressure, as well as a decrease in the body's immune system's ability to combat various diseases. Chronic stress in older people may result in a decreased caloric intake, a lowered body weight, and a lowered lymphocyte count. In addition, older individuals who have experienced this stress response will show an increased systolic pressure and mean arterial pressure, and some degree of left ventricular hypertrophy.[116]

Stress can be both good and bad, and Selye describes both.[114] Eustress is good stress and can be used for growth. A lack of eustress can be exemplified by an older person who sits all day and does nothing, with little initiative or interest. They have no need or desire to adapt or respond to their environment. A possible intervention is placing a hungry, lonely kitten in the same environment. When the older patient begins to take care of this kitten, they will adapt to the new stimulus, and the kitten will give the person something to work for and with. Therefore, the kitten could be considered a eustress.

Bad stress is called distress.[114] The same kitten could be an example of distress if, one month later, it was run over by a truck. The older person would experience loss and a negative need to adapt.

Before evaluating stress, retirement deserves special mention. Retirement is also an example of a lifestyle adaptation that can prove to be good or bad. Retirement presents an emotion-laden change because work fulfills many social needs, and perhaps most importantly, work bestows a status. A physical or occupational therapist, for example, knows their status at a social gathering, with patients, and within the medical community. What is the status of a retiree? Work also fixes associations. For example, the physical therapist knows that they will see Bob, the nurse, Jane, the social worker, etc. Who does the in-home retiree see on a regular basis?

Work also regulates activity. The rehabilitation therapist knows that she or he works from nine to

Facts on Aging Quiz

Please take this short "Facts on Aging Quiz"

T F **1.** The majority of old people (past age 65) are senile (i.e., defective memory, disoriented, or demented).

T F **2.** All five senses tend to decline in old age.

T F **3.** Most old people have no interest in, or capacity for, sexual relations.

T F **4.** Lung capacity tends to decline in old age.

T F **5.** The majority of old people feel miserable most of the time.

T F **6.** Physical strength tends to decline in old age.

T F **7.** At least one-tenth of the aged are living in long-stay institutions (i.e. nursing homes, mental hospitals, homes for the aged, etc.)

T F **8.** Aged drivers have fewer accidents per person than drivers under age 65.

T F **9.** Most older workers cannot work as effectively as younger workers.

T F **10.** About 80% of the aged are healthy enough to carry out their normal activities.

T F **11.** Most old people are set in their ways and unable to change.

T F **12.** Old people usually take longer to learn something new.

T F **13.** It is almost impossible for most old people to learn new things.

T F **14.** The reaction time of most old people tends to be slower than reaction time of younger people.

T F **15.** In general, most old people are pretty much alike.

T F **16.** The majority of old people are seldom bored.

T F **17.** The majority of old people are socially isolated and lonely.

T F **18.** Older workers have fewer accidents than younger workers.

T F **19.** Over 15% of the US population are now age 65 or older.

T F **20.** Most medical practitioners tend to give low priority to the aged.

T F **21.** The majority of older people have incomes below the poverty level (as defined by the Federal Government).

T F **22.** The majority of old people are working or would like to have some kind of work to do (including housework and volunteer work).

T F **23.** Older people tend to become more religious as they age.

T F **24.** The majority of old people are seldom irritated or angry.

T F **25.** The health and socioeconomic status of older people (compared to younger people) in the year 2000 will probably be about the same as now.

Figure 4–2. Facts on Aging: a short quiz. *(Reprinted with permission Palmore E. Facts on aging: a short quiz.* Gerontologist. *Aug 1977; 17:3150320. © The Gerontology Society of America.)*

five, five days a week. The retiree often does not have the same amount of regulated activity. Work also bestows meaningful life experience. A physical or occupational therapist helps people to gain independence and to improve the quality of their lives. What is the retiree doing to get meaning in life? These types of questions and issues have spawned the field of preretirement and retirement planning. For a successful retirement, the previously listed attributes of work must continue to be fulfilled. This may mean that the retiree volunteers or participates in strong social programs to meet these needs.[117]

STRESS EVALUATION

Stress can be evaluated in several ways. In Chapter 6, the Life Events Scale and Geriatric Social Readjustment Scale are explained in detail. These two tools provide some information on an older person's stress level. In addition, a complex array of symptoms may indicate stress. For example, on the physiological level an increase in skin temperature, blood pressure, temperature, heart rate, respiration, and autonomic system activity all indicate stress. Impairment in problem-solving ability, social responsiveness, judgment, reality interpretation, and thoughts are all cognitive changes. Motor changes affected by stress are tremor, speech disturbance, and muscle tension. Finally, an older person under stress may display anger, guilt, depression, or anxiety.[116]

The following are the most frequent cues to stress in the elderly: decreased productivity, lack of awareness to the outside environment, decreased interest, rumination, preoccupation, lack of concentration, irritability and angry outbursts, withdrawal, tendency to cry (sobbing without tears), suspiciousness, and critical of self and others.[118]

Stress management or lifestyle adaptation techniques for older adults are different from those suggested for younger persons. Since older persons may have experienced an accumulation of stressors, the intervention itself should impose as few changes as possible. The geriatric physical or occupational therapist may overload the person's system by suggesting an entire lifestyle modification for energy conservation, as well as a medication and exercise program. Some additional considerations in planning adaptations for older persons are:

1. If a person is about to experience a high stress situation (a grandchild's wedding, for example) advise them to improve nutrition and increase rest.
2. Respect the individual's time clock. Choose the person's peak performance time to introduce change.
3. Try to encourage continuity of personnel.
4. Explain stress concepts to older persons. Let them know it may take longer to feel the effects of stress management if they are experiencing multiple

stress or if they have been experiencing the current stress for a long time.
5. If a person has been experiencing chronic stress, it may be a sign that change is needed (e.g., the kitten and eustress example).

Before suggesting specific stress management techniques, there are several factors that affect coping patterns of older persons. The first is social support. Older persons who believe that they are loved, esteemed, and mutually obligated to a support system have better coping mechanisms.[119] The older person's inner resources have also been found to improve coping responses, and the most important of these are flexibility, past experiences with successful coping, nonavoidance, and resumption of daily activities as soon as possible.[120] Finally, older persons with improved problem-solving ability respond better to stressful events than poor problem solvers.[121]

Stress control techniques range from cognitive to physical.[115,122] Some examples of cognitive techniques are medication, selective awareness, and systematic desensitization; a few examples of physical techniques are progressive neuromuscular relaxation, biofeedback, physical activity, and breathing control. (Refer to references 115 and 122 for specific information on these techniques).

The technique that is simplest to learn and most useful for other activities is breathing control. Teaching breathing control for relaxation involves deep diaphragmatic breathing. The older person should breathe in slowly and visualize calmness and relaxation with each inhalation and exhalation. This should be done for two to three minutes three to four times a day. A final note on stress management comes from Hans Selye, who was himself an excellent example of a healthy older person. He lived until his 90s, swam and rode his bike daily, and wrote, researched, and lectured until the day he died. Dr Selye's personal recipe for stress was that people should strive to their highest level, but never strive in vain. Second, they should find their minimum daily requirement of stress, because he viewed stress as the spice of life. Finally, he advocated "Altruistic-egoism," which means taking care of oneself by taking care of others.[118]

CONCLUSION

This chapter has reviewed the psychosocial theories of aging, the cognitive changes in late life, as well as multiple situations requiring coping mechanisms. Important problems, such as depression, delirium, and dementia, were discussed with treatment implications for the physical and occupational therapist. Finally, the end of the chapter focused on the aspects of lifestyle adaptation and society's belief system toward aging and older persons.

PEARLS

- Full life development theories, such as Erickson's and Maslow's, discuss accomplishment stages throughout life for successful aging.
- Late life theories, such as those described by Peck, Neugarten, and Havighurst, focus on the state of late life and the older person's role in adopting to this stage of life.
- Memory loss can be assisted by classes and educational interventions.
- Intellectual performance in the aged can be enhanced by the therapist in many ways, including the mode of information presented, pacing, and feedback.
- Depression in its many forms is very common in the elderly and can impact performance. Treatment ranges from behavioral to pharmacological to electroconvulsion shock therapy.
- Social isolation, including geographic, presentation, behavioral, and attitudinal types of isolation, can bar older persons from effectively interacting with their surroundings.
- Institutionalization causes changes in behavior and affects a person's performance. These effects can be countered with recognition of symptoms and behavioral and environmental interventions.
- Anxiety disorders, such as adjustment disorders, anxiety states, and phobic states, are often underreported and missed in the aged.
- Death, dying, grief and multiple loss can be a very different phenomenon in the older person. Recognizing different behavioral interventions can help the older person to die with dignity.
- Dementia affects millions of older persons and can be classified as acute disorders, chronic disorders, and presenile dementias. Assessment and treatment modification for working with these patients is based on behavioral and environmental modification by the therapist.
- Recognizing one's belief systems via the 'Facts on Aging Quiz' can help the therapist work better with the aged.
- Numerous signs, such as a decreased interest in productivity and awareness, may be signs of stress that will respond to rehabilitation interventions, such as life-style adaptations and stress control techniques.

REFERENCES

1. Mossey J, Murtan E, Knott K, et al. Determinants of recovery 12 months after hip fracture: the importance of psychosocial factors. *Am J Public Health.* March 1989; 79:279–286.
2. Magaziner J. Predictions of functional recovery one year following hospital discharge for hip fracture: a prospective study. *J Gerontol.* 1990; 45: 101–107.
3. Gilford, DM, ed. *The Aging Population in the Twenty-First Century.* Washington, DC: National Academy Press; 1998.
4. Erikson EH. *Identity, Youth & Crisis.* New York: Norton; 1968
5. Lewis CB. Psychological aspects of aging. In: Lewis CA, ed. *Aging: Health Care's Challenge.* Philadelphia: FA Davis; 1985.
6. Jung CG: *The Stages of Life. The Structure and Dynamics of the Psyche.* New York, Pantheon, 1960.
7. Buehler C. Theoretical observations about life's basic tendencies. *Am J Psychother.* 1959; 13: 561–581.
8. Maslow A. *Motivation and Personality.* New York: Harper & Row; 1954.
9. Maslow A. *Toward a Psychology of Being.* Princeton, Van Nostrand Co., Inc.; 1962.
10. Peele B. Psychological developments in the second half of life. In: Neugarten B, ed. *Middle Age and Aging.* Chicago: University of Chicago Press; 1975.
11. Neugarten B. *Middle Age and Aging.* Chicago: University of Chicago Press; 1975.
12. Cummings E, Henry W. *Growing Old: The Process of Disengagement.* New York: Basic Books; 1961.
13. Lipman A. Latent function analysis in gerontological research. *Gerontologist.* 1969; 5:256–259.
14. Lipman A, Smith KJ. Functionality of disengagement in old age. *J Gerontol.* 1968; 23:517–521.
15. Perls TT, Burbrick E, Wager CG, Vijg J, Kruglyak L. Siblings of centenarians live longer. *Lancet.* 1998; 351(3):1560.
16. Brodsky DM. The conflict perspective and understanding aging among minorities. In: Manual RC, ed. *Minority Aging.* Westport, Conn: Greenwood Press; 1982.
17. De Beauvoir S. *The Coming of Age.* New York: Putnam Books; 1972.
18. Estes CL. *The Aging Enterprise.* San Francisco: Jossey-Bass; 1979.
19. Lipman A. Minority aging from the exchange and structural-functionalist perspectives. In: Manual RC, ed. *Minority Aging.* Westport, Conn. Greenwood Press, 1982.
20. Homans G. *Social Behavior in Elementary Forms.* New York, Harcourt Brace & World, 1961.
21. Dowd JJ. Aging as exchange: A test of the distributive justice proposition. *Pacific Sociol Rev.* 1978; 21:351–375.
22. Havighurst R, Neugarten B, Tobin S. Disengagement and patterns of aging. In: Neugarten B, ed. *Middle Age & Aging.* Chicago: University of Chicago Press; 1975.
23. Butler R, Lewis M. *Aging and Mental Health.* St. Louis: Mosby-Year Book, Inc.; 1982;33–35.
24. Havighurst RJ. Flexibility and the social role of the retired. *Am J Sociol.* 1954; 59:399.
25. Neuhaus R, Neuhaus R. *Successful Aging.* New York: John Wiley & Sons; 1982:9–12.
26. Havighurst RJ. *Developmental Tasks and Education.* New York: David McKay Pubs.; 1972.
27. Levinson D. *Seasons of a Man's Life.* New York: Knopf; 1978.

28. Schaie KW. *Intellectual Development in Adulthood: The Seattle Longitudinal Study.* New York: Cambridge University Press, 1996.

29. Bolla KI, Lindgren KN, Bonaccorsy C, Bleecker ML. Memory complaints in older adults: fact or fiction? *Arch Neurology.* 1991; 48:61–64.

30. Crook TH, Feher EP, Larrabee GJ. Assessment of memory complaint in age-associated memory impairment: The MAC–Q. *International Psychogeriatrics.* 1992; 4:165–176.

31. Linn RT, Wolf PA, Bachman DL, Knoefel JE, Cobb JL, Belanger AJ, Kaplan EF, D'Agostino RB. The 'preclinical phase' of probable Alzheimer's disease. *Arch Neurol.* 1995; 52:485–490.

32. Sliwinski M, Lipton RB, Buschke H, Stewart W. The effects of preclinical dementia on estimates of normal cognitive functioning in aging. *J Gerontol.* 1996; 518:217–225.

33. Riley KP. Cognitive development. In: Bonder BR, Wagner MB, eds. *Functional Performance in Older Adults.* Philadelphia, PA: FA Davis Company; 1994.

34. Cockburn J, Smith P. The relative influence of intelligence and age on everyday memory. *J Gerontol.* 1991; 46(l):31–35.

35. Hultoch D, Masson M, Small B. Adult age differences in direct and indirect test of memory. *J Gerontol.* 1991; 46(l):22–30.

36. Craik F, Masani P. Age differences in the temporal integration of language. *Brit J Psychology.* 1967; 58:291–299.

37. Botwinck J. *Aging and Behavior.* 2nd ed. New York: Springer; 1978.

38. Larrabee GJ, Crook TH. Estimated prevalence of age-associated memory impairment derived from standardized tests of memory function. *International Psychogeriatric.* 1994; 6:95–104.

39. Feher EP, Larrabee GJ, Sudilovsky A, Crook, TH. Memory self-report in Alzheimer's disease and age-associated memory impairment. *J Geriatr Psych and Neurol.* 1993; 6:58–65.

40. American Psychiatric Association. *Diagnostic and Statistical Manual of Mental Disorders,* 4th ed. Washington DC: American Psychiatric Association. 1994:124.

41. Kral VA. Senescent forgetfulness: Benign and malignant. *J Canadian Med Assoc.* 1962; 86: 257–260.

42. Kahn R, Miller N, Zarit S, et al. Memory complaint and impairment in the aged. *Arch Gen Psychiatry.* 1975; 32:1569–1573.

43. Gurland B. The comparative frequency of depression in various adult age groups. *J Gerontol.* 1976; 31:283–292.

44. Youngjohn JR, Larrabee GJ, Crook TH. Discriminating age-associated memory impairment from Alzheimer's disease. *Psychol Assess.* 1992; 4: 54–59.

45. King DA, Cox C, Lyness JM, Conwell Y, Caine ED. *Quanitative* and *qualitative* differences in the verbal learning performance of elderly depressives and healthy controls. *J Int Neuropsychol Soc.* 1998; 4(2):115–126.

46. McEnte W, Crook TH. Age associated memory impairment: a role for catecholamines. *Neurology.* 1990; 40:526–530.

47. Oscar–Berman M, Pulsaski JL. Association learning and recognition memory in alcoholic Korsakoff patients. *Neuropsychology.* 1997; 11(2): 282–289.

48. Wolf DS, Gearing M, Snowdon DA, Mori H, Markesbery WR, Mirra SS. Progression of regional neuropathology in Alzheimer disease and normal elderly: findings from the Nun Study. *Alzheimer Did Assoc Disord.* 1999; 13(4): 226–231.

49. Riley KP, Snowdon DA, Saunders AM, Roses AD, Mortimer JA, Nanayakkara N. *J Gerontol B Psychol Sci Soc Sci.* 2000; 55(2):S69–S75.

50. Snowdon DA. Aging and Alzheimer's disease: lessons from the Nun Study. *Gerontologist.* 1997; 37(2):150–156.

51. Snowdon DA, Tully CL, Smith CD, Riley KP, Markesbery WR. Serum folate and the severity of atrophy of the neocortex in Alzheimer disease: finding from the Nun Study. *Am J Clin Nutr.* 2000; 71(4):993–998.

52. Johansson B, Allen–Burge R, Zarit SH. Self-reports on memory functioning in a longitudinal study of the oldest old: relation to current, prospective, and retrospective performance. *J Gerontol.* 1997; 52: 139–146.

53. Labouvie–Vief G. Intelligence and cognition. In: Birren JE, Schaie KW, eds. *Handbook of the Psychology of Aging.* New York: Van Nostrand Reinhold; 1985.

54. Cattell RB. Theory of fluid and crystallized intelligence: a clinical experiment. *J Educ Psychol.* 1963; 54:1.

55. Knox AB. *Adult Development and Learning.* San Francisco: Jossey-Bass; 1977.

56. Botwinick J. *Aging and Behavior: A Comprehensive Integration of Research Findings.* New York: Springer Publishing; 1978.

57. Hayslip B, Kennelly KJ. Cognitive and noncognitive factors affecting learning among older adults. In: Lumsden BD, ed. *The Older Adult as a Learner.* Washington, DC: Hemisphere Publishing; 1985.

58. Eisdorfer C, Nowlin F, Wilke F. Improvement of learning in the aged by modification of autonomic nervous system activity. *Science.* 1970; 170:1327.

59. Schultz NR, Hoyer WJ. Feedback effects on spacial egocentrism in old age. *J Gerontol.* 1976; 31:72.

60. Bettes S. Depression: the "common cold" of the elderly. *Generations.* Spring 1979; 3:15.

61. Epstein L. Symposium of age differentiation in depressive illness: depression in the elderly. *J Gerontol.* 1976; 31:278.

62. Gurland B. The comparative frequency of depression in various adult age groups. *J Gerontol.* 1976; 31:283–292.

63. Ferucci LI, Guralnik J, Marchionni N, et al. Aging and prevalence of depression. *Gerontologist.* October 1990; 30:314A.

64. Starksteen S, Robinson R, Rice T. Comparison of patients with and without major stroke depression

matched for size and location of lesion. *Arch Gen Psychiatry.* 1988; 45:247.

65. Nemiroff R, Colarusso C. *The Race Against Time: Psychotherapy and Psychoanalysis in the Second Half of Life.* New York: Plenum Press; 1985.

66. Pettinati H, Bonner K. Cognitive functioning in depressed geriatric patients with a history of ECT. *Am J Psychiatry.* January 1984; 141:1.

67. Goffman E. *Stigma: Notes on the Management of Spoiled Identity.* Englewood Cliffs, NJ: Prentice Hall, Inc.; 1963.

68. Ebersole P, Hess P. *Towards Healthy Aging: Human Needs and Nursing Response.* St. Louis: Mosby Co.; 1981:382.

69. Goffman E. *Asylums: Essays on the Social Situations of Mental Patients and Other Inmates.* Garden City, NY: Doubleday; 1961.

70. Shader R, Goodman M. Panic disorders: current perspectives. *J Clin Psychopharmacol.* 1982; 2:2–105.

71. Carey G, Gottesman I, Robins E. Prevalence and rates for the neurosis: pitfalls in the evaluation of familiarity. *Psychol Med.* 1980; 10:437–443.

72. Kleen D, Robkin J, eds. *Anxiety: New Research and Changing Concepts.* New York: Raven Press; 1981.

73. Tumball J, Tumball S. Management of specific anxiety disorders in the elderly. *Geriatrics.* 1985; 40:875–81.

74. Weg R. *The Aged: Who, Where, How Well.* Los Angeles: Ethel Percy Andrus Gerontology Center; 1979.

75. Frankle V. *Man's Search for Meaning.* Boston: Beacon Press; 1959.

76. Ebersole P, Hess P. *Towards Healthy Aging: Human Needs and Nursing Response.* St. Louis: Mosby Co.; 1981; 384.

77. Kalish R. *Death, Grief and Caring Relationships.* Monterey, Calif.: Brooks/Cole; 1981.

78. Kübler–Ross E. *On Death and Dying.* New York: Macmillan; 1969.

79. Bowlby J. Process of mourning. *Int J Psychoanal.* 1961; 42:317.

80. Engel G. Grief and grieving. *Am J Nursing.* 1964; 64:93.

81. Harper B. *Death: The Coping Mechanisms of the Health Professional.* Greenville, NC: Southeastern University Press; 1977.

82. Shua–Haim JR, Sabo MR, Ross JS. Delirium in the elderly. *Clin Geriatr.* 1999; 7(3):47–64.

83. Dobmeyer K. Delirium in elderly medical patients. *Clin Geriatr.* 1996; 4:43–68.

84. Berkow R. Cognitive failure: Delirium and dementia. In: Abrams WB, Beers MH, Berkow R, eds. *The Merck Manual of Geriatrics,* 2nd ed. Whitehouse Station, NJ: Merck & Co, Inc., 1995; 1139–1146.

85. Pompei P, Casall CK. Delirium in hospitalized elderly patients. *Hosp Proc.* 1993; July 15:49–56.

86. Jahnigan DW. Delirium in the elderly hospitalized patient. *Hosp Pract.* 1990; August 15:135–157.

87. Tueth MJ, Cheong JA. Delirium: Diagnosis and treatment in the older patient. *Geriatrics.* 1993; 48:75–80.

88. O'Keefe S, Lavan J. The prognostic significance of delirium in older patients. *J Am Geriatr Soc.* 1994; 42:252–256.

89. Sunderland T. Anticholinergic sensitivity in patients with dementia of the alzheimer type and age-matched controls. *Arch Gen Psychiatr.* 1987; 44:418–426.

90. Goodwin J. Association between nutritional status and cognitive functioning in a healthy elderly population. *JAMA.* 1983; 249:2917–2921.

91. Glenner G. Alzheimer's disease (senile dementia) a research update and critique with recommendations. *J Am Ger Soc.* 1982; 30:59–62.

92. Rocca W, Amaducci LA, Shoenberg BS, et al. Epidemiology of clinically diagnosed Alzheimer's disease. *Ann Neurol.*1981; 19:415.

93. Gurland B, Cross P. Epidemiology of psychopathology in old age: some implications for clinical services. *Psychiatric Clinics in N Am.* 1982; 5:11–26.

94. Hay J, Ernst R. The economic costs of Alzheimer's disease. *Am J Public Health.* 1987; 77:1169.

95. Rossman J. *Clinical Geriatrics.* 2nd ed. Philadelphia: Lippincott Co.; 1979.

96. Eisdorfer C, Cohen D. The cognitively impaired elderly: differential diagnosis. In: Storandt M, Seigler I, Elias M, eds. *The Clinical Psychology of Aging.* New York: Plenum Publishing Corp.; 1985.

97. Delaney P. Dementia: the search for reversible causes. *South Med Journal.* 1982; 75:707–709.

98. Clarfield A. The reversible dementias: do they reverse? *Ann Intern Med.* September 1988; 476–486.

99. Snowdon DA, Greiner LH, Markesbery WR. Linguistic ability in early life and the neuropathology of Alzheimer's disease and cerebrovascular disease. Findings from the Nun Study. *Ann N Y Acad Sci.* 2000 Apr; 903:334–38.

100. Gregg EW. Diabetes a significant risk factor for cognitive decline in older women. *Arch Intern Med.* 2000; 160,174–180.

101. Forsyth E, Ritzline PD. An overview of the etiology, diagnosis, and treatment of Alzheimer disease. *Phys Ther.* 1998; 78(12):1325–1331.

102. Hayter J. Patients who have Alzheimer's disease. *Am J Nurs.* 1974; 74:1460.

103. Luxemborg J, Feigenbaum L. Cognitive impairment on a rehabilitative service. *Arch Phys Med Rehab.* 1986; 67:796–798.

104. Lazarus LW, Newton N, Cohler B, et al. Frequency and presentation of depressive symptoms in patients with primary degenerative dementia. *Am J Psychiatry.* January 1987; 41–45.

105. Teschendorf B. Cognitive impairment in the elderly: delirium, depression, or dementia? *Focus on Geriatric Care and Rehab.* September 1987; 1:4.

106. Blessed G, Tominson BE, Roth M, et al. The association between quantitative measures of dementia and of senile change in the grey matter of elderly subjects. *Br J Psychiatry.* 1968; 114:797.

107. Pfeiffer E. A short portable mental status questionnaire for the assessment of brain deficit in elderly patients. *J Am Ger Soc.* 1975; 23:433.

108. Folstein MF, Folstein SE, McHugh PR. Mini-Mental State. A practical method for grading the cognitive state of patients for the clinician. *J Psychiatric Res.* 1975; 12:189–198.

109. Mace NL, Rabins PV. *The 36-Hour Day.* 3rd ed. Baltimore, MD: John Hopkins University Press; 1999.

110. Butler R. Agen-ism: another form of bigotry. *Gerontologist.* 1969; 9:243.

111. Palmore E. Facts on aging—a short quiz. *Gerontologist.* 1977; 17:4.

112. Kemp B. The psychosocial context of geriatric rehabilitation. In: Kemp B, Brummel–Smith K, Ramsdell JW, ed. *Geriatric Rehabilitation.* Boston: Little, Brown & Co.; 1990.

113. Kvitek S, Dr Shaver BJ, Blood H, et al. Age bias: physical therapists and older patients. *J Gerontol.* 1986; 41:702.

114. Selye H. *The Stress of Life.* New York: McGraw-Hill; 1959.

115. Allen R, Hyde D. *Investigations in Stress Control.* Minneapolis: Burgess Publishing; 1982.

116. Lakatta E. Hemodynamic adaptions to stress with advancing age. *Acta Med Scand.* 1986; 711(suppl): 39–52.

117. Neres M. Coping with stress in nursing. *Am Nurse.* September 15, 1977; 9:4.

118. Selye H. Stress and aging. *J Am Ger Soc.* September 1970; 18:9.

119. Cobb S. Social support as a moderator of life stress. *Psychosom Med.* 1976; 38:300.

120. Henry J, Stephans P. *Stress, Health and the Social Environment.* New York: Springer-Verlag; 1977.

121. Fry P. Mediators of perception of stress among community-based elders. *Psychological Reports.* 1989; 65:307–314.

122. Iglarsh A. Stress and aging. In: Lewis CB, ed. *Aging: Health Care's Challenge.* Philadelphia: FA Davis Co; 1990.

CHAPTER 5

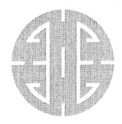

Pathological Manifestations of Aging

PATHOLOGICAL MANIFESTATION OF AGING

Aging is considered a normal physiological process because of its universality. As much as the aging process may influence the predisposition to disease, aging in and of itself is not considered to be pathological. This distinction seems conceptually clear, however, the fine line between aging and disease is often blurred when applied to specific cases, and some degree of decreasing biological, physiological, anatomical, and functional capabilities occur as one ages. (See Chapter 3, Comparing and Contrasting Age-Related Changes in Biology, Physiology, Anatomy, and Function.) Some degree of atrophy is evident in all tissues of the body. A variety of degenerative processes are called "normal aging" until they proceed far enough to cause clinically significant disability.

Recent epidemiological genetic study findings indicate pathologic significance of age-related changes such as vascular stiffening and loss of muscle mass[1] which are genetically driven and were, until recently, considered normal aging. Genes with effects on unrecognized pathologies could be detected through genome scans to identify loci affecting broader outcomes.

Genetic factors may influence not only physiologic functions, but also their rates of change with age, which can influence whether and when disease occurs. Rates of change with age in many physiologic functions directly affect risk of age-related morbidity (e.g., changes in bone density, vital capacity, cognitive function, lens opacity, and blood pressure). Another important group includes rates of decline in homeostatic functions, such as glucose tolerance, blood pressure stability, and balance. Rates of change in cellular biochemical properties implicated in age-related pathologies could also be studied, as data is needed on the predictive validity of such changes for mortality, age related diseases, or functional status.

The incidence of many diseases is influenced markedly as age advances (Figure 5–1).[2] The death rates for atherosclerosis, myocardial degeneration, hypertension, and cancer all increase more steeply than the overall death rate, which arouses the suspicion that aging predisposes an individual either to the development of the condition or to a fatal outcome. With some conditions, such as respiratory infections, the incidence is not increased in the elderly, but the likelihood of fatality from the insult is greater than in younger persons.[3] In a child or young adult, death is most commonly caused by some form of accident (Figure 5–2); however, in the elderly, the main problems are coronary heart disease, cerebrovascular accidents, respiratory diseases, diabetes, peripheral vascular diseases, and neoplasms.[4]

The purpose of this chapter is to review those pathologies that are manifested in the aged population, but will not cover a detailed consideration of every possible geriatric pathology; rather, it will examine some of the more common conditions that afflict the elderly and affect functional activities of daily living. The format of this chapter follows that of

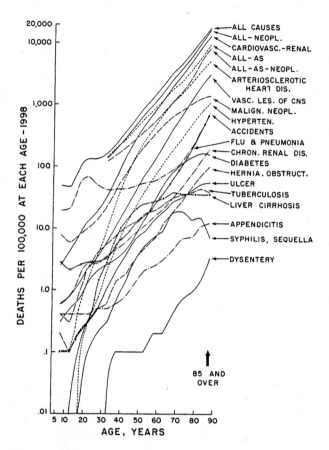

Figure 5–1. *Age-specific death rates from selected causes. (Created graph from statistics garnered from: US Bureau of the Census. Statistical Abstract of the United States. Profiles of Older Americans: 1999. Washington DC: Bureau of the Census. 2000.)*

Chapter 3, Comparing and Contrasting Age-Related Changes in Biology, Physiology, Anatomy, and Function for convenient comparison between age-related and pathological changes with aging.

AGING AS DISEASE

There is always the tacit implication that aging, like growth and development, is a normal physiological process lying outside the domain of disease. Though aging may not be considered a disease process, the time-dependent loss of structure and function in all organ systems leads to pathological end states. There is a general decline in structure, function, and number of many kinds of cells with age. Cellular aging is accompanied by denaturation of extracellular proteins. The collagen and elastin of the skin become irreversibly crystalline and broken. The hyaline cartilage on articular surfaces of joints becomes fibrillar and fragmented, and the beautifully ordered structure of the lens of the eye becomes brittle and chaotic as lens protein is gradually denatured.

The aging process proceeds slowly and ubiquitously over the life course resulting in a loss of structure and function within every organ or tissue. Countless microtraumas occur and accumulate in small

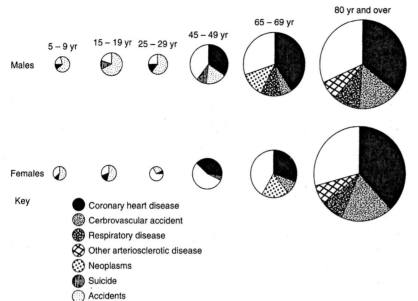

Figure 5–2. Principle causes of death for each sex at different ages. (*Created from statistics garnered from: Administration on Aging. Older Americans 2000: Key Indicators of Well-Being. Federal Interagency. Forum on Aging-Related Statistics. Washington DC: Bureau of the Census. 2000.*)

increments as imperceptible injuries. Over a lifetime, the skin elastin is exposed to microinsults from ultraviolet rays from the sun, repetitive mechanical stresses cause degeneration of articular cartilage, and reactions with metabolites diminish the opacity of the lens of the eye. The most important aging changes occur at the molecular level, as reviewed in Chapter 2, Comparing and Contrasting the Theories of Aging. Small injuries occurring within the cell result in the loss of genetic memory and progressive cross-linking of collagen, the chief structural protein in the body.

Wiley Forbus, a pathologist, defined disease as the reaction to injury.[5] If aging is a gradual accumulation of incompletely repaired injuries due to microtrauma through the life course, it may not be normal, despite its universality. Perhaps "aging" is a pathological process resulting from tissue reactions to imperceptible, avoidable injuries.

Physical and occupational therapists could play a major role in preventing the disabilities that result from these insidious microtraumas. Preventive strengthening and conditioning exercises, positioning, joint and tissue mobilization, and the numerous modalities that could be employed all impact functional capabilities, especially in an aged population. From the authors' clinical perspective, preventing disabilities that can result from pathological processes greatly improves the level of function and the quality of life. There are certainly changes that occur in aging that don't need to be inevitable.

CARDIOVASCULAR MANIFESTATIONS OF AGING

There are no clinically significant effects on heart function which can be ascribed to aging alone. Cardiovascular dysfunction attributed to the aging process closely mimics the decline in cardiac function seen with inactivity.[6–8] Arteriosclerosis is a generally used term to describe any form of vascular degeneration associated with a thickening and loss of resilience in the arterial wall.[9] Atherosclerosis is a more specific type of degeneration that is associated with an accumulation of fat in the intimal lining of the blood vessels and an increase of connective tissue in the underlying subintima.[9] Almost all animal species show some degree of atherosclerosis, and, for this reason, it has been considered an inevitable accompaniment of aging. The pathological consequences depend on the site. Weakness in the aorta can cause an aneurysm; ischemic heart disease can result from atherosclerotic changes in the coronary arteries; and cerebrovascular accidents can result from involvement of the cerebral vessels.[10]

Other cardiovascular pathologies increase in incidence with age in addition to ischemic heart disease, and these include cardiomyopathies, conductive system diseases, valvular heart disease, and peripheral vascular disease.[11] The result is that the heart is less effective as a pump and has less reserve to meet increased activity needs. Functional abilities of the individual become more and more restricted as the severity of heart disease increases. Cerebral vascular problems resulting from cardiovascular conditions need consideration and are dealt with more extensively in a subsequent section of this chapter, along with other neuromuscular pathologies.

Ischemic Heart Disease

Ischemic heart disease, commonly called coronary artery disease (CAD), results from blockage of blood flow to cardiac muscle. Some 40% of those aged 65 to 74 years and 50% of those aged 75 years and older have evidence of heart disease.[9] When there is a reversible lack of oxygen in the cardiac muscle in response to an increased activity level or emotional stress, anginal pain results from atherosclerotic changes in the coronary arteries. The effect of ischemia can be reversible, and the muscle cells will gradually regain their ability to contract as circulation is restored. A rapid loss of blood flow lasting 30 to 60 minutes can cause death of the myocardial cells.[10] Irreversible damage to a part of the heart muscle from vascular narrowing can result from plaque formation that totally blocks the coronary vessel, such as an embolus or a thrombus, the consequence of which is a myocardial infarction. Myocardial degeneration can progress with repeated minor episodes of irreversible oxygen depletion in the cardiac muscle. As degeneration progresses, the heart muscle functions poorly and congestive heart failure can be the result. Furthermore, muscle deprived of its blood supply becomes prone to chaotic and unregulated contractions, which can result in life-threatening arrhythmias.

Oxygen extraction in the coronary circulation is relatively complete even at rest.[9] When work demands are increased on the heart, additional oxygen is required to meet the energy needs of the cardiac muscle cells. This oxygen is obtained through the dilatation of the coronary vessels. With rigid, atherosclerotic vessels, dilatation does not readily occur. Vascular resistance is increased due to the inelastic quality of the vessels and blood flow is impeded by plaque obstruction.

Gross obstruction of the major coronary vessels results in anginal pain typically brought on by vigorous exercise.[12] In the elderly, however, anginal pain is not a consistent symptomatic indicator of ischemia of the cardiac tissue. The elderly more commonly report dyspnea (shortness of breath). Clinically, shortness of breath is a much more reliable indicator of ischemia than anginal pain in the elderly individual.[13] There is a general correlation between ST segment depression on the EKG and the onset of anginal symptoms,[9] though in the elderly, marked ST segment depression occurs with dyspnea without the development of the characteristic anginal pain.[13]

Early intervention in ischemic heart disease takes several forms. The most important is to reduce the risk factors that predispose individuals to the development of coronary artery disease, such as cigarette smoking, high blood pressure, and serum cholesterol. Secondary prevention of heart attacks, once CAD is established, requires the reduction of risk factors as well as the use of aspirin to prevent platelet aggregation, which may initiate obstruction of a coronary artery, and beta blockers, which appear to limit the extent of muscle injury. Management of symptomatic coronary artery disease is similar in all age groups, and consists of medical and surgical interventions. Since the pathophysiology of coronary artery disease is the mismatch between the metabolic demands of the heart muscle and the ability of the coronary arteries to supply blood, interventions are directed at de-

creasing the metabolic needs of the heart muscle or increasing the ability of the coronary arteries to carry blood. The metabolic demands of heart muscle can be reduced by lowering the pressure against which the heart has to push, by reducing the rate at which the heart contracts, and by reducing the overall metabolic demands of the body by correcting hyperthyroidism, anemia, low oxygen, or elevated temperature. Calcium channel blocking agents and beta blockers reduce the metabolic demands on heart muscle, and nitroglycerine reduces the pressure against which the heart has to pump by causing dilitation of the coronary vessels. Beta blockers[14] and calcium channel blockers[15] often improve function by reducing myocardial contractility, however, this may leave the elderly individual vulnerable to cardiac failure. It is still debated how far the effectiveness and toxicity of these drugs is modified by aging.[16] Exercise is still the treatment of choice for cardiovascular diseases.

There are a number of reasons why exercise is helpful to the patient with angina.[9] Development of an enhanced "collateral" flow has not been established.[17] However, the cardiac oxygen demand is decreased by a drop in both heart rate and blood pressure at a given work load. The lengthening of the diastolic phase facilitates coronary perfusion.[9] Though progress is slow in the elderly, dramatic gains of maximum oxygen intake can be achieved if the exercise periods are of sufficient lengths.[9,18] Many activities of daily living can be brought below the anginal threshold by exercise training. Strengthening of the skeletal muscles may help to reduce blood pressure, and, therefore, to reduce the likelihood of developing anginal symptoms during functional activities of daily living.

Surgical intervention is directed at increasing the capacity of the coronary arteries to provide blood to the heart muscle. Critically narrowed sections of arteries can be identified by cardiac catheterization and angiography. Obstructions can be circumvented by grafts or removed by transluminal angioplasty if the narrowing occurs in larger branches of the coronary arteries. The results of coronary artery bypass graft (CABG) surgery and angioplasty are determined more by the preoperative function of the patient's heart than by the patient's age.[19] In the absence of other severe coexisting disease, the elderly are good candidates for cardiac surgery.

Treatment of acute myocardial infarctions in the aged runs the gamut from infarct reduction (e.g., the use of enzymes such as streptokinase) and emergency angioplasty to comfort measures only. The determination of where in the spectrum of care the individual is most appropriately treated is a decision made jointly by the patient, physician, and family. In this area of medicine, as in few others, the conflict is so stark between the potentially dehumanizing technologic imperative of modern treatment and the need to make treatment decisions on the basis of the patient's wishes and preferences. There are appropriate limits to treatment which are often lost in the attempt to apply the latest technology. Further discussion of this important issue is found in the Chapter 17, Attitudes and Ethics in Gerontology.

Rehabilitation following myocardial infarction involves an integration of physical and occupational therapy to achieve maximal physical functioning, in addition to nutritional and medical interventions to control the progression of coronary artery disease. Much research has examined the interactions between physical activity and myocardial infarction, however, the general focus has been on middle-aged males even though infarction is more frequent in older age groups.[9,18,20] Two major risk factors, diabetes and hypertension, also become more prevalent with aging.[9]

Some of the postulated mechanisms of infarction (hemorrhage into an atherosclerotic plaque, impaction of an embolus from a fragmented plaque, and development of severe relative oxygen insufficiency) could be induced by vigorous physical activity.[19] However, other pathologies such as the formation of a thrombus on an ulcerated plaque seem more likely to occur when an individual is asleep. The histories obtained in nonfatal incidents of myocardial infarction suggest that about 25% were precipitated by physical activity, with exercise increasing the immediate risk by a factor of 6 to 12.[9,21-23] The potential risk during exercise is outweighed by the benefits of exercise.[18] In older age groups, a smaller proportion of ischemic heart disease deaths occur suddenly, and, if all age groups are considered, the association between strenuous activity and death is rare.[9,24] A more extensive discussion of exercise intervention following myocardial infarction is provided in Chapter 13, Cardiopulmonary and Cardiovascular Treatment Considerations.

Cardiomyopathy/Congestive Heart Failure

Cardiomyopathies are conditions in which the heart muscle hypertrophies and cardiac function is impaired often resulting in congestive heart failure.[10] The muscle of the heart weakens because of poor nutrition, toxins, infections, or genetic factors.[5] The weakening results in dilation of the heart and can lead to congestive heart failure because the heart cannot contract strongly enough to empty a sufficient amount of blood into the peripheral vasculature to meet the body's needs. Hypertrophy of cardiac muscle tissue can be the end results of hypertension, outflow obstruction, or genetic factors.[10] The cardiovascular changes imposed by cardiomyopathies impairs function through several pathological mechanisms. The hypertrophied heart is stiff and does not easily fill with blood. As a result, the heart contracts vigorously but there is little forward circulation to show for the effort and the body's energy and oxygen needs are not met. In hypertrophic cardiomyopathy, the

muscle abnormally contracts, actually creating an obstruction to the outflow of blood from the heart. The more strongly the heart contracts, the greater is the obstruction.

Exercise has historically been contraindicated in the patient with cardiomyopathy, however, as research discussed in Chapter 13, Cardiopulmonary and Cardiovascular Treatment Considerations indicates, that perspective is rapidly changing as the benefits of exercise in this condition are documented and acknowledged.[25-27] Medical treatment is directed at correcting or ameliorating the pathophysiology of the underlying cause of the heart failure. Rehabilitative efforts need to be directed towards maintaining and improving the maximal functional capabilities of the elderly individual and preventing the debilitating effects of immobility.

In dilated cardiomyopathies, the heart is not strong enough to move blood against the pressure in the blood vessels.[28] As a result, fluid builds up in the pulmonary circulation causing pulmonary edema, difficulty breathing, low blood oxygen, and further stress on the metabolic needs of the contracting cardiac muscle. Medical intervention is directed toward strengthening the heart's contraction using medications, such as digoxin. More effective emptying of the heart can be achieved if the pressure against which the heart has to move blood is decreased. This is called afterload reduction.[29] Agents that reduce afterload include nitrates, peripheral vasodialators (e.g., prazosin, hydralazine), and other blood pressure-lowering agents. Diuretics, which reduce the amount of fluid systemically (termed a preload reduction), also help to reduce pulmonary edema and improve cardiac efficiency.[18] In hypertrophic cardiomyopathy, the problem is the inability of the heart to adequately fill. The rapid, wormy contractions of the hypertrophic heart obstruct the outflow of blood. Dyastolic dysfunction arises when the heart does not adequately fill during diastole, the heart's relaxation phase.[10] Two classes of medication have been found to be effective in improving the efficiency of the cardiac pump. Beta blockers (e.g., propranolol, metoprolol, timolol) and calcium channel blockers (e.g., diltiazem, nifedipine, verapamil) reduce the intensity and speed of cardiac muscle contraction, activating the slow twitch, anaerobic muscle fibers, and thereby improving the strength of muscle contraction. The beta blockers work by blocking the effect of epinephrine on heart muscle, because epinephrine promotes rapid and vigorous contractions. Calcium channel blockers affect the way in which calcium flows into and out of cardiac muscle. Calcium plays an essential role in regulating the force of contractions.[30]

Conduction System Diseases

Conduction system diseases are those which affect the rate and rhythm of the heart's contractions.[10] The propagation of the electrical wave which results in the coordinated contraction of the heart muscle is initiated in the two pacemaker sites in the heart and carried initially along specialized pathways that spread the wave throughout the heart, also known as the conduction system. These pacemakers and pathways can be damaged by many different agents, including those that result in cardiomyopathies and myocardial infarction.[30] The most common consequences of pacemaker dysfunction are extremely rapid (tachycardic) contractions, poorly coordinated (dysrhythmic) contractions, or extremely slow (bradycardic) contractions that are less effective in moving blood and result in diminished cardiac output.[9] Low cardiac output can result in confusion, fatigue, poor exercise tolerance, and congestive heart failure. Rapid reductions in cardiac output can cause syncope.

Tachycardias and poorly coordinated rhythms, such as atrial fibrillation, are usually treated with medication to control the rate and convert the rhythm back to normal. Occasionally, electrical cardioversion is required.[10] Bradycardia is usually managed by surgical implantation of an artificial pacemaker, which can be set to trigger a heartbeat at a predetermined rate. Age, per se, is not a contraindication to pacemaker therapy, and the surgery is minor and well tolerated.

Valvular Disease of the Heart

The heart valves, which function to keep the blood flowing in one direction, tend to withstand many microtraumas throughout the life course. Defects of the heart valves are of two types. Stenosis or narrowing of the valve restricts blood flow,[10] and insufficiency or regurgitation results in the backward flow of blood. Both conditions increase the work load on the heart and greatly reduce its efficiency.[9] Two valves are most frequently involved. The mitral valve between the left atrium and ventricle, and the aortic valve, which moves the blood into the systemic circulation.

Rheumatic valve disease, caused by earlier episodes of rheumatic fever, is the most common cause of mitral stenosis and insufficiency in the aged.[30] Congestive heart failure, arrhythmias, and embolization of blood clots from the heart to the brain and other organs are the most common complications of mitral valve disease. These patients require attentive medical management, which includes the use of anticoagulants to prevent emboli, diuretics to control congestive heart failure, and digitalis or other medications to control the heart rate.[10] Nutritional support is often required to assure compliance with a low sodium diet. Because of the potentially serious side effects from too much anticoagulant (bleeding, herorrhagic stroke) and digoxin (arrhythmias), the narrow range of effective dosages, and the deleterious effect of inadequate dosage, exercise must be gradually implemented and progressed slowly. Protective intervention should focus on skin protection and maintenance of maximal functional capabilities, with close monitoring of the individual's vital signs and subjective responses of perceived tolerance to increasing activity levels.

Surgical intervention to correct mitral stenosis needs to precede the development of fixed pulmonary hypertension and right heart failure.[10] Valve replacement and valvulotomy (where the valve is widened but not replaced) are done through open heart surgery. Transluminal valvulotomy, in which the valve is widened by using catheter-guided balloons, offers significantly lower operative risk in selected patients. Almost all patients continue to require medication for control of heart rate, prevention of emboli, and treatment of congestive heart failure. The response to gradually increasing levels of physical activity following surgery is usually favorable.[10]

Aortic valve disease is common in the aged and results from rheumatic valve disease, increasing damage to a congenitally misformed valve, or the progression of age-related injury to an otherwise normal valve.[30] The latter results from the gradual buildup of scar tissue and calcium on the valve leaflets as part of the normal aging of the valve. The most clinically significant lesion is stenosis of the aortic valve. This results in a progressive increase in the resistance to the flow of blood out of the heart, and, as a result, the heart pumps blood against increasingly great afterload.[10] Patients can experience angina without coronary artery disease, because even normal coronary arteries are unable to deliver sufficient blood to meet the metabolic demands of the overtaxed heart muscle. As the stenosis increases, transient decreases in cardiac output due to arrhythmias or ischemia result in syncope.[9] Finally, when the heart is no longer able to compensate by hypertrophy for the increasing resistance to flow, congestive heart failure supervenes. Unlike previously discussed situations in which congestive heart failure occurs and is amenable to medical intervention, congestive heart failure in aortic stenosis carries a grave prognosis and can be effectively managed only by surgical replacement of the damaged valve.[10] Efforts need to be directed toward maintaining the maximal functional capabilities through exercise programs utilizing activities of daily living as the exercise mode.

Infection of the heart valve, or endocarditis, is a rare but significant illness in the aged.[10] This is due not only to its potential for causing death or severe disability, but also to its subtle presentation. Lethargy, fatigue, anorexia, failure to thrive, anemia, worsening congestive heart failure, progressive renal failure, low grade fever, embolic stroke or transient ischemic attack, worsening control of diabetes, and development of a new heart murmur are all potentially caused by bacterial endocarditis.[30] Early antibiotic therapy can be lifesaving. Exercise is contraindicated during the acute phase of endocarditis, but gradual resumption of activities of daily living (ADLs) can begin once the infection has been medically controlled.[9]

Hypertension

Hypertension is another common condition affecting the cardiovascular system. It is clear that the aged with systolic blood pressures above 160 mm Hg and diastolic pressures above 95 mm Hg are at increased risk for stroke, congestive heart failure (hypertensive cardiomyopathy), and renal failure. Isolated systolic hypertension carries a similar risk,[10] because much of the cardiovascular morbidity and mortality in the elderly is related to hypertension.[2] This is true for both isolated systolic hypertension and systolic-diastolic blood pressure elevations.[31] In addition to accelerated atherogenesis (myocardial infarction and congestive heart failure), hypertension adversely affects cardiac performance, renal function, and cerebral blood flow. It also increases aortic aneurysm rupture and dissection, and increases the incidence of cerebrovascular bleeding.[32]

Treatment to lower blood pressure significantly reduces the risks of developing these complications. Medical and dietary management are important in controlling hypertension. In the elderly, most recommendations are for drug treatment for blood pressure readings in excess of 160/95.[32] There is little proof that antihypertensive drug therapy alters the course of asymptomatic elderly individuals without evidence of end-organ damage from isolated systolic hypertension.

Nevertheless, isolated systolic hypertension doubles the risk of cardiovascular complications, so that the risk, expense, and inconvenience of drug therapy must be compared with the benefits of lower systolic blood pressure. Compliance with medication and the early identification and avoidance of drug-induced side effects, such as dizziness, hypokalemia, depression, syncope, and confusion, are major challenges to the health care team. Complications of antihypertensive therapy are more frequent in the elderly individual, both because the diminution of renal function increases the incidence of drug toxicity and because the aged patient with less sensitive baroreceptor responses is more susceptible to the orthostatic complications of volume depletion. Assuming the upright posture gradually may help avert dizziness and syncope. Exercise has been shown to have positive effects in reducing high blood pressure and is discussed extensively in Chapter 13, Cardiopulmonary and Cardiovascular Treatment Considerations. Control of hypertension has the potential to decrease cardiovascular morbidity and mortality.

Myocardial Degeneration

The general decline of cardiac performance with age and with inactivity affects the ability of elderly individuals to function at their maximum. The recognized changes in cardiac function include a decrease in right ventricular work rate and a variable change of left ventricular work rate depending on the relative magnitudes of the reduction in maximum cardiac output and the increase of systemic blood pressure.[9,33] While a young person readily accepts a sustained increase of cardiac work rate, in old age an equivalent relative stress may give rise to cardiac failure, particularly if there are other circulatory problems such as a high systemic blood pressure, a minor disorder of the heart valves, or an excessive intake of fluids. Complaints of shortness of breath in the elderly frequently reflect problems with getting enough oxygen to the working muscle through a failing circulatory system.

The exact reason for a reduction in myocardial function has not been determined. Some authors suggest that it is part of the normal aging process and can be attributed to the wasting of the heart muscle, loss of elasticity with slowing of cardiac relaxation,[34] the fibrotic changes in the heart valves, and a modification of catecholamine production or sensitivity.[33] Others suggest that amyloidosis (tissue proteinosis) may precipitate degeneration of cardiac muscle tissue and lead to failure. Pomerance[35] found amyloid material in the hearts of 12% of subjects who died after the age of 80 years from cardiac failure. Other authors have argued that lack of oxygen by numerous repetitive microtraumas to the myocardium leads to myocardial degeneration.[36] They found that cardiac function was well preserved in those with a good myocardial oxygen supply, however, a high proportion of their sample population failed to satisfy that criteria and had chronic oxygen supply problems according to EKG and scintigraphic evidence. On autopsy, most older people showed both atheromatous plaques and small myocardial scars, so ischemic changes over a lifetime could be responsible for impaired cardiac function.[35]

Individuals with a seriously reduced cardiac reserve report a marked need for rest even after mild physical activity.[37] In addition to persistent and undue fatigue, an inadequate cardiac response to exercise usually causes acute shortness of breath (dyspnea), while a restriction of blood flow to the heart itself may produce anginal pain. Inadequate blood flow to the peripheral tissues may give the skin a bluish hue (peripheral cyanosis). The pulse rate typically rises over the day, with a slow and incomplete recovery during rest pauses.[9] Activities of daily living are notably difficult for these elderly individuals. Lying down can induce a sharp reoccurrence or increase of dyspnea and create a "fear of sleeping" that further adds to the severe fatigue experienced on minimal activity by an individual with myocardial degeneration.

The ankle edema of cardiac failure needs to be distinguished from problems of venous drainage. Improper application of modalities, such as a Jobst intermittent compression boot, or elevation of the lower extremities above the horizontal plane could be detrimental to the elderly individual in cardiac failure, where they would be quite effective in positively modifying the problems encountered with venous return pathologies. In cardiac failure, a delay in the S3 sound, a so-called "gallop rhythm," is indicative of a delay in left ventricular filling.[10]

Adverse reactions to exercise in the individual with congestive heart failure (cardiac failure) include an absence of the anticipated rise of systemic blood pressure, an accumulation of a substantial oxygen debt, and a slow recovery of heart rate and ventilation after cessation of the effort.[9] Cardiac stroke volume decreases rather than increases as the intensity of work is augmented. Myocardial contractility is also impaired.

While there is probably merit in persuading subjects with diffuse myocardial disease to preserve existing function through cautiously prescribed effort, the intensity of such activity must be held below the level at which left ventricular failure begins to occur. Once failure has developed, there is little alternative to a combination of traditional medical therapy and rest until the heart is again operating on the favorable (compensated) portion of its pressure/volume reserve.[9] The reduction of muscle mass and decrease of renal function increases the circulatory half-life of digoxin,[38] although the inotropic effect on the heart is diminished with aging.[39] Beta-blocking agents may worsen the tendency to cardiac failure, as may alcohol abuse.[40]

Peripheral Vascular Disease

Peripheral vascular disease is frequently the result of untreated hypertension, cigarette smoking, diabetes mellitus, and elevated serum cholesterol.[30] Atherosclerosis and other forms of peripheral vascular disease can lead to partial or complete obstruction of the main arterial supply to the limbs. The consequences are intermittent claudication with walking and skin lesions which may lead to amputation.[9] When early intervention to reduce risk factors is unsuccessful, management is through the modification of diet to reduce weight and cholesterol, medications to enhance blood flow and reduce blood pressure, and behavior modifications to reduce cigarette consumption. Exercise is particularly helpful in treating peripheral vascular disease from a preventative perspective.[9,41–44] Buerger-Allen exercises improve the vitality of the peripheral vascular system and impact on back and lower extremity flexibility and strength. They also serve to decrease the debilitating effects of postural hypotension by facilitating adjustment to postural positional changes. (See Chapter 13 for a detailed description of exercise rational and protocol.) Surgical intervention is effective in cases of symptomatic peripheral vascular disease that results in rest pain, claudication, or nonhealing ulcers.[10,45] As in coronary artery disease, partial obstructions of peripheral arteries, most commonly in the lower extremities, can be treated with bypass grafting or by dilating the obstructed section of the artery using transluminal angioplasty.

Intermittent claudication is muscular pain which, analogous to anginal pain, reflects an acute lack of oxygen to the working muscles. The level of discomfort depends on the level of peripheral vascular obstruction.[46,47] The condition is seen most often in the elderly, and the subsequent mortality of the claudicant patient is high. A minor orthopaedic anomaly such as a hammer or claw toe can develop a lesion which can lead to a gangrenous lesion due to the absence of an adequate blood supply in the affected extremity.[46] Immobility created by a gangrenous lesion can lead to depression and renal complications and death is frequently the result of a coronary thrombosis or hemorrhage.[48–50]

Amputation is required for the relief of pain and to stop the spread of infection (gangrene) in those patients for whom other surgical procedures are impossible. When an individual has both diabetes and peripheral vascular disease, there is about a 5% incidence of amputations per year.[46] Because the patient's ability to ambulate is greatly affected by the level at which the amputation is performed, the most distal site is preferred. However, the amputation must be performed at a level where there is sufficient blood supply to assure adequate healing. Progressive amputations, and severely restricted mobility is usually required if the amputation is below the area of adequate blood supply and the incision does not heal. The result is that the patient is exposed to the risks of surgery again.

Loss of a limb is a traumatic event. Often the process of grieving must begin before the actual surgery and is helped by contributions from social service, psychiatry, nursing, and rehabilitative services. Depression is a major impediment to the successful rehabilitation of these patients and must be addressed if intensive nursing and physical and occupational therapy are to be successful.

PULMONARY MANIFESTATIONS OF AGING

The respiratory system functions to assure the exchange of oxygen and carbon dioxide between the air and the blood within the lungs. This system can be thought of as having several related but separate components: movement of air into and out of the lungs, the exchange of oxygen and carbon dioxide, and the defense of the lung from infection. Changes with age affect every aspect of the respiratory system.

The chest wall becomes a less efficient bellows with age. The anteroposterior diameter of the chest increases and the rib cage becomes more rigid as progressive curvature of the spine, calcification of costal cartilage, and osteoporosis limit the compliance of the chest wall. The chest muscles atrophy with age and also contribute to the gradual decline in the efficiency with which air is moved into and out of the lungs. The collapse of small airways due to the loss of elasticity of lung tissue with age results in increasing resistance to air flow. As a result, the amount of physical effort that must go into breathing increases by 20% between the ages of 20 and 70 years.[28]

Although the bronchi are not usually affected by normal aging, the surface area of the alveoli decreases by 4% each decade of life.[20] The alveolar wall is also thinner and contains fewer capillaries for the delivery of blood. The size of the alveoli increases due to the loss of elasticity and recoil. It is the loss of recoil that creates an increased susceptibility to airway collapse, the major factor contributing to the altered distribution of air within the lungs.

Ideally, each area of the lung where blood is available for gas exchange would be ventilated giving a perfect match of ventilation and perfusion. With age, larger areas of the lung are perfused but not ventilated because of airway collapse and redistribution of blood flow.[9] This results in the return of unoxygenated blood to the general circulation and decreased efficiency of the respiratory system. Pulmonary circulation may also decline with age, further reducing the capacity of the system to respond to the demand for increased supply of oxygen to tissues.

Changing mechanics within the lung and chest wall also make the lung more susceptible to infection with age. The gag reflex is diminished, thereby increasing the risk of aspiration. Concurrently, the cough reflex is also diminished and the effectiveness of the cough reduced because of reduced chest wall compliance and chest muscle strength. Ciliary action, which normally moves secretions up and out of the lungs, also declines, particularly in smokers. These factors combine to compromise the lung's ability to defend against infection. Some drugs play important roles in depressing the respiratory system. Sedatives and analgesics, such as alcohol and narcotics, are known to depress respiration and dull the cough and gag reflexes, thus predisposing the elderly person to the risks of hypoxia and aspiration pneumonia.

The two most common types of disease affecting the respiratory system are pneumonias, which compromise gas exchange and serve as a source of sepsis, and diseases that affect the amount of air flow in the lungs such as asthma, chronic obstructive lung disease (COPD), and emphysema.

Pneumonia

Pneumonia is the most common infectious cause of death in the elderly[51] and the most common infection requiring hospitalization. It is often the means of death for patients with other serious conditions, such as diabetes, cancer, stroke, congestive heart failure, dementia, and renal failure. The increased incidence of pneumonia with aging is due in part to the weakening of the local pulmonary defenses; however, the high mortality of pneumonia is largely due to its more subtle presentation in the elderly. Typical symptoms such as a productive cough, fever, and pleuritic chest pain are frequently absent, but subtler symptoms, such as confusion, alteration of sleep-wake cycles, increased congestive heart failure, anorexia, and failure to thrive, are more common. A

typically lower core temperature in an older, inactive adult, results in a failure to recognize that the individual has a fever. Misdiagnosis and late diagnosis are common and contribute to the high mortality of pneumonia in the elderly.[51]

Successful treatment of pneumonia requires early recognition and institution of proper antibiotic therapy. The identification of causative bacteria in the examination of a sputum sample is the single most important diagnostic test for determining initial antibiotic therapy. Unfortunately, such samples are often difficult to obtain in a dehydrated and confused elderly patient, and, as a result, therapy is often empirical and not as specifically directed or effective as possible. Hydration, nutritional support, chest physical therapy, and treatment of complicating illnesses are often required in addition to antibiotics.

Obstructive and Resistive Lung Disease

Conditions that cause obstruction to air flow within the lungs are called obstructive airway diseases, while conditions that result in resistance to air flow are called resistive airway diseases. They share the common characteristic of increased resistance to air flow within the airways.[28] Asthma is a reversible resistive airway disease characterized by episodic increases in airway resistance due to spasm and narrowing of airways in response to infection, allergic reactions, and environmental conditions. Chronic obstructive pulmonary disease (COPD) denotes conditions of increased airway resistance which are irreversible because of permanent structural damage and obstruction resulting from cigarette smoking, infections, toxic exposures, or any combination of these.

Emphysema is a term used to describe the permanent destruction of aveoli with the resulting expansion of the remaining aveoli. A consequence of emphysema is a reduction in the area in which gas exchange can occur. This results in perfusion/ventilation mismatch and hypoxia. Emphysema is associated with increased airway resistance due to collapse of small airways.

Chronic bronchitis is a different disease process in which there is chronic inflammation of the small airways with resulting increased mucus, airway plugging, and destruction of small airways.[51,52,53] As a consequence, airflow is reduced because of permanent narrowing of the small airways. There is often a reversible component of the airway obstruction superimposed on the chronic changes. Cigarette smoking is the leading cause of chronic bronchitis and multiplies the deleterious effects of other environmental agents such as asbestos, silica, coal dust, and fibers. Frequently, emphysema and chronic bronchitis coexist.

Patients with obstructive airway diseases usually manifest disabilities that result either from hypoxia, hypercapnia, or dyspnea. Both hypoxia and hypercapnia can cause confusion, fatigue, and worsening heart failure. Breathlessness, or dyspnea, is usually the most limiting symptom of COPD. Functional impairment due to COPD can be severe, and COPD is often fatal. Over half of the patients die within two years of their first episode of respiratory failure.[52] These patients require extensive therapeutic and supportive interventions.

The treatment goal of individuals with COPD is to prevent smoking and maintain optimum functioning for as long as possible. This usually involves chest physical therapy, medication, oxygen therapy, and environmental changes designed to conserve energy and reduce exertion. The depression that accompanies chronic illness of all types can be particularly significant in COPD patients, many of whom feel that they have brought it on themselves by smoking. Because of its complexity, COPD is an excellent example of a health problem that requires an interdisciplinary approach.

MUSCULOSKELTAL MANIFESTATIONS OF AGING

The musculoskeletal system is comprised of muscles and tendons, the fascia, the bony skeleton, and joints (including ligaments and cartilage). The individual experiences gradual decrease in strength, control, and mobility as the components of this system age.

Muscle Changes with Aging

Muscle alterations are complex and poorly understood, because the composition of muscles changes over time with replacement of myofibrils by fat, collagen, and scar tissue. Individual muscle fibriles also change with age and become more permeable to water, sodium, and chloride.[9] Blood flow to muscles decreases with age thereby reducing the amount of nutrients and energy available to the muscle, and muscle strength declines.[54] This process begins early in life and accelerates rapidly after the fifth decade, especially when overshadowed by inactivity. By age 60, the total loss in lean muscle mass, referred to as sarcopenia, represents 10% to 20% of the maximum muscle power attained at age 30.[9] (See Chapter 3, Comparing and Contrasting Age-Related Changes in Biology, Physiology, Anatomy, and Function for a detailed description of muscle changes with aging.)

Myopathy and Myositis

Muscle dysfunction in the aged is usually the result of toxic or metabolic factors acting on muscle, rather than due to any intrinsic disease of the muscle.[55] Symptoms suggesting myopathy include weakness in the hip girdle muscles, made apparent by the person's increasing difficulty rising from a chair, and the development of a waddling gait or shoulder girdle weakness, manifested by inability to lift objects above shoulder level. Muscle soreness is not a usual finding with myopathy and is more common with myositis, where there is infiltration of muscles by inflammation.[56] Polymyositis can be ideopathic or related to the presence of underlying carcinoma. Myositis usually responds to steroids or other anti-inflamatory agents.

Muscle weakness can result from several correctable causes including hyperthyroidism, alcoholism, adrenocortical steroid excess (Cushing's disease or administration of steroids), and hypokalcemia (from diarrhea or diuretic use). Correction of the underlying cause usually results in resolution of the weakness.[54]

Fibromyalgia/Myofibralgia

Fibromyalgia, also called myofibralgia, is a common form of nonarticular rheumatism with diffuse musculoskeletal aching and multiple tender points at characteristic sites.[57] Diffuse pain syndromes are common in older persons. Fibromyalgia and polymyalgia are the most common connective tissue disorders in the elderly population. Fibromyalgia may be a secondary phenomenon associated with some of the other diffuse pain syndromes. Pathophysiologic mechanisms in fibromyalgia are not fully understood, however, it is likely to be multifactorial and include poor sleep and psychological factors.[58] However, recent evidence suggests that only a minority of fibromyalgia patients are depressed or have psychological problems, and based on laboratory findings, this connective tissue pain syndrome is more likely a biochemical imbalance. Yaron and associates[59] evaluated serum levels of hyaluronic acid in patients with fibromyalgia. They found that hyaluronic acid serum levels were significantly elevated compared to healthy controls and patients with rheumatoid arthritis. This observation suggests that fibromyalgia is associated with a biochemical abnormality and that serum hyaluronic acid could be a laboratory marker for its diagnosis.[59]

Exercise has been found to be the most effective modality in the treatment of fibromyalgia. Wigers and colleagues[60] compared short- and long-term effects of aerobic exercise, stress management, and treatment-asusual in elderly fibromyalgia patients. Outcome measures included a patient-made drawing of pain distribution, dolorimetry of tender points, ergometer cycle test, global subjective improvement and registration of pain scales, disturbed sleep, lack of energy, and depression scores. Both aerobic exercise and stress management showed positive short-term effects. However, aerobic exercise was overall the most effective treatment, despite being subject to the most skeptical patient attitude prior to the study. At follow-up, symptom severity was remarkably less in the aerobic exercise group and the decreased diffuse pain appeared to be the motivator for compliance with the exercise program.[60] In comparing an evidence-based clinical fibromyalgia program, referred to as Fibro-Fit, with results of controlled clinical trials, Bailey and associates[61] found improvements in all outcome measures (e.g., self-efficacy, pain, physical fitness, function, and coping skills). The results suggest that Fibro-Fit is effective in improving physical impairments and function. The advantage of this program for an older population is that it is not aerobic. Submaximal endurance activities are utilized in addition to strengthening (e.g., weight lifting and theraband) and stretching activities.[61] To evaluate the efficacy of a six-week exercise and educational program for elderly patients with fibromyalgia, Gowans and coresearchers[62] implemented a walking, strengthening, and stretching program, in additional to an educational component. The outcome measures were compared to a nonexercising control group of elders with the same diagnosis. The program produced significant improvements in the six-minute walk test, well-being, perceived fatigue, self-efficacy (for controlling pain and other symptoms), and knowledge. This study is yet another example of the benefits of activity and exercise in fibromyalgia. Short-term exercise and educational programs can produce immediate and sustained benefits for patients with fibromyalgia.[62]

SKELETAL MANIFESTATIONS OF AGING

Aging brings with it many complex and poorly understood changes in bone structure. Until about the age of 45, bone mass increases in both men and women, but for the next 25 years both sexes show a progressive decline in bone mass, with women losing about 25% and men approximately 12%.[63] Although bone growth continues into old age, reabsorption of the interior of the long and flat bones (trabecular bone) increases until it occurs at a greater rate than the formation of new bone. As a result bone strength and stability decline. This is particularly true of trabecular bone, which is found in the highest proportions in vertebral bodies, wrists, and hips. This correlates with the clinical observation of increased incidence of fractures at these sites with age.[64]

Bone is a living tissue that undergoes a continuous cycle of bone formation (involving osteocytes and osteoblasts) and bone resorption (osteoclasts).[65] Factors affecting bone remodeling include: (1) the impact of mechanical forces on the skeleton; (2) circulating hormones, including estrogen, testosterone, calcitonin, parathyroid hormone, and 1,25 dihydroxyvitamin D; and (3) local humoral factors, such as interleukin-1 and interleukin-6, transforming growth factors, and tumor necrosis factor.[65,66] During bone development, chondrocyte proliferation and differentiation may be influenced by the number of cytokines, signaling molecules, and transcription factors. Osteoblastic proliferation may also be affected by these factors. There is increasing research and investigation into the relationship between osteoblast differentiation and other cell lineages as well as the role of regulation of osteocytes.[66]

Determination of bone health requires consideration of two factors: namely, the development of maximum peak bone mass in early life and the rate of bone loss in the later years, particularly around the menopausal and andropausal stage.[67] Peak bone mass and postmenopausal, postandropausal bone loss are principally determined by four factors: genetics, mechanical loading, nutrition, and hormones.[68]

Osteoporosis

Osteoporosis is a heterogeneous condition characterized by an absolute decrease in the amount of normal bone (i.e., loss of bone). Osteoporosis is defined as a metabolic bone disease "characterized by low bone mass and microarchitectural deterioration of bony tissue leading to enhanced bone fragility and a consequent increase in fracture risk."[69] Osteoporosis results when the production of new bone mass is exceeded by the reabsorption of old bone, in other words, osteoporosis is the failure of bone formation to keep pace with bone resorption. This is termed coupling. The result is that bone becomes structurally weakened. There is a normal mineral: collagen ratio unlike that of other metabolic bone diseases, such as osteomalacia, which is a disease characterized by relative deficiencies of mineral in relation to collagen.[70] Osteoporosis is due neither to a lack of dietary calcium nor defective bone mineralization,[63,70] rather it is caused by endosteal resorption, which is greater than the formation of new osteons or bone units.[70–72] Age related trabecular bone loss starts at age 35, and cortical bone loss from about age 40. The loss proceeds at about 0.5% per year; but, at female menopause, the accelerated rate is 2% to 8% due directly or indirectly to lowered estrogen production.[63] The greater the bone mass attained at the time resorption exceeds the creation of new bone, the more time is needed before significant structural changes result. This, in part, accounts for the higher incidence of clinically significant osteoporosis in women than men because men have greater bone mass to start with.

The reasons for the differential rates of demineralization of bone between men and women are not understood, but there are several factors that appear to have a role in the process for both sexes. For example, estrogen deficiency occurring with menopause leads to accelerated bone loss and is partially reversed by replacing estrogen.[63] Clinical hypogonadism is a well-established cause of osteoporosis in men as well. In fact, vertebral fractures, once considered uncommon in men, actually occur at a rate equal to that of women until late in life, when the incidence in women increases rapidly. In both sexes, bone mass is lower in those who have vertebral deformities.[73] A major gender difference is that women more frequently experience severe vertebral fractures with the attendant complications (e.g., pain, kyphotic deformity).[74] However, when men do sustain fractures, they suffer adverse outcomes to the same (if not greater) extent as do women.[75]

Especially consequential are systemic diseases, medications, and lifestyles that may increase the risk of bone loss. Other factors contributing to skeletal weakness include malabsorption of calcium leading to poor bone mineralization (osteomalacia) which affects both sexes. A negative calcium balance can result from calcium deficiency in the diet, malabsorption, and accelerated loss. Impaired absorption of calcium from the intestine can be due to insufficient vitamin D because of diet, or renal or hepatic disease. Calcium absorption can be affected as part of intestinal malabsorption syndromes, such as sprue and regional enteritis.[76] Endocrine disorders affecting calcium balance include hyperthyroidism; excess corticosteroids, as in Cushing's disease or steroid administration; and hyperparathyroidism leading to excess bone resorption as well as hypoparathyroidism resulting in poor calcium absorption. Immobility for any reason and at any age can lead to marked negative calcium balance. When a limb is immobilized, localized osteoporosis occurs.[8]

Thus, for the elderly, decreased mobility adds to the already abundant factors present for the development of osteoporosis. The presence of osteoporosis requires a thorough review of potentially treatable causes. Treatment is a judicious balance of exercise, medication, and dietary manipulation. (See Chapter 11, Orthopedic Treatment Considerations).

Although important, age-related bone loss explains only part of the problem of osteoporosis. A wide variety of other factors appears to affect bone health in men and women.[77,78] Weight contributes substantially to the variation in bone mass, with heavier individuals having greater bone density,[78,79] and weight loss seems to be associated with greater rates of bone loss and higher rates of fractures.[80] Tobacco smoking exerts a negative effect on bone.[80]

The importance of osteoporosis relates to the incidence of bone fracture in postmenopausal females and postandropausal males. Women are postmenopausal for 40% of their lives. Symptomatic osteoporosis affects one in three of the older female population and results in more than 175,000 femur fractures and 500,000 vertebral fractures per year in American women starting in the fifth and sixth decades of life.[78,81] The incidence of fractures is similar for men, but starts later—in the seventh and eighth decades of life.[74] Fracture of the femur is a major contributor to mortality in the elderly. Activity, particularly weight-bearing activity; prescription of medications such as calcitonin or sodium flouride, dietary supplements of calcium intake of 1500 mg/day, and vitamin D 400–600IU/day may possibly retard further bone loss.[81] Boron supplementation may reduce the urinary excretion of calcium and magnesium and elevate the concentration of 17 beta-estradiol,[82] thus, inhibiting normal bone loss of aging. Calcium supplementation is thought to inhibit immunoreactive and parathyroid hormone (PTH) secretion as levels of PTH increase with age in response to diminished levels of extracellular fluid calcium. Estrogen replacement therapy may retard the "normal" bone loss of aging, but, the protective effect may last no longer than two to three years after termination of treatment.[83] Chapter 7, Exploring Nutritional Needs covers dietary modifications that impact bone health. Chapter 11, Orthopedic Treatment Considerations covers hormone replacement therapy for osteoporosis in depth.

Although the entire skeleton loses mass with aging, the distribution of bone loss is not uniform. Those areas of the skeleton with the highest content of trabecular bone, such as vertebral bodies, and bones of the wrist and hip, will lose the greatest amount of their mass.[71,72]

Calcium supplementation and dietary modification for the prevention and management of osteoporosis, and drugs used to treat osteoporosis are discussed in Chapter 7, Exploring Nutritional Needs and Chapter 8, Pharmacology, respectively.

Bone mineral density (BMD) as measured by dual x-ray absorptiometry (DXA) is expressed as absolute BMD (g/cm^2) and may be designated by either the number of standard deviations (SD) from the mean of age-matched controls (known as Z score) or the number of SD from the young normal mean (T score).[84] The World Health Organization (WHO) developed guidelines for the clinical diagnosis of osteoporosis, which are based on the T score, with a T score of less than −1.0 being defined as osteopenic and a T score of less than −2.5 being referred to as osteoporosis. An outline of these diagnostic criteria for osteoporosis is shown in Table 5–1.[85]

The WHO guidelines for T scores are as follows: (1) a T score above −1.0 is defined as "normal;" (2) T score between −1.0 to −2.5 is defined as "osteopenic;" (3) a T score below −2.5 is define as "osteoporotic;" and (4) a T score below −2.5, plus one or more fragility fractures, is defined as "severely osteoporotic." This classification is particularly important for the physical or occupational therapist prescribing exercise and determining levels of risk for fractures and frailty. The authors of the book have added preventive "actions" to those prescribed by WHO in Table 5–1, in addition to expanding the criteria to provide suggested prescriptions for rehabilitative interventions.

Osteopenia

The term osteopenia describes an evenly systemic decrease in bone density below an expected level. Therefore, bone loss is not unilateral or limited to one area of the skeleton. Osteopenia is the prelude to osteoporosis. Table 5–1 indicates the BMD range that differentiates osteopenia from osteoporosis.

Osteomalacia

Osteomalacia is a softening of bone owing to poor mineralization. Pain, tenderness, and weakness are often symptoms, as is concurrent weight loss. Vitamin D and calcium deficiencies are usually present. Osteomalacia most often presents in patients with

TABLE 5-1. MODIFIED WHO CRITERIA FOR OSTEOPOROSIS (ADDED ENHANCED "ACTION" AND "REHABILITATION PRESCRIPTION")[85]

Category	Fracture Risk	Action	Rehabilitation Prescription
Normal BMD < 1 SD below young adult reference range	Below average	Be watchful for "clinical triggers" Preventive interventions: Diet & exercise	Trunk extension exercises Resistive exercises Weight-bearing exercises Deep breathing exercises Aerobic exercise
Osteopenia BMD 1 - 2.5 SD below young adult reference range	Above average	Consider hormone replacement therapy Be watchful for "clinical triggers" Nutritional supplements Drug therapy as warranted Repeat investigations 2-3 years	Trunk extension exercises Resistive exercises Weight-bearing exercises Deep breathing exercises Aerobic exercise Functional activities Environmental modifications Fall prevention program
Osteoporosis BMD > 2.5 SD below young adult reference mean	High	Exclude secondary causes Therapeutic intervention indicated: Diet, exercise, supplementation, drug therapy as warranted Hormone replacement therapy	Trunk extension exercises Resistive exercises Weight-bearing exercises Deep breathing exercises Functional activities Environmental modifications Fall prevention program
Severe Osteoporosis BMD > 2.5 SD below young adult reference mean, plus 1 or more fragility fractures	Extremely high	Exclude secondary causes Therapeutic intervention indicated: Diet, exercise, supplementation, drug therapy as warranted Established osteoporosis	Trunk extension exercises Weight-bearing exercises Deep breathing exercises Functional activities Environmental modification Fall prevention program Protective clothing as warranted

Source: World Health Organization (see ref 85)

biliary tract or intestinal disease, in whom vitamin D absorption is decreased.

Osteomalacia (and rickets) can be due to one or a combination of abnormalities of calcium, vitamin D, phosphate, or alkaline phosphatase. The most common pathogenesis is a disorder of vitamin D availability, activation, or action.[70] Vitamin D abnormalities cause osteomalacia by resulting in inadequate amounts of calcium and phosphorus to support the normal mineralization of the bone matrix. Similarly, primary or secondary calcium and phosphate deficiency states cause osteomalacia when their reduced ambient concentration leads to an inadequate supply of minerals for proper matrix mineralization. Disorders that produce phosphaturia also limit the availability of phosphate for mineralization of bone and thus can cause osteomalacia and rickets. A rare cause is an inherited defect in the synthesis of alkaline phosphatase, an enzyme important in the mineralization process. Certain drugs in excess, including the bisphosphonates and sodium flouride, also cause osteomalacia by their toxicity to the mineralizing osteoblast and mineralizing front.[70]

Osteonecrosis

Osteonecrosis, or avascular necrosis, is the death of bone and is primarily caused by a disruption in blood supply to the bone, most commonly affecting the femoral head in the elderly.[71] This may occur when a fracture of the pelvis or femur results in perforation of the arteries that supply the femoral head. It may also occur secondary to other conditions that disrupt femoral head blood supply. Some examples include long-term steroid use or multiple steroid injection history, alcohol abuse, gout, and failure of an internal fixation of an intracapsular hip fracture.

Death of bone and bone marrow cellular components occurs in osteonecrosis in the absence of infection. Necrosis of the osteocytes occurs as a result of ischemia. Pain is the initial symptom. If the hip joint is involved, pain will be exacerbated by weight-bearing activities. An antalgic gait is common, and pain is provoked by specific movements, especially hip adduction, internal rotation, and hip flexion.

Treatment in the elderly is generally total joint replacement. Rehabilitation in the elderly with osteonecrosis focuses on joint protection preoperatively, maintaining strength and functional activities, and postoperative reconditioning.

Paget's Disease

Paget's disease (PD, also called osteitis deformans) is a disorder of bone remodeling characterized by increased bone resorption and increased formation. It usually presents after the fourth decade of life and its prevalence increases with age to affect 1% to 2% of individuals over age 60 in the United States, with a slight male predominance.[65] It is usually a focal disease involving one bone (monostotic), but it can involve several bones (polystotic). In rare cases, PD can become generalized, especially in familial disease. Osteogenic sarcoma is a dreaded complication of PD in the elderly.[65]

Increased and abnormal osteoclastic bone resorption is the initiating event in PD. There is accumulating evidence that a slow virus plays a role in its pathogenesis. Increased interleukin-6 (IL-6) production may be a contributing factor to the development of PD. Genetic mechanisms are also likely to be important in familial cases, with possible linkage to chromosome 6 or 18.[65,71]

The rate of bone resorption in PD can be as much as ten-fold to twenty-fold the normal rate. This is reflected in increased biochemical indices of bone resorption, including urinary excretion of collagen catabolites, like hydroxyproline and collagen cross-linked peptides, and osteoclast products, notably serum acid phosphatase. Osteoblastic new bone formation responds appropriately to the increased resorption, and this is reflected in increased osteoblast products such as alkaline phosphatase and osteocalcin. The increased cellular activity produced highly vascular and cellular bone, and collagen is deposited by overworked osteoblasts in an abnormal and disorganized pattern of "woven bone."[71]

Because the tight coupling of formation and resorption is maintained in PD despite the increased skeletal turnover, systemic mineral homeostasis is usually unperturbed and serum calcium is usually normal. However, when patients with PD are immobilized, as can occur upon fracture or surgery, they may become hypercalciuric or even hypercalcemic. This occurs because muscle stimulation of bone formation is decreased and bone resorption proceeds relatively unopposed. Hypercalcemia may also signal the presence of hyperparathyroidism, which is commonly reported with an increased level of calcium in the serum plasma of a patient with PD.[71]

JOINT CHANGES WITH AGING

Degenerative changes in joints begin as early as the second or third decade, and after age 40 progress more rapidly.[86] These changes occur mainly in the weight-bearing joints such as the ankles, knees, hips, and lumbar spine. Cartilage forms the weight-bearing surfaces of these joints. By age 30, it begins to crack, shred, and fray. Over time, deep vertical fissures appear, and the cartilage-producing cells die or become less effective. Ultimately, the cartilage layers are eroded exposing the bone beneath to direct contact with the opposing bone.[87] This contact causes pain and produces the physical sign of crepitus, or grinding, when the joint is moved. New bone formation is stimulated, but the bone growth is irregular. Often, it interferes with joint mobility as the resulting osteophytes enlarge. Synovial membranes, which surround and protect joints, also exhibit changes due to age. With age, the synovial lining thickens and the synovial fluid becomes more viscous. Other changes include the shrinkage of the intervertebral discs in the lumbar spine due to loss of water content in the discs.[87] Coupled with vertebral body collapse, disc shrinkage can produce a significant loss of height. The aging changes associated with bone, cartilage, and synovial membranes are dealt with extensively in Chapter 3, Comparing and Contrasting-Age Related Changes in Biology, Physiology, Anatomy, and Function.

Degenerative Arthritis/Osteoarthritis

Arthritis is an inflammation within the joint space which causes pain, loss of mobility, and deformity of the joint. There are several different types of arthritis, but all lead to a common final pathway known as degenerative joint disease (DJD) or osteoarthritis.[88] Recurrent joint trauma leads to intra-articular damage, resulting in the release of proteolytic enzymes, which often causes bleeding. A cycle is set up with increased cartilage damage, bleeding, and the release of potentially distructive enzymes. Over time, cartilage is eroded, new bone growth stimulated, and the joint gradually loses its ability to respond to trauma, making it even more susceptible to additional trauma and damage.[87] Pain develops because of irritation of the periostium, joint capsule, and fibrotic changes of the periarticular muscles. Unlike rheumatoid arthritis, the synovial membrane in osteoarthritis is not the primary site of involvement. However, over time it can become fibrotic as a result of the primary degenerative process.[88]

The joints most often affected by DJD are the hands, knees, hips, lumbar, and cervical spine. It is manifested clinically by stiffness and pain that increase with use. Impaired mobility makes it difficult to accomplish routine activities of daily living (ADLs).[89]

The onset of symptoms in osteoarthritis can occur insidiously or suddenly. Generally, joint destruction occurs gradually and progresses slowly. Pain is described as a deep ache, can occur at rest, and often awakens the individual at night with nocturnal discomfort. Stiffness of the involved joint(s) after periods of inactivity occurs and usually is resolved in a relatively short period of movement. Loss of flexibility is associated with soft tissue contractures, intra-articular loose bodies, osteophytes, and loss of joint surface congruity.[90]

The development of effective anti-inflammatory medications and improvement of surgical interventions in joint disease has changed the current management of end stage DJD. Joint replacement can be very effective in restoring function and limiting pain, and joint fusion and anti-inflammatory medications are often effective in pain control.

Rehabilitative treatment is focused on protection of the involved joint from excessive mechanical stresses with the use of an assistive ambulatory device, foot orthotics that provide shock absorption and proper joint positioning, and patient education on nutrition, hydration, and reduction of wear and tear on the joint. Maximizing joint function through flexibility and strengthening exercises is important.

Rheumatoid Arthritis

Rheumatoid arthritis (RA) can occur at any age and is characterized by the abrupt onset of symmetrical joint swelling, erythema, and pain. Inflammation of the synovial membrane results in the release of proteolytic enzymes which perpetuate inflammation and joint damage.[87] A biochemical marker for RA is a positive rheumatoid factor, which is an antibody that reacts with immunoglobulin antibodies found in the plasma. Rheumatoid factor is also often found in the synovial fluid and synovial membranes of individuals with the disease. It is hypothesized that the interaction between rheumatoid factor and the immunoglobulin triggers events that initiate an inflammatory reaction. The leukocytes, monocytes, and lymphocytes phagocytes attracted in the immune system response lead to the release of lysosomal enzymes, which cause articular cartilage destruction and synovial hyperplasia. These changes also result in the development of destructive vascular granulation tissue called pannus. This tissue proliferates, gradually diminishing the joint space.[90] The pannus contains inflammatory cells which destroy the cartilage, bone, and periarticular tissues leading to joint instability, deformity, or ankylosis.

Symptoms are usually insidious and progress slowly as the disease progresses. Complaints of joint pain, muscle fatigue and weakness, weight loss, and general loss of stamina are common. Inflammation and musculoskeletal symptoms are localized to the specific joint, though multiple joints are usually involved. Morning stiffness is more pronounced and of longer duration than in osteoarthritis. Intense pain can occur following periods of rest. The involved joints tend to be the small joints of the hands and feet, the wrists, shoulders, elbows, hips, knees, and ankles. Essentially every joint is involved in this autoimmune, systemic condition. Eventually deformities occur affecting mobility and basic ADLs. Rheumatoid arthritis is a systemic disease, therefore, other signs and symptoms are often present, including: fever, fatigue, malaise, poor appetite, weight loss, nutritional deficiencies, weakness, anemia, enlarged spleen, and lymphadenopathy (disease of the lymph nodes).[88]

Response to therapy is usually quite good. Treatment needs to focus on reducing pain, maintaining mobility and minimizing joint restrictions, edema, and joint damage. Given the ease with which the aged develop muscle atropy with disuse, aggressive physical therapy is essential to maintain strength and joint mobility during phases of remission, and occupational therapy is required to focus on joint protection and basic ADLs. During exacerbation, physical and occupational therapy should be directed toward pain management through decreasing swelling in the joint (ice, electrical stimulation), maintaining joint mobility and decreasing discomfort (oscillation joint mobility techniques, active motion), and encouraging participation in functional ADL. Foot orthotics are recommended to reduce shock and reposition the foot to lessen the stresses on the involved lower extremity joints.[91]

Gout

Gout is a form of arthritis that usually affects only a few joints. Needle-like crystals of uric acid (monosodium urate crystals), are deposited in joints, tendons, and bursae, and they incite a rapidly progressive inflammatory reaction. The result is the abrupt onset of severe pain, and development of an acutely tender and inflamed joint which can incapacitate the individual very rapidly. In middle age, gout is episodic, but, in later years it tends to occur with greater frequency and in more joints.[28] Gout tends to affect men more than women. It occurs spontaneously or as a result of other illnesses or treatments. Some diuretics used to treat congestive heart failure or hypertension may cause gout because they interfere with the secretion of uric acid from the kidney, thereby causing an elevated uric acid level. Other causes of gout include rapid tissue turnover such as seen in lymphoma, leukemia, thalassemia, psoriasis, and pernicious anemia. Acidosis of any cause, such as diabetes, alcohol, or renal failure can also precipitate gout. When crystals other than monosodium urate crystals are found, such as calcium pyrophosphate dihydrate crystals, the condition is called *pseudogout*.

Treatment is medical and directed at eliminating and preventing acute attacks and correcting the hyperuricemia. The prognosis for preventing permanent joint deformity is good if treatment is undertaken early in the course of chronic gout.[86] NSAIDs or colchicine are medications used during the acute phases, and the involved joints should be rested, elevated, and protected with assistive ambulation devices and protective splints or othotics. Dietary changes, weight loss, and moderation of alcohol intake are important modifications. Medications such as allopurinol are utilized to reduce hyperuricemia, which is key to preventing acute inflammation.

Temporal Arteritis/Polymyalgia Rheumatica

Inflammation of small- and medium-sized arteries that derive from the aortic arch give rise to a condition called giant cell arteritis or temporal arteritis

(TA). It is part of a spectrum of conditions that include the entity of polymyalgia rheumatica (PMR), which is only seen in individuals over the age of 50.[28] Neck and hip girdle stiffness and pain, an elevated sedimentation rate, low grade anemia, fever, weight loss, elevated globulins, and rapid response to steroids are the characteristics of polymyalgia rheumatica. Of the greatest clinical significance is the high incidence of sudden monocular blindness, which can occur from the obliteration of the opthalmic artery by the arteritis.[92] This potential outcome requires the early and aggressive evaluation and treatment of anyone suspected of having PMR/ TA. Diagnosis is established by biopsy of the temporal artery, looking for evidence of arteritis. The biopsy is positive in approximately 50% of cases[11]; however, a negative result on biopsy does not exclude the presence of PMR/ TA. It is a relapsing, systemic disease which usually responds to steroids and resolves over one to two years. It is one of the most common preventable causes of blindness in the aged.

Spondyloarthropathies

Spondyloarthopathies are a group of disorders that include ankylosing spondylitis, Reiter's syndrome, and psoriatic arthritis. These conditions are all more prevalent in an older adult population.[90]

Ankylosing spondylitis is an inflammatory arthopathy which involves the sacroiliac joints, apophyseal joints, intervertebral disk articulations, and the costovertebral joints. This pathology can also affect the large peripheral joints, including the hip, knee, and shoulder.[90] Ultimately, this disorder leads to fibrosis, calcification, and ossification of the involved joints and is associated with a marked loss in functional mobility. The onset is insidiuous back pain and stiffness with pain described as an ache. These individuals experience considerable morning stiffness that is decreased with activity and increased with rest. The recumbent position is not tolerated well. As the disease progresses, the cervical and thorasic spines and the chest cage become involved. Radiating pain is generally reported in the lower and upper extremities as spinal mobility is compromised. Complaints of pain are usually accompanied by non-mechanical complaints of weight loss, fever, and fatigue.

Nonsteroidal anti-inflammatory drugs (NSAIDs) are used to control pain and inflammation. Heat modalities provide temporary relief of stiffness. Severe postural deformities are associated with inactivity, so exercise, inclusive of range-or-motion and strengthening exercises, to minimize thoracic kyphosis is critical. Due to thoracic structural changes, respiratory status needs to be monitored. The more severe the kyphosis, the more likely that pulmonary status will be compromised. Deep breathing exercises should be accompanied by mobilization of all thoracic articulations. Stretching and strengthening exercise are particularly important in addressing muscle imbalances. Extension of the trunk needs to be emphasized, although aggressive stretching should be avoided during periods of inflammation.

Reiter's syndrome is a reactive arthritis in which an inflammatory arthropathy follows an infective process, such as bacillary dysentary or venereal disease. There is a triad of symptoms associated with this syndrome, which include urethrits and conjunctivitis, early on in the disease, and arthritis, which is typically asymmetrical and involves the joints of the lower extremities.[93] The digits, especially the toes, can become swollen and distended (dactylitis). The arthritis can progress and spread to the spine and the upper extremities. Other potential manifestations include mouth ulcers, skin rashes, and inflammation of the glans penis or clitoris. Low back pain is a common complaint.[93] Treatment is directed at the symptoms with NSAIDs for pain and inflammation, joint protection, and functional mobility exercises. Immobilization and inactivity should be aggressively discouraged with an emphasis on range-of-motion and stretching exercises.

Psoriatic arthritis is an inflammatory joint disorder affecting individuals with psoriasis. It leads to erosion of the periarticular bone and significant joint destruction. There is a lymphocyte infiltration into the synovium and the appearance of edematous granulation tissue which leads to thickening of the synovium. As the disease progress, the joint space is often lost to the build-up of dense fibrous tissue. The distal interphalangeal joints of the hands and feet are most commonly involved with concommitant joint deformities (e.g., claw deformity) and flexor tenosynovitis. Pitting of the nail beds is also commonly associated with psoriatic arthritis. The sacroiliac joint can also be involved and typically occurs unilaterally. Other problems associated with psoriasis include inflammatory eye disease, including conjunctivitis and iritis; renal disease; mitral valve prolapse; and aortic regurgitation.

The emphasis of treatment is the control of the psoriasis and symptomatic interventions inclusive of NSAIDs for pain and inflammation, corticosteroid injections, and functional mobility exercises to maintain the joint space. Orthotics are often helpful in providing relief to painful joints of the feet.

NEUROMUSCULAR MANIFESTATIONS OF AGING

Central Nervous System

Central nervous system (CNS) impairment is a leading cause of functional disability in the aged.[30] The normal process of aging results in the gradual diminution of size and number of cells in all locations within the CNS.[11] The size and weight of the brain declines with age as demonstrated by autopsy and computed axial tomography (CAT) scan results.[94] Metabolic activity declines as measured by oxygen consumption and blood flow, and the conduction rate of peripheral nerves declines steadily.[9] Of great interest, however, is the observation that the changes of normal aging do not result in significant neurological impairment.[30] Although there is a steady diminution of the components of the CNS over time, there is no associated neurological deficit that can be ascribed solely to aging.

Unimpaired, normal aging occurs in the majority of elderly persons. The development of chronic, severe, cognitive impairment, however, occurs in nearly 30% of individuals over the age of 80.[30] The functional impairments resulting from CNS dysfunction can be severe. It is useful to think of them as resulting from changes in cognition (such as judgment, comprehension, memory), changes in sensory input (blindness, deafness, neuropathy), and changes in ability to execute actions (paralysis, gait disorders, loss of coordination, incontinence, aphasia). Alterations of capacity in any of these spheres can result from and cause alterations in psychiatric performance as well.

The final common pathways of neurological dysfunction are the transcortical tracts. They involve cognitive functioning, movement, sensation, and sensory integration of movement. A multiplicity of specific diseases and conditions result in dysfunction within these realms. Some are preventable, and early medical intervention is essential. Others are relentlessly progressive and do not respond to disease-specific interventions. In these conditions, interventions are directed at achieving the individual's maximal functional level. The following sections are a brief and greatly simplified survey of the more common types of neurological disease in the aged.

Confusion/Delirium

Cognitive disorders of all types account for nearly two thirds of nursing home admissions and a significant majority of those elderly persons who are incapacitated by illness.[95] Severe cognitive dysfunction may not impair an individual's longevity, especially with meticulous attention to treatable complicating illnesses. As a result, the aged with cognitive dysfunction make up the largest group of functionally disabled individuals.

Those conditions resulting in alterations in cognitive function can be divided into several groups on the basis of reversibility and chronicity. Acute cognitive dysfunction of rapid onset without underlying damage to brain tissue carries the best prognosis for recovery. This usually results from toxic or metabolic derangements, which affect the normal functioning of the brain, or from psychiatric illness, such as depression, that also has a metabolic basis. The term delirium is used to describe these acute confusional states. Susceptibility to toxic/metabolic delirium (toxic encephalopathy) is not limited to the elderly; however, the more limited metabolic reserve of the aging brain makes the elderly person more sensitive than younger persons to minor stresses.

Confusion, restlessness, agitation, poor attention span, reversal of sleep-wake cycles, hallucinations, and paranoia can all be manifestations of delirium. Subtle changes resulting from correctable toxic/metabolic abnormalities can persist for extended periods before they are recognized as resulting from potentially reversible causes. Appropriate interventions are frequently delayed. It is particularly important for these reversible conditions to be identified by the health care team because failure to intervene in a timely manner can result in permanent cognitive dysfunction. Equally important is the risk that inappropriate treatment will result in further functional impairment or a greatly increased risk of injury. Pathological brain dysfunction resulting from toxic/metabolic causes usually has a good prognosis for recovery when the underlying abnormality is corrected. Table 5–2 lists the more common causes of toxic confusion/delirium in the elderly.

TABLE 5–2. COMMON CAUSES OF TOXIC/METABOLIC CONFUSION/DELIRIUM IN THE ELDERLY.[95]

Drugs	Metabolic Abnormalities
Alcohol	Hypoglycemia
Psychotropics (tranquilizers, antipsychotics, antidepressants)	Hyponatremia
Over-the-counter sleep, cold, and allergy medications	Hypocalcemia
Analgesics	Hypothermia
Antihypertensives	Hypothyroidism
Beta-blockers (propranolol)	Hypoxia
Antiparkinsonian medications	Vitamin B_{12} deficiency
Anticonvulsants (phenobarbital, phenytoin, carbamazepine)	Hepatic failure (elevated ammonia)
Digoxin	Renal failure (elevated BUN, creatine)
H_2 blockers (cimetadine)	Elevated cortisol
Amphetamines	Cortisol deficiency
	Pulmonary failure (elevated carbon dioxide)

Source: Wedgewood (see ref 95)

Interventions are directed at identifying and correcting the underlying metabolic abnormality. Although the prognosis for return to baseline CNS function is usually good with correction of the abnormality, the patient's overall prognosis is often determined by the underlying disease that causes the metabolic abnormality rather than the degree of brain dysfunction. During a confusional state, however, the individual is more prone to accidental injury, complications such as aspiration pneumonia, and further cognitive dysfunction due to inappropriate use of sedatives that may aggravate rather than relieve the agitation. The occurrence of any of these complications may worsen the overall prognosis for recovery. Acute toxic/metabolic delirium may coexist with chronic progressive forms of brain dysfunction, such as Alzheimer's disease.

Dementias

Dementias are characterized by slow onset of increasing intellectual impairment, including disorientation, memory loss, diminished ability to reason and make sound judgments, loss of social skills, and the development of regressed or antisocial behavior.[96] Frequently, depression is superimposed on dementia as a reaction to the perceived loss of intellectual skills, which leads to further cognitive impairment.[97]

Alzheimer's disease and multi-infarct dementia are the two most common forms of irreversible dementia. Each has a fairly characteristic pattern of onset and findings. Alzheimer's disease is usually slowly progressive and begins insidiously. It is not associated with focal neurological deficits or abrupt changes in severity. Patients typically begin with short-term memory deficits that progress to severely regressed behavior, an inability to learn or remember new tasks, and loss of ability to perform ADLs.[98] Multi-infarct dementia is usually of more rapid onset, occurs in younger individuals, and progresses in a step-wise fashion with abrupt worsening and subsequent plateaus of function. Frequently, there are focal neurological deficits such as paresis and parethesias.[99] Often, the individual is hypertensive, diabetic, or both. He or she may also show evidence of generalized atherosclerosis.[100]

It is important to distinguish between Alzheimer's and multi-infarct dementias. The prevention of recurrent cerebral infarction may arrest the progression of multi-infarct dementia, which has as its pathophysiological basis irreversible brain damage resulting from repetitive ischemic injury caused by emboli or bleeding. Normalization of blood pressure is the most effective intervention known. Other types of reversible dementia, such as those resulting from hypothyroidism, vitamin B_{12} deficiency, and normal pressure hydrocephalus, can become "fixed" and unresponsive to treatment unless identified and treated at an early stage. Early identification of these correctable dementias is essential. Unfortunately, though no such therapeutic imperative currently exists for Alzheimer's disease, recent research on Alzheimer's has produced promising results and the potential for delaying, and perhaps preventing the onset of this dreaded dementia looms on the horizon.

Regardless of the etiology of dementia, once reversible causes have been ruled out, the main tasks of the clinical team are to minister to the patient's emotional needs, assist in the act of grieving for lost function, alter the environment so that the patient's remaining skills can be used, augment the patient's capacity to successfully undertake ADLs, educate the family, provide emotional and physical support for the family and caretakers, and provide the patient and family with a realistic prognosis. Any superimposed illness can cause a rapid and prolonged decline in mental status, which may totally resolve as the underlying illness is treated.

Alzheimer's Disease: A Special Consideration

Striking with cruel randomness across an increasingly elderly population, Alzheimer's disease (AD) afflicts some 4 million Americans, most of them over the age of 65.[101] They may range from a former president to a neighbor next door, but the ailment is always the same: it clutters the brain with tiny bits of protein, slowly robbing victims of their mental power until they are no longer able to do even the simplest chores or recognize their closest friends and kin. So far, medical science has been stymied, unable to treat the disease or slow its fatal progression. However, recent research is encouraging. Strategies to prevent or delay the onset of symptoms, as well as to prevent the decline into the advanced stage of AD are being explored. While these strategies do not yet exist in a proven and clinically applicable form, the science is progressing rapidly.[102] There may yet be a light at the end of that long, dark tunnel called Alzheimer's.

Alzheimer's disease is the form of dementia that is most common in the elderly population. Currently it has been diagnosed in approximately 4 million Americans, and if the present trend continues, it is projected that the number will increase to 14 million by the year 2050. Women are more likely to suffer from AD, with a women to men ratio of 2.8:1.0 for those aged 75 and older. Alzheimer's is the fourth leading cause of death following heart disease, cancer, and stroke.[103–105] One in every ten persons over the age of 65 has Alzheimer's, and approximately half those over the age of 85 are diagnosed with AD.[103,104]

Alzheimer's disease is a progressive, degenerative disease that affects the hippocampus, neocortex, and transcorticol pathways of the spinal cord, resulting in impaired memory and thinking, behavioral changes, and progressive return of primitive motor patterns that were encephalized during late fetal and early childhood development. The classic appearance of neurofibrillary plaques and tangles progressively impedes synaptic connections and results in neuronal death.[106] The neuritic plaques are comprised of amyloid precursor protein (APP) that is encoded for by a gene on chromosome 21. Smaller fragments of APP called amyloid beta peptides (Aß) have also been identified.[107] The gene carries the code for APP and appears to be one link in the chain of events that leads to deposits of beta amyloid. The neurofibrillary tangles are composed of paired helical filaments that consist of tau proteins and develop in the cytoplasm of pyramidal cells.[107] Neuritic plaques and neurofibrillary tangles are located in the areas of the cerebral cortex linked to intellectual function and sensory integration (just posterior to Wernicke's area) and the hippocampus and neocortex, the two most primitive areas of the brain.[101,108,109]

Some scientists believe that as many as half of all cases of Alzheimer's may have a genetic component. In addition to the abnormality on chromosome 21, chromosome 14 defects have also been identified in individuals with early-onset AD. Further support of this theory is the recent discovery of a gene on chromosome 19 that appears to be defective in many people with the more common, late-onset form AD. It has also been found that one form of the apolipoprotein E4 (APOE4) gene is inherited at an increased rate among patients with late-onset Alzheimer's.[107,110] This apolipoprotein is involved in cholesterol metabolism. Chromosome 1 has also been identified to carry a "presenile" gene associated with early-onset AD.[110]

The protease theory of Alzheimer's is also being explored. An enzyme called protease has been identified and isolated in individuals with AD and may play a key role in creating the biochemical chaos in the brain that causes Alzheimer's. This enzyme has become the target of many drug designers. Just as protease inhibitor medications are currently used to block the activity of the autoimmune deficiency (AIDS) virus by targeting proteins (e.g., beta-secretase), it is hypothesized that protease inhibitors may also be effective in blocking amyloid plaque formation.[109] Protease has long been postulated to act as a chemical scissors that helps snip away excess protein from brain cells, thereby inhibiting the buildup of protein debris that accumulates into amyloid plaques.

Nongenetic, environmental factors, such as an infectious agent (e.g., virus), nutritional components, or toxic environmental substances (e.g., metals or industrial chemicals) are also being evaluated for their potential roles in the development of this disease. An example of potential nutritional factors in AD is provided by the Nun Study. Previous studies suggested that low concentrations of folate in the blood are related to poor cognitive function, dementia, and Alzheimer's disease-related neurodegeneration of the brain. Nutrients, lipoproteins, and nutritional markers were measured in participants of the Nun Study who later died between the ages of 78 and 101 years old (mean: 91 years). At autopsy, several neuropathic indicators of AD were determined including atrophy of the neocortex (frontal, temporal, and parietal) and the number of neocortical lesions (senile plaques and neurofibrillary tangles). There was a strong correlation between serum folate and severity of atrophy of the neocortex. Low serum folate was associated with atrophy of the cerebral cortex.[111] Other nutrients, such as the low circulating levels of antioxidants, have been identified as potentially contributing to the development and progression of the disease.

Scientists have now learned that Alzheimer's disease begins at least 20 years before symptoms appear, and prevention and early intervention could potentially improve the quality of life of people predisposed to this disease. Some of the major scientific discoveries related to Alzheimer's disease over the past few years include

- Genes associated with Alzheimer's have been identified on four chromosomes;
- Diagnostic techniques have improved to a 90% accuracy rate (without autopsy);
- The Food and Drug Administration has approved several drugs for the treatment of Alzheimer's, an effective first step toward effective therapies;
- Mounting evidence that readily available treatments, such as estrogen, vitamin E, folate, ibuprofen, and exercise may help slow or prevent Alzheimer's;
- Associations between higher levels of education and reduced risk of Alzheimer's has been observed;[107] and
- Scientists have learned that Alzheimer's is not caused by a single factor but probably by a number of genetic and environmental factors.

Sister Mary, the gold standard for the Nun Study, was a remarkable woman who had high cognitive test scores before her death at 101 years of age. What is more remarkable is that she maintained this high status despite having abundant neurofibrillary tangles and senile plaques. Findings from Sister Mary and all 678 participants in the Nun Study may provide unique clues about the etiology of aging and Alzheimer's disease, exemplify what is possible in old age, and show how clinical expression of some diseases may be averted.[112]

Further discussion of the evaluation, staging, and intervention in AD is provided in Chapter 12, Neurological Treatment Considerations.

Cerebrovascular Diseases

In contrast to the dementing illnesses which result in "global" brain dysfunction, cerebrovascular disease more commonly results in focal brain dysfunction.[100] There are several different types of cerebrovascular disease, each with a different pathophysiological mechanism, prognosis, and treatment. The mechanisms include the rupture of small blood vessels from hypertension; abrupt blockage of vessels by emboli from the heart or atheramatous plaques in the large arteries leading to the brain; and spontaneous formation of blood clots within the blood vessels due to local increases in coaguability. The pathophysiology of cerebrovascular disease is the interruption of blood flow to brain tissue with resultant cell damage or death from ischemia.[9] Decreases in the heart's ability to pump blood can lead to ischemia, as can blockage of the blood vessels to or within the brain from atheromatous plaque, emboli, or inflammation of the lining of the blood vessels. Uncontrolled hypertension, diabetes mellitus, smoking, and elevated cholesterol contribute to cerebrovascular disease directly by affecting the entire circulatory system.

Preventive interventions must be specifically directed at the underlying pathophysiology. Hypertension can be controlled by medication, diet, and exercise. The prevention of emboli usually requires the use of anticoagulants such as aspirin, diperiadamole, and warfarin. The risk of bleeding, both into the brain and into other organs, increases with the use of these agents and often limits their use in certain patients. If emboli result from cardiac arrhythmias, prevention results from a return to normal sinus rhythm through the use of electrical cardioversion or antiarrhythmics such as quinidine, procainamide, and digoxin.[30] Because of the heightened risk of intracerebral bleeding, anticoagulants are avoided in the presence of hypertension and in cerebral vascular accidents resulting from bleeding into brain tissue.

Recurrent, small cerebral vascular accidents can result in multi-infarct dementia. More commonly, however, limited areas of the brain are damaged and result in more focal disabilities, including loss of motor or sensory function over the right or left side of the body, alterations in vision, speech, and the ability to interpret sensory inputs. The extent of the deficit following a stroke depends on the location and function of the injured part of the brain, the degree of damage, and the availability of unaffected regions of the brain which can assume the lost function. Residual effects can be so subtle as to be functionally negligible or so extensive that only the most basic brain functions, such as the control of respiration and blood pressure, are preserved.

Parkinson's Disease

Parkinson's disease (PD) is the most prevalent type of parkinsonism, a clinical syndrome caused by lesions in the basal ganglia, predominantly in the substantia nigra, that produce deficits in motor behavior.[113] Parkinsonism is a clinical rather than an etiologic entity, since it is associated with several pathological processes that damage the extrapyramidal system. Its many causes are divided into four categories:[113]

- Primary, or idiopathic (PD)
- Secondary parkinsonism (associated with infectious agents, drugs, toxins, vascular disease, trauma, brain neoplasm)
- Parkinson-like syndromes
- Heredodegenerative diseases.

Parkinson's disease is a progressive degenerative disease of unknown cause resulting in the loss of melanin-containing brain cells in the substantia nigra and locus caeruleus and a decrease of dopamine in the caudate nucleus and putamen. The term Parkinson's disease is reserved for those cases of unknown etiology.[114] Parkinson's disease makes up approximately 80% of cases of parkinsonism.[113] The syndrome results in a reduction in muscle power, rigidity and slowness of movement (akinesia), crucial to the characteristic tetrad known as **TRAP**:

Resting **T**remor
Cogwheel **R**igidity
Bradykinesia/**A**kinesia
Postural reflex impairment

Of this tetrad, only resting tremor is truly suggestive of PD, an early sign that may remain prominent even late in the disorder.[115] The others occur in varying degrees in other forms of parkinsonism.

Parkinson's syndrome is used to describe the same constellation of anatomical, motor, and intellectual deficits which result from specific agents and cause Parkinson-like symptoms. These include post encephalitic (von Economo's disease), posttraumatic (boxer's parkinsonism), and toxin induced parkinsonism (e.g., haloperidal). Similar movement disorders often result from the use of neuroleptics or reserpine but are not associated with any anatomical changes. Parkinsonism is a commonly occurring syndrome of the aged.[113,114] When fully developed, there is characteristic increased limb rigidity, stooped posture, shuffling gait, decreased mental acuity, difficulty initiating movement, and tremor which is usually symmetrical, rhythmic, and abolished by intentional movement. Early in its course, however, parkinsonism may give an asymmetrical tremor, slight increase in muscle tone with associated decrease in spontaneous movement, masking of the face with loss of spontaneous expression, and generalized rigidity in muscle tone. As these restrictions on voluntary movement progress, they result in significant functional impairment. Associated incontinence and constipation further complicate the management of these individuals.

Benign familial tremor is often mistaken for Parkinson's disease early in its course. Characteristically, the tremor is more rapid (seven to nine per second) and increases with movement. As a result, patients complain of an inability to lift a spoon or cup without spilling its contents. There is no associated hypokinesia or gait disorder. Alcohol, sedatives, and beta-blockers (such as propranolol) effectively reduce the amplitude of the tremor.[115,116]

In parkinsonism, drug treatment and intensive physical and occupational therapy are frequently helpful, however, these interventions do not change the relentless progression of functional impairments. Drug therapy is directed at the amelioration of symptoms at the lowest effective dose. Drugs are of three general classes: (1) those that are anticholenergic; (2) those that mimic the effects of dopamine (such as bromocryptine); and (3) those that replete dopamine (L-dopa). (Refer to Chapter 8, Pharmacology) Physical and occupational therapy to maintain strength, improve posture, prevent contractures, and maintain the maximal functional capabilities of the individual with Parkinsonism is crucial. Since the onset of PD is typically in the fifth or sixth decade of life, and is progressive, the complications of the aging process are superimposed on the progression of this disease. Lack of mobility, loss of balance, and weakness result in more falls and the complications of immobility, such as osteoporosis, cardiovascular deconditioning, muscle weakness, and loss of flexibility are other considerations in the treatment of patients with PD. Despite the progressive nature of this illness, many patients can maintain full function for several decades with a combination of physical and occupational therapy and drug intervention.[113,117] Refer to Chapter 12, Neurological Treatment Considerations for a comprehensive review of treatment interventions in Parkinson's disease patients.

Stimulation of the brain with electrodes implanted in the brain shows promise in control of the tremor in PD.[118] Stereotactic surgery in the lateral ventral nucleus of the thalamus has also proved to be helpful in the treatment of dyskinesia and tremor that is not controlled through drugs.[113] Despite the ethical considerations inherent in fetal cell transplantation and genetic remodeling, these are the two areas of scientific investigation that hold the most hope for patients with PD. Fetal cell transplantation has proven to be effective in enhancing motor function in persons with advanced PD. Additionally, in early animal studies, the use of glia-derived neurite-promoting factor (GdNPF) in conjunction with fetal cell transplant, appears to promote survival of dopamine neurons in fetal cells, which may protect mature dopamine neurons from damage induced by PD.[119]

Huntington's Disease

Huntington's disease (HD), a progressive hereditary disorder, affects 25% of its victims after the age of 50.[120,121] It is characterized by abnormalities of movement, personality disturbances, and dementia. HD is associated with choreic movement which is brief, explosive, purposeless, involuntary, and random. While the cause remains unknown, there is a specific pattern of tissue damage in the brain. The ventricles are enlarged as a result of atrophy of the adjacent basal ganglia, specifically the caudate nucleus and putamen, collectively referred to as the striatum.[120,121] The volume of the brain decreases and the dementia is ascribed to the dysfunction of the striatum.[120] There is a reduction in the amount of neurotransmitters, including GABA, acetylcholine, and metenkephalin. This re-

sults in an imbalance of neurotransmitters with relatively higher levels of dopamine and norepinephrine. The normal balance of inhibition and excitation responses of the basal ganglia and thalamus that usually provide controlled, smooth movement is disrupted. Excess dopamine results in overexcitation of the thalamocortical pathway, explaining the abnormal movement patterns of chorea. As the disease progresses, rigidity and bradykinesia, or slowness of movement occurs.[120,121]

The clinical manifestations of HD include chorea, dysdiadochokinesia (inability to make rapid alternating movements), abnormal eye movements (small jerky saccadic movements), an unsteady gait, dysarthria (decreased rate and rhythm of speech), dysphagia, cachexia (wasting of muscle mass with weight loss), sleep disorders, and urinary incontinence. Muscle strength and tone will usually be normal in the early phases, however, as the disease progresses, there is a significant reduction in muscle strength and the tone becomes rigid.[120,121]

In addition to the physical manifestations, the mental disturbances in persons with HD include personality and behavioral changes such as irritability, apathy, depression, decreased work performance, violence, impulsivity, and emotional lability.[120] The neuropsychological profile characteristically includes a type of memory disturbance that affects information retrieval. Short-term recall is poor, and motorically, when a physical command is given, patients are unable to recall the movement and have difficulty with organization, planning and sequencing, even when all the information is provided.[120] Additionally, individuals with HD have visuospatial deficits, impaired judgment, and ideomotor apraxia (the inability to perform previously learned tasks).

The primary treatment is medical management. Drugs for symptomatic relief of chorea are often used, inclusive of anticonvulsants or antipsychotic drugs that block dopamine neurotransmission. There is a high incidence of side effects associated with these drugs including acute dystonias, pseudoparkinsonism, and akathisia (uncontrolled physical restlessness). Tardive dyskinesia resulting in involuntary movement of the face, tongue, and lips may also occur with long-term use of these pharmaceutical agents. Surgical procedures to remove the medial globus pallidus, thought to be overactive due to the neuronal loss in the striatum, have been tried with inconsistent results. Implantation of adrenal medullary grafts have proved to offer only transient improvement. As with PD, techniques using electrotherapeutic procedures are being explored.

From a rehabilitation perspective, treatment is directed toward safety and maintenance of the highest possible level of functional capabilities. Education of the individual and their caregivers, including gait and safety in mobility is the basis for therapeutic intervention. Patients with HD frequently fall, so the environment needs to be safety proofed. The use of protective clothing, such as hip protectors (this author uses ice hockey shorts and shirts which are well padded) may be warranted. Chorea may throw an individual off balance. Likewise, those individuals with brady- kinesia have a tendency to "freeze," especially when they are fearful of falling, and this may also precipitate falls.

The inability to perform skilled or purposeful movements, apraxia, leads to significant problems in the performance of ADLs. Self-care activities become increasingly difficult, despite cueing from caregivers. Instruction in transfer techniques for caregivers is particularly important.

It is crucial that soft tissue deformities be prevented through proper positioning. The ability to intervene with neurotherapeutic techniques, may be limited in the face of progressive motor system impairments and the concomitant decline in cognitive functioning. However, techniques that reduce tone may also reduce choriform movements. Increasing stability about the shoulders, trunk, neck, and hips will help maintain function. The treatment of HD patients has some parallels with the treatment of cerebral palsy athetosis. Maintaining the optimal quality of life is the most important goal for treatment of individuals with HD and their families.[122]

At present, the best hope for the person with Huntington's disease lies in a better understanding of the genetic mechanisms causing the destruction of the GABA-containing cells in the striatum and in the cerebral cortex.

Amyotrophic Lateral Sclerosis

Amyotrophic lateral sclerosis (ALS), commonly known as "Lou Gehrig's disease," is a degenerative disease affecting both the upper and lower motor neurons. It is a progressive disease with an adult onset between the ages of 50 and 70 years, and as a result is a disease seen in an older adult population. There is a massive loss of anterior horn cells of the spinal cord and the motor cranial nerve nuclei in the brainstem resulting in muscle atrophy and weakness (amyotrophic). Demyelination and gliosis of the corticospinal tracts and corticobulbar tracts caused by degeneration of the Betz cells in the motor cortex results in upper motor neuron symptoms (lateral sclerosis).[123] Numerous theories abound related to the etiology of ALS because of its similarity to poliomyelitis, which affects the anterior horn cells, however, the true cause is still unknown. Some theories proport a viral origin, while other theories suggest toxicity (increased lead and aluminum levels and abnormalities in calcium and magnesium concentration). Other theories suggest that ALS may be related to an accelerated form of normal aging, the loss of androgen receptors in motor neurons, a lack of neurothrophic hormone, abnormal DNA in motor neurons, excess oxidative stress due to free radicals, or problems with thyrotropin-releasing hormone.[124] A more recent theory is that there is a decrease in the level of glutamate and an increase in intracellular calcium leading to "excitotoxicity" and causing an autoimmune response whereby an antibody to calcium channels leads to motor neuron destruction. However, the evidence of autoimmunity is not conclusive.[125]

The clinical manifestations are variable depending on the extent of involvement of the upper or lower motor neurons. There is an insidious development of asymmetrical weakness, usually in the distal aspect of one extremity in the initial phases of the disease. The individual reports stiffness and cramping with volitional movement, especially after periods of rest. Weakness with resultant wasting and atrophy of the muscles occurs and patients experience fasciculations, or spontaneous twitching of muscle fibers (reflective of lower motor neuron involvement). Generally the extensor muscles weaken faster than flexor muscles, especially in the hands. Spasticity occurs when there is upper motor neuron involvement. Cranial nerve involvement is heralded by tongue fasciculations and weakness, facial and palatal weakness, and swallowing difficulties. Occulomotor and bowel and bladder function are usually spared. There is an unremitting spread of weakness to other muscle groups leading to total paralysis of spinal musculature and muscles innervated by the cranial nerves. Death is usually related to respiratory failure.[126]

A historically consistent diagnostic criteron for ALS is the absence of sensory involvement. However, some researchers have found sensory dysfunction, particularly in somatosensory-evoked potentials transmitted in the posterior columns of the spinal cord.[127] Autonomic nervous system involvement has also been quantified by the sweat test (sympathetic) and parasympathetic vascular reflex testing of heart rate changes during Valsalva and deep breathing. Patients with ALS show symptoms of autonomic dysfunction and this suggests the problems would appear to be associated with atrophy and bulbar changes.[128] There is also evidence of pyramidal tract dysfunction (e.g., hyperreflexia, spasticity, and Babinski and Hoffmann reflexes)[123] reflective of upper motor neuron involvement.

Emphasis of intervention is to maintain the highest level of function throughout the course of the disease.[129] Symptomatic measure may include the use of anticholinergic drugs to control drooling, and antispasmotic drugs such as diazepam, quinine, or baclofen. Due to the difficulty with chewing and swallowing, nutrition needs to be monitored. A dysphasia program may be warranted in the presence of jaw weakness, loss of tongue mobility, difficulty in lip closure, and impairment of the swallowing reflex. Respiratory complications can occur due to aspiration, so the consistency and texture of foods should be monitored. Use of chest physical therapy inclusive of incentive spirometry, intermittent positive pressure breathing, postural drainage, segmental expansion and diaphragmatic excursion exercises should be employed, even in the early stages of the disease.

Respiratory failure and malnutrition are generally part of the terminal stages of ALS.

Exercise and activity programs should be based on function and in line with the patient's personal goals. Despite physical and occupational therapy interventions, the disease is progressive and treatment will need to be modified and staged to incorporate diminished motor abilities. Specific therapeutic goals may include maintaining maximal muscle strength within the limits imposed by ALS and minimizing/preventing secondary consequences of inactivity, such as contractures, thrombophlebitis, decubiti, and respiratory infections. It is very important that the patient not be overworked as there is anecdotal evidence that too much muscle activity exacerbates the loss of muscle strength in poliomyelitis,[129,130] and this can probably be extrapolated to include the patient with ALS due to the similarities in these diseases. A primary consideration for the therapist working with a patient with ALS is to prevent further deconditioning and disuse atrophy beyond that imposed by the disease, so maintainance of the strength and flexibility to accomplish ADLs is appropriate. Older, newly diagnosed patients with ALS who have led a sedentary lifestyle prior to diagnosis should be encouraged to increase their activity levels. In the final stages of ALS, palliative care including pain management, positioning, basic ADLs, feeding, and chest physical therapy will be necessary.[123]

Normal Pressure Hydrocephalus

Normal pressure hydrocephalus is common in the elderly.[30] It presents with the clinical triad of dementia, slow, shuffling gait, and urinary incontinence. Dilation of the ventricles with hydrocephalus is thought to affect the function of the surrounding brain tissue which controls lower extremity movement and bladder function. Computerized axial tomography (CAT) scan of the head can establish the presence of ventricular enlargement but cannot determine whether it is due to atrophy of brain tissue or enlargement of the ventricles. However, in selected cases that have shown clinical improvement after repeated removal of cerebrospinal fluid, placement of a surgical shunt occasionally results in resolution of the dementia, incontinence, and gait disorder.[28]

Cervical Spondylosis

Cervical spondylosis is caused by the bony spurs from severe degenerative arthritis impinging on the cervical spinal cord.[28] Patients usually develop a clumsy, spastic, and stiff gait, incontinence, and diminished sensation in the lower extremities. Cervical CAT scanning, myelograms, and magnetic resonance imaging (MRI) can establish the location and extent of spinal cord impingement. Surgical decompression of the spinal cord may be necessary to interrupt the progression of this condition and its associated severe disabilities.[30]

Spinal Cord Injury

Living with a spinal cord injury (SCI) is challenging enough, then comes age to complicate the situation. With its abrupt demand for extreme courage and determination, SCI is a sizable adversary affecting any individual who, up until the point of injury to the spinal cord, no matter what the cause, has enjoyed full physical function without giving it a second thought. Acceptance is essential for emotional healing, but, dealing with the initial SCI-induced limitations isn't the only bridge SCI patients will have to cross. Somewhere along the journey, aging comes into the picture, too, as it does for all of us. The patient with SCI is going to age like we all age. And, just as it's important for us to stay healthy and in good physical shape, it's also important for patients with SCI. All of the complications they have had from day one of their spinal cord injury, they are going to have throughout their life—and their level of independence could be greatly affected.

This is not to suggest that all spinal cord injuries happen in youth, and that a SCI patient then ages. Some older individuals suffer from SCI due to accidents and falls, fractures from osteoporosis, complications of surgeries, infections, tumors, and multiple other pathologies. But, for the most part, patients who sustained SCI early in life, because of better medical and surgical interventions, are living longer and aging in wheelchairs. There are numerous problems, superimposed on the aging process, that result.

Overuse conditions are extremely common in the shoulders of older patients with SCI who use wheelchairs. While performing transfers, patients with SCI rely on their shoulders to bear the body weight. The problem is, the shoulder isn't made to be the sole weight-bearing joint. Problems with impingement syndromes and rotator cuff impairments frequently occur, in addition to osteoarthritic changes in the shoulder joint. Wrist problems are also common in an older adult SCI population for the same reason.

Postural changes occur due to trunk inactivity. Without active muscle contraction in the trunk, the spine is prone to osteoporotic changes. When a weak trunk is combined with a sling-back or low-back wheelchair, the patient's body tends to collapse into a more stable position. Over time, this can lead to scoliosis, kyphosis, pain syndromes, and breathing and gastrointestinal problems. To provide additional support for the trunk, avoiding the use of low-back and sling-back chairs and using, instead, chairs that have a padded, higher, board-like back is advisable. In severe cases, a custom-made back may be warranted.

Fragile skin combined with static sitting and laying position is frequently a problem with the elderly SCI patient. With aging comes a change in skin quality. The membrane loses its padding of fat, skin becomes less elastic, thinner, and more fragile. The loss of the level of protective sensation eliminates the ability to know when too much pressure is occurring in one place, especially over bony prominences. This increases the potential for pressure sores and ulceration. Pressure ulcers can occur over the trochanters, ischial tuberosity, and the coccyx in sitting. The same areas are prone to break down in patients who spend long periods of time in bed. These patients are more likely to have problems with the sacrum, heels, ankles, knees, elbows and shoulders. Positioning with frequent changes, seating cushions, and special mattresses can be helpful.

Due to the changes in the quality of tissues of the tendons, muscles, and cartilages discusssed in Chapter 3, Comparing and Contrasting Age-Related Changes in Biology, Physiology, Anatomy and Function, the inactivity inherent with SCI increases the risk for contractures at any of the extremity joints. A consistent stretching regimen and splinting as deemed necessary is required to prevent the need for casting or surgical releases. Patient education regarding positioning and stretching are crucial components of a rehabilitation program.

To combat the muscle loss associated with aging coupled with the inactivity imposed by SCI, patients need to understand the importance of regular exercise. In general, muscle maintenance is even more important for older patients with SCI than people who are able-bodied, because the former relies on the concentrated muscle bulk to retain independence. Adaptive devices to make a task easier and less frustrating are helpful in encouraging movement and functional activities.

Fatigue is another issue associated with aging and sedentary lifestyles. To prevent the loss of energy reserve from robbing patients of their independence, therapists can suggest changes in daily activities and equipment that decrease the demands. Heavier wheelchairs can be exchanged for light-weight chairs, which require less effort for mobilization. For longer distances, the use of motorized chairs may be warranted. Changing from a car to a van with a lift is another recommendation that can save patients both time and energy. With a van, an individual isn't burdened with having to load a wheelchair into a small vehicle, and the lift eliminates the strain of a chair-to-vehicle transfer.

As older individuals with SCI age, so do their family members. It is not unusual to have a caregiver who is within the same age range as the patient and who is the sole source of assistance for that individual. Instead of having to move to an assisted living or rehab facility, patients with SCI can usually remain at home by taking advantage of home health services. A trained caregiver coming into the home three or four times a week to help with baths and other needs can provide the extra support a family needs to ensure a loved one can continue to live at home.

Peripheral Nervous Systems

With aging, the number and size of peripheral nerve fibers diminish with a concomitant decrease in conduction velocity.[131] There is often a clinically insignificant decrease in touch and vibration sense. The peripheral nerves, however, are easily affected by nutritional deficiencies, toxins, and endocrine disorders.[30] The resulting neuropathies can cause marked loss of position sense, resulting in instability, falls, chronic pain, and dysesthesia (painful and persistent sensation induced by even a gentle touch of the skin).

The common nutritional deficiencies which lead to neuropathy are folic acid (caused by poor diet or folic acid antagonists, such as diphenylhdantoin, sulfonamides), vitamin B_{12} (caused by pernicious anemia due to malabsorption of B_{12}), and alcohol-related deficiencies of thiamine, pyridoxine, and other B vitamins.[28,132] Toxic neuropathies can result from heavy metal exposure (such as lead and arsenic), medications (such as nitrofurantoin, disulfiram, diphenylhydantoin), or from uremia. Replacement of the deficiency and removal of the toxin are the cornerstones of therapy. Prognosis is good for resolution.[133]

Diabetic neuropathy can take several forms. There is a distal sensory polyneuropathy which affects the hands and feet with diminished sensation and burning pain; a proximal motor neuropathy resulting in proximal muscle wasting and weakness; and a diffuse autonomic neuropathy resulting in orthostatic hypotension, neurogenic blad- der, obstipation (intractable constipation), and bowel immotility.[134] In addition to these diffuse forms of neuropathy, single nerves can be affected. The resulting mononeuropathies can cause loss of ocular muscle function and painful nerve root and branch dysfunction wherever an involved nerve travels.[135] Treatment is symptomatic and may involve analgesics, specific physical therapy, and possible splinting. Relief from painful dysesthesias may be obtained in some cases with the use of diphenylhydantoin, amitriptyline, or carbamazepine. Tight control of the blood sugar appears neither to prevent nor lessen diabetic neuropathy.[136] Rarely, another endocrine disease, hypothyroidism, can present with neuropathy. It responds to thyroid hormone replacement. Other causes of neuropathy in the aged include paraneoplastic syndromes (lung, ovary, multiple myeloma) and amyloid.[137]

NEUROSENSORY MANIFESTATIONS OF AGING

Vestibular Problems

Vestibular complaints have been reported in over 50% of elderly people.[138] The central mechanisms that are involved in the control of balance do not appear to change excessively with age, but are more likely to be affected by degenerative neurologic diseases such as Alzheimer's or Parkinson's disease. However, there are age-related changes in the peripheral vestibular system. Hair cell receptors decrease in number and there is a loss of the vestibular receptor ganglion cells. The myelinated nerve cells of the vestibular system decrease by as much as 40%. There is a reported increase in the incidence of benign paroxysmal positioning vertigo (BPPV) with complaints of dizziness with head movements. This may be due to an increase in the deposits in the posterior semicircular canal. Partial loss of vestibular function in the elderly can lead to complaints of dizziness, with less ability of the nervous system to accommodate to positional changes.[138]

Coupled with the vestibular losses, there is concomitant loss in vision and somatosensation, which severely affects sensory input necessary for the maintenance of balance. In addition, there are longer response latencies and delayed reaction times. Vision changes include loss of acuity, decreased peripheral fields, and loss of depth perception. The loss of input from this combination is slow, with compensation developing through the years. Therefore, compensatory strategy in response to postural instability is not the same as in the person with acute vestibular insufficiency. There is an overall loss of functional reserve so that the threshold for clinical loss is lowered. This is demonstrated by the increased number of falls in older people with a history of falls compared to an age-matched groups with no history of falls when they are tested with increased challenges to balance.[139] There is an apparent decrease in the ability to integrate the conflicting sensory information to determine appropriate postural responses. Since there are changes as well in motor output, the loss of balance, in addition to lack of sensory organization, may be due to a poor response to vestibulospinal stimulation.[139]

Various pathological conditions will affect the peripheral vestibular system to produce vertigo or disequilibrium. Benign paroxysmal positional vertigo is the most common cause of vertigo with changes in head position in an older adult population. Generally, BPPV is associated with the deposition of otoconial material in the cupula of the posterior semicircular canal. The otoliths adhere to the cupula in some cases and retard its return to a resting position after head rotation, or obstruct the flow of endolymph, producing symptoms from the affected posterior semicircular canal by impeding or ceasing stimulation to the vestibular nerve. It can be unilateral or bilateral. Prolonged inactivity can also lead to symptoms of BPPV. Habituation exercises (placing the person in positions that provoke vertigo) and balance exercises have been found to be very effective in the treatment of this disorder. These exercises are discussed in Chapter 12, Neurological Treatment Considerations.

Acute vestibular neuritis, also known as *labyrinthitis*, is the second most common cause of vertigo in the elderly.[140] It is associated with a viral infection causing inflammatory changes of branches of the vestibular nerve. In the elderly, onset is usually preceded by upper respiratory or gastrointestinal tract infections. The chief complaint is the acute onset of prolonged severe rotational vertigo that is exacerbated by movement of the head. Symptoms include spontaneous horizontal-rotatory nystagmus beating toward the good ear, postural imbalance, and nausea.[140] Antiviral medications are used in this condition, and habituation exercises help to quickly resolve this condition once the infection clears.

Ménière's disease is a disorder of the inner-ear function that can cause hearing problems and vestibular symptoms in the elderly.[140] The patient complains of a sensation of fullness of the ear, a reduced ability to hear, and tinnitus. These symptoms are accompanied by rotational vertigo, postural imbalance, nystagmus, and nausea and vomiting that can last for extended periods of time. A phenomenon identified in Ménière's disease is endolymphatic hydrops, a condition in which malabsorption of endolymph results in an increase in endolymphatic fluid pressure in the endolyphatic duct and sac. Medical intervention includes a salt-restricted diet and the use of diuretics to maintain the fluid balance in the ear. Vestibular suppressant medication is sometimes used during the acute phases and the patient is advised to avoid caffeine, alcohol, and tobacco. In severe cases surgical intervention is to insert a shunt to drain excess fluid from the ear, however, the effectiveness of this procedure is questionable.[140] Ménière's disease presents a challenge to rehabilitation efforts. Until the fluid imbalance is controlled, patients with this disease do not respond well to typical vestibular rehabilitation programs. Emphasis should be on safety and balance exercises.[141] Challenging the balance to recruit the other systems, such as the cervico-ocular reflex and proprioceptive and visual mechanisms for controlling posture during stance and ambulation may be effective.

Bilateral vestibular disorders may occur secondary to other diseases in the elderly or could be drug induced. Conditions that may lead to vestibular problems include meningitis, labyrinthine infections, oteosclerosis, Paget's disease, polyneuropathy, bilateral tumors (acoustic neuromas in neurofibromatosis), endolymphatic hydrops, bilateral vestibular neuritis, cerebral hemosiderosis, ototoxic drugs, inner-ear autoimmune disease, or congenital malformations of the inner ear.[140] Autoimmune conditions such as rheumatoid arthritis, psoriasis, ulcerative colitis, and Cogan's syndrome (iritis accompanied by vertigo and sensorineural hearing loss) can lead to a progressive, bilateral sensorineural hearing loss often accompanied by bilateral loss in vestibular function. Additionally, alcohol may cause an acute vertigo as the dehydration created by alcoholic substances can change the specific gravity of the endolymph. Other agents that may cause vertigo include organic compounds of heavy metals and aminoglycosides.[140,142] Controlled physical exercises can improve the condition in patients with bilateral vestibulopathy by recruiting nonvestibular sensory capacities such as the cervico-ocular reflex and proprioceptive and visual control of stance and gait. (See Chapter 12, Neurological Treatment Considerations).

Skin Pathologies

The skin is the largest organ of the body and functions to protect the interior of the body from the effects of pathogens, toxins, environmental extremes, trauma, and ultraviolet irradiation. With age, and often as the result of the accumulated effects of repeated injury, the skin changes. It grows and heals more slowly, becomes more sensitive to most toxins, and is less able to resist injury.[143] It becomes less effective as a barrier to infections. The specialized appendages, such as sweat and sebum glands, pressure and touch sensors, and hair follicles, atrophy. This results in dryness, a decrease in ability to alter body temperature through sweating, and loss of hair. The small blood vessels in the skin diminish with age, which contributes to less effectiveness as a barrier to infection, diminished reserve for repair, and altered ability to assist in thermoregulation.[144]

There are several skin diseases that are common in the aged and which have significant effects on function. These include malignant tumors, herpes zoster, and decubitus ulcers. A great deal of data has accumulated to demonstrate an association between cutaneous aging and the development of skin cancers, infections, and ulcers.[143] Many of the factors that appear to predispose individuals to the development of pathological manifestations in the aged are similarly operative in the development of skin problems.[145] These include cumulative exposure to carcinogens, diminished DNA repair capacity, and decreased immunosurveillance. In addition, the reduced epidermal density in the skin that is seen with senescence is likely to play a role in the development of skin lesions, infections, and ulcerations.

Malignant Tumors

Skin cancer is the most common malignancy known to the human race.[145] As with most malignant diseases, its incidence increases exponentially with age, however, there are few cancers that are as age-dependent as cutaneous malignant disease. The three most important malignant tumors of the skin in the aged are basal cell carcinoma, squamous cell carcinoma, and malignant melanoma.

Basal cell carcinomas arise in areas of sun-exposed skin and increase with the intensity and duration of sun exposure as well as genetic background. This type of nonmelanoma skin cancer accounts for approximately 50% of all cancers reported each year in the United States[146]; 80% of all skin cancers fall into the category of basal cell carcinomas.[147] Though basal cell carcinomas occur in all races, the prevalence increases with fair skin and decreases with more intensely pigmented skin. The most common sites are the face, tops of the ears, neck, anterior chest, arms, and hands. Treatment is virtually always successful in eradicating the tumor unless there has been extensive local invasion of muscle and bone. These tumors rarely ever metastasize but can be locally invasive and deforming if not treated early. Fortunately, they are slow growing and seldomly get large enough to be more than a cosmetic problem.

Squamous cell carcinomas arise from chronically irritated skin. Sun damage is the most common cause but other irritants include tobacco (lip and mouth), snuff (nose), coal tar, soot, and X-rays. Chronically traumatized scars following burns or surgery are other sites of predeliction.[145] These cancers are locally invasive and frequently metastasize to regional lymph nodes, brain, and lung, and therefore, carry a higher mortality rate than basal cell carcinomas. Early detection and excision result in higher cure rates. Extensive surgery with excision of all regional lymph nodes and radiation therapy are frequently employed to cure these tumors. They are poorly responsive to chemotherapy.[148]

Malignant melanoma is also the result of sun damage.[149] It is estimated that approximately 17,700 people develop a new primary malignant melanoma each year.[146] This means that approximately 1 in every 185 individuals living an average life span will develop malignant melanoma in this country.[150] Furthermore, the incidence of this disease is doubling every 10 to 15 years.[150] Despite constantly improving cure rates over the years, the death rate is over 5500 per year and increasing.[146] Although malignant melanoma affects all age groups, the highest age-specific incidence rates occur in the population over the age of 60 years of age.[151] In the elderly, lentigo maligna melanomas and acral-lentiginous melanomas (occurring on the plantar surface of the foot, most commonly on the weight-bearing areas of the heel and forefoot[152]) occur disproportionately in the geriatric population. Both present as flat areas of increased, multicolored (brown, black, red, and blue) pigmentation. Occasionally, white areas are also present within the lesion, presumably related to foci of spontaneous regression of the tumor. Because the prognosis for survival with melanoma is related to the depth of skin invasion at the time of excision, these melanomas have a good prognosis if removed early. Nonetheless, deaths occur from lentigo maligna melanoma at the same rate as other melanomas when matched for similar anatimic site and thickness.[153] Other forms of melanoma are also found in the elderly and require early detection and excision to avoid the increasingly poor prognosis with lesion depth. As time goes on, particularly if the tumor becomes invasive, nodularity may develop at the surface of the lesion and ulceration may occur. The nodular melanoma, which is more aggressive in nature, comprises approximately 20% of malignant melanomas.[146] Melanomas metastasize early and extensively to brain, lung, liver, and bone tissue.

Skin cancer is a major concern in geriatric populations. Both cumulative exposure to carcinogens and age-related factors contribute to the high prevalence of cutaneous malignancy in the elderly. Although mortality rates from skin cancer are relatively low, morbidity can be significant, particularly if lesions are neglected. Physical and occupational therapists could have a major impact on the early detection of skin cancers by assessing skin status during physical evaluation, not only for obvious ulcerations or lesions, but the more subtle presentations of skin changes as well.

Herpes Zoster

Herpes zoster results from the reactivation of a dormant varicella virus (chicken pox), which had been sequestered for a long time in a sensory nerve root. The result is an intensely painful and pruritic eruption over the area innervated by one sensory nerve root. Immunocompromised hosts, such as those on steroids, or with chronic diseases that alters the immune response, such as cancer and renal failure, have a greater incidence of herpes zoster.[154] Healthy individuals also get herpes zoster, however, the reasons for its reactivation are obscure.

Two types of disability result from this infection. First, the eruption itself requires local care to prevent superinfection by bacteria, and the associated pain inhibits mobility, appetite, and sleep. Second, there is a high incidence of postherpetic neuralgia in the aged.[137] A severe burning pain can persist for months—long after the local eruption has resolved. Although there are some medications which lessen the severity of the initial pain, the patient with postherpetic neuralgia usually requires narcotics for relief. Rehabilitative efforts with herpes zoster is in maintaining mobility through functional exercise and ambulation. In an elderly individual, pain-imposed restriction of activity can lead rapidly to the devastating effects of bed rest, especially when a neuralgia exists.

Decubitus Ulcers

Decubitus ulcers result from prolonged pressure and shear force induced damage to the skin. Usually occurring over bony prominences, pressure and shear forces impair circulation to the area, resulting in ischemic changes in the tissue and in ulcer formation.[155] They are most common in situations in which there is forced immobility due to illness or injury, diminished response to pain because of altered sensorium or inability to move, and altered nutritional status, usually as the result of some other illness or injury. Chronic weight loss leads to a decrease in subcutaneous fat, fragile epidermis, decreased blood flow to the dermal vessels, and a depressed immune function. Although aging skin has altered healing properties, decubitus ulcers are the result of other illnesses and are not simply the result of aging. They are rarely seen in otherwise healthy elderly persons.

Decubitus ulcers are potentially serious in frail elderly who are chronically ill. The patients most susceptible are those who are among the most debilitated and are confined to bed or chair.

It takes less than an hour of unrelieved pressure exceeding that of the capillary blood flow to induce pressure necrosis.[155] Bony prominences, such as over the coxa, lateral hips, heels, ankles, elbows, and scapulae, are frequently subjected to pressure high enough to cause ischemic injury. Malnutrition and diminished cutaneous blood flow contribute to the genesis and the perpetuation of these ulcers. Once the skin has broken down, irritation due to incontinence, exposure to bacterial contaminants, and compromised blood flow will contribute to further skin, subcutaneous fat, and muscle breakdown.[156]

Decubitus ulcers are easier to prevent than they are to cure. Prevention requires meticulous attention to potential pressure areas and development of treatment strategies to assure that pressure is distributed evenly and no spot has pressure applied too long. Once a pressure sore develops, it must be kept free from any further pressure in order to heal.

Treatment also includes debridement of any dead skin, either surgically or through dressing changes designed to remove necrotic tissue. In order for the ulcer to heal, the base of the ulcer must be free of necrotic debris and bacteria and it must provide a suitable environment for the growth of new skin. It must also be kept pressure free. Furthermore, the patient must receive adequate nutrition, including trace elements and vitamins such as zinc and vitamin C. Restoration of nutritional status is essential to healing decubitus ulcers. Achieving nitrogen balance by providing sufficient protein to make new tissue (with adequate levels of calories to protect the protein from being used for energy) is a primary goal. Surgical closure is sometimes required. Given the intensity and duration of the required treatment to heal an established decubitus ulcer, every effort should be made to prevent the occurrence of pressure sores through careful positioning and turning, air and water mattresses to distribute pressure, and attention to nutrition.

Physical therapy intervention includes low intensity current or nonthermal ultrasound.[157] Debridement can be accomplished using a whirlpool, though prolonged immersion in water in the dependent position should be avoided as it emaciates the tissues and increases the risk of further tissue breakdown. Functional activity and therapeutic exercise should be employed to maintain physical condition and capabilities of avoiding prolonged pressure. Further discussion of integumentary problems and treatment approaches is provided in Chapter 14, Integumentary Treatment Consideration.

Disturbances of Touch

Touching provides one with important information about one's environment. It is also an important method of communication. The aging process often leads to a general decline in tactile sensitivity,[143] but the degree of loss is highly variable. Some situations are more profound than others due to underlying pathological conditions, declining circulation, or injury. A loss or decline in tactile acuity will affect the older person's ability to localize and properly identify stimuli. It also reduces the patient's response time due to the reduction in speed and intensity with which the stimuli is perceived.

The skin is a very important element in the ability to sense touch. The dermis thins, loses elasticity, and has a diminished vascularity with age.[145] Loss of tissue support for remaining capillaries results in fragility and easy bruising (senile purpura).

The most common appearance of aging skin is dryness, scaling, and an atrophic appearance.[143] These changes may be related to systemic disease or functional problems, but are considered part of the normal process of aging. The changes are associated with diminished sebaceous activity, a decrease in hydration of the horny layers, alterations in the metabolic and nutritional components associated with skin production and repair, and a dysfunction in keratin formation.[145] The skin loses its elasticity. Hair loss is related to vascular insufficiency.[30] The associated involvement of the peripheral arterial and venous systems produces pigment changes and an increased deposit of hemosiderin in the soft tissues, adding to the disturbed keratin formation. In general, the skin appears dry and yellowish with a wrinkled, inelastic and parchment-like appearance. The decline in cellular division with age results in a slower rate and efficiency of tissue repair following any trauma.[145]

As with the other senses, touch acuity declines with age. Peripheral receptors provide the neurosensory input for the sense of touch, pressure, pain, and temperature. The receptors are found within the dermis and epidermis of the skin. Receptors can be free-standing or arranged in small corpuscular masses. Meissner's corpuscles (touch-texture receptors), Pacini's corpuscles (pressure-vibration receptors), and Krause's corpuscles (temperature receptors), as well as peripheral nerve fibers are noted to decline in transmission, but the ability to sense pain remains intact because there are few age-related changes that occur in the free nerve endings. Sensitivity to touch, temperature, and vibration, however, frequently decline with age, therefore, the elderly person must take special care to avoid injury from concentrated pressures or excessive temperature on the skin.[157]

Vibratory sensitivity loss is sometimes related to certain nervous system disorders. Reliable data exists, however, to indicate that there is a clear decline in vibratory sense that may begin as early as age 50 and that has no underlying pathology.[143] The decline appears to be greater in the lower extremities, and is thought to be the result of undetected microchanges in the circulation in the legs or lower spinal cord.

Stereognosis is the ability to recognize an object by touching and manipulating it. A decline in this area is not thought to be related to aging but rather to an impairment of the central neurological processes, such as that seen in cerebral vascular accidents.

Ocular Pathologies with Age

Low vision is an extremely common problem in the elderly, which may have devastating consequences for functional independence and health status. It ranks only behind heart disease and arthritis as the etiology for impaired function in those over the age of 70.[158] Vision is the sense that human beings seem to depend on the most, because our society relies heavily on visual cues. Much of our communication is via visual images, such as the written word, facial expressions and body language, billboards, and television. Identification of much that is in one's environment occurs through vision. It is a major tool for environmental safety, independence, and mobility.

With aging, several structural changes occur in the eye that evolve into pathologies, all of which result in a decline in visual acuity. Many of these changes begin at an early age and progress steadily, but slowly, over time. The slowness of this process allows for the individual to gradually accommodate to the changes and to continue functioning. At some point, however, the cumulative effects of the process will result in some loss of independence and mobility.

The lens ages early so that by the age of 50 most people will exhibit some signs of aging in their vision.[92] With age, the cytoplasm of transparent crystalline cells that form the lens throughout life become discolored, opaque, and rigid. Additionally, certain ligaments and muscles weaken, thereby limiting the ability of the anterior-posterior diameter of the lens to expand.[159] Gradually, the lens becomes set in size and flat. This condition, known as presbyopia, leads to a decline in both visual acuity and field. As the lens ages, thickens, and becomes yellow and somewhat opaque, the risk of cataracts also increases.[92] Because the lens is clouded, light rays entering through the lens scatter as they move through the visual system. This is the primary cause of the glare that can be so disorienting for the aged person. Also, as the lens thickens, the chamber becomes more shallow. The major danger in such a case is the onset of acute angle glaucoma. With increasing age, less light reaches the retina because the pupil becomes smaller.[159] There is a linear decrease in the amount of light reaching the retina from the age of 20 to the age of 60.[92] This results in the need for increasing available light in order to see, and an increase in the time needed to adapt to sudden changes from bright to diminished light or darkness. Further, it should be noted that the eye requires approximately double the illumination for each thirteen years of adult life.[92] Thus, the final level of vision in diminished lighting, after time allowed for accommodation, is less for the aged person than for the younger.

Color vision is also affected by age. While the mechanism is still not entirely understood, it is believed that the discoloration of the lens leads to color filtering and a decline of color intensity, especially with greens and blues.[92] It is thought that as the lens yellows with age, the shorter light waves of the greens and blues are more completely filtered out, while the longer-waved half of the color spectrum retains the capacity to pass through the lens to the retina. Yellows, oranges, and reds have been found to stimulate the sympathetic nervous system responses in the elderly.[160] It is not necessarily that profound that elderly individuals tend to develop a "taste" for brighter- colored clothes. Conversely, an individual with cataracts may lose the longer-waved rays, and the related ability to see red.[160]

Over time there is atrophy of orbital fat, which occurs with the pattern of general wasting.[92] This leads to the loss of the normal fat cushion behind the globe and may produce some recession of the eye and the characteristic sunken eye appearance known as *enophthalmos*. Enophthalmos is often accompanied by a deepening of the upper lid fold and a slight obstruction of the peripheral visual fields. The skin of the upper lid also tends to relax, causing the upper lid to drop onto the lashes resulting in some restriction of the lid, and leading to an upper lid ptosis. When severe, such a condition will limit vision for objects above eye level, such as traffic lights and stop signs.

The production of tears also declines with age.[92] If there has been sufficient relaxation of the lid, the direction of the tear duct (the lacrimal puncta) will also change. Normally, the direction is inward, toward the eye itself, but with relaxation the direction is changed so that it is focused away from the eye and is thus exposed to the air. This leads to excessive tearing. This condition, if pronounced enough, leads to senile ectropion, a physical state in which the lower lid is physically unable to cover the lower portion of the eye.[159] This leaves no opportunity for the palpebral conjunctiva to be bathed in tears. This causes chronic dryness, which will lead to metaplasia and keratinization of the epithelial layer. The opposite situation may also occur, that of senile entropion may also occur. This a turning inward of the lower lid leading to irritation of the cornea and lower conjunctiva by the lashes. Severe cases of either ectropion or entropion will require plastic surgery.

The vitreous body also undergoes changes with aging. The gel-like substance undergoes some amount of shrinkage after the age of 60.[159] The primary role of the vitreous is to support the retina, and this becomes compromised as the amount of available fluid decreases. By the age of 70 or 80, most people develop some degree of detachment of the vitreous body from the posterior aspect of the globe. This occurrence is often heralded by transient flashes of light or by a small number of dark, floating opacities. These flashes are noted most often when turning in bed, not noted when sitting quietly. A sudden shower of dark spots or floating opacities are strongly suggestive of a retinal break

and should be treated as an emergency to decrease the possibility of actual retinal detachment. Frequently, prophylactic surgery will be suggested for the uninvolved eye.[92]

Age-related macular degeneration (AMD) causes loss or blurriness of central vision creating a blind spot. Peripheral vision remains intact. Age-related macular degeneration results in an inability to see fine details, such as colors or a person's facial features.[158] Age-related macular degeneration is a progressive, degenerative disorder of the retina, and it is the leading cause of new cases of blindness in people aged 65 and older. In this country, nearly 11% of the population between 65 and 74 have AMD to some degree, as do 28% of those older than 75.[161]

Immediately beneath the sensory retina lies a single layer of cells called the retinal pigment epithelium. These cells provide nourishment to the portion of the retina where they are in contact. In AMD, the maintenance of this contact is threatened. A small hemorrhage may break through and accumulate between the retinal pigment epithelium and the sensory retina. This leads to disruption of the photoreceptor cells' nutrition and to their death, with attendant loss of central vision.[162] This type of age-related maculopathy is referred to as the *wet type* because of the leaking vessels and edema or blood that detaches the retina. The *dry type* consists of disintegration of the retinal pigment epithelium because of nutritional loss. The light-sensitive cells of the macula break down over time and a yellow deposit called drusen accumulates under the retina.[163]

A *cataract* is an opacity of the lens that reduces visual acuity (to 20/30 or less).[164] An early sign is the complaint of "glare" from bright lights at night or even during the day, the result of rays of light being scattered by the opacities. Over time, the lens opacities progress and eventually interfere with vision so that reading becomes difficult even with glasses. The hallmark of all cataracts is painless, progressive loss of vision. Though the cause has not been elucidated, there appears to be a strong nutritional link related to low levels of antioxidants.[165] Cataract surgery, the removal of the lens from the eye, is the treatment of choice.[166]

Glaucoma is a disorder characterized by increased intraocular pressure that can lead to irreversible damage to the optic nerve, with the accompanying impairment of blindness. It is a pathological process in the eye that anatomically or functionally blocks the outflow channels. The most common type of glaucoma in the elderly is the open-angle glaucoma accounting for 90% of all cases.[167] Onset is insidious and usually asymptomatic causing slow loss of visual field, affecting both eyes, and occurring more commonly in blacks.[168] Secondary glaucoma is associated with diabetes (diabetic retinopathy), uveitis, and with occular tumors that affect the optic nerve.[168]

The leading causes of visual impairment are age related, but appropriate care can preserve useful vision for most older adults.[169] Vision loss due to macular degeneration cannot be delayed in all patients, however, it can sometimes be postponed through laser therapy. Low-vision rehabilitation can maximize the usefulness of remaining sight. Cataract surgery is highly successful. Early detection and treatment of glaucoma can prevent vision loss. Laser treatment is remarkably effective in treating diabetic retinopathy.[169] Otherwise, the low vision state is best addressed with vision-enhancing devices, adaptive equipment, and patient education available through occupational therapy. Referral to a low-vision rehabilitation program is needed for a comprehensive evaluation and intervention. Individual adaptation and supportive services often result in a significant improvement in function and quality of life for those elders with low vision.

Hearing Pathologies with Age

Changes in the morphological structures in the ear with age can lead to pathological changes. Briefly, these changes are: atrophy and degeneration of hair cells and supporting cells in the basal coil of the cochlea leading to sensory presbyacusis; loss of auditory neurons causing neural presbyacusis; atrophy of the stria vascularis in the scala media with corresponding deficiencies in bioelectric and biochemical properties of the endolymphatic fluids, known as metabolic presbyacusis; atrophic changes in structures associated with vibration of the cochlear partition, known as cochlear conductive presbyacusis; loss of minute vessels that supply the spiral ligament, stria vascularis and tympanic lip, which causes vascular presbyacusis; and a loss of neurons from the cochlear nucleus leading to central presbyacusis.[170] While each of these entities has been separately identified and studied, it is important to note that they seldomly happen independently of each other.

Hearing loss may result from dysfunction of any component of the auditory system. In conductive hearing loss, the dysfunction affects the orderly transmission of sound from the external environment to the inner ear and may involve any of the structures lateral to the oval window (e.g., the tympanic membrane or stapes). Sensorineural hearing loss is due to dysfunction of the sensory elements (hair cells) or neural structures (fibers of the cochlear nerve). A mixed hearing loss combines both sensorineural and conductive elements. In central hearing loss, the dysfunction is localized to higher auditory centers of the brain.

The hearing losses that occur with presbyacusis affect the higher, pure tone frequencies.[170] Basically, the individual loses the hard sounds of language. This leads to a decrease in ability to understand speech where parts of words or whole words are lost because of higher tones as well as the interference of background noise. The use of hearing aids and surgical implants has provided relief for some, but the process of presbyacusis is such that these steps can only blunt the effects of the problem. Because most cases of presbyacusis are of mixed etiology, as has already been noted, intervention will not completely correct the loss. Thus, the clinical focus should be on improving and maintaining as much of the hearing capability as possible and helping the older person, and the family adapt to the limitations necessitated by substituting other forms of communication and environmental stimuli to compensate for the loss that remains.[171]

The clinician needs to be mindful of the effects of hearing loss on all aspects of the older patient's life. Failure to consider the effects of hearing loss when evaluating such problems as depression, confusion, possible attention span deficits, and a variety of other clinical problems may lead to less than adequate clinical intervention.

Tinnitus is the diagnosis given to a variety of "ear noise" disorders. A small percentage of the elderly suffer from this condition to varying degrees,[170] and it is an annoying problem. Patients often report constant or intermittent noises, such as buzzing, ringing, or hissing, that result in a distortion of accurate reception of environmental sounds and voices. If patients complain of tinnitus, considerations for a quiet treatment environment should be made to decrease the bombardment of external noise sources superimposed on the internal sources.

Otalgia is ear pain that results from an otologic process or may be referred along neural pathways, including the trigeminal, glossopharyngeal, vagus, and cervical nerves. Inflammation of the pinna, external auditory canal, tympanic membrane, or middle ear can result in otalgia. With eustachian tube obstruction, negative pressure in the middle ear may produce painful retraction of the tympanic membrane. In the elderly, it is common for pain in the temporomandibular joint (TMJ) to be referred to the ear.

Massive accumulation of cerumen (wax) is frequently seen in the elderly. The individual is usually dehydrated, complains of hearing loss and a feeling of fullness in the ear, and often reports dizziness.

An effusion in the middle ear, usually related to obstruction of the eustachian tube is called serous otitis media. In the elderly, this condition generally occurs unilaterally and the patient perceives a sensation of aural fullness and hearing loss.

Dizziness, encompassing the sensations of vertigo, dysequilibrium, and unsteadiness, is a common complaint in elders with ear disorders. Evaluation of balance problems should include an assessment of hearing pathologies.

Proprioceptive and Vestibular Dysfunction

Proprioception or kinesthesia are affected by changes in the neurosensory mechanisms. Though a greater degree of sensory or perceptual loss results from local system changes (e.g., impaired vision from increased lens density), cerebral cortex cell loss may result in less cellular availability for sensory interpretation.

This is important when evaluating an elderly individual's gait pattern and balance. Peripheral vascular disease and diabetes may affect proprioceptive input. Vibratory sense is diminished or lost in the early stages of type II diabetes.

There is scant research on proprioception in the aged population. Skinner and co-workers[172] reported that the ability to replicate passive knee motion and the ability to detect motion diminished with increasing age. Older subjects detect motion less well at low frequencies of movement, though they still accurately report joint motion sensation.[173] Compared to younger individuals, people over the age of 50 required passive movement thresholds of perception that were twice as high in the lower extremities, but there was no difference in the upper extremities.[174] Impairment of proprioception rarely occurred in a neurologic screening of a sample of subjects ranging in age from 67 to 87.[175] On the other hand, perception of passive knee movement in individuals 65 years of age and older showed an age-related decline in position sense.[176] Perhaps proprioceptive loss is joint specific. Clinically, it appears to decline in the lower extremities with advancing age and is an important consideration when working with the elderly. Loss of proprioception is usually an irreversible deficit and contributes a great deal to falls in the elderly. Barrett and associates[176] found that proprioception was improved by almost 40% by applying an Ace bandage around the knee. It is often helpful to use light cuff weights (i.e., > 1 pound) around the ankles for facilitating increased proprioceptive awareness when pathologies manifest in proprioceptive loss. Though the prospect of reversing proprioceptive deficits is low, the elderly individual can be taught to compensate for a decrease in position sense by visual input.

Degeneration occurs in the sensory receptors in both the otoliths and semicircular canals affecting the vestibular system. The function of this system is to monitor head postion and to detect head movements. When an individual is deprived of visual and lower extremity somatosensory information, the vestibular system is left to control balance. Healthy young adults are able to balance without meaningful visual or support surface information, but healthy elderly adults with normal amounts of vestibular degeneration lose their balance and are at risk for falls when vestibular input is the only spatial orientation information available. Diseases of the neuromuscular system further compound this problem. Balance problems or the "fear of falling" may severely compromise ambulatory capabilities in the elderly. Patients with vestibular lesions can be potentially treated with specific exercises to improve vestibualr function or can be taught compensatory techniques using vision.[177,178]

Sensory Changes in Smell

There is a close association between the sense of smell and human behavior. The olfactory memory is a very powerful one, and it can elicit strong emotions. The sense of smell is also key in recognizing what is occurring in the environment. The effects of aging alone on the ability to smell are minimal, and any decline in the sense of smell is probably related to an underlying pathology. Research has shown that there is a wide variation among elderly individuals' ability to smell.[171,179] There does appear to be a decline in fiber in the olfactory bulb, and by the age of 80, almost three-fourths of the fiber are lost.[180] It is recognized that women have greater olfactory acuity than men;[180] however, postmenopausal women exhibit decreased ability to smell, which is thought to be the result of a decline in estrogen levels following menopause. Eating is perhaps the most directly affected activity when olfactory acuity is involved. In order to detect the flavor of food, one must be able to smell it. Thus, the aged person with a loss of smell may complain that food is tasteless. For the person with olfactory loss, hot foods are more easily perceived than are cold foods. As with all of the senses, smell serves as an environmental safety factor. The inability to smell will raise certain safety concerns that can be resolved using alternative methods, such as ensuring that there are smoke detectors in the house to compensate for the loss of ability to smell smoke.

Sensory Changes in Taste

The sense of taste is closely associated with the senses of smell and vision. How food looks and smells enhances or detracts from its taste. There are four basic sensations in taste perceived by the taste buds: bitter, salty, sweet, and sour. Taste buds located in different areas of the tongue are responsible for perceiving the different sensations. Thus, any pathology affecting the tongue will also affect the ability to perceive the sensation for that area. Research indicates that there is a decline in taste sensitivity with age.[171,179] While it is not fully understood, there is a clear decline in the number of taste buds. Taste buds have the ability to rapidly regenerate, but the speed with which they do so declines with age. Eventually, the rate of loss exceeds the rate of replacement. There is some research that indicates that cigarette and pipe smoking is a factor in this decline.[180] While there are other age-related changes, such as the decline in flow of saliva, these changes are not considered significant until they are well advanced. It is unlikely that age-related changes will affect the ability to taste prior to the age of 70. When these changes do occur, the older person seems to have an increased sensitivity to bitterness, and a decreased sensitivity to sweetness and saltiness.

Compensation for these losses revolves around recognizing how to enhance the senses that are involved senses. It is beneficial to make food visually more appealing, to serve hot foods hot, to increase the use of herbs and spices to enhance flavor, to create an enjoyable social and physical environment, and to aggressively maintain good oral hygiene. Refer to Chapter 7, Exploring Nutritional Needs for further discussion of feeding programs and nourishment.

GASTROINTESTINAL PATHOLOGIES IN AGING

Age-related changes in function are apparent in the gastrointestinal system, and these changes, combined with poor nutrition, can lead to pathological states.[154] This is important to physical and occupational therapy, because without an adequate energy source, functional capabilities of any individual become restrained and limited. For example, the loss of dentition and dimunition of salivary gland activity with age impairs mastication and deglutition, thereby affecting the overall function of the system. There are no significant changes in bowel function that can be ascribed solely to aging;[181] however, the aging gastrointestinal system is more susceptible to cancer, vascular insufficiency, and chronic degenerative conditions. Common gastrointestinal problems encountered in the elderly include dysphagia; ulcer disease; pernicious anemia; cancer of the pancreas, stomach and large intestine; constipation; and cholelithiasis. Gastrointestinal complaints are extremely common in the aged, and gastrointestinal disease accounts for over a quarter of hospital admissions.[182]

Dysphagia

Dysphagia is difficulty in swallowing. It commonly results from neuromuscular disorders, such as cerebral vascular accident, Parkinson's disease, diabetes, or other neuropathies. Malnutrition results from decreased intake; aspiration of oral contents is a common accompaniment that frequently leads to pneumonia. Siebens and colleagues[183] have identified a fairly high incidence of swallowing problems involving the mouth, pharynx, and upper esophageal sphincter in the elderly population. It is common to classify dysphagia according to the lesions causing the abnormal movement of food through the mouth, pharynx, and upper esophageal sphincter as *oropharyngeal dysphagia*. Those abnormalities producing difficulty with the passage of ingested material through the smooth muscle portion of the esophagus as *esophageal dysphagia*.[184] Oropharyngeal dysphagia is characterized clinically by difficulty initiating the process of swallowing, and physically by impaired ability to transfer food from the mouth into the upper portion of the esophagus. This process involves a closely coordinated central mechanism between the sensory nerves from afferent receptors (cranial nerves V, IX, and X) and the efferent nerves (V, VII, IX, X, and XII) that supply the muscles in this area. Many lesions of the central nervous system and muscle apparatus of the mouth and upper esophageal sphincter can produce oropharyngeal dysphagia. Cerebrovascular accidents and Parkinson's disease frequently result in dysphagia. Pathologies that affect the motor end plates, such as myasthenia gravis, can inhibit proper muscle functioning. Muscle problems such as those seen in metabolic myopathy (e.g., thyroid disease, steroid therapy), primary myositis, and amyloidosis can create swallowing difficulties.[181] Tumors or surgical scarring can cause local obstruction to the passage of food, and motility disorders like abnormal upper esophageal sphincter relaxation or pharyngeal/ upper esophageal sphincter incoordination can cause oropharyngeal dysphagia.

True esophageal dysphagia, where the transport of the ingested material down the esophagus is impaired, is common in the elderly.[184] Carcinoma of the esophagus, which occurs with increasing frequency in the elderly, usually presents with dysphagia. The most common symptom is the sensation of food "hanging up" in the esophagus. It has a poor prognosis for cure and usually requires extensive palliative treatment. Hiatus hernia, another cause of dysphagia, is also increasingly common in the aged. Few, however, are symptomatic, and medical management with antacids and H_2 blockers is effective.[182] It is important to understand that achalasia can initially present in the elderly, and that other motility disorders, such as diffuse esophageal spasm and scleroderma, do occur in these individuals.[184] Another cause of esophageal dysphagia that is unique to the elderly population is dysphagia aortica, in which the transport of material down the esophagus is impaired by a markedly tortuous and enlarged aorta, heart, or both.[181]

The role of the physical and occupational therapist in treating dysphagia is to coordinate the team efforts of speech pathology, dietary, and nursing to provide a comprehensive positioning and feeding program. The physical therapist is involved in evaluating and treating head and trunk control; neck range of motion; neck weakness; sitting balance; abnormal postural reflex activity interfering with head control, sitting balance, or both; gross facial muscle test; ability to handle secretions; voluntary deep breathing ability, breath control and voluntary cough; and gross motor upper extremity ability. The occupational therapist is involved in some of the same interventions, and additionally provides adaptive equipment as warranted. Specific emphasis needs to be placed on wheelchair and bed positioning, and respiratory status.

Ulcer Disease

Ulcer disease is common in the elderly; and the presentation is often atypical,[181] because the complications of obstruction, bleeding, and perforation are more common in older patients than in younger individuals. Emergency surgical treatment for bleeding in the elderly carries up to a 20% mortality.[154] Medical management is effective in uncomplicated cases and rests on the use of antacids, avoidance of salicylates, and other nonsteroidal and steroidal anti-inflammatory agents and H_2 blockers, such as cimetadine. Cimetadine-induced confusion is a common complication in the aged, and a reduced dose may be necessary to prevent this.

The difficulties encountered in rehabilitation of the aged with ulcer disease are centered around the poor nutritional status and resulting decline in activity level. Focus needs to be on the maintainance of maximal functional capabilities and adequate nutrition.

Pernicious Anemia

Pernicious anemia results from a common age-related decline in the absorption of vitamin B_{12}. This usually occurs in the setting of chronic inflammation of the lining of the stomach called *atrophic gastritis*.[181] Not only can impaired B_{12} absorption cause significant disease (e.g., dementia, neuropathy, anemia), but it is associated with a higher incidence of carcinoma of the stomach. Replacement of vitamin B_{12} through monthly injections, in addition to monitoring B_{12} intake through dietary means, effectively prevents or corrects the deficiency. The most clinically significant findings in patients with pernicious anemia are low energy levels, confusion, and peripheral neuropathies resulting in proprioceptive problems.

Cancer

Gastrointestinal malignancies account for the second largest number of cancer deaths behind lung cancer.[154] The esophagus, stomach, pancreas, and large intestine are the most common sites. Cancer of the stomach is more common with advancing age, has its peak incidence in the eighth and ninth decades, and has a poor five-year survival rate. Cancer of the pancreas has a similar five-year survival rate, but its peak incidence is in the sixth decade.[181] Late diagnosis due to atypical, vague, or misleading symptoms, such as depression or altered mental status, is the rule. Cancer of the colon accounts for half of all gastrointestinal malignancies. Because they are not usually "clinically silent," as with other malignancies, intervention can be earlier and more successful. Rectal bleeding, anemia, weight loss, and altered bowel habits are the common presenting complaints. However, weakness, depression, fatigue, anorexia, and decreased functional competence are also early nonspecific clues to colon cancer. Unless the elderly person's condition makes it likely that they will soon die from some other cause, surgery is often required to cure the patient and to prevent intestinal obstruction. The five-year survival rate for colon cancer varies widely depending on the extent of the tumor at the time of initial treatment, but complete cures and long remissions are common.

Biliary Tract Disease

Cholelithiasis increases with age and occurs in nearly one-third of those over the age of 70.[181] Although most gallstones are "silent," infection and biliary obstruction due to stones are increasingly common in the elderly. Emergency surgery for cholecystitis in the elderly carries a 25% mortality. This has spurred some to advocate prophylactic cholecystectomy in those elderly with multiple small stones because they are at highest risk for passing a stone and causing an obstruction. Nonoperative techniques are being developed such as endoscopic papillotomy in which the bile duct is widened from within the intestine by use of an endoscope, which avoids anesthesia and surgery. This technique is useful for some elderly people who would otherwise not tolerate surgery.

BOWEL AND BLADDER PROBLEMS

Urinary Incontinence

Urinary incontinence can affect both men and women. It afflicts more than half of nursing home residents and is often the reason for admission.[185] The causes of incontinence can be divided into two broad categories: established and transient.[186] Established incontinence is usually the result of neurological damage or intrinsic bladder or urethral pathology. By contrast, incontinence caused by transient causes, such as a medication or diet, is generally reversible if the underlying problem can be addressed adequately.

Incontinence is not a normal sequela of aging and characteristics of what is commonly called "overactive bladder" include decreases in bladder capacity, urethral compliance, maximal urethral closure pressure, and urinary flow rate.[186] In both sexes, postvoid residual volume and the prevalence of involuntary detrusor contractions probably increase, while urethral resistance increases in men.[187]

The various types of urinary incontinence identified are stress, urge, mixed, overflow, and functional incontinence. Stress incontinence refers to the loss of bladder control due to the physical stress of increased pressure in the abdomen from such activities as coughing, sneezing, laughing, jogging, or straining on a lift or during a bowel movement. Urge incontinence is defined as the sudden urge to urinate without the ability to hold the urine long enough to reach a bathroom. Mixed incontinence is a combination of stress and urge incontinence. Overflow incontinence is the accidental loss of urine from a chronically full bladder. This may occur as the result of a cystocele (a vaginal hernia or bulge due to weakened vaginal muscles), an enlarged prostrate, or a tumor, all of which block the flow of urine through the urethra. Other causes of overflow incontinence might include damage to the bladder nerves from diabetes, loss of adequate estrogen or progesterone,[188] or a herniated lumbar disc. Functional incontinence is the inability to get to the bathroom because of physical limitations, or the inability to manage clothing once the individual has made it to the bathroom. In the older adult, a combination of these conditions may exist.

The causes of transient incontinence may be denoted by the mnemonic DIAPPERS:[189]

- **D**elirium
- **I**nfection (especially urinary tract infection)
- **A**trophic vaginitis
- **P**harmaceuticals
- **P**sychological factors (e.g., depression, poor motivation)
- **E**xcess fluid output (e.g., diuretics, diabetes)
- **R**estricted mobility (e.g., Parkinson's disease, arthritis)
- **S**tool (constipation or impaction)

Any condition that impairs cognition, mobility, or the ability to hold urine can contribute to functional incontinence. Although such causes potentially may be reversible, in reality, many patients' functional status may not improve, and therefore incontinence becomes established. Many of the causes of established incontinence involve urinary tract dysfunction. These include overactivity of the bladder with involuntary contraction; failure of the bladder to contract at the appropriate time or as strongly as it should; low resistance to urinary flow when it should be high (stress incontinence); and high resistance to urinary flow when it should be low (urinary obstruction).[190] Detrusor instability is characterized by a sudden and urgent need to empty the bladder. The volume emptied is variable but may be large. Often in the elderly, the detrusor muscle contracts, but the bladder does not empty completely leaving residual urine and an increased risk for urinary tract infection.[186]

There are numerous interventions for urinary incontinence that rehabilitation therapists can offer the older person with this condition.[191,192] Behavioral treatments are considered appropriate for patients with stress, urge, and mixed incontinence. Physical therapy may include biofeedback, therapeutic exercise, neuromuscular reedu- cation, therapeutic activity, and gait training. Instruction in pelvic floor exercises, commonly known as Kegels, is helpful in regaining strength of the pelvic floor musculature.[191] Occupational therapy may be involved in training for functional activities that facilitate toileting as well as the modification of clothing (i.e., replacing buttons or zippers with velcro) to enhance the ease of disrobing and eliminate incontinence resulting from functional limitations.

Fecal Incontinence

The inability to control bowel movements is termed fecal incontinence. This condition may have psychological causes such as depression, anxiety, confusion, or disorientation. Physiologic contributors to fecal incontinence that are most commonly seen in the elderly include neurological impairments that involve sensory and motor function (such as cerebral vascular accident, Parkinson's, spinal cord injury, or later stages of Alzheimer's disease), anal dysfunction resulting from giving birth, hemorrhoids, rectal prolapse, anal dilatation, altered levels of consciousness, and severe diarrhea. Diabetes and autonomic neuropathy may produce internal sphincter dysfunction as well. Fecal impaction is a common cause of diarrhea in the geriatric population. The stool proximal to the obstructing fecal mass becomes liquefied and oozes around the obstruction. Since elders with long-standing constipation cannot sense the movement of stool in the rectal vault and the fecal impaction tonically inhibits the internal anal sphincter, this may lead to fecal incontinence. The preservation of continence is complex, and its failure is usually multifactoral.[193]

Treatment includes hydration and in the presence of a fecal impaction an enema may be warranted. From a medical perspective, nonspecific diarrhea is treated with bulking agents and antidiarrheal drugs. Physical therapy may implement sphincter exercises to restrengthening the weakened muscle. Biofeedback treatment is very successful in the treatment of fecal incontinence. The visual or auditory feedback provides sufficient sensory input (for a patient with good cognition) to often resolve the problem in one treatment session. Biofeedback has been found to be helpful in more than 70% of individuals with incontinence due to sensory or motor impairment.

Diverticulosis/Irritable Bowel Syndrome

Diverticulosis refers to outpouchings (diverticula) in the wall of the small or large intestines causing a condition in which the mucosa and submucosa herniate through the muscular layers of the colon.[193] Diverticulitis is the inflammatory condition of these pouches in the intestines.[193] The causes include atrophy or weakness of the bowel muscle, increased intraluminal pressure, obesity, and chronic constipation. One hypothesis is that diverticular disease results from a low fiber diet, which decreases stool bulk and predisposes an individual to constipation. The subsequent increased intraluminal pressure pushes the mucosa through connective tissue, weakening bowel muscle.

Clinically the condition is asymptomatic in approximately 80% of people affected. When the diverticula become inflamed, diverticulitis develops, and the person experiences severe abdominal pain. The mechanism of pain is most likely the result of increased tension in the colonic wall.

Irritable bowel syndrome (IBS) is a group of symptoms that represent the most common disorder of the gastrointestinal tract. This is a chronic condition that is often associated with stress. Unlike conditions such as colitis, there is no inflammation associated with this disorder. Irritable bowel is a functional disorder of motility of the intestines as a result of the digestive tract's reaction to stress or diet. Episodes of emotional stress, fatigue, smoking, alcohol intake, or eating an especially large meal with high fat content, roughage, or fruit, can aggravate or precipitate symptoms. Intolerance of lactose and other sugars is also associated with IBS.[194]

Both diverticulosis and IBS are treated with dietary modifications. Increases in bran and bulk foods are encouraged. Exercise does wonders in improving motility and increasing muscular tone. Additionally, relaxation techniques, psychotherapy, biofeedback training, and pharmacologic treatment may be helpful. Often, anticholinergic agents are given prior to meals to help control symptoms.

Constipation

Constipation is increasingly common with advancing age.[193] Although bowel transit times are normal in otherwise healthy adults, many other age-related factors can contribute to having fewer than three stools per week. Inactivity, inadequate dietary fiber, inadequate fluids, drug side effects (e.g., narcotics, iron, sedatives, anticholinergics), oversedation, confusion, and prior laxative abuse can all contribute to constipation. Alterations in the intestine due to local disease, such as hemorrhoids, strictures, diverticulitis, and cancer, can also contribute to constipation. Correction of contributory factors, use of regular periodic laxatives, and patient education are usually effective. For those patients who are too confused to respond to the urge to stool, regular disimpaction is important.

The best intervention for constipation is hydration and movement (e.g., walking).

Diarrhea

Frequent, soft, watery stools, termed diarrhea, results in poor absorption of water and nutritive elements, electrolytes, fluid volume, and acidosis may result due to potassium depletion.[193] Weight loss is often an accompanying symptom of chronic diarrhea. Diarrhea can be the result of food intolerance or could be drug induced (commonly accompanies the use of antibiotics).

KIDNEY PROBLEMS

Renal Disease

The kidneys are the major modulators of the amount of water, sodium, and potassium found in the extracellular fluid of the body. They also are a major route of drug excretion and are important in maintaining an appropriate blood pressure.[154] Alterations in renal function can have profound effects on all of these essential functions.

With age, the amount of blood that can be filtered by the kidneys declines steadily.[181] This is in part due to a decline in the amount of blood that arrives at the kidney because of heart disease or narrowing of the blood vessels. It is also caused in large part to the decrease in the number and size of the glomeruli, which are the areas of the kidney that filter plasma. The ability of the kidney to reabsorb water and solutes from the filtered plasma also declines.[195] Although these reabsorptive capacities remain, they are at a significantly lower level in the aged and help to account for the decreased capability of the aged person to excrete an excessive amount of water or to prevent the loss of water in the face of dehydration.

There are eight commonly encountered problems in the aged to which altered renal function contributes: too much or too little water; too much or too little sodium; too much potassium; drug intoxication; and acute and chronic renal failure.[196] All of these disruptions of body homeostasis can result in altered mental status and can be life threatening.

Acute and Chronic Renal Failure

Acute cessation of renal function can occur at any age, but the diminished blood supply of the aging kidney renders it more susceptible to injury.[196] Hypotension is the usual precipitating cause and can result from dehydration, over-medication, surgery, or sepsis. Acute injury from certain antibiotics or from contrast dye used in radiology can also result in acute renal shut down.

Acute renal failure is associated with the rapid buildup of toxic waste products and drugs, fluid overload, and elevation of serum potassium. Any of these complications can be fatal if not managed correctly. In addition, the immune system is impaired, and patients with acute renal failure frequently die with infections.[197,198]

Chronic renal failure is marked by the slow deterioration of renal function and is usually detected when the presence of another illness stresses the renal system and elevated blood urea nitrogen (BUN), hyponatremia, or increased fluid retention lead to an evaluation of renal function.[199] The functional side effects of chronic renal failure result primarily from anemia and congestive heart failure. Patients with renal disease severe enough to cause significant chronic mental status changes have a poor prognosis and often require dialysis or transplantation—a touchy subject in light of possible rationing of health care imposed by health care reforms.

The clinical implications of problems in the kidney in relation to exercise and activity tolerance center around the electrolyte balance and the potential inability of the kidney to facilitate homeostasis. Increasing energy expenditure through exercise is positively correlated with an improvement in mortality and morbidity through a number of mechanisms.[200] Despite these benefits some are relevant, especially for the elderly with renal failure, to recommend fitness programs because of the fear that exercising too intensely will provoke cardiac arrhythmias, myocardial infarction, or increased blood pressure.[201] Regular eccentric training can increase protein turnover (37% higher muscle catabolism) in older people and can require a higher protein intake.[202]

Combined with a calorie-appropriate diet, regular exercise maintains a reasonable body weight, delays loss of lean muscle mass, and promotes good physical performance. Activity level is a predictor of survival for people aged 60 years and beyond.[203,204]

Sodium and Water Balance

The aging kidney has a diminished capacity for excreting a water load because of its inability to excrete a very diluted urine.[197] The resulting water excess leads to a dilution of serum sodium, which in turn results in fatigue, lethargy, nonspecific weakness, and confusion. In extreme cases, seizures and coma can result. Excess water frequently is retained from the use of hypotonic solutions during intravenous therapy. It may also result from the syndrome of inappropriate antidiuretic hormone secretion (SIADH), which causes the kidneys to excrete a concentrated urine. Head trauma, stroke, pneumonia, and certain drugs can cause SIADH. Several commonly used medications can also induce hyponatremia including aspirin, haloperidol, chlorpropamide, acetaminophen, barbituates, and amitriptyline.[198]

Regardless of the mechanism, the results of low serum sodium can be life threatening, and require immediate intervention to reverse sodium decline. Since the problem is usually one of excess water rather than decreased sodium, treatment usually consists of restricting free water or promoting the excretion of dilute urine. The addition of sodium through the use of hypertonic solutions is reserved for the most severe cases.[199]

At the other extreme of water balance is dehydration, in which the aging kidney has a diminished capacity to conserve water by making a more concentrated urine.[205] The consequence of this deficit is that the aged individual is much more susceptible to dehydration in the presence of fever. Because of the resulting changes in mental status, the effect of fever and mild dehydration may be enough to initiate a vicious cycle in which the elderly patient becomes progressively dehydrated with the resulting confusion and loss-of-thirst mechanism.[199,206] Significant dehydration is often an associated finding in elderly persons presenting with other illnesses, such as pneumonia, colds, flu, urinary tract infections, and strokes. The inability to maintain adequate hydration is often the deciding factor that precipitates admission to the hospital for the elderly person.

Intravenous fluid replacement is often required to regain fluid balance. Frequently the mental status changes resulting from dehydration and elevated serum sodium last long after the fluid imbalance has been corrected.

Increasing the amount of sodium presented to the aging kidney results in retention of sodium because the excess load cannot be as effectively excreted as it is in younger individuals.[197,205] Because retention of water follows the retention of sodium, the result of an increased sodium load is an expansion of the total extracellular fluid. This results in congestive heart failure, edema, and elevated blood pressure.[198,205]

Alternatively, the aging kidney cannot correct for a decrease in the amount of sodium presented to the kidneys. The aging kidney loses sodium and, therefore, is less able to maintain homeostasis with a limited sodium load. What results is a steady decline in the total extracellular fluid and associated hypotension, dizziness, weakness, and falling. The lessened functional reserve of the aging kidney makes it less able to correct for alterations of water and salt, which would not stress the younger individual.[196] The resulting abnormalities of sodium and water accompany other illnesses and increase both morbidity and mortality in the aged.

Potassium

Excess potassium, or hyperkalemia, can cause fatal cardiac arrhythmias.[207] It is more common in the aged because of several age-related changes in renal function. Aldosterone is the hormone responsible for maintaining potassium balance, and it affects the kidney by causing potassium to be exchanged for sodium in the urine. The net result is that potassium is excreted and sodium retained. With age, the amount of aldosterone diminishes, as does the kidney's capacity to excrete potassium.[199] The presence of potassium-sparing drugs or diabetes amplifies these effects. In the setting of dehydration, when there is both decreased renal blood flow and acidosis, there is a marked decrease in the excretion of potassium and a significant shift of potassium from within the cells into the extracellular space. The resulting severe hyperkalemia can cause life-threatening arrythmias.[205]

Drug Intoxication

The kidneys are one of the major routes of drug detoxification and excretion,[196] and a progressive decline in renal function results in lower clearances for many different types of drugs. Higher serum levels are reached and maintained longer in the elderly than in younger individuals using the same amount of drug.[198] For many compounds, this means that standard adult dosages result in toxic blood levels in the elderly. Among the most important drugs that are retained are digitalis, several types of antibiotics, sedatives and psychotrophic drugs, and oral diabetic agents. As a consequence, drug dosages need to be adjusted downward in the elderly. Chapter 8, Pharmacology, discusses this in greater detail.

ENDOCRINE DISEASES

The endocrine system encompasses a diverse group of organs and specialized glands that produce hormones. Hormones are chemical messengers which instruct cells with complementary receptors to perform a specific metabolic act.[208] The islet cells of the pancreas produce insulin, which helps regulate glucose metabolism. The thyroid gland elaborates thyroxine, which in turn modulates the overall metabolic rate of cells within the organism. Parathyroid glands elaborate parathyroid hormone, which is central to regulation of calcium metabolism. Three hormones help modulate the fluid and electrolyte balance of the body: the posterior pituitary gland makes antidiuretic hormone (ADH); the kidneys produce renin; and the adrenal glands produce aldosterone.[209]

Although many other hormones exist, excess or deficiency of the previously listed hormones account for most of the clinically significant endocrine diseases encountered in the aged. With aging, there appears to be a reduction in the sensitivity of the target cells to the hormone messenger.[210] This is due, in some cases, to a reduction in the number of hormone receptors found on the target cells.

Glucose Metabolism and Diabetes Mellitus

The number of insulin receptors found on cell membranes decreases with age.[211] Reflecting this change, the incidence of glucose intolerance increases with age and reaches nearly 25% by age 80.[212] In the aged, it is important to identify glucose intolerance, not only to prevent the complications of untreated diabetes (neuropathy, retinopathy, nephropathy, and accelerated atherosclerosis) but, even more so, to identify those individuals at risk for nonketotic hyperosmolar coma or severe hyperglycemia, which can be precipitated by infection, dehydration, or other physiologic stress.

Nonketotic hyperosmolar coma is exclusively a disease of aged diabetics.[211] It is characterized by extremely high blood sugar and osmolarity (hyperosmolar). Patients present with mental status changes which range from lethargy to coma. They are severely dehydrated and frequently hypotensive. It is often easy to overlook the precipitating event (e.g., pneumonia, urinary tract infection, or myocardial infarction) because the severity of the neurological changes suggests a primary neurological event.

Dehydration and hypotension are more significant clinical problems than the hyperglycemia. Treatment consists of fluid replace- ment and very low dose insulin therapy to slowly bring down the elevated blood sugar.[213] Prevention of this syndrome involves the early identification of diabetic patients who are slipping into the cycle of infection, decreased oral intake, dehydration, increased blood sugar, and the resulting acceleration of dehydration through the forced excretion of water when the kidneys cannot reabsorb all of the glucose presented to it and glucose is lost in the urine. Rehydration and treatment of the primary illness will usually prevent the development of nonketotic hyperosmolar coma.

Diabetes mellitus is a chronic disease that affects approximately 12 million people in the United States.[103,104] Insulin is needed for glucose to be transferred from the blood to the muscle and fat cells.[134] People who suffer from diabetes cannot produce enough insulin (Type I) or cannot properly use the insulin they do produce (Type II), causing hyperglyemia.[214]

The complex nature of diabetes creates a broad spectrum of physical complications and reactions that can make the condition extremely dangerous. Diabetes is the leading cause of blindness, and can cause glaucoma and cataracts. People with diabetes are twice as likely to have heart attacks and strokes, five times more prone to foot ulceration with the development of gangrene, and seventeen times more prone to kidney disease when compared to the general population.[214] Complications of diabetes also affect the mouth; reproductive system; nervous and vascular systems; the muscular system; and the skin. They also reduce an individual's defense mechanisms in the presence of infection.

Symptoms of diabetes include increased urination, thirst, hunger, fatigue, and lethargy; weight loss; and numbness or tingling in the feet and hands. Though no clear understanding of the cause of diabetes has been found and there is no cure, the disease can be controlled by achieving and maintaining normal blood glucose levels.[135] This requires a carefully balanced utilization of four critical components: diet, exercise, education for self-monitoring, and drug therapy.

By its very nature, diabetes is a condition in which food is improperly metabolized, thereby producing too much glucose. Therefore, diet control is critical to diabetes control, especially in Type II diabetes.[135] Patients with diabetes should be encouraged to eat less in general, to consume fewer calories, and to eat less fat and simple sugars.

The second area of control is exercise. Exercise improves blood glucose control, improves circulation, reduces cardiovascular risk, and keeps the patient fit.[215,216] Daily exercise increases the tissue sensitivity to insulin for two to three days, thereby decreasing the need for insulin injection.[216] Exercise and the diabetic will be dealt with more extensively in the Chapter 13, Cardiopulmonary and Cardiovascular Treatment Considerations.

Patients with diabetes should receive a thorough education about the disease, its complications, and the specific steps that must be taken to keep it under control. Self-monitoring involves a routine check of glucose levels, either by checking the urine or blood. Blood glucose monitoring is the method of choice since it is a more accurate measurement of glucose levels. In addition, self-monitoring of skin condition, especially in the lower extremities, is a vital component of diabetic education.

Drug therapy for diabetes consists of oral agents (Type II only) and insulin. Insulin is obtained from animal sources, such as cows and pigs, or from a biosynthesis process that results in insulin products that are the same as human insulin.[214] The synthesized insulin has gained popularity in recent years because it causes the formation of fewer insulin antibodies and is less likely to trigger allergic reactions. Insulin requirements may change in patients who become ill, especially with vomiting or fever.

Signs of hyperglycemia may be caused by a missed insulin dose, overeating, not following the diabetic diet, or a fever or infection. These signs include excessive thirst, urination, dry mouth, drowsiness, flushed dry skin, fruitlike breath odor, stomach ache, nausea, vomiting, and difficulty breathing.

Signs of hypoglycemia may be caused by too much insulin, missing a snack or meal, sickness, too much exercise, drinking alcoholic beverages, or taking medications that contain alcohol. Symptoms include anxiety, chills, cold sweats, cool pale skin, confusion, drowsiness, excessive hunger, headache, nausea, nervousness, shakiness, vision changes, and unusual tiredness or fatigue. If these symptoms occur, the consumption of a sugar-containing food (e.g., orange juice or honey) should reverse the symptoms.

Thyroid Disease

Clinically, significant disease can result from both excess and deficiency of thyroid hormone. In both hyper- and hypothyroidism, the presentation of the syndrome can be very different in the aged than it is in younger patients. As is the rule in most illnesses in the aged, the presentation is usually more subtle, and the symptoms and signs less specific.[210] With advancing age, there is no change in the circulating levels of total thyroxine or triiodothyronine or the free hormone values.[208] However, there is a decreased production of thyroid hormones with aging that is counterbalanced by a decrease in thyroid hormone degradation. In addition, there is a tendency for diminished feedback of thyroid hormones, leading to a mild increase in thyrotropin levels, particularly in women. In older men, there is an increased prevalence of failure for thyroid-stimulating hormone (TSH) to respond to thyrotropin-releasing hormone (TRH).

Hypothyroidism is common in the aged and results from failure of the thyroid gland to elaborate sufficient thyroid hormone despite maximum stimulation of the gland by TSH. The incidence of hypothyroidism increases from approximately 1% below the age of 60 to 4% to 7% after the age of 60.[217] Vague symptoms abound: dry skin, chronic muscle and joint pains, lethargy, confusion, weight gain, edema, depression, apathy, sensitivity to sedatives, and cold intolerance. Patients with severe hypoglycemia develop hypothermia and have cognitive dysfunction resembling dementia. These hypofunctions are seen most commonly in the hospitalized elderly patient who experiences the stress of surgery or other acute illness.[218] More subtle abnormalities, such as pseudodementia, depres-

sion, and lethargy, are more common in ambulatory patients.

Untreated hypothyroidism places the individual at increased risk of death from concurrent illness. Treatment involves the gradual replacement of thyroid hormone on a daily basis until the TSH value becomes normal. This usually requires dosage adjustments monthly for several months.

In the aged, hyperthyroidism results most commonly from an excess of thyroid hormone released from a multinodular goiter. Between 7% and 12% of patients with hyperthyroidism are over the age of 60.[208] Although many symptoms of hyperthyroidism in the aged are similar to those in the younger patient, they are usually more subtle. Common manifestations include the development of glucose intolerance (diabetes mellitus), congestive heart failure, atrial fibrillation, muscle weakness, weight loss, diarrhea, and agitation. However, there is a small group of the aged with "apathetic hyperthyroidism" in which the presentation of disease is diametrically different from the usual.[219] These individuals show depression, apathy, failure to thrive, and constipation. Although their symptoms are similar to patients with hypothyroidism, correction of the elevated thyroid hormone level abolishes the symptoms.

Surgical ablation of the thyroid gland is rarely done and is usually reserved for situations in which the enlarged gland compromises the patient's airway. The use of radioactive iodine, which is selectively concentrated in the gland, produces the most lasting reduction in hormone levels.[210] It is so effective that virtually all patients treated with this modality develop hypothyroidism requiring hormone replacement. Medications, such as propylthiouracil, that block the production of thyroid hormone are effective alternatives to radioactive iodine. Their use is complicated by the development of bone marrow suppression and a significant relapse rate when the medication is withdrawn. In the majority of cases, both types of treatment produce excellent results.

Antidiuretic Hormone Imbalance

Antidiuretic hormone (ADH) increases the reabsorption of water from the kidney, and its release is stimulated by a decrease in circulating fluid volume or an increase in osmolarity. It is an important part of the endocrine system, which maintains fluid balance.[208] Under certain circumstances, the pituitary makes excessive amounts of ADH, which results in SIADH. Several intracranial processes, such as stroke, meningitis, and subdural hematoma, and intrathoracic conditions, such as pneumonia, tuberculosis, and bronchiectasis, can cause SIADH. Recurring episodes of SIADH precipitated by acute viral illness have been reported as well. This syndrome results in excess water retention, which in turn causes a severe dilution of serum sodium.[210] This results in lethargy, confusion, and seizures. It usually responds to restricting free water and correcting the precipitating factors, and it can be intermittent or chronic.

Parathyroid Disease

Parathyroid hormone maintains calcium balance by stimulating the absorption of calcium from the intestine, reabsorption from the urine, and mobilization from bone.[210] The amount of circulating parathyroid hormone increases with age because of age-related decreases in the amount of calcium absorbed from the intestine. Part of this decrease results from lower levels of calcium and vitamin D (essential for absorption of calcium) in the diet and less sunlight-mediated conversion of vitamin D to more active forms.[220]

A decrease in the circulating levels of ionized calcium triggers the release of parathyroid hormone. In situations such as renal failure, serum calcium levels decrease because of binding with retained phosphates normally excreted in the urine. The resulting decrease in calcium triggers the release of parathyroid hormone and often raises its level out of the normal range. This is called secondary hyperparathyroidism.[210] Parathyroid hormone levels usually return to normal when the stimulus for lowering calcium is removed. Occasionally, however, the parathyroid glands continue to overproduce hormone even after the stimulus is removed. The result is autonomous, hyperfunctioning parathyroid glands that raise the serum calcium level and lead to clinically apparent hyperparathyroidism. A more common cause of hyperparathyroidism is the development of a single parathyroid adenoma which produces excess hormone.[209,210] In either situation, the elevated calcium level causes profound mental status changes, including confusion, lethargy, and coma. Elevated calcium is a reversible cause of altered mental status in the aged. Osteomalacia, renal stones, and peptic ulcer disease are also associated with hyperparathyroidism. However, in the aged, they are less common than mental status changes.

Parathyroid surgery is an effective treatment. Conservative management using high sodium diets, phosphate supplements, and diuretics, such as furosemide, is also effective in patients who cannot tolerate surgery.[221] Hypoparathyroidism can result from surgery, or develop spontaneously. It is rare, and the main symptom, tetany, can usually be prevented by calcium supplements and agents, such as hydrocholorothiazide, which retard calcium loss by the kidneys.

CANCER

As the U.S. population becomes increasingly elderly, cancer rates have gone up and are expected to continue that increase. Currently 50% of all malignancies occur in the 12% of the population aged 65 and older.[222] While mortality from cardiovascular disease has been declining in this age group over the past two decades, cancer-related mortality has remained constant.[223] Age is the single most significant risk factor for cancer. Cancer incidence and mortality rates increase exponentially with age until the age of 84 years. At this point, it has been found that the occurrence of cancer plateaus (survival of the fittest?).

Simply defined, cancer refers to a large group of diseases characterized by uncontrolled cell growth and spread of abnormal cells. Cancer is called by many other terms, including malignant neoplasm, malignancy, carcinoma, and tumor. In its various forms it is a genetic disease, characterized by changes in the normal genetic mechanisms that regulate cell growth and division.[224] *Differentiation* is the process by which normal cells undergo physical and structural changes as they develop into different tissues with specialized physiologic function. In malignant cells, differentiation is altered and may be entirely lost so that the cell no longer resembles its parent cell. When this occurs it is called an undifferentiated or *anaplastic* malignancy. *Dysplasia* is a category of tumor in which there is a disorganization of cells from their normal shape, size, or organization. *Metaplasia* is the first stage of dysplasia, which is reversible and benign. This stage is the stage targeted for early detection screenings. *Hyperplasia* refers to an increase in the number of cells in tissue resulting in an increase in tissue mass. *A tumor,* or a *neoplasm,* is a new growth and may be benign or malignant.

Two, nonmutually exclusive hypotheses may account for higher cancer rates among the older population. First, carcinogenesis is a time-consuming process. Therefore, cancer is more likely to become detectable in older individuals.[223] Second, a number of molecular changes occur with aging. These changes are similar to those of carcinogenesis and prime the aging cells to the effects of late-stage carcinogens.[224,225] Aging cells, when copying their genetic material, may begin to err, giving rise to mutations, but the aging immune system may not recognize these mutations as foreign, thus allowing them to proliferate and form a malignancy. Research has reported findings that indicate that mutations linked with lymphoma and leukemia accumulate with age.[225] For example, individuals 60 years of age and older have a 40-fold risk of developing non-Hodgkin's lymphoma compared to younger populations. Older individuals are more likely to develop cancer after exposure to environmental carcinogens than younger individuals. Both experimental and epidemiological data support this hypothesis.[225,226] The clinical consequences are important. Increased likelihood of developing cancer makes older persons ideal candidates for preventative interventions. The older individual may be a candidate for all forms of primary cancer prevention, from elimination of environmental carcinogens, increased activity, modification of diet, and in some cases, chemoprevention.

Cancers that exhibit the most consistent increases in rate with age are leukemia and cancers of the digestive system, breast, prostrate, and urinary tract.[222] The incidence of myelodysplastic syndrome (MDS), a group of hematopoietic stem cell disorders leading to leukemia, appears to be increasing in the aging population.[224,225] Several neoplasms may behave differently in the older patient. Simply put, older people may develop "different" cancers. In addition, patient age may influence tumor growth and affect the individual's responsiveness to treatment.[227]

Two primary approaches to the treatment of elderly cancer patients include curative and palliative interventions.[223] Curative cancer treatment includes surgery, radiation, chemotherapy, biotherapy, and hormone therapy. Surgery, aimed at tumor removal is frequently used in combination with other treatment modalities listed above. Adjuvant therapy used following surgery is used to decrease the potential proliferation of any residual cancer cells. Surgical interventions in the elderly carry the negative consequences of confusion and weakness related to the use of anesthesia and prolonged bed rest and immobility following the procedure (see Chapter 9, Principles and Practices in Geriatric Rehabilitation, for an extensive review of the ramifications of bed rest in the older population). Radiation therapy is used to irradicate cancer cells. The success of this intervention is dependent on the localization of the tumor and the fact that malignant cells respond differently to radiation depending on blood supply, oxygen satuation, previous irradiation, and immune system status. Side effects may include nausea and vomiting leading to more attention to nutrition, and overall weakness results in functional declines. Chemotherapy is generally used when there is widespread metastatic disease, such as in leukemia, with the aim of destroying cancer cells through the use of potent chemical agents. The side effects are similar to those of radiation. In addition, chemotherapy usually dramatically alters the status of red blood cell and platelet counts, leaving the individual in a particularly compromised immune state.[223] Patients often are required to reside in protective environments (significantly limiting functional activities) in order to protect them from exposure to potential infectious agents. Biotherapy, also called immunotherapy, relies on biologic response modifiers (BRM) to change or modify the relationship between the tumor and the host by strengthening the host's immune system response.[224,225] The most widely used agents include interferons (which have a direct antitumor effect) and interleukin-2 (one of the cytokine proteins released by the macrophage to trigger the immune response). Other forms of biotherapy include bone marrow transplantation (used for cancers that are unresponsive to high levels of chemo or radiation therapy), monoclonal antibody therapy (ß lymphocytes that bind to and destroy cancer cells), the injection of colony-stimulating factors (used as hematopoietic growth factors which guide the division and differentiation of normal cells in individuals with

particularly low blood counts) and hormonal therapy (used in cancers that are affected by specific hormones). Hormonal therapy is being utilized more and more to good effect in an older population. For example, the luteinizing-release hormone leuprolide is used in the treatment of prostrate cancer. It has been found that this hormone inhibits testosterone release and tumor growth. Likewise, the use of tamoxifen, an antiestrogen hormonal agent, is used in breast cancer to block estrogen receptors in tumor cells that require estrogen to survive.[224,225]

Palliative care, providing symptomatic relief, may include radiation or chemotherapy, physical therapy (e.g., physical agents, exercise, positioning, relaxation techniques, biofeedback, manual therapy), medications, acupuncture, chiropractic care, alternative medicine (e.g., homeopathic and naturopathic treatment), nutritional therapy, and hospice care. It is primarily end-of-life care with the emphasis on minimizing pain and helping to make patients as comfortable as possible as they approach their impending death.

Numerous symptoms and functional losses in the older cancer patient require attention by physical and occupational therapy. The management of pain and a minimization of functional loss are imperative in treating the elderly cancer patient. Treatment approaches for the management of pain by the rehabilitation professional may include noninvasive physical agents, such as cyrotherapy, thermotherapy, electrical stimulation, immobilization, exercise, massage, biofeedback, and relaxation techniques. Often functional mobility exercises are helpful in relieving pain and improving a cancer patients outlook. As the individual becomes older the level of frailty increases dramatically. In frail elderly patients, functional reserves are exhausted and tolerance of physical stress is poor.[228] Although chronological age alone cannot be used to make a clinical assessment of patient age, in the majority of people over the age of 75 with a cancer diagnosis, frailty needs to be addressed.[228] It has been determined that, even in the frailest elderly patient newly diagnosed with cancer, the life expectancy is greater than two years.[228] While frail patients seem candidates only for palliative measures, exercise and pain management have been found to not only improve functional capabilities and decrease pain, but also to serve to improve the quality of life. These patients require continuous and effective treatment of their symptoms no matter what the prognosis.

IMMUNE SYSTEM DISEASES

Aging impacts the efficiency and effective response of the immune system.[229–231] The immune system is comprised of several cell types, which form a network of interacting elements that together generate *humoral immunity* (ß lymphocytes), *cell-mediated immunity* (thymus-derived or T lyphocytes) and *non-specific immunity* (monocytes and polymorphonuclear neutrophil leukocytes).[230,231] A variety of regulatory and effector T lymphocytes are activated in the immune response. T helper cells, T suppressor and T cytotoxic cells, all of which are dependent on the production of soluable mediators. The inflammatory response is the result of the secretion of interleukin-1 (IL-1) by macrophages. This substance produces fever, increased vascular permeability, and other signs of inflammation. IL-1 facilitates the activation of T cells, which in turn produce the T cell growth factor interleukin-2 (IL-2). IL-2 stimulates the proliferation of additional T lymphocytes and other lymphokines (γ-interferon, ß cell growth factor) and differentiation factors, which promote the expansion of ß lymphocyte populations and the production of antibody. T suppressor cells down-regulate the immune response, maintain self-tolerance, and provide a regulatory counterbalance to the action of T helper lymphocytes. Other T cells, large granular lymphocytes, have natural killer activity. It has been found that in an older population, especially if nutrition is compromised, the interaction of these compounds is slower and not always harmonious.[229–131]

Aging is accompanied by immune dysregulation as immune function declines. Involution of the thymus (the central lymphoid organ for T cell development) is a universal accompaniment of aging. The thymus contributes to immune function by providing a microenvironment in which T cells mature, and by producing a family of polypeptide hormones that induce further maturation of T lymphocytes. Thymic hormone levels in the serum have been noted to decline to a barely detectable level by the age of 60. As a result, there is a remarkable loss of functional capacity of cell-mediated immunity in older individuals with a delayed and often insufficient reaction to antigens.[230,231] Age-related increase in autoimmune activity is both a cellular and humoral phenomenon and research indicates that in the elderly there is a reduced humoral and cellular immunocompetence, reduced suppressor cell activity, and increased autoantibody activity, all of which are associated with reduced survival.[229]

Several factors affect the immune system, in addition to aging. Nutritional status has a profound effect on immune function (See Chapter 7, Exploring Nutritional Needs). Severe deficits in caloric and protein intake or vitamins such as vitamins A or E lead to deficiencies in T cell function and numbers.[229] Zinc is required as a cofactor in the production of approximately seventy enzymes, some of which are found in lymphocytes. Deficient zinc can profoundly depress both T and B cell function. Secondary zinc deficiencies, associated with malabsorption syndromes, chronic renal disease, chronic diarrhea, burns or psoriasis (loss of zinc through the skin) can also impact immunity. Some medications (such as chemotherapeutic agents) suppress blood cell formation and compromise

immune response.[229] Drugs, such as analgesics, antithyroidal medications, anticonvulsants, antihistamines, antimicrobial agents, and tranquilizers, induce immunologic responses that destroy mature granulocytes. Other drugs that suppress immune system response are corticosteroids and chemotherapeutic agents. Surgery and anesthesia can suppress both T and B cell function for as much as one month following intervention. Burns increase susceptibility to bacterial infections as a result of decreased neutrophil function, decreased complement levels, decreased cell-mediated immunity, and decreased primary humoral responses. Even stress, psychological well-being, and socioeconomic status have been linked to susceptibility of disease through depressed immune function.[230,231]

Human immune function undergoes adverse changes with aging, including the T cells, which have a central role in cellular immunity. The T cells show the largest age-related differences in distribution and function, with thymus involution the underlying cause. The immune responses to exercise affect the status of thymus and subsequent T cell health.[232] Immunity is greatly enhanced with exercise. Exercise-associated changes in numbers and function of lymphocytes and granulocytes, and in levels of immunoglobins and the implications for interactions with viral infections have been positive in numerous research studies.[230] The immune responses to acute exercise indicate that the natural killer (NK) cell response to a single exercise challenge is normal in older individuals, but immediately after exercise the elderly subjects manifest less suppression of phytohemagglutinin (PHA)-induced lymphocyte proliferation than younger individuals.[232] In contrast, strenuous exercise seems to induce a more sustained postexercise suppression of cellular immunity in older subjects.[232,233] Therefore, the intensity of exercise is important. Epidemiologic and experimental studies have shown that an increase in frequency and severity of infections may occur after intense, long-term exercise.[233] Bruunsgaard and associates[233] found that cell-mediated immunity was impaired in the first days after prolonged, high-intensity exercise, whereas there was no impairment in antibody production after a two-week rest period. A few cross-sectional comparisons of immune status between physically fit elderly individuals and young sedentary controls suggest that habitual physical activity may enhance NK cell activity, checking certain aspects of the age-related decline in T cell function, such as reduced mitogenesis in response to plant lectins and decreases in the production of certain types of cytokine.[232] Shepard[234] found that both physical activity and exposure to environmental stressors such as cold, heat, and high altitudes modify various component of immune function. T cell counts, NK cell counts, and cytolytic activity, cytokine secretion, lyphocyte proliferation, and immunoglobin levels are affected by these factors. Light physical activity or a moderate level of environmental stress stimulate the immune response, but exhausting physical activity or more severe environmental stress have a suppressant effect, manifested by a temporary increase in susceptibility to viral infections.[234] Combinations of physical activity and environmental stress appear to have an additive effect. Thus, an intensity of physical activity or of environmental stress that is beneficial in itself can readily cause immunosuppression if the body is challenged by the two stimuli simultaneously.[234] In exercising the older adult then, the therapist needs to incorporate a moderate level of exercise in moderate environmental conditions to enhance the functioning and effectiveness of the immune system.[232–234 Sheppard98]

The number of older individuals with acquired immunodeficiency syndrome (AIDS) has increased steadily since the epidemics began in the early 1980s.[235] In the late 1980s, 10% of AIDS cases were in individuals more than 50 years of age, and 3% were in people more than 60 years of age.[236] The risk factors for contracting the human immunodeficiency virus (HIV) infection in the older population shifted slowly from intravenous drug use and homosexuality to transfusion-related and heterosexual causes. The clinical presentation of AIDS in older people tends to be nonspecific and is often attributed to the aging process.[237] The natural history of HIV infection is often worse, possibly related to delayed diagnosis and attributable to less experience with HIV in older adults. As AIDS becomes more common in older people, the issue of the feasibility of screening arises. Because it is so difficult to recognize AIDS encephalopathy among patients with dementia and the fact that older people are rarely questioned about drug abuse or sexual history, screening for AIDS in this portion of the population becomes particularly challenging. A tragic part of the increased development of AIDS in older people is their shorter survival time compared to younger populations. This greater mortality may reflect actual damage by the HIV virus itself, or the comorbid conditions of AIDS superimposed on the aging process and multisystem involvement unrelated to this disease. It may reflect a different mix of opportunistic infections, increased sensitivity to and severity of the tuberculosis problem, a decrease in compliance with treatment, and a decreased choice of aggressive treatment by older people.

From a rehabilitation perspective, HIV is considered a chronic illness on a continuum (i.e., from being asymptomatic to exhibiting mild to severe symptoms) rather than as a terminal illness. In addition to physical fitness and strength training, therapists need to address activities of daily living and work simplification. Programs for an older population must be simple and easily incorporated into activities of daily living. For the individual with neurological involvement, proprioceptive neuromuscular facilitation (PNF) and Bobath techniques may be beneficial. The presence of peripheral neuropathies may signal nutritional deficiencies requiring dietary support. Without proper nutrition, therapy involving balance training, extremity strengthening and stretching, and motor skills may have limited benefit. For individuals with painful myopathy, progressive resistive training with weights or theraband may be helpful. Muscle spasms accompanying myopathy may respond to gentle but consistent stretching exercises. Longer rest periods between exercises may be necessary. Muscle and joint mobilization techniques as well as breathing exercises are important components of rehabilitation efforts. Poor posture and improper body mechanics related to muscle weakness and fatigue generally accompany the progression of the disease process, malnutrition, or muscle wasting. Instruction in postural awareness, stretching and strengthening of specific muscle groups, as well as attention to nutrition are important.

HYPOTHERMIA

Hypothermia is an often fatal environmental emergency. Deaths due to hypothermia are usually accidental and are the result of exposure to extreme environmental temperatures.[238] Exposure to cold, together with the elderly person's decreased ability to cope with the effects of changes in ambient temperature because of decreased metabolism and body fat, less efficient peripheral vasocontriction, often poor nutrition, and concomitant medical disorders, presents a problem of significant dimensions.[239] Other factors contributing to the development of hypothermia are drugs, alcohol, metabolic disorders, stroke, and sepsis.

The ability to perceive cold diminishes with age. The ability to detect environmental temperature differences varies between 2.5° and 10° C (4.8° and 18° F) in the elderly as compared with a discrimination threshold of 0.8° C (1.4° F) in the young.[239] Due to lower activity levels and poor circulation, the elderly individual's basal metabolic rate is often significantly decreased, and this is reflected in a lower core temperature. Body water acts as a thermal buffer and heat reservoir, but in the elderly, total body water is decreased, reducing this protective mechanism. Shivering occurs in only 10% of the elderly and, coupled with decreased resting metabolic rate, results in an inability to maintain normal core temperature.[239] These problems, together with concomitant problems (e.g., heart failure, diabetes mellitus, hypothyroidism, movement disorders, and drugs) result in a mortality rate of approximately 50% in the elderly with hypothermia.[238]

Determining that an elderly individual is suffering from hypothermia requires a certain degree of suspicion in conjunction with physical and laboratory examination. Because standard clinical thermometers do not record temperatures below 34.4° C (94° F), a special thermometer may be required to establish core temperature. Skin color is usually pale and cold to the touch, and the individual may be experiencing sleepiness, confusion, and disorientation. Often hypothermia is accompanied with cardiovascular changes, such as hypotension, bradycardia, artrial flutter, and ventricular tachycardia. Pulmonary manifestations are slow, shallow breathing and a decreased cough reflex. Hypothermic individuals frequently present with atelectasis and pneumonia.[238] Changes in laboratory and diagnostic tests include electrolytes (decreased CO_2), creatinine and glucose (increased), CBC (increased Hb, Hct, and WBC), platelets (decreased), PT and PTT (decreased), and arterial blood gases (increased PO_2 and PCO_2 and decreased pH). Neurological symptoms include thick, slow speech, ataxic gait, and depressed reflexes.[239]

Therapy for accidental hypothermia can be divided into primary intervention by rewarming and secondary treatment of the direct effects and complications of hypothermia. From a rehabilitation perspective, activity above the resting level helps to enhance circulation and promote warming of the tissues.

It is not uncommon to see an elderly person wearing a sweater on a hot summer day. With advancing age, the efficiency of mechanisms that regulate heat production and loss declines, placing many older people at high risk for cold discomfort and hypothermia, even in warm environments. Whereas healthy elders compensate by turning up the thermostat and adding extra clothing, the frail elders with impaired environmental awareness, physical abilities, and communication may be dependent on caregivers to provide the extra warmth they require. Education of the caregiver is crucial.

HYPERTHERMIA

Abnormally high body temperature due to pathologic changes, inadequate or inappropriate responses of heat-regulating mechanism, and high environmental temperature represent an important health risk for older people.[240–242] Both chronic diseases exacerbated by heat and heat stroke itself can lead to death in an elderly population. Under usual environmental conditions, convection and radiation, as well as evaporation from skin and lungs provide adequate heat loss. The hypothalamus regulates heat loss via neuroendocrine and autonomic mechanisms.[240,241] Heat causes blood vessels of the skin to dilate, and increased sweating due to cholinergic discharge occurs. Vasodilation, in turn, increases heart rate and cardiac output (CO).[240] When environmental temperature exceeds body surface temperature, heat loss by convection and radiation stops and heat absorption begins. Evaporation of sweat becomes a means of heat loss, but increased humidity prevents cooling by this mechanism.

Aging appears to reduce the effectiveness of sweating in cooling the body. The sweat glands become fibrotic, and surrounding connective tissue becomes less vascular. In addition, the remaining anatomically normal glands may not function normally. Older individuals require a higher core temperature to initiate sweating and produce lower maximal sweat output.[240,241] Because physiologic responses to heat include vasodilation and associated increases in cardiac work and output, the high prevalence of heart disease in older persons increases their risk of heat stress. Heart failure worsens this problem when ambient heat and humidity are increased. Thus, changes seen both with normal aging and as the consequence of diseases more common in the elderly combine to impair optimal heat regulation.[240,241]

Risk factors for hyperthermia include ambient temperature and humidity, low socioeconomic status (can't afford airconditioning for home), impaired ability to perform self-care, alcoholism (dehydration), cognitive decline, and concomitant disorders (e.g., cardiovascular or cerebral vascular disease, diabetes, COPD). Some drugs predispose the elderly to heat stroke. Anticholinergic agents, phenothiazines, tricyclic antidepressants, antihistamines, to name a few, impair both hypothalamic function centrally and sweat output peripherally. By altering awareness of heat, these drugs, as well as narcotics, sedative-hypnotics, and alcohol, diminish the ability to respond to heat stress. Amphetamines can increase body temperature by direct action on the hypothalamus. Diuretics (by causing fluid loss) and β-adrenergic blockers (by impairing cardiovascular responsiveness) can increase the risk of heat stroke.[241] Therefore, it is important that the therapist pay close attention to the drugs that their exercising elderly individual is on. Hyperthermia is often a complication of activity and exercise, especially in a hot environment. Sensible environmental manipulation includes having the patient wear light clothing and monitoring the ambient temperature. Adequate fluid intake and avoidance of overexercise are important. Prevention is preferable to treatment, since morbidity and mortality are high due to hyperthermia.

CONCLUSION

The incidence of disease increases as one ages. Disease states seem to be the result of microinsults over one's lifetime that are universal in all systems of the body, though the end-state pathology may be different and the progression may be at varying speeds. The question arises: Are these small, cumulative injuries avoidable? Free radicals are unavoidable byproducts of our own metabolism. Background radiation is a universal fact of life (about one-third of it comes from our own intracellular potassium).[5] A temperature of 37° C is hot as far as molecular stability is concerned, and no chemical bond is immune from rupture by thermal perturbations.[5] In this context, aging, like the microinsults which cause it, may also be ubiquitous and inevitable and lead to pathological problems.

Genetic epidemiologic studies on diseases of aging are increasing rapidly, and will increase understanding of how genetic factors affect risks for them.[243] Individuals vary not only in whether or not they develop a disease, but also in the ages when they do, and in the rate at which premorbid changes progress to disease. Studying age-specified traits can identify protective factors as well as risk factors. The identification of the contribution of genetic factors to successful aging, such as extended survival without an adverse outcome, or lack of decline in function, is an important potential outcome of genetic studies.

This chapter has reviewed those pathologies that are commonly manifested in the aged population, and examined some of the conditions that are likely to afflict the elderly and affect functional activities of daily living.

PEARLS

- The death rate for certain diseases increases more steeply than the overall death rate, which arouses the suspicion that aging predisposes one to the development of the condition or a fatal outcome.
- There are no clinically significant effects on heart function that can solely be ascribed to aging. Therefore, the numerous pathologies seen in the cardiovascular system (e.g., ischemic heart disease, cardiomyopathy, conductive system disease, valvular disease, hypertension, myocardial degeneration, and peripheral vascular disease) account more for the decrements in the function of the system.
- The two most common types of diseases affecting the respiratory system are pneumonias, which compromise gas exchange and serve as a source for sepsis, and chronic obstructive lung disease and emphysema, which affect the amount of airflow in the lungs.
- Muscle alterations are complex and poorly understood, because the composition of muscle changes over time with replacement of myofibrils by fat, collagen, and scar tissue. The total loss in lean muscle mass that accompanies aging is commonly referred to as sarcopenia. Other conditions seen include myopathy, myositis, fibromyalgia, and myofibralgia.
- The most commonly seen conditions affecting bone in older adults include osteoporosis, osteopenia, osteomalacia, Paget's disease, and joint changes (e.g., degenerative arthritis or osteoarthritis, rheumatoid arthritis, gout, temporal arteritis or polymyalgia, and spondyloarthropathies).
- Diseases of the neuromuscular system (e.g., CNS and peripheral nervous system dysfunction, confusion, dementia and delirium, Alzheimer's disease, cerebrovascular disease, Parkinson's disease, Huntington's disease, amyotrophic lateral sclerosis, normal pressure hydrocephalus, cervical spondylosis, spinal cord injury, and peripheral nervous system problems), like those of the cardiovascular system, are much more responsible for the decrements seen in aging than the effects of aging.
- Vestibular problems in the elderly are numerous and include benign paroxysmal positional vertigo, acute vestibular neuritis or labyrinthitis, Ménière's disease, and bilateral vestibular disorders.
- Diseases of the sensory system affect all of the body's functions involving the skin (the largest organ in the body) proprioception, and pain, touch, thermal and vibratory sensation.
- Pathological changes in vision (presbyopia, glaucoma, enophthalmos, senile ectropia or entropia, macular degeneration, and cataract); hearing (presbyacusis, conductive hearing loss, tinnitis, otalgia, and serous otitis media); smell; and taste greatly impact functional capabilities and safety in the older adult population.
- Age-related changes in function are apparent in the gastrointestinal system, and these changes, combined with poor nutrition, can lead to pathological states including dysphagia, ulcer disease, pernicious anemia, cancer of the gastrointestinal tract, and biliary tract disease.
- Bowel and bladder problems generally encountered in the elderly include urinary incontinence, fecal incontinence, diverticulosis and irritable bowel syndrome, constipation, and diarrhea.
- The kidneys are the major modulators of the amount of water, sodium, and potassium found in the extracellular fluid of the body, and are a major route of drug excretion and maintaining blood pressure. Alterations in renal function can have profound effects on all of these essential functions.
- Excess or deficiencies of hormones account for most of the clinically significant endocrine diseases encountered in the aged.
- Age is the single most significant risk factor for cancer.
- Aging impacts the efficiency and effective response of the immune system.
- Two life-threatening conditions, hypothermia and hyperthermia, need to be recognized and treated in the elderly. The regulation of body temperature will greatly impact an individual's homeostatic well-being during activity and exercise and must be considered when prescribing exercise.

REFERENCES

1. Holloszy JO, ed. Workshop on sarcopenia: muscle atrophy in old age. *J Gerontol A Biol Sci Med Sci.* 1995; 50A(special issue):1–161.
2. US Bureau of the Census. *Statistical Abstract of the United States. Profiles of Older Americans: 1999.* Washington DC: Bureau of the Census. 2000.
3. Kohm RR. Human aging and disease. *J Chron Dis.* 1963; 16:5–21.
4. Administration on Aging. Older Americans 2000: Key Indicators of Well-Being. Federal Interagency.

Forum on Aging-Related Statistics. Washington DC: Bureau of the Census. 2000.

5. Johnson HA. Is aging physiological or pathological? In: Johnson HA, ed. *Relations Between Normal Aging and Disease.* Aging Series Vol. 28. New York: Raven Press; 1985: 239–247.

6. Dieftick JE, Whedon GD, Shorr E. Effects of immobilization upon various metabolic and physiologic functions of normal men. *Am J Med.* 1948; 4:3–9.

7. Lamb LE, Stevens PM, Johnson RL. Hypokinesia secondary to chair rest from 4 to 10 days. *Aerospace Med.* 1965; 36:755.

8. Miller PB, Johnson RL, Lamb LE. Effects of four weeks of absolute bed rest on circulatory functions in man. *Aerospace Med.* 1964; 35:1194.

9. Shepard RJ. *Physical Activity and Aging.* 2nd ed. Gaithersburg, Md: Aspen Publishers, Inc.; 1987.

10. Ragen PB, Mitchell J. The effects of aging on the cardiovascular response to dynamic and static exercise. In: Weisfelt ML, ed. *The Aging Heart.* New York: Raven Press; 1980: 269–296.

11. Ham RJ, Marcy ML, Holtzman JM. The aging process: biological and social aspects. In: Wright J, ed. *Primary Care Geriatrics.* Boston: PSG, Inc.; 1983.

12. Ellestad MH. *Stress Testing—Principles and Practice.* 2nd ed. Philadelphia: Davis; 1985.

13. Ewing DJ, Campbell IN, Clarke BF: Heart-rate response to standing as a test for automatic neuropathy. *Brit Med J.* 1978; 1(6128):1700.

14. Thadani U, Davidson C, Singleton W, Taylor SH. Comparison of the immediate effects of five beta-adrenoceptor blocking drugs with different ancillary properties in angina pectoris. *N Engl J Med.* 1989; 300:750–755.

15. Cairns JA. Current management of unstable angina. *Can Med Assoc J.* 1988; 119:477–480.

16. Gerstenblith G, Weisfeldt ML, Lakatta EG. Disorders of the heart. In: Andres R, Bierman EL, Hazzard WR, eds. *Principles of Geriatric Medicine.* New York: McGraw-Hill; 1985; 515–526.

17. Kattus A, Grollman J. Patterns of coronary collateral circulation in angina pectoris: relation to exercise training. In: Russek HI, Zohman BL, eds. *Changing Concepts of Cardiovascular Disease.* Baltimore, Md: Williams and Wilkins; 1972; 352–376.

18. Larson EB, Bruce RA. Health benefits of exercise in an aging society. *Arch Intern Med.* 1987; 147:353.

19. Astrand PO. Exercise physiology and its role in disease prevention and in rehabilitation. *Arch Phys Med Rehabil.* 1987; 68:305.

20. Kohl HW, Moorefield DL, Blair SN. Is cardiorespiratory fitness associated with general chronic fatigue in apparently healthy men and women? *Med Sci Sports Exerc.* 1987; 19(S6).

21. Shepard RJ. Sudden death—a significant hazard of exercise. *Brit J Sports Med.* 1974; 8:101–110.

22. Shepard RJ. Do risks of exercise justify costly caution? *Phys Sports Med.* 1977; 5(2):58–65.

23. Shepard RJ. *Ischemic Heart Disease and Exercise.* Chicago: Croom Heim, London and Year Book Medical Publishers, Inc.; 1981.

24. Romo M. Factors related to sudden death in acute ischemic heart disease. A commununity study in Helsinki. *Acta Med Scand.* 1972; 547(suppl): 7–92.

25. Webb-Peploe KM, Chua TP, Harrington D, Henein MY, Gibson DG, Coats AJ. Different response of patients with idiopathic and ischaemic dilated cardiomyopathy to exercise training. *Int J Cardiol.* 2000; 74(2–3):215–224.

26. Thomson HL, Morris-Thurgood J, Atherton J, McKenna WJ, Frenneaux MP. Reflex responses of venous capacitance vessels in patients with hypertrophic cardiomyopathy. *Clin Sci.* 1998; 94(4): 339–346.

27. Harrington D, Clark AL, Chua TP, Anker SD, Poole-Wilson PA, Coats AJ. Effects of reduced muscle bulk on the ventilatory response to exercise in chronic congestive heart failure secondary to idiopathic dilated and ischemic cardiomyopathy. *Am J Cardiol.* 1997; 80(1):90–93.

28. Kenney RA. *Physiology of Aging: A Synopsis.* Chicago: Year Book Medical Publishers, Inc; 1982.

29. Baker PB, Arn AR, Unverferth DV. Hypertrophic and degenerative changes in human hearts with aging. *J Coll Cardiol.* 1985; 5:536A.

30. Schneider EL, Reed JD. Modulations of aging processes. In: Finch CE, Schneider EL, eds. *Handbook of the Biology of Aging.* New York: Academic Press; 1985.

31. NIH. *National High Blood Pressure Education Program Coordinating Committee, 1989: Statement on Hypertension in the Elderly.* Bethesda, Md: National Institutes of Health; 1989.

32. Abrams WB. Pathophysiology of hypertension in older patients. *Am J Med.* 1988; 85(suppl 3b):7–13.

33. Toscani A. Physiology of muscular work in the aged. In: Huet JA, ed. *Work and Aging.* Second international course in social gerontology. International Centre of Social Gerontology, Paris, 1971.

34. Harrington TR, Dixon K, Russell RO, et al. The relation of age to the duration of contraction, ejection and relaxation of the normal human heart. *Amer Heart J.* 1984; 67:189–199.

35. Pomerance A. Pathology of the heart with and without failure in the aged. *Brit Heart J.* 1965; 27: 697–710.

36. Weisfeldt ML, Gerstenblith ML, Lakatta EG. Alterations in circulatory function, In: Andres R, Bierman EL, Hazzard WR, eds. *Principles of Geriatric Medicine.* New York: McGraw-Hill; 1985: 248–279.

37. Bruce RA. Evaluation of functional capacity in patients with cardiovascular disease. *Geriatrics.* 1957; 12:317–328.

38. Triggs EJ, Nation RL. Pharmacokinetics in the aged: a review. *J Pharm Biopharmacol.* 1975; 3:387.

39. Gerstenblith G, Spurgeon HA, Froelich JP, et al. Diminished inotropic responsiveness to ouabain in aged rat myocardium. *Circ Res.* 1979; 44: 517–523.

40. Reeves WC, Nanda NC, Gramiak R. Echocardiography in chronic alcoholics following prolonged periods of abstinence. *Amer Heart J.* 1978; 95: 578–583.

41. Garner AW, Poehlman ET. Exercise rehabilitation programs for the treatment of claudication pain. *JAMA*. 1995; 274:975–980.

42. Patterson RB, Pinto B, Marcus B, Colucci A, Braun T, Roberts M. Value of a supervised exercise program for the therapy of arterial claudication. *J Vasc Surg*. 1997; 25(2):312–319.

43. Regensteiner JG, Steiner JB, Hiatt WR. Exercise training improves functional status in patients with peripheral arterial disease. *J Vasc Surg*. 1996; 23(1):104–115.

44. Ubels FL, Links TP, Sluiter WJ, Reitsma WD, Smit AJ. Walking for training for intermittent claudication diabetes. *Diabetes Care*. 1999; 22(2): 198–201.

45. Kuntz RE. Importance of considering progression when choosing a coronary revascularization strategy: The diabetes-percutaneous transluminal coronary angioplasty dilemma. *Circulation*. 1999; 99 (7):847–851.

46. Thiele BL, Strandness DE. Disorders of the vascular system: peripheral vascular disease. In: Andres R, Bierman EL, Hazzard WR, eds. *Principles of Geriatric Medicine*. New York: McGraw-Hill; 1985: 527–535.

47. McDermott MM, Mehta S, Liu K, Guralnik JM, Martin GH, Criqui MH, Greenland P. Leg symptoms, the ankle-brachial index, and walking ability in patients with peripheral arterial disease. *J General Intern Med*. 1997; 14:173–181.

48. Berman ND. *Geriatric Cardiology*. Lexington, Ky: Collamore Press; 1982:1–244.

49. Meijer WT, Hoes AW, Rutgers D, Bots ML, Hofman A, Grobee DE. Peripheral arterial disease in the elderly: The Rotterdam study. *Arteriosclerosis, Thrombosis, and Vasc Biol*. 1998; 18(2): 185–192.

50. Murphy TP. Medical outcomes studies in peripheral vascular disease. *J Vasc Interventional Radiol*. 1998; 9(6):879–889.

51. Gladman JRF, Barer D, Venkatesan P, et al. The outcome of pneumonia in the elderly: a hospital survey. *Clin Rehab*. 1991; 5:201–204.

52. Cummings G, Semple SG. *Disorders of the Respiratory System*. Oxford, England: Blackwell; 1973.

53. Wynne JW. Pulmonary disease in the elderly. In: Rossman I, ed. *Clinical Geriatrics*. 2nd ed. Philadelphia: Lippincott Co.; 1979.

54. Grimby G, Saltin B. The aging muscle. *Clin Physiol*. 1983; 3:209–218.

55. Cress ME, Schultz E. Aging muscle: functional, morphologic, biochemical, and regenerative capacity. *Top Geriatric Rehab*. 1985; l(l):11–19.

56. Mense S. Physiology of nociception in muscles. Advances in pain research and therapy. In: Friction JR, Awad EA, eds. *Myofascial Pain and Fibromyalgia*. New York: Raven Press; 1990; 17.

57. Gowin KM. Diffuse pain syndromes in the elderly. *Rheum Dis Clin North Am*. 2000; 26(3): 673-682.

58. Bennett RM. Fibromyalgia: the commonest cause of widespread pain. *Compr Ther*. 1995; 21(6): 269–275.

59. Yaron I, Buskila D, Shirazi I, Neumann L, Elkayam O, Paron D, Yaron M. Elevated levels of hyaluronic acid in the sera of women with fibromyalgia. *J Rheumatol*.1997; 24(11):2221–2224.

60. Wigers SH, Stiles TC, Vogel PA. Effects of aerobic exercise versus stress management treatment in fibromyalgia. A 4.5 year prospective study. *Scand J Rheumatol*. 1996; 25(2):77–86.

61. Bailey A, Starr L, Alderson M, Moreland J. A comparative evaluation of a fibromyalgia rehabilitation program. *Arthritis Care Res*. 1999; 12(5): 336–340.

62. Gowans SE, de Hueck A, Voss S, Richardson M. A randomized, controlled trial of exercise and education for individuals with fibromyalgia. *Arthritis Care Res*. 1999; 12(2):120–128.

63. Dowd T. The female climacteric. *Nat OB-GYN Group*. 1990; 6(l):32–54.

64. Dawson-Huges B, Dallal G, Krall E. A controlled trial of the effect of calcium supplement on bone density in postmenopausal women. *N Eng J Med*. 1990; 329(13):878–883.

65. Mundy G. Bone remodeling. In: Favus MJ, ed. *Primer on the Metabolic Bone Diseases and Disorders of Mineral Metabolism*. American Society for Bone and Mineral Research. 4th ed. Philadelphia, PA: Lippincott Williams and Wilkins; 1999: 30–38.

66. Francis RM, Sutcliffe AM, Scane AC. Pathogenesis of osteoporosis. In: Stevenson JC, Lindsay R, eds. *Osteoporosis*. Philadelphia, PA: Chapman & Hall Medical; Lippincott Williams and Wilkins; 1998: 29–52.

67. Johnston CC Jr, Slemenda CW. Pathogenesis of postmenopausal osteoporotic fractures. In: Stevenson JC, Lindsay R, eds. *Osteoporosis*. Philadelphia, PA: Chapman & Hall Medical; Lippincott Williams and Wilkins; 1998:53-64.

68. Goltzman D. The contribution of basic science to the field of osteoporosis. *Osteoporosis Int*. 2000; 11(suppl 2):S43-S46.

69. Consensus Development Conference. Diagnosis, prophylaxis and treatment of osteoporosis. *Am J Med*. 1993; 94:646–650.

70. Eastell R. Pathogenesis of postmenopausal osteoporosis. In: Favus MJ, ed. *Primer on the Metabolic Bone Diseases and Disorders of Mineral Metabolism*. American Society for Bone and Mineral Research. 4th ed. Philadelphia, PA: Lippincott Williams and Wilkins; 1999: 260–262.

71. Deftos W. *Clinical Essentials of Calcium and Skeletal Disorders*. Caddo, OK: Professional Communications Inc.; 1998.

72. Giansiracusa DF, Kantrowitz FG. Metabolic bone disease. In: Keiber JB. *Manual of Orthopaedic Diagnosis and Intervention*. Baltimore: Williams and Wilkins Co.; 1978.

73. Mann DR, Rudman CG, Akinbami MA. Preservation of bone mass in hypogonadal female monkeys with recombinant human growth hormone administration. *J Clin Endocrinol Metab*. 1992; 74(11): 1263–1269.

74. Burger H, Van Daele PLA, Grashuis K. Vertebral deformities and functional impairment in men and women. *J Bone Miner Res*. 1997; 12(1): 152–157.

75. Matthis C, Weber U, O'Neill TW. Health impact associated with vertebral deformities: results from

the European Vertebral Osteoporosis Study (EVOS). *Osteoporos Int.* 1998; 8:364–372.

76. Fujiswawa Y, Kida K, Matsuda H. Role of change in vitamin D metabolism with age in calcium phosphorous metabolism in normal subjects. *J Clin Endocrinol Metab.* 1984; 59:719–726.

77. Nguyen TV, Eisman JA, Kelly PJ. Risk factors for osteoporotic fractures in elderly men. *Am J Epidemiol.* 1996; 144(2):258–261.

78. Felson DT, Zhang Y, Hannan MT. The effect of postmenopausal estrogen therapy on bone density in elderly women. *N Engl J Med.* 1993; 329: 1141–1146.

79. Mussolino ME, Looker AC, Madans JH. Risk factors for hip fracture in white men: The NHANES I epidemiologic follow-up study. *J Bone Miner Res.* 1998; 13(7):918–924.

80. Nguyen TV, Kelly PJ, Sambrook PN. Lifestyle factors and bone density in the elderly: Implications for osteoporosis prevention. *J Bone Miner Res.* 1994; 9(11):1339–1346.

81. Harrington TR. Preventing osteoporosis in menopausal women. *J MSSK Med.* June 1990.

82. Nielson F, Hunt C, Mullen L, Hunt J. Effect of dietary boron on mineral, estrogen, and testosterone metabolism in postmenopausal women. *FASEB J.* 1987; 1:394–397.

83. Pogrund H, Bloom R, Menczel J. Preventing osteoporosis: current practices and problems. *Geriatrics.* 1986; 41(5):55–71.

84. Lees B, Banks LM, Stevenson JC. Bone mass measurements. In: Stevenson JC, Lindsay R, eds. *Osteoporosis.* Philadelphia, PA: Chapman & Hall Medical; Lippincott Williams and Wilkins; 1998: 137–160.

85. World Health Organization Study Group on Assessment of Fracture Risk and Its Application to Screening and Postmenopausal Osteoporosis. Report of a WHO Study Group. Technical Report Series (No. 84), 1994.

86. Chesworth B, Vandervoort A. Age and passive ankle stiffness in healthy women. *Phys Ther.* 1989; 69(3):217–224.

87. Walker J. Connective tissue plasticity: issues in histological and light microscopy studies of exercise and aging in articular cartilage. *JOSPT.* 1991; 14(5):189–197.

88. Klein FA, Rajan RK. Normal aging: effects on connective tissue metabolism and structure. *J Gerontol.* 1985; 40(5):579–585.

89. Donatelli R, Owens-Burkart H. Effects of immobilization on the extensibility of periarticular connective tissue. *JOSPT.* 1981; 3(2):67–71.

90. Schiller AL. Bones and joints. In: Rubin E, Farber JL, eds. *Pathology.* 2nd ed. Philadelphia, PA: JB Lippincott. 1994; 1273–1347.

91. Herman HH, Bottomley JM. Anatomical and biomechanical considerations of the elder foot. *Top Geriatr Rehabil.* 1992; 7(3):1–13.

92. Boyer GG. Vision problems. In: Camevali E, Patrick C, eds. *Nursing Management for the Elderly.* Philadelphia: Lippincott Co.; 1989.

93. Hellman DB. Arthritis and musculoskeletal disorders. In: Tierney LM, McPhee SJ, Papadakis MA, eds. *Current Medical Diagnosis and Treatment.* 34th ed. Norwalk, CT: Appleton & Lange, 1995; 726–732.

94. Payton OD, Roland JL. Aging process: Implications for clinical practice. *Phys Ther.* 1983; 63(l): 41–48.

95. Wedgewood, J. The place of rehabilitation in geriatric medicine: an overview. *Int Rehabil Med.* 1985; 7:107.

96. Molsa PK, Paljarvi L, Rinne JO, et al. Validity of clinical diagnosis in dementia: a prospective clinicopathologic study. *J Neurol Neurosurg Psychiatry.* 1985; 48:1085–1090.

97. Alexopoulos GS, Abrams RC, Young RC, Shamoian CA. Cornell scale for depression in dementia. *Biol Psychiatry.* 1988; 23:271–284.

98. Hughes CP, Berg L, Danziger WL, et al. A new clinical scale for the staging of dementia. *Br J Psychiatry.* 1982; 140.-566–572.

99. Cummings JL, Miller B, Hill MA, Neshkes R. Neuropsychiatric aspects of multi-infarct dementia and dementia of the Alzheimer type. *Arch Neurol.* 1987; 44:389–393.

100. Hachinski VC, Illiff LD, Zilhka E, et al. Cerebral blood flow in dementia. *Arch Neurol.* 1975; 32: 632–637.

101. Gilman S. Alzheimer's disease. *Perspect Bio Med.* 1997; 40:230–245.

102. Post SG. Future scenarios for the prevention and delay of Alzheimer disease onset in high-risk groups. An ethical perspective. *Am J Prev Med.* 1999; 16(2):105–110.

103. National Center for Health Statistics. *Health, United States, 1999, with Health and Aging Chartbook.* Hyattsvill, MD: National Center for Health Statistics, 1999; 36–37.

104. National Center for Health Statistics. *Health, United States, 1999, with Health and Aging Chartbook.* Hyattsvill, MD: National Center for Health Statistics, 1999; 34–35.

105. Centers for Disease Control and Prevention. *Unrealized Prevention Opportunities: Reducing the Health and Economic Burden of Chronic Disease.* Atlanta, GA: Centers for Disease Control and Prevention, National Center for Chronic Disease Prevention and Health Promotion. 1997.

106. Forsyth E, Rizline PD. An overview of the etiology, diagnosis, and treatment of Alzheimer disease. *Phys Ther.* 1998; 78:1325–1331.

107. Snowdon DA, Greiner LH, Markesbery WR. Linguistic ability in early life and the neuropathology of Alzheimer's disease and cerebrovascular disease. Finding from the Nun Study. *Ann N Y Acad Sci.* 2000; 903:34–38.

108. Small GW, Rabins PV, Barry PP. Diagnosis and treatment of Alzheimer disease and related disorders. *JAMA.* 1997; 278:1363–1371.

109. Wolf DS, Gearing M, Snowdon DA, Mori H, Markesbery WR, Mirra SS. Progression of regional neuropathology in Alzheimer disease and normal elderly: findings from the Nun Study. *Alzheimer Dis Assoc Disord.* 1999; 13(4): 226–231.

110. Riley KP, Snowdon DA, Saunders AM, Roses AD, Mortimer JA, Nanayakkara N. Cognitive function and apolipoprotein E in very old adults: findings from the Nun Study. *J Gerontol B Psychol Sci Soc Sci.* 2000; 55(2):S69–S75.

111. Snowdon DA, Tully CL, Smith CD, Riley KP, Markesbery WR. Serum folate and the severity of atrophy of the neocortex in Alzheimer disease: finding from the Nun Study. *Am J Clin Nutr.* 2000; 71(4):993–998.

112. Snowdon DA. Aging and Alzheimer's disease: lessons from the Nun Study. *Gerontologist.* 1997; 37(2):150–156.

113. Waters CH. *Management of Parkinson's Disease.* 2nd ed. Caddo, OK: Professional Communications Inc. 1999.

114. Schoenberg BS. Epidemiology of movement disorders. In: Marsden CD, Fahn S, eds. *Movement Disorders.* London: Butterworth; 1987:17–32.

115. Adams RD, Victor M, Ropper AH. *Principles of Neurology.* 6th ed. New York, NY: McGraw-Hill 1997; 1067–1078.

116. Quinn NP, Rossor MN, Marsden CD. Dementia and Parkinson's disease-pathological and neurochemical considerations. *Br Med Bulletin.* 1986; 42: 86–92.

117. Homykiewicz O. Brain neurotransmitter changes in Parkinson's disease. In: Marsden CD, Fahn S, eds. *Movement Disorders.* London: Butterworth; 1987:41–58.

118. Phillips P. New surgical approaches to Parkinson disease. *JAMA.* 1999; 282(12):1117–1118.

119. Tsui JC. Treatment of Parkinson's disease. In: Calne DB, ed. *Neurodegenerative Disease.* Philadelphia, PA: WB Saunders, 1994; 573–582.

120. Wojecieszek JM, Lang AE. Hyperkinetic movement disorders. In: Coffey CE, Cummings JL, eds. *Textbook of Neuropsychiatry.* Washington DC: American Psychiatric Press, 1994; 406–415.

121. Harper PS, Morris M. The epidemiology of Huntington's Disease. In: Harper PS, ed. *Huntington's Disease.* Philadelphia, PA: WB Saunders; 1991: 1–36.

122. Peacock IW. A physical therapy program for Huntington's disease patients. *Clin Management.* 1987; 7:22.

123. Hallum A. Neuromuscular diseases. In: Umphred DA, ed. *Neurological Rehabilitation.* 3rd ed. St. Louis, MO: Mosby-Year Book, Inc.; 1995: 375–393.

124. Hasson SM. Progressive and degenerative neuromuscular diseases and severe muscular dystrophy. In: Hasson SM, ed. *Clinical Exercise Physiology.* St Louis, MO: Mosby-Year Book, Inc.; 1994.

125. Caroscio JT. Amyotrophic lateral sclerosis: the disease. In Caroscio JT, ed. *Amyotrophic Lateral Sclerosis.* New York, NY: Thieme Medical Publishers; 1986.

126. Ringle SP. The natural history of amyotrophic lateral sclerosis. *Neurology.* 1993; 43:1316.

127. Tashiro K. Sensory findings in amyotrophic lateral sclerosis. In: Tsubaki T, Yase Y, eds. *Amyotrophic Lateral Sclerosis.* Amsterdam: Elsevier Science Publishers; 1988.

128. Daube JR. Classification of ALS by autonomic abnormalities. In: Tsubaki T, Yase Y, eds. *Amyotrophic Lateral Sclerosis.* Amsterdam: Elsevier Science Publishers; 1988.

129. Sinaki M. Exercise and rehabilitation measures in amyotrophic lateral sclerosis. In: Tsubaki T, Yase Y, eds. *Amyotrophic Lateral Sclerosis.* Amsterdam: Elsevier Science Publishers; 1988.

130. Bennett RL, Knowlton GC. Overwork weakness in partially denervated skeletal muscle. *Clin Orthop.* 1958; 12:22.

131. Baloh RW. Neurology of aging: vestibular system. In: Albert ML, ed. *Clinical Neurology of Aging.* New York: Oxford University Press; 1984.

132. Batata M, Spray GH, Bolton FG, et al. Blood and bone marrow changes in elderly patients, with particular reference to folic acid, vitamin B_{12}, iron and ascorbic acid. *Brit Med J.* 1967; 2: 667–669.

133. Burchinsky, SG. Neurotransmitter receptors in the central nervous system and aging: pharmacological aspects (review). *Experimental Aging.* 1984; 19: 227–239.

134. Gambert SR. *Diabetes Mellitus in the Elderly: A Practical Guide.* New York: Raven Press; 1990.

135. Bergman M. *Principles of Diabetes Management.* New York: Medical Examination Publishing Co.; 1987.

136. Riddle MC. Diabetic neuropathies in the elderly: management update. *Geriatrics. 1990;* 45(9):32–36.

137. Gutmann E, Hanzlikova V. Basic mechanisms of aging in the neuromuscular system. *Mech Ageing Dev* 1972; 1:327–349.

138. Chandler JM, Duncan PW. Balance and falls in the elderly: issues in evaluation and treatment. In: Guccione AA, ed. *Geriatric Physical Therapy.* St. Louis, MO: Mosby-Year Book; 1993; 237–252.

139. Shumway-Cook A, Woollacott MH. *Motor Control: Theory and Function.* Baltimore, MD: Williams & Wilkins; 1995.

140. Fetter M. Vestibular system disorders. In: Herdman SJ, ed. *Vestibular Rehabilitation.* Philadelphia, PA: FA Davis; 1994: 80–89.

141. Allison L. Balance disorders. In: Umphred DA, ed. *Neurological Rehabilitation.* 3rd ed. St Louis, MO: Mosby-Year Book, Inc.; 1995: 802–837.

142. Epley JM. Aberrant coupling of otolithic receptors: manifestations and assessment. In: Arenberg IK, ed. *Dizziness and Balance Disorders.* New York, NY: Kugler Publications; 1993: 183–202.

143. Gilchrest BA. *Skin and Aging Processes.* Boca Raton, Fla: CRC Press, Inc.; 1984: 67–81.

144. Silverberg N, Silverberg L. Aging and the skin. *Postgrad Med.* 1989; 86:131–136.

145. Pollack SV. Skin cancer in the elderly. In: Cohen FU, ed. Cancer II: Specific Neoplasms. *Clin Geriatr Med.* 1987; 3(4):715–728.

146. Silverberg E. Cancer statistics, 1984. *CA.* 1984; 34: 7–23.

147. Scotto J, Fears TR, Fraumeni JF, Jr. Incidence of nonmelanoma skin cancer in the United States. US

Department of Health and Human Services Pub. No. (NIH) 82–2433, Washington, DC: US Government Printing Office; 1981.

148. Albright SD III. Treatment of skin cancer using multiple modalities. *J Am Acad Dermatol.* 1982; 7:143–171.

149. Kopf AW. Malignant melanoma in humans. In: *Causes and Effects of Changes in Stratospheric Ozone: Update 1983.* National Research Council, National Academy of Sciences. Washington, IDC: National Academy Press; 1984.

150. Kopf AW. Prevention of malignant melanoma. *Dermatol Clin.* 1985; 3:351–360.

151. McLeod GR, Davis NC, Little JH. Melanoma: experience of the Queensland Melanoma Project. In: Balch CM, Milton GW, eds. *Cutaneous Melanoma.* Philadelphia: Lippincott; 1985.

152. Feldman DE, Stoll H, Maize JC. Melanomas of the palm, sole, and nail bed: a clinicopathologica study. *Cancer.* 1980; 46:2492–2504.

153. Koh HK, Michalik E, Sober AJ. Lentigo maligna melanoma has no better prognosis than other types of melanoma. *J Clin Oncol.* 1984; 2:994–1001.

154. Andres R. Normal aging versus disease in the elderly. In: Andres EL, Bierman EL, Hazzard WR, eds. *Principles in Geriatric Medicine.* New York: McGraw-Hill; 1985:38–41.

155. Bennett L, Lee B. Pressure versus shear in pressure sore causation. In: Lee B, ed. *Chronic Ulcers of the Skin.* New York: McGraw-Hill; 1985:39–56.

156. Kosiak M. Prevention and rehabilitation of ischemic ulcers. In: Kottke F, Stillwell G, Lehman J, eds. *Krusen's Handbook of Physical Medicine and Rehabilitation.* 3rd ed. Philadelphia: Saunders; 1982:881–888.

157. McCulloch J, Hovde J. Treatment of wounds due to vascular problems. In: Kloth L, McCulloch J, Feedar J, eds. *Wound Healing: Alternatives in Management.* Philadelphia: Davis; 1990:177–195.

158. Swagerty DL Jr. The impact of age-related visual impairment on functional independence in the elderly. *Kans Med.* 1995; 96(1):24–26.

159. Kasper RL. Eye problems of the aged. In: Reichel RJ, ed. *Clinical Aspects of Aging.* Baltimore, Md: Williams and Wilkins; 1988.

160. Andreasen MK. Making a safe environment by design. *J Gerontol Nurs.* 1985; 11(6):18–22.

161. Hawkins BS, Bird A, Klein R, West SK. Epidemiology of age-related macular degeneration. *Mol Vis.* 1999; 5:26.

162. Fong DS. Age-related macular degeneration: update for primary care. *Am Fam Physician.* 2000; 61(10):3035–3042.

163. Silvestri G. Age-related macular degeneration: genetics and implication for detection and treatment. *Mol Med Today.* 1997; 3(2):84–91.

164. McCarty CA, Nanjan MB, Taylor HR. Attributable risk estimates for cataract to prioritize medical and public health action. *Invest Ophthalmol Vis Sci.* 2000; 41(12):3720–3725.

165. Taylor A. Nutritional influences on risk for cataract. *Int Ophthalmol Clin.* 2000; 40(4):17–49.

166. Storr-Paulsen A, Bernth-Petersen P. Combined cataract and glaucoma surgery. *Curr Opin Ophthalmol.* 2001; 12(1):41–46.

167. Elolia R, Stokes J. Monograph series on aging-related diseases: XI. Glaucoma. *Chronic Dis Can.* 1998; 19(4):157–169.

168. Willis A, Anderson SJ. Effects of glaucoma and aging on photopic and scotopic motion perception. *Invest Ophthalmol Vis Sci.* 2000; 41(1): 325–335.

169. Kalina RE. Seeing into the future. Vision and aging. *West J Med.* 1997; 167(4):253–257.

170. Zegeer LJ. The effects of sensory changes in older persons. *J Neuroscience Nurs.* 1986; 18:325–332.

171. Christenson MA. Designing for the older person by addressing the environmental attributes. *Phys Occup Ther Geriatrics.* 1990; 8:31–48.

172. Skinner HB, Barrack RL, Cook SD. Age-related decline in proprioception. *Clin Orthop.* 1984; Apr (184):208–211.

173. Kokmen E, Bossemeyer RW, Williams WJ. Quantitative evaluation of joint motion perception in an aging population. *J Gerontol.* 1978; 33:62.

174. Laidlaw RW, Hamilton MA. A study of thresholds in perception of passive movement among normal control subjects. *Bull Neurol Inst.* 1937; 6:268–340.

175. Benassi G, D'Alessandro R, Gallassi R, et al. Neurological examination in subjects over 65 years: an epidemiological survey. *Neuroepidemiology.* 1990; 9:27–38.

176. Barrett DS, Cobb AG, Bently G. Joint proprioception in normal, osteoarthritic and replaced knees. *J Bone Joint Surg.* 1991; 73B:53–56.

177. Herdman SJ. Exercise strategies in vestibular disorders. *Ear Nose Throat J.* 1989; 68:961–964.

178. Herdman SJ. Assessment and treatment of balance disorders in the vestibular deficient patient. In: Duncan P, ed. *Balance.* Proceedings of the American Physical Therapy Association Forum. Alexandria, Va: APTA Publications; 1990:87–94.

179. Hayteir J. Modifying the environment to help older persons. *Nurs Health Care.* 1983; 4:265–269.

180. Maloney CC. Identifying and treating the client with sensory loss. *Phys Occup Ther Geriatrics.* 1987; 5:31–46.

181. Bartol MA, Heitkemper M. Gastrointestinal problems. In: Carnevali P, and Patrick, B eds. *Nursing Management for the Elderly.* Philadelphia: Lippincott Co.; 1989.

182. Bidlack WR, Kirsch A, Meskin MS. Nutritional requirements of the elderly. *Food Technology.* 1988; 40:61–70.

183. Siebens H, Trupe E, Siebens A, et al. Correlates and consequences of eating dependency in institutionalized elderly. *J Am Geriatr Soc.* 1986; 34(3): 192–198.

184. Castell DO. Dysphagia in the elderly. *J Amer Ger Soc.* 1986; 34(3):248–249.

185. Brandeis GH, Baumann MM, Hossain M, Morris JN, Resnick NM. The prevalence of potentially remediable urinary incontinence in frail older people: A study using the Minimum Data Set. *J Am Geriatr Soc.* 1997; 45(2):179–184.

186. Dillon L, Fonda D. Medical evaluation of causes of lower urinary tract symptoms and urinary incontinence in older people. *Top Geriatr Rehabil.* 2000; 15(4):1–15.

187. Fonda D. Nocturia: a disease or normal ageing? *Br J Urol Int.* 1999; 84(1):13–15.

188. Vliet EL. Hormone connections in urinary incontinence in women. *Top Geriatr Rehabil.* 2000; 15(4): 16–30.

189. Resnick NM. Urinary incontinence in the elderly. *Medical Grand Rounds.* 1984; 3:281–290.

190. Resnick NM. Urinary incontinence. *Lancet.* 1995; 345:94–99.

191. Meadows E. Physical therapy for older adults with urinary incontinence. *Top Geriatr Rehabil.* 2000; 16(1):22–32.

192. Fantl JA, Newman DK, Colling J. *Urinary Incontinence in Adults: Acute and Chronic Management. Clinical Practice Guideline No. 2, 1996 Update.* Rockville, MD: US Department of Health and Human Services, Agency for Health Care Policy and Research; 1996. AHCPR Pub No. 96–0682.

193. Snape WJ. Disorders of gastrointestinal motility. In: Wyngaarden JB, Smith LH, Bennett JC, eds. *Cecil Textbook of Medicine,* ed 19. Philadelphia: WB Saunders; 1992: 671–680.

194. Schuster MM. Irritable bowel syndrome. In: Sleisenger MH, Fordtran JS, eds. *Gastrointestin Disease,* ed 5. Philadelphia: WB Saunders; 1993: 917–929.

195. Goldman R. Decline in organ function with age. In: Rossman I, ed. *Clinical Geriatrics.* 2nd ed. Philadelphia: Lippincott Co.; 1979.

196. Goyal VK. Changes with age in the human kidney. *Exp Gerontol.* 1982; 17:321–331.

197. Lindeman RD, Goldman R. Anatomic and physiologic age changes in the kidney. *Exp Gerontol.* 1986; 21:379–406.

198. Lindeman RD, Tobin JD, Shock NW. Longitudinal studies on the rate of decline in renal function with age. *J Amer Ger Soc.* 1985; 33:278–285.

199. Fine LG. Preventing the progression of human renal disease: have rational therapeutic principles emerged? *Kidney Int.* 1988; 33: 116–128.

200. Nieman DC. *The Sports Medicine Fitness Course.* Palo Alto, Calif.: Bull Publishing Co.; 1986.

201. Drinkwater BL: *The Role of Nutrition and Exercise in Health. Continuing Dental Education.* Seattle: University of Washington; 1985.

202. Suominen H, Heikkinen E, Liesen H. Effect of 8 weeks endurance training on skeletal muscle metabolism in 56–70 year old men. *Eur J Appl Physiol.* 1987; 37:173–180.

203. Kaplin GA, Seemah TE, Cohen RD. Mortality among the elderly in the Alameda County study: behavioral and demographic risk factors. *Am J Public Health.* 1987; 77(3):307–312.

204. Stones MJ, Dorman B, Kozma A. The prediction of mortality in elderly institution resident. *J Gerontol Psychol Sci.* 1989; 44(3):72–79.

205. Weinberg AD, Minaker KL. Dehydration. Evaluation and management in older adults. Council on Scientific Affairs, American Medical Association. *JAMA.* 1995; 274(19):1552–1556.

206. Phillips PA, Rolls BJ, Ledingham JJG: Reduced thirst after water deprivation in healthy elderly men. *N Engl J Med.* 1984; 311:753–759.

207. Lindeman RD. Hypokalemia: causes, consequences, and correction. *Am J Med Sci.* 1976; 272:5–17.

208. Mooradian AD, Morley JE, Korenman SG. Endocrinology in aging. *Dis Mon.* 1988; 34:395–461.

209. Greenblatt RB. *Geriatric Endocrinology.* Aging Series Vol. 5, New York: Raven Press; 1978.

210. Morley JE. Geriatric endocrinology. In: Mendelsohn G, ed. *Diagnosis and Pathology of Endocrine Disease.* Philadelphia: Lippincott Co.; 1988.

211. Lipson LG. Diabetes in the elderly: diagnosis, pathogenesis and therapy. *Am J Med.* 1986; 80 (suppl 5A):10–21.

212. Morley JE, Mooradian AD, Rosenthal MJ, et al. Diabetes mellitus in elderly patients: Is it different? *Am J Med.* 1987; 83:533–544.

213. Rosenthal MJ, Hartnell JM, Morley JE, et al. UCLA geriatric grand rounds: diabetes in the elderly. *J Am Geriatr Soc.* 1987; 35:435–447.

214. Jackson RA. Mechanisms of age-related glucose intolerance. *Diabetes Care. 1990;* 13(suppl 2):9–19.

215. Jette DU. Physiological effects of exercise in the diabetic. *Phys Ther.* 1984; 64(3):339–342.

216. Kohl HW, Villegas JA, Gordon NF, Blair SN. Cardiorespiratory fitness, glycemic status, and mortality risk in men. *Diabetes Care.* 1992; 15(2):184–192.

217. Robuschi G, Safran M, Braverman LE. Hypothyroidism in the elderly. *Endocr Rev.* 1987; 8: 142–153.

218. Morley JE, Slag MF, Elson MK, et al. The interpretation of thyroid function tests in hospitalized patients. *JAMA.* 1983; 249:2377–2379.

219. Morley JE. The aging endocrine system. *Postgrad Med.* 1983; 73:107–120.

220. Chapuy MC, Chapuy P, Meunier PJ. Calcium and vitamin D supplements: effects of calcium metabolism in elderly people. *Am J Clin Nutr.* 1987; 46: 324–328.

221. Chernoff R. *Geriatric Nutrition: The Health Professional's Handbook.* Gaithersburg, Md: Aspen Publishers, Inc.; 1991.

222. Yancik R, Ries LA. Cancer in the older person: magnitude of the problem. In: Balducci L, Lyman GH, Ershler WB. *Comprehensive Geriatric Oncology.* The Netherlands: Harwood Academic Publishers; 1998:95–104.

223. Duthie EH. Physiology of aging: relevance to symptoms, perceptions, and treatment tolerance. In: Balducci L, Lyman GH, Ershler WB. *Comprehensive Geriatric Oncology.* The Netherlands: Harwood Academic Publishers; 1998:247–262.

224. Campisi J. Aging and cancer: the double edged sword of proliferative senescence. *J Am Ger Soc.* 1997; 45(4):482–490.

225. Anisimov V. Age as a risk factor for multistage carcinogenesis. In: Balducci L, Lyman GH, Ershler WB. *Comprehensive Geriatric Oncology.* The Nether-

lands: Harwood Academic Publishers; 1998: 157–178.

226. Barbone F, Bonvenzi M, Cavallieri F. Air pollution and lung cancer in Trieste, Italy. *Am J Epidemiol.* 1995; 141:1161–1169.

227. Balducci L. Prevention and Treatment of Cancer in the Elderly. *Oncol Issues.* 2000; 15:26–28.

228. Balducci L, Beghe C. The application of the principles of geriatrics to the management of the older person with cancer. *Crit Rev Oncol Hematol.* 2000; 35(3):147–154,

229. Brink JJ, Reichel W. Cell biology and physiology of aging. In: Reichel W, ed. *Care of the Elderly: Clinical Aspects of Aging.* ed 4. Baltimore: Williams & Wilkins; 1995:472–475.

230. Chen HX, Ryan PA, Ferguson RP. Characteristics of acquired immunodeficiency syndrome in the elderly. *J Am Ger Soc.* 1998; 46(2):153–156.

231. Terpenning M. AIDS in older people. *J Am Ger Soc.* 1998; 46(2):244–245.

232. Shinkai S, Konishi M, Shephard RJ. Aging and immune response to exercise. *Can J Physiol Pharmacol.* 1998; 76(5):562–572.

233. Bruunsgaard H, Hartkopp A, Mohr T, Konradsen H, Heron I, Mordhorst CH, Pedersen BK. In vivo cell-mediated immunity and vaccination response following prolonged, intense exercise. *Med Sci Sports Exerc.* 1997; 29(9):1176–1181.

234. Shepard RJ. Immune changes induced by exercise in an adverse environment. *Can J Physiol Pharmacol.* 1998; 76(5):539–546.

235. Le TP, Tuazon CU. Human immunodeficiency virus (HIV) in the elderly: a case report. *J Am Ger Soc.* 1998; 46(2):249–250.

236. Shipp AJ, Wolff A, Selik R. Epidemiology of acquired immune deficiency syndrome in persons aged 50 years or older. *J Acquir Immune Defic Syndr.* 1991; 4(1):84–88.

237. Wallace JI, Paauw DS, Spach DH. HIV infections in older patients: When to suspect the unexpected. *Geriatrics.* 1993;48(1):61–70.

238. Ward ME, Cowley AR. Hypothermia: a natural cause of death. *Am J Forensic Med Path.* 1999; 20(4):383–386.

239. Worfolk JB. Keep frail elders warm! *Geriatr Nurs.* 1997; 18(1):7–11.

240. Stauss HM, Morgan DA, Anderson KE, Massett MP, Kregel KC. Modulation of baroreflex sensitivity and spectral power of blood pressure by heat stress and aging. *Am J Physiol.* 1997; 272(2 Pt 2): H776–784.

241. Vassallo M, Gera KN, Allen S. Factors associated with high risk of marginal hyperthermia in elderly patients living in an institution. *Postgrad Med J.* 1995; 71(834):213–216.

242. Fehrenbach E, Niess AM. Role of heat shock proteins in the exercise response. *Exerc Immunol Rev.* 1999; 5:57–77.

243. Cauley JA, Dorman JS, Ganguli M. Genetic and aging epidemiology. The merging of two disciplines. *Neurol Clin.* 1996; 14:467–475.

CHAPTER 6

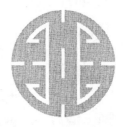

Assessment Instruments

The demands in health care for cost-effective care are pushing rehabilitation and medical professionals to prove the efficacy and efficiency of the care provided. The obvious place for caregivers to begin this process is in the area of assessment. The evolution of medicine and rehabilitation has been a mixture of science, philosophy, sociology, and intuition. Some of the finest practitioners may be some of the worst scientists. However, they may have an extraordinary intuitive sense. Because of this fine mixture, it is difficult to quantify assessments, treatments, and outcomes. Nevertheless, this needs to be done. The work in health care assessment has grown exponentially in the last twenty years, and more tools are being developed and more scrutiny is being applied to treatment interventions and outcomes.

In the area of aging, these efforts are extremely timely. As was noted in Chapter 1, the number of older persons is growing dramatically. In addition, the National Long-Term Care Survey noted 3.0 million older persons with impairment in one or more daily activities.[1] The Supplement on Aging portion of the National Interview Survey showed 6.0 million impaired elderly,[2] and the *Journal of Gerontology: Medical Sciences* noted recently that the "quality of life is judged more by the level of functioning and ability to remain independent than by specific diseases diagnosed by the physician."[3]

The implications of improved, appropriate, and standard measures also impact the clinician by im-

proving communication among practitioners, fostering consistency, and reaffirming knowledge and skill.

This chapter will discuss three important components of the physical therapist's assessment of the elderly. The first section will discuss mental status measures for older persons; the second will discuss the most common functional assessment tools for the elderly; and the third will discuss the modifications needed when assessing the older person using accepted physical measures, such as goniometry, manual muscle tests, and nerve conduction velocity.

MENTAL STATUS MEASURES

Mini-Mental State Examination

The Mini-Mental State Examination (MMSE) was published in 1975 by Folstein[4] and it has been widely used since then to assess cognitive changes in older patients. The MMSE was developed to assess patients who have deficits in memory, language, or both. These deficits correlate to intellectual impairment that may indicate Alzheimer's disease. The test indicates impairment, though it does not make a diagnosis.[5] The MMSE correlates with Wechsler Intelligence Scales and the Wechsler Memory Test, as well as to cerebral lesions detected by CAT scan.[4,5]

The test is relatively easy to administer and takes between five and ten minutes. The test and its instructions for administration can be found in Figure 6–1.

Mini-Mental State Exam

Orientation:	Maximum Score	Score	Instructions
What is the (year) (season) (date) (day) (month)?	5	_____	Ask for the date. Then proceed to ask other parts of the question. One point for each correct segment of the question.
Where are we: (state) (county) (town) (hospital) (floor)?	5	_____	Ask for the facility then proceed to parts of the question. One point for each correct segment of the question.

Registration:			
Name three objects (bed, apple, shoe). Ask the patient to repeat them.	3	_____	Name the objects slowly, one second for each. Ask him to repeat. Score by the number he is able to recall. Take time here for him to learn the series of objects, up to 6 trials, to use later for the memory test.

Attention and Calculation:			
Count backwards by 7s. Start with 100. Stop after 5 calculations.	5	_____	Score the total number correct. (93, 86, 79, 72, 65)

Alternate question:			
Spell the word "world" backwards.	5	_____	Score the number of letters in correct order. (dlrow = 5. dlorw = 3)

Recall:	Maximum Score	Score	Instructions
Ask for the three objects used in question 2 to be repeated.	3	_____	Score one point for each correct answer. (bed, apple, shoe)

Language:			
1. Naming: Name this object. (watch, pencil)	2	_____	Hold the object. Ask patient to name it. Score one point for each correct answer.
2. Repetition: Repeat the following– "No ifs, ands or buts."	1	_____	Allow one trial only. Score one point for correct answer.
3. Follow a 3-stage command: "Take the paper in your right hand, fold it in half, and put it on the floor."	3	_____	Use a blank sheet of paper. Score one point for each part correctly executed.
4. Reading: Read and obey the following: Close your eyes.	1	_____	Instruction should be printed on a page. Allow patient to read it. Score by a correct response.
5. Writing: Write a sentence.	1	_____	Provide paper and pencil. Allow patient to write any sentence. It must contain a noun, verb, and be sensible.
6. Copying: Copy this design.	1	_____	All 10 angles must be present. Figures must intersect. Tremor and rotation are ignored.
	Total Score	_____	(Max. 30) Test is not timed.

Figure 6–1. *(Reprinted with permission from Folstein MF, Folstein SE, McHugh PR. Mini mental state. A practical method for grading the cognitive state of patients for the clinician. J Psychiatr Res. 1975; 12:189–198.)*

The maximum score possible on this test is 30. A score below 24 indicates cognitive impairment and is not considered normal for older persons. A score of 21 to 24 is considered mild intellectual impairment, a score of 16 to 20 reflects moderate impairment, and a score below 15 is considered severely impaired.[4] The MMSE also relates to depression, and is indicative of depression at a score of 19. Patients show improvement on the MMSE scores as the depression is ameliorated.[6]

The Mental Status Questionnaire

The Mental Status Questionnaire (MSQ) is composed of ten questions and, therefore, is quick and easy to administer. Because of its ease of use and its validity and reliability, it has been used extensively for the past three decades.[7] This test does show a correlation between low scores and impaired cognition.

Despite the test's convenience and research strength, however, it does have several clinical weaknesses. It lacks sensitivity and may show false positives because it does not pick up impairment until the scores are in the high range. It also omits several important domains of cognitive functioning, including reasoning, visual-spatial relationships, and many aspects of language. Table 6–1 shows the MSQ.[7] The MSQ has also been criticized for a lack of relevancy of its questions to institutional residents.[6]

Depression Scales

Despite the high prevalence of depression in the older population, the diagnosis of depression may be missed.[8] However, when screening instruments are used, the recognition of depression is increased.[9]

The Zung Self-Rating Scale   The Zung Self-Rating Depression Scale is widely used for screening for depression. However, this scale may not be the best choice for older persons. The validity on this test was tested on a university outpatient population,[10] and elderly persons scored higher on it. Because of this, the elderly may be considered "borderline" even when they are not depressed.[11]

The test is composed of ten negative and ten positive statements, with the respondent giving an answer that correlates with a one to four rating. The scores can be expressed as a percentage of 80, with 80 being the highest score and most indicative of severe depression[12] (Fig. 6–2).

Popoff Index of Depression   The Popoff Index of Depression may be more applicable to the older patient who is seen in the community. This test allows for more covert responses, which can help to identify persons who are not ready to make obvious statements about their depression. It is slightly more sensitive to patients who are somatizing as well.[13] The test consists of fifteen groups of statements. Each

group has a covert, overt, and healthy response. If the respondent chooses either the covert or the overt response, he or she will get a point. A score higher than 10 is indicative of depression. This test, as well as the Zung test, has been shown to have sensitivity and reliability when compared to other tests and population studies (Fig. 6–3).[14]

Beck Depression Inventory   The Beck Depression Inventory (Fig. 6–4) is another very popular instrument for depression screening. The test was initially administered by interview, but it is also adaptable for self-administration.[15] The original form has twenty-one sets of statements with a scoring mechanism from zero to three. In a primary care setting, a cutoff score of 13 was indicative of depression with a high sensitivity and specificity.[16] In elderly patients, it was found that using a cutoff score of 10 only missed 3% of the depressed patients.[17]

The short form of the Beck's Depression Inventory correlates as well as the long version and only takes the patient 5 minutes to complete. The 13 questions for the short version are taken from Figure 6–4[18] as follows: A,B,C,D,E,G,I,L,M,N,O,Q,R. In addition, in the short version the responses are reversed so that the patient reads the most negative response first.[16]

The Geriatric Depression Scale   The final tool to be described for assessing depression is the Geriatric Depression Scale. This 30 item, yes-or-no questionnaire determines that a score of over 8 has a 90% sensitivity and an 80% specificity in detecting depression in the older population.[19] There is also a short version consisting of the following 15 questions: 1–4, 7, 9, 10, 12, 14, 15, 17, and 21–23. A score of over 5 on this form may indicate depression.[20] The test and the method of scoring is shown in Figure 6–5.[20]

TABLE 6–1.   MENTAL STATUS QUESTIONNAIRE (MSQ)

The patient gets a point for every error when asked the following questions, and the scores show the severity of brain syndrome as follows:
0–2 = none or minimal
3–8 = moderate
9–10 = secvere

1. What is this place?
2. Where is this place located?
3. What day of the month is it today?
4. What day of the week is it?
5. What year is it?
6. How old are you?
7. When is your birthday?
8. In what year were you born?
9. What is the name of the president?
10. Who was the president before this one?

Reprinted with permission from Kahn RL, et al. Brief objective measures for the determination of mental status in the aged. *Am J Psychiatry.* 1960; 117:326.

The Zung Self-Rating Depression Scale

1. (–) I feel down-hearted and blue.
2. (+) Morning is when I feel the best.
3. (–) I have crying spells or feel like it.
4. (–) I have trouble sleeping at night.
5. (+) I eat as much as I used to.
6. (+) I still enjoy sex.
7. (–) I notice that I am losing weight.
8. (–) I have trouble with constipation.
9. (–) My heart beats faster than usual.
10. (–) I get tired for no reason.
11. (+) My mind is as clear as it used to be.
12. (+) I find it easy to do the things I used to.
13. (–) I am restless and can't keep still.
14. (+) I feel hopeful about the future.
15. (–) I am more irritable than usual.
16. (+) I find it easy to make decisions.
17. (+) I feel that I am useful and needed.
18. (+) My life is pretty full.
19. (–) I feel that others would be better off if I were dead.
20. (+) I still enjoy the things I used to do.

Statements are answered "a little of the time," "some of the time," "a good part of the time," or "most of the time." The responses are given a score of 1 to 4, arranged so that the higher the score, the greater the depression: the statements designated with (+) are given "1" for response "most of time," while those with (–) are given a "4" for "most of the time."

Figure 6–2. (Adapted and reprinted with permission from Zung A. A self-rating depression scale. Arch Gen Psychiatry. 1965; 12:63–70.)

Popoff Index of Depression

1. O. Everything is an effort.
   H. I have a lot of energy.
   C. Maybe I'm just getting older.

2. H. I've got a lot of pep.
   C. I tire easily.
   O. I'm tired all the time.

3. C. I'm in a rut.
   O. Things are not going well.
   H. I'm pleased with the way things are going.

4. O. I don't have much to look forward to.
   H. I look forward to the future.
   C. I go along as best I can.

5. H. I enjoy getting up in the morning.
   C. I push myself to get going in the morning.
   O. I find it hard to face the day.

6. C. I don't feel rested after sleeping.
   O. I've been having trouble sleeping lately.
   H. I sleep fine and feel rested.

7. O. I haven't been eating as well lately.
   H. I enjoy eating.
   C. Food doesn't taste as good as it used to.

8. H. Sex is pleasurable to me.
   C. Sometimes I'm too tired for sex.
   O. I've lost some interest in sex lately.

9. C. I force myself to do my work.
   O. I don't have much ambition.
   H. I am ambitious.

10. O. I don't feel like doing much lately.
    H. I enjoy doing lots of things.
    C. I don't go out much because I am too tired.

11. H. Things are going good.
    C. Sometimes everything goes wrong.
    O. I can't cope with things very well lately.

12. C. I'd do better if I felt better.
    O. Sometimes I can't do anything right.
    H. Things are running smoothly.

13. O. I'm depressed.
    H. I'm happy.
    C. I don't let myself get depressed.

14. H. I'm happy with the way I'm doing things.
    C. Everybody feels they could do better.
    O. I'm not doing things as well as I used to.

15. O. Sometimes I feel like giving up.
    H. I'm enjoying my life.
    C. I fight it when I feel discouraged.

In the questionnaire, "C" indicates a "covert" response, "O" an overt response, and "H" a healthy response.

Figure 6–3. (Adapted and reprinted with permission from Popoffs. A simple method for diagnosis of depression by the family physician. Clin Med.1969; 76:26.)

The Beck Depression Inventory

A Mood
0 I do not feel sad.
1 I feel blue or sad.
2a I am blue or sad all the time and I can't snap out of it.
2b I am so sad or unhappy that it is very painful.
3 I am so sad or unhappy that I can't stand it.

B (Pessimism)
0 I am not particularly pessimistic or discouraged about the future.
1 I feel discouraged about the future.
2a I feel I have nothing to look forward to.
2b I feel that I won't ever get over my troubles.
3 I feel that the future is hopeless and that things cannot improve.

C (Sense of Failure)
0 I do not feel like a failure.
1 I feel I have failed more than the average person.
2a I feel I have accomplished very little that is worthwhile or that means anything.
2b As I look back on my life all I can see is a lot of failures.
3 I feel I am a complete failure as a person (parent, husband, wife).

D (Lack of Satisfaction)
0 I am not particularly dissatisfied.
1a I feel bored most of the time.
1b I don't enjoy things the way I used to.
2 I don't get satisfaction out of anything any more.
3 I am dissatisfied with everything.

E (Guilty Feelings)
0 I don't feel particularly guilty.
1 I feel bad or unworthy a good part of the time.
2a I feel quite guilty.
2b I feel bad or unworthy practically all the time now.
3 I feel as though I am very bad or worthless.

F (Sense of Punishment)
0 I don't feel I am being punished.
1 I have a feeling that something bad may happen to me.

2 I feel I am being punished or will be punished.
3a I feel I deserve to be punished.
3b I want to be punished.

G (Self Hate)
0 I don't feel disappointed in myself.
1a I am disappointed in myself.
1b I don't like myself.
2 I am disgusted with myself.
3 I hate myself.

H (Self Accusations)
0 I don't feel I am any worse than anybody else.
1 I am very critical of myself for my weaknesses or mistakes.
2a I blame myself for everything that goes wrong.
2b I feel I have many bad faults.

I (Self-punitive Wishes)
0 I don't have any thought of harming myself.
1 I have thoughts of harming myself, but I would not carry them out.
2a I feel I would be better off dead.
2b I have definite plans about committing suicide.
2c I feel my family would be better off if I were dead.
3 I would kill myself if I could.

J (Crying Spells)
0 I don't cry any more than usual.
1 I cry more now than I used to.
2 I cry all the time now. I can't stop it.
3 I used to be able to cry but now I can't cry at all even though I want to.

K (Irritability)
0 I am no more irritated now than I ever am.
1 I get annoyed or irritated more easily than I used to.
2 I feel irritated all the time.
3 I don't get irritated at all at the things that used to irritate me.

L (Social Withdrawal)
0 I have not lost interest in other people.
1 I am less interested in other people now than I used to be.

— Continued —

Figure 6–4. *(Reprinted with permission from Inventory for measuring depression. Arch Gen Psychiatry. 1961; 4:561–571.)*

─── *Continued from previous page* ───

2 I have lost most of my interest in other people and have little feeling for them.
3 I have lost all my interest in other people and don't care about them at all.

M (Indecisiveness)
0 I make decisions about as well as ever.
1 I am less sure of myself now and try to put off making decisions.
2 I can't make decisions any more without help.
3 I can't make any decisions at all any more.

N (Body Image)
0 I don't feel I look any worse than I used to.
1 I am worried that I am looking old or unattractive.
2 I feel that there are permanent changes in my appearance and they make me look unattractive.
3 I feel that I am ugly or repulsive looking.

O (Work Inhibition)
0 I can work about as well as before.
1a It takes extra effort to get started at doing something.
1b I don't work as well as I used to.
2 I have to push myself very hard to do anything.
3 I can't do any work at all.

P (Sleep Disturbance)
0 I can sleep as well as usual.
1 I wake up more tired in the morning than I used to.
2 I wake up 1 to 2 hours earlier than usual and find it hard to get back to sleep.
3 I wake up early every day and can't get more than 5 hours sleep.

Q (Fatigability)
0 I don't get any more tired than usual.
1 I get tired more easily than I used to.
2 I get tired from doing anything.
3 I get too tired to do anything.

R (Loss of Appetite)
0 My appetite is no worse than usual.
1 My appetite is not as good as it used to be.
2 My appetite is much worse now.
3 I have no appetite at all anymore.

S (Weight Loss)
0 I haven't lost much weight, if any, lately.
1 I have lost more than 5 pounds.
2 I have lost more than 10 pounds.
3 I have lost more than 15 pounds

T (Somatic Preoccupation)
0 I am no more concerned about my health than usual.
1 I am concerned about aches and pains or upset stomach or constipation or other unpleasant feelings in my body.
2 I am so concerned with how I feel or what I feel that it's hard to think of much else.
3 I am completely absorbed in what I feel.

U (Loss of Libido)
0 I have not noticed any recent change in my interest in sex.
1 I am less interested in sex than I used to be.
2 I am much less interested in sex now.
3 I have lost interest in sex completely.

Items with "a" or "b" are scored the same as the corresponding number.

Figure 6–4. (Continued)

Geriatric Depression Scale

1. Are you basically satisfied with your life? (no)

2. Have you dropped many of your activities and interests? (yes)

3. Do you feel that your life is empty? (yes)

4. Do you often get bored? (yes)

5. Are you hopeful about the future? (no)

6. Are you bothered by thoughts that you just cannot get out of your head? (yes)

7. Are you in good spirits most of the time? (no)

8. Are you afraid that something bad is going to happen to you? (yes)

9. Do you feel happy most of the time? (no)

10. Do you often feel helpless? (yes)

11. Do you often get restless and fidgety? (yes)

12. Do you prefer to stay home at night, rather than go out and do new things? (yes)

13. Do you frequently worry about the future? (yes)

14. Do you feel that you have more problems with memory than most? (yes)

15. Do you think it is wonderful to be alive now? (no)

16. Do you often feel downhearted and blue? (yes)

17. Do you feel pretty worthless the way you are now? (yes)

18. Do you worry a lot about the past? (yes)

19. Do you find life very exciting? (no)

20. Is it hard for you to get started on new projects? (yes)

21. Do you feel full of energy? (no)

22. Do you feel that your situation is hopeless? (yes)

23. Do you think that most persons are better off than you are? (yes)

24. Do you frequently get upset over little things? (yes)

25. Do you frequently feel like crying? (yes)

26. Do you have trouble concentrating? (yes)

27. Do you enjoy getting up in the morning? (no)

28. Do you prefer to avoid social gatherings? (yes)

29. Is it easy for you to make decisions? (no)

30. Is your mind as clear as it used to be? (no)

Score one point for each response that matches the yes or no answer after the question.

Figure 6–5. *(Adapted and reprinted with permission from Yesavage JA, Brink TL. Development and validation of a geriatric depression screening scale: A preliminary report. J Psych Res. 1983; 17:41.)*

Stress Measures

A final area of psychosocial assessment is stress.

The Holmes and Rahe Life Events Scale The most widely used tool for evaluating stress is the Holmes and Rahe Life Events Scale.[21] This scale is shown in Figure 6–6. In administering this tool, the therapist asks the patient to circle the events that have occurred in the last year or will occur in the coming year. The therapist adds up the scores, and the total score is compared to the following scale. A score of below 180 points indicates mild stress or less than a 40% chance of a serious illness in the next year; a score of 180 to 300 indicates moderate stress or a 40% chance of developing a serious illness in the next year; and a score above 300 indicates severe stress or an 80% chance of a serious illness in the next year.[21]

FUNCTIONAL ASSESSMENT

The word function is repeated eighty-eight times in the current Center for Medicare and Medicaid Services (CMS) regulations on rehabilitation.[22] This fact should encourage rehabilitation professionals to think about and use functional measures, because CMS uses these regulations as requirements for payment.

Functional measurement is also important because it differs from the current methods physical therapists and occupational therapists use to assess patient status, and they may not truly reflect a patient's functional level. These measures, such as range of motion, strength, and other musculoskeletal parameters, may be important to assessment, but they do not always relate to function. If rehabilitation professionals are to show efficacy in what they do, it is important that they assess function in conjunction with musculoskeletal parameters. Combining these two assessments will make a truly comprehensive rehabilitation evaluation possible.

A recent study by Mary Tinetti scrutinizes the use of musculoskeletal measures.[23] Her study showed very little relationship between musculoskeletal measures and functional outcomes of older patients.[23]

A third factor contributing to the importance of functional evaluation is the ability to give a beginning and end point based on a functional outcome, as well as a relationship of this outcome to a patient's independence. For example, the Barthel Index (see Fig. 6–7) can rate a patient's difficulty with bathing or walking. The patient's ability to perform these tasks is assigned a level that is indicated by a number. As the person progresses with treatment, they are moved to higher levels. If they regress, they are ranked at a lower level. In addition, the total scoring on this index indicates to the assessor when the patient is able to go home or is in need of assistance.

These numbers translate to a patient's specific ability to function and can be very helpful in making decisions related to disposition and the need for continued care. On the other hand, a muscle strength measure indicating normal (5/5) muscle strength means nothing if the person cannot get in and out of a tub or eat independently. The combination of strength and function measures is extremely helpful, however, when assessing cause and outcome.

The purpose of this section is to encourage the health professional to avoid doing unnecessary and time-consuming tests. Many of these functional tests can be done by the patient with paper and pencil prior to the treatment program and on discharge without unnecessarily monopolizing the health professional's time.

A final justification of functional evaluation comes from an article written by Robert Kane, Dean of the School of Public Health at the University of Minnesota.[24] Dr Kane is a well-respected researcher in gerontology and health care and an advocate for functional assessment for geriatricians. In his article, he states that a specialty is not truly a specialty until it has its own instrument. He gave radiology as an example. This discipline would not have its current credibility or base if it were not for x-rays. Also, cardiology would not have evolved into a specialty if it were not for heart catheterization. He then asserts that geriatrics will truly not be accepted as a specialty until the professionals in that area have a similar tool. He believes that the tool for geriatrics is functional assessment.[24]

By extrapolating on his thoughts, it can be seen that rehabilitation is an area where functional assessment is a tool, especially for rehabilitation professionals in the area of geriatrics. The following sections follow this argument and advocate functional assessment for rehabilitation professionals, particularly for those working in geriatrics.

What is Functional Assessment?

Functional assessment differs from traditional assessment in several ways. For example, it targets specific behaviors and tasks a patient wishes to accomplish. If a therapist were to ask a patient, "What do you want from physical therapy?," the patient would not say, "I want my muscles to test normal or 5/5." Rather, they would answer, "I want to increase the strength in my legs," or "I want to run 10 miles pain free." These responses are rarely indicated in rehabilitation notes or incorporated into work goals. Instead, many notes state that the goal of treatment is to increase strength or function. This is not enough. A goal stated in slightly more specific functional terms is, "Increase strength so that the patient is able to run a marathon without pain," or "the patient is able to walk from bed to bathroom unassisted, without falling or losing balance." An even better functional statement would be a quantified response, such as, "The patient scores 80 on the Barthel and can return home independently."

The Holmes and Rahe Social Adjustment Scale

Rank	Life Event	Mean Value
1	Death of spouse	100
2	Divorce	73
3	Marital separation	65
4	Jail term	63
5	Death of close family member	63
6	Personal injury or illness	53
7	Marriage	50
8	Fired at work	47
9	Marital reconciliation	45
10	Retirement	45
11	Change in health of family member	44
12	Pregnancy	40
13	Sex difficulties	39
14	Gain of new family member	39
15	Business readjustment	39
16	Change in financial state	38
17	Death of close friend	37
18	Change to different line of work	36
19	Change in number of arguments with spouse	35
20	Mortgage over $10,000	31
21	Foreclosure of mortgage or loan	30
22	Change in responsibilities at work	29
23	Son or daughter leaving home	29
24	Trouble with in-laws	29
25	Outstanding personal achievement	28
26	Wife begin or stop work	26
27	Begin or end school	26
28	Change in living conditions	25
29	Revision of personal habits	24
30	Trouble with boss	23
31	Change in work hours or conditions	20
32	Change in residence	20
33	Change in schools	20
34	Change in recreation	19
35	Change in church activities	19
36	Change in social activities	18
37	Mortgage or loan less than $10,000	17
38	Change in sleeping habits	16
39	Change in number of family get-togethers	15
40	Change in eating habits	15
41	Vacation	13
42	Christmas	12
43	Minor violations of the law	11

Figure 6–6. (Reprinted with permission from Holmes T, Rahe R. The social readjustment rating scale. J Psychosom Res. 1967; 11:213–218.)

Barthel Index

The following presents the items or tasks scored in the Barthel Index with the corresponding values for independent performance of the tasks:

	"Can do by myself"	"Can do with help of someone else"	"Cannot do at all"
Self-Care Index			
1. Drinking from a cup	4	0	0
2. Eating	6	0	0
3. Dressing upper body	5	4	0
4. Dressing lower body	7	4	0
5. Putting on brace or artificial limb	0	2	0 (Not applicable)
6. Grooming	5	0	0
7. Washing or bathing	6	0	0
8. Controlling urination	10	5 (Accidents)	0 (Incontinent)
9. Controlling bowel movements	10	5 (Accidents)	0 (Incontinent)
Mobility Index			
10. Getting in and out of chair	15	7	0
11. Getting on and off toilet	6	3	0
12. Getting in and out of tub or shower	1	0	0
13. Walking 50 yards on the level	15	10	0
14. Walking up/down 1 flight of stairs	10	5	0
15. If not walking: propelling or pushing wheelchair	5	0	0 (Not applicable)

Barthel Total: Best score is 100; worst score is 0.

NOTE: Tasks 1–9, the Self-Care Index (including control of bladder and bowel sphincters), have a total possible score of 53. Tasks 10–15, the Mobility Index, have a total possible score of 47. The 2 groups of tasks combined make up the total Barthel Index with a total possible score of 100.

Figure 6–7. *(Reprinted with permission from Mahoney FI, Barthel DW. Functional evaluation: the Barthel Index. Md Med J. 1965; 14(2):61–65.)*

Katz ADL Index

The Index of Independence in Activities of Daily Living is based on an evaluation of the functional independence or dependence of patients in bathing, dressing, going to the toilet, transferring, continence, and feeding. Specific definitions of functional independence and dependence appear below the index.

A   Indpendent in feeding, continence, transferring, going to toilet, dressing, and bathing.

B   Independent in all but one of these functions.

C   Independent in all but bathing and one additional function.

D   Independent in all but bathing, dressing, and one additional function.

E   Independent in all but bathing, dressing, going to toilet, and one additional function.

F   Independent in all but bathing, dressing, going to toilet, transferring, and one additonal function.

G   Dependent in all six functions.

Other   Dependent in at least two functions, but not classifiable as C, D, E, or F.

Independence means without supervision, direction, or active personal assistance, except as specifically noted below. This is based on actual status and not on ability. A patient who refuses to perform a function is considered as not performing the function, even though he is deemed able.

Bathing (sponge, shower, or tub)
Independent: assistance only in bathing a single part (as back or disabled extremity) or bathes self completely.
Dependent: assistance in bathing more than one part of body; assistance in getting in or out of tub or does not bathe self.

Dressing
Independent: gets clothes from closets and drawers, puts on clothes, outer garments, braces, manages fasteners, act of tying shoes is excluded.
Dependent: does not dress self or remains partly undressed.

Going to toilet
Independent: gets to toilet, gets on and off toilet, arranges clothes, cleans organs of excretion (may manage own bedpan used at night only and may or may not be using mechanical supports).
Dependent: uses bedpan or commode or receives assistance getting to and using toilet.

Transfer
Independent: moves in and out of bed independently and moves in and out of chair independently (may or may not be using mechanical supports).
Dependent: assistance in moving in or out of bed and/or chair, does not perform one or more transfers.

Continence
Independent: urination and defecation entirely self-controlled.
Dependent: partial or total incontinence in urination or defecation, partial or total control by enemas, catheters, or regulated use of urinals and/or bedpans.

Feeding
Independent: gets food from plate or its equivalent into mouth (precutting of meat and preparation of food, as buttering bread, are excluded from evaluation).
Dependent: assistance in act of feeding (see above), does not eat at all or parenteral feeding.

Figure 6–8. *(Reprinted with permission from Katz S, et al. Studies of illness in the aged. The Index of ADL: a standardized measure of biological and psychosocial functions. JAMA. 1963; 185:914–919.)*

Richard Bohannon and colleagues, in an article in the *International Journal of Rehabilitation Research,* showed that the number one priority when rehabilitating stroke patients is the patient walking independently.[25] Physical therapists may forget this when implementing various measures and techniques. Therefore, if the focus is on function, therapists will not lose sight of patients' needs.

The goal of rehabilitation is to assist people in achieving their highest level of function, but confusion often interferes with this. Instead of focusing on the goal, therapists focus on the signs and symptoms. When measuring and treating range of motion, strength, or endurance, the goal of function must be maintained. The second area of confusion and poor implementation of function is the use of function to mean different things (for example, the function of a knee or a hip). Instead, function must be examined in terms of the whole individual[26] and, more specifically, how that person functions versus how his or her shoulder functions.

If function is defined as the normal or characteristic performance of the individual,[27] the individual is the unit of analysis rather than the body part or organ system. It is not just a shoulder or a kidney that is being studied, it is a whole person. Can the patient reach up into the cabinet even if they have a rotator cuff tear, and do they need to? Is there some modification that they should be taught to adapt to their environment?

Understanding function includes more than understanding physical function, because there are four components of function.[28] The first is physical function, which is the component that physical therapists work with the most. This subsection of function includes sensory motor performance, walking, climbing stairs, and other activities of daily living. The second component is mental function, including intelligence, cognitive ability, and memory. The third is emotional function defined as coping with life's stressors, anxieties, and satisfactions. The fourth is social function. This area looks at a person's interaction with family members and the community, and any economic considerations. A good reference for functional assessment tools in older persons is Kane and Kane's *Assessing the Elderly.*[26] The next section will examine examples of different functional tools; the majority will be dedicated to physical scales, but some will be multidimensional.

Functional Assessment Tools

The Barthel Index The Barthel Index is one of the most widely known and well-established physical functional parameters assessment tools.[29] It measures toileting, bathing, and ambulation (Fig. 6–7).[29] On the Barthel Index, the best score is 100 and the worst is 0. Tasks 1 through 9 have a possible score of 53, and tasks 10 through 15 have a possible score of 47, for a total possible score of 100.

Exploring a few items on this index will demonstrate how it is scored. If a patient can drink from a cup independently, they get 4 points. If, however, they need someone's help or they cannot do it at all, they get 0. The reason this scoring mechanism seems strange is because it is a weighted scale. Weighted scales were developed to correlate with other measures. In a weighted scale, the accomplishment of one item may be more important to a specific measure and is, therefore, scored higher than others. Because of this weighing, it is imperative to use the numbers shown on the tool.

To administer this test, give a patient the form without the numbers, and allow the patient to check the appropriate column. Later, the scorer can add up the numbers. This test is more reliable, however, if a health professional assesses and grades each task as the patient performs it.[29]

What do the numbers mean? The test reflects the patient's ability to perform activities of daily living (ADLs) without an attendant.[29] It correlates well with clinical judgment and mortality, as well as with discharge to a less restrictive environment.[29] A score of 60 or above means that a person can be discharged home but will require at least two hours of assistance in ADLs. If they score 80 or above, it means that the person can be discharged home but will require assistance of up to two hours in self-care. When working with a patient that has been assessed as independent in self-care and scores a 50 on the Barthel Index, this would indicate the contrary.

The Katz ADL Index The Katz ADL Index was one of the first attempts at standardizing functional assessment. This tool includes six major areas of ADLs: bathing, feeding, dressing, toileting, transferring, and continence. The index is shown in Figure 6–8, and it can be scored in two ways. The first way that is shown uses letter ratings from A to G on a Guttman type scale. The rater chooses the most accurate assessment of the individual's performance. There is also a Likert-type of rating for this scale. Here, each activity is given a score from 0 to 3, where 0 is complete independence, 1 is a use of a device, 2 is the use of human assistance, and 3 is complete dependence. The scores are added up and averaged. This index has been used in various settings, from institutional to community.[30,31] The reliability in the Guttman version ranges from 0.948 to 0.976, there are no reliability measures for the Likert version.

Kenny Self-Care Index The Kenny Self-Care Index reports professional judgment of six major ADLs (see items listed in the scale shown in Fig. 6–9). The professional rates the patient on all items on a 5 point scale as follows: 0 = complete dependence, 1 = uses extensive assistance, 2 = moderate assistance, 3 = minimal assistance, 4 = total independence. The scores are added and averaged for each category and all are summed for a basic physical function score. This

---

List of Items in the Kenny Self-Care Index

1. Bed
   a. Move in bed
   b. Rise and sit
2. Transfers
   a. Sitting
   b. Standing
   c. Toilet
3. Locomotion
   a. Walking
   b. Stairs
   c. Wheelchair

4. Dressing
   a. Upper trunk and arms
   b. Lower trunk and legs
   c. Feet
5. Personal hygiene
   a. Face, hair, arms
   b. Trunk, perineum
   c. Lower extremities
   d. Bowel program
   e. Bladder program
6. Feeding

Figure 6–9. *(Reprinted with permission from Schoening H, Anderson L, Bergstrom D, et al. Numerical scoring of self-care status of patients. Arch Phys Med Rehab. Oct 1965; 46:689.)*

index can be used to show improvement as evidenced by a higher score. There are no studies on reliability or validity as of yet.[32]

Instruments of Daily Living The instruments described so far have assessed basic ADLs. Instrumental ADLs are also important to independent living, but they are more complex. Examples of these types of activities are using the telephone, shopping, and managing money. The Instruments of Activities of Daily Living (IADL) identifies seven items and then provides the rater with rankings for independence (see instrument Table 6–2 for items and rankings).[33] Despite the lack of reliability and validity measures for this scale, it can be useful in indicating what services may be needed by the patient. For example, deficits in an area will dictate if a person needs transportation assistance or meal preparation.

PULSES The PULSES profile is an acronym for six multidimensional areas of function. These areas are P = physical condition, U = upper limb function, L = lower limb function, S = sensory components, E = excretory function, and S = support factors. The PULSES Profile is shown in Table 6–3. Each of the six items is rated according to the description listed below each item. The PULSES has not been shown to be reliable. However, it has been shown to correlate to other functional measures.[34,35] This tool has been used with a variety of patient settings and patient groups, and it is probably best used in a situation where a significant degree of change is expected.[36]

Functional Independence Measure The next measure is the Functional Independence Measure (FIM). The Functional Independence Measure is copyrighted and is available from the Research Foundation, State University of New York (SUNY).[36] It is an extensive work containing several scales on transferring, feeding, dressing, bowel and bladder control,

TABLE 6–2. INSTRUMENTAL ACTIVITIES OF DAILY LIVING[33]

1. Telephone:
   I: Able to look up numbers, dial, receive, and make calls without help.
   A: Able to answer or dial operator in an emergency, but needs special phone or help in getting number or dialing.
   D: Unable to use the telephone.
2. Traveling:
   I: Able to drive own car or travel alone on bus or taxi.
   A: Able to travel but not alone.
   D: Unable to travel.
3. Shopping:
   I: Able to take care of all shopping with transportation provided.
   A: Able to shop but not alone.
   D: Unable to shop.
4. Preparing meals:
   I: Able to plan and cook full meals.
   A: Able to prepare light foods but unable to cook full meals alone.
   D: Unable to prepare any meals.
5. Housework:
   I: Able to do heavy housework (e.g., scrub floors).
   A: Able to do light housework, but needs help with heavy tasks.
   D: Unable to do any housework.
6. Medication:
   I: Able to take medications in the right dose at the right time.
   A: Able to take medications, but needs reminding or someone to prepare it.
   D: Unable to take medications.
7. Money:
   I: Able to manage buying needs, writes checks, pays bills.
   A: Able to manage daily buying needs, but needs help managing checkbook, paying bills.
   D: Unable to manage money.

I, Independent; **A,** assistance; **D,** dependent.
Reprinted with permission and adapted from Multidimensional Functional Assessment Questionnaire. ed 2. Duke University: Duke University Center for the Study of Aging and Human Development; 1978; 169–170
Reprinted with permission and adapted from Multidimensional Functional Assessment Questionnaire. Ed 2. Duke University: Duke University Center for the Study of Aging and Human Development; 1978; 169–170.

TABLE 6–3. MODIFIED PULSES PROFILE

P—*Physical condition:* Includes diseases of the viscera (cardiovascular, gastrointestinal, urologic, and endocrine) and neurologic disorders:
1. Medical problems sufficiently stable that medical or nursing monitoring is not required more often than 3 month intervals.
2. Medical or nurse monitoring is needed more often than 3 month intervals but not each week.
3. Medical problems are sufficiently unstable as to require regular medical and/or nursing attention at least weekly.
4. Medical problems require intensive medical and/or nursing attention at least daily (excluding personal care assistance only).

U—*Upper limb functions:* Self-care activities (drink/feed, dress upper/lower, brace/prothesis, groom, wash, perineal care) dependent mainly on upper limb function:
1. Independent in self-care without impairment of upper limbs.
2. Independent in self-care with some impairment of upper limbs.
3. Dependent on assistance or supervision in self-care with or without impairment of upper limbs.
4. Dependent totally in self-care with marked impairment of upper limbs.

L—*Lower limb functions:* Mobility (transfer chair/toilet/tub or shower, walk, stairs, wheelchair) dependent mainly on lower limb function:
1. Independent in mobility without impairment of lower limbs.
2. Independent in mobility with some impairment in lower limbs, such as needing ambulatory aids, a brace or prosthesis, or else fully independent in a wheelchair without significant architectural or environmental barriers.
3. Dependent on assistance or supervision in mobility with or without impairment of lower limbs, or partly independent in a wheelchair, or there are significant architectural or environmental barriers.
4. Dependent totally in mobility with marked impairment of lower limbs.

S—*Sensory components:* Relating to communication (speech and hearing) and vision:
1. Independent in communication and vision without impairment.
2. Independent in communication and vision with some impairment, such as mild dysarthria, mild aphasia, or need for eyeglasses or hearing aid, or needing regular eye medication.
3. Dependent on assistance, an interpreter, or supervision in communication or vision.
4. Dependent totally in communication or vision.

E—*Excretory functions* (bladder and bowel):
1. Complete voluntary control of bladder and bowel sphincters.
2. Control of sphincters allows normal social activities despite urgency or need for catheter, appliance, suppositories, etc. Able to care for needs without assistance.
3. Dependent on assistance in sphincter management or else has accidents occasionally.
4. Frequent wetting or soiling from incontinence of bladder or bowel sphincters.

S—*Support factors:* Consider intellectual and emotional adaptability, support from family unit and financial ability:
1. Able to fulfill usual roles and perform customary tasks.
2. Must make some modification in usual roles and performance of customary tasks.
3. Dependent on assistance, supervision, encouragement, or assistance from a public or private agency due to any of the above considerations.
4. Dependent on long-term institutional care (chronic hospitalization, nursing home, etc.) excluding time-limited hospital for specific evaluation, treatment, or active rehabilitation.

Reprinted with permission from Granger C, Albrecht G, Hamilton B. Outcome of comprehensive medical rehabilitation: measurement by PULSES Profile and the Barthel Index. *Arch Phys Med Rehab.* 1979; 60:145.

communication, and so forth. The whole package together makes up the FIM.

One of the FIM's scales measures locomotion scale. The numbers to the left (1 through 7) indicate the need for assistance. For example, number 7 on the scale would be complete independence defined as a patient that "walks a minimum of 150 feet without assistance/assistive device and does not use a wheelchair and performs it safely." Scores of 6 and 7 are considered no help required. Scores of 5 and below mean that the person does require a helper.

Please remember that insurance reviewers may not feel that a helper is someone who is a skilled care helper, like a physical therapist, and this must be taken into consideration when filling out the form. For example, when treating a patient who scores a 5, it is not obvious that the skilled care of a physical therapist is necessary. Interpret numbers of 4 and 5 to be in questionable need of skilled care, unless the

therapist is providing specific skilled services. The rating of 4 and 5 is not enough to justify care. In contrast, a score of 1, 2 and 3 may justify need of care.

This particular test is good for showing a person's improvement through percentages of assistance required. As the patient improves, grade them on this scale accordingly. The therapist can also establish goals based on this scale. A patient may score a 2 initially, but may achieve a 5 later on. Simply state, "on the FIM that the patient has gone from level 2 to level 5." This lends credibility to the treatment application.

Again, this is just one part of a larger tool encompassing many physical and social parameters. It is a huge battery of tests, and it is available for a minimal amount of money from SUNY[37] (Fig. 6–10).

Functional Status Index The next tool is the Functional Status Index (Table 6–4). This differs from pre-

Functional Independence Measure (FIM)

Locomotion   Includes walking, once in a standing position, or using a wheelchair, once in a seated position, on a level surface.

Check most frequent mode of locomotion. If both are about equal, check W *and* C. If initiating a rehabilitation program, check the mode for which training is intended.

(   ) W = walking   (   ) C = wheelchair

No Helper

7. Complete Independence–*Walks* a minimum of *150* feet without assistive devices. Does not use a wheelchair. Performs safely.

6. Modified Independence—*Walks* a miniumum of *150* feet but uses a brace (orthosis) or prosthesis on leg, special adaptive shoes, cane, crutches, or walkerette; takes more than reasonable time or there are safety considerations.

    If not walking, operates manual or electric wheelchair independently for a minimum of 150 feet; turns around; maneuvers the chair to a table, bed, toilet; negotiates at least a 3 percent grade; maneuvers on rugs and over door sills.

5. Exception (Household Ambulation)—Walks only short distances (a minimum of 50 feet) with or without a device. Could take more than reasonable time, or there are safety considerations, or operates a manual or electric wheelchair independently only short distances (a minimum of 50 feet).

Helper

5. Supervision—*If walking,* requires standby supervision, cuing, or coaxing to go a minimum of *150* feet.

    If not walking, requires standby supervision, cuing, or coaxing to go a minimum of *150* feet in wheelchair.

4. Minimal Contact Assistance—Subject performs 75% or more of locomotion effort to go a minimum of *150* feet.

3. Moderate Assistance—Performs 50% to 74% of locomotion effort to go a minimum of *150* feet.

2. Maximal Assistance—Performs 25% to 49% of locomotion effort to go a minimum of *50* feet. Requires assistance of one person only.

1. Total Assistance—Performs less than 25% of effort, or requires assistance of two people, or does not walk or wheel a minimum of *50* feet.

Figure 6–10. *(Reprinted with permission from Uniform Data System for Medical Rehabilitation. Research Foundation of the State University of New York, Buffalo, NY.)*

TABLE 6-4. FUNCTIONAL STATUS INDEX

Suggested Response Lists		
List I	List II	List III
1. No help	1. Extremely easy	1. No pain
2. Use equipment	2. Somewhat easy	2. Mild pain
3. Use human assist	3. Neither easy nor difficult	3. Moderate pain
4. Use human assist & equipment	4. Somewhat difficult	4. Severe pain
5. Unable to do	5. Extremely difficult	

Reprinted with permission from Jette AM. Functional status index: Reliability of a chronic disease evaluation instrument. *Arch Phys Med Rehab.* 1980; 61(9):395–401.

vious tools because it looks at pain—an important component of many patient pro- grams. The Functional Status Index measures the degree of independence, the degree of difficulty, and the amount of pain experienced when performing ADLs.[37] This test was originally developed for patients with arthritis and is, therefore, particularly good for evaluating those patients. The test evaluates gross mobility, hand activities, personal care, and home chores. The best way to administer this test is for the evaluator to ask the patient the questions and give the respondent a list of responses.[38]

The evaluator will say, "Take a look at your assistance sheet and assess your ability when walking outside." The person would look at the assistance list and may say, "My son always has to help me, but I do not use a cane. I guess I am a 3." The evaluator would then say, "Thinking about how you walk inside, would you say that it is extremely easy, somewhat easy . . . ," thus going through the difficulty list. Then finally, the evaluator repeats the same procedure with the pain list (Fig. 6–11). This is very time consuming for the health care professional, but with some sacrifice of validity, a patient can fill out the form by themselves. The advantage of this test is its inclusion of pain. Many older patients may be able to perform most activities, but they experience pain while they are doing them. In many cases, this could be the justification for treatment. None of the previous measures assesses pain, which makes this test a useful tool.[38]

Functional Status Questionnaire The final functional tool to be discussed here is the Functional Status Questionnaire (FSQ). This tool has been shown to have reliability and construct validity,[38] and it provides a comprehensive assessment of physical, psychological, and social functions. The clinician can use the report to screen and monitor a patient's status. Figure 6–12 is an example of one of the subscales. This form is quite easy for the older person to fill out. The scoring of the scale is extremely complicated, but it provides a visual analog scale of the patient's functioning in terms of maximum function and a warning zone for delineation of functional disability. This information is easily generated from the software package.[39]

Functional Assessment Scales and Indices

Unfortunately, there is not enough room in this chapter to discuss all the available functional assessment tools, though Table 6–5 provides information and references for additional tools that are available.[39] This section is meant to provide an overview of the available tools. After the therapist reviews the separate tools, three important points must be made about functional assessment. They are

1. Why is it so important?
2. What are the differences in the tools?
3. When should these tools be used?

In addition, measures of ADLs have been shown to correlate with the following:

1. Admission to a nursing home.[40]
2. Use of physician services.[41]
3. Insurance coverage.[42]
4. Living arrangements.[40]
5. Use of hospital services.[43]
6. Use of paid home care.[44]

As mentioned earlier, therapists must begin to correlate standard measurements, such as a goniometry, to functional assessment for productive values of these parameters.

The biggest problem in functional tools and surveys is that, depending on what is measured, the outcomes can vary greatly.[45] Wiener showed in one comparison a 60% difference in ADL problem identification from one study to another.[45] The reasons stated for this were

1. Methods used to collect data.
2. Age comparison.
3. How the ADLs were classified in terms of difficulty, length of problem, and type of assistance.
4. Which ADLs were used.
5. Sampling method.[46]

Table 6–6 is a list of surveys studied by Wiener and information reviewed on ADLs.[45]

Applegate has also done an excellent comparison of some of the more widely used functional tools[46] (see Table 6–7).

Functional Status Index

Activity	Assistance	Pain	Difficulty	Comment
Mobility				
Walking inside	☐	☐	☐	_____
Climbing up stairs	☐	☐	☐	_____
Transferring to & from toilet	☐	☐	☐	_____
Getting in & out of bed	☐	☐	☐	_____
Personal care				
Combing hair	☐	☐	☐	_____
Putting on pants	☐	☐	☐	_____
Buttoning clothes	☐	☐	☐	_____
Washing all parts of the body	☐	☐	☐	_____
Putting on shoes/slippers	☐	☐	☐	_____
Home chores				
Vacuuming a rug	☐	☐	☐	_____
Reaching into high cupboards	☐	☐	☐	_____
Doing laundry	☐	☐	☐	_____
Washing windows	☐	☐	☐	_____
Doing yardwork	☐	☐	☐	_____
Hand activities				
Writing	☐	☐	☐	_____
Opening containers	☐	☐	☐	_____
Turning faucets	☐	☐	☐	_____
Cutting food	☐	☐	☐	_____
Vocational				
Performing all job responsibilities	☐	☐	☐	_____
Avocational				
Performing hobbies requiring hand work	☐	☐	☐	_____
Attending church	☐	☐	☐	_____
Socializing with friends & relatives	☐	☐	☐	_____

Figure 6–11. (Reprinted with permission from Jette AM. Functional status index: Reliability of a chronic disease evaluation instrument. Arch Phys Med Rehab. 1980; 61(9):395–401.)

Daily Activities

This group of questions refers to many types of physical and social activities. We would like to know how **difficult** it was for you to do each of these activities, on the average, **during the past month**. By difficult, we mean how hard it was or how much physical effort it took to do the activity **because of your health**. Circle the number:

    4   if you usually had **no difficulty** doing it;
    3   if you usually had **some difficulty** doing it;
    2   if you usually had **much difficulty** doing it;
    1   if you usually **did not do the activity because of your health**; or
    0   if you usually **did not do the activity for other reasons**.

During the Past Month, How Much Physical Difficulty Did You have . . .	Usually Did With No Difficulty	Usually Did With Some Difficulty	Usually Did With Much Difficulty	Usually Did Not Do Because of Health	Usually Did Not Do For Other Reasons
1. Taking care of yourself, that is, eating, dressing, or bathing?	4	3	2	1	0
2. Moving in and out of a bed or chair?	4	3	2	1	0
3. Walking *several* blocks?	4	3	2	1	0
4. Walking *one* block or climbing *one* flight of stairs?	4	3	2	1	0
5. Walking indoors, such as around your home?	4	3	2	1	0
6. Doing work around the house such as cleaning, light yard work, home maintenance?	4	3	2	1	0
7. Doing errands, such as grocery shopping?	4	3	2	1	0
8. Driving a car or using public transportation?	4	3	2	1	0
9. Visiting with relatives or friends?	4	3	2	1	0
10. Participating in community activities, such as religious services, social activities, or volunteer work?	4	3	2	1	0
11. Taking care of other people such as family members?	4	3	2	1	0
12. Doing vigorous activities such as running, lifting heavy objects or participating in strenuous sports?	4	3	2	1	0

Figure 6–12. *(Reprinted with permission from Jette A, Davies A, Cleary P, Rubenstein LV, et al. Functional status questionnaire reliability and validity when used in primary care. J Gen Intern Med. May/June 1986; 1:143–149.)*

TABLE 6–5. FUNCTIONAL ASSESSMENT SCALES AND INDICES

Scale Index	Domain	Assessor	Mode	Rel/Val[a]
Katz ADL	Eating Bathing Dressing Transfer Continence Toileting	Professional	Performance self-report	X X
Modified ADL Scale	Eating Ambulation Bathing Dressing Transfer Personal grooming Continence Toileting	Lay	Self, proxy, performance	X X
PULSES	Physical condition Upper limbs Lower limbs Sensory Excretory Social function	Lay	Performance	X
Kenny Self-Care	Bed activities Transfers Locomotion Continence Dressing Feeding	Professional	Performance	X
Philadelphia Geriatric Center Scale (PGC)	Toileting Feeding Dressing Grooming Ambulation Bathing	Lay	Self, proxy	X X
Philadelphia Geriatric Center Scale II (PGCII)	Telephone Shopping Food Preparation Housekeeping Laundry Public Transport Medications Finances	Both	Self, proxy	X X
Functional Health Scale	Heavy work Current illness Limitation in activities Walk ½ mile Climb stairs Socialize	lay	Self, proxy	
PACE II	Telephone Finances Shopping Housekeeping Meal preparation	Both	Self, proxy	
OARS II	Telephone Shopping Transportation Meal preparation Medication Finance	Both	Self	X
PACE II	7 ADL 17 range of motion 8 strength Balance Coordination	Both	Self, proxy, performance	

(continued)

TABLE 6–5. (CONTINUED)

Scale Index	Domain	Assessor	Mode	Rel/Val[a]
OARS	Eating Dressing Grooming Walking Transfer Bathing Continence Toileting	Both	Self, proxy	X
Functional Health of the Institutionalized Elderly	Transfer Eating Walking Bathing Dressing Toileting	Professional	Self, performance	X X
Functioning for Independent Living	Vision Hearing Speech Continence Behavior Orientation Communication Wandering	Professional	Self, proxy, performance	X
Performance Activities of Daily Living (PADL)	Shave Wipe nose Drink from cup Comb hair File nails Eat with spoon Turn faucet Switch lights Button on and off Slippers on and off Brush teeth Telephone Sign name Turn key Tell time Stand and sit	Professional	Performance	X X

[a]Rel/Val: Reliability and validity.

The final question to be answered is when should these tools be used. The most efficient way to use these tools is to have a goal in mind for its use, such as to establish a baseline to show improvement, to screen for problems, to set rehabilitation goals, or to monitor the patient's progress.[47]

The medical community in general is developing a keen interest in functional assessment. Lachs and Williams, in the *Annals of Internal Medicine,* urge general practitioners to use functional assessments.[47,48] In addition, this article specifically delineates physical therapy as an appropriate referral once functional deficits are noted. Table 6–8 is a procedural chart on functional assessment from Lachs and Williams' work.[48]

Therapists in geriatrics must get involved in functionally assessing patients not only for the efficacious assessment potential, but also for continuity of care from medical peers.

MODIFIED PHYSICAL THERAPY MEASURES

Musculoskeletal Parameters

Strength It is widely accepted that strength decreases with age. However, no studies exist to date that show a difference in the strength decline with age using simple manual muscle test techniques. This makes it difficult for a practitioner to use the current knowledge of age's strength changes in the clinical setting.

In the realm of dynamometer and muscle hypertrophy, some clinically useful information has been generated. The best sources on muscle hypertrophy are Tomanek and Woo, and Goldspink and Howells.[49,50] Basically, these resources contend that older muscle does hypertrophy but not to the same extent. Figure 6–13 contains some formulas for assessing hy-

TABLE 6–6. TYPE OF INFORMATION ON ADL ITEMS IN NATIONAL SURVEYS

Survey	Population	Number of ADLs[a]	Minimum Duration of Disability	Needs Assistance	Receives Human Assistance	Uses Special Equipment	Receives Standby Help	Level of Difficulty
National Long-Term Care Survey (1982)	Noninstitutionalized, functionally impaired elderly	9	Yes	Yes	Yes	Yes	Yes	No
New Beneficiary Survey (1982)	New Social Security beneficiaries (between mid-1980 and mid-1981)	4	No	No	Yes	No	No	Yes
National Health and Nutrition Examination Survey I Followup (1982–1984)	Persons aged 25–74 (between 1971–1974 and 1974–1975) examined in NHANES I	6	No	No	Yes	Yes	No	Yes
National Long-Term Care Survey (1984)	Functionally impaired elderly, age 65+	9	Yes	Yes	Yes	Yes	Yes	No
National Health Interview Survey Supplement on Aging (1984)	Elderly persons, age 55+	9	No	No	Yes	Yes	No	Yes
Survey of Income and Program Participation—Disability Module (1984)	Noninstitutionalized population	4	No	Yes	Yes	No	No	No
Longitudinal Study of Aging (1984–1986)	Noninstitutionalized persons aged 70+ in 1984	9	No	No	Yes	Yes	No	Yes
National Nursing Home Survey (1985)	Current residents of nursing homes	6	No	No	Yes	Yes	No	No
National Mortality Followback Survey (1986)	Persons aged 25 and over who died in 1986	5	No	No	Yes	Yes	No	No
National Medical Expenditure Survey-Household (1987)	Noninstitutionalized population	7	Yes	No	Yes	Yes	No	No
National Medical Expenditure Survey-Institutional (1987)	Persons in nursing homes and personal care facilities	6	No	No	Yes	Yes	No	No

[a]Some surveys have a different number of ADLs on the instrument that screens for disability than on the detailed survey. Where that occurs, the larger of the two numbers is reported. Reprinted with permission from Wiener J, Hanley N, Clark R, Van Nostrand J. Measuring the activities of daily living: Comparisons across national surveys. *J Gerontol Soc Sci.* 1990; 45(6)229–237. © The Gerontological Society of America.

TABLE 6–7. COMPARISON OF WIDELY USED FUNCTIONAL TOOLS

Instrument	Function Assessed	Range or Sensitivity	Administration	Strengths	Weaknesses
Katz ADL Scale	Basic self-care	Limited to basic activities; not sensitive to small changes	By patient or interviewer; based on judgments	Simple assessment of basic skills; useful in rehabilitative setting	Limited range of activities assessed; ratings subjective
Barthel Index	Self-care and ambulation	Slightly broader range than Katz ADL Scale; includes stair climbing, wheel chair use	By interviewer; based on judgment or observation	Range of activities useful in rehabilitational setting	Range not useful for small impairments; ratings subjective
Kenny Self-Care Scale	Self-care and ambulation	Similar to Barthel Index	By interviewer; based on judgment or observation	Range useful in rehabilitational setting	Range narrow for small impairments; ratings subjective
Instrumental ADL Scale	More complex activities: food preparation, shopping, housekeeping	Higher range of performance than Katz ADL Scale; not sensitive to small changes	By interviewer or patient; based on judgment	Assesses functions important for independent living	Ratings subjective
Timed Manual Performance	Timed assessment of performance of structured manual tasks	Broad range, from signing name to lifting latches	By interviewer; based on observation; requires special props	Assesses actual performance; sensitive to small changes[7]	Difficult to use in patients who are seriously ill or cognitively impaired
Performance Test of ADL	Self-care, mobility, and transfers	Ranges from ADL and instrumental ADL to mobility and transfers	By professional or trained interviewer; requires observation of patient performing specific activities; requires props	Direct observation of range of functions; useful in variety of clinical settings	Time consuming; difficult to use in seriously ill patients
Framingham Disability Scale	Self-care and physical activities	Broad range of activities, from self-care to lifting objects; not sensitive to small changes	By interviewer	Assesses broad range of activities; detects persons with less serious disabilities	Complex scoring; summary scores may hide important problems observed in individual tasks

Reprinted with permission from Applegate W, Blass J, Williams F. Instruments for the functional assessment of older patients. *N Engl J Med.* 1990; 322(17):1207–1214.

pertrophy and charts illustrating the comparison in muscle hypertrophy.[51]

It is apparent from these formulas that the calculation for the difference in muscle hypertrophy is rather cumbersome and not easily applicable in the clinic. The authors suggest being wary of using muscle hypertrophy measures (i.e., girth) as the only criteria for assessing muscle strength increases with age.

Dynanomomter testing of strength can be replicated in the clinic. Rice carried out a simple assessment of numerous joints' strength using a modified sphygmomanometer.[52] Table 6–9 is his chart of absolute strength measures.[52]

Borges and associates also showed the torque changes with age in the knee using the Cybex dynamometer (see Table 6–10).[53]

Finally, Vandervoort and Hayes found a 71% decrease in plantarflexor muscle isometric strength in the elderly as compared with the young.[54] This study was done on both young and old healthy women.[55] Their findings revealed strength development for the young of 0.16 nm per second and 0.09 nm per second in the elderly group.

TABLE 6–8. PROCEDURE FOR FUNCTIONAL ASSESSMENT SCREENING IN THE ELDERLY

Target Area	Assessment Procedure	Abnormal Result	Suggested Intervention
Vision	Test each eye with Jaeger card while patient wears corrective lenses (if applicable)	Inability to read greater than 20/40	Refer to ophthalmologist
Hearing	Whisper a short, easily answered question, such as "What is your name?" in each ear while the examiner's face is out of direct view	Inability to answer question	Examine auditory canals for cerumen and clean if necessary. Repeat test; if still abnormal in either ear, refer for audiometry and possible prosthesis
Arm	Proximal: "Touch the back of your head with both hands" Distal: "Pick up the spoon"	Inability to do task	Examine the arm fully (muscle, joint, and nerve), paying attention to pain, weakness, limited range of motion. Consider referral for physical therapy
Leg	Observe the patient after asking: "Rise from your chair, walk ten feet, return, sit down"	Inability to walk or transfer out of chair	Do full neurologic and musculoskeletal evaluation, paying attention to strength, pain, range of motion, balance, and traditional assessment of gait. Consider referral for physical therapy
Urinary incontinence	Ask: "Do you ever lose your urine and get wet?"	Yes	Ascertain frequency and amount. Search for remediable causes including local irritations, polyuric states, and medications. Consider urologic referral
Nutrition	Weigh the patient. Measure height	Weight is below acceptable range for height	Do appropriate medical evaluation
Mental status	Instruct: "I am going to name three objects (pencil, truck, book). I will ask you to repeat their names now and then again a few minutes from now." [See text discussion.]	Inability to recall all three objects after 1 minute	Administer Folstein Mini-Mental Status Examination. If score is <24, search for causes of cognitive impairment. Ascertain onset, duration, and fluctuation of overt symptoms. Review medications. Assess consciousness and affect. Do appropriate laboratory tests
Depression	Ask: "Do you often feel sad or depressed?"	Yes	Administer Geriatric Depression Scale. If positive (normal score, 0 to 10), check for antihypertensive, psychotropic, or other pertinent medications. Consider appropriate pharmaceutical or psychiatric treatment
ADL-IADL[a]	Ask: "Can you get out of bed yourself?"; "Can you dress yourself?"; "Can you make your own meals?"; "Can you do your own shopping?"	No to any question	Corroborate responses with patient's appearance; question family members if accuracy is uncertain. Determine reasons for the inability (motivation compared with physical limitation). Institute appropriate medical, social, or environmental interventions
Home environment	Ask: "Do you have trouble with stairs inside or outside of your home?"; ask about potential hazards inside the home with bathtubs, rugs, or lighting	Yes	Evaluate home safety and institute appropriate countermeasures
Social support	Ask: "Who would be able to help you in case of illness or emergency?"	. . .	List identified persons in the medical record. Become familiar with available resources for the elderly in the community

[a]ADL-IADL: activities of daily living-instrumental activities of daily living.
Reproduced with permission from Lachs M, Feinstein A, Cooney L, et al. A simple procedure for general screening for functional disability in elderly patients. *Ann Intern Med.* 1990, 112:699–704.

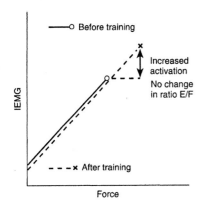

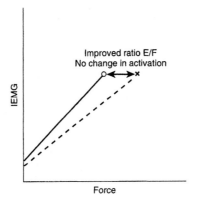

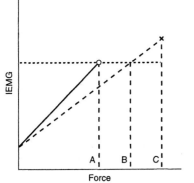

$$\% \ MH = \frac{B - A}{C - A} \times 100$$

$$\% \ NF = \frac{C - B}{C - A} \times 100$$

Figure 6–13. Hypertrophy in older men. **A.** Strenth gain due to neural factors. **B.** Strength gain due to hypertrophy. **C.** Evaluation of percentage contributions of neural factors (NF) vs. hypertrophy (MH). *(Reprinted with permission from Moritani T, Devries HA. Potential for gross muscle hypertrophy in older men. J Gerontology. 1980; 35(5):673.)*

In conclusion, the clinical implications of the information noted in the arzea of strength changes with age are

1. Be wary of girth measures as a means of reflecting strength gains.
2. Compare outcomes to the norms noted. For example, compare knee extension torques to Borges's measures versus measures of torque on younger persons.
3. Compare strength measures to Rice's norms versus the classic manual muscle test for more comparable findings.

Range of Motion The literature on range of motion norms is still somewhat controversial. For example, Walker et al. showed no significant differences in range of motion in 28 joints of young and old subjects[55] (Table 6–11).

TABLE 6–9. ABSOLUTE AND RELATIVE STRENGTH MEASUREMENTS

Muscle Groups	Men			Women		
	Strength (kg)	Strength/Body Weight (kg/kg)	n	Strength (kg)	Strength/Body Weight (kg/kg)	n
Shoulder abductors	12.4 ± 5.0^{a}	0.17 ± 0.07	37	9.3 ± 3.3	0.15 ± 0.05	81
Shoulder flexors	12.7 ± 5.0^{a}	0.17 ± 0.07	37	9.3 ± 3.4	0.14 ± 0.05	81
Elbow extensors	14.9 ± 4.6^{a}	0.20 ± 0.06	37	11.2 ± 3.3	0.19 ± 0.06	81
Elbow flexors	15.2 ± 5.1^{a}	0.21 ± 0.07	37	10.9 ± 3.9	0.18 ± 0.06	81
Hip extensors	14.4 ± 5.8^{a}	0.19 ± 0.08	31 (2)	11.6 ± 4.0	0.19 ± 0.06	69 (1)
Hip flexors	16.2 ± 6.7^{a}	0.23 ± 0.09	31 (2)	10.8 ± 3.3	0.18 ± 0.06	74 (1)
Knee extensors	19.1 ± 5.7^{a}	0.27 ± 0.09	31 (5)	16.7 ± 4.8	0.28 ± 0.08	77 (2)
Dorsiflexors	15.1 ± 4.5^{a}	0.21 ± 0.07	37	12.6 ± 4.1	0.21 ± 0.06	79
MS grip	23.2 ± 4.4	0.33 ± 0.08	20 (17)	20.1 ± 5.7	0.31 ± 0.09	74 (7)
Dynamometer grip	30.8 ± 6.6^{a}	0.43 ± 0.1^{a}	37	21.6 ± 6.1	0.36 ± 0.08	64

Values are means ± SD, 1 kg = 9.806 newtons. MS = modified spygmomanometer. Parentheses indicate the number of measurements that exceeded the upper limit of the MS.
[a]Indicates significant difference ($p \leq 0.05$) between men and women for absolute or relative strength measurements.
Reprinted with permission from Rice C. Strength in an elderly population. *Arch Phys Med Rehabil.* 1989; 70:391–397.

TABLE 6-10. KNEE EXTENSION TORQUE AT 90 DEGREES PER SECOND

	Age (Years)	Torque
MEN	20	122
	70	78
WOMEN	20	68
	70	38

Reprinted with permission from Borges O. Isometric and isokinetic knee extension and flexion torque in men and women aged 20–70. *Scand J Rehab Med.* 1989; 21:45–53.

Frekany and Leslie showed that even if an older group did have motion limitation, it could be normalized with appropriate stretching exercises.[56] James and Parker give probably the most comprehensive and recent reference on joint range of motion norms of the lower extremity[57] (Fig. 6–14).

Information also exists on upper extremity and spinal norms for range of motion. These are listed in chart form in Tables 6–12 through 6–15. These findings, even though controversial, can assist the therapist to set more appropriate goals. If, for example, as was stated in Bassey's chart, the norms for shoulder flexion are 129, then a goal of 170 is inappropriate. Keeping these charts for review can help to design appropriate programs.

Postural Changes with Age Posture changes with age. Perfect posture demonstrates a plumb line that bisects the ear, just anterior to the acromion process, through the greater trochanter, just posterior to the patella and just anterior to the lateral malleolus (see Fig. 6–15).[58]

Changes in posture with age include[58]

1. Forward head.
2. Rounded shoulders.
3. Change in lordotic curve (either flatter or more curved).
4. Increased hip flexion.
5. Increased knee flexion.

TABLE 6-11. UPPER AND LOWER LIMB RANGE OF MOTION MEAN VALUES AND STANDARD DEVIATIONS FOR AGE GROUPS COMBINED BY SEX AND FOR SEXES COMBINED[a] (AGES 60-84)

Upper Limb Motion	Men (age groups combined)		Women (age groups combined)		Diff. Between M/W	p^b	Sexes Combined	
	X̄	s	X̄	s	M/W	p^b	X̄	s
Shoulder abduction	155	22	175	16	−20[c]	<0.001	165	21
flexion	160	11	169	9	−9	<0.001	165	11
extension	38	11	49	13	−11[c]	<0.001	44	13
medial rotation	59	16	66	13	−7	NS	62	15
lateral rotation	76	13	85	16	−9	0.02	81	15
Elbow beginning flexion	6	5[d]	1	3	−5[d]	<0.001	4	5
flexion	139	14	148	5	−9	0.002	143	11
Radioulnar pronation	68	9	73	12	−5	NS	71	11
supination	83	11	65	11	+18	<0.001	74	14
Wrist flexion	62	12	65	8	−3	NS	64	10
extension	61	6	65	10	−4	0.05	63	9
radial deviation	20	6	17	6	+3	NS	19	6
ulnar deviation	28	7	23	7	+5	0.01	26	7
Hip beginning flexion	11	3	11	5	0	NS	11	4
flexion	110	11	111	12	−1	NS	111	11
abduction	23	9	24	6	−1	NS	23	7
adduction	18	4	11	4	+7	<0.001	14	5
medial rotation	22	6	36	7	−14[c]	<0.001	29	10
lateral rotation	32	6	30	7	+2	NS	31	7
Knee beginning flexion	2	2	0	1	+2	<0.001	1	2
flexion	131	4	135	7	−4	0.01	133	6
Ankle plantar flexion	29	7	40	6	−11[c]	<0.001	34	8
dorsiflexion	9	5	10	5	−1	NS	10	5
Subtalar inversion	31	11	29	10	+2	NS	30	10
eversion	13	6	12	5	+1	NS	12	6
First metatarsophalangeal beginning flexion	3	7	1	4	+2	NS	2	5
extension	62	17	59	8	+3	NS	61	17
flexion	5	7	8	16	−3	NS	6	8

[a] All values reported in integers.
[b] Univariate *t* tests, *df* = 1, 58 (*t* values can be obtained from any statistical text with table of critical values for *t* distribution).
[c] Difference > intertester error.
[d] One man deleted because of the presence of pathologically restricted ROM, n = 29.
Reprinted with permission from Walker J, Sue D, Miles-Elkousy N, Ford G, Trevelyan H: Active mobility of extremities in older subjects. *Phys Ther.* 1984; 64(6):919–923. Reprinted with permission of the American Physical Therapy Association.

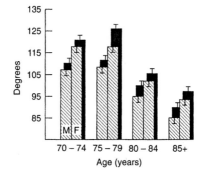

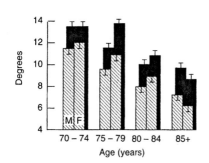

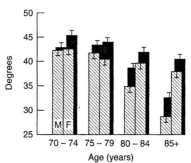

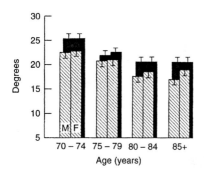

Figure 6–14. Lower extremity range of motion. **A.** Knee flexion. **B.** Ankle dorsiflexion (knee extended). **C.** Ankle plantar flexion (knee extended). **D.** Ankle dorsiflexion (knee flexed). E. Ankle plantar flexion (knee flexed). *(Reprinted with permission from James B, Parker A. Active & passive mobility of lower limb joints in elderly men and women. Lower extremity range of motion. Am J Phys Med Rehabil. 1989; 68(4):162–167.)*

TABLE 6–12. SPINAL RANGE OF MOTION: MEANS AND STANDARD DEVIATIONS IN 10-YEAR INTERVALS FOR LUMBAR RANGE OF MOTION[80]

	Shöber (cm)				Extension (°)				R Lat Flexion (°)				L Lat Flexion (°)			
	$\overline{X}$	s	CV	n[a]	$\overline{X}$	s	CV	n	$\overline{X}$	s	CV	n	$\overline{X}$	s	CV	n
20–29	3.7	0.72	19.5	31	41.2	9.6	23.3	31	37.8	5.8	15.4	31	38.7	5.7	14.7	31
30–39	3.9	1.00	25.6	42	40.0	8.8	22.0	44	35.3	6.5	18.4	44	36.5	6.0	16.4	44
40–49	3.1	0.81	26.1	16	31.1	8.9	28.6	16	27.1	6.5	24.0	16	28.5	5.2	18.2	16
50–59	3.0	1.10	36.7	43	27.4	8.0	29.2	43	25.3	6.2	24.5	44	26.8	6.4	23.9	44
60–69	2.4	0.74	30.8	26	17.4	7.5	43.1	27	20.2	4.8	23.8	27	20.3	5.3	26.1	27
70–79	2.2	0.69	31.4	9	16.6	8.8	53.0	10	18.0	4.7	26.1	10	18.9	6.0	31.7	10

[a]Different "n's" appear in some age groups because of the difficulty in measuring patients with various medical conditions (e.g., rash).
Reprinted with permission from Fitzgerald GK, Wynveen KJ, Rheault W, Rothschild B. Objective assessment with establishment of normal values for lumbar spinal range of motion. *Phys Ther.* Nov 1983; 63(11):1778. Reprinted with permission of the American Physical Therapy Association.

TABLE 16–13. SPINAL/NECK RANGE OF MOTION[81]

	Age		
	10	30	80
Flexion	35°	30°	27°
Lateral Flexion	63°	50°	30°
Extension	60°	50°	35°
Rotation	165°	150°	130°

Reprinted with permission from Lind B, et al. Normal range of motion of the cervical spine. *Arch Phys Med Rehab.* Sept 1989; 70:692–695.

TABLE 6–14. SHOULDER FLEXION RANGE OF MOTION[82]

Age	Male	Female
65–74 years old	129°	124°
75+ years old	121°	114°

Reprinted with permission from Bassey E, et al. Flexibility of the shoulder joint measured as range of abduction in a large representative sample of men and women over 65 years of age. *Eur J Appl Physiology.* 1989; 58:353–360.

TABLE 6–15. SHOULDER RANGE OF MOTION[83]

60–74 years old
Flexion: 159°
Abduction: 159°
75+ years old
Flexion: 159°
Abduction: 154°

Reprinted with permission from Boyle S. Geriatric shoulder range of motion. Master's thesis. Philadelphia: University of Pennsylvania, February 1989.

Standard means of assessing posture are acceptable for older persons. The clinician must be sure to align the plumb line from the malleoli and up, otherwise a false alignment will be noted.

A good tool for rating and screening posture is the REEDCO Posture Score Sheet (see Fig. 6–16).

This evaluation tool is self-explanatory, and it is not singular to older persons. It can be used on young and old to provide a quantitative approach to posture analysis. Since posture can be an important variable in movement, balance, and gait of older persons, it is imperative that the clinician assess it as objectively as possible.[59]

Gait Assessment

Gait changes with age are as variable as many of the other characteristics listed in this section are. What will be given here are norms or averages.

To begin the examination of the gait cycle, motion will be discussed. The first place that a change is noted in the old versus the young is in the preswing phase. Older persons show 5° less motion in plantarflexion when compared to young (i.e., 15° as compared to

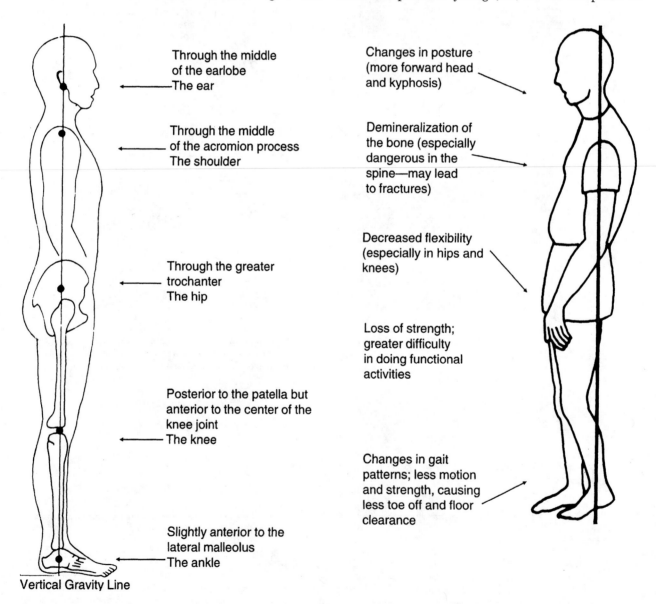

Through the middle of the earlobe
—The ear

Through the middle of the acromion process
The shoulder

Through the greater trochanter
The hip

Posterior to the patella but anterior to the center of the knee joint
— The knee

Slightly anterior to the lateral malleolus
— The ankle

Vertical Gravity Line

Changes in posture (more forward head and kyphosis)

Demineralization of the bone (especially dangerous in the spine—may lead to fractures)

Decreased flexibility (especially in hips and knees)

Loss of strength; greater difficulty in doing functional activities

Changes in gait patterns; less motion and strength, causing less toe off and floor clearance

Figure 6–15. Posture changes with age. (*Reprinted with permission from Lewis C, Musculoskeletal changes with age. In: Lewis, C, ed.* Aging: The Health Care Challenge. *Philadelphia: F.A. Davis; 1990.*)

POSTURE SCORE SHEET	Name _____			SCORING DATES				
	GOOD - 10	FAIR - 5	POOR - 0					
HEAD LEFT RIGHT	HEAD ERECT GRAVITY LINE PASSES DIRECTLY THROUGH CENTER	HEAD TWISTED OR TURNED TO ONE SIDE SLIGHTLY	HEAD TWISTED OR TURNED TO ONE SIDE MARKEDLY					
SHOULDERS LEFT RIGHT	SHOULDERS LEVEL (HORIZONTALLY)	ONE SHOULDER SLIGHTLY HIGHER THAN OTHER	ONE SHOULDER MARKEDLY HIGHER THAN OTHER					
SPINE LEFT RIGHT	SPINE STRAIGHT	SPINE SLIGHTLY CURVED LATERALLY	SPINE MARKEDLY CURVED LATERALLY					
HIPS LEFT RIGHT	HIPS LEVEL (HORIZONTALLY)	ONE HIP SLIGHTLY HIGHER	ONE HIP MARKEDLY HIGHER					
ANKLES	FEET POINTED STRAIGHT AHEAD	FEET POINTED OUT	FEET POINTED OUT MARKEDLY ANKLES SAG IN(PRONATION)					
NECK	NECK ERECT, CHIN IN, HEAD IN BALANCE DIRECTLY ABOVE SHOULDERS	NECK SLIGHTLY FORWARD, CHIN SLIGHTLY OUT	NECK MARKEDLY FORWARD, CHIN MARKEDLY OUT					
UPPER BACK	UPPER BACK NORMALLY ROUNDED	UPPER BACK SLIGHTLY MORE ROUNDED	UPPER BACK MARKEDLY ROUNDED					
TRUNK	TRUNK ERECT	TRUNK INCLINED TO REAR SLIGHTLY	TRUNK INCLINED TO REAR MARKEDLY					
ABDOMEN	ABDOMEN FLAT	ABDOMEN PROTRUDING	ABDOMEN PROTRUDING AND SAGGING					
LOWER BACK	LOWER BACK NORMALLY CURVED	LOWER BACK SLIGHTLY HOLLOW	LOWER BACK MARKEDLY HOLLOW					
			TOTAL SCORES					

Figure 6–16. Posture score sheet. *(From REEDCO, Auburn, NY. Copyright 1974. Reprinted with permission.)*

Modified Functional Ambulation Profile

Patient: _____

STATIC WEIGHT-BEARING CAPACITY

Date ___ ___ ___ ___ ___ ___ ___ ___ ___ ___

Bilateral Time ___ ___ ___ ___ ___ ___ ___ ___ ___ ___

Left Unilat. Time ___ ___ ___ ___ ___ ___ ___ ___ ___ ___

  with eyes closed ___ ___ ___ ___ ___ ___ ___ ___ ___ ___

Right Unilat. Time ___ ___ ___ ___ ___ ___ ___ ___ ___ ___

  with eyes closed ___ ___ ___ ___ ___ ___ ___ ___ ___ ___

DYNAMIC (in place) WEIGHT TRANSFER RATE

Date ___ ___ ___ ___ ___ ___ ___ ___ ___

Time to complete ___ ___ ___ ___ ___ ___ ___ ___ ___

4 transfers (8 steps) ___ ___ ___ ___ ___ ___ ___ ___ ___

BASIC AMBULATION EFFICIENCY

Date ___ ___ ___ ___ ___ ___ ___ ___

Through//bars
holding on time/steps ___ ___ ___ ___ ___ ___ ___ ___

Twelve foot distance
outside//bars time/steps ___ ___ ___ ___ ___ ___ ___ ___

COMMENTS

Figure 6–17. *(Reprinted with permission from Nelson AJ. Function ambulation profile. Physical Ther. 1974; 54:1059–1065.)*

20°).[60] The knee range of motion shows no difference. However, the hip exhibits 5° more flexion (i.e., 35° versus 30° in the younger population).[61] Gait velocity is also less in older persons. Average velocity in the young is 82.6 m/min, and it is 78.6 m/min in the 60 to 87 age range.[62] Stride length is also shorter in the older population. Healthy older persons have a stride length of 1.39 m and younger persons have an average stride length of 1.5 m.[63]

All of the changes noted are the only significant differences noted in healthy older persons. If other pathological factors are taken into consideration, then other gait abnormalities will be noted.

Functional Ambulation Profile   Two tools are particularly good for assessing gait in older persons. The first tool is the Functional Ambulation Profile (FAP) by Dr. Arthur Nelson (Fig. 6–17).[64] This tool is particularly useful for older patients who have suffered from a stroke. To use this assessment tool, enter the date and the patient's bilateral time; that is, how long the person can stand on both feet. Some patients cannot stand for 30 seconds without dizziness or support. The longest anyone needs to be timed is 2 minutes. The next entry on the FAP is unilateral time: how long the person can stand on the left leg. Repeat for the right leg. Next, conduct the test with patient's eyes closed, and add the score code for this variation. According to Bohannon, the norms for persons over 70 years old are that they can stand with the eyes open for 14.2 seconds and with the eyes closed for 4.3 seconds.[65]

Begin the notes for the basic ambulation section of this tool by entering the distance needed for functional independence. It may be the distance from bed to bathroom, for example this may measure 50 feet. Count the steps as the patient walks, however. The distance of 12 feet shown on the form is arbitrary; whatever distance is used must be used each time the measurement is recorded in order for it to be consistent and reliable.

A watch will also be needed with a second hand to administer this test. To modify this test for someone using an assistive device, just note the use of the device in the comments. Also note pain with a star or other code.

Gait Abnormality Scale   Another excellent tool is the Gait Abnormality Rating Scale (GARS) by Wolfson and associates.[66] This tool was developed to detect fallers. It is, however, an excellent tool for quantifying aspects of gait patterns for older persons (see Table 6–16).

The GARS is quite easy to score. The patient is given the corresponding numerical value to each item listed, and the scores are added to get the individual's GARS score. Wolfson and co-workers found that persons scoring higher than 18 were more likely to fall. Not only is this a good tool for assessing gait, it also can be used to predict patients who are more vulnerable to falling.[66]

In addition, the classic methods of assessing gait, such as the evaluation of shoe wear and standard gait analysis, are still applicable to the older population. The tools that have just been presented are extra ways of assessing gait that are specific to the older population.

Cardiopulmonary Tests

Chapters 5 and 13 provided background information on the complex array of physiological changes in the cardiopulmonary system with age. This section will discuss modifications in the assessment parameters that will be needed to account for these changes. The chart of normal changes found in Figure 6–18 offers an explanation for the parametric change seen in a typical cardiopulmonary assessment.[67] Table 6–17 is an outline of the typical assessment process for a patient interview and physical examination.[67]

In these assessments several changes can be noted for the average older person. These are

1. There may be an increase in the anterior-posterior diameter of the chest with age. This should be very slight. If it is excessive, then it may indicate pathology (e.g., emphysema).
2. There may be a slight use of accessory muscles for breathing. Again, a slight use of these muscles is acceptable, however, as noted previously, more than that is indicative of pathology
3. Note that the following are signs of abnormal pathology or deconditioning: an elevated heart rate over 84 BPM prior to start of the exam,[68] a rise of over 20 BPM with the initial evaluation,[68] orthostatic hypotension, anxiety, arrhythmias, or fatigue during or later in the day.[68]

Exercising testing of the cardiovascular system was developed for younger populations, however, the tests can be modified for older persons. Table 6–18 lists five of the more common exercising-testing protocols.

The tests, even with modification and slowing for the older person, may be too vigorous. Table 6–19 gives low-level functional protocol.[67]

One more exercise test protocol was developed by Everett Smith.[69] This test is useful for the very low-level patient that is either unable to get out of a chair or performs better in a chair. This is the Chair Step Test shown in Figure 6–19. This test was developed by Smith and attempts to tax the cardiovascular system while controlling for those patients who may be unsafe on other cardiopulmonary exercise tests.[69] To perform this test, the patient sits in a chair and extends to touch, with alternating feet, boxes of various heights (as listed in Fig. 6–19). Each stage lasts 5 minutes, with the last stage involving alternately raising the arms on the same side of the body to shoulder level. The therapist monitors the patient at 2 minutes and 5 minutes. This test progresses the patient from 2.3 to 3.9 metabolic equivalents (METS).[68]

TABLE 6-16. COMPONENTS OF THE GAIT ASSESSMENT RATING SCORE (GARS)

A. General Categories
  1. Variability—a measure of inconsistency and arrhythmicity in stepping and arm movements.
    0 = fluid and predictably paced limb movements.
    1 = occasional interruptions (changes in velocity), approximately <25% of time.
    2 = unpredictability of rhythm approximately 25–27% of time.
    3 = random timing of limb movements.
  2. Guardedness—hesitancy, slowness, diminished propulsion and lack of commitment in stepping and arm swing.
    0 = good forward momentum and lack of apprehension in propulsion.
    1 = center of gravity of head, arms, and trunk (HAT) projects only slightly in front of push-off, but still good arm-leg coordination.
    2 = HAT held over anterior aspect of foot, and some moderate loss of smooth reciprocation.
    3 = HAT held over rear aspect of stance-phase foot, and great tentativity in stepping.
  3. Weaving—an irregular and wavering line of progression.
    0 = straight line of progression on frontal viewing.
    1 = a single deviation from straight (line of best fit) line of progression.
    2 = two to three deviations from line of progression.
    3 = four or more deviations from line of progression.
  4. Waddling—a broad-based gait characterized by excessive truncal crossing of the midline and side-bending.
    0 = narrow base of support and body held nearly vertically over feet.
    1 = slight separation of medial aspects of feet and just perceptible lateral movement of head and trunk.
    2 = 3–4″ separation feet and obvious bending of trunk to side so that cog of head lies well over ipsilateral stance foot.
    3 = extreme pendular deviations of head and trunk (head passes lateral to ipsilateral stance foot), and further widening of base of support.
  5. Staggering—sudden and unexpected laterally directed partial losses of balance.
    0 = no losses of balance to side.
    1 = a single lurch to side.
    2 = two lurches to side.
    3 = three or more lurches to side.
B. Lower Extremity Categories
  1. % Time in Swing—a loss in the percentage of the gait cycle constituted by the swing phase.
    0 = approximately 3:2 ratio of duration of stance to swing phase.
    1 = a 1:1 or slightly less ratio of stance to swing.
    2 = markedly prolonged stance phase but with some obvious swing time remaining.
    3 = barely perceptible portion of cycle spent in swing.
  2. Foot Contact—the degree to which heel strikes the ground before the forefoot.
    0 = very obvious angle of impact of heel on ground.
    1 = barely visible contact of heel before forefoot.
    2 = entire foot lands flat on ground.
    3 = anterior aspect of foot strikes ground before heel.
  3. Hip ROM—the degree of loss of hip range of motion seen during a gait cycle.
    0 = obvious angulation of thigh backwards during double support (10°).
    1 = just barely visible angulation backwards from vertical.
    2 = thigh in line with vertical projection from ground.
    3 = thigh angled forward from vertical at maximum posterior excursion.
  4. Knee Range of Motion—the degree of loss of knee range of motion seen during a gait cycle.
    0 = knee moves from complete extension at heel-strike (and late-stance) to almost 90° (@ 70°) during swing phase.
    1 = slight bend in knee seen at heel-strike and late-stance and maximal flexion at midswing is closer to 45° than 90°.
    2 = knee flexion at late stance more obvious than at heel-strike, very little clearance seen for toe during swing.
    3 = toe appears to touch ground during swing, knee flexion appears constant during stance, and knee angle during stance, and knee angle during swing appears 45° or less.
C. Trunk, Head, and Upper Extremity Categories
  1. Elbow Extension—a measure of the decrease of elbow range of motion.
    0 = large peak-to-peak excursion of forearm (approximately 20°), with distinct maximal flexion at end of anterior trajectory.
    1 = 25% decrement of extension during maximal posterior excursion of upper extremity.
    2 = almost no change in elbow angle.
    3 = no apparent change in elbow angle (held in flexion).
  2. Shoulder Extension—a measure of the decrease of shoulder range of motion.
    0 = clearly seen movement of upper arm anterior (15°) and posterior (20°) to vertical axis of trunk.
    1 = shoulder flexes slightly anterior to vertical axis.
    2 = shoulder comes only to vertical axis or slightly posterior to it during flexion.
    3 = shoulder stays well behind vertical axis during entire excursion.
  3. Shoulder Abduction—a measure of pathological increase in shoulder range of motion laterally.
    0 = shoulders held almost parallel to trunk.
    1 = shoulders held 5–10° to side.
    2 = shoulders held 10–20° to side.
    3 = shoulders held greater than 20° to side.

(continued)

TABLE 6–16. **(CONTINUED)**

4. Arm-Heel Strike Synchrony—the extent to which the contralateral movements of an arm and leg are out of phase.
    0 = good temporal conjunction of arm and contralateral leg at apex of shoulder and hip excursions all of the time.
    1 = arm and leg slightly out of phase 25% of the time.
    2 = arm and leg moderately out of phase 25–50% of time.
    3 = little or no temporal coherence of arm and leg.
5. Head Held Forward—a measure of the pathological forward projection of the head relative to the trunk.
    0 = earlobe vertically aligned with shoulder tip.
    1 = earlobe vertical projection falls 1″ anterior to shoulder tip.
    2 = earlobe vertical projection falls 2″ anterior to shoulder tip.
    3 = earlobe vertical projection falls 3″ or more anterior to shoulder tip.
6. Shoulders Held Elevated—the degree to which the scapular girdle is held higher than normal.
    0 = tip of shoulder (acromion) markedly below level of chin (1–2″)
    1 = tip of shoulder slightly below level of chin.
    2 = tip of shoulder at level of chin.
    3 = tip of shoulder above level of chin.
7. Upper Trunk Flexed Forward—a measure of kyphotic involvement of the trunk.
    0 = very gentle thoracic convexity, cervical spine flat, or almost flat.
    1 = emerging cervical curve, more distant thoracic convexity.
    2 = anterior concavity at mid-chest level apparent.
    3 = anterior concavity at mid-chest level very obvious.

Reprinted with permission from Wolfson L, Whipple R, Amerman P. Gait assessment in the elderly. A gait abnormality rating scale and its relation to falls. *J Gerontol Med Sci.* 1990; 45(1):M14. © The Gerontological Society of America.

As noted in the previous sections, classic measures of cardiopulmonary functions are still appropriate for the older person. However, the clinician must be aware of changes that will affect those tests and choose to use more age-suitable ones.

Nerve Conduction Velocity

This section will discuss the manifestation of these systems in terms of nerve conduction velocities. (Again Chapters 5 and 12 describe the normal and pathological changes in the nervous system with age.) In all of the extremities, sensory nerve action potentials proprogate at a slower velocity and decrease in amplitude.[75] This decrement begins in the third decade and progresses in to the eighth decade.[70] The amplitude of sensory potentials drops from 43 to 21 μv, and sensory velocity in digital nerves steadily declines from 57 to 48 m/sec.[71] Despite these changes, the refractory period is relatively unaffected in the older person.[70] Conduction velocity in the dorsal column shows little change before the age of 60; however, it declines sharply after 60 at a rate of ± 0.78 m/sec each year.[72] Tables 6–20 and 6–21 compare young and old conduction velocities.[72]

Motor conduction velocities slow at an even greater rate as do sensory nerves. The rate of decline of these nerves is 1 m/sec per decade after 15 to 24 years of age.[70] Several tables (see Tables 6–20 through 6–23) show the motor nerve conduction velocity changes with age.[72] Nerve conduction velocity can only be assessed by a therapist or physician specifically trained in this area. Nevertheless, all clinicians should be aware of changes with age that will affect the results of those tests.

Assessing Ethnicity

This final section on assessment deals with the concept of assessing ethnicity.[73] Rempusheski makes a strong plea to health professionals to recognize bias and differences in ethnic views of health care providers and recipients. Table 6–24 is a copy of her assessment cate-

Parameter	Change with Increased Age	
Vital capacity (VC)	Decreased	
Functional residual capacity (FRC)	Increased	
Residual volume (RV)	Increased	Change dependent on size and sex
Forced expiratory volume (FEV$_{1.0}$ liter)	Decreased	
Forced expiratory flow (FEF$_{25-75\%}$ liter/sec)	Decreased	
		Standard Values/Age-related change
Partial pressure of arterial oxgen (Pa$_{o2}$)	Decreased	80–100 mmHG:104–0.42 × age
Partial pressure of arterial carbon dioxide (Pac$_{o2}$)	Unchanged	35–45 mmHG
pH	Unchanged	7.35–7.45

CARDIAC RESERVE: EFFECTS OF AGE AND DISEASE

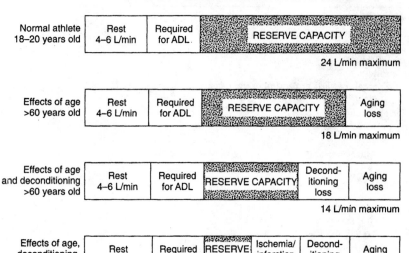

Figure 6–18. Normal changes seen with aging. (*Reprinted with permission from Irwin S, Zadai C. Cardiopulmonary rehabilitation of the geriatric patient. In: Lewis C, ed. Aging: The Health Care Challenge. Philadelphia: F.A. Davis; 1990.*)

TABLE 6–17. ASSESSMENT PROCESS FOR PATIENT INTERVIEW AND PHYSICAL EXAMINATION

Patient Interview	**Observation**
Patient perception of problem/disease process	Patient position
Specific didactic knowledge	use of upper extremities
Emotional reaction	use of musculature
embarrassment	Thoracic cage
anxiety	symmetry
preoccupation	ratio of AP to Lat diameter
denial	Breathing
Family perception of problem/disease process	rate and depth
Patient description of disease progress and physical	rhythm
performance ability	pattern
Patient history of dyspnea/orthopnea	**Palpation**
	subcostal angle/AP to Lat diameter
Chart Review	localized expansion/symmetry
Medical history	excursion/mobility
Previous admissions and diagnosis	locate painful areas
Present medical problems: active/inactive	**Auscultation**
present medications	Normal breath sounds
admitting diagnosis/objectives/care plan	Abnormal breath sounds
Laboratory studies	Adventitious breath sounds
pulmonary function tests/ABGs	
metabolic studies/blood work	
recent EKG	
significant radiographic findings	
Work/Social History	
Present and past jobs/working environment	
Present and past living locations	
Social habits	
smoking	
alcohol	
physical activity	

Reprinted with permission from Irwin S, Zadai C. Cardiopulmonary rehabilitation of the geriatric patient. In: Lewis C, ed. *Aging: The Health Care Challenge.* Philadelphia: F.A. Davis; 1990.

TABLE 6–18.   EXERCISE TESTING PROTOCOLS

12-Minute Walk[a]	Level walking for 12 min distance recorded.	No equipment necessary yet correlates well with study results of more complex tests; can be used for patients who cannot accomplish either treadmill walking or bike riding because of dyspnea.
Low Level Functional	See Table 6–19.	Intermittent walk test for use with moderate to severely impaired patients. Allows flexibility of workload assignment and establishes an accurate baseline.
Balke Test[b]	Treadmill: speed constant at 3.0 mph; grade initially 0% increased by 3.5% every 2 min.	Slight increase in speed for patient with less impairment allows pulmonary and cardiovascular stress to come before leg fatigue.
Bruce[b]	Treadmill: speed initially 1.7 mph; grade initially 10%; both are increased every 3 min in a specified manner.	Can be used with relatively fit individuals to stress accurately all systems' response to exercise. Good to assess exercise-induced bronchospasm in fit individuals.
Bicycle Test[c]	Specific workload (i.e., watts or Kg/min) patient rides for a preset time, next workload determined by patient response.	Intermittent subjective test based on patient response. Requires lower extremity strength and endurance to reach high metabolic response level.

[a]McGavin CR, Cupta SP, McHardy GJR. Twelve-minute walking test for assessing disability in chronic bronchitis. *Br Med J.* 1976; 1:822.
[b]From Physician's handbook for evaluation of cardiovascular and physical fitness, Tennessee Heart Association, 1972.
[c]Ellestad NH. *Stress Testing: Principles and Practice.* Philadelphia: F.A. Davis, 1979.
Reprinted with permission from Irwin S, Zadai C. Cardiopulmonary rehabilitation of the geriatric patient. In: Lewis C, ed. *Aging: The Health Care Challenge.* Philadelphia: F.A. Davis; 1990.

gories.[74] These categories can be used by the practitioner interested in evaluating and planning programs most relevant and acceptable to the older person.

CONCLUSION

Assessment is not simply a range of motion test. Assessment of the older person involves not only modification of the norms of classically used tools such as goniometry or nerve conduction velocities, but it also involves a thorough assessment, which requires evaluation of functional parameters as well. In addition, psychosocial and ethnic concerns may need to be addressed. This chapter has presented several valuable tools for each of these areas. It is the practitioner's responsibility to choose the one's best suited for their practice.

Chair Step Test

		HR/BP	HR/BP	HR/BP
6″	2 min	———	———	———
12″	2 min	———	———	———
18″	2 min	———	———	———
18″	2 min	———	———	———

Figure 6–19. *(Adapted from Serfass RC, Agre JC, Smith EL. Exercise testing for the elderly.* Top Ger Rehab. *Oct 1985; 1(1):58–67, with permission.)*

TABLE 6–19. LOW-LEVEL FUNCTIONAL PROTOCOL

Collect resting data supine and sitting	ECG, BP, RR, HR, O_2sat, PFTs
Stage I	Objective assessment of dyspnea/1.5–2 mph, 0% grade
	Walk 6 min = 4 min stabilization + 2 min gas collection
	Rest: Patient returns to baseline HR, RR, and O_2sat
Stage II	Functional ambulation assessment/treadmill set at speed and incline equal to functional work capacity based on physiologic and symptomatic response to Stage I
	Walk 6 min = 4 min stabilization + 2 min gas collection
	Rest: Patient returns to baseline HR, RR, and ABGs
Stage III	Maximum exercise tolerance/treadmill set to produce HR of 70–85% max or predicted ventilatory max ($35 \times FeV_1$)
	Walk 6 min = 4 min stabilization + 2 min gas collection
	Rest: Patient returns to baseline HR, RR, and ABGs
Criteria to terminate test	85% predicted or HR_{max}, desaturation to 85% or lower SaO_2, reaching a ventilatory maximum ($35 \times FEV_1$), development of significant cardiac arrhythmias, or development of significant symptoms

Reprinted with permission from Irwin S, Zadai C. Cardiopulmonary rehabilitation of the geriatric patient. In: Lewis C, ed. *Aging: The Health Care Challenge.* Philadelphia: F.A. Davis; 1990.

TABLE 6–20. ELECTROPHYSIOLOGIC MEASUREMENTS IN THE YOUNG AND OLD SUBGROUPS AND IN THE COMBINED NORMAL CONTROL POPULATION. FIGURES REPRESENT MEAN ± 1 SD

	Unit	Young Adults	Old Adults	Combined Population
Number of measurements		30	30	60
Age	years	31.6 ± 14.1	74.1 ± 7.5	52.8 ± 24.2
Height	cm	171.4 ± 9.2	163.4 ± 9.9	167.4 ± 10.3
Median motor CV	m/sec	59.4 ± 2.6	52.6 ± 4.0	56.0 ± 4.8
Median sensory CV	m/sec	64.3 ± 3.2	56.9 ± 5.0	60.6 ± 5.6
Median F-wave latency (F)	msec	26.7 ± 2.0	28.4 ± 2.3	27.5 ± 2.3
Tibial F-wave latency (F)	msec	48.5 ± 4.2	55.8 ± 6.7	52.1 ± 6.4
Median SEP latency (SEP)	msec	16.0 ± 1.4	16.2 ± 1.1	16.1 ± 1.3
Tibial SEP latency (SEP)	msec	34.4 ± 4.2	38.2 ± 3.8	36.3 ± 3.8
Spinal conduction (CV)	m/sec	55.8 ± 12.1	42.4 ± 13.1	48.4 ± 12.4

Reprinted with permission from Dorfman L, Bosley T. Age-related changes in peripheral and central nerve conduction in man. *Neurology.* 1979; 29:40.

TABLE 6–21. CONDUCTION VELOCITY AND LATENCY (NORMALIZED BY HEIGHT) CHANGES WITH AGE CORRESPONDING TO THE LINEAR REGRESSION EQUATION
$y = a \times AGE + b$[11]

Variable	Change with age (a)	y Intercept (b)	SD^a $\frac{y/x}{y}$	SD^b $\frac{y/x_1, x_2}{y}$
Median motor CV	−0.15 m/sec/yr	63.9 m/sec		
Median sensory CV	−0.16 m/sec/yr	69.2 m/sec		
Spinal conduction (CV)	−0.24 m/sec/yr	60.8 m/sec		
Median F-wave latency (F)	+0.04 msec/m/yr	14.4 msec/m	0.056	0.054
Tibial F-wave latency (F)	+0.12 msec/m/yr	24.9 msec/m	0.076	0.067
Median SEP latency (SEP)	+0.015 msec/m/yr	8.8 msec/m	0.050	0.045
Tibial SEP latency (SEP)	+0.08 msec/m/yr	17.6 msec/m	0.078	0.071

[a]Normalized average standard error of y corrected for x in the single linear regression analysis y = ax + b.
[b]Normalized average standard error of y corrected for x_1 and x_2 in the multiple linear regression analysis.
$y - a_1 x_1 + a_2 x_2 + a_3 x_1 x_2 = b.$ (x_1 = age, x_2 = height.)
Reprinted with permission from Dorfman L, Bosley T. Age-related changes in peripheral and central nerve conduction in man. *Neurology.* 1979; 29:40.

TABLE 6–22. MAXIMUM SENSORY CONDUCTION VELOCITY IN DISTAL AND PROXIMAL SEGMENTS OF SUPERFICIAL PERONEAL, SURAL, AND POSTERIOR TIBIAL NERVE IN 34 SUBJECTS 15 TO 33 YEARS OLD, AND 37 SUBJECTS 40 TO 65 YEARS OLD (TEMPERATURE ON SKIN 35° TO 37°C)[84]

Age Segment	(yr)	n[a]	A Conduction Velocity (m/sec) Mean	95%	SD	n[a]	B Conduction Velocity (m/sec) Mean	95%	SD
N, peroneus superficialis									
Bit toe—	15–25	19	46.1	39.0	4Ã1				
sup. ext. retinac.	40–65	17	42.2	36.0	6.3				
Sup. ext. retinac.	15–33	24	55.9	50.0	3.8	12	55.9	47.0	5.0
-capitul. fibul	40–65	23	52.9	47.0	3.7				
Sup. ext. retinac.	15–30	15	56.3	50.0	3.7				
-poplit. fossa	40–65	11	53.0	48.0	2.9				
Capitul. fibul.	15–25					13	55.8	47.0	4.7
-poplit. fossa	40–65					11	53.5	46.0	5.2
N. suralis									
Dors. ped.-	15–30	16	51.2	42.0	4.5				
lat. malleol.	40–65	15	48.3	40.0	5.3				
Lat. malleol.	15–30	21	56.5	51.0	3.4	16	55.9	49.0	4.2
-sura	40–65	16	54.8	46.5	4.5	12	56.3	47.0	5.5
Lat. malleol.	15–30	19	57.3	52.0	3.5				
-poplit. fossa	40–65	12	53.3	47.5	4.1				
Sura-	15–30					18	57.6	52.0	3.0
poplit. fossa	40–65					10	54.3	47.0	4.8
N. tibialis posterior									
Bit toe-	15–30	23	46.1	39.0	3.5				
med. malleol.	40–65	10	43.4	37.0	3.8				
Med. malleol.	15–30	17	58.6[b]	52.5	3.8	22	56.4	51.0	4.0
-poplit. fossa	40–52	7	57.4[b]	51.5	4.5	6	54.0	47.0	4.4

A: calculated from the latency measured between onset of the stimulus and the initial peak of the sensory potential.
B: calculated from the difference of latencies, measured at two sites of recording.
[a]Number of nerves.
[b]Conduction velocity in fibers of mixed nerve.
Reprinted with permission from Behse F, Buchtal F. Normal sensory conduction in the nerves of leg in man. *J Neurol Neurosurg Psychiatry.* 1971; 34:408.

TABLE 6–23. MAXIMUM CONDUCTION VELOCITIES OF ULNAR NERVE FIBERS TO MUSCLES OF THE HYPOTHENAR EMINENCE AT VARIOUS AGES[85]

Age in Years	N[a]	Average Conduction Velocity	Standard Deviation
		m/sec	
3.5–10	8	61.5	6.30
10–20	8	57.1	6.19
20–30	35	58.4	4.28
30–40	7	57.4	6.45
40–50	2	56.8	—
50–60	3	49.7	—
60–70	10	51.3	5.26
70–82[b]	10	51.5	7.26

[a]If more than one measurement was made on a single individual, the average only was used.
[b]Includes only one case above 80 years of age.
Reprinted with permission from Wagman I, Lesse H. Conduction velocity of ulnar nerve in human subjects of different ages & sizes. *Fed. Proc.* 1950; 9:130.

TABLE 6–24. ASSESSMENT CATEGORIES WITH WHICH TO ELICIT RITUALS, BELIEFS, AND SYMBOLS OF CARE ACTIVITIES

Sleep

Condition of room/environment: occupancy of room and bed/sleeping surface, kind of bed/sleeping surface and other furniture, condition of room (temperature, lights, doors and windows open or closed, other artifacts/symbols in room).

Kinds of covering, comforting materials: pillow/head support (height/number of supports used, type, positioning), covering (blanket type, sheet type, other).

Sleepwear: covering on head, body, legs, feet (type and variation by season or event).

Care of bed linen: kind of cleaning, frequency, how, by whom.

Bedtime ritual: time, tasks, others involved, food or liquid consumed, sensory stimulation, symbols/icons used.

Rules for sleeping: when, with whom, how, in what positions, where, beliefs related to rules.

Rules for awakening: by whom/what, how, mechanisms used.

Awakening rituals: time, tasks, others involved, food or liquid consumed, sensory stimulation, symbols/icons used.

Personal Hygiene

Tending one's body: rituals for mouth care (tools and substances used, time, who can assist); rituals for body and hair care (how, when, where, how often, substances used, taboos, gender rules, symbols, beliefs associated with aspects of ritual).

Associations with health/illness: care associated with body fluids/excretions, symbolism, body temperature, activities of tending one's body, substances used in rituals, seasonal/climate taboos, kinds of activities, time of day/year, gender rules, beliefs.

Eating

Kinds of foods: preferences, dislikes, specific to an event, ritual, specific to time of day/week/month/year, seasonal, rules or taboos for hot foods, cold foods, rules for amount, type, composition, beliefs, and symbolism associated with specific foods.

Schedule of foods: rules for when/when not to eat; amount related to time of day; healthy/ill status; associated with certain rituals, beliefs, symbols; before/after meal rituals, symbols/icons used/present.

Environment for eating: place, people, position, taboos/rules, symbols/icons used/present.

Implements/utensils: kind, number, rules for use of each, taboos, utensils as symbols.

Reprinted with permission from Rempusheski V. The role of ethnicity in elder care. *Nurs Clin N Am.* Sept 1989; 24(3):717–724.

PEARLS

- Sample tools for assessing cognitive changes in mental status of the elderly are the Mini-Mental State Examination (MMSE) and the Mental Status Questionnaire (MSQ).
- The Zung, Popoff, Beck, and Geriatric Depression Scales are all useful tools for assessing depression in the elderly.
- The Holmes and Rahe Life Events Scale is one of the best known tools for assessing stress levels.
- Functional assessment is a method of measuring an individual's performance.
- Numerous functional assessment tools are available for evaluating older persons. Choose the tool best suited to the setting, clientele, mode of administration, and domain to be evaluated.
- Standard physical therapy measures, such as strength, range of motion, posture, and gait, change with age and may be better assessed with specific tools and norms designed for the elderly.
- Cardiopulmonary parameters, as well as nerve conduction velocity, change with age and require different normative values for assessment comparison.
- Assessing ethnicity of the elderly will help health professionals recognize bias and differences that may obstruct care.

REFERENCES

1. Manton KG. A longitudinal study of functional change and mortality in the United States. *J Gerontol Soc Sci.* 1988; 53:S153–161.
2. Kasper JD. Using the long-term care surveys: longitudinal and cross-sectional analyses of disabled older people. *Proceedings of the 1987 Public Health Conference on Records and Statistics.* DHHS Pub. No. 88–1214. Hyattsville, Md: National Center for Health Statistics; 1988: 353–358.
3. Guralnik JM, Branch LG, Cummings SR, et al. Physical performance measures in aging research. *J Gerontol Med Sci.* 1989; 44:M141–146.
4. Folstein M. Mini-mental state: a practice of method for grading the cognitive state of patients for the clinician. *J Psychiatr Res.* 1975; 12:189–198.
5. Folstein M, Rabins P. Psychiatric evaluation of the elderly patients. Primary Care. September 1979; 6(3):609–619.
6. Kane R, Kane R. Measuring mental status. In: Kane R, Kane R: *Assessing the Elderly.* Lexington, Mass: Lexington Books, 1981.
7. Kahn RL, Goldfarb AI, Pollack M, et al. Brief objective measures for the determination of mental status in the aged. *Am J Psychiatry.* 1960; 117:326.
8. Prestidge B, Lalle C. Prevalence and recognition of depression among primary care outpatients. *J Family Pract.* 1987; 25:67–72.

9. German P, Shapiro S, Skinner EA. Use of health and mental health services. *J Am Ger Soc.* 1985; 33: 246–252.

10. Zung W, Richard D, Shrot M. Self-rating depression scale in an outpatient clinic. *Arch Gen Psychiatry.* 1965; 13:508–515.

11. Freedman N, Bucci W, Elkowitz E. Depression in a family practice elderly population. *J Am Ger Soc.* 1982; 30:372–377.

12. Zung A. A self-rating depression scale. *Arch Gen Psychiatry.* 1965; 12:63–70.

13. Popoff S. A simple method for diagnosis of depression by the family physician. *Clin Med.* 1969; 76: 24–29.

14. Okimoto J, Barnes R, Yoith R, et al. Screening for depression in geriatric medical patients. *J Am Psy.* 1982; 139:799–802.

15. Gallagher D. The Beck depression inventory and older adults review of its development and utility. In: Brink T, ed. *Clinical Gerontology: A Guide to Assessment and Intervention.* New York: Haworth Press; 1986:149–163.

16. Nielson A, Williams T. Depression in ambulatory medical patients prevalence by self-report questionnaire and recognition by non-psychiatric physicians. *Arch Gen Psychiatry.* 1980; 37:999–1004.

17. Kamerow D, Campbell T. Is screening for mental health problems worthwhile in family practice? *Postgrad Med.* 1972; 1:37–43.

18. Beck A, Beck R. Screening depressed patients in family practice: a rapid technique. *Postgrad Med.* 1972; 52:81–85.

19. Brink T, Yesavage J, Lum D, et al. Screening tests for geriatric depression. *Clin Gerontologist.* 1982; 1: 37–42.

20. Yesavage J. The use of self-rating depression scales in the elderly. In: Poon E, ed. *Clinical Memory Assessment of Older Adults.* Washington, DC: American Psychological Association; 1986.

21. Holmes T, Rahe R. The social readjustment rating scale. *J Psychosom Res.* 1967; 11:213–218.

22. Intermediary Manual Part 3—Claims Process. Section 3904 Medical Review (MR) of Part 3 Intermediary Outpatient Physical Therapy (OPT) Bills [Edit], HCFA; 1988.

23. Tinetti M. Performance oriented assessment of mobility problems in elderly patients. *J Am Ger Soc.* 1986; 34(2):119–126.

24. Kane RL. Beyond caring: the challenge to geriatrics. *J Am Ger Soc.* 1988; 36(5):467–472.

25. Bohannon R, Andrews A, Smith M. Rehabilitation goals of patient with hemiplegia. *Int J Rehabil Res.* 1988; 11(2):181–183.

26. Kane RL, Kane RA. *Assessing the Elderly.* Lexington, Mass: Lexington Books; 1981.

27. *Dorland's Medical Dictionary,* 26 ed. Philadelphia: Saunders; 1981.

28. Jette AM. State of the art of functional status assessment. In: Nothstein J, ed. *Measurement in Physical Therapy.* New York: Churchill Livingstone; 1988.

29. Mahoney FI, Barthel DW. Functional evaluation: the Barthel Index. *Md Med J.* 1965; 14(2):61–65.

30. Katz S, Downs TD, Cash HR, et al. Progress in the development of the Index of ADL. *Gerontologist.* 1970; 10:20.

31. Katz S, Ford AB, Moskowitz RW, et al. Studies of illness in the aged. The Index of ADL: a standardized measure of biological and the psychosocial functions. *JAMA.* 1963; 185:914–919.

32. Schoening H, Anderson L, Bergstrom D, et al. Numerical scoring of self-care status of patients. *Arch Phys Med Rehab.* October 1965; 46:689.

33. Filenbaum G. Screening the elderly: a brief instrumental activities of daily living measure. *J Am Ger Soc.* 1985; 33:698–706.

34. Moskovitz E, McCann C. Classification of disability in the chronically ill and aging. *J Chron Dis.* 1957; 5:342.

35. Granger C, Greer DS. Functional status measure and medical rehabilitation outcomes. *Arch Phys Med Rehab.* 1976; 57:103.

36. Functional Independence Measure (FIM). *Uniform Data System for Med Rehab.* Buffalo, NY: Research Foundation of SUNY; 1990.

37. Jette AM. Functional status index: reliability of a chronic disease evaluation instrument. *Arch Phys Med Rehab.* 1980; 61(9):395–401.

38. Jette A, Cleary PD, Rubenstein LV, et al. Functional status questionnaire reliability and validity when used in primary care. *J Gen Intern Med.* May/June 1986; 1:143–149.

39. Branch LG, Meyers AR. Assessing physical function in the elderly. *Clin Geriatric Med.* 1987; 3(1):29–51.

40. Bishop C. Living arrangement choices of elderly singles. *Health Care Financing Review.* 1986; 7:65–73.

41. Wan TTH, Odell BG. Factors affecting the use of social and health services for the elderly. *Aging and Society.* 1981; 1:95–115.

42. Branch LG, Jette AM. A prospective study of long-term care institutionalization among the aged. *Am J Pub Health.* 1982; 72:1373–1379.

43. Branch LG, Jette AM, Evashwick C. Toward understanding elders' health service utilization. *J Comm Health.* 1981; 7:80–92.

44. Macken CL. A profile of functionally impaired elderly persons living in a community. *Health Care Financing Review.* 1986; 7:33–50.

45. Wiener JM, Hanley RJ, Clark R, et al. Measuring the activities of daily living: comparisons across national surveys. *J Gerontol Soc Sci.* 1990; 45(6): 229–237.

46. Applegate W, Blass J, Williams F. Instruments for the functional assessment of older patients. *N Eng J Med.* 1990; 322(17):1207–1214.

47. Lachs M, Feinstein AR, Cooney LM, et al. A simple procedure for general screening for functional disability in elderly patients. *Ann Intern Med.* May 1990; 112(9):699–704.

48. Williams M. Why screen for functional disability in elderly persons? *Ann Intern Med.* May 1990; 112(9): 639.

49. Tomanek R, Woo Y. Compensatory hypertrophy of the plantare muscle in relation to age. *J Gerontol.* 1970; 25(1):23–29.
50. Goldspink G, Howells K. Work induced hypertrophy in exercised normal muscles of different ages and the reversibility of hypertrophy after cessation of exercise. *Am J Physiol.* 1974; 239:179–193.
51. Moritani T, Devries HA. Potential for gross muscle hypertrophy in older men. *J Gerontol.* 1980; 35 (5):673.
52. Rice C. Strength in an elderly population. *Arch Phys Med Rehabil.* 1989; 70(5):391–397.
53. Borges O. Isometric and isokinetic knee extension and flexion torque in men and women aged 20–70. *Scand J Rehab Med.* 1989; 21:45–53.
54. Vandervoort A, Hayes K. Plantarflexor muscle function in young and elderly women. *Eur J Appl Physiol.* 1989; 58:389–394.
55. Walker JSD, Walker JM, Sue D, et al. Active mobility of the extremities in older subjects. *Phys Ther.* 1984; 64(6):914–923.
56. Frekany G, Leslie D. Effects of an exercise program on selected flexibility measurements of senior citizens. *Gerontologist.* 1975; 182–183.
57. James B, Parker A. Active and passive mobility of lower limb joints in elderly men and women. *Am J Phys Med Rehab.* August 1989; 68(4): 162–167.
58. Lewis C. Musculoskeletal changes with age. In: Lewis C, ed. *Aging: The Health Care Challenge.* Philadelphia: Davis; 1990: 135–160.
59. REEDCO Research. *REEDCO Posture Score Sheet.* Auburn, NY; 1978.
60. Murray MP. Gait as a total pattern of movement. *Am J Phys Med.* 1976; 46:290.
61. Murray MP, Kory RC, Clarkson BH. Walking patterns in healthy old men. *J Gerontol.* 1969; 24:169.
62. Andriacchi TP, Ogle JA, Galante JO. Walking speed as a basis of normal and abnormal gait measurements. *J Biomech.* 1977; 10:261.
63. Findley FR, Cody KA, Finizie RV. Locomotion patterns in elderly women. *Arch Phys Med Rehabil.* 1967; 50:140.
64. Nelson A. Function ambulation profile. *Phys Ther.* 1974; 54:1061–1064.
65. Bohannon R, Larken PA, Cook AC, et al. Decrease in timed balance test scores with aging. *Phys Ther.* 1989; 64:1067.
66. Wolfson L, Whipple R, Amerman P. Gait assessment in the elderly. A gait abnormality rating scale and its relation to falls. *J Gerontol Med Sci.* 1990; 45(1): M14–M15.
67. Irwin S, Zadai C. Cardiopulmonary rehabilitation of the geriatric patient. In Lewis C, ed. *Aging: The Health Care Challenge.* 2nd ed. Philadelphia: Davis; 1990; 181–210.
68. Siebens H, Deconditioning. In: Kemp B, Brummel-Smith K, Ramsdell JD, eds. *Geriatric Rehabilitation.* Boston, Little, Brown & Co.; 1990: 177–191.
69. Serfass RC, Agre JC, Smith E. Exercise testing for the elderly. *Top Geriatric Rehab.* October 1985; 1(1): 58–67.
70. Schaumburg H, Spencher P, Ochoa T. The aging human peripheral nervous system. In Katzman R, Terry R (eds).: *The Neurology of Aging.* Philadelphia: Davis: 1975; 442–444.
71. Buchtal F, Rosenflack A, Behse F. Sensory potentials of normal and diseased nerves. In Dyck P, Thomas P, Lambert E. *Peripheral Neuropathy.* Philadelphia: Saunders; 1975: 433–446.
72. Dorfman L, Bosley T. Age-related changes in peripheral and central nerve conduction in man. Neurology. 1979; 29:38–44.
73. Rempusheski V. The role of ethnicity in elder care. *Nursing Clinics of North America* 24(3):717–724, September 1989.
74. Fitzgerald GK, Wynveen KJ, Rheult W, Rothschild B. Objective assessment with establishment of normal values for lumbar spine range of motion. *Phys Ther.* November 1983; 63(11):1778.

CHAPTER 7

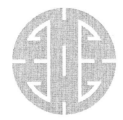

Exploring Nutritional Needs

With improvements in health care, living standards, and socioeconomic status, more adults are living to old age. As the population ages, it is increasingly important to understand the factors that affect the nutritional status and thus the health status of older adults. Many factors contribute to inadequate nutrition, including health status, financial capacities, mobility, exercise, and physiologic needs.[1,2]

Nutrition is an area that is rarely considered when exercise is prescribed and functional levels are deter-

mined for activity in the elderly. Nutritional manifestations often overlap normal aging and disease and facilitate their progression. In fact, nutritional deficits frequently mimic and exacerbate the aging process. With the elderly, under- and overnutritional problems and concerns are of great importance in accurately determining overall fitness and functional levels of activity. In the Surgeon General's report of 1979, the goals for the 1980s were improved health and quality of life for all individuals over the age of 65.[3] This was hoped to be accomplished by encouraging healthy exercise and nutritional practices. It was anticipated that by providing a coordinated educational effort on federal, regional, state, and local levels that the average annual number of days of restricted activity resulting from acute and chronic health problems could be reduced by 20% (or to fewer than 30 days per year) by 1990.[4] With the turn of the century and the start of a new millennium in January, 2000, the Department of Health and Human Services (DHHS) has continued these efforts with *Healthy People 2010*. The benefits of better nutrition (in addition to increased levels of physical activity) have been realized with resulting increases in longevity and a compression of morbidity.[2,5]

This chapter will address the changes related to aging that affect the nutritional well-being of the elderly by looking at common deficiencies and risk factors. Guidelines for good nutrition in the elderly and the impact of poor nutrition on the physical, emotional and cognitive well-being of the elderly will also be addressed. In addition, components of nutritional programs for the elderly will be presented to provide the necessary guidelines for nutritional measures and the insights essential to assessing the nutritional status of the elderly to promote health, prevent or reduce risks of certain diseases, support other medical interventions, and improve the quality of life in old age.

There is no clear demarcation to indicate where on the spectrum of "healthy old age" nutrition begins and ends. There is clearly a state produced by normal aging, but there is great difficulty in identifying this conceptually "healthy" state in the absence of overt or occult disease. As each cohort ages there is a progressive variability in biological efficiency. This variability is a result of a combination of the disparate influences of activity, disease, environment, time, genetic profile, and nutrition on an individual's aging process.

AGE-RELATED CHANGES IN THE GASTROINTESTINAL SYSTEM

Changes in the digestive system will have the most impact on nutritional status as the gastrointestinal tract is most directly involved in ingestion, absorption, transport, and excretion of food products.[1,6]

Changes in the Oral Cavity

The theoretical link between food choice and masticatory efficiency has long been established. It has been found that there is a progressive alteration in food choice with decreasing number of teeth, with the greatest effect being among those who are edentulous. This altered food selection results in significant differences in the hematological status for some key nutrients. Therefore, changes in oral cavity status affecting diet is a risk factor for systemic diseases, such as atherosclerosis, osteoporosis, and cancer.[7]

Several changes associated with aging affect the oral cavity. There are decreasing amounts of saliva in the mouth coupled with the loss of natural teeth or ill-fitting dentures, which inhibit the chewing of foods. It is estimated that approximately 50% of individuals are edentulous by the age of 65.[7] Poor dentition and decreased saliva can cause discomfort and poor mastication. As a result, the elderly tend to pick softer and moister foods to compensate. They eat fewer raw fruits and vegetables and less meat that requires chewing. These changes in eating patterns appreciably diminish the gratification of eating. The inability to chew foods properly is often an embarrassment for the older person reducing the desire to eat with others, and thus decreasing socialization.

The decrease in saliva also compromises the digestive process. Many of the foods that we ingest require the components of saliva to initiate the breakdown of nutrients for absorption along the remainder of the integumentary digestive tract. Failure to commence this digestive process results in malabsorption of many vital nutrients.[7]

Sensory Changes in Taste and Smell

There is a decrease in sensory input with aging.[8,9] Atrophy of gustatory papillae decrease taste, and a decrease in olfaction affects the sense of smell.[10] Sensory losses in taste and smell may potentiate a poor appetite. Loss of dentition not only decreases chewing ability, thereby affecting appetite, but dentures also detract from the perceptual response and can negatively affect the desire to consume certain foods. In addition, depression, smoking, and medications can have an effect on sensory input, diminishing the pleasure of eating.[11] Mulligan suggests that sensory changes may be the result of misuse, disuse, or pathology, and challenges the concept of sensory loss as a normal, age-related change.[12]

Elderly individuals who experience changes in any of the five senses, including sight, hearing, touch, taste, and smell, may also experience a decreased ability or willingness to eat, which may lead to malnutrition. If unchecked, malnutrition can lead to or complicate cognitive, speech and language deficits, and functional losses. Malnutrition from sensory deficits can result in dysphagia by increasing the risk of aspiration from weakened oral-pharyngeal muscle tone. Lack of appetite leads to malnutrition, which contributes to dysphagia.

Esophageal Changes

The esophagus shows little change with age. Esophageal changes are generally related to pathology, such as a hiatal hernia. Swallowing and peristalsis remain relatively intact. Khan[13] suggests that the peristaltic amplitude and velocity of the upper third of the esophagus may decrease with advanced age. Impaired swallowing is common in elderly individuals, but available evidence indicates that this is due more to the effects of associated diseases, such as cerebrovascular accident, neoplasia, stricture or spasm of the esophagus, hiatal hernia, or esophagitis, than to the intrinsic effects of aging per se.[1] Dysphagia and eating dependence can have a profound impact on nutrition. Common disorders result in malnutrition because of oropharyngeal and esophageal dysphagia.[1]

The symptoms of oropharyngeal dysphasia include reflux of fluid out through the nose, persistent cough, a wet hoarseness, overt choking, and a persistent sense of the need to clear the throat. Clinical signs include progressive wasting, dehydration, and recurrent bronchitis. Oropharyngeal dysphagia occurs in elderly individuals because of underlying neurologic disease, muscle weakness, or atrophy. Typically, liquids are handled less well than soft foods. Dysphagia for solid foods is strongly suggestive of anatomic narrowing of the lower esophageal ring.[1]

Esophageal dysphagia is due to a disturbed swallowing mechanism in the body of the esophagus, usually causing a lodgment of food or an awareness of the passage of food through the chest, occasionally with pain. Most often dysphagia is caused by anatomic rather than functional changes. Many elderly individuals with motility abnormalities attributed to presbyesophagus demonstrate features most consistent with esophageal spasm. This is often related to other conditions, such as diabetes mellitus, senile dementia, and peripheral neuropathy, which most likely account for these abnormalities on the basis of neuromuscular functioning. In very old persons, there is a marked decline in the magnitude of esophageal contractions, suggesting smooth muscle weakness.[1] The result is gastroesophageal reflux and reported heartburn.

Gastric Changes

The gastric mucosa shows age-related atrophy.[1] As a result of this, fewer chief and parietal cells remain to provide sufficient pepsin, hydrochloric acid, and gastric mucus. These elements are essential for the absorption of vitamin B_{12} and iron, which are required to initiate protein digestion.[14] Horowitz[14] reported that there is a delay in gastric emptying of both solids and liquids with advancing age, though no clinical significance was found. The parietal cells of the stomach lose their ability to secrete hydrochloric acid, and there is a general reduction in the secretion of digestive juices in old age. There is some evidence from testing with large amounts of gastric and intestinal material that aging causes a relative insufficiency in the capacity to digest protein.[1,15] The clinical significance of this is the unavailability of protein for energy production and maintenance of healthy muscle tissue. The inability of the body to efficiently utilize ingested protein also impacts wound healing and tissue repair.

One of the most remarkable changes with aging is the frequent development of atrophic gastritis and the inability to secrete gastric acid.[1] Though the older adult population tends to be the largest body of consumers purchasing over-the-counter antacid compounds, the majority of elders do not have enough acid in their stomachs to break foods down. The gastric discomfort elders experience is generally the result of poor motility rather than acid indigestion. It has been found that the lack of acid is due to an infection by H. pylori in the majority of cases.[1] The lack of gastric acid in atrophic gastritis may lead to small intestinal bacterial overgrowth and influences the absorption of a variety of micronutrients, including iron, folate, calcium, vitamin K, and vitamin B_{12}.

Intestinal Changes

There is a reduction in the intestinal mobility and in the amount of digestive enzymes as a function of age, which are both associated with a reduction in carbohydrate absorption.[1] With a possible decrease in gastric emptying, reduced carbohydrate absorption, and a decrease in lipase excretion by the pancreas, absorption of dietary fat becomes very inefficient.[16] This decrease in the overall efficiency of the gastrointestinal tract can result in constipation and diverticular disease. The colon remains functionally intact,[17] though some changes appear to be age related. These changes include an increase in diverticula and decreases in motility, rectal wall elasticity, and sphincter tone.[18] The effect that aging might have on the absorption of food has been tested by using xylose as a marker substance. Though there is a gradual decrease in absorption of xylose after the age of 60, the most significantly impeded age group is over 80 years of age when the intestinal capacity to absorb xylose is significantly influenced and diminished. Calcium absorption has been found to decrease with age.[15,19] Undernutrition or excesses in nutrient intake can contribute to these physiological gastrointestinal changes.[20] Psychologically, changes in the gastrointestinal tract can trigger overconcern and undue anxiety, especially about bowel function, to the extent that essential foods are excluded from the daily diet.

Lactose maldigestion is a frequent condition in older adults. The intolerance of dairy products leads to avoidance of these foods and likely contributes to the development of osteopenia.[1]

Because passive absorption is dependent on the surface area of the small intestine, a decrease in the number of villi, villus atrophy, and abnormal villus shape with advancing age affects nutrient absorption. With age, the older individual may have functional abnormalities in the intestine because of altered enzyme activity of epithelial cells.[1] This leads to poor absorption of carbohydrates, fat, protein, and micronutrients inclusive of vitamins D, A, K, C, iron, zinc, and B_{12}.[1]

Changes in Renal Function

The kidneys show changes related to aging that directly affect the nutritional status of the elderly. Though not considered a part of the digestive system, the renal nephron is responsible for the provision of some essential nutrients to the blood.[20] With age, there is a decrease in renal blood flow affecting the return of nutrients. In addition, there is a decrease in glomerular filtration, sodium retention, urine concentration capacity (an increased water output decreasing hydration), and daily creatinine excretion. Combining these changes with a loss of nephrons with aging results in a decrease in efficiency and possible kidney insufficiency. Diminished glucose resorption occurs, and often there is either excessively low or high sodium blood levels, reflections of the decrease in efficiency in kidney functioning.

Poor hydration may further lead to a suppression in kidney function. An individual requires between 1.5 liters to 2.0 liters of fluid per day. Inadequate fluid intake can lead to chronic dehydration and electrolyte imbalances. Physiologic alterations that occur with aging contribute to the increased likelihood of dehydration. As people get older, osmoreceptors (cells that influence the release of vasopressin) decrease. Vasopressin, a hormone released from the posterior pituitary gland, increases the absorption of water by the kidneys, thereby preventing excess water loss.

Renal insufficiency is common in old age. Glomerular filtration rates, renal blood flow, and renal tubular function all decline in efficiency. Atrophy of renal mass is usual and especially pronounced in the cortex by a decline in the number of nephrons and hypertrophy and sclerosis in the remaining nephrons. In addition, chronic degenerative diseases, including hypertension, diabetes mellitus, and kidney disease, also often give rise to kidney damage. In end stage renal disease, therapeutic diets are often prescribed to decrease the symptomatology and blood biochemistry disturbances. These include limitation of protein, sodium and phosphorus.[21] The possibility that age-related deterioration in kidney function is not inevitable but that it results in part from chronic protein overnutrition is receiving much attention.[22,23] The theory that protein restriction can decrease progression of chronic renal insufficiency is currently being studied.

Changes in the Liver

There is a decrease in the liver enzyme activity with aging. This directly affects the metabolism of carbohydrates and the breakdown of drugs and alcohol in the system. Alterations in synthetic, excretory, or metabolic processes can affect the response to disease and the disposition of drugs. This is more thoroughly covered in the subsequent chapter on pharmacology. (Chapter 8, Pharmacology).

Liver weight decreases and this parallels the anthropometric changes of decreased body weight and muscle mass. In advanced age, the liver becomes disproportionately small and there is a reduction in the numbers of hepatocytes. Other changes in liver morphology are nonspecific and may be due to extrahepatic processes. There is an increase in portal and periportal fibrosis, and liver cells tend to be larger. It is suggested that the enlargement of the liver cells may be due to compensatory hypertrophy.[1] An increased amount of lipofuscin pigment is present in the Kupffer's cells, and changes in the Golgi apparatus and rough and smooth endoplasmic reticulum may parallel hepatic functional changes seen in older individuals.[24]

Decreases in liver blood flow occur with age resulting in the potential for changes in drug metabolism. Levels of albumin, a product of hepatic synthesis, are frequently reduced in the elderly and result in a decreased rate of total body protein synthesis.[1]

Other Age-Related Changes

Other age-related changes or chronic diseases influencing food habits are those affecting the musculoskeletal, neuromuscular, and cardiovascular, and pulmonary systems. Problems creating pain, weakness, paralysis, breathing difficulties, or fatigue create loss of function and resulting immobility. Shopping, opening food containers and cooking can often become insurmountable obstacles.

Changes in body composition and weight and a decline in physical exercise and activity levels also influence nutritional needs. With aging, as with inactivity, there is an increase in adipose tissue, a decrease in lean body mass, a decrease in basal metabolism (only a problem from the prospective of obesity), a decrease in caloric requirements, and a decrease in total body water.[25]

Predictors of potential malnutrition include recent weight loss, depression, bereavement, loneliness, multiple medications and long-term medication use, and functional losses.

AGE-RELATED CHANGES THAT AFFECT NUTRITION

The biological, anatomical, and physiological changes that occur with aging were discussed in Chapter 3 and will only be discussed in this chapter as they relate to the nutritional status of the elderly. A progressive decline in the efficiency of many physiological organ functions and an inability to restore homeostasis once it is disrupted are both related to aging.[18] There are extraneous factors complicating the nutritional and homeostatic situation, such as age, frequency of disease and disabilities, multiple medications, and hereditary and genetic predispositions. The decline in physiological functioning shows considerable variation from one individual to the next, and it varies even among cells, tissues, and organs of the same individual.[6] For instance, in calculating body water content, there is significant but normal change with age, and these changes can be compounded by dehydration or edema secondary to inflammatory processes from diseases or social factors. Table 7–1 summarizes the common physiological changes accompanying aging, their potential functional outcome, and the probable clinical manifestations that may affect the nutritional status of an elderly individual.

BASAL METABOLIC RATE

The basal metabolic rate (BMR) declines rapidly from the time of birth to the age of 20. Further decreases in the BMR gradually occur until approximately the age 80. Cell mass and muscle mass slowly decline with age, and muscle mass is partially replaced by fat and connective tissue.[26–28] It is not known whether the slowing of the BMR is the result of a decline in cell mass or if it reflects an actual decrease in metabolic activity. Of interest is the fact that the decline in lean body mass is reflected in a 15% to 20% decrease in exchangeable potassium per kilogram from age 20 to 75.[29,30] This exchangeable body potassium is viewed as an indicator of lean body mass. The decline of BMR with advancing age parallels that of exchangeable potassium. Thus, energy requirements, as a reflection of BMR, appear proportional to lean body mass at all ages.[31]

In conjunction with the BMR decline, there is a gradual reduction in physical activity from the approximate age of 20 to 65.[26,27] Further advances in age do not appear to significantly influence energy expenditure unless there are additional variables, such as arthritis, cerebral vascular accident, cardiovascular or pulmonary diseases. An elderly person involved in moderately strenuous exercise requires significantly more energy output compared to younger individuals.[28,30] It has been hypothesized that this occurs because of the decrease in neuromuscular coordination and the resulting increase in muscular inefficiency. The consequence is "wasted energy."[28] This potential for greater energy loss is balanced by a reduction in extraneous movements and less indulgence in activity on the part of the older person. Overall, the decrease in energy requirement superimposed on the decrease in demand on a reduced lean body mass results in decreasing caloric requirements with advancing age.[31]

Other age-related changes occur in body composition and function. On a cellular level there is a decrease in nutrient uptake by cells, glucose and lipid metabolism decrease, and protein synthesis declines.[32] These changes have a direct effect on BMR as well as altering the energy requirements of activity in the elderly.

The optimal level of physical activity varies because of differences among the elderly in their lifestyles, disabilities, and severity of disease. Evidence is rapidly accumulating that marked declines in physical activity among the aged are undesirable from a health standpoint.[5] Reasonable levels of physical activity improve physical conditioning, may improve some aspects of endocrine function, contribute positively to bone health, increase cerebral oxygenation and alertness, and prevent muscle atrophy.[33,34] Exercise can improve work capacity and cardiovascular function when it is undertaken with sufficient frequency, intensity, and duration. Body fat decreases, lean body mass increases, and endurance increases on aerobic exercise programs with improvement in oxygen delivery and use.[18,35] Exercise also contributes to psychological and social health.

Absorption of nutrients ingested has been shown to be enhanced with physical activity.[36,37] In fact, at a cellular level, the cell absorbs nutritional compounds and elements according to what the "cell's brain" thinks it needs. If someone is sedentary, the cell will only absorb enough nutrient substances for maintenance of homeostasis and physiological efficiency at that level of activity. Therefore, if the nutrients are not absorbed, when the body is then stressed beyond its dormant level, it obtains required nutrients from the bodies storehouses. For instance, protein, which is essential for the production of ATP within the Kreb cycle, is obtained from the muscle, further decreasing muscle mass. Calcium, a fundamental component for cardiac muscle contraction, skeletal muscle contraction, transmission of nerve impulses, synaptic connections within the central nervous system, as well as bone strength, is drawn from the skeleton if adequate circulating calcium is not available to meet the cellular needs at increasing levels of activity.[34]

AGE-RELATED CHANGES IN MUSCLE METABOLISM

Advancing age is associated with a remarkable number of changes in body composition, including reduction in lean body mass and an increase in body fat. Decreased lean body mass occurs primarily as a result of losses in skeletal muscle mass. This age-related loss in muscle mass is termed *sarcopenia*. As discussed above, loss in muscle mass accounts for the age-associated decreases in basal metabolic rate, muscle strength, and activity levels, which, in turn are the cause of the decreased energy requirements of the elderly.[34]

The decline in skeletal muscle mass with advancing age is paralleled by a decrease in the total ribonucleic acid (RNA) concentration in muscle tissue,[34,38] which affects protein metabolism and production of essential amino acids for energy production. Additionally, it has been reported that there is a reduction in the protein-synthetic activity of muscle ribosomes with increasing age, a decrease in the proportion of polyribosomes, and a decline in the pH enzyme frac-

TABLE 7-1. PHYSIOLOGICAL CHANGES AND FUNCTIONAL NUTRITIONAL CONSIDERATIONS

Physiological Changes With Aging	Potential Functional Outcome	Probable Clinical Outcome
Musculoskeletal		
Decreased number and size of muscle fibers	Decrease in lean body mass	Decreased muscular strength, decreased mobility
Decreased bone density	Osteoporosis	Increased risk of fractures
Decreased joint mobility	Narrowing of joint space	Impaired mobility
Central Nervous System		
Cerebral atrophy, senile plaques, neurofibrillary tangles	Parkinson-like symptoms, supranuclear palsy	Confusion, diminished response and perception, memory loss, decreased ADL, poor nutritional compliance
Decreased sensory function	Decreased reaction to pain, touch, heat, and cold	Decreased perception leading to accidental injury
Impaired proprioception	Diminished mechanisms controlling balance	Increased susceptibility to falls
Skin		
Thinning of epithelial and subcutaneous layer	Tissue and vascular fragility	Increased susceptibility to abrasions, bruises, and burns
Eye		
Sclerosis of lens	Cataract, decreased peripheral vision	Impaired peripheral vision, susceptibility to accidents
Degeneration of muscles of accommodation	Smaller pupils	Impaired visual acuity, decreased socialization
Degenerative changes in vitreous, retina, and choroid vision	Decreased color vision and decreased night vision	Susceptibility to accidents
Degeneration of intrinsic/extrinsic ocular muscles	Impaired upward gaze	Susceptibility to falling
Hearing		
Degeneration of organ of corti	Loss of high frequency tones	Decreased hearing, decreased socialization
Smell		
Atrophy of olfactory mechanism	Impaired sense of smell	Decreased appreciation of food
Oral Cavity		
Decreased salivary flow	Dry mouth	Poor oral hygiene, gingivitis, impaired food bolus formation
Resorption of gums and bony tissue surrounding	Tooth loss, impaired force of bite	Preference for softer foods, malfunctioning dentures
Diminished taste bud sensory input	Increased salt and sugar consumption	Diet high in sugar and salt
Gastrointestinal		
Decrease in esophageal smooth muscle, dysfunction of lower esophageal sphincter	Decreased esophageal mobility	Difficulty swallowing, high-bulk foods, hiatus hernia
Decreased intestinal blood flow, decreased liver size	Impaired intestinal absorption and liver metabolism	Subclinical malnutrition
Decreased contractile function of smooth intestinal muscle	Decreased intestinal motility	Constipation
Decreased HCL secretion, decreased number of absorbing cells	Defective absorption of calcium and iron	Pernicious anemia, iron deficiency anemia, osteoporosis
Decreased gallbladder motility	Gallstones	Gastrointestinal upsets, fatty food intolerance
Renal		
Decrease in nephrons, atherosclerosis in combination with decreased cardiac output	Decreased ability to dilute and concentrate urine, diminished renal blood flow	Renal insufficiency, increased potential for dehydration
Endocrine		
Pancreatic beta cells, function and insulin end-organ responsiveness diminish	Progressive glucose intolerance with advancing age	Diabetes mellitus, susceptibility of hypoglycemia if on insulin or oral hypoglycemic drugs
Psychological		
Role changes	Retirement, loss of productivity, increased leisure time	Depression, decreased nutritional intake, decreased finances
Loss	Multiple physical, cognitive, financial, and social loss	Depression, isolation, decreased nutrient intake

Modified and used with permission: Foley CJ and Tideiksaar R (1980)[202]

tion, all contributing to alterations in tissue protein synthesis and energy production in muscle tissue with advancing age.[39]

Ultimately, studies of protein metabolism at the cellular and organ level have been evaluated in reference to the status of whole body protein metabolism. In this context, Waterlow and Stephen[40] observed that with increased age and body weight, the turnover of body protein decreased affecting both liver and muscle cells. They concluded that there was a marked reduction in total body protein turnover in older subjects. Numerous studies have been undertaken to determine body protein in humans, and a few of these studies have dealt with the changes in body protein content with advancing years. Of special importance to the clinician is the catabolic and corresponding anabolic component of metabolism in the presence of infection. Anabolic responses occur not only during recovery but also in the early phase of illness when anabolism is associated with increased production of phagocytes and other leucocytes and the induction of several tissue enzymes and of several immunoglobulins. Overall liver protein synthesis is increased and skeletal muscle protein synthesis is decreased in response to an infectious episode.[9]

Cross-sectional, as well as longitudinal studies, reveal that there is a progressive decline in body potassium and a fall in intracellular fluid as aging progresses.[9] Because of possible changes in the intracellular concentration of potassium with age, the precise physiological significance of body potassium loss in the later years is uncertain. Tissues with a high potassium content, such as skeletal muscle, may decrease relative to those with a lower potassium concentration, and the relative amount of connective tissue, which contains little potassium, may become greater. However, a loss of total body potassium is generally taken to indicate a decrease in total cellular protein mass, and this may be due, to a large extent, to a decrease in skeletal muscle protein mass with age.[29,36]

The motor function of the human declines with age. It has already been noted that the number of functioning motor units decreases with age (see Chapter 3) and this decrease is exacerbated with inactivity. The decline in number of muscle fibers is also associated with a decrease in speed of contraction and myofibrillar and myosin ATPase activity. The rate of calcium transport by the sarcoplasmic reticulum increases with age, which might relate to the muscle dysfunction by making it difficult to obtain sufficient calcium in the myoplasm for the contractile requirements of the actomyosin system.[41] The age-related decline in bone mass (osteoporosis) is highly correlated with loss of skeletal muscle. Calcium is one of the most important elements in the body, with essential functions in muscle contraction, nerve conduction, and membrane transport. For body function at rest, maintaining a serum calcium level greater than 6.0 mg/dL is far more important than maintaining skeletal mass. Ideally, a circulating serum calcium should be around 9.8mg/dL for an active older adult.[31] Although the body supply of calcium is almost exclusively from bone, calcium can be obtained from the diet. Calcium balance for homeostasis is therefore dependent on the skeletal mass and on the dietary intake of calcium.

Creatinine excretion has been used as an index of muscle mass in children and adults and should have the same meaning in the elderly, even though creatine clearance is reduced with aging.[21] The total body protein synthesis per gram of creatinine excretion is considerably higher in the aged subject compared to that of young adults. Because muscle mass is reduced, the higher turnover per unit of creatinine excretion in the elderly may be interpreted to reflect a greater contribution by the active visceral tissues relative to whole body protein metabolism in the elderly. Research data suggests that not only is there a shift in the distribution of body protein synthesis with increasing age, but the rate of muscle protein breakdown and synthesis may decline at the same time. The net result of these concurrent changes is an increase in total body protein synthesis per unit of creatinine with a maintenance of the total body protein synthesis rate when expressed per unit of body cell mass (BCM).

This hypothesis of the changes in the quality and quantity of total body protein metabolism can be further supported by comparing urinary nitrogen and its related amino acid (3-methylhistidine) excretion in young adults and elderly subjects. This unusual amino acid is present in actin of all muscles and in myosin of "white" muscle fibers. It is quantitatively excreted in the urine and unlike the common amino acids of body proteins it is not reused for purposes of protein synthesis. Preliminary comparative findings on the urinary output of this amino acid in young adults and elderly subjects suggest that the daily output of 3-methylhistidine is much lower in the elderly. This reflects the decreased muscle mass. In addition, when normalized for differences in creatinine excretion the output of 3-methylhistidine is still quite different for the elderly. This observation suggests that, per unit of muscle mass, the rate of muscle protein breakdown appreciably declines with age.[9]

A relationship between the nutritional state and skeletal muscle function has long been suspected. During periods of either partial or total starvation, body protein is broken down to supply the required amino acids. As a labile pool of body protein is unavailable for this purpose, all the protein that is broken down serves either a functional or structural role, resulting in a loss of the BCM. Body cell mass represents the total mass of living, functioning cells, the component of the body composition that is metabolically active, and, therefore, the source for oxygen consumption and carbon dioxide production. Skeletal muscle accounts for 60% of BCM and is the largest source of endogenous amino acids. As a result, protein-calorie malnutrition is invariably accompanied by skeletal muscle wasting.[42] A relationship has been demonstrated between skeletal muscle function and nutritional state, and the validity of skeletal muscle function as a functional measure of nutritional state has been demonstrated.[42–45]

CHRONIC DISEASE AND NUTRITION IN THE ELDERLY

Aging processes and lifelong eating patterns are often associated with diseases and disorders that influence the life span, such as atherosclerosis, hypertension, osteoporosis, diabetes, cancer, Alzheimer's disease, renal disease, dental disease, obesity, and immunity.[46] The prevalence of many chronic degenerative diseases increases with advancing age. These disease states may have synergistic negative effects on individuals whose physiological function is already compromised by the aging process. Many chronic conditions have dietary implications that alter the need for nutrients, the physical and metabolic form in which nutrients are delivered, and the activities of daily living related to food and eating. Modifications in the type or amount of energy, or in the energy-providing nutrients, vitamins, and minerals may all be called for in order to provide nutritional support or to control the progression of chronic degenerative diseases.

Unfortunately, manifestations of malnutrition, such as cracks in the mouth or a bright red tongue, are overt signs of a problem that is far advanced. For example, physical signs of dehydration are usually not apparent until it's in the advanced stages. With decreased nutrient intake, there is gradual tissue depletion with evolving biochemical abnormalities before an overt deficiency surfaces. Table 7–2 summarizes the most frequently encountered conditions and the related nutritional problems.

Nutrition and Heart Disease in the Elderly

The association between nutrition and coronary heart disease (including hypertension) is mainly due to the effect of nutrients on serum lipids and lipoproteins.[47] Cholesterol intake does not play a very important role for plasma cholesterol although there are strong interindividual differences in response. The intake of saturated fatty acids negatively affects plasma low-density lipoprotein cholesterol concentration, while mono- and polyunsaturated fatty acids are generally regarded as beneficial.[47,48] Omega-3 fatty acids mainly decrease triglyceride concentration while omega-6 polyunsaturated fatty acids mainly affect low-density lipoprotein cholesterol.[49] Omega-3 fatty acids have been found to reduce the thrombogenetic risk factors in cardiovascular disease.[50] There is evidence that the genetic makeup of an individual may

TABLE 7–2. CHRONIC CONDITIONS AND RELATED NUTRITIONAL PROBLEMS

Chronic Condition	Related Nutritional Problems
Alzheimer's disease, other dementias	Cachexia and emaciation due to poor eating habits and self-care
Celiac sprue	Malabsorption, diarrhea, weight loss, malabsorption with secondary vitamin deficiencies
Cerebral vascular accident	Suppressed cough reflex, increased risk of choking, dysphagia
Chronic mesenteric ischemia	Abdominal pain after eating, weight loss, malabsorption
Constipation	Prolonged transit time especially with immobility, decreased colonic motility
Gastroenteritis	Malabsorption, protein and vitamin B complex deficiencies, poor absorption of calcium and all other nutrients, loss of appetite
Colitis	Decreased elasticity of rectal wall, abdominal discomfort, fecal impaction
Coronary artery disease	Dyspnea, drugs lead to suppressed appetite and constipation
Diabetes mellitus	Glucose intolerance, poor energy utilization
Diverticular disease	Gastrointestinal pain, bowel discomfort, possible bleeding, infection, lack of appetite, weight loss
Emphysema	Dyspnea leading to lack of appetite and difficulty eating
Gallbladder disease	Gallstones, cholecystitis, pancreatitis, food restriction, some foods repugnant, undernutrition
Gastritis/duodenitis	Malabsorption of proteins, vitamin B_{12} and iron, some food restrictions, other foods repugnant, undernutrition
Hiatal hernia	Gastroesophageal reflux, heartburn, dysphagia
Liver diseases	Foods repugnant, restricted protein, drug level changes
Obesity	Energy intakes usually low, need for essential nutrient intake
Osteoarthritis	Difficulty in food shopping and preparation
Osteoporosis	Dyspnea with vertebral collapse, distortion of thorax and abdominal compression, lack of appetite, difficulty eating, decreased intake
Peptic ulcer	Obstruction, bleeding, and perforation, dysphagia, dyspepsia, retrosternal discomfort, antacid overuse and undernutrition
Pernicious anemia	B_{12} deficiency, spinal cord degeneration
Renal disease	Limited ability to handle protein, sodium, potassium, and water

Modified and used with permission: Dwyer JT (1993)[406]

influence dietary risks for cardiovascular disease and blood serum lipid levels.[51] Lipoprotein A, a genetic risk factor for coronary artery disease, diabetes, and cerebrovascular disease, is influenced by dietary factors. Antioxidant vitamins, coenzyme Q10, and omega-3 fatty acids have beneficial influences, whereas linoleic acid, saturated fats, and sugars have an adverse effect on phenotype expression.[51] There is significant evidence that genes are involved in determining enzymes, receptors, cofactors, and structural components involved in regulation of blood pressure, the metabolism of lipids, lipoproteins, and inflammatory and coagulation factors that are involved in determining an individual's risk.[51,52] In a study by Loktionov and associates,[52] the researchers found that total cholesterol concentrations were positively related to saturated fat intake, but elevated low-density lipid cholesterol levels associated with high saturated fat intake can be expected particularly in those individuals who combine 'risky' (high fat diet) dietary behavior with the presence of the apolipoprotein E (ApoE) genotype.

Other nutrients that affect risk for cardiovascular disease are dietary fiber, calcium, magnesium, iron, and antioxidants. Dietary fiber decreases intake of calories and fat, while iron and antioxidants play a role in oxidative modification of low-density lipoproteins. A low intake would lead to an accelerated uptake of low-density lipoprotein into the macrophage.[47]

Intervention studies have not shown conclusively the benefit of high-dose supplementation of the antioxidants vitamin E or beta-carotene on coronary heart disease. However, it has been shown that vitamin E is an antioxidant that serves to protect the vessels from oxidative damage.[53,54] Quercetin, a bioflavonoid, also appears to play a protective role against low-density lipid damage.[55]

Blood levels of an amino acid called homocysteine have been linked to cardiovascular disease. Homocysteine plasma concentration is influenced by folate as well as vitamin B_6 and B_{12}. Higher blood levels of folic acid, B_6, and B_{12} are associated with low levels of homocysteine. Whether a high-dose supplementation with these substances decreases plasma concentrations of homocysteine and positively influences the course of coronary heart disease is currently being studied.[55] Rimm and coworkers[56] examined supplementary intakes of folate and vitamin B_6 and found these dietary nutrients, when taken above the current recommended daily allowance, had an important role in the primary prevention of coronary heart disease.[56]

Vitamin C (another antioxidant) intake has been linked to prevention of heart disease. A protective response to low-density lipid damage[57] and a reversal of dysfunction caused by increases in homocysteine[58] have been demonstrated in clinical research.

A review of the National Health and Nutrition Examination Survey (NHANES I) to assess the relationship of coronary heart disease with modifiable dietary elements and behavioral characteristic emphasized the association of these factors with causation and prevention of heart disease. The survey determined that the following factors, independently and inversely, were associated with coronary heart and vascular disease deaths and hospitalizations: alcohol intake, dietary riboflavin, dietary iron, serum magnesium, leisure time exercise, habitual physical activity, and female gender. Positive significant independent determinants of coronary events also included cigarette smoking, sedimentation rate, Quetelet's rule (body weight in kilograms should be the same as the number of centimeters over 100 of the body length), maximum body weight, and age.[59]

Nutrition and Osteoporosis in the Elderly

Osteoporosis is a heterogeneous condition characterized by an absolute decrease in the amount of normal bone (i.e., loss of bone mass). It results from the failure of bone formation to keep pace with bone resorption. This is termed coupling. It is due neither to a lack of dietary calcium nor defective bone mineralization,[60] but rather to endosteal resorption, which is greater than the formation of new osteons or bone units.[61] Loss of bone is an almost universal accompaniment of aging that proceeds at an average rate of 0.5% to 1% per annum from midlife on.[19] Age-related trabecular bone loss starts at age 35, and cortical bone loss from about age 40. The loss proceeds at about 0.5% per year, until at female menopause and male andropause, the rate of loss is accelerated to 2% to 8% due (directly or indirectly) to lower estrogen (females) and testosterone (males) production.[60]

There are at least four nutrients involved in this process: calcium, salt, protein, and vitamin D. Dietary substances, such as caffeine and carbonated drinks, have also been linked to an increase in bone loss.

The pathogenesis of osteoporosis in men (at andropause) and women (at menopause) is exacerbated by low calcium intake. Calcium is a positive risk factor because calcium requirements increase when hormonal levels decrease due to an increase in obligatory calcium loss and a small reduction in calcium absorption that persists to the end of life. Nordin and associates[19] did a meta-analysis of twenty calcium trials and demonstrated that, based on the evidence in these studies, the progression of osteoporosis can generally be arrested by calcium supplementation, although there is some doubt about its effectiveness in the first few years after menopause in women. Many other trials have investigated the effects of calcium supplementation on bone health. Although insufficient when used as the only intervention, calcium in combination with other nutritional or hormonal substances, has helped to prevent or stall the progression of osteoporosis.[62] Though some of the research remains controversial, the protective effect of calcium (800 to 1500 mg per day) on bone mass is one of the few health claims permitted by the U.S. Food and

Drug Administration. In women who are post-menopausal by six or more years, calcium citrate malate can significantly reduce bone loss at a dosage of 800 mg/day.[63] In several studies, calcium intake has not correlated with protection. For example, in men[62] or women[64] shortly after becoming menopausal, little effect occurs on the relative density of bone. Moreover, even most positive studies focusing on the effects of isolated calcium supplementation on bone mass show only minor effects. Nonetheless, a review of research shows that calcium supplementation plus hormone replacement therapy, or calcium in combination with one or more nutritional substances (vitamin D, magnesium, zinc, copper, manganese, silicon, strontium, folic acid, vitamin B_6, vitamin B_{12}, or vitamin K) has been found to have a significant impact on the health of bone.

Salt is a negative risk factor because it increases essential calcium loss; every 100 mmol of sodium takes 1 mmol of calcium out of the body. Restricting salt intake lowers the rate of bone resorption in both sexes.[19,62,65] Short-term increases in dietary salt result in increased urinary calcium loss, which is resolved with the removal of salt from the diet.[66]

Though bone formation requires protein, too much protein is another negative risk factor for the development of osteoporosis.[67,68] Increasing animal protein intake from 40 to 80 grams daily increases urine calcium by about 1 mmol/day. Low protein intake in third world, or developing, countries may partially protect against osteoporosis.[19] Additionally, although high animal protein correlates with an increased risk of osteoporosis, protein supplementation following a fracture in elderly people appears to result in better bone and overall health compared with no protein supplement.[67]

Vitamin D is important because age-related vitamin D deficiency leads to malabsorption of calcium, accelerated bone loss, and increased risk of hip fracture. Vitamin D supplementation has been shown to retard bone loss and reduce hip fracture incidence in elderly women.[19] Vitamin D increases calcium absorption and when supplemented in combination with calcium, enhances bone health. Supplementary D reduces bone loss in women who consume insufficient amount of the vitamin from food.[69] While people who get outdoors regularly and live in sunny climates are unlikely to need vitamin D supplementation, it is recommended that a diet rich in vitamin D (between 400 to 800 IU per day) be consumed to ward off bone loss.

Other nutrient substances are important for the maintenance of bone health. Among these are magnesium, zinc, copper, boron, manganese, silicon, strontium, folic acid, vitamin B_6, vitamin B_{12}, and vitamin K. Both bone and blood levels of magnesium have been reported to be low in people with osteoporosis.[70,71] Supplemental magnesium (between 250 and 750 mg per day) has reduced markers of bone loss in men[70] and has been shown to increase circulating

levels of this substance in both men and women.[71] Levels of zinc in both blood and bone have been found to be low in individuals with osteoporosis.[72,73] Urinary loss of zinc is high in osteoporotic people[72] and elderly individuals consuming 10 mg or less per day of zinc are twice as likely to sustain a hip fracture compared to those whose diets contain more than 10 mg per day.[72,73] Combining supplemental minerals including zinc (10 to 30 mg) with calcium enhances the absorption of calcium. Copper is needed for normal bone synthesis. A recent controlled study reported that 3 mg per day prevented bone loss.[74] Of interest is the fact that elderly individuals who are taking zinc supplements deplete copper nutriture. Thus, people on zinc supplements need to supplement copper as well. All minerals discussed so far (calcium, magnesium, zinc, and copper) can be found at appropriate levels in high potency multivitamin/mineral tablets.

A preliminary trial found that supplementation with 3 mg per day of the trace mineral boron reduced urinary loss of both calcium and magnesium.[75] However, the effect was achieved by significantly increasing estrogen and testosterone levels, so supplemental boron, above and beyond a daily multivitamin, is most likely unnecessary. Interest in the effect of manganese and bone health began when famed basketball player Bill Walton's repeated fractures were prevented with manganese supplementation.[76] A subsequent study reported manganese deficiency in osteoporotic women and found that a combination of mineral, including manganese was reported to stop bone loss.[77] Silicon plays a significant role in bone formation.[78] Supplementation with silicon has increased bone formation in preliminary bone density studies in osteoporotic women, although the optimum levels remain unknown. Strontium, a mineral that is considered to be nonessential, is also believed to play a role in bone formation; preliminary evidence suggests that women with osteoporosis may have reduced absorption of this trace mineral.[79] Increased bone formation and decreased bone pain have also been reported in osteoporotic people given 600 to 700 mg per day.[62] Although levels used in research have been quite high, optimal intakes have yet to be established and the recommended daily dosage is 1 to 3 mg, less than many people consume in their daily diets.[62] Folic acid, vitamin B_6, and vitamin B_{12} are known to reduce blood levels of the amino acid homocysteine, while homocysteinuria, a condition associated with high homocysteine levels, frequently causes osteoporosis. For the purpose of lowering homocysteine, amounts of folic acid and vitamins B_6 and B_{12} found in high potency B-complex supplements and multivitamins have been found to be sufficient.[62] Finally, vitamin K is required for bone formation and has been found to be low in both blood and bone levels in people with osteoporosis.[80] One study found that postmenopausal women have reduced urinary loss of calcium after taking 1 mg per day of vitamin K.[81] In controlled studies, people with osteoporosis given large amounts of vitamin K (45 mg per day) showed an increase in bone density after six months and decreased bone loss after one year.[82] In a group of estrogen-deficient women, evidence of increased bone formation occurred when they were given 10 mg of vitamin K per day for one month.[83]

Activity (particularly weight-bearing activity), calcitonin, sodium fluoride, calcium intake of 1500 mg/day, and vitamin D 400 to 600 IU/day may retard bone loss.[84] Boron supplementation may reduce the urinary excretion of calcium and magnesium and elevate the concentration of 17 beta-estradiol,[85] thus, inhibiting "normal" bone loss of aging. Calcium supplementation is thought to inhibit immunoreactive and parathyroid hormone (PTH) secretion as levels of PTH increase with age in response to diminished levels of extracellular fluid calcium. Estrogen replacement therapy may retard the normal bone loss of aging, but, the protective effect may last no longer than two to three years after termination of treatment.[86]

Caffeine has been linked to fractures and, like salt, increases the urinary excretion of calcium. Research indicates that two to three cups per day may accelerate bone loss in individuals (especially postmenopausal women) who have calcium intakes of less than 800 mg per day.[87,88] Caffeine consumption becomes less of a risk as dietary intake of calcium increases.[88] Carbonated drinks are associated with increased bone loss. This appears to be connected to the presence of phosphoric acid, a substance found in sugar and sugar substitute-containing soft drinks. Calcium binds to phosphoric acid and is carried out in greater amounts in the urine. Preponderance of evidence suggests that there is a benefit to limiting drinks that contain sugar, phosphoric acid, and other chemicals, and a dietary change in that direction may reduce urinary loss of calcium.[89]

Nutrition and Diabetes Mellitus in the Elderly

Approximately 18% of the population between the ages of 65 and 75 years have diabetes mellitus.[90,91] In general, elderly individuals tend to have impaired glucose tolerance when compared with younger individuals. Data suggest that only about 10% of the variance in total serum glucose response to an oral glucose load is arributable to age.[92] Body weight and the level of physical activity appear to have a more important role in the pathogenesis of hyperglycemia with aging. The major factors involved in hyperglycemia and the development of type II diabetes mellitus include a poor second-phase insulin secretion, failure to inhibit glucose production, a defect in the insulin receptor and postreceptor sites, obesity, and lack of physical activity. Regardless of the etiology of diabetes mellitus in the elderly, evidence reveals that control of glucose levels improves the quality of life, and decreases morbidity and mortality rates in older patients.

Impaired glucose tolerance associated with aging has been shown in cross-sectional studies to be related to the level of physical activity and fitness.[93] In a prospective trial of the effects of exercise on glucose tolerance, Seals and associates[94] found that while glucose levels did not change, both insulin and C peptide levels decreased. In addition, high-density lipoprotein cholesterol levels increased and triglyceride levels decreased. In elderly patients with type II diabetes mellitus, short-term exercise programs do not show a major advantage over dietary control of glucose intake.[95] However, long-term exercise programs did result in improvements of glucose tolerance.[96,97] In combination with dietary control, the possible benefits of exercise on glucose tolerance are evident. In addition, exercise may also improve cardiovascular function, lipid profiles, hypertension, osteopenia, and psychological components in diabetic elders.

There are a number of effects on vitamin and mineral status in diabetes mellitus.[98] Many of these changes parallel those seen with aging. Diabetes mellitus is associated with decreased zinc absorption and hyperzincuria.[99] Zinc deficiencies are associated with poor wound healing, poor immune function, immune dysfunction, and anorexia.[100] Supplementary zinc administration has been shown to improve immune function[101] and facilitate wound healing[102] in patients with zinc deficiencies. This is particularly important given the poor healing capabilities in individuals with diabetes mellitus.

Chromium plays a role in normal glucose homeostasis. Deficiency of chromium has been implicated in the glucose intolerance with aging.[103] Copper levels are elevated in type II diabetes mellitus.[104] The clinical significance of this is not clearly known, however, Klevay[104] demonstrated that experimentally induced copper deficiency resulted in elevation of cholesterol levels. Thiamine is essential for the transport of metabolized glucose into the Krebs cycle. In type II diabetes mellitus, erythrocyte transketolase activity, an indirect measure of thiamine status, is elevated, which may be related to poor availability of intracellular glucose. Diabetes mellitus is also associated with pernicious anemia. Vitamin B_{12} deficiency is common in the diabetic patient and is associated with posterior column neuropathy and dementia.

Nutrition and Cancer in the Elderly

The National Cancer Institute (NCI)[105] estimates that about 7.3 million Americans alive today have a history of cancer and that one third of cancer deaths are related to diet. The NCI has supported research covering the gamut from basic mechanisms of the action of dietary constituents, human metabolic studies, clinical trials of dietary modifications and chemopreventive potential of individual nutrients to population-based studies, with a steadfast commitment to defining the roles that diet and nutrition have in the development of cancer.[105] Sixty percent of cancers in the United States are diagnosed in people 65 years of age or older.[106] Older people have ten times a greater risk of developing cancer than those under 65 years of age. Compared with the rest of the US population, older people suffer disproportionately from morbidity, adversity, and hardship caused by cancer. Sixty-seven percent of all cancer mortality occurs in people 65 years of age and older.[106]

Cancer is in large part a disease of the elderly. The parallel increase in cancer risk with advancing age is well recognized, and several pathophysiological mechanisms common to both conditions have been proposed to explain this interrelationship.[107] The importance of nutrition, both in delaying the aging process and in protecting against cancer is also well recognized, and it is therefore of interest to compare the relative impact of several of the more widely studied dietary manipulations on each of these conditions. For example, caloric restriction, which putatively reduces oxidative stress and effectively increases life span in animals also seems to reduce the incidence of many cancers, possibly due to diminished mitogenesis.[107,108] Likewise, oxidative damage to DNA appears to be common to both processes but may be more important in the mitochondria with respect to aging and in the nucleus in relation to cancer.[107] Inadequate dietary folate and impaired DNA methylation status are closely associated with increased cancer risk, and recently defective somatic cell methylation and accumulated genetic instability have been proposed as key mechanisms contributing to senescence.[108,109] (See Chapter 2, Comparing and Contrasting the Theories of Aging for further discussion related to these theories.) Several other well-established anticancer dietary strategies, which include increased fiber intake and the consumption of more fruits and vegetables, have not been studied extensively in relation to aging, although many of the phytochemicals considered important as chemopreventive agents for cancer may well contribute to delaying the aging process.[107,109,110] Closely related to nutrition is the role of physical activity, which has been strongly linked to a reduction in risk of some cancers as it alters metabolism of nutrients in a positive way (absorption and utilization of nutrients is more efficient in a fit individual). Although less is known with respect to exercise and biological markers of aging, physical activity does retard age-related decline in muscle strength and in bone density and plays a preventive role in warding off cancer.[110]

In addition to the theories discussed above, a number of other external factors (smoking, alcohol, sun exposure, viruses) and internal factors (hormones, immunocompetence, genetic mutations) contribute to cancer. For the majority of Americans who don't smoke or drink alcohol to excess, dietary choices and physical activity are the most important modifiable determinants for cancer risk.[111] It is currently estimated that about 32% of cancers may be avoided by changes in diet with 20% to 42% of cancer deaths avoidable by dietary modifications.[112]

Evidence from both animal and epidemiologic studies indicate that, throughout life, excessive energy intake in relation to requirements increases risk of human cancer. Rapid growth rates in childhood lead to earlier age at menarche, which in turn increases risk of breast cancer, and accumulation of body fat in adulthood is related to cancers of the colon, kidney, and endometrium as well as postmenopausal breast cancer.[112] Higher intake of vegetables and fruits has been associated with lower risks of many cancers.[112] The constituents responsible for these apparent protective effects remain uncertain, although evidence supports the contribution of folic acid and antioxidant vitamins (e.g., vitamins C, E, and A).[108,112] Recent evidence suggests that the percentage of energy from fat in the diet is not a major cause of cancers of the breast or colon, however, higher intake of meat and dairy products has been associated with greater risk of prostate and kidney cancer, which may be related to saturated fat content.[108,113] Also, red meat consumption has been associated with risk of colon cancer in numerous studies.[112–114] Excessive consumption of alcohol increases risks of upper gastrointestinal tract cancers, and even moderate intake appears to increase cancers of the breast and large bowel.[112–115] Although many details remain to be learned, evidence is strong that remaining physically active and lean throughout life, consuming an abundance of fruits and vegetables, and avoiding high intakes of red meat, foods high in animal fat, and excessive alcohol will substantially reduce risk of human cancers.[112–115]

It is now widely accepted that diet is as important as tobacco as a cause of human cancer. However, whereas we can dispense with tobacco altogether with general benefits to health, we cannot do without food. It is, therefore, necessary to determine the pattern of nutrition that is associated with the lowest cancer risk. This is made more difficult by the fact that some kinds of cancer are associated with overnutrition (e.g., colon, breast, prostate, kidney), and some with poor nutrition (e.g., esophagus, stomach, liver). The major nutrition factors associated with increased cancer risk are: (1) overweight (as a surrogate for excess energy intake); (2) low intake of fresh fruit; (3) low intake of vegetables; and (4) low intake of whole grains.[113]

The presence of cancer as well as the various antineoplastic regimens used in its treatment (surgery, radiation therapy, chemotherapy) can have a profound impact on nutritional status. Cachexia is a common cause of morbidity and mortality in cancer patients.[116,117] Nutritional comorbidities related to treatment interventions with cancer include:

- Anorexia/cachexia with progressive weight loss and undernutrition
- Sensory changes (taste, smell) that alter food intake
- Tumor-induced alterations in nutrient metabolism
    - protein, fat and/or carbohydrate

- hypercalcemia
- hypophosphatemia/osteomalacia
- hypo-/hyperglycemia
- Increased energy expenditure irrespective of body weight and activity level
- Impaired food intake and malnutrition secondary to
  - bowel obstruction
  - tumor-induced intestinal dysmotility
- Malabsorption secondary to
  - deficiency/inactivation of pancreatic enzymes
  - deficiency/inactivation of bile salts
  - small bowel fistula
  - infiltration of small bowel, lymphatic system, or mesentery by malignant cells
  - blind loop syndrome (bacterial overgrowth)
  - small bowel hypoplasia induced by malnutrition
- Protein-losing enteropathy
- Anemia secondary to
  - chronic blood loss
  - bone marrow suppression
- Fluid and electrolyte disturbances secondary to
  - persistent vomiting
  - diarrhea, fistula
  - intestinal secretory abnormalities with hormone-secreting tumors
  - inappropriate antidiuretic hormone secretion
  - hyperadrenalism (tumors producing corticosteroids/corticotrophin)

Of all the environmental factors associated with cancer, dietary components appear to play an important role in the initiation and progression of the disease. Nutrients and nonnutrients in the diet can influence the carcinogenic process at various stages, from initiation to overt manifiestations.[115,116] Disease prevention is desirable and nutrition habits/food choices that impact the development of cancer include the type of food eaten (plant versus animal sources), method of food preparation (low fat, limit smoked or pickled or processed foods), serving size (moderate), variety (maximize vitamin/mineral intake from food sources), total caloric intake (less is best, BMI of 22–27), and alcoholic beverage intake (moderate consumption, if at all).[115,116] For many individuals, a daily multivitamin that contains folic acid and antioxidants is recommended as part of a reasonable overall cancer prevention strategy.[116]

With the unprecedented expansion of the segment of the population aged 65 and older, it is expected that by the year 2030, one in five older Americans will be diagnosed with cancers of all sorts. Because cancer incidence and mortality rates are highest in this group it is of great importance for rehabilitation professionals to provide treatment to older aged cancer patients. In addition, older aged cancer patients are likely to have preexisting conditions at diagnosis, creating a special clinical challenge.[106,115,116]

Nutrition and Alzheimer's Disease

As research progresses in the area of Alzheimer's disease (AD) and its etiology, it has become apparent that there is a nutritional basis for the accumulation of beta amyloid, a genetic name for a class of sticky proteins, associated with the neurofibrillary plaques and tangles characteristic of this disease. Although this accumulation appears to have a genetic basis, the question as to whether modification of the diet may impede the initiation or progression of Alzheimer's is currently a topic of great interest in this field of study. Preliminary evidence has linked populations at high risk for AD with higher levels of dietary fat and calories; similarly, fish intake has been linked with low-risk populations.[118–121] Whether these foods can actually increase or reduce the risk of Alzheimer's disease, however, remains unknown.

Aluminum in the diet, an unnecessary and potentially toxic metal, has been implicated as causal in the etiology of AD, though this remains controversial.[122,123]

Many nutrients or indices of nutritional status are associated with cognitive functioning. For instance, results from recent studies indicate that supplementation with beta-carotene (vitamin A), alpha-tocopherol (vitamin E) or both can be beneficial to cognitive function in elderly people.[118,120] Folate rather than B_{12} appears to be associated with cognitive functioning as well.[119,120] Furthermore, the daily intake of ginkgo biloba extract, a herbal remedy, can enhance cognitive performance and has been proven to delay cognitive decline in dementia. A proper dietary composition with regard to the ratio of carbohydrates to proteins, as well as the inclusion of sufficient micronutrients, seems to have a favorable effect in the maintenance of cognitive function in the elderly. Glucose can enhance cognitive function, and it has been shown that a rapid decline of glucose levels may impair cognitive ability and induce feelings of lack of energy. Low doses of caffeine have also been shown to enhance cognitive functioning in older individuals. The effects of nutritional supplements may be modest, but they do not seem to be very different from those medicinal or investigational cognitive-enhancing or antidementia drugs currently being studied.

Phosphatidylserine, which belongs to a special category of fat-soluble substances called phospholipids, is related to lecithin, and is an essential component of cell membranes. It is a naturally occurring compound present in the brain, and it has been determined that this substance is often diminished in patients with AD. Researchers have shown that supplementation with phosphatidylserine improves mental function, such as ability to remember names and other types of recall, in individuals with AD.[124,125]

Large amounts of vitamin E may slow the progression of Alzheimer's disease, according to researchers from the Alzheimer's Disease Cooperative Study. A two-year double-blind study of individuals with AD of moderate severity found that 2,000 IU per day of vitamin E extended the time the patients were able to care for themselves (e.g., bathing, dressing, eating), compared with those taking a placebo.[126] Preliminary evidence has linked people who use antioxidant supplements (vitamins E or C) to a lower risk of AD compared with people not taking supplements.[127] Other research shows that higher blood levels of vitamin E correlate with better brain functioning in older adults.[127,128] The link between antioxidants and protection may make sense because in conditions related to AD, oxidative damage appears to be part of the disease process.[129]

It has been found that a choline-like substance, 2-dimethylaminoethanol (DMAE), may increase levels of the brain neurotransmitter acetylcholine. One trial demonstrated that AD individuals given supplemental DMAE showed changes in memory (ability to remember faces, numbers, and names) but did not affect behavioral characteristics (e.g., agitation, pacing, sleeplessness) of AD patients.[130] Subsequent research in a double-blind, placebo-controlled study did not, however, find a significant benefit from the use of DMAE in people with AD.[131]

The acetyl group that is part of acetyl-L-carnitine contributes to the production of the neurotransmitter acetylcholine. Several clinical trials suggest that acetyl-L-carnitine delays the progression of AD,[132] improves memory,[133] and enhances overall performance in some individuals with AD.[134] One double-blind study found that acetyl-L-carnitine slowed progression of the disease in people under the age of 65 but paradoxically appeared to have the opposite effect in older people with AD.[135] Overall, however, most research indicates improvement in short-term studies and reduction in the rate of deterioration in longer studies (lasting one year or more).[136]

Mitochondrial function appears to be impaired in people with AD. Due to its effect on mitochondrial functioning, one group of researchers has given coenzyme Q_{10}, along with iron and vitamin B_6, to subjects with AD and reported that the progression of the disease was prevented by up to two years compared to nonsupplemented controls.[137]

Some researchers have found links between AD and evidence of vitamin B_{12} and folic acid deficiencies,[138] while others consider the problem to be of only minor significance.[139] Little is known about whether supplementation with either vitamin would benefit individuals with AD, nonetheless, it makes sense for people with AD to be tested for vitamin B_{12} and folate deficiencies and to be treated if they are deficient.

Nutrition and Renal Disease in the Elderly

It has been suggested that the high and continuous protein intake common in current Western societies increases renal blood flow, glomerular filtration rate, and the transcapillary pressure gradient in the glomerulus.[140,141] These changes contribute to and are associated with an increase in extracellular matrix[141] and ultimately with age-related glomerular sclerosis. Although the reduction in functioning glomeruli seen in humans between the fourth and eighth decades does not cause significant renal insufficiency by itself, it may be very important when combined with intrinsic renal disease.

Recent studies support a relationship between protein intake and age-related decrease in renal function.[140,141] With renal disease, low-protein diets slow the decline in renal function, histologic damage, and mortality.[140,142] Low-protein (and phosphorus) diets can also ameliorate uremic symptoms, secondary hyperparathyroidism, and metabolic acidosis in patients with chronic renal failure (CRF).[140,141] Albeit controversial, evidence also suggests that dietary protein restriction can slow the rate of progression of renal failure and the time until end-stage renal failure.[140] These dietary regimens appear to be safe in patients with CRF, and appear to activate normal compensatory mechanisms designed to conserve lean body mass when dietary protein intake is restricted.[140,141] Control of hypertension with angiotensin-converting enzyme (ACE) inhibitors or angiotensin II receptor blockers, and antioxidative therapy, in addition to a reduction of protein and fat intake, reduce the progression of renal damage.[141,142] Metabolic acidosis, a condition commonly encountered in CRF and end-stage renal disease, is often accompanied by complications inclusive of bone lesions, depression of myocardial contractility, and growth retardation.[143] Correction of acidosis through dietary means has been found to improve serum albumin concentration in elderly patients on hemodialysis and this correction induced a decrease in renal hypertension.[143,144]

The principle of nutritional interventions, which are to maintain lean body mass, stimulate immunocompetence, and repair functions, such as wound healing, are similar for patients with acute renal failure (ARF) and other catabolic clinical conditions.[145] However, in ARF the multiple metabolic consequences of acute uremia need to be taken into account. These not only affect fluid, electrolyte, and acid-base balance, but also the metabolism of amino acids, proteins, carbohydrates, and lipids. In addition, these metabolic alterations are modified by the acute disease process of associated complications, such as severe infections.[143,145]

In addition to renal disease associated with metabolic dysfunction, epidemiologic evidence directly links nutrition to renal cell cancer.[146] Kidney cancer specifically renal cell parenchymal cancer (RCC), comprising 1.7% of all malignant diseases in the older adult, is strongly related with obesity. Studies suggest that diet may be an important factor in the etiology of this malignancy.[146] A positive association of protein and fat intake, as well as the main food sources of nutrition from meat, milk, and fats increases the risk of renal cancer.[108,113,146] There appears to be a strong protective effect from fruits and vegetables in case-control studies and an increased risk of RCC associated with consumption of fried and sauteed foods, excessive alcohol and coffee consumption, and low intakes of magnesium, vitamin E, and overall high energy consumption.[108,113,146]

From a rehabilitation perspective, resistance or strength training may help reverse the malnutrition common among patients in chronic renal failure, delay the progression of renal disease,[147] and have a protective effect on the development of renal cancer.[110] Resistive training results in muscle mass accretion, improved physical function, and slowed progression of muscle wasting. In addition, significant increases in muscle mass, muscle strength, and muscle function in frail elders greatly improves functional capabilities and the quality of life for renal patients.[147] States of malnutrition leading to muscle wasting directly affect lean tissue mass and functional capacity. Even at dietary protein intake below the recommended dietary allowances, resistance training appears to exert an anabolic effect by improving energy intake and protein use allowing nitrogen retention.[147] The potential benefits of resistance exercise extend beyond this direct impact on protein metabolism. They include improvements in functional capacity such as gait, balance, mobility, strength, exercise tolerance, improved glucose uptake, insulin sensitivity, and self-esteem. As an adjunct to current treatment modalities for ARF and CRF, exercise may serve as a cost-effective, noninvasive approach to counteract malnutrition and improve the quality of life.

Nutrition and Urinary Incontinence

The role of nutrition in incontinence is somewhat controversial, but it is clear that a diet inadequate in basic nutrients can contribute to repeated bladder infections and poor muscle tone and bladder control. Changes in the kidney with age can lead to acidity and under- or overconcentration of urine which can irritate the bladder. Inadequate intake of water can also lead to dehydration and overconcentration of urine which can irritate the bladder, result in bladder infections and in constipation or fecal impaction, all of which can cause or contribute to urinary incontinence. Additionally, the effects of drugs on nutrient absorption, metabolism, and excretion may impact the concentration of urine, loss of specific nutritional elements, and irritation of the bladder. Nutrient deficiencies can create changes in the connective tissues of the body and result in poor bladder tone, poor quality muscle contraction, poor nerve conduction, and decreases in overall fitness levels as measured by strength, flexibility, and endurance. All of the above circumstances can directly or indirectly impact the presence of "stress," "urge," "mixed," and/or "functional" incontinence.[148]

Urinary incontinence is a common problem with a possibly simple and non-invasive solution—hydration. Although many individuals restrict fluid intake to reduce incontinent episodes, clinical studies suggest that adequate hydration is more useful in the management of urinary incontinence.[149,150] A study by Dowd and associates[150] was conducted in older community-dwelling women to determine the effects of hydration on the number of urinary incontinent episodes. Subjects were randomly assigned to one of three groups: increase fluid intake by 500 cc, maintain fluid intake at baseline level, or decrease fluid intake by 300 cc. Caffeine-containing substance (e.g., coffee, soft drinks) and alcohol consumption were avoided. Fluid intake and output diaries were kept for five weeks. Adherence to the fluid intake protocols was monitored closely. The results were significant. For those individuals who increased their fluid intake, there was a reported decrease in daily urinary incontinent episodes, fewer changes of absorptive pads, and subjectively, the subjects felt that the most significant learning was their recognition of the need to increase fluid intake when they initially thought that fluid restriction was necessary to prevent wetting incidences. Those who did not change fluid intake levels reported no change in episodes of incontinence, and those who decreased fluid intake actually experienced an increase in the number of incidences of incontinence on a daily basis.[23] These results strongly indicate that hydration should be encouraged to prevent episodes of urinary incontinence.

Nutritional deficits could potentially explain some of the problems associated with urinary incontinence. For instance, protein malnutrition causes muscle wasting, edema, hypoalbuminemia, and poor wound healing. Muscle mass declines and is paralleled by a decrease in the total RNA concentration in muscle tissue. This affects protein metabolism and production of essential amino acids for energy production.[151] The decline in number of muscle fibers is associated with a decrease in speed of contraction and myofibrillar and myosin ATPase activity. This would clearly impact the contractility of the pelvic floor musculature. Therefore, it can be hypothesized that the lack of adequate protein in the diet could directly be linked to the presence of urinary incontinence.

Poor protein availability also results in muscle dysfunction by making it difficult to obtain sufficient calcium in the myoplasm for the contractile requirements of the actomyosin system.[41] The effects of protein malnutrition coupled with a deficiency in calcium availability will affect all of the muscles of the body, including the pelvic floor.

Vitamin C is a crucial element in the synthesis of collagen which makes up all of the tissues of the body. Vitamin C is also a potent nonenzymatic, antioxidant protector against free radical damage[152] and is touted as an immune system enhancer. Vitamin C in combination with zinc increases the strength of contraction cf muscles.[153,154] A deficiency in this element leads to poor quality of connective tissues including muscles, blood vessels, and smooth connective tissue and has the potential of increasing the likelihood of the development of urinary tract infections and inflammation. It will influence the health of the bladder and kidneys, the integrity of the circulation to the kidney, bladder, and pelvic floor, and the contractility of the pelvic floor muscles.

One approach to controlling urinary infections is to increase the acidity of urine. Supplemental vitamin C enhances urinary acidity. Vitamin C can also help when inflammation, but not infection, is present as in the case of urethritis, an irritation of the male urethra caused by phosphoric crystals.[155] In a study by Rous,[155] men suffering from this painful disorder were given 3,000 mg of vitamin C for four days with complete relief of symptoms. It is hypothesized that the irritating phosphoric crystals form in the urine because of insufficient acidity. The large dose of vitamin C was a safe way of introducing enough acidity to form the crystals back into solution.[155] It is interesting to note that what was working was the "wasted" vitamin C, the part that could not be used by the body and spilled into the urine. But, far from being wasted, the excess vitamin C in their urine was exactly what was needed to protect and restore health.

Zinc deficiencies are common in an older population. In the absence of zinc, muscle cell permeability of glucose is severely retarded and results in poor muscle homeostasis, a decrease in O_2 and CO_2 exchange and sluggish, ineffective muscle contraction.[153] Research suggests its importance in enhancing muscle function and strength of muscle contraction.[156] Zinc is a constituent of enzymes involved in most major metabolic pathways. Supplementation of zinc in the presence of a deficiency could therefore support and enhance the surviving muscle fibers in the older adult and maximize the health and function of the remaining muscle tissue. This would surely impact the pelvic floor muscles.

Interestingly, Hamilton[157] provides evidence that vitamin C promotes the absorption of zinc by enhancing mitochondrial enzymatic reactions associated with increased physical demands for energy production. Though the evidence is limited in relation to the interaction of vitamin C and zinc in muscle functioning, the available research indicates that both vitamin C and zinc are effective at increasing the contractile strength of the muscles.[158] Paying attention clinically to the presence of vitamin C and/or zinc deficiencies, and supplementing when necessary, may not only impact the quality of contraction of the pelvic floor muscle, but could influence overall functional capabilities often associated with functional incontinence.

Magnesium deficiencies have been reported to contribute to bladder instability and also to bone health and muscle fitness.[159,160] In a prospective, randomized, double-blind, placebo-controlled study of women with sensory urgency or detrusor instability, and an associated magnesium deficiency, the researchers randomly assigned magnesium hydroxide (study group) or placebo (control group).[159] Pre- and post-treatment symptoms, frequency-volume charts, and cystometry results were compared. The women receiving magnesium reported a subjective improvement in their urinary symptoms compared with the women receiving placebo, who experienced little to no improvement in symptoms. There was not, however, a statistically significant difference in pre- and post-treatment urodynamic parameters despite the reported symptomatic improvement in the study group. Magnesium supplements were well tolerated without any side effects reported. These results suggest that magnesium hydroxide may be beneficial for detrusor instability or sensory urgency in women.[159]

Interestingly, in insulin-resistant patients with mild to moderate decrease in kidney function there is a high prevalence of magnesium deficiency. In a study by Sebekova,[160] the potential pathogenic role of magnesium deficiency in insulin-resistant individuals was studied in skeletal muscle free magnesium concentrations in patients with impaired kidney function. It was found by comparing the patient group with healthy controls that those in the study group had acidic pH levels in serum measures which were more expressed as measures of insulin resistance went up. Acidity of urine was substantially elevated in the study group with reduced kidney function. Serum creatinine levels and creatinine clearance correlated with intracellular pH in the patient group.[160] This suggests that the acidity of urine, and subsequent irritation of the bladder wall, could be a factor in urinary incontinence in individuals who are deficient in magnesium.

A relationship between vitamin B_{12} deficiency and incontinence has been established in older people.[161] It has been suggested that this is due to the neurological symptoms of sensory loss and mild dementia associated with this deficiency. A vitamin B_{12} deficiency may lead to diminished neurosensory input as to bladder fullness or inappropriate neurological stimulation of the bladder, causing instability. Dementia has also been implicated as a causal factor in the presence of urinary incontinence.

Many foods, food substances, dyes and chemical preservatives contained in foods, drug-nutrient interactions, nonfood substances such as tobacco, and overall composition of the diet have effects on the bladder.[148] Certain foods and nonfood substances are irritants to the wall of the bladder. These substances include caffeine, alcohol, tobacco (nicotine), chocolate, spices and spicy foods, acidic foods (tomatoes, citrus fruits), sugar substitutes (NutraSweet), sharp cheeses, coffee, tea, carbonated beverages, and chemical preservatives found in many foods and beverages. These foods may irritate the lining of the bladder and increase the urge and frequency to void. Consumption of these food substances and nonfood substances such as alcohol, nicotine, dyes, and chemical preservatives have been found to aggravate urinary incontinence causing bladder pain and spasms in many patients/ clients.

Nutrition and Dental Disease in the Elderly

Nutritional status has an important role in oral health. There is a sophisticated system of nutrient interaction that is essential to the formation of healthy teeth and the maintenance of oral and circumoral tissues throughout life.[162,163] The systemic effects of nutrients on oral health, growth and development, cell integrity and renewal, proper function of the tissues and saliva, tissue repair, and resistance and susceptibility to oral diseases are all important factors in the maintenance of adequate nutrition in the older adult.[164–166] Due to the extensive impact nutrition has on the oral cavity, the authors have summarized systemic effects of nutrients on oral health in Table 5–3.[162–167] Inadequate amounts of nutrients can result in fragile, friable oral tissues with a loss of adaptability and tolerance to irritants, and a loss of repair potential.[167] For many nutrient deficiencies, the oral cavity serves as an early warning system. Although not all nutrient deficiencies have oral manifestations, the most common ones are included in Table 7–3.

The theoretical link between food choices and masticatory efficiency has long been established. Recent evidence has confirmed this, demonstrating a progressive alteration in food choice with decreasing numbers of teeth, with the greatest effect being among those who are edentulous.[162,165,166] This altered food selection results in significant differences in the hematological status for some key nutrients. As diet is a risk factor for numerous systemic diseases, identifying where altered food choice is a consequence of reduced ability to chew might assist in addressing nutritional alternatives to prevent life-threatening consequences of deficiencies.[162,163,167] Adequate food and fluid intake and nutritional health are requisites for sustaining life. Though many oral functions remain intact in healthy older adults, significant alterations arise from oral and systemic diseases and their treatments. These may have a profound effect on eating, drinking, chewing, and swallowing, therefore negatively impacting the nutritional status of older individuals.[168] The care of older persons with smell, taste, dental or alveolar, oral mucosal, chewing, and swallowing problems requires a multidisciplinary team of health care providers.

Obesity and Nutrition In the Elderly

Obesity is common in persons aged 65 years or older. A diet that is higher in calories than required for the body's energy needs leads to energy storage and fat deposition. Excess calories from fat, carbohydrate, and protein foods leads to obesity. Some drugs promote appetite (hyperphagic drugs) leading to obesity because of increased food intake. Alcohol intake, in addition to a diet that provides sufficient food-energy to meet caloric needs, can also lead to obesity. Reduction in body weight in obese persons is commonly retarded or impeded by a disinclination for exercise. Exercise may also be restricted as a result of secondary effects of obesity, such as osteoarthritis and cardiovascular dysfunction leading to physical disabilities.

Obesity is associated with numerous medical disabilities. Causal relationships have been identified between obesity and the development of late-onset diabetes, essential hypertension, and hypertensive heart disease. Obesity increases the risk of cardiovascular disease. Data from the Framingham Heart Study demonstrate a continuous relationship between obesity and coronary morbidity and mortality (greater in men than in women). Obesity is associated with increased blood pressure and serum lipoprotein levels.[169] The effects of weight change on blood lipid profiles are considerable. The Framingham Study has shown that weight reduction results in modest increases in high-density lipoprotein (HDL) cholesterol.[170] It appears that both blood lipids and blood pressure are sensitive to the degree of obesity.

Obesity is the most common nutritional problem of public health concern in the United States.[171] While gross obesity is uncommon in the very old (because persons who are morbidly obese are more likely to die at an earlier age), obesity is still a serious disability in the elderly.

Obesity is also associated with the development of abdominal hernias. Gallbladder disease and gout are more common in obese individuals, and most importantly, obesity is associated with increased symptoms of degenerative osteoarthritis. Other complications include varicose veins with stasis dermatitis and stasis ulcers and bacterial and yeast infections between fat folds.[169,170]

In general, obesity is a hindrance to independent living in the elderly. Despite the limitations of modern actuarial reports and experimental finding, the data do show that obesity shortens life span and that limitation in food or caloric intake can result in a longer life.[91]

Nutrition and Immunity in the Elderly

Immune function declines with age, leading to increased infection and cancer rates in aged individuals.[106,172] In fact, recent progress in the study of immune system aging has introduced the idea that rather than a general decline in the functions of the immune system with age, immune aging is mainly characterized by a progressive appearance of immune dysregulation throughout life.[172,173] Nutritional factors play a major role in the immune responses of aged individuals and are of great consequence even in the very healthy elderly.

Systemic studies have confirmed that nutrient deficiencies impair immune system response and lead to frequent severe infections resulting in increased mortality, especially in the elderly.[173–176] Protein-energy

TABLE 7–3.   SYSTEMIC EFFECTS OF NUTRIENTS ON ORAL HEALTH AND ORAL MANIFESTATIONS OF NUTRITIONAL DEFICIENCIES

Nutrient	Systemic Effect on Oral Health	Oral Manifestations of Deficiency
Vitamin A	Oral epithelial integrity Tooth development Wound healing Taste bud development Saliva production	Candidiasis Gingiva hypertrophy, inflammation Peridontal disease Decreased taste acuity Diminished saliva production
Vitamin B complex	Wound healing	Fissures, dry, scaly lips Leukoplakia of oral mucosa (white thickened patches with fissures) Peridontal disease Papillary hypertrophy, magenta color, fissuring, glossitis of tongue
Vitamin B_1	Wound healing	
Vitamin B_2 (riboflavin)	Wound healing	Atrophic/enlarged papillae tongue Shiny, red, dry, fissured lips Magenta color of tongue
Vitamin B_3 (niacin)	Wound healing	Dry, scaly, fissured lips Irritated, inflammed, ulcerated, red, painful, denuded oral mucosa Tongue—glossitis, glossodynia Red, swollen, beefy tip and border of tongue Dorsum of tongue smooth and dry Ulcerative gingivitis
Vitamin B_6	Poor wound healing Sensation	Burning/sore mouth Dry, scaly, fissured lips Tongue—glossitis, glossodynia
Vitamin B_{12}	Poor wound healing Sensation Saliva production	Osteopenia/Osteoporosis Burning/sore mouth Bleeding gums Halitosis Dry, scaly, fissured lips Epithelial dysplasia of mucosa Oral paresthesias (burning, numbness, tingling) Loss or distortion of taste Ulcerations Beefy, red, glossy, smooth tongue
Vitamin C	Epithelial integrity Periodontal maintenance Tooth Formation Poor wound healing	Blood vessel fragility/bleeding Osteopenia/Osteoporosis; abnormal osteoid formation, fragility, loss Burning/sore mouth Gingivitis Oral infections Peridontal disease Tooth mobility/loosening
Vitamin D	Bone formation and maintenance Tooth formation and maintenance	Peridontal disease Osteopenia/Osteoporosis
Vitamin K		Candidiasis Bleeding gums
Calcium	Bone formation and maintenance Muscle tone maintenance Nerve impulse transmission Tooth formation and maintenance	Excess bone resorption, loss of mineral density, fragility Osteopenia/Osteoporosis Bleeding tendencies Periodontal disease Loss, mobile teeth/edentulous
Copper	Bone formation and maintenance Collagen synthesis Peridontal maintenance Wound healing	Decreased trabeculae/bone fragility
Folic acid	Epithelial integrity Wound healing Circulatory integrity	Burning/sore mouth Candidiasis/Mucositis/Stomatitis Atrophy or loss of papillae Gum inflammation Dry, scaly, fissured lips

(continued)

TABLE 7–3. (Continued)

Nutrient	Systemic Effect on Oral Health	Oral Manifestations of Deficiency
Folic acid (cont)		Glossitis of tongue Swollen, red tip/borders of tongue Slick, bald, pale, or fiery tongue Ulcerations Bleeding of gums and mucosa
Iron	Epithelial integrity Peridontal maintenance Sensation	Burning/sore mouth Bleeding of gums and mucosa Candidiasis Dental caries Dysphagia Atrophic papillae Dry, scaly, pale lips Oral infections and ulcerations Pale oral mucosa Oral paresthesias Atrophic, pale, glossitis tongue
Magnesium	Bone formation and maintenance Tooth formation and maintenance Wound healing Prevents tooth decay	Bone fragility/Osteoporosis Dental caries Swollen, bleeding gums
Phosphorus	Bone formation and maintenance Tooth formation and metabolism Prevents tooth decay	Dental decay Peridontal disease Tooth loss
Calcium-phosphorus	Bone maintenance Periodontal maintenance	Osteopenia/Osteoporosis Tooth loss
Protein	Epithelial integrity Taste bud renewal Tooth formation Wound healing Muscle integrity	Poor bone repair Fragility, burning sensation of epithelium of mouth Dry, scaly, fissured lips Oral infections with poor healing Periodontal disease Delayed wound healing
Protein-calorie	Maintenance of bone health Epithelial integrity	Bone loss Epithelial fragility Candidiasis Necrotizing ulcerative gingivitis Peridontal disease
Water	Epithelial integrity	Burning/sore mouth Dehydrated, fragile epithelium Diminished muscle strength Glossopytosis of tongue Dimished saliva production Dry mouth
Zinc	Epithelial integrity/metabolism Peridontal maintenance Taste bud renewal Wound healing	Candidiasis Dental caries Epithelial thickening Atrophic mucosa Peridontal disease Decreases smell acuity Decreased taste acuity Delayed wound healing Diminished saliva production

malnutrition results in reduced number and function of T cells, phagocytic cells, and secretory immunoglobin A antibody response. In addition, levels of many complement components are reduced.[173,175] Similar findings have been reported for moderate deficiencies of individual nutrients such as trace minerals and vitamins, particularly zinc, iron, selenium, vitamins A, B_6, C, and E.[173,174] For example, zinc deficiency is associated with profound impairment of cell-mediated immunity such as lymphocyte stimulation response and decreased chemotaxis of phagocytes. In addition, the level of thymulin, which is a zinc-dependent hormone, is markedly decreased.[173,177] The use of nutrient supplements, singly or in combination, stimulates immune response and may result in fewer infections in the elderly, as well as reducing the problems associated with malnourished, critically ill elderly patients.

Malnutrition is often one of the consequences of chronic and neoplastic diseases.[174–176] Additionally, secondary immunological changes occur as the result of environmental factors other than diet, including drug intake, physical activity, and stress, or are alternatively due to underlying diseases. For instance, the effects of high lipid intake as well as the impact of diseases, such as Alzheimer's disese and atherosclerosis, underline the complexity of immunological alterations to be expected in old age.[177] Because aging and malnutrition exert cumulative influences on immune responses, many elderly people have poor cell-mediated immune responses and are therefore at greater risk for infection and complications associated with an immunosuppressed response.[178]

Both excessive thinness[179] and severe obesity are associated with impaired immune responses, and obesity increases the risk of infection.[180] All forms of sugar (including honey) interfere with the ability of white blood cells to destroy bacteria. Diets high in sucrose impair immune system response.[181,182] Alcohol intake, including single episodes of moderate consumption, has an immunosuppresive effect.[183,184]

Excessive intake of total dietary fat impairs immune response, but some types of fat (monounsaturated fats, as found in olive oil) have no detrimental effects and may even be beneficial.[185,186] Research on the effect of the omega-3 fats abundant in fish, fish oils, and flaxseed oil, have been shown to improve immune system function and reduce infections in critically ill patients.[187] The positive effects of omega-3 fats have been demonstated to be further improved with the addition of antioxidants, especially vitamin E.[188]

As previously discussed, zinc supplements have been reported to increase immune function and this effect is particularly potent in the elderly, most of whom have zinc deficiencies.[189,190] Vitamin A plays an important role in immune system function and helps mucous membranes, including those in the lungs, resist invasion by microorganisms.[191] Beta-carotene and other carotenoids have increased immune cell numbers and activity in human research, an effect that appears to be separate from their role as precursors to vitamin A.[192] In the elderly, supplementation may increase natural killer cell activity.[193] Vitamin C stimulates the immune system by elevating interferon[194] levels and enhancing the activity of immune cells.[195] Vitamin E enhances all measures of immune cell activity in the elderly.[196] A combination of antioxidant vitamins A, C, and E has been found to significantly improve immune cell number and activity compared to placebo in a group of hospitalized elderly people.[197] Most double-blind studies find that elderly people have better immune function and reduced infection rates when taking a multivitamin.[198,199]

CLINICAL EVALUATION OF NUTRITIONAL STATUS

There are several physical findings related to nutritional status, and many of the normal changes of aging mimic clinical findings described as pathognomic of malnutritive states in the elderly.[2] Clinically overt malnutrition is rarely caused by a primary deficit in nutritional intake, rather it is more likely associated with gastrointestinal tract dysfunctions, or with one of the chronic debilitating illnesses common to the elderly. In contrast, subclinical malnutrition,[200] by definition, undetectable by physical findings on clinical evaluation, is probably frequent in certain at-risk elderly populations. These subgroups might include those who are institutionalized, those with mental disturbances or gross central nervous system disease, or those at or below the poverty level. In subclinical malnutritive states, an elderly individual may manifest depleted nutritional reserves as a failure to thrive. Diminished nutritional reserves may contribute to postoperative confusion, delayed recovery times of homeostatic function, slow wound healing, and increased susceptibility to infection.[201]

Anthropometric variables provide estimates of body composition that can be utilized as indicators of nutritional status. The most relevant of anthropometric measures are weight and skin-fold thickness.[202] Weight is a measure of all the constituents of the body. Weight, however, does not reflect any of the alterations or changes in the relative proportions of body constituents which accompany aging, specifically the increase in fat and decline in lean muscle mass. Variables, such as food or fluid intake, constipation, or problems producing edema are not accounted for by weight measures.[203,204] *Weight/height* measures have been standardized to define "ideal" weights. Another measure utilizing weight is a *weight/stature* measure. This measure provides a moderate correlation with percent of body fat and a high degree of correlation with total body fat in the elderly.[205] A third weight measure is *relative weight*. Height decreases approximately 3 cm during an average life span as a result of loss of bony mass secondary to osteoporosis, loss of joint space resulting from intervertebral disk shrinkage and wearing of articular cartilage, and postural changes, such as kyphosis due to anterior vertebral wedge fractures. Because of the potential inaccuracies in the estimation of height, other related measures are employed. For example, recumbent length or arm span measures are used for comparison to actual height measures. Arm span is a reasonable equivalent to height during all stages of the life span. The measure of "wing span" reflects the height prior to loss of stature with age. Relative weight is then determined utilizing adjusted height tables which have been standardized to account for possible height reduction adjusted for age.[206,207]

Other anthropometric measures include triceps/subscapular skin-fold thickness and upper arm circumference. The accuracy of skin-fold thickness measures in the elderly is questionable due to age-related changes in the skin and altered skin compressability. Upper arm circumference is a good measure of total body fat in edematous patients in cases where weight might be misleading. There are, however, progressive muscular changes associated with aging, specifically an increase in fibrous tissue, loss of muscle fibers, and an increase in intramuscular fat, that may confound the accuracy of this measure. Measuring skin-fold thickness at the inferior angle of the scapula is more precise than triceps caliper measures as a result of these confounding factors. It is important to recognize that all of these anthropometric measures do not actually measure nutritional status, rather, they provide an indicator of nutritional status. When compared with standardized norms, these measures provide a percentile nutritional rank for the individual patient.[209,210]

Laboratory evaluations that may contribute to nutritional evaluation or appropriate nutritional intervention include assessment of visceral protein status (serum transferrin or albumin), renal and liver function, pancreatic endocrine function (glucose), serum electrolytes and minerals (calcium, magnesium, and phosphorus), and hematologic evaluation (total lymphocyte count and red cell indices). Although not routinely used, delayed cutaneous hypersensitivity testing (skin test antigens) may be helpful to gauge systemic immune function. Determination of nitrogen balance by 24-hour urinary urea nitrogen (UUN) is helpful in nutritional intervention regimens, particularly in the use of enteral or parenteral nutrition. The aim of nutritional intervention is to minimize the degree of negative nitrogen balance (i.e., excessive loss of body protein not compensated by adequate nutritional intake). If nitrogen intake is less than output, the patient is considered to be in negative nitrogen balance, with a net loss of body protein. This contributes to progressive muscle wasting, fatigue, and immune compromise. Therefore obtaining this information is imperative in comprehensive nutritional assessment of elderly individuals.[209,210]

Functional assessment tools are also valuable in assessing the elderly individual's nutritional status. Increasingly, attention has been paid to the importance of maintaining essential activities of daily living among the aged. Simple questionnaires have been developed that appear to be closely associated with nutritional risk.[203,208-210] These provide another type of assessment tool important in assessing the overall nutrition-related functional status. Functional assessment tools such as those evaluating basic activities of daily living and instrumental activities of daily living provide important insights into the well-being of the aged.[203,209,211]

The clinical or physical examination may reveal findings associated with nutritional deficiencies.[209,210] The history and physical examination are the most important components of assessment of nutritional status. This should include weight history (current,

usual, and ideal); assessent of oral intake changes (type and duration); symptoms impacting nutrition (including anorexia, nausea and vomiting, diarrhea, constipation, stomatitis/mucositis, dry mouth, taste/olfactory abnormalitites, and pain); medications that may affect intake or metabolic requirements; other medical conditions that may affect nutritional intake or nutrition intervention options; and performance status evaluation. Physical examination entails a general assessment of physical condition, including evidence of weight loss, loss of subcutaneous fat, muscle wasting, presence of sacral or tibial edema, or ascites.

Table 7–4 provides possible clinical manifestations of nutritional deficiencies that can occur in the aged. It is important to keep in mind that before ascribing any physical findings elicited on physical examination to nutritional problems, the clinician should consider whether the findings are consistent with normal aging or with an underlying disease state.

Obtaining a quantitative as well as a qualitative dietary history can be helpful in dietary assessment, especially as a means of demonstrating to the elderly person or his or her family or caregiver that changes can be made to increase calorie, protein, and micronutrient intake. Useful data also include specific likes, dislikes, and intolerance of specific foods by the person. The latter may help to determine the need for specific supplemental nutients or enzymes (lactase, other disaccharidases, or pancreatic enzymes).

Malnutrition is an important predictor of morbidity and mortality. In the elderly, various subjective nutritional assessments have been developed that provide high inter-rater agreement, correlate with other measures of nutritional status, and predict subsequent morbidity. Familiarizing the rehabilitation professional with the information garnered from such tools is helpful in synchronizing nutritional with functional goals. Standardized staging criteria for degree of nutritional deficit or risk have been developed and validated in two commonly utilized tools.[210,212-214]

The Subjective Global Assessment (SGA) is a reproducible and valid tool for determining nutritional status in the institutional-[212] and community-dwelling elderly.[209] This evaluation tool has been validated in a number of patient populations including surgical, human immunodeficiency virus (HIV), acquired immunodeficiency syndrome (AIDS), renal dialysis, and cancer populations.[214] With appropriate training, the method is sensitive, specific, and has little interobserver variability. Figure 7–1 provides an example of information obtained by the SGA.[213] It is comprised of a patient survey and clinician evaluation that correlates with physical measures of skinfold caliper, weight, and height measures and nutritional status and has been determined to be highly predictive for morbidity and mortality.[209] The SGA has been found to be particularly sensitive in identifying elderly individuals who are undernourished or

TABLE 7–4. PHYSICAL MANIFESTATIONS OF MALNUTRITION

Nutrient Deficiency	Physical Manifestation
Protein	Edema; hypoalbuminemia; enlarged liver; diarrhea
Protein/Energy	Muscle wasting; sparse, thin, dry, brittle hair; dry, inelastic skin; muscle weakness
Vitamin A	Poor visual accommodation to dark; Bitot's spots (eyes); dryness of the eyes; hair loss; impaired taste; gooseflesh
Vitamin D	Bowed legs, beading of ribs, and other skeletal deformities (Rickets)
Vitamin K	Bleeding (poor coagulation of blood)
Thiamin (B_1)	Cardiac enlargement; mental confusion; irritability; calf muscle tenderness and foot drop; hypoflexia; hyperesthesia; paresthesia
Riboflavin (B_2)	Fissures around mouth; reddened, scaly, greasy skin around the nose and mouth; magenta-colored tongue
Niacin (B_3)	Bright red, swollen, painful tongue; pellagrous dermatitis; Depression, insomnia, headaches, dizziness; dementia; diarrhea
Pyridoxine (B_6)	Neuropathies; glossitis; nasolabial seborrhea
Folic Acid	Red, painful, shiny, smooth tongue; skin hyperpigmentation
Vitamin B_{12}	Mild dementia; sensory losses in hands and feet; red, smooth, shiny, painful tongue; mild jaundice; optic neuritis; anorexia; diarrhea
Vitamin C	Joint tenderness and swelling; hemorrhages under the skin; spongy gums that bleed easily; poor wound healing; petechiae
Essential Fatty Acids	Sparse hair growth; dry, flaky skin; depression and psychosis, dementia
Calcium	Poor reflexes; poor cardiovascular accommodation to activity; slow mental processing; depression; dementia
Magnesium	Lethargy and weakness; anorexia and vomiting; tremor; convulsions
Iodine	Goiter
Iron	Pallor; pale, atrophic tongue; spoon-shaped nails; pale conjunctivae
Zinc	Sluggish muscle contraction; poor wound healing; diminished taste and appetite; der-matitis, hair loss, diarrhea

at risk for developing undernutrition.[213] Similarly, the Mini Nutritional Assessment (MNA) is designed and validated to provide a single, rapid assessment of nutritional status in elderly patients in outpatient clinics, hospitals, and nursing homes.[210] The MNA has been found to be an efficient method for detecting malnutrition in the elderly, and also accurately predicts the one-year mortality.[215] It has been translated into several languages and validated in many clinics around the world. The MNA is composed of simple measurements and brief questions that can be completed in about ten minutes. Figure 7–2 provides a sample of the information collected by the MNA in its various formats.[215,126] Like the SGA, the MNA scale has also been found to be predictive of mortality as well as predictive of hospital cost.[210] Most important it is possible to identify people at risk for malnutrition before severe changes in weight or albumin levels occur. These individuals are more likely to have a decrease in caloric intake that can be easily corrected by nutritional intervention.[210]

NUTRITIONAL REQUIREMENTS OF THE ELDERLY

Many studies have been done on nutrition in institutionalized elders, but there are inherent difficulties in assessing the nutritional status of community elderly. As a group, there is very little information available relating to the nutritional quality of diets consumed by the elderly compared to any other age group.

Major nationwide surveys such as the USDA Food Consumption Surveys, the Department of Health and Human Services Ten State Nutrition Survey, and the National Health and Nutrition Examination Survey (NHANES), have been used to assess the nutritional status of the elderly. Findings vary depending on the age, sex, and economic status characteristics of the group surveyed and the methods used for study (e.g., clinical signs, biochemical measurements, or dietary intake surveys). These studies are hampered by the lack of anthropometric, biochemical, and clinical norms that are specific to the elderly.

In spite of this, some generalizations can be made. Diets of the elderly living independently in the community have been found to be more nutritionally adequate than those who are institutionalized or in nursing homes.[217,218] Dietary intake data reveal that a substantial portion of diets for the elderly are low in vitamins C and A, thiamine, calcium, iron, folate and zinc compared to the recommended dietary allowances (RDA). The prevalence of nutritional problems among the aged arising from low dietary intakes appears to be quite high. In national population and community-based surveys, intakes were low among those 65 years of age, especially among the poor, for protein, calcium, thiamine, vitamin D, folic acid, vitamin B_6 and zinc.[219] Many diets were found to have very low caloric intakes. Twenty-one percent of the white population and 36% of the black population had daily intakes of less than 1000 calories. Conversely, 25% of the lower income black and white women aged 45 to 75 years of age were found to be

---

Patient Name (last name, first name):_____ **Date:**_____

History

1. <u>Weight change</u>: Overall loss in past 6 months: amount = _____kg _____%
           Change in past 2 weeks: ☐ increase ☐ no change ☐ decrease

2. <u>Dietary intake change</u> (relative to normal) ☐ no change
           ☐ change   duration = _____weeks
       type: ☐ suboptimal solid diet   ☐ full liquid diet
           ☐ hypocaloric liquids   ☐ starvation

3. <u>Gastronintestinal symptoms</u> (that persisted for > 2 weeks)
     ☐ none   ☐ nausea   ☐ vomiting   ☐ diarrhea   ☐ anorexia

4. <u>Functional capacity</u> ☐ no dysfunction (i.e., full capacity)
       ☐ dysfunction   duration = _____weeks
       type: ☐ working suboptimally   ☐ ambulatory   ☐ bedridden

Physical (for each trait specify: 0 = normal, 1+ = mild, 2+ = moderate, 3+ = severe)
_____ loss of subcutaneous fat (triceps, chest)
_____ muscle wasting (quadriceps, deltoids)
_____ ankle edema
_____ sacral edema
_____ ascites (accumulation of fluid in the peritoneal cavity of abdomen)

Subjective Global Assessment rating (select one)
  YA = well nourished
  YB = moderately (or suspected of being) malnourished
  YC = severely malnourished

Figure 7–1. Subjective Global Assessment (SGA) (*Source: Sacks GS, Dearman K, Replogle WH, Cora VL, Meeks M, Canada T. Use of Subjective Global Assessment to identify nutrition-associated complications and death in geriatric long-term care facility residents. J Amer Coll Nutrition. 2001; 19(5):570–577.*)

obese. Protein was reported to be near or above the RDA with the exception of some low income groups. In fact, the elderly appear to maintain approximately the same ratio of protein, fat, and carbohydrate in their diets compared to younger cohorts, namely: 13% to 30% protein; 50% to 55% carbohydrate; and 30% to 35% fat. When biochemical methods were used, vitamins C, A, and B_6, thiamine, riboflavin, iron, zinc and calcium were most likely to be below RDA standards.[2] Despite the reporting of the inadequate dietary intake of these nutrients, there was a relative lack of clinical symptoms indicating nutrient deficiencies. Clinical signs other than iron deficiency were infrequently found. This leads one to question the appropriateness of RDA standards for good nutrition in an elderly population.

The aged are highly vulnerable to malnutrition because there is little direct experimental evidence available from which to establish nutritional standards or necessary dietary intake, especially for those aged 85 years and over. Information on the nutritional needs of the elderly have been derived by extrapolation from investigations using young adults.[171] Table 7–5 provides the most recent RDAs for individuals aged 40 years and older.

Because elderly adults have distinct metabolic characteristics that alter various nutrient requirements, simple extrapolations of nutrient requirements for younger adults are not warranted. Gastrointestinal function is well preserved with aging regarding the digestion and absorption of macromutrients, but the aging gastrointestinal tract becomes less efficient in absorbing vitamin B_{12}, vitamin D, and calcium.[31,220] The new dietary reference intakes considered recent studies in aging adults and concluded that the RDAs should be between 1200 mg to 1500 mg and 15 microg for calcium and vitamin D, respectively, for persons over the age of 70 years.[31,220,221] The new RDAs for riboflavin, niacin, thiamine, folate, vitamin B_6, and vitamin B_{12} are not different for persons in the oldest age category (> 70 years) than those aged 40 to 70 years.[31,220,221] Because this line of study

Last name:	First name	Sex:	Date:

Age:	Weight, kg:	Height, cm:	I.D. Number:

Complete the screen by filling in the boxes with the appropriate numbers. Add the numbers for the screen. If score is 11 or less, continue with the assessment to gain a Malnutrition Indicator Score.

Screening

Has food intake declined over the past 3 months due to loss of appetite, digestive problems, chewing or swallowing difficulties?

☐ 0 = severe loss of appetite
1 = moderate loss of appetite
2 = no loss of appetite

Weight loss during the last 3 month?

☐ 0 = weight loss greater than 3 kg (6.6 pounds)
1 = does not know
2 = weight loss between 1 and 3 kg (2.2 and 6.6 pounds)
3 = no weight loss

Mobility

☐ 0 = bed or chair bound
1 = able to get out of bed/chair but does not go out
2 = goes out

Has suffered psychological stress or acute disease

☐ 0 = yes 2 = no

Neuropsychological problems

☐ 0 = severe dementia or depression
1 = mild dementia
2 = no psychological problems

Body Mass Index (BMI) (weight in kg)/(height in m)^2

☐ 0 = BMI less than 19
1 = BMI 19 to less than 21
2 = BMI 21 to less than 23
3 = BMI 23 or greater

Screening score (subtotal max. 14 point)
12 points or greater = Normal—not at risk—no need to complete assessment
11 points or below = Possible malnutrition—continue assessment

Assessment

Lives independently (not in a nursing home or hospital)

☐ 0 = no 1 = yes

Takes more than 3 prescription drugs per day

☐ 0 = no 1 = yes

Pressure sore or skin ulcers

☐ 0 = no 1 = yes

Continued

—— *Continued from previous page* ——

How many full meals does the patient eat daily?

☐ 0 = 1 meal
1 = 2 meals
2 = 3 meals

Select consumption markers for protein intake

☐•☐ —At least one serving of dairy products (milk, cheese, yogurt) per day? ☐ yes ☐ no
—Two or more servings of legumes or eggs per week? ☐ yes ☐ no
—Meat, fish, or poultry every day? ☐ yes ☐ no

0.0 = if 0 or 1 yes
0.5 = if 2 yes
1.0 = if 3 yes

Consumes two or more servings of fruits or vegetables per day

☐ 0 = no   1 = yes

How much fluid (water, juice, coffee, tea, milk . . .) is consumed per day?

☐•☐ 0.0 = less than 3 cups
0.5 = 3 to 5 cups
1.0 = more than 5 cups

Mode of feeding

☐ 0 = unable to eat without assistance
1 = self-fed with some difficulty
2 = self-fed without any difficulty

Self view of nutritional status

☐ 0 = views self as being malnourished
1 = is uncertain of nutritional state
2 = views self as having no nutritional problem

In comparison with other people of the same age, how does the patient consider his/her health status?

☐•☐ 0.0 = not as good
0.5 = does not know
1.0 = as good
1.0 = better

Mid-arm circumference (MAC) in cm

☐•☐ 0.0 = MAC less than 21
0.5 = MAC 21 to 22
1.0 = MAC 22 or greater

Calf circumference (CC) in cm

0 = CC less than 31
1 = CC 31 or greater

Assessment (max. 16 points)	☐ ☐•☐
Screening score	☐ ☐
Total Assessment (max. 30 points)	☐ ☐•☐

Malnutrition Indicator Score

17 to 23.5 pints   at risk of malnutrition   ☐

Less than 17 points   Malnourished   ☐

Figure 7–2. Mini Nutritional Assessment (MNA) *(Sources: Riogo SP, Sanchez-Vilar O, Gonzalez de Villar N. Geriatric nutrition: studies about MNA. Nutr Hosp. 1999; 14(5)suppl 2:32S–42S. Guigoz Y, Vallas B, Garry PJ. Mini Nutritional Assessment: A practical assessment tool for grading the nutritional state of elderly patients. Facts and Research in Gerontology. 1994; Suppl 2:15–59.)*

Table 7–5. RECOMMENDED DAILY ALLOWANCES (REVISED 2000)

Males	40-50 yrs	51-70 yrs	70+ yrs
Weight (kg)[a]	70	70	70
Height (cm)[a]	173	171	170
Energy (kg)	2600	2400	2200
Protein (gr)	65	65	65
Fat Soluble Vitamins			
Vitamin A (I.U.)	5000	5000	5000
Vitamin D (I.U.)	400	400	400
Vitamin E (I.U.)	30	30	30
Vitamin C (mg)	60	60	60
Folate acid (mg)	0.4	0.4	0.4
Niacin (mg equiv)	18	17	17
Riboflavin (mg)	1.7	1.7	1.7
Thiamine (mg)	1.3	1.2	1.2
Water Soluble Vitamins			
Vitamin B_6 (mg)	2.0	2.0	2.0
Vitamin B_{12} (µg)	5	5	5
Calcium (mg)	800	800	800
Phosphorus (gm)	0.8	0.8	0.8
Iodine (µg)	125	110	100
Iron (mg)	10	10	10
Magnesium (mg)	350	350	350
Zinc (µg)	15	15	15
Selenium (µg)	60	60	60
Females			
Weight (kg)	58	58	60
Height (cm)	160	157	154
Energy (kg)	1850	1700	1650
Protein (gr)	55	55	55
Fat Soluble Vitamins			
Vitamin A (I.U.)	5000	5000	5000
Vitamin D (I.U.)	400	400	400
Vitamin E (I.U.)	25	25	25
Vitamin C (mg)	60	100	100
Folate acid (mg)	0.4	0.4	0.4
Niacin (mg equiv)	13	12	12
Riboflavin (mg)	1.5	1.5	1.5
Thiamine (mg)	1.0	1.0	1.0
Water Soluble Vitamins			
Vitamin B_6 (mg)	2.0	2.0	2.0
Vitamin B_{12} (µg)	5	6	6
Calcium (mg)	1500	1500	1500
Phosphorus (gm)	1.5	1.5	1.5
Iodine (µg)	100	90	80
Iron (mg)	18	10	10
Magnesium (mg)	300	300	300
Zinc (µg)	15	15	15
Selenium (µg)	55	55	55

Weights and heights represent actual median weights and heights for age groups derived from national data collected by the National Center for Health Statistics. From Committee on Dietary Allowances of the Food and Nutrition Board of the National Academy of Science/Nutrition Research Council, 2000.

is a quickly advancing field, it will be important to closely follow new research on nutrient requirements and aging over the next several years.

The increasing relative and absolute number of elderly in most countries and the high prevalence of disease in the higher age groups make the lack of nutritional standards an important concern. Both the aging process per se and the effects of disease on nutritional status add difficulties to determining RDAs based on chronological age. Not only disease, but also factors such as impaired vision, presbycusis, oral health, smoking, and alcohol use or misuse may complicate nutrition in the elderly. Cohort differences may have a marked impact on nutrition regarding several factors. In many countries meal habits and intake of energy and nutrients in at least young elderly are on average acceptable.[218] However, variation is marked. Standardizing nutient requirements from the perspective of prevention and dietary habits becomes an ominous task.

Lowenstein[222] reviewed the problem of lack of nutrient standards for the aged. It was found that the quality of the diet required by the aged is higher. Caloric needs decrease because of reduced metabolic rates and lower levels of physical activity, while needs for protein, vitamins and minerals stay more or less constant. Thus, nutrient density (i.e., nutrients per calorie) necessary to fulfill recommended dietary allowances is higher for the aged when compared to younger adults.[222] The fact that separate guidelines have not been established for advancing age (except for extrapolations for the 55 and over age group) reflects the lack of solid knowledge of the needs of the elderly. When this is coupled with the fact that (1) the elderly are much less uniform compared to other age groups with respect to biological, anatomical and physiological aging; (2) the elderly have an increased susceptibility to disease and chronic illness; and (3) there are a variety of other social and psychological influences that affect diet, which makes it unlikely that a specific standard can be devised that accounts for all these factors.[218]

The aged are vulnerable and at high risk of developing nutritional problems because of various social, psychological, and physical factors,[171] including living alone (especially if there has been a recent bereavement or significant negative life event), lack of an effective family or community support network, and low income. Psychological factors such as depression, mental deterioration, and impaired self-concept, increase the risk of nutritional deficiencies. Physical factors, such as functional dependence, sensory impairment, and limited mobility (especially when they are associated with severe chronic degenerative diseases), also have a negative influence. Indices of nutritional risk using these factors are proving useful in identifying the aged with more nutritional deficits than their hospitalized or institutionalized peers.[209]

The elderly generally have a progressive decline in exercise levels and a proportional decrease in energy expenditure, which, when linked to the decrease in their BMR, suggests the need to progressively reduce caloric intake.[223]

Recommendations for dietary intake according to the food pyramid have been altered for those individuals aged 70 and older. Figure 7–3 is the modified food pyramid for the mature (70 and over) adult.

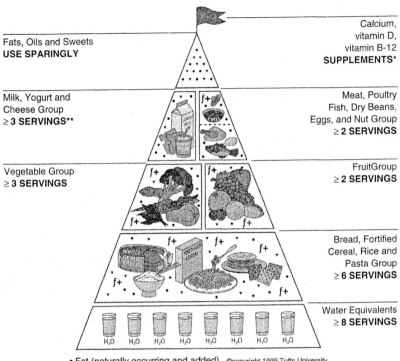

Fats, Oils and Sweets
USE SPARINGLY

Calcium,
vitamin D,
vitamin B-12
SUPPLEMENTS*

Milk, Yogurt and
Cheese Group
≥ 3 SERVINGS**

Meat, Poultry
Fish, Dry Beans,
Eggs, and Nut Group
≥ 2 SERVINGS

Vegetable Group
≥ 3 SERVINGS

FruitGroup
≥ 2 SERVINGS

Bread, Fortified
Cereal, Rice and
Pasta Group
≥ 6 SERVINGS

Water Equivalents
≥ 8 SERVINGS

• Fat (naturally occurring and added)   ©copyright 1999 Tufts University
▼ Sugars (added)
ƒ +Fiber (should be present)
These symbols show fat, added sugars, and fiber in foods
* Not all individuals need supplements, consultyour healthcare provider
** ≥ Greater than or equal to

Figure 7–3.   Modified Food Pyramid
for Mature (70+) Adults

COMMON NUTRITIONAL DEFICIENCIES IN THE AGED

The need for the forty-two essential nutrients remains qualitatively similar over the life span. However, quantitative changes for some nutrient requirements are of importance to the elderly individual. When diet-related disorders are present, additional alterations in nutrients may also be necessary. When mean population intakes of a nutrient are below a standard, such as the RDA, nutritionists regard it as a "problem nutrient." Surveys of the aged reveal that mean intakes of calories and calcium are low and often problematic, and that, while mean intakes of protein are adequate, at least a third of those surveyed have intakes below the standard, especially in certain subgroups of the population.[219,224] Other vitamins and mineral present special problems for certain groups of the aged and will be discussed. Although vitamin and mineral deficiencies are presumed to be more common in the elderly, there is little experimental data on which to estimate exact daily requirements of these so-called micronutrients in the diet. Increased need, with age, for vitamins and minerals may result from less efficient absorption, altered metabolism and excretion, and increasing use of certain medications. It is important to remember that any nutrient may be insufficient or in excess and can constitute a problem for the elderly.

Calories/Energy Intake

The RDA for energy intake is just enough kilocalories to maintain an energy balance. As indicated in Table 7–5 the specific recommendations for calories in people aged 51 to 70 is 2400 kcalories for men, and 1700 kcal for women. The unstated range is from 2000 to 2800 kcal and 1200 to 2000 kcal for men and women, respectively. For those aged 70 and older, the recommendation is for 2200 kcal for men (range 1650 to 2450) and 1650 kcal for women (range 1200 to 2000).

Four major factors influence energy needs: (1) resting energy expenditure, (2) physical activity, (3) growth, and (4) thermogenesis (heat production secondary to food consumption, exercise, or cold stress). Resting energy expenditure and physical activity both decline with age, and therefore, energy needs are lower. Linear growth does not occur in the aged organism, although during recovery, healing, and rehabilitation, lean body mass and fat may be synthesized, which requires energy. Thermogenesis (heat production), a relatively minor contributor to energy needs at any age, is not known to differ between aged and younger persons. Resting metabolic rate differs with age chiefly because lean body mass, which is metabolically active tissue, decreases by about 3 kg per decade after age 50. Cellular metabolic rate also decreases with age. It is assumed that energy allowances should decrease by 6% from ages 51 to 70 years, and by another 6% after age 76 to account for reductions in resting metabolism. Energy output in the form of physical activity declines with age. Currently a decrease of 300 kcal for men and 200 kcal for women is recommended for ages 51 to 70 years, with an additional 500 kcal for men and 400 kcal for women substracted after age 70 years to account for reduced activity levels.

The effects of aging on energy requirements and energy balance suggest that current RDAs underestimate the usual energy needs of adults of all ages, including older adults.[225] Investigations have found a significant negative association between body fatness and energy expenditure for physical activity, and a signigicant position association between energy expenditure for physical activity and fat-free mass.[225] Surveys report that energy intakes among the aged are so low as to be inadequate for a significant proportion of the population.[224–227] One might conclude that, in view of such low intakes, a large proportion of the aged are extremely lean if not emaciated. However, median weights at age 70 are 5 kg higher in men and 7 kg higher in women compared to younger cohorts.[225]

Certainly this argues against widespread starvation among the aged. One explanation for this discrepancy is that the energy intake standards are too high. Some evidence suggests that, in healthy individuals of desirable weight, energy intake recommendations and outputs closely agree.[228] Many elderly are ill, and with increasing age and illness interindividual differences in energy requirements and body weight become more pronounced.[229] Limitations on physical activity caused by chronic diseases, such as arthritis, hip fractures, emphysema, osteoporosis, congestive heart failure, cerebral vascular accidents, peripheral vascular disease, and other degenerative conditions, limit physical activity, and consequently, reduce energy needs in at least one tenth of the population over 65 years of age.[217] Among the very old, especially those who are in nursing homes, energy needs are often only slightly above basal metabolic rate. While the energy need is lower for some aged, it is extremely high for others. When neuromuscular coordination declines, mechanical efficiency is reduced, and difficulties in balance control are increased, the energy cost of movement is greatly increased.

Age-related changes in body composition can be considered the consequence of changes in energy and protein metabolism, while also having a leverage effect on protein and energy requirements.[24] Changes in organ and systems weights obviously affect energy balance regulation. Considered at the system level, age-related changes are numerous, but it is still debated whether they are related to aging per se or to conditions (such as poor nutrition, disease, drug treatments, etc.) that prevail in elderly persons. It is likely that most changes occurring in the gastrointestinal, circulatory, and immune system do not af-

fect energy and protein requirements at rest. However, aging is associated with difficulties in adapting to new environmental conditions that lead to stress. Repeated episodes of stress might lead to accumulation of deficits that can affect energy and protein balances.[24]

Protein/Energy Malnutrition

The RDA for protein is 0.8 g per kilogram of high quality protein per day. On average this amounts to approximately 56 g for men and 44 g for women.[222,230] The latest RDA shoots for a slightly higher consumption of protein for the average weight, healthy older adult as established in Table 7–5.[31,220] On average, a healthy adult requires approximately .36 grams of protein per pound of body weight. Using this formula, a 140-pound person would need 50 g (or less than 2 ounces) of protein per day.[231] Protein requirements are more likely to be affected by stresses, such as disease, that may increase dietary protein requirements by two or more times. The reduced contribution of muscle to body protein metabolism in the aged may decrease the ability of the individual to adapt during periods of restricted dietary energy or protein intake, when protein synthesis in vital organs is maintained by mobilization of amino acids from the periphery.[232,233] The reduction in energy intake is likely to increase protein needs because the efficiency of protein utilization depends on energy balance. An allowance of 12% to 14% of the total energy needs of the elderly should come from protein sources.[233]

Clinical correlates of nutritional indicators for protein intake used in large surveys have not been well established. For example, a decrease in serum albumin does not occur early in states of protein deficiency states, however, declines are significant when a pure deficiency state exists. There is a gradual decline in serum albumin that normally accompanies advancing age,[234] but, a drop in serum albumin does not usually occur in the initial stages of protein deficiency, rather, it shows significant declines only in the advanced stages of severe deficiency. This makes interpretation of lab results of serum albumin levels difficult with respect to the elderly. A serum albumin below the normal range for adults could be an indication of a normal age-related change or protein malnutrition.

Chronic protein-energy malnutrition is synonymous with cachexia. Cachexia usually results from low food intake secondary to anorexia. In the elderly, common causes of cachexia are cancer, chronic neurological disease with associated paralysis, end stage hepatic or renal disease, and cardiac cachexia resulting from high dosage digitalis therapy. While cachexia is mainly due to reduced energy and protein intake, additional causes are the catabolic effects of disease and excessive losses of nutrients by malabsorption or through protein-losing enteropathy (any disease of the intestine).

Amino Acids

Amino acids are the building blocks of protein. Twenty amino acids are needed to build the various proteins used in the growth, repair, and maintenance of body tissues. Eleven of these amino acids can be made by the body itself, while the other nine (called essential amino acids) must come from the diet. The classification of an amino acid as essential or nonessential does not reflect its importance because all twenty amino acids are necessary for health. Rather, this classification system simply reflects whether or not the body is capable of manufacturing a particular amino acid.[233]

The essential amino acids are isoleucine, leucine, lysine, methionine, phenylalanine, threonine, tryptophan, histidine, and valine. The nonessential amino acids are arginine, alanine, asparagine, aspartic acid, cysteine, glutamine, glutamic acid, glycine, proline, serine, and tyrosine.

Foods of animal origin, such as meat, fish, poultry, eggs, and dairy products, are the richest dietary sources of the essential amino acids. However, the outdated belief that vegetarians need to be concerned about combining certain foods to obtain enough essential amino acids has been disproved.[233] Simply by consuming enough calories it appears that adequate nutrients for the production of amino acids are provided. In fact the term *protein malnutrition* has been replaced by the term *protein-calorie malnutrition.* Nutritionists recommend that protein, as a source of amino acids, account for 10% to 12% of calories in a balanced diet. An appropriate range of protein intake for healthy older adults, dependent on activity level, would be between 45 and 65 g daily. Most diets provide more protein than the body needs, however, in the elderly, protein food sources (meats, dairy products, legumes, etc) are often omitted from the diet, placing the older individual at higher risk for protein-calorie malnutrition.

Calcium/Vitamin D

Calcium is the most abundant mineral in the human body. Calcium is needed to form bones and teeth and is also required for blood clotting, transmission of signals in nerve cells, and muscle contraction. Although calcium plays at least some minor role in lowering blood pressure, the mechanisms involved appear complex and remain somewhat unclear.[235] Calcium also appears to partially bind some fats and cholesterol which positively influences overall cholesterol levels.[236] The importance of calcium for preventing osteoporosis is probably its most well-known role.

Nutrient requirements, according to the RDAs, remain relatively constant with advancing age. Studies have revealed, however, that calcium intake should more closely approximate 1500 mg/day, especially in women.[63] This will aid in preventing postmenopausal osteoporosis. In addition, since calcium maintains an inverse relationship to phosphorus, the ingestion of foods that have high levels of phosphorus, such as carbonated drinks and meats, should be reduced. A reduction in dietary phosphorus could result in higher total body calcium and perhaps delay or reduce the rate of development of osteoporosis. Exercise has been shown to have a further beneficial effect on calcium absorption and utilization. This is discussed in Chapter 11, Orthopedic Treatment Considerations.

Several factors negatively influence adequate calcium nutrition in the elderly. Intake of calcium among the aged is low and frequently does not meet the RDA.[227] Absorption of dietary calcium in the gut is poor,[237] and the ability to adapt to a low calcium diet decreases with age.[238] There are several possible explanations for this. Decreased sensitivity to parathyroid hormone decreases thyroid production of the polypeptide hormone calcitonin, which decreases serum levels of this endrocrine component ultimately decreasing calcium absorption from the gut.[239] Calcitonin regulates the balance of calcium and phosphate in the blood by direct action on bone and kidney. Since passive absorption accounts for only half of calcium absorbed by the gut and the active transport process of calcium absorption requires calcitrol (the dietary nutrient product of conversion of calcitonin), decreases in this nutrient decrease absorption with advancing age.[240] Thus, dietary calcium absorbed by the gut contributes less to the maintenance of serum calcium, and bone is resorbed to maintain serum calcium.

Other factors that enhance the risk of poor calcium nutrition are large amounts of protein in the diet, which increases urinary calcium losses,[241] and high levels of phosphorus, which increase calcium fecal losses.[242] Protein has profound effects on urinary calcium levels and on calcium nutriture. Doubling of dietary protein has been found to increase urinary calcium by as much as 50%.[241] Since the kidney filters as much as 10 g of calcium per day, these differences may be of great consequence in calcium metabolism.[243] Protein increases the obligatory renal loss of calcium, and its sulphur-containing amino acids are oxidized to sulfate during metabolism. The sulfates are then eliminated by a compensatory decrease in the tubular reabsorption of calcium. Even in the presence of large amounts of phosphorus in the diet, the effect that phosphorus has on decreasing urinary calcium is not enough to prevent protein's negative effect.[240]

Sodium also increases urinary calcium loss at the tubualar level,[240] and very high levels of dietary fiber intake (e.g., >30 g) may affect the absorption of calcium as well. Both dietary fiber and phytic acid, which is often associated with the bran portion of cereals, decrease calcium absorption. Oxalic acid (found in rhubarb and spinach) also decreases calcium absorption.

Caffeine increases both the amount of calcium secreted in digestive juice and the amount of renal calcium losses. Alcohol also increases urinary calcium losses, and at very high levels, it may have an adverse effect on bone cell metabolism.

One significant hormonal event that influences calcium nutrition is menopause. Estrogens increase calcium absorption and decrease renal losses, so that on the same calcium intake, the estrogen-replete female utilizes dietary calcium better. Postmenopausal estrogen replacement therapy is often considered for preventing negative calcium balance and osteoporosis in women who have poor dietary intake of calcium and have low activity levels or are sedentary. Growth hormones and hormonal events such as pregnancy also increase absorption and decrease renal lossess. Men are not excluded from the hormonal influences on bone loss. With andropause, the lower levels of testosterone and progesterone influence calcium absorption similar to that seen in menopausal and postmenopausal women. (See Chapter 3, Comparing and Contrasting Age-Related Changes in Biology, Physiology, Anatomy, and Function for further discussion of menopause and andropause).

Dietary supplements may contain one of several different forms of calcium. Calcium carbonate supplements have been found to contain higher levels of elemental calcium compared with calcium citrate, and as a result, fewer tablets are required to supplement calcium.[244] Calcium carbonate appears to be as bioavailable as the calcium found in milk and is readily absorbed.[244] Hydrochloric acid is required to break calcium down in the stomach. Therefore, products (often touted as the best sources of calcium) that decrease gastric acid (i.e., antacids) may actually inhibit the breakdown and subsequent absorption of calcium.[245,246] Of interest is that research has found that adding hydrochloric acid in acid-deplete elderly actually restores calcium absorption.[247] It must additionally be noted that consumption of a meal along with calcium supplementation and the introduction of hydrochloric acid can improve absorption of this nutrient even more. It has also been shown that consumption of a meal without addition of hydrochloric acid results in better absorption of calcium.[245] Often the discomfort elders experience is the result of gastric immotility rather than acid indigestion. As discussed in previous sections of this chapter, the poor production of gastric acids is often a bigger problem for older individuals than too much acid. Besides what sort of calcium supplements are best absorbed, when to take calcium is also important. As mentioned above, better absorption occurs when taken with a meal. It has also been shown that supplementing calcium in the evening appears better for osteoporosis prevention than taking calcium in the morning, based on the circadian rhythm of bone loss.[248]

The current RDA for vitamin D is 400 IU per day. The most important role for vitamin D is maintaining blood levels of calcium, which it accomplishes by increasing calcium absorption and reducing urinary calcium loss. It also plays a role in immunity and blood formation,[249] and helps cells "differentiate"—a process that may reduce the risk of cancer. Vitamin D is needed for adequate blood levels of insulin[250] and has been reported to help the body process sugar.[251]

Bone loss is significantly increased during the winter months secondary to the decrease in ultraviolet rays of the sun. One hypothesis says this is a result of a lack of vitamin D necessary for calcium absorption. A vitamin D deficiency is defined biochemically as levels of calcitrol below 3.8 µg/mL. Among institutionalized and housebound aged who are not taking vitamin D supplements, this biochemical indicator of vitamin D deficiency is relatively prevalent.[252] Osteomalacia, or undermineralized bone, sometimes contributes to the increase incidence of fractures among the aged.[253] Because several foods are fortified with vitamin D, however, intakes are higher and deficiencies somewhat rarer in the United States compared with other countries.[254] It has been shown that an individual can get enough vitamin D from milk. The causes of osteomalacia include vitamin D disturbances due to inadequate exposure to sunlight, dietary deficiency, and altered absorption or metabolism of the vitamin due to disease.

Iron

Iron is part of hemoglobin, the oxygen-carrying component of the blood. Iron-deficient individuals tire easily because their bodies are starved for oxygen. Iron is also part of myoglobin, which helps muscle cells store oxygen. Without enough iron, adenosine triphosphate (ATP, the fuel the body runs on) cannot be properly synthesized. As a result, iron deficiency leads to fatigue.

The current RDA for iron is 10 mg/day for individuals 51 years and older. The need for iron declines with age among females. This is a postmenopausal event since iron is no longer lost through menstrual bleeding and childbearing. Counterbalancing decreased iron loss, there is some evidence that the efficiency of iron absorption may be decreased among the aged. This is due to the presence of atrophic gastritis, which makes the body less able to use the hydrochloric acid available to reduce iron from the oxidized (ferric) form to the absorbable form (ferrous).[255] Other factors that decrease iron absorption among the aged are frequent use of antacids, calcium supplements, and tea, all of which form complexes with iron in the gut and decrease absorption. Some elderly individuals decrease their intake of red meat and other animal flesh foods rich in highly bioavailable iron because of dental difficulties or limited incomes. Instead they rely on plant foods, which are generally lower in bioavailable iron. Some aged also decrease their intakes of ascorbic acid-rich foods and protein-rich foods, thereby decreasing intakes of ascorbic acid and amino acids, two enhancers of iron absorption.

Concerns about iron in the elderly usually focus on its role in blood production. Lack of iron is a causation factor of anemia, however, evidence that iron deficiency anemias are a normal part of aging is weak, though the incidence of anemia increases with age. Experimental animal models do not show that aging is accompanied by anemia, although hematopoeitic reserve capacity, or the time it takes for hematocrit to recover after stress is increased.[256] Reductions in hematocrit which are not associated with dietary iron deficiency, chronic disease, or blood loss are usually a result of an abnormality in cellular proliferation.[257] Anemias due to other causes are common. Indeed, in contrast to popular belief, iron deficiency anemia is not the sole or major cause of anemia in the aged. In addition to lack of iron, nutritional anemias due to deficiency of ascorbic acid, vitamin B_6, vitamin B_{12}, folic acid, and protein-calorie malnutrition are also observed.[258] Blood losses of iron may be due to alcohol abuse, frequent use of aspirin, infection, neoplasms, and renal disease.

Vitamin B_{12}

Vitamin B_{12} is needed for nerve cell activity, DNA replication, and works with folic acid to control homocysteine levels. A vitamin B_{12} deficiency can cause fatigue.

Different surveys have found either no change or decreased levels of vitamin B_{12} in the elderly.[259,260] Achlorhydria, which decreases B_{12} absorption, occurs in 15% to 20% of persons over age 40.[261] In the elderly, a vitamin B_{12} deficiency is commonly due to lack of gastric intrinsic factor, which causes malabsorption of vitamin B_{12}. In pernicious anemia, a disease common in the elderly, the production of gastric intrinsic factor ceases and there is a complete lack of gastric acid production (achlorhydria).[262] Pernicious anemia is an autoimmune disease in which megaloblastic and neurological signs are caused by vitamin B_{12} deficiency. Vitamin B_{12} from the diet cannot be absorbed in the absence of gastric intrinsic factor. The aging process increases the risk of autoimmune disease within the gut. B_{12} deficiency produces both megablastic anemia and neurologic symptoms including mild dementia, sensory losses in the hands and feet, and a painful, red, smooth and shiny tongue. In addition, a mild jaundice appearance is commonly seen in an individual with a vitamin B_{12} deficiency. Pernicious anemia represents one of the conditions associated with the syndrome of polyglandular failure (as described by Addison in 1955).[263] Thus, in elderly patients with B_{12} deficiency other associated diseases, such as hypothyroidism, diabetes mellitus, and Addison's disease (adrenal failure), are often found.

Folic Acid

Folic acid, a part of the vitamin B complex, is needed for DNA synthesis. DNA allows cells, including cells in the fetus when a woman is pregnant, to replicate normally. Adequate intake of folic acid early in pregnancy is important for preventing most neural tube birth defects.[264] Folic acid is also needed to keep homocysteine levels in blood from rising. Folic acid is required by the body to utilize vitamin B_{12}. Proteolytic enzymes and antacids inhibit folic acid absorption.[265,266]

Low folic acid levels have been found in depressed institutionalized elderly and elderly in general hospitals as well as among elderly living at home. Serum folate levels less than 3.0 mg/mL or red cell folate less than 140 mg/mL are indicative of folate deficiency which may be caused by inadequate dietary intake due to poor food choices that is often related to alcoholism; use of drugs, such as anticonvulsants that interfere with the absorption or metabolism of folate; the increased use of heat processed foods (i.e., TV dinners) with reduced folate content; a restricted intake associated with poor dentition; gastrointestinal surgery that reduces folate absorption; or impaired folate metabolism. Intakes of 400 μg per day are usually sufficient to meet the needs of the older population. Garry and co-workers[259] found that among healthy elderly subjects low plasma folate and erythrocyte folate levels were common. The subjects, however, did not have significantly increased mean corpuscular volumes, which is a pathological consequence of folate deficiency (e.g., increased red blood cell production). Other studies in elderly people with low incomes or physical or mental deterioration have shown that folate deficiency is not uncommon in this group.[267] Further, Elsborg[268] has shown that in elderly subjects with nutritional folate deficiency, folate absorption is impaired. This malabsorption of folate appears to be related to the folate deficiency itself and can be reversed by treatment with folic acid. Besides its effect on red blood cells, it has been suggested that folate deficiency may produce mental dysfunction in the elderly.[269,270]

Vitamin B_1

Vitamin B_1 (thiamine) is needed to process carbohydrates, fat, and protein. Every cell of the body requires vitamin B_1 to form ATP—the fuel the body runs on. Nerve cells require vitamin B_1 in order to function normally. Deficiency is most commonly found in alcoholics, people with malabsorption conditions, and those eating a poor quality diet.[271]

Vitamin B_2

Vitamin B_2 (riboflavin) is needed to process amino acids and fats, activate vitamin B_6 and folic acid, and help convert carbohydrates into ATP. Under some circumstances, vitamin B_2 can act as an antioxidant. Vitamin B_2 deficiency can occur in alcoholics, and may be more likely in people with cataracts[271] or sickle cell anemia.[272]

Vitamin B$_3$

The body uses vitamin B$_3$ (niacin, niacinamide) in the process of releasing energy from carbohydrates. Vitamin B$_3$ comes in two basic forms—niacin (also called nicotinic acid) and niacinamide (also called nicotinamide). It is needed to form fat from carbohydrates and to process alcohol. The niacin form of vitamin B$_3$ also regulates cholesterol,[273] though niacinamide does not. An example of a severe vitamin B$_3$ deficiency is pellegra, a chronic disease characterized by gastrointestinal disturbances, skin eruptions, and mental disorders resulting from a lack of nicotinic acid in the diet.

Vitamin B$_5$

Pantothenic acid, sometimes called vitamin B$_5$, is involved in the Krebs cycle of energy production and is needed to make the neurotransmitter acetylcholine. It is also essential in producing, transporting, and releasing energy from fats. Synthesis of cholesterol (needed for vitamin D and hormone synthesis) depends on pantothenic acid. Pantothenic acid also activates the adrenal glands.[274] Pantethine, a variation of pantothenic acid, has been reported to lower blood levels of cholesterol and triglycerides.[275] Vitamin B$_5$ deficiencies may occur in people with alcoholism but are generally believed to be rare.

Vitamin B$_6$

Vitamin B$_6$ (pyridoxine) is the master vitamin in the processing of amino acids, the building blocks of all proteins and some hormones. Vitamin B$_6$ helps to make and take apart many amino acids and is also needed to make serotonin, melatonin, and dopamine. Vitamin B$_6$ also aids in the formation of several neurotransmitters and is therefore an essential nutrient in the regulation of neurological and mental processes and possibly mood.[276] Vitamin B$_6$ lowers homocysteine levels to a small degree. Vitamin B$_6$ deficiencies cause impaired immunity, peripheral neuropathy, and mental confusion. Deficiencies have been noted to occur in individuals with diabetes mellitus and in women on either hormone replacement therapy or on oral contraceptives. Alchoholics and renal failure patients also experience marginal vitamin B$_6$ deficiencies.[277]

Biotin

Biotin, a water-soluble B vitamin, acts as a coenzyme during the metabolism of protein, fats, and carbohydrates. Certain rare genetic diseases can leave people with depletion of biotin due to the inability to metabolize the vitamin normally. A dietary deficiency of biotin, however, is quite uncommon, even in those consuming a diet low in this B vitamin. Nonetheless, if someone eats large quantities of raw egg whites, a biotin deficiency can develop, because a protein found in raw egg white inhibits the absorption of biotin. Cooked eggs do not present this problem. Long-term antibiotic use can interfere with biotin production in the intestine and increase the risk of deficiency symptoms, such as dermatitis, depression, hair loss, anemia, and nausea. Long-term use of antiseizure medications may also lead to biotin deficiency.[278] Alcoholics, people with inflammatory bowel disease, and those with diseases of the stomach have been reported to show evidence of poor biotin status.[278]

Vitamin C

Vitamin C is a water-soluble vitamin that functions as a powerful antioxidant. In this capacity vitamin C functions to protect LDL cholesterol from oxidative damage (only when LDL is damaged does cholesterol appear to lead to heart disease).[279] Vitamin C is needed to make collagen, the "glue" that strengthens many parts of the body, such as muscles and blood vessels. Vitamin C also plays important roles in wound healing and as a natural antihistamine. Vitamin C is a primary component in the synthesis of synovial fluid, and as such, plays an important role in the maintenance of joint health. This vitamin also aids in the formation of liver bile and helps to fight viruses and to detoxify alcohol and other substances.[280] Although vitamin C appears to have only a small effect in preventing the common cold, it reduces the duration and severity of a cold.[281] Recently, researchers have shown that vitamin C improves nitric oxide activity.[282] Nitric acid is needed for the dilation of blood vessels, potentially important in lowering blood pressure and preventing spasm of arteries in the heart that might otherwise lead to heart attack. Vitamin C has reversed dysfunction of cells lining blood vessels.[283] The normalization of the functioning of these cells may be linked to prevention of heart disease.

Evidence indicates that vitamin C levels in the eye decrease with age and that supplementing with vitamin C prevents this decrease, leading to a lower risk of developing cataracts.[284] Vitamin C has also been reported to reduce activity of the enzyme aldose reductase, an enzyme responsible for accumulation of sorbital in eyes, nerves, and kidneys of people with diabetes.[285] Therefore, interference with the activity of aldose reductase protects diabetics from the rapid progression of devastating consequences of this disease.

Ascorbic acid is a potent nonenzymatic protector against free radical damage.[286] Spurred by the proclamations (and longevity) of Linus Pauling, megadoses of vitamin C have been touted as playing a protective role in upper respiratory tract infections[287] and neoplasm.[108,109,111–114] Schorah and associates[288] found that elderly individuals receiving vitamin C had small but statistically significant increases in body weight and plasma albumin, and a reduction in purpura and petechial hemorrhages. No changes in mood or mobility were observed. The risks of megadoses of vitamin C include rebound scurvy when ascorbic acid is reduced to the RDA, reduced vitamin B[12] absorption, oxalic acid renal calculi, false-negative fecal occult blood results (which could lead to delayed diagnosis of colonic cancer), and excessive absorption of dietary iron.[280] It has been concluded that taking too much vitamin C is not worth these risks.[280,289]

An association between ascorbic acid and arteriosclerosis has been made. Early intimal changes seen in the arteries of patients with atherosclerosis are similar to those observed in patients with scurvy.[290] Coupled with the finding of low leukocyte ascorbic acid levels in patients with coronary atherosclerosis and acute myocardial infarction, these findings have led to the suggestion that vitamin C may be involved in the pathogenesis of atherosclerosis.[279,289] Numerous studies have documented lower ascorbic acid levels in plasma, leukocytes, and platelets in older subjects.[288,291,292] Not only do ascorbic acid levels fall with age, but the levels of free radicals associated with ascorbate also fall.[293] The decline in ascorbate radical levels with age may indicate a decline in the free radical defense mechanism.

Spindler[294] studied vitamin C status in elderly people with and without cognitive impairment. Leukocyte vitamin C levels were found to be unacceptably low in the impaired subjects but less so in the unimpaired subjects, though levels were still below those recommended. All of the subjects with low vitamin C levels were consuming at least 100% of the Recommended Dietary Intake (RDI)* of vitamin C. Vitamin C levels were lower in men than in women, but in women the degree of cognitive impairment was related to their poor vitamin C status. The author suggests that the proposed RDA for vitamin C is below intake levels required to support acceptable nutritional status in healthy elderly and that the RDA might be hazardous if applied indiscriminately as a standard for those who are cognitively impaired.[294]

Vitamin E

Early studies established that vitamin E levels decline with aging.[295] Vitamin E is necessary for the action of glutathione peroxidase, which prevents the formation of the hydroxyl radical by converting hydrogen peroxide to water. Besides its role as an antioxidant, vitamin E has been suggested to have some

*The Recommended Dietary Intake (RDI) also referred to as the Dietary Reference Intake (DRI) are nutrient based reference values for use in planning and assessing diets. They are intended to replace the Recommended Dietary Allowances (RDA) which are based on the amounts needed to protect against deficiency diseases. The RDIs reflect a shift in emphasis from preventing deficiency to decreasing the risk of chronic disease through nutrition. They refer to average daily intake over one or more weeks.

effect in the management of intermittent claudication.[296] Vitamin E is a powerful antioxidant that protects cell membranes and other fat-soluble parts of the body, such as LDL cholesterol.[297–299]

Vitamin E appears to play a central role in maintaining the structure and function of the human nervous system.[300] According to Sokol,[301] vitamin E deficiency initiates and perpetuates a progressive neuromuscular degeneration with irreversible neurologic consequences if treatment is delayed.

Vitamin E may also be useful in the treatment of neurological disorders not associated with vitamin E deficiency.[300] Its use is being investigated in Parkinson's disease, and it appears that vitamin E may help to prevent or retard the degeneration of nerves that occurs in Parkinson's disease.[301]

The names of all types of vitamin E begin with either "d" or "dl," which refer to differences in chemical structure. The "d" form is natural and "dl" is synthetic. The natural form is more active, and as a result better absorbed and utilized.

Vitamin A

Vitamin A helps cells reproduce normally, a process called differentiation. Cells that have not properly differentiated are more likely to undergo precancerous changes.[300] Vitamin A, by maintaining healthy cell membranes, helps prevent invasion by disease-causing microorganisms. Vitamin A also stimulates immunity and is needed for formation of bone, protein, and growth hormone. Beta carotene is a substance from plants that the body can convert to vitamin A.

The main functions of vitamin A are its role in the eye's adaptation to the dark, maintaining epithelial integrity, and hemoglobin synthesis. A significant decline in light threshold in relation to aging has been demonstrated; however, this does not correlate with serum vitamin A levels and is not improved by vitamin A administration.[302] Follicular hyperkeratosis, a classic sign of vitamin A deficiency, is often seen in elderly subjects, but does not appear to be related to a vitamin A deficiency.[303] There is no evidence that plasma vitamin A or the absorption of vitamin A is affected by aging. Vitamin A, however, is the second most commonly used nutritional supplement.[304]

In contrast to the rarity of symptoms from vitamin A deficiency in the elderly, vitamin A toxicity is more commonly seen. Symptoms include general malaise, headaches, dry skin, bone loss, liver dysfunction, leukopenia, and hypercalcemia.[305]

Beta-Carotene

Beta-carotene, a substance from plants that the body can convert into vitamin A, also acts as an antioxidant and immune system booster. Other members of the antioxidant carotene family include cryptoxanthin, alpha carotene, xanthine, lutein, and lycopene; however, unlike beta carotene, most of these nutrients do not convert to significant amounts of vitamin A.

The type of beta carotene consumed appears to be of great importance. Researchers originally believed that there was no meaningful difference between natural (from food) and synthetic (from supplements) beta carotene. This view was questioned when the link between beta carotene-containing foods and lung cancer prevention[306] was not duplicated in studies using synthetic pills.[307] In smokers, synthetic beta carotene resulted in an increased risk of lung cancer in double-blind research.[308,309] It appears that natural beta carotene may possibly have activity that is distinct from the synthetic form. For example, the natural form (found in foods and made of two molecules) has antioxidant activity that the synthetic form (consisting of only one molecule) lacks.[310] As a result of the potential precancerous effects caused by synthetic beta carotene, it is advisable that beta carotene be obtained from dark green vegetables and orange-yellow fruits and vegetables.

Elderly individuals who limit their consumption of beta carotene-containing vegetables could be at higher risk of developing a vitamin A deficiency; however, because beta carotene is not an essential nutrient (i.e., it can be synthesized so doesn't need to come from dietary sources), deficiencies are rare.

Zinc

Zinc is a component of more than 300 enzymes that are needed to repair wounds, maintain fertility, synthesize protein, help cells reproduce, preserve vision, boost immunity, and protect against free radicals.

Zinc deficiency in humans can lead to anorexia, impaired immune function, poor wound healing, decreased strength of muscle contraction, and possibly, altered taste acuity. The RDA for zinc in persons over 51 is set at 15 mg. On the basis of an analysis of the literature, Sandstead and colleagues[311] estimated that the average daily intake of zinc in elderly persons in the United States ranged from 7 to 13 mg. The average diet frequently provides less than the RDA for zinc. Zinc deficiencies are more common in alcoholics and individuals with sickle cell anemia, malabsorption problems, and chronic kidney disease.[312] On balance, it appears that serum zinc levels decrease with aging.[311,313,314] Decreases in hair zinc levels have also been demonstrated with aging.[311,315] Other studies have found that zinc concentration in bone[316] and kidney[317] also fall after the age of 50 years.

Zinc has been demonstrated to be necessary for adequate functioning of T cell lymphocytes.[318] Aging is associated with a progressive deterioration in T lymphocyte function.[319] The role of zinc in wound healing is now well established,[320] and zinc supplementation has been shown to accelerate healing of leg ulcers in elderly subjects.[102,321]

The effect of zinc supplementation on enhancing appetite in elderly subjects has been clearly demon-strated,[322] and zinc deficiency may play a role in the anorexia of aging. Zinc deficiency decreases the responsiveness of neurotransmitters (including the opioid peptide dynorphin) that are potent stimulators of food intake.[322,323]

Impotence is extremely common in the elderly, and a strong correlation has been established between hyperzincuria, low serum zinc levels, and impotence in this population.[324] Zinc supplementation restored potency in a significant percentage of the elderly subjects studied.

It appears that zinc levels decline with age, possibly as the result of chronic, long-term marginal zinc intake. This situation can be further aggravated by the hyperzincuria associated with chronic diseases, such as diabetes mellitus, to which the elderly are particularly prone. Burnet[325] has hypothesized that zinc deficiency may also play a role in the pathogenesis of dementia based on zinc's essential role in enzyme production, such as DNA polymerases that are necessary for DNA replication, repair, and transcription. Research continues to substantiate lower levels of zinc in the central nervous system and brain in patients with Alzheimer's disease.[325]

Copper

Copper serves as a catalyst in the biochemistry of every organ system. In particular, copper plays a role in iron absorption and mobilization, which as previously discussed, is particularly relevant to aging.[326] It is also part of the antioxidant enzyme superoxide dismutase. Copper is a catalyst for lysyloxidase, an enzyme important for the cross-linking of collagen and elastin,[327] and it plays a role in the conversion of dopamine to norepinephrine.[328] Copper is needed to make ATP; the synthesis of some hormones requires copper, as does collagen. Klevay[104] found that copper deficiency increases serum cholesterol levels, possibly by increasing the rate of cholesterol released from the liver to the circulation. As high dietary zinc accentuates copper deficiency, Klevay[104] suggested that atherosclerosis is related to the ratio of zinc to copper. Despite the great theoretic interest in the role of copper in the aging process, there is little information concerning copper in the aged population. Yunice and associates[329] reported a small but significant increase in serum copper levels with aging. Bunker and coworkers[314] also found an increase in plasma copper with aging but no change in leukocyte copper levels. Copper absorption appears similar in aged and young subjects.[314,329]

Chromium

Chromium is an essential trace mineral that helps the body maintain normal blood sugar levels.[330] Chromium also plays a role in increasing HDL,[331] and lowers overall cholesterol levels.[332]

Chromium deficiency leads to hyperglycemia, hypercholesterolemia, and corneal opacities.[333] Tissue chromium levels decline with age and may do so more dramatically in Western societies where people eat refined foods, which are deficient in chromium.[334] Preliminary studies have suggested that chromium-rich brewer's yeast improves glucose tolerance, insulin sensitivity, and cholesterol levels in elderly subjects.[335] Serum chromium levels have been reported to be lower in subjects with coronary artery disease.[336] At present, a role for chromium in diabetes mellitus or atherosclerosis have not been proved, although available studies have raised intriguing possibilities concerning chromium's role in some of the degenerative diseases of developed countries.

Chromium, in a form called chromium picolinate, has been studied for its potential role in altering body composition. Preliminary research suggests that chromium picolinate increases fat loss and lean muscle tissue gain.[337–339]

Iodine

Iodine is needed to make thyroid hormones, which are necessary to maintain normal metabolism in all cells of the body. Reports suggest that iodine may have a number of important functions in the body unrelated to thyroid function that might help people with a wide variety of metabolic conditions.[340] Iodine deficiency can cause hypothyroidism, goiter, and cretinism. People who avoid dairy food, seafood, and iodized salt may be at risk for a deficiency, though deficiencies are now uncommon in Western societies.

Magnesium

Magnesium is needed for bone, protein, and fatty acid formation, making new cells, activating B vitamins, relaxing muscles, clotting blood, and forming ATP. Insulin secretion and function also require magnesium. Magnesium also acts in a way related to calcium channel blocker drugs. This effect may be responsible for the fact that under certain circumstances, magnesium has been found to potentially improve vision in people with glaucoma[341] and to lower blood pressure.[342] Magnesium deficiency is common in people taking potassium-depleting prescription drugs, or in individuals overutilizing laxatives. Alcoholism, severe burns, diabetes, and heart failure are other potential causes of deficiency. Chronic diarrhea and other conditions of malabsorption are also associated with magnesium deficiency. Almost two-thirds of elderly individuals who are hospitalized are found to be deficient.[343] Symptoms severely affect function and include fatigue, abnormal heart rhythms, muscle weakness and spasm, depression, loss of appetite, and listlessness.[343]

Manganese

Manganese is needed for healthy skin, bone, and cartilage formation, as well as glucose tolerance. It also helps activate superoxide dismutase, an important antioxidant. Clear deficiencies are rare, however, manganese deficiency is evident in individuals with osteoporosis, so this deficit becomes important in the older adult population.[344]

Phosphorus

Selective phosphorus deficiency induced in normal subjects by an inadequate diet or by ingestion of large quantities of phosphate-binding antacids leads to a distinctive clinical syndrome characterized by anorexia, weakness, and bone pain.[9] Severe hypophosphatemia has been documented in association with alcohol withdrawal, diabetes mellitus, excessive antacid ingestion, recovery from burns, unsupplemented hyperalimentation, and severe respiratory alkalosis. Patients with a phosphorus deficiency may develop a metabolic encephalopathy (irritability, muscle weakness, hypothesias and parasthesias, dysarthria, confusion, seizures, and coma), hemolysis, leukocyte dysfunction, and platelet dysfunction. To avoid deficiency, a one-to-one ratio with calcium is recommended.[9] Calcium is a natural binder to phosphorus and they work in harmony to create bone mass.

Of interest is that soft drinks, both diet and regular, are phosphonated to create the bubbles and perserve the sugars.[89] This nonbiological form of phosphorus links to calcium and causes the loss of calcium via the urine. As discussed in Chapter 11, Orthopedic Treatment Considerations, the avoidance of phosphonated drinks is important as a preventive measure for osteoporosis.

Potassium

Potassium is needed to regulate water balance, levels of acidity, blood pressure, and neuromuscular function. It is also required for carbohydrate and protein metabolism. Deficiencies, termed hypokalemia, are associated with diets low in fruits and vegetables, prolonged vomiting, diarrhea, or use of potassium-depleting diuretic drugs. The most frequent cause of hypokalemia in the elderly is diuretic therapy used for treatment of edematous and hypertensive conditions. Multiple pathophysiologic mechanisms occur to explain the development of hypokalemia in older individuals. For example, the patient who vomits has a reduction in potassium in addition to loses of hydrogen ions, producing a metabolic alkalosis that in turn shifts potassium intracellularly and augments urinary potassium losses. The resulted contracted intravascular volume increases renal reabsoption of sodium and bicarbonate, which further enhances the metabolic alkalosis that increase urinary potassium losses. So, this can become an escalating, life-threatening deficiency. The need for replacement potassium in elders on diuretics is very important. Low potassium can precipitate cardiac arrhythmias and sudden death.[9]

Potassium and sodium work together in the body to maintain muscle tone, blood pressure, water balance, and other functions.

Selenium

Selenium activates an antioxidant enzyme called glutathione peroxidase, which may help protect the body from cancer.[345,346] Selenium has also been found to induce apoptosis (programmed cell death) in cancer cells.[346] Selenium is also essential for healthy immune functioning.[347] Even in a nondeficient population of elderly people, selenium supplementation has been found to stimulate the activity of white blood cells, the primary component of the immune system.[348] Selenium is also needed to activate thyroid hormones.

Water Intake

Many elderly adults experience dehydration from age-related changes in organ function. Dehydration reduces the amount of electrolytes, such as sodium, potassium, calcium, magnesium, chloride and phosphate, which are important for conducting neurological impulses to the brain. The recommended daily amount of fluid consumption is between 2000 mL to 2500 mL. In the case of elderly individuals, cognitively impaired, dependent and incontinent individuals tend to be underhydrated. Many drugs that patients take also decrease water intake.[349]

Dehydration is the most common fluid and electrolyte disturbance in the elderly.[350] The threshold for recognition of thirst is higher in the elderly. In many instances, cognitive or physical disabilities also reduce the ability to recognize thirst, express thirst, or obtain access to water.[351] In addition, healthy elderly individuals seem to have reduced thirst in response to fluid deprivation.[350] Elderly individuals also produced less concentrated urine following fluid deprivation. Since elderly subjects had higher vasopressin levels in response to dehydration, the decreased capacity to concentrate the urine is most likely at the renal level.[350] Fluids, as well as solid foods, are essential to life. Approximately 2.0 to 2.5 liters of water or other fluid per day is a reasonable goal to strive for in the aged. Diuretic fluids, such as coffee and soft drinks, should be avoided.

An increase in serum sodium concentration results from a loss of body water in excess of salt loss. Among elderly patients, hypernatremia (dehydration with elevated sodium levels in the serum) is most common in those who are bedridden and not provided with sufficient water to satisfy their thirst or in those whose thirst sensation is diminished by impaired central nervous system functioning. A net deficit of water is associated with vomiting, diarrhea, diabetes insipidus, and hyperpyrexia (excessive sweating). In general, older patients appear to be predisposed to the development of hypernatremia. Surgery, febrile illnesses, infirmity, and diabetes mellitus account for most of these incidences.[352] Chapter 5, Pathological Manifestations of Aging, deals more extensively with the physiological and functional ramifications of dehydration.

DRUGS' EFFECTS ON NUTRITION

The frequent use of pharmacologic agents increases the vulnerability of the elderly to malnutrition. Drug-diet interactions occur at all ages, but are more common in the elderly because of prescription and over-the-counter drug use on a regular basis. In addition, age related changes in gastrointestinal function, liver and renal function, and body composition alter drug and nutrient metabolism. Coexisting disease, undernutrition, and malnutrition may further complicate these interactions.[353,354]

Drugs may affect nutritional status in the simplest sense by their effects on appetite, but more commonly, absorption, metabolism, and excretion of dietary constituents are altered. Dietary factors such as water consumption, amount of food consumed, timing of meals in relation to drug intake, and the constituents consumed may affect absorption and oxidative drug metabolism.[353]

Drugs cause malabsorption of nutrients by exerting an effect on the ability of the gastrointestinal mucosa to absorb. These effects can be limited and specific for a particular nutrient, or they may affect an entire class of nutrients, such as fat-soluble vitamins or trace minerals. For instance, drugs may decrease nutrient bioavailability by repelling the nutrient, therefore inhibiting the intestinal phase of fat digestion and absorption.[355] Drugs may also interfere with nutrient absorption through secondary mechanisms. For example, drugs can impair absorption of nutrients by adverse effects on gastric or intestinal, pancreatic or hepatic bile secretion. H_2 blockers (such as cimetidine) inhibit gastric acid production, thereby reducing the liberation of vitamin B_{12} from its protein-bound state, making it less available for association with intrinsic factors.[355] This could result in vitamin B_{12} deficiency and resulting pernicious anemia.

Several over-the-counter drugs may induce adverse nutritional effects. Antacids are associated with impaired absorption of riboflavin, copper, and iron, and may induce hypophosphatemia[356] with the development of proximal limb muscle weakness, malaise, paresthesias, anorexia, and secondary syndromes of hypomagnesemia/ tetany,[357] and osteomalacia.[358] Excessive use of sodium bicarbonate can result in sodium overload and render the pH of the gut sufficiently alkaline to decrease the absorption of folic acid.[359] Commonly used drugs that increase calcium need include aluminum-containing antacids, which decrease phosphorus absorption, lowering plasma phosphorus and ultimately increasing calcium excretion.[360] Thiazide diuretics, on the other hand, decrease calcium needs by decreasing urinary calcium losses and may have a positive effect on bone mass.[361]

Laxatives, if taken at mealtime or in the postprandial absorptive period, prevent absorption of carotenes and fat-soluble vitamins via solubilization. Overuse of stool softeners may result in malabsorption of glucose, calcium, potassium, vitamin D, and protein. Laxative use has been linked to an increased incidence of osteomalacia.[362] In the elderly patient, the risks of hypokalemia and potassium deficiency, with the attendant hazards of cardiac arrhythmias, digitalis toxicity, and hyperglycemia, are associated with concurrent use of laxatives and diuretics.[355]

Anti-inflammatory drugs, commonly used by elderly individuals, produce small hemorrhages of the gastrointestinal mucosa, leading to iron-deficiency anemia and decreased absorption of vitamin C. Chronic aspirin use is associated with folic acid deficiency and macrocytic anemia.[355]

Drugs may act to inhibit the essential intermediary metabolism of a nutrient or to promote its catabolism. For example, drug interference of vitamin D metabolism with a secondary impairment of calcium absorption can result in osteomalacia. Drugs that increase hepatic enzymes for drug metabolism (e.g., sedatives, hypnotics, and anticonvulsants), may increase the demand for specific nutrients, such as folic acid, B_6, and B_{12}.

Drugs may also increase the excretion of some nutrients by displacement from plasma protein-binding sites, chelation, or reduction of renal reabsorption. For example, aspirin competes for folic acid-binding sites on serum proteins and enhances the vitamin's excretion.[363] Long-term use of aspirin results in chelation of essential minerals such as copper and zinc. Although diuretic therapy effectively decreases the resorption of sodium, it also reduces renal absorption enhances renal excretion of calcium, chromium, magnesium, potassium, and zinc.[355]

Table 7–6 provides a summary of drug-induced effects on nutrient absorption, metabolism, and excretion.[355]

Drugs have an effect on nutrition and conversely, diet has been shown to affect the metabolism and response to many drugs. Food may influence both the absorption and the presystemic metabolism of drugs. These effects may be caused by food intake or by different nutrients or additives, food/fluid volume, or polycyclic hydrocarbons present in grilled foods.

Food and its constituents can influence drug absorption as a result of physical or chemical interactions between the food product and the drug or because of physiologic changes in the gastrointestinal tract. The net effect of this interaction may be that drug absorption is reduced, slowed, or increased by food intake.[364] Food can act to alter the rate of gastric emptying and drug dissolution. It can act as a mechanical barrier, preventing drug access to the mucosal surface. For example, acetaminophen absorption is more rapid after fasting than after consumption of a high-carbohydrate meal containing pectin.[355] Foods interfere with the mucosal transfer of drugs, such as

levodopa, a drug whose chemical structure is similar to that of amino acids. Competition for transport between the drug and amino acids from protein in the diet diminishes drug uptake and appears responsible for the "on-off" phenomenon of levodopa in Parkinson's patients.[365]

Nutritional influences on drug distribution may be limited in the elderly who are poorly nourished because of a reduction in plasma albumin. Even in well-nourished, healthy elders, albumin concentrations have been found to be lower compared to younger adults.[355] As a result, the extensively protein-bound drugs, such as warfarin and diazepam, are not as readily distributed due to a reduced binding capacity in old age.

Metabolism of drugs may also be affected by nutrient intake, particulary the composition of the diet. Research indicates that the total caloric input and the percentage of calories obtained from different sources (e.g., carbohydrates, proteins, fats) will influence pharmacokinetics of various drugs.[366,367] For example, the rate of drug breakdown and elimination is affected by the type of diet consumed. Comparing high-carbohydrate, high-fat, or high-protein diets, the rate of drug elimination is slowest with the high-carbohydrate diet and fastest with the high-protein diet.[355] Reduced drug clearance is demonstrated in elders whose diets are low in protein.[355]

Specific dietary constituents such as cruciferous vegetables and charcoal-broiled beef can also alter drug metabolism.[368] Certain foods should not be ingested when specific drugs are on board. As one among many examples, fermented cheese and wine inhibit the monoamine oxidase enzymes (MAO inhibitors). High amounts of tyramine contained in these foods stimulate the release of catecholamines (norepinephrine, epinephrine), which confounds the action of MAO inhibitors whose purpose is to suppress these elements. As a result, consumption of tyramine-containing foods in the presence of MAO inhibitors can cause a dramatic and life-threatening increase in blood pressure.[367]

Under normal circumstances, most vitamin-rich foods are good for us. However, as discussed above, certain medications can have an increased or decreased absorption when taken with food, thereby affecting their efficiency. For example, tetracycline antibiotics are not effective when taken within an hour of milk or dairy products. Hismanal (astermizole), Plendil (felodipine) or Procardia/Adalat (nifedipine), should not be taken with acid-containing juices, such as grapefruit juice, which may increase blood levels of these drugs and result in harmful side effects.[355,368] Individuals taking blood pressure medications, particularly ACE inhibitors or potassium-sparing diruetics, should avoid potassium salt substitutes because of the danger of potassium overload. One of the most serious interactions occurs when Coumadin (warfarin) is taken with foods high in vitamin K. Coumadin interferes with the body's

TABLE 7–6. MECHANISM OF DRUG EFFECTS ON SPECIFIC NUTRIENT ABSORPTION, METABOLISM, AND EXCRETION

Drug Group	Nutrient Influenced	Mechanism of Nutritional Alteration	Kinetic Alteration
Anticoagulants			
Warfarin (Coumadin)	Vitamin K	⇓ Reductase/carboxylation	Metabolism
Antibiotics (general)	Vitamin B_1, B_2, B_6, B_{12}, K, biotin	Δ Bacterial flora	Absorption
Cephalosporins	Vitamin K	⇓ Reductase/carboxylation	Metabolism
Tetracyclines	CA	Chelation	Absorption
Isoniazid/INH (Isoniazid)	Vitamin B6	⇓ Pyridoxal kinase	Metabolism
		⇓ Hepatic/renal vitamin D hydroxylation	
Trimethoprim/TMP	Folic acid	Folate antagonist	Metabolism
Anticonvulsants			
Phenobarbital	Vitamin D, CA	Δ Vitamin D metabolites	Metabolism
	Folic acid	⇑ Hepatic microsomal enzymes	
Phenytoin (Dilantin)	Vitamin D, CA	Δ Vitamin D metabolites	Metabolism
	Folic acid	⇑ Hepatic microsomal enzymes	
Antihypertensives			
• Vasodilators	Vitamin B_6	⇓ Pyridoxal kinase	Metabolism
Hydralazine (Apresoline)			
• Loop diuretics	Na, K, CA, Cr, Mg, Zn,	⇑ Renal excretion	Excretion
Furosemide (Lasix)	Vitamin B_1, B_6		
• Thiazide diuretics	Na, K, Mg, Zn	⇑ Renal excretion	Excretion
Hydrochlorothiazide (HydroDIURIL)			
• Triamterene/			
hydrochlorothiazide	Na, CA	⇑ Renal excretion	Excretion
(Dyazide)	Folic acid	⇓ Dihydrofolate reductase	Metabolism
Antihyperlipidemics			
Cholestyramine (Questran)	Vitamin A, D, E, K, B_{12}, beta-	Adsorption to anion exchange resin	Absorption
Colestipol (Colestid)	carotene, folic acid, CA, Fe, Zn		
Anti-Inflammatory Agents			
Prednisone (Deltasone)	Vitamin D, CA	⇓ Hepatic/renal vitamin D hydroxylation	Metabolism
Colchicine	Vitamin B_{12}	Mucosal injury	Absorption
Sulfasalazine (Azulfidine)	Folic acid	⇓ Dihydrofolate reductase	Metabolism
Indomethacin (Indocin)	Vitamin C, Fe	Mucosal injury	Absorption
Sulindac (Clinoril)	Folic acid	⇓ Dihydrofolate	Metabolism
Naproxen (Naprosyn)			
Ibuprofen (Motrin)			
Aspirin	Vitamin C, Fe	Mucosal injury	Absorption
	Folic acid	Competition for binding sites	Excretion
Antineoplastics (general)	Most nutrients	Mucosal injury	Absorption
Methotrexate	Folic acid	Folate antagonist	Metabolism
Antiulcer Agents			
• H_2 receptor antagonists	Vitamin B_{12}, folic acid, Fe, Zn	⇓ Gastric acid secretion	Absorption
Cimetidine (Tagamet)			
Ranitidine (Zantac)			
Famotidine (Pepcid)	Vitamin D, Ca	⇓ Hepatic/renal vitamin D hydroxylation	Metabolism
Proton pump inhibitors	B_{12}, folic acid, Fe, Zn	⇓ Gastric acid secretion	Absorption
Omeprazole (Prilosec)			
Lansoprazole (Prevacid)	Vitamin D, CA	⇓ Hepatic/renal vitamin D hydroxylation	Metabolism
Antacids			
Aluminum and magnesium	Phosphate	Precipitation	Absorption
hydroxides (Amphogel,	Vitamin B_{12}, folic acid, Fe, Zn	⇓ Gastric acid secretion	
Maalox, Mylanta)			
Na bicarbonate (Alka-Seltzer)	Vitamin B_{12}, folic acid, Fe, Zn	⇓ Gastric acid secretion	Absorption
Laxatives			
• Lubricants			
Mineral oil (Haley's M-O)	Vitamins A, D, E, K, beta carotene	Solubilization	Absorption
• Stimulant cathartics			
Phenolphthalein (Ex-Lax)	CA, Vitamins D, K	⇑ GI motility	Absorption
Bisacodyl (Dulcolax)			

(Continued)

TABLE 7–6. (Continued)

Drug Group	Nutrient Influenced	Mechanism of Nutritional Alteration	Kinetic Alteration

Psychotherapeutics
• Tricyclic antidepressants
  Amitriptyline (Elavil)
  Nortriptyline (Pamelor)
  Imipramine (Tofranil)
  Desipramine (Norpramin)
  Doxepin (Sinequan)
	Vitamin B$_2$	⇓ Flavin adenine dinucleotide	Metabolism

Neuroleptics
  Chlorpromazine (Thorazine)
  Thioridazine (Mellaril)
  Fluphenazine (Prolixin)
  Thiothixene (Navane)
	Vitamin B$_2$	⇓ Flavin adenine dinucleotide	Metabolism

KEY: ⇓ = inhibit or decrease; ⇑ = induce or increase; Δ = change

ability to make blood clots. Vitamin K helps the body form blood-clot factors, thus it decreases the effectiveness of Coumadin.

ALCOHOL'S EFFECTS ON NUTRITION

Alcohol is both a drug and a food which provides substantial amounts of energy. It is widely abused by individuals of all ages. Among the aged, its abuse is especially easy since the risks of intoxication from a given dose of alcohol are elevated because lean body mass and total body water decrease with age. The consequence is that the total volume of distribution of alcohol is smaller and peak blood alcohol levels are higher than in younger persons.[369] Greater physiological sensitivity to the effects of alcohol and greater psychological vulnerability to alcohol abuse due to depression, loneliness, and lack of meaningful roles combine to make alcohol abuse risks high in the aged. Alcohol use should be avoided entirely among the elderly with known dementia, chronic medication with psychoactive drugs, a previous history of alcohol abuse, or chronic and extreme depression.

Moderate alcohol use (one or two drinks per day) has been associated with some health benefits. Alcohol in moderation is an appetite stimulant, enhancing the taste of food. It increases HDL cholesterol levels, thereby lowering atherosclerotic risks. Moderate alcohol intake is also associated with lowered congestive heart failure rates.[370] Since elderly energy intakes are already low, however, care must be taken to ensure that calories from alcohol do not displace other items in the diet which provide not only energy, but protein, vitamins, and minerals.

THEORIES OF AGING RELATED TO NUTRITION

Though the mechanisms of aging are not clearly understood, there is evidence suggesting that nutrition influences the aging process.[371] Aging, and related diseases, viewed from a nutritional perspective, results from the influence of different nutrients on immunological, genetic, neurological, and endocrinological functions. For example, oxidative mechanisms may play an important role in the aging process. It is important, therefore, to emphasize the relationship between health and nutrition in the elderly.

Since nutrients are obtained from the food we eat and utilized by the cells of the body, nutritional factors have been directly credited for their role in longevity. Malnutrition can contribute to chronic diseases. A combination of good nutrition and exercise leads to better health and energy levels and notably improves an individual's capability to withstand psychological and physical stresses.

Theories related to nutrition and longevity abound; for example, obesity has been correlated to shorter lifespan. In humans there is evidence that the restriction of total caloric intake appears to be more important than the restriction of any particular macronutrient in increasing longevity.[91] With advancing age and the occurrence of concomitant illness, there is an increased risk of developing nutritional deficiencies. Altered nutritional status, especially the extremes of under- and overnutrition, is associated with the pathogenesis of any number of common diseases of the elderly. Thus, it would appear that nutritional modulation and manipulation represents one possible approach to successful aging and healthy longevity. (see Chapter 2, Comparing and Contrasting the Theories of Aging) Several studies have attempted to determine relationships between specific food components, chronic disease and longevity. In 1935, a classic study by McCay demonstrated that laboratory rats lived significantly longer when their caloric intake was restricted at an early age.[372] Subsequent studies have confirmed that the leaner rats lived longer and that the onset of age-related diseases was significantly later in the undernourished laboratory animals.[373,374]

There are many molecular theories of aging that relate specifically to nutrition. It has been proposed that degenerative changes associated with age may be from free radical reactions, with resulting damage to cell membranes and cell organelles.[375] Mechnikova hypothesizes that the accumulation of toxins secreted by intestinal bacteria can in fact facilitate the aging process.[376]

Some theories attribute aging to the gradual oxidation of lipid membranes throughout life and therefore promote the consumption of foods with antioxidant properties. A number of in vivo and in vitro studies have explored the effects of both natural and synthetic sources of antioxidants, including vitamins A, C, E and selenium, in prolonging average maximal lifespan.[373] An increase in the average life span was observed; however, there is no evidence that any of these antioxidants delay the aging process or significantly extend the maximum lifespan.[374] Conversely, Richard and associates[371] report that particularly with regard to antioxidant micronutrient requirements, accelerated aging may in fact be related to a deficit in the intakes of antioxidant vitamins (tocopherols, carotenoids, and vitamin C) and trace elements (zinc and selenium, as well as to an impaired adaptive mechanism against oxidative stress.[371] Antioxidants have been demonstrated to decrease the effects of certain environmental and nutritional factors on average lifespan.[371,377,378] Physiological modifications occurring during the lifetime and environmental influences are significant factors contributing to the impairment of micronutrient status. These factors have to be considered when defining the specific requirements of the elderly. For example, there is no evidence that supplementation of the micronutrient iron alone has any benefit in altering the aging process or impacting the incidence of disease. However, combined supplementation, including iron, zinc, selenium, vitamins C and E and carotenoids, has been found to potentially prevent accelerated aging and reduce the risk of several common age-related diseases.[371]

There is substantial and long-standing literature linking the level of general nutrition to longevity. Reducing nutrition below the amount needed to sustain maximun growth increases longevity in a wide range of organisms. Oxidative damage has been shown to be a major feature of the aging process. Telomere shortening is now well established as a key process regulating cell senescence in vitro.[379] There is some evidence that the same process may be important for aging in vivo (see Chapter 2). Very recently it has been found that oxidative damage accelerates telomere shortening. It is therefore possible to propose that the level of nutrition determines oxidative damage which in turn determines telomere shortening and cell senescence and that this pathway is important in determining aging and longevity in vivo.[379]

Energy produced from plant and animal nutrients is potential energy obtained by oxidation of carbohydrates, fats or lipids, and proteins.[380] This potential energy is converted by metabolic reactions to various forms of energy within the body systems. In essence, theories related to energy in nutrition and aging deal with the energy balance or homeostatic mechanisms. Electrical energy provides conduction of nerve impulses, mechanical energy for muscle contraction, chemical energy for anabolism and catabolism, and heat for the regulation of body temperature and the maintenance of homeostasis. Temperature regulation requires as much as 60% of the energy obtained from food, whereas anabolic processes require 30% to 40%.[381]

The body reaches a state of energy balance when the amount of energy expended is equal to the amount of energy consumed. If the energy intake exceeds the energy expended, a positive energy state exists and energy is stored as glycogen or fat. When the expenditure of energy exceeds the amount of energy consumed, a negative energy state exists. This becomes an important consideration in the elderly as the ratio of intake to output is often unbalanced. The incidence of undernourishment in elderly is quite high as is the other end of the spectrum: obesity. In the elderly, physical activity and BMR decrease. Without a concommitant decrease in food intake, the chances of weight gain and diseases associated with inactivity increase substantially. Nutritional needs will vary according to body size and composition, rate of growth and physical activity.[9]

At cell maturity, there is a cessation of growth. With aging the catabolic rate (cell breakdown) slightly exceeds the anabolic rate (cell growth). The result of this is a gradual decrease in the total number of body cells.[382] Young[383] hypothesizes that at the cellular level, translational or posttranslational processes in protein metabolism may influence aging. The energy balance important in physical functioning is, therefore, affected by progressive loss of cells, a decrease in mitotic capacity (protein metabolism), and an overall decrease in lean body mass. Enzymes and hormones also play a key role in metabolism. Genetics may influence enzyme activity, and hormonal activity changing the rate of metabolism in the elderly.

Although it appears that genetic factors play an important role in nutrition of the elderly, environmental factors are also important. These include psychological, socioeconomic, cultural, and ecological factors. The nutritional adequacy of an older person could be affected by a number of factors, such as:

1. The ability to select appropriate nutrient sources (physical, cognitive, socioeconomic factors);
2. The ability to prepare meals (physical or cognitive problems);
3. The ability to ingest food (oral health, physical or cognitive changes);
4. The ability to digest ingested food;
5. The ability to absorb digested food;
6. The ability to metabolize absorbed nutrients;
7. The ability to utilize or store nutrients;
8. The ability to excrete waste products of metabolism.

Another predominant theory in aging is that modulation of the age-associated immune dysfunctions commonly occurring with advancing age can be altered by nutritional intervention. Nutrition has a strong influence on the immune system of the elderly. Aging induces dysregulation of the immune system, mainly as a result of changes in cell-mediated immunity.[178,384] Aging is associated with changes to the equilibrium of peripheral T and B lymphocyte subsets, such as decrease in the ratios of mature to immature cells. As a consequence, cell-mediated immune responses are weaker and neither cell-mediated nor humoral responses are as well adapted to antigen stimulus.[385] Undernutrition, common in aged populations, also induces lower immune responses, particularly in cell-mediated immunity.[178,384] Protein-energy malnutrition is asso- ciated with decreased lymphocyte proliferation, reduced cytokine release, and lower antibody response to vaccines. Micronutrient deficits, namely zinc, selenium, and vitamin B_6, all of which are prevalent in aged populations, have the same influence on immune reponses.[178,371] Because aging and malnutrition exert cumulative influences on immune responses, many elderly people have poor cell-mediated immune responses and are therefore at a high risk for infection.[178] It has been hypothesized that many of the changes in immune response that have been attributed to aging may, in fact, be related to nutrition and not aging.[384] Exercise has been found to influence the immune system response (mild to moderate exercise enhances it; severe exercise impairs it) as well as mediates how efficiently ingested nutrients are absorbed, metabolized, and excreted.[386,387] The immune theory of aging is covered extensively in Chapter 2, Comparing and Contrasting the Theories of Aging.

Age-related changes in lifestyle, socioeconomic status, and decreased basal metabolism make homeostasis a difficult state to achieve. Recent studies have begun to examine the specific affect of environmental factors influence on nutritional requirements of the elderly.[388]

Preventively oriented nutritional strategies for the aged differ from those most effective in earlier years.[217] For instance, drug-diet interactions rarely cause malnutrition in younger adults, but, they may in the elderly, and such causes of malnutrition are preventable. Several measures can keep the adverse interactions of nutrients and drugs to a minimum.[389] Review of medication schedules and over-the-counter drug use can eliminate harmful drug-drug and drug-diet effects. It is important to consider the abuse of antacids, drugs, or alcohol. Avoidance of drugs that are associated with unwanted nutritional effects is recommended, especially among the aged who are already malnourished due to disease processes.

Many nutritional measures involving health promotion will act at the level of primary prevention as previously discussed. Secondary prevention with early detection and nutritional support and treatment for various chronic degenerative diseases, developing sensory deficits, cognitive and emotionally related eating and drinking problems, drug-diet interactions, and failures of the social support system for the aged are vital components in preventive intervention.[390] Special risk factors for nutritional problems include severe chronic illnesses, especially if house-bound or confined to an institution; social isolation, depression, and other mental disability; severe dental and periodontal disease; and low socioeconomic status.[391,392]

Finally, nutritional support is an important part of tertiary prevention (rehabilitation). Since most of the aged suffer from one or more chronic degenerative diseases, this type of prevention is especially important.

EXERCISE, NUTRITION, AND AGING

Advancing age is associated with a remarkable number of changes in body composition, including reduction in lean body mass and increase in body fat. Decreased lean body mass occurs primarily as a result of losses in skeletal muscle mass. This age-related loss in muscle mass, or sarcopenia, accounts for the age-associated decrease in BMR, muscle strength, and activity levels, which, in turn are the cause of decreased energy requirements of the elderly.[34] A reduction in the body's major protein pool requires that adequate dietary protein to replace obligatory nitrogen loss and to support protein turnover is essential for maintaining muscle mass. Sedentary lifestyle also contributes to this loss and exercise helps to preserve muscle fibers.[35] In sedentary persons, the main determinant of energy expenditure is fat-free mass.[34,393] It also appears that declining energy needs are not matched by an appropriate decline in energy intake in many older adults, with the ultimate result being increased body fat content. Increased body fat and increased abdominal obesity are linked to the greatly increased incidence of non-insulin dependent diabetes and heart disease among the elderly. Regular exercise can affect nutrition needs and functional capacity in the elderly.[34,394] (Refer to Chapter 13, Cardiopulmonary and Cardiovascular Treatment Considerations, for a more extensive review of the benefits of exercise and nutrition, and exercise prescription).

SUPPLEMENTING NUTRIENTS

It is well known by nutritionists that the best sources of vitamins and minerals are natural sources. A balanced diet, in moderate amounts, is more trustworthy than nutritional supplements. Nutrients from ingested foods, because of their biocompatability with the metabolic makeup of humans, are more readily absorbed, metabolized, and utilized than supplemental doses of vitamins and minerals. With the aging gastrointestinal tract, often vitamin pills are not actually broken down or utilized. Supplements are often taken ad lib without consideration of their interaction with other supplements. Table 7–7 provides a summary by this author of the importance of specific nutrients, where to find them naturally, and what nutrients supplements should concomitantly be taken to enhance in the metabolism of each vitamin or mineral. Rule of thumb: If you take vitamins, a multivitamin is the best recommendation. Mixing and matching supplements could lead to devastating consequences.

Despite the fact that the way to get an abundant supply of nutrients is through healthy eating (a variety of foods on a daily basis) many elderly individuals do not consume a balanced diet. There are conditions and illnesses that deplete vitamins from their systems and need to be replenished. Many elders are on chronic drug regimens that increase the risk of progressive nutrient depletion. Appropriate levels of vitamin supplementation have been proposed for specific drug therapies in the elderly.[389] It is fairly common for drug-related depletion of nutrients in geriatric patients to be complicated by dietary inadequacy or by disease states that induce nutrient deficiencies.[355]

Notwithstanding such well-justified therapeutic needs for nutrient supplementation, it is important to recognize the extensive nature of self-prescribed supplement use among older aduts. The estimated prevalence of nutrient supplementation in the eldery ranges from 30% to 70%.[355] While several of the factors discussed above suggest that there may be valid reasons to recommend nutrient supplementation for older adults, current trends indicate that their supplementation regimens are not always appropriate. Self-selected supplements are not often based on individual needs, but on something the person heard or read, along with their belief that their choice of supplements will have a beneficial effect.

NUTRITIONAL PROGRAMS FOR THE ELDERLY

Federal food assistance programs were the result of the Surgeon General's 1979 report. Excellent references are available on community nutrition services for the aged.[395,396] They include food and nutrition services for the healthy aged, such as the elderly meals program, meals for maintaining the dependent aged at home, and food and nutrition services for the aged in group care and health care facilities.

Under the auspices of the Older Americans Act, the federal government's Administration on Aging provides congregate and home-delivered meals to over 2.5 million Americans 65 years of age and older. Those who participate in the "Meals on Wheels" program for the homebound aged are often economically poor and have multiple diseases, with a relatively high prevalence of nutritional deficiencies which are correctable by provision of adequate food and nutritional supplements.[397–404] The meals provide a minimum of a third of the RDA, and in this sense, are helpful in sustaining the nutrition of the aged.

In addition, the opportunity for social interaction provided by congregate dining or regular visits to deliver meals to the homebound elderly is also important and may increase food intake as well as improve the quality of life. The elderly who attend congregate meals tend to be healthier than those receiving home-delivered services.[397] In addition to providing substantial amounts of daily nutrient intakes, the elderly who attend congregate meal sites can also be screened for referral to other preventive services.

The federal food stamp program, which provides coupons that increase food purchasing power, are available for the poor elderly. While only about 30% of the aged now participate in the program and the program benefits are only about $60 per month, the availability of this extra food money may be a great help in increasing diet quality. At present, many eligible elderly individuals fail to apply for or use this program.[398,405]

The aged who reside in group care or health care facilities are in especially fragile health and often have special nutritional needs or feeding requirements. Conditions of participation in the Medicare and Medicaid programs require that the institutions maintain certain standards with respect to food and nutrition services in order to obtain certification and licensure.[399] Dietary and institutional consultants can assure that these standards are met, and plan to implement more extensive nutrition services in these institutions, including appropriate menus which meet the RDA and therapeutic diet needs, dining rooms that are available and accessible for those who use them, feeding assistance where needed, and the attainment of food safety regulations.[396,399]

Unfortunately, undernutrition is prevalent in long-term care facilities.[400] It has been determined that a combination of behavioral, environmental, and disease-related factors greatly influence nutrition status. Our efforts as health care prefessionals must be directed toward influencing some of these factors to minimize undernutrition in the institutionalized elderly.

Scientific evidence increasingly supports that good nutrition is essential to the health, self-sufficiency, and quality of life of older adults.[171,401–403] With the population of the United States living longer than ever before, the older adult population will be more diverse and heterogeneous as we move forward in the 21st century. The oldest-old and minority populations will grow more quickly than the young-old and non-Hispanic white populations, respectively. For the 34-plus million adults 65 years of age and older living in the United States, a broad array of culturally appropriate food and nutrition services, physical activities, and health and supportive care customized to accommodate the variations within this expanding population is needed. With changes and lack of coordination in

TABLE 7–7. NUTRIENT ROLE, NATURAL SOURCES, AND COMPLEMENTARY VITAMINS AND MINERALS

Vitamins	Role of Nutrient	Natural Sources	More Effective With . . .
A	Need for normal growth/vision, for healthy teeth, nails, bones, glands; powerful antioxidant	Fish liver oils, dairy products, liver dark--green & yellow vegetables	B-Complex, C, D, E, Calcium Phosphorus, Zinc
Beta Carotene (Pro Vitamin A)	Converted into vitamin A only as the body needs it; antioxidant	Yellow and orange fruits & vegetables	B-Complex, C, D, E, Calcium Phosphorus, Zinc
B_1 (Thiamine)	Needed for healthy nervous system, muscle tone, normal digestion,energy; processes carbohydrates, fat, protein	Brewer's yeast, wheat germ, liver, whole-grain cereals, nuts, pork beef peas/beans, fish, peanuts	B-Complex, B_2, Folic acid, Niacin C, E, Manganese, Sulfur
B_2 (Riboflavin)	Necessary for good vision, skin, nails, hair; converts carbohydrates to ATP; processes amino acids & fats; folic acid and B_6 activation; antioxidant	Brewer's yeast, liver, leafy vegetables, whole-grain breads, milk	B-Complex, B_6, Niacin, C
B_3 (Niacin)	Helps release energy, necessary for healthy nervous and digestive systems; regulates cholesterol	Lean meats, poultry, fish, nuts	B-Complex, B_1, B_2, C
B_5 (Pantothenic Acid)	Important for healthy skin/nerves, energy release,healthy digestive tract; activates adrenal gland; energy from fats; makes acetylcholine; synthesis of cholesterol	Organ meats, brewer's yeast, egg yolks, whole-grain cereals, salmon, diary products, meat	B-Complex, B_1, B_{12}, C, Sulfur, Biotin
B_6 (Pyridoxine)	Essential for production of antibodies, nerve tissue, red blood cells and for metabolism of fats.Helps regulate body fluids; building block for all proteins & some hormones; synthesis of neurotransmitters	Organ meats, whole-grain cereals, bananas, potatoes, raisin bran, lentils, turkey, tuna	B-complex, B_1, B_2, B_5, C, sodium, magnesium, potassium, linoleic acid
B_{12} (Cobalamin)	Essential for normal function all body cells including brain & nerve cells; DNA replication	Liver, kidney, muscle meats, fish, dairy products, eggs, poultry	B-complex, B_6, folic acid, C, potassium, sodium
Biotin	Essential to metabolism of fats, carbohydrates, and proteins	Organ meat, egg yolks, whole-grain cereals, brewer's yeast, milk, oatmeal, mushrooms, bananas, peanuts, soy	B-complex, B_{12}, folic acid, B_5 sulfur
C (Ascorbic Acid)	Essential for healthy teeth, bones, joints, red blood cells, immune system, muscle contraction	Citrus fruits/juices, tomatoes, green peppers, strawberries, all other fruits and vegetables	All vitamins/ minerals, calcium, magnesium
D	Important for health of bones, teeth, collagen, cartilage, nervous system, heart and aids blood-clotting	Fish liver oil, eggs, sunshine (reacts with skin to form D internally)	A, C, calcium, phosphorus
E (Trocopherol)	Helps protect unsaturated fats from abnormal breakdown & prolongs life of red blood cells, nerve/brain tissue	Vegetable oils, wheat germ, whole-grain cereals, green vegetables, seeds, nuts	A, B-complex, B_1, C, Selenium Manganese
Folic Acid	Part of B-complex. Essential for normal metabolism of growing cells/ tissues, red blood cells, heart h ealth	Green leafy vegetables, liver, brewer's yeast	B-complex, B_{12}, biotin, B_5, C

Minerals

Calcium	Essential for strong teeth/bones. Health and functioning of nerve, brain, heart tissue	Milk, dairy products, green leafy and green vegetables, soy products, dried peas, other beans, sardines	A, C, D, Fe, Magnesium, Boron, Phosphorus, manganese

(Continued)

TABLE 7–7. (Continued)

Vitamins	Role of Nutrient	Natural Sources	More Effective With...
Copper	Needed to utilize iron and for health of bones, nerves & connective tissue	Liver, whole-grain cereals, almonds, green leafy vegetables, dried peas/beans, seafoods, kidney, egg yolk	Cobalt, iron, zinc
Iodine	Helps regulate metabolism. Normal functioning of thyroid gland	Seafood, iodized salt, kelp, seaweed, vegetables grown in iodine-rich soil	Not established
Iron	Quality of blood, oxygenation, increases resistance to stress/disease, enhances immune system, important for proper muscle functioning	Liver, oysters, heart, lean meat, egg yolk, wheat germ, fish, leafy green vegetables	B_{12}, folic acid, C
Magnesium	Essential for healthy nerves/muscles and for producing energy. Healthy collagen, bones, and teeth; muscle relaxation; cell production; clotting of blood; formation of ATP; activates all B vitamins	Green vegetables, wheat germ, soy beans, figs, corn, apples, almonds, grains, nuts, beans, fish, meat	B_6, C, D, calcium, phosphorus, protein
Manganese	Activates enzymes in body. Important for health of reproductive organs; glucose tolerance; antioxidant	Whole-grain cereals, egg yolks, green vegetables, wheat germ, nuts, beans, bran, beet tops, pineapple, seeds	B_1, E, calcium, phosphorus
Phosphorus	Cell growth/ maintenance, energy production, tooth/bone/muscle health, kidney function, nerve conduction	Meat, fish, poultry, eggs, whole grains, seeds, nuts, milk, cheese	A, D, calcium, iron, manganese, protein
Potassium	All tissue growth, muscle contraction; O_2 to brain; H_2O & pH balance; blood pressure regulation & neuromuscular function; metabolism of carbohydrates and protein	All fruits & vegetables, oranges, whole grains, sunflower seeds, nuts, meats, mint leaves, potatoes, bananas, melons, beans, milk	B_6, sodium, phosphorus
Selenium	A natural antioxidant regulates various metabolic processes; immune system function; activates hormones	Cereal bran/germ, broccoli, onions, tomatoes, tuna, brewer's yeast, corn oil, nuts, whole grains, seafood	Vitamin E
Zinc	Tissue growth, muscle contraction, bone health	Shellfish, nuts, liver, kidney, egg yolks,	A, calcium, copper, phosphorus

health care and social support systems, health care professionals must be proactive, and collaborate with existing services for the elderly to improve policies, interventions, and programs that support older adults throughout the continuum of care to ensure nutritional well-being and quality of life.

CONCLUSION

Although the majority of the elderly are not undernourished, they represent a particularly vulnerable segment of the population with a precarious nutritional balance that can easily be disturbed by illness, decreased mobility, or increased economic hardship. As such, it is essential that health professionals pay particular attention to the components of nutritional status of the elderly. This includes patients in institutional settings where refusal of food or fluids may lead to unexpected nutritional deficiencies. Adequate nutrition is not a panacea. It is most useful as a preventive

and therapeutic tool in combination with exercise, stress management, and education.[404,406] It appears clear that the significance of nutritional adequacy will grow as it adds increasingly to the rehabilitation of community and institutionalized elders.

Much research is needed, and specific nutritional regimens for those elderly individuals in the community and those in institutions should be implemented and evaluated for benefits, effectiveness, and harmful effects. Nutritional education should be on the top of the agenda for the population at large, for the elderly, and for health care professionals. Major recommendations from the National Research Council of the National Academy of Sciences on diet and health have suggested social, scientific, and clinical environments for implementation of dietary changes. What remains is to fill the gaps with research, look at nutrition from different perspectives, and translate these findings into improved health. Health promotion and disease prevention can delay, or possibly even eliminate, chronic disorders and the so-called "normal" aging process. Nutrition appears to have proved itself as a crucial ally in rehabilitation of the elderly.

PEARLS

- The age-related changes in the gastrointestinal system, such as decreased saliva, poor dentition, decrements of taste and olfaction, gastromucosal atrophy, and reduced intestinal mobility will have the most impact on nutritional status because this system is directly involved in digestion.
- Basal metabolic rate declines rapidly from birth to age 20 and then gradually until age 80, when it tends to plateau.
- Decreased lean body mass occurs primarily as a result of losses in skeletal muscle mass. This age-related loss in muscle mass is termed sarcopenia.
- Numerous chronic diseases that are more prevalent in the elderly, such as Alzheimer's disease, cerebral vascular accidents, heart disease, osteoporosis, obesity, cancer, urinary incontinence, and diabetes, demonstrate related nutritional problems.
- Obesity is common in the aged and can be due to decreased activity, medication, and poorly balanced diet. This problem is associated with numerous medical disabilities, such as osteoarthritis, diabetes, hypertension, and heart disease, and can greatly hinder an older person's independence.
- The clinical evaluation of nutritional status can be done by the use of anthropometric measures, functional assessment tools, physical signs of nutrition deficiencies, or a combination of these.
- Malnutrition is an important predictor of morbidity and mortality.
- The elderly require a higher qualtiy, more nutrient dense (i.e., more nutrients per calorie) diet.
- The recommended daily allowance of nutrients changes with advancing age.
- Drugs may affect nutritional status in the simplest sense by their effect on appetite, but more commonly, absorption, metabolism, and excretion of dietary constituents are altered.
- Though the mechanisms of aging are not clearly understood, there is evidence suggesting that nutrition influences the aging process.
- Age-related loss in muscle mass accounts for the age-associated decrease in BMR, muscle strength, and activity levels, which, in turn are the cause of decreased energy requirements of the elderly.
- Despite the fact that the way to get an abundant supply of nutrients is through healthy eating (a variety of foods on a daily basis) many elderly individuals do not consume a balanced diet and require supplementation.
- Programs such as the Federal Food Assistance program, federal food stamps, and congregate and home-delivered meals can assist the older person in attaining adequate nutrition.

REFERENCES

1. Saltzman JR, Russell RM. The aging gut. Nutritional issues. *Gastroenterol Clin North Am.* 1998; 27(2):309–324.
2. Steen B. Preventive nutrition in old age—a review. *J Nutr Health Aging.* 2000; 4(2): 114–119.
3. US Department of Health, Education and Welfare. *Public Health Service. Healthy People: The Surgeon General's Report on Health Promotion and Disease Prevention 1979.* Washington, DC: Government Printing Office; 1979.
4. Wartow NJ. The national initiative on health promotion for older persons: the role of the administration on aging. *Top Geriatr Rehabil.* 1990; 6(l): 69–77.
5. de Jong N. Nutrition and senescence: healthy aging for all in the new millennium? *Nutrition.* 2000; 16(7–8):537–541.
6. Steen B. Body composition and aging. *Nutr Rev.* 1988; 46:45–51.
7. Walls AW, Steele JG, Sheiham A, Marcenes W, Moynihan PJ. Oral health and nutrition in older people. *J Public Health Dent.* 2000; 60(4): 304–307.
8. Bidlack WR, Kirsch A, Meskin MS. Nutritional requirements of the elderly. *Food Technology.* 1988; 40:61–70.
9. Chernoff R. *Geriatric Nutrition: The Health Professionals Handbook.* 2nd Edition. Gaithersburg, Md: Aspen Publishers; 1999.
10. Schiffman SS. Chemosensory impairment and appetite commentary on "Impaired sensory functioning in elders: the relation with its potential determinants and nutritional intake." *J Gerontol A Biol Sci Med Sci.* 1999; 54(8):B332–335.
11. Murphy C. Chemical senses and nutrition in the elderly. In: Kare MR, Brand TG, eds. *Interaction of the Chemical Senses with Nutrition.* New York: Academic Press; 1986.
12. Mulligan R. Oral health: effect on nutrition and rehabilitation in older persons. *Top Geriatr Rehabil.* 1989; 5(1):27–35.
13. Khan TA, Shragge BW, Crispen JS, et al. Esophageal mobility in the elderly. *Am J Digestive Dis.* 1977; 22:1049–1054.
14. Horowitz M, Maddern GT, Chateron BE, et al. Changes in gastric emptying rates with age. *Clin Sci.* 1984; 67:213–218.
15. Werner I, Hambraeus L. Protein digestion insufficiency with aging. *Acta Soc Med Upsal.* 1970; 76:239.
16. Webster SGP, Wilkinson EM, Gowland E. A comparison of fat absorption in young and old subjects. *Age Ageing.* 1977; 6:113–117.
17. Berman PM, Kirsner TB. The aging gut. II. Diseases of colon, pancreas, liver, and gallbladder, functional bowel disease, and iatrogenic disease. *Geriatrics.* 1972; 27(4):117–124.
18. Shepard RJ. Nutrition and the physiology of aging. In: Young EA, ed. *Nutrition, Aging and Health.* New York: Alan R Liss; 1986.

19. Nordin BE, Need AG, Steurer T, Morris HA, Chatterton BE, Horowitz M. Nutrition, osteoporosis, and aging. *Ann NY Acad Sci.* 1998; 854:336–351.

20. Weg RB. Nutrition: a crucial "given" in rehabilitation. *Top Geriatr Rehabil.* 1989; 5(1):1– 26.

21. Walser M. Renal system. In: Paige DM, ed. *Clinical Nutrition.* 2nd ed. St Louis: Mosby; 1988: 227–241.

22. Rudman D. Kidney senescence: a model for aging. *Nutr Rev.* 1088; 46:209–214.

23. Mitch WE. Protein metabolism and the aging kidney. In: Mitch WE, Klahr S, eds. *Nutrition and the Kidney.* Boston: Little, Brown and Co.; 1988.

24. Ritz P. Physiology of aging with respect to gastrointestinal, circulatory, and immune system changes and their significance for energy and protein metabolism. *Eur J Clin Nutr.* 2000; 54(Suppl 3):S21–S25.

25. Chernoff R. Aging and nutrition. *Nutrition Today.* 1987; 22(2):4–11.

26. Tzanoff SP, Norris AH. Effect of muscle mass decrease on age related BMR changes. *J Appl Physiol.* 1977; 43:1001–1006.

27. Tzanoff SP, Norris AH. Longitudinal changes in basal metabolism in man. *J Appl Physiol.* 1973; 45:536–539.

28. Roberts SB, Dallal GE. Effects of age on energy balance. *Am J Clin Nutr.* 1998; 68(4):975S–979S.

29. Shizgal HM, Spanier AH, Humes J, Wood CD. Indirect measurement of total exchangeable potassium. *Am J Physiol.* 1977; 233(3):F253–259.

30. Forbes GB, Reina JC. Adult lean body mass declines with age: some longitudinal observations. *Metabolism.* 1980; 19:633–663.

31. Russell RM. The aging process as a modifier of metabolism. *Am J Clin Nutr.* 2000; 72(2 Suppl): 529S–532S.

32. Uauy R, Winterer JC, Bilmazes C, et al. The changing pattern of whole body protein metabolism in aging humans. *J Gerontol.* 1978; 33: 663–671.

33. Shepard RJ. *Physical Activity and Aging.* Gaithersburg, Md: Aspen Publishers; 1987.

34. Evans WJ, Cyr-Campbell D. Nutrition, exercise, and health aging. *J Am Diet Assoc.* 1997; 97(6): 632–638.

35. Butler RN. Fighting frailty. Prescription for healthier aging includes exercise, nutrition, safety, and research. *Geriatrics.* 2000; 55(2):20.

36. Bonnefoy M, Constans T, Ferry M. Influence of nutrition and physical activity on muscle in the very elderly. *Presse Med.* 2000; 29(39): 2177–2182.

37. Sonn U, Rothenberg E, Steen B. Dietary intake and functional ability between 70 and 76 years of age. *Aging.* 1998; 10(4):324–331.

38. Young VR. Impact of aging on protein metabolism. In: Armbrecht HJ, Prendergast JM, Coe RM, eds. *Nutritional Intervention in the Aging Process.* New York: Springer Verlag; 1984:27–48.

39. Shizgal HM. Body composition. In: Fischer JE, ed. *Surgical Nutrition.* Boston, Little, Brown & Co.; 1983:3–17.

40. Waterlow JC, Stephen JML. The turnover of protein with aging. *Clin Sci.* 1967; 33:489–496.

41. Astrand PO, Rodahl K. *Textbook of Work Physiology.* San Francisco, London: McGraw-Hill Book Co., 1970.

42. Shizgal HM, Vasilevsky CA, Gardiner PF, et al. Nutritional assessment and skeletal muscle function. *Am J Clin Nutr.* 1986; 44:761–771.

43. Russell DM, Leiter LA, Whitwell J, et al. Skeletal-muscle function during hypocaloric diets and fasting: a comparison with standard nutritional assessment parameters. *Am J Clin Nutr.* 1983; 37: 133–138.

44. Lopes J, Russell DM, Whitwell J, Jeejeebhoy KN. Skeletal muscle function in malnutrition. *Am J Clin Nutr.* 1982; 36:602–610.

45. Kelly SM, Roza A, Field S, et al. Inspiratory muscle strength and body composition in patients receiving total parenteral nutrition. *Am Rev Resp Dis.* 1984; 130:33–37.

46. McGee M, Jensen GL. Nutrition in the elderly. *J Clin Gastroenterol.* 2000; 30(4):372–380.

47. Klor HU, Hauenschild A, Holback I, Schnell-Kretschmer H, Stroh S. Nutrition and cardiovascular disease. *Eur J Med Res.* 1997; 2(6):243–257.

48. Katan MB, Zock PR, Mensink RP. Dietary oils, serum lipoproteins, and coronary heart disease. *Am J Clin Nutr.* 1995; 61(6 Suppl):1368S–1373S.

49. Nestel PJ. Controlling coronary risk through nutrition. *Can J Cariol.* 1995; 11(Suppl G):9G–14G.

50. Hrboticky N, Sellmayer A. Nutrition in prevention of coronary heart disease. *Z Arztl Fortbild (Jena).* 1996; 90(1):11–18.

51. Singh RB, Niaz MA. Genetic variation and nutrition in relation to coronary heart disease. *J Assoc Physicians India.* 1999; 47(12):1185–1190.

52. Loktionov A, Scollen S, McKeown N, Bingham SA. Gene-nutrient interactions: dietary behavior associated with high coronary heart disease risk particularly affects serum LDL cholesterol in apolipoprotein E epsilon4-carrying free-living individuals. *Br J Nutr.* 2000; 84(6):885–890.

53. Belcher JD, Balla J, Balla G. Vitamin E, LDL, and endothelium: Brief oral vitamin supplementation prevents oxidized LDL-mediated vascular injury in vitro. *Arterioscler Thromb.* 1993; 13: 1779–1789.

54. Stephens NG, Parsons A, Schofield PM. Randomized controlled trial of vitamin E in patients with coronary disease: Cambridge Heart Antioxidant Study (CHAOS). *Lancet.* 1996; 347:781–786.

55. Pandya DP. Nutrition and coronary heart disease. *Compr Ther.* 1998; 24(4):198–204.

56. Rimm EB, Willett WC, Hu FB, et al. Folate and vitamin B6 from diet and supplements in relation to risk of coronary heart disease among women. *JAMA.* 1998; 279(5):359–364.

57. Frei B. Ascorbic acid protects lipids in human plasma and low-density lipoprotein against oxidative damage. *Am J Clin Nutr.* 1991; 54: 1113S–1118S.

58. Chambers JC, McGregor A, Jean-Marie J. Demonstration of rapid onset vascular endothelial dysfunction after hyperhomocysteinemia. An effect

reversible with vitamin C therapy. *Circulation.* 1999; 99:1156–1160.

59. Gartside PS, Glueck CJ. The important role of modifiable dietary and behavioral characteristics in the causation and prevention of coronary heart disease hospitalization and mortality: the prospective NHANES I follow-up study.

60. Dowd TT. The female climacteric. *Nat OB/GYN Group.* 1990; 6(1):32–54.

61. Giansiracusa DF, Kantrowitz FG. Metabolic bone disease. In: Keiber JB. *Manual of Orthopaedic Diagnosis and Intervention.* Baltimore, Md: Williams and Wilkins Co.; 1978.

62. Gaby AR. *Preventing and Reversing Osteoporosis.* Rocklin, Ca: Prima Publishing, 1994.

63. Dawson-Hughes B, Dallal G, Krall E. A controlled trial of the effect of calcium supplement on bone density in postmenopausal women. *N Eng J Med.* 1990; 329(13):878–883.

64. Riis B, Thomsen K, Christiansen C. Does calcium supplementation prevent postmenopausal bone loss? *N Eng J Med.* 1987; 316(4):173–177.

65. Zarkadas M, Geougeon-Reyburn R, Marliss EB. Sodium chloride supplementation and urinary calcium excretion in postmenopausal women. *Am J Clin Nutr.* 1989; 50(10):1088–1094.

66. Evans CEL, Chughtai AY, Blumsohn A. The effect of dietary sodium on calcium metabolism in premenopausal and postmenopausal women. *Eur J Clin Nutr.* 1997; 51(4):394–399.

67. Feskanich D, Willett WC, Stampfer MJ, Colditz GA. Protein consumption and bone fractures in women. *Am J Epidemiol.* 1996; 143(4): 472–479.

68. Abelow BJ, Holford TR, Insogna KL. Cross-cultural association between dietary animal protein and hip fracture: a hypothesis. *Calcif Tissue Int.* 1992; 50(1):14–18.

69. Dawson-Hughes B, Dallal GE, Krall EA. Effect of vitamin D supplementation on wintertime and overall bone loss in healthy postmenopausal women. *Ann Intern Med.* 1991; 115:505–512.

70. Dimai HP, Porta S, Wirnberger G. Daily oral magnesium supplementation suppresses bone turnover in young adult males. *J Clin Endocrinol Metab.* 1998; 83:2742–2748.

71. Stendig-Lindberg G, Tepper R, Leichter I. Trabecular bone density in a two year controlled trial of per-oral magnesium in osteoporosis. *Magnesium Res.* 1993; 6(2):155–163.

72. Relea P, Revilla M, Ripoll E. Zinc, biochemical markers of nutrition, and type I osteoporosis. *Age Ageing.* 1995; 24:303–307.

73. Elmståhl S, Gulberg B, Janzon L. Increased incidence of fractures in middle-aged and elderly men with low intakes of phosphorus and zinc. *Osteoporos Int.* 1998; 8(3):333–340.

74. Eaton-Evans J, McIlrath EM, Jackson WE. Copper supplementation and bone-mineral density in middle-aged women. *Proc Nutr Soc.*1995; 54: 191A

75. Nielson FH, Hunt CD, Mullen LM, Hunt JR. Effect of dietary boron on mineral, estrogen, and testosterone metabolism in postmenopausal women. *FASEB J.* 1987; 1(4):394–397.

76. Gold M. Basketball bones. *Science.* 1980; 80(1): 101–102.

77. Strause L, Saltman P, Smith KT. Spinal bone loss in postmenopausal women supplemented with calcium and trace minerals. *J Nutr.* 1994; 124(11): 1060–1064.

78. Eisinger J, Clairet D. Effects of silicon, fluoride, etidronate and magnesium on bone mineral density: a retrospective study. *Magnes Rev.* 1993; 84 (3):247–249.

79. Ferrari S, Zolezzi C, Savarino L. The oral strontium load test in assessment of intestinal calcium absorption. *Minerva Med.* 1993; 84(5): 527–534.

80. Tamatani M, Morimoto S, Nakajima M. Decreased circulating levels of vitamin K and 25-hydroxyvitamin D in osteopenic elderly men. *Metabolism.* 1998; 47(2):195–199.

81. Knapen MHJ, Hamulyak K, Vermeer C. The effect of vitamin K supplementation on circulating osteocalcin (Bone Gla protein) and urinary calcium excretion. *Ann Intern Med.* 1989; 111:1001–1005.

82. Iwamoto I, Kosha S, Noguchi S. A longitudinal study of the effect of vitamin K_2 on bone mineral density in postmenopausal women: a comparative study with vitamin D_3 and estrogen-progestin therapy. *Maturitas.* 1999; 31(2): 161–164.

83. Cracium AM, Wolf J, Knapen MJH. Improved bone metabolism in female elite athletes after vitamin K supplementation. *Int J Sports Med.* 1998; 19(5): 479–484.

84. Harrington T. Preventing osteoporosis in menopausal women. *J MSSK Med.* June, 1990.

85. Nielsen F, Hunt C, Mullen L, Hunt J. Effect of dietary boron on mineral, estrogen and testosterone metabolism in postmenopausal women. *FASE B J.* 1987; 1:394–397.

86. Pogrund H, Bloom R, Menczel J. Preventing osteoporosis: current practices and problems. *Geriatrics.* 1986; 41(5):55–71.

87. Kynast-Gales SA, Massey LK. Effect of caffeine on circadian excretion of urinary calcium and magnesium. *J Am Coll Nutr.* 1994; 13(4): 467–472.

88. Harris SS, Dawson-Hughes B. Caffeine and bone loss in healthy postmenopausal women. *Am J Clin Nutr.* 1994(5):573–578.

89. Kim SH, Morton DJ, Barrett-Conner EL. Carbonated beverage consumption and bone mineral density among older women: The Rancho Bernardo Study. *Am J Public Health.* 1997; 87(2): 276–279.

90. Harris MI, Hadden WC, Knowler WC, et al. Prevalence of diabetes and impaired glucose tolerance and plasma glucose levels in US population aged 20–74 years. *Diabetes.* 1987; 4: 523–534.

91. Ivan L. Nutrition, aging, old age. *Orv Hetil.* 1998; 139(49):2951–2956.

92. Zavaroni I, Dall'Aglio E, Bruschi F. Effect of age and environmental factors on glucose tolerance and insulin secretion in a worker population. *J Am Geriatr Soc.* 1986; 34:271–278.

93. Rosenthal MJ, Hartnell JM, Morley JE, et al. UCLA geriatric rounds: diabetes in the elderly. *J Am Geriatr Soc.* 1987; 35:435–447.

94. Seals DR, Hagberg JM, Hurley BF, et al. Effects of endurance training on glucose tolerance and plasma lipid levels in older men and women. *JAMA.* 1984; 252:645–649.

95. Krotkiewski M, Lonnroth P, Mandroukas K, et al. The effects of physical training on glucose metabolism in obesity in type II diabetes mellitus. *Diabetologia.* 1985; 28:881–390.

96. Saltin B, Lindgarde F, Houston M, et al. Physical training and glucose tolerance in middle-aged men with chemical diabetes. *Diabetes.* 1979; 28(suppl): 30–32.

97. Bogardus C, Ravussin E, Robbins DC, et al. Effects of physical training and diet therapy on carbohydrate metabolism in patients with glucose intolerance and non-insulin dependent diabetes mellitus. *Diabetes.* 1984;33:311–318.

98. Mooradin AD, Morley JE. Micronutrient status in diabetes mellitus. *Am J Clin Nutr.* 1987; 45: 877–895.

99. Kinlaw WB, Levine AS, Morley JE, et al. Abnormal zinc metabolism in type II diabetes mellitus. *Am J Med.* 1983; 75:273–277.

100. Morley JE. Nutritional status of the elderly. *Am J Med.* 1986; 81:679–695.

101. Niewoehner CB, Allen JI, Boosalis M, et al. The role of zinc supplementation in type II diabetes mellitus. *Am J Med.* 1986; 81:63–68.

102. Hallbook T, Lanner E. Serum-zinc and healing of venous leg ulcers. *Lancet.* 1972; 11:780–782.

103. Wallach S. Clinical and biochemical aspects of chromium deficiency. *J Am Coll Nutr.* 1985; 4: 107–120.

104. Klevay LM. Hypercholesterolemia produced by an increase in the ratio of zinc to copper ingested. *Am J Clin Nutr.* 1978; 26:1060–1065.

105. Greenwald P, Milner JA, Clifford CK. Creating a new paradigm in nutrition research within the National Cancer Institute. *J Nutr.* 2000; 130(12): 3103–3105.

106. Yancik R. Cancer burden in the aged: an epidemiologic and demographic overview. *Cancer.* 1997; 80(7):1273–1283.

107. Dreosti IE. Nutrition, cancer, and aging. *Ann NY Acad Sci.* 1998; 854(11):371–377.

108. Basdevant A. Nutrition and cancer. *Ann Pharm Fr.* 2000; 58(6 Suppl):448–451.

109. Boutwell RK. Nutrition and carcinogenesis: historical highlights and future prospects. *Adv Exp Med Biol.* 1995; 369:111–123.

110. Rockhill B, Willett WC, Hunter DJ. A prospective study of recreational physical activity and breast cancer risk. *Arch Intern Med.* 1999; 159: 2290–2296.

111. American Cancer Society. Guidelines on diet, nutrition, and cancer prevention: reducing the risk of cancer with healthy food choices and physical activity. The American Cancer Society 1996 Advisory Committee on Diet, Nutrition, and Cancer Prevention. *CA Cancer J Clin.* 1996; 46(6): 325–341.

112. Willett WC. Nutrition and cancer. *Salud Pulica Mex.* 1997; 39(4):298–309.

113. Hill MJ. Nutrition and human cancer. *Ann NY Acad Sci.* 29(12):68–78.

114. Willett WC. Diet, nutrition, and avoidable cancer. *Environ Health Perspect.* 1995; 108(Suppl 8): 165–170.

115. Krishnaswamy R, Polasa K. Diet, nutrition and cancer—the Indian scenario. *Indian J Med Res.* 1995; 102(11):200–209.

116. Willett WC. Goals for nutrition in the year 2000. *CA Cancer J Clin.* 1999; 49(6):331–352.

117. Nixon DW. Cancer, cancer cachexia, and diet: lessons from clinical research. *Nutrition.* 1996; 12(1 Suppl):S52–S56.

118. Riedel WJ, Jorissen BL. Nutrients, age, and cognitive function. *Curr Opin Clin Nutr Metab Care.* 1998; 1(6):579–585.

119. Grant WB. Dietary links to Alzheimer's disease. *Alz Dis Rev.* 1997; 2(1):42–55.

120. Smith MA, Petot GJ, Perry G. Diet and oxidative stress: a novel synthesis of epidemiological data on Alzheimer's disease. *Alz Dis Rev.* 1997; 2(1): 58–59.

121. Kalmijn S, Lauher LJ, Ott A. Dietary fat intake and the risk of incident dementia in the Rotterdam study. *Ann Neurol.* 1997; 42:776–782.

122. Munoz DG. Is exposure to aluminum a risk factor for the development of Alzheimer disease?—No. *Arch Neurol.* 1998; 55:737–739.

123. Forbes WF, Hill GB. Is exposure to aluminum a risk for the development of Alzheimer disease?—Yes. *Arch Neurol.* 1998; 55:740–741.

124. Crook T. Effects of phosphatidylserine in Alzheimer's disease. *Psychopharmacol Bull.* 1992; 28 (1):61–66.

125. Gindin J, Novickov M, Kedar D. The effect of plant phosphatidylserine on age-associated memory impairment and mood in the functioning elderly. *Psychopharmacol Bull.* 1995; 31(2): 136–144.

126. Sano M, Ernesto C, Thomas RG. A controlled trial of selegiline, alpha-tocopherol, or both as treatment for Alzheimer's disease. *N Engl J Med.* 1997; 336:1216–1222.

127. Morris MC, Beckett LA, Scherr PA. Vitamin E and vitamin C supplement use and risk of incident Alzheimer disease. *Alz Dis Assoc Disorders.* 1998; 12(1):121–126.

128. Schmidt R, Hayn M, Reinhart B. Plasma antioxidants and cognitive performance in middle-aged and older adults: results of the Austrian Stroke Prevention Study. *J Am Geriatr Soc.* 1998; 46(12): 1407–1410.

129. Letham R, Orrell M. Antioxidants and dementia. *Lancet.* 1997; 349:1189–1190.

130. Ferris SH, Sathananthan G, Gershon S. Senile dementia. Treatment with Deanol. *J Am Ger Soc.* 1977; 25(3):241–244.

131. Fisman M, Mersky H, Helmes E. Double-blind trial of 2–dimethylaminoethanol in Alzheimer's disease. *Am J Psych.* 1981; 138(9):970–972.

132. Pettegrew JW, Klunk WE, Panchalingam K. Clinical and neurochemical effects of acetyl-L-carnitine in Alzheimer's disease. *Neurobio Aging.* 1995; 16(1):1–4.

133. Salvioli G, Neri M. L-acetyl-carnitine treatment and mental decline in the elderly. *Drugs Exp Clin Res.* 1994; 20(2):169–176.

134. Cucionotta D. Multicenter clinical placebo-controlled study with acetyl-L-carnitine (LAC) in the treatment of mildly demented elderly patients. *Drug Development Res.* 1988; 14(2): 213–216.

135. Thal LJ, Carta A, Clarke WR. A 1–year multi-center placebo-controlled study of aceyl-L-carnitine in patients with Alzheimer's disease. *Neurol.* 1996; 47(6):705–711.

136. Calvani M, Carta A, Caruso G. Action of acetyl-L-carnitine in neurodegeneration and Alzheimer's disease. *Ann NY Acad Sci.* 1992; 663(5): 483–486.

137. Imagawa M, Naruse S, Tsuji S. Coenzyme Q_{10}, iron, and vitamin B_6 in genetically-confirmed Alzheimer's disease. *Lancet.* 1992; 340:671.

138. Clarke R, Smith D, Jobst KA. Folate, vitamin B_{12}, and serum total homocysteine levels in confirmed Alzheimer disease. *Arch Neurol.* 1998; 55(12): 1449–1455.

139. Joosten E, Lesaffre E, Riezler R. Is metabolic evidence for vitamin B-12 and folate deficiency more frequent in elderly patients with Alzheimer's disease? *J Gastroenterol.* 1997; 52A:M76–M79.

140. Maroni BJ, Mitch WE. Role of nutrition in prevention of the progression of renal disease. *Annu Rev Nutr.* 1997; 17:435–455.

141. Drukker A. The progression of chronic renal disease: immunological, nutritional and intrinsic renal mechanisms. *Isr J Med Sci.* 1997; 33(11): 739–743.

142. Lusvarghi E, Fantuzzi AL, Medici G, Barbi L, Amelio A. Natural history of nutrition in chronic renal failure. *Nephrol Dial Transplant.* 1996; 11(Suppl 9):75–84.

143. Brady JP, Hasbargen JA. A review of the effects of correction of acidosis on nutrition in dialysis patients. *Semin Dial.* 2000; 13(4):252–255.

144. Owen WF. Nutritional status and survival in end-stage renal disease patients. *Miner Electrolyte Metab.* 1998; 24(1):72–81.

145. Druml W. Nutritional management of acute renal failure. *Am J Kidney Dis.* 2001; 37(1 Suppl 2): S89–S94.

146. Wolk A, Lindblad P, Adami HO. Nutrition and renal cell cancer. *Cancer Causes Control.* 1996; 7(1):5–18.

147. Castaneda C, Grossi L, Dwyer J. Potential benefits of resistance exercise training on nutritional status in renal failure. *J Ren Nutr.* 1998; 8(1): 2–10.

148. Bottomley JM. Complementary nutrition in treating urinary incontinence. *Top Geriatr Rehabil.* 2000; 16(1):61–77.

149. Reiff TR. Water and aging. In: Watkin DM. *Nutrition in Older Persons. Clinics in Ger Med.* 1987;3(2):403–411.

150. Dowd TT, Campbell JM, Jones JA. Fluid intake and urinary incontinence in older community-dwelling women. *J Community Health Nurs.* 1996;13 (3):179–186.

151. Young VR. Impact of aging on protein metabolism. In: Armbrecht HJ, Prendergast, JM, Coe RM, eds: *Nutrition in the Aging Process.* New York: Springer Verlag; 1984:27–48.

152. Leibovitz BE, Siegel BV. Aspects of free radical reactions in biological systems: aging. *J Gerontol.* 1990;35:45–56.

153. Isaacson A, Sandow A. Effects of zinc on responses of skeletal muscle. *J Gen Physiol.* 1978; 46: 655–677.

154. Garry PJ, Goodwin JS, Hunt WC, Gilbert BA. Nutritional status in a healthy elderly population: Vitamin C. *Am J Clin Nutr.* 1982;36:332–339.

155. Rous SN. Administration of vitamin C in men with urethritis. *NY State J of Med.* 1991;82: 118–123.

156. Krotkiewski M, Gudmundsson M, Backstrom P, Mandrovkas K. Zinc's relationship to muscle strength and endurance. *Acta Physiol Scand.* 1982; 116:309–311.

157. Hamilton EM, Whitney E. *Nutrition: Concepts and Controversies.* 2nd Edition. New York: West Publishing Co; 1982.

158. Gey GO, Cooper KN, Bottenberg RA. Effect of ascorbic acid and zinc and endurance performance and athletic injury. *JAMA.* 1970;211:105–109.

159. Gordon D, Groutz A, Ascher-Landsberg J, Lessing JB, David MP, Razz O. Double-blind, placebo-controlled study of magnesium hydroxide for treatment of sensory urgency and detrusor instability: preliminary results. *Br J Obstet Gynaecol.* 1998; 105(6):667–669.

160. Sebekova K. Investigation of free intracellular magnesium, pH and energy balance in striated msucle of patients with kidney disease: relation to insulin resistance. *Gratisl Lek Listy.* 1999 100(8): 411–416.

161. Rana S, D'Amico F, Merenstein JH. Relationship of vitamin B_{12} deficiency with incontinence in older people. *J Am Geriatr Soc.* 1998; 46(7): 931–932.

162. Walls AW, Steel JG, Sheiham A, Marcenes W, Moynihan PJ. Oral health and nutrition in older people. *J Public Health Dent.* 2000; 60(4): 304–307.

163. Saunders MJ. Nutrition and oral health in the elderly. *Dent Clin North Am.* 1997; 41(4):681–698.

164. Lessard GM. Discussion: nutritional aspects of oral health—new perspectives. *Am J Clin Nutr.* 1995; 61(2):446S.

165. Mojon P, Budtz-Jorgensen E, Rapin CH. Relationship between oral health and nutrition in very old people. *Age Ageing.* 1999; 28(5):463–468.

166. Walls AW. Oral health and nutrition. *Age Ageing.* 1999; 28(5):419–420.

167. Drury TF, Winn DM, Snowden CB, Kingman A, Kleinman DV, Lewis B. An overview of the oral health component of the 1988–1991 National Health and Nutrition Examination Survey (NHANES III—Phase 1). *J Dent Res.* 1996; 75 Spec No:620–630.

168. Ship JA, Duffy V, Jones JA, Langmore S. Geriatric oral health and its impact on eating. *J Am Geriatr Soc.* 1996; 44(4):456–464.

169. Bosch JP, Saccaggi A, Lauer A, et al. Renal functional reserve in humans, effect of protein intake on glomerular filtration rate. *Am J Med.* 1984; 75: 943–950.

170. Uchida S, Tsutsumi O, Hise MK, et al. Role of epidermal factor in compensatory renal hypertrophy in mice. *Kidney Int.* 1988; 33:387–392.

171. American Dietetic Association. Position of the American Dietetic Association: nutrition, aging, and the continuum of care. *J Am Diet Assoc.* 2000; 100(5):580–595.

172. Lesourd B, Mazari L. Nutrition and immunity in the elderly. *Proc Nutr Soc.* 1999; 58(3): 685–695.

173. Chandra RK. Nutrition and immunology: from clinic to cellular biology and back again. *Proc Nutr Soc.* 1999; 58(3):681–683.

174. Proceeding of a conference on nutrition and immunity. Altlanta, Georgia, May 5–7, 1997. *Nutr Rev.* 56(1 Pt 2):S1–S186.

175. Turczynowski W, Szczepanik AM, Klek S. Nutritional therapy and the immune system. *Przegl Lek.* 2000; 57(1):36–40.

176. Macallan DC. Nutrition and immune function in human immunodeficiency virus infection. *Proc Nutr Soc.* 1999; 58(3):743–748.

177. Wick G, Grubeck-Loebenstein B. Primary and secondary alterations of immune reactivity in the elderly: impact of dietary factors and disease. *Immunol Rev.* 1997; 160(12):171–184.

178. Lesourd BM. Nutrition and immunity in the elderly: modification of immune responses with nutritional treatments. *Am J Clin Nutr.* 1997; 66(2): 478S–484S.

179. Chandra RK. Nutrition and the immune system: an introduction. *Am J Clin Nutr.* 1997; 66(2): 460S-463S.

180. Stallone DD. The influence of obesity and its treatment on the immune system. *Nutr Rev.* 1994; 52(1):37–50.

181. Sanchez A. Role of sugars in human neutrophilic phagocytosis. *Am J Clin Nutr.* 1973; 26(5): 1180–184.

182. Nutter RL, Gridley DS, Kettering JD. Modification of a transplantable colon tumor and immune responses in mice fed different sources of protein, fat, and carbohydrate. *Cancer Lett.* 1983; 18(1): 49–62.

183. Szabo G. Monocytes, alcohol use, and altered immunity. *Alcohol Clin Exp Res.* 1998; 22(2): 216–219S.

184. MacGregor RR, Louria DB. Alcohol and infection. *Curr Clin Top Infect Dis.* 1997; 17(2):291–315.

185. Kelley DS, Daudu PA. Fat intake and immune response. *Prog Food Nutr Sci.* 1993; 17(1):41–63.

186. Yaqoob P. Monounsaturated fats and immune function. *Proc Nutr Soc.* 1998; 57(3):511–520.

187. Tashiro T, Yamamori H, Takagi K. n-3 versus n-6 polyunsaturated fatty acids in critical illness. *Nutrition.* 1998; 14(4):551–553.

188. Wu D, Meydani SN. n-3 polyunsaturated fatty acids and immune function. *Proc Nutr Soc.* 1998; 57(3):503–509.

189. Fortes C, Forastiere F, Agabiti N. The effect of zinc and vitamin A supplementation on immune response in an older population. *J Am Geriatr Soc.* 1998; 46(1):19–26.

190. Girodon F, Lombard M, Galan P. Effect of micronutrient supplementation on infection in institutionalized elderly subjects: a controlled trial. *Ann Nutr Metab.* 1997; 41(1):98–107.

191. Macknin ML. Zinc lozenges for the common cold. *Cleveland Clin J Med.* 1999; 66(1):27–32.

192. Semba RD. Vitamin A, immunity, and infection. *Clin Infect Dis.* 1994; 19(3):489–499.

193. Santos MS, Meydani SN, Leka L. Natural killer cell activity in elderly men is enhanced by beta-carotene supplementation. *Am J Clin Nutr.* 1996; 64(4):772–777.

194. Gerber WF. Effect of ascorbic acid, sodium salicylate, and caffeine on the serum interferon level in response to viral infection. *Pharmacology.* 1975; 13(2):228–232.

195. Anderson R. The immunostimulatory, anti-inflammatory and antiallergic properties of ascorbate. *Adv Nutr Res.* 1984; 9(1):19–45.

196. Meydani SN, Barklund MP, Liu S. Vitamin E supplementation enhances cell-mediated immunity in healthy elderly subjects. *Am J Clin Nutr.* 1990; 52(3):557–563.

197. Penn ND, Purkins L, Kelleher J. The effect of dietary supplementation with vitamins A, C and E on cell-mediated immune function in elderly long-stay patients: a randomized controlled trial. *Age Ageing.* 1991; 20(2):169–174.

198. Pike J, Chandra RK. Effect of vitamin and trace element supplementation on immune indices in healthy elderly. *Int J Vitam Nutr Res.* 1995; 65(1): 117–127.

199. Girodon F, Lombard M, Galan P. Effect of micronutrient supplementation on infection in institutionalized elderly subjects: a controlled trial. *Ann Nutr Metab.* 1997; 41(1):98–107.

200. Exton-Smith AN. The problem of subclinical malnutrition in the elderly. In: Exton-Smith AN, Scott DL, eds. *Vitamins in the Elderly.* Briston: Wright and Sons, Ltd.; 1968; 12–18.

201. Gambert SR, Guansing AR. Protein-calorie malnutrition in the elderly. *J Am Geriatr Soc.* 1980; 28: 272–275.

202. Foley CJ, Tideiksaar R. Nutritional problems in the elderly. In: Cambert SR, ed. *Contemporary Geriatric Medicine.* New York: Plenum; 1980; I.

203. Vellas B, Guigoz Y, Baumgartner M, Garry PJ, Lauque S, Albarede JL. Relationships between nutritional markers and the Mini-Nutritional Assessment in 155 Older Persons. *J Am Geriatr Soc.* 2000; 48(10):1300–1309.

204. Sacks GS, Dearman K, Replogle WH, Cora VL, Meeks M, Canada T. Use of subjective global assessment to identify nutrition-associated complications and death in geriatric long-term care

facility residents. *J Am Coll Nutr.* 2000; 19(5): 570–577.

205. Natlow AB, Heslin J. *Geriatric Nutrition.* Boston: CBI Publishing Co.; 1980.

206. Dyer AR, Stamler J, Berkson DM, Lindberg HA. Relationship of relative weight and body mass index to 14-year mortality in the Chicago People Gas Co. study. *J Chronic Dis.* 1975; 28:109–123.

207. Master AM, Lasser RP, Beckman G. Tables of average weight and height of Americans aged 65–94 years. *JAMA.* 1960; 172:658–662.

208. Wolinsky FD, Coe RM, Chavez MN, et al. Further assessment of the reliability and validity of a nutritional risk index: analysis of a three wave panel to study elderly adults. *Health Services Res.* 1986; 20:977–990.

209. Duerksen DR Yeo TA, Siemens JL, O'Connor MP. The validity and reproducibility of clinical assessment of nutritional status in the elderly. *Nutrition.* 2000; 16(9):740–744.

210. Vellas B, Guigoz Y, Garry PJ, Nourhashemi F, Bennahum D, Lauque S, Albarede JL. The Mini Nutritional Assessment (MNA) and its use in grading the nutritional state of elderly patients. *Nutrition.* 1999; 15(2):116–22.

211. Fillenbaum GG. *The Well-being of the Elderly: Approaches to Multidimensional Assessment.* Geneva: World Health Organization; 1984. WHO Offset Publication No. 34.

212. Sacks GS, Dearman K, Replogle WH, Cora VL, Meeks M, Canada T. Use of Subjective Global Assessment to identify nutrition-associated complications and death in geriatric long-term care facility residents. *J Amer Coll Nutrition.* 2001; 19(5): 570–577.

213. Detsky AS, McLaughlin JR, Baker JP. What is subjective global assessment of nutritional status? *J Parenteral Enteral Ntrition.* 1987; 11(1): 8–13.

214. Hirsh S, de Obaldia N, Petermann M. Subjective global assessment of nutritional status: further validation. *Nutrition.* 1991; 7(1):35–38.

215. Riogo SP, Sanchez-Vilar O, Gonzalez de Villar N. Geriatric nutrition: studies about MNA. *Nutr Hosp.* 1999; 14(5)suppl 2:32S–42S.

216. Guigoz Y, Vallas B, Garry PJ. Mini Nutritional Assessment: A practical assessment tool for grading the nutritional state of elderly patients. *Facts and Research in Gerontology.* 1994; Suppl 2:15–59.

217. Branch LG, Jette AM. Personal health practices and mortality among the elderly. *Am Public Health.* 1984; 74:1126–1129.

218. Steen B, Rothenberg E. Aspects of nutrition of the elderly at home—a review. *J Nutr Health Aging.* 1998; 2(1):28–33.

219. O'Hanlon P, Kohrs MB. Dietary studies of older Americans. *Amer J Clin Nutr.* 1988; 31: 1257–1269.

220. Russell RM, Rasmussen H, Lichtenstein AH. Modified Food Guide Pyramid for people over seventy years of age. *J Nutr.* 1999; 129(3): 751–753.

221. National Research Council. *Committee Report on Dietary Allowances of the Food and Nutrition Board.* Washington, DC: National Academy of Sciences Publication; 1989.

222. Lowenstein FW. Nutritional requirements of the elderly. In: Young EA, ed. *Nutrition, Aging and Health.* New York: Alan R Liss Publishers; 1986; 61–89.

223. Wolinsky FD, Coe RM, Miller DK, et al. Measurement of global and functional dimensions of health status in the elderly. *J Gerontol.* 1984; 39: 88–92.

224. Korhs MB, Czajka-Narins D. Assessing nutrition of the elderly. In: Young EA, ed. *Nutrition, Aging and Health.* New York: Alan R Liss Publishers; 1986: 25–59.

225. Roberts SB, Dallal GE. Effects of age on energy balance. *Am J Clin Nutr.* 1998; 68(4):975S–979S.

226. Abraham S. Dietary intake findings, United States 1971–1974. In: *National Health Survey, Vital and Health Statistics.* US Department of Health, Education and Welfare, Public Health Service; 1977.

227. Carroll MD, Abraham S, Dresser CM. Dietary intake source data: United States 1976–1980. In: *The National Health Survey.* Washington, DC: Department of Health & Human Services; 1983. Series 11, NO. 231. DHHS Publication No. PHS-83-1681.

228. Calloway DH, Zanni E. Energy requirements and energy expenditure of elderly men. *Am J Clin Nutr.* 1980; 33:2088–2092.

229. Widdowson EM. How much food does man require? An evaluation of human energy needs. *Experientia.* 1983; 44(suppl):11–25.

230. Munro HN, Suter PM, Russell RM. Nutritional requirements of the elderly. *Am Rev Nutr.* 1987; 7: 23–49.

231. Lemon P. Is increased dietary protein necessary or beneficial for individuals with a physically active life? *Nutr Rev.* 1996; 54(1):S169–S175.

232. Cahill GF. Starvation in man. *N Engl J Med.* 1970; 282:668–675.

233. Young VR, Pellett PL. Plant proteins in relation to human protein and amino acid nutrition. *Am J Clin Nutr.* 1994; 59(suppl):1203S–1212S.

234. Greenblatt DJ. Reduced albumin concentration in the elderly: a report from the Boston collaborative drug surveillance program. *J Am Geriatr Soc.* 1979; 27:20–23.

235. Osborne CG, McTyre RB, Dudek J. Evidence for the relationship of calcium to blood pressure. *Nutr Rev.* 1996; 54(2):365–381.

236. Bell L, Halstenson CE, Halstenson CJ. Cholesterol-lowering effects of calcium carbonate in patients with mild to moderate hypercholesterolemia. *Arch Intern Med.* 1992; 152(12):2441–2444.

237. Bullamore JR, Gallagher JC, Wilkinson R, Nordin BEC. Effect of age on calcium absorption. *Lancet.* 1990; 11:535–537.

238. Ireland P, Fordtran JS. Effects of dietary calcium and age on jejunal calcium absorption in humans studied by intestinal perfusion. *J Clin Invest.* 1983; 52:2671–2681.

239. Armbrecht HJ. Changes in calcium and vitamin D metabolism with age. In: Armbrecht HJ, Prender-

gast JM, Coe RM, eds. *Nutritional Intervention in the Aging Process*. New York: Springer Verlag; 1984:69–86.

240. Heaney RP. Calcium intake, bone health, and aging. In: Young EA, ed. *Nutrition, Aging and Health*. New York: Alan R Liss Publications; 1986: 165–186.

241. Johnson NE, Alcantara EN, Linksweiler HN. Effect of level of protein intake on urinary and fecal calcium retention of young adults. *J Nutr.* 1990; 100: 1425–1430.

242. Draper HH, Sie TL, Bergen JC. Osteoporosis in aging rats induced by high phosphorus diet. *J Nutr.* 1984; 102:1113–1142.

243. Heaney RP, Recker RR. Effects of nitrogen, phosphorus and caffeine on calcium balance in women. *J Lab Clin Med.* 1982; 99:46–55.

244. Mortensen L, Charles P. Bioavailability of calcium supplements and the effect of vitamin D: Comparisons between milk, calcium carbonate, and calcium carbonate plus vitamin D. *Am J Clin Nutr.* 1996; 63(3):354–357.

245. Serfaty-Lacrosniere C, Woods RJ, Voytko D. Hypochlorhydria from short-term omeprazole treatment does not inhibit intestinal absorption of calcium, phosphorus, magnesium or zinc from food in humans. *J Am Coll Nutr.* 1995; 14(3): 354–358.

246. Knox TA, Kassarhian Z, Dawson-Hughes B. Calcium absorption in elderly subjects on high- and low-fiber diets: effect of gastric acidity. *Am J Clin Nutr.* 1991; 53(7):1480–1486.

247. Ivanovich P, Fellows H, Rich C. The absorption of calcium carbonate. *Ann Intern Med.* 1967; 9(2): 271–285.

248. Blumsohn A, Herrington K, Hannon RA. The effect of calcium supplementation on the circadian rhythm of bone reabsorption. *J Clin Endocrinol.* 1994; 79(4):730–735.

249. Dawson-Hughes B, Harris SS, Krall EA. Rates of bone loss in postmenopausal women randomly assigned to one of two dosages of vitamin D. *Am J Clin Nutr.* 1995; 61(8):1140–1145.

250. Labriji-Mestaghanmi H, Billaudel B, Garnier PE, Sutter BCJ. Vitamin D and pancreatic islet function. Time course for changes in insulin secretion and content during vitamin deprivation and repletion. *J Endocrine Invest.* 1988; 11(5):577–587.

251. Boucher BJ. Inadequate vitamin D status: does it contribute to disorders comprising syndrome 'X'? *Br J Nutr.* 1998; 79(2):315–327.

252. McKenna MJ, Freaney R, Meade A, Muldowney FP. Hypovitaminosis D and elevated serum alkaline phosphatase in elderly people. *Am J Clin Nutr.* 1985; 41:101–108.

253. Slovik DM, Adams JS, Weer RM, et al. Deficient production of 1,25 dihydroxyvitamin D in elderly osteoporotic patients. *N Eng J Med.* 1991; 305: 372–374.

254. Baker MR, Peacock R, Nordin BEC: The decline in vitamin D status with age. *Age Ageing.* 1980; 9: 249–256.

255. Freiman R, Johnston FA. Iron absorption in the healthy aged. *Geriatr.* 1983; 18:716–720.

256. Lipschitz DA, Mitchell CO, Thompson D. The anemia of senescence. *Am J Hematol.* 1986; 11:47–54.

257. Lipschitz DA, Udupa KB, Milton KY, Thompson D. The effect of age on hematopoiesis in man. *Blood.* 1984; 63:502–509.

258. Lipschitz DA, Mitchell CO. The correctability of the nutritional, immune and haematopoietic manifestations of protein-calorie malnutrition in the elderly. *J Amer Coll Nutr.* 1982; 1:17–25.

259. Garry PJ, Goodwin JS, Hunt WC. Folate and vitamin B12 status in a healthy elderly population. *J Am Geriatr Soc.* 1984; 32:719–726.

260. Bailey LB, Wagner PA, Christakis GJ, et al. Vitamin B12 status of elderly persons from urban low-income households. *J Am Geriatr Soc.* 1990; 28: 276–278.

261. Comfort MW. Gastric acidity before and after development of gastric cancer. Its etiologic, diagnostic and prognostic significance. *Ann Intern Med.* 1991; 34:1331–1336.

262. Steinberg WM, Toskes PP. A practical approach to evaluating mal-digestion and mal-absorption. *Geriatrics.* 1988; 33:73–85.

263. Trence DL, Moriev JE, Handwerger BS. Polyglandular auto-immune syndromes. *Am J Med.* 1984; 77:107–116.

264. Daly LE, Kirke PN, Molloy A. Folate levels and neural tube defects. *JAMA.* 1995; 274:1698–1702.

265. Russell RM, Golner BB, Kransinski SD. Effect of antacid and H2 receptor antagonists on the intestinal absorption of folic acid. *J Lab Clin Med.* 1988; 112(4):458–463.

266. Russel RM, Dutta SK, Oaks EV. Impairment of folic acid absorption by oral pancreatic extracts. *Dig Dis Sci.* 1980; 25(3):369–373.

267. Read AE, Cough KR, Pardge JL, et al. Nutritional studies on the entrants to an old people's home, with particular reference to folic acid deficiency. *Br Med J.* 1985; 11:843–848.

268. Elsborg L. Reversible malabsorption of folic acid in the elderly with nutritional folate deficiency. *Acta Haematol,* 1986; 55:140–147.

269. Batata M, Spray GH, Bolton FG, et al. Blood and bone marrow changes in elderly patients, with special reference to folic acid, vitamin B12, iron and ascorbic acid. *Br Med J* 1987; 2:667–669.

270. Fox JH, Topel JL, Huckman MS. Dementia in the elderly—a search for treatable illnesses. *J Gerontol.* 1985; 30:557–564.

271. Bhat KS. Nutritional status of thiamine, riboflavin and pyridoxine in cataract patients. *Nutr Rep Internat.* 1987; 36:685–692.

272. Varma RN, Mankad VN, Phelps DD. Depressed erythrocyte glutathione reductase activity in sickle cell disease. *Am J Clin Nutr.* 1983; 38(5): 884–887.

273. Brown WV. Niacin for lipid disorders. *Postgrad Med.* 1995; 98(2):185–193.

274. Fidanza A. Therapeutic action of pantothenic acid. *Int J Vit Nutr Res.* 1983; supple 24:53–67 [review].

275. Avogaro P, Bon B, Fusello M. Effect of pantethine on lipids, lipoproteins and apolipoproteins in man. *Curr Ther Res.* 1983; 33(4):488–493.

276. Parry G, Bredesen DE. Sensory neuropathy with low-dose pyridoxine. *Neurology.* 1985: 35(12): 1466–1468.

277. Gaby AR. Literature review and commentary: Vitamin B-complex. *Neurology.* 1990; 40(4): 338–339.

278. Zempleni J, Mock DM. Biotin biochemistry and human requirements. *J Nutr Biochem.* 1999; 10(1): 128–138.

279. Balz F. Antioxidant vitamins and heart disease. Paper presented at the 60th Annual Biology Colloquium, Oregon State University, Corvallis, Oregon, February 25, 1999.

280. Levine M, Conry-Cantilena, Wang Y. Vitamin C pharmacokinetics in healthy volunteers: evidence for a recommended dietary allowance. *Proc Natl Acad Sci USA.* 1996; 93:3704–3709.

281. Hemilä H. Does vitamin C alleviate the symptoms of the common cold? A review of current evidence. *Scand J Infect Dis.* 1994; 26(1):1–6.

282. Taddei S, Virdis A, Ghaidoni L. Vitamin C improves endothelium-dependent vasodilation by restoring nitric oxide activity in essential hypertension. *Circulation.* 1998; 97:2222–2229.

283. Chambers JC, McGregor A, Jean-Marie J. Demonstration of rapid onset vascular endothelial dysfunction after hyperhomocysteinemia. An effect reversible with vitamin C therapy. *Circulation.* 1999; 99:1156–1160.

284. Taylor A. Cataract: relationship between nutrition and oxidation. *J Am Coll Nutr.* 1993; 12(1):138–146.

285. Vincent TE, Menditatta S, May JM. Inhibition of aldose reductase in human erythrocytes by vitamin C. *Diabetes Res Clin Pract.* 1999; 43(1):1–8.

286. Leibovitz BE, Siegel BV. Aspects of free radical reactions in biological systems: aging. *Gerontol.* 1990; 35:45–56.

287. Pauling LC. Vitamin C and the common cold. San Francisco: Freeman; 1970.

288. Schorah CJ, Tormev WP, Brooks GH, et al. The effect of vitamin C supplements on body weight, serum proteins, and general health of an elderly population. *Am J Clin Nutr.* 1981; 34:871–876.

289. Sauberlich HE. Ascorbic acid. In: Olson RE, ed. *Nutrition Reviews: Present Knowledge in Nutrition.* Washington, DC: Nutrition Foundation; 1984; 269–272.

290. Sulkin NM, Sulkin DF. Tissue changes induced by marginal vitamin C deficiency. *Ann NY Acad Sci.* 1975; 258:317–328.

291. Attwood EC, Robey E, Kramer JJ, et al. A survey of the haematological, nutritional, and biochemical state of the rural elderly with particular reference to vitamin C. *Age Aging.* 1988; 7:46–56.

292. Burr ML, Elwood PC, Hole DJ, et al. Plasma and leucocyte ascorbic acid levels in the elderly. *Am J Clin Nutr.* 1984; 27:144–151.

293. Susaki R, Kurokawa T, Tero-Kubota S. Ascorbate radical and ascorbic acid level in human serum and age. *J Gerontol.* 1983; 38:26–30.

294. Spindler AA. The role of vitamin C in cognitive impairment in the elderly. *Nutr Rep Internatl.* 1989; 39:713–717.

295. Vatassery GT, Johnson GJ, Krezowski AM. Changes in vitamin E concentrations in human plasma and platelets with age. *J Am Coll Nutr.* 1983; 4: 369–375.

296. Haeger K. Long-time treatment of intermittent claudication with vitamin E. *Am J Clin Nutr.* 1984; 27:1179–1181.

297. Rimm EB, Stampger MJ, Ascherio A. Vitamin E consumption and the risk of coronary heart disease in men. *N Engl J Med.* 1993: 328: 1450–1456.

298. Stampfer MJ, Hennekens CH, Manson JE. Vitamin E consumption and the risk of coronary heart disease in women. *N Engl J Med.* 1993: 328: 1444–1449.

299. Stephans NG, Parsons A, Schofield PM, et al. Randomized controlled trial of vitamin E in patients with coronary disease: Cambridge Heart Antioxidant Study (CHAOS). *Lancet.* 1996; 347(4):871–786.

300. Azais-Braesco V, Winklhoffer-Roob B, Ribalta J, et al. Vitamin A, vitamin E and carotenoid status and metabolism during ageing: functional and nutritional consequences. *Endocr Regul.* 2000; 34(2): 97–98.

301. Sokol RJ. Vitamin E deficiencies in the elderly. *Free Radical Bio Med.* 1989; 6:189–193.

302. Birren JE, Bick MW, Fox C. Age changes in the light threshold of the dark-adapted eye. *J Gerontol.* 1988; 43:267–271.

303. Watkin DM. *Handbook of Nutrition, Health and Aging.* Park Ridge, NJ: Noyes Publications; 1983.

304. Read MH, Graney AS. Food supplement usage by the elderly. *J Am Diet Assoc.* 1982; 80:250–253.

305. Bendich A, Langseth L. Safety of vitamin A. *Am J Clin Nutr.* 1989; 49(3):358–371.

306. Shekelle RB, Lepper M, Liu S. Dietary A and risk of cancer in the Western Electric Study. *Lancet.* 1981; 11:1185–1190.

307. Hennekens CH, Burning JE, Manson JE. Lack of effect on long-term supplementation with beta carotene on the incidence of malignant neoplasms and cardiovascular disease. *N Engl J Med.* 1996; 334:1145–1149.

308. Albanes D, Heinone OP, Taylor PR. Alpha-tocopherol and beta-carotene supplements and lung cancer incidence in the Alpha-Tocopherol, Beta Carotene Cancer Prevention Study: effects of baseline characteristics and study compliance. *J Natl Cancer Inst.* 1996; 88:1560–1570.

309. Omenn GS, Goodman GE, Thornquiest MD. Effects of a combination of beta carotene and vitamin A on lung cancer and cardiovascular disease. *N Engl J Med.* 334:1150–1155.

310. Ben-Amotz A, Levy Y. Bioavailability of a natural isomer mixture compared with synthetic all-trans beta-carotene in human serum. *Am J Clin Nutr.* 1996; 63(6):729–734.

311. Sandstead HH, Henriksen LK, Greger JL, et al. Zinc nutriture in the elderly in relation to taste acuity, immune response and wound healing. *Am J Clin Nutr.* 1982; 36:1046–1059.

312. Prasad A. Discovery of human zinc deficiency and studies in an experimental human model. *Am J Clin Nutr.* 1991; 53(3):403–412.

313. Lindman RD, Clark ML, Colmore JP. Influence of age and sex on plasma and red-cell zinc concentrations. *J Gerontol.* 1991; 26:358–363.

314. Bunker VW, Hinks LJ, Lawson MS, et al. Assessment of zinc and copper status of healthy elderly people using metabolic balance studies and measurement of leucocyte concentrations. *Am J Clin Nutr.* 1984; 40:1096–1102.

315. Wagner PA, Krista ML, Bailey LB, et al. Zinc status of elderly black Americans from urban low-income households. *Am J Clin Nutr.* 1990; 33: 1771–1777.

316. Alhava EM, Oikkonen H, Puittinen J, et al. Zinc content of human cancellous bone. *Acta Orthop Scand.* 1987; 48:1–4.

317. Schroeder HA, Nelson AP, Tipton TH, et al. Essential trace metals in man: zinc. Relation to environmental cadmium. *J Chronic Dis.* 1987; 20: 179–210.

318. Blazsek I, Mathe G. Zinc and immunity. *Biomed Pharmacother.* 1984; 38:187–193.

319. Makinodan T, Yunis E, eds. *Immunology and Aging.* New York: Plenum Press; 1977; 1.

320. Wacker WEC. Role of zinc in wound healing: a critical review. In: Prasad AS, ed. *Trace Elements in Human Health and Disease.* New York: Academic Press; 1986:107–114.

321. Haeger K, Lanner E, Magnusson PO. Oral zinc sulfate in the treatment of venous leg ulcer. In: Pories WJ, Strain WH, Hsu JM, Woosley RL, eds. *Clinical Applications of Zinc Metabolism.* Springfield, Ill: Charles C. Thomas; 1974: 158–167.

322. Essatara M'B, Morley JE, Levine AS, et al. The role of the endogenous opiates in zinc deficiency anorexia. *Physiol Behav.* 1984; 32:475–478.

323. Morley JE, Levine AS. The pharmacology of eating behavior. *Ann Rev Pharmacol Toxicol.* 1985; 25: 127–146.

324. Billington CJ, Levine AS, Morley JE. Zinc status in impotent patients. *Clin Res.* 1983; 31(abstr):714A.

325. Burnet FM. A possible role of zinc in the pathology of dementia. *Lancet.* 1991; 1:186–188.

326. Cartwright GE, Wintrobe MM. The question of copper deficiency in man. *Am J Clin Nutr.* 1984; 15:94–110.

327. Harris HD, O'Dell BL. Copper and amine oxidases in connective tissue metabolism. Protein-metal interaction. *Adv Exp Med Biol.* 1984; 48: 267–284.

328. O'Dell BL. Biochemistry of physiology and copper in vertebrates. In: Prasad AS, ed. *Trace Elements in Human Health and Disease.* New York: Academic Press; 1986; 1:391–413.

329. Yunice AA, Linedman RD, Czerwinski AW, et al. Influence of age and sex on serum copper and ceruloplasmin levels. *J Gerontol.* 1984; 29: 277–281.

330. Saner G, Yüzbasiyan V, Neyzi O. Alterations of chromium metabolism and effect of chromium supplementation in Turner's syndrome patients. *Am J Clin Nutr.* 1983; 38(4):574–578.

331. Riales R, Albrink MJ. Effect of chromium chloride supplementation on glucose tolerance and serum lipids including high-density lipoprotein of adult men. *Am J Clin Nutr.* 1998; 34(12): 2670–2678.

332. Wang MM, Fox EZ, Stoecker BJ. Serum cholesterol of adults supplemented with brewer's yeast or chromium chloride. *Nutr Res.* 1989; 9: 989–998.

333. Schroeder HA. Serum cholesterol and glucose levels in rats fed refined and less refined sugars and chromium. *J Nutr.* 1989; 97:237–242.

334. Schroeder HA, Nason AP, Tipton IH. Chromium deficiency as a factor in atherosclerosis. *J Chronic Dis.* 1990; 23:123–142.

335. Offenbacher EG, Pi-Sunyer FX. Beneficial effects of chromium rich yeast on glucose tolerance and blood lipids in elderly subjects. *Diabetes.* 1980; 29:919–925.

336. Newman HAI, Leighton RF, Lanese RR, et al. Serum chromium and angiographically determined coronary artery disease. *Clin Chem.* 1978; 24:541–544.

337. Page TG, Ward TL, Southern LL. Effect of chromium picolinate on growth and carcass characteristics of growing-finishing pigs. *J Animal Sci.* 1991; 69(3):356–359.

338. Lefavi R, Anderson R, Keith R. Efficacy of chromium supplementation in athletes: Emphasis on anabolism. *Int J Sport Nutr.* 1992; 2(1): 111–122.

339. McCarty MF. The case for supplemental chromium and a survey of clinical studies with chromium picolinate. *J Appl Nutr.* 1991; 43(1): 59–66.

340. Kunin RA. Clinical uses of iodide and iodine. *Nutr Healing.* 1998; 1(7):7–10.

341. Gasper AZ, Gasser P, Flammer J. The influence of magnesium on visual field and peripheral vasospasm in glaucoma. *Ophthalmologica.* 1995; 209 (1):11–13.

342. Kawano Y, Matsuoka H, Takishita S, Omae T. Effects of magnesium supplementation in hypertensive patients. *Hypertension.* 1998; 32(2): 260–265.

343. Weisinger JR, Bellorin-Front E. Magnesium and phosphorus. *Lancet.* 1998; 352(3):391–396.

344. Raloff J. Reasons for boning up on manganese. *Science.* 1986; 199 [review issue].

345. Clark LC, Combs GF, Turnbull BW. Effects of selenium supplementation for cancer prevention in patients with carcinoma of the skin. *JAMA.* 1996; 276:1957–1963.

346. Yoshizawa K, Willett WC, Morris SJ. Study of prediagnostic selenium levels and risk of advanced prostate cancer. *J Natl Cancer Inst.* 1998; 90: 1219–1224.

347. Yu SY, Li WG, Zhu YJ. Chemoprevention trial of human hepatitis with selenium supplementation in China. *Biol Trace Element Res.* 1989; 20(1): 15–20.

348. Peretz A, Néve J, Desmedt J. Lymphocyte response is enhanced by supplementation of elderly subjects with selenium-enriched yeast. *Am J Clin Nutr.* 1991; 53(12):1323–1328.

349. Armstrong-Esther CA, Browne KD, Armstrong-Esther DC, Sander L. The institutionalized elderly: dry to the bone! *Int J Nurs Stud.* 1996; 33(6): 619–628.

350. Phillips PA, Rolls BJ, Ledingham JGG, et al. Reduced thirst after water deprivation in healthy elderly men. *N Engl J Med.* 1984; 311:753–759.

351. Miller PD, Krebs RA, Neal BJ, et al. Hypodipsia in geriatric patients. *Am J Med.* 1982; 73: 354–356.

352. Lavizzo-Mourey R, Johnson J, Stolley P. Risk factors for dehydration among elderly nursing home residents. *J Am Geriatr Soc.* 1988; 36: 213–218.

353. Roe DA. Therapeutic effects of drug-nutrient interactions in the elderly. *J Am Diet Assoc.* 1985; 85: 174–178.

354. Smith CH, Bidlack WR. Dietary concerns associated with the use of medications. *J Am Diet Assoc.* 1984; 84:901–908.

355. Blumberg J, Couris R. Pharmacology, nutrition, and the elderly: interactions and implications. In: Chernoff R. *Geriatric Nutrition: The Health Professional's Handbook.* 2nd Edition. Gaithersburg, MD: Aspen Publishers, Inc. 1999; 342–365.

356. Lotz M, Zisman E, Bartter C. Evidence for phosphorus depletion syndrome in man. *N Engl J Med.* 1968; 278:409–415.

357. Rud RK, Singer FR. Magnesium deficiency and excess. *Annual Rev Med.* 1981; 32(2):245–259.

358. Insogna KL, Bordley DR, Caro JF. Osteomalacia and weakness from excessive antacids. *JAMA.* 244:2544–2546.

359. Benn A, Swan CJH, Cooke WT. Effect of intraluminal pH on the absorption of pteroylmonoglutamic acid. *Cr Med J.* 1971; 16(1):148–150.

360. Spencer H, Lender M. Adverse effects of aluminum-containing antacids on mineral metabolism. *Gastroenterol.* 1989; 76:603–606.

361. Wasnich R, Benfante R, Yanok-Heilbrun L, Vogel J. Thiazide effect on the mineral content of bone. *N Eng J Med.* 1983; 309:344–347.

362. Frame B, Guiang HL, Frost HN. Osteomalacia induced by laxative ingestion. *Arch Intern Med.* 1971; 128:794–796.

363. Lawrence VA, Lowenstein JE, Eichner ER. Aspirin and folate binding: in vivo and in vitro studies of serum binding and urinary excretion of exogenous folate. *J Lab Clin Med.* 1984; 103(6): 944–948.

364. Welling P. Nutrient effects on drug metabolism and action in the elderly. *Drug Nutr Interact.* 1985; 4(1):183–193.

365. Nutt JG, Woodward WR, Hammerstad JP. The "on-off" phenomenon in Parkinson's disease: relation to levodopa absorption and transport. *N Engl J Med.* 1984; 310:483–488.

366. Hathcock JN. Metabolic mechanisms of drug-nutrient interactions. *Fed Proc.* 44(1):124–129.

367. Ciccone CD. Pharmacokinetics II: drug elimination. In: Ciccone CD. *Pharmacology in Rehabilitation.* 2nd Edition. Contemporary Perspectives in Rehabilitation. Philadelphia, PA: F.A. Davis. 1996; 32–43.

368. Anderson KE. Nutrient regulation of chemical metabolism in humans. *Fed Proc.* 44(1):130–134.

369. Vestal RE, Norris AH, Tobin JD, et al. Antipyrin metabolism in man: influence of age, alcohol, caffeine and smoking. *Clin Pharm Ther.* 1975; 18: 425–432.

370. Alderman E, Coltart D. Alcohol and the heart. *Br Med Bull.* 1982; 38:77–81.

371. Richard MJ, Roussel AM. Micronutrients and ageing: intakes and requirements. *Proc Nutr Soc.* 58 (3):573–578.

372. McCay CM, Crowell MF, Maynard LA. The effect of retarded growth upon length of life span and ultimate body size. *J Nutr.* 1935; 10:63–79.

373. Young VR. Diet as modulator of aging and longevity. *Fed Proc.* 1979; 38:1994–2000.

374. Porta EA. Nutritional factors and aging. In: Robin RB, Mehlman MA, eds. *Advances in Modern Human Nutrition.* Park Forest South, II: Pathotox; 1980; 1:106–118.

375. Harman D. Free radical of aging: dietary implications. *Am J Clin Nutr.* 1972; 25:839–943.

376. Mechnikova O. *Life of Elie Metchnikoff.* London: Constable and Company; 1921.

377. Kohn RR. *Principles of Mammalian Aging.* Englewood Cliffs, NJ: Prentice Hall; 1978.

378. Shamberger RJ, Andreone TL, Willis CE. Antioxidants and cancer, I.V. initiating activity of maignaldehyde as a carcinogen. *J Natl Cancer Inst.* 1963; 53:316–326.

379. Jennings BJ, Ozanne SE, Hales CH. Nutrition, oxidative damage, telomere shortening, and cellular senescence: individual or connected agents of aging? *Mol Genet Metab.* 2000; 71(1–2):32–42.

380. Ordy JM. Nutrition as modulator of rate of aging, disease, and longevity. In: Ordy JM, Harman D, Alin-Slater RB, eds. *Nutrition in Gerontology.* New York: Raven Press; 1994; 26:1–17.

381. Hegsted DM. Energy needs and energy utilization. *Nutr Rev.* 1974; 32:33–45.

382. Kreutler PA. *Nutrition in Perspective.* Englewood Cliffs, NJ: Prentice Hall; 1980.

383. Young VR. Protein metabolism with aging. In: Munro HN, ed. *Mammalian Protein Metabolism.* New York: Academic Press; 1980; IV.

384. Mazari L, Lesourd BM. Nutritional influences on immune response in healthy aged persons. *Mech Aging Dev.* 1998; 104(1):25–40.

385. Lesourd BM. Nutrition and immunity in the elderly: modification of immune responses with nutritional treatments. *Am J Clin Nutr.* 1997; 66(2): 478S–484S.

386. Pedersen BK, Bruunsgaard H, Jensen M, Toft AD, Hansen H, Ostrowski K. Exercise and the immune system—influence of nutrition and ageing. *J Sci Med Sport.* 1999; 2(3):234–252.

387. Nieman DC. Exercise immunology: future directions for research related to athletes, nutrition, and the elderly. *Int J Sports Med.* 2000; 21(Suppl 1): S61–S68.

388. Weg RB. *Nutrition and the Later Years.* Los Angeles: University of Southern California Press; 1979.

389. Roe DA. *Handbook: Interactions of Selected Drugs and Nutrients in Patients.* Chicago, IL: American Dietetic Association. 2001.

390. Stultz BM. Preventive health care for the elderly. *Western J Med.* 1984; 141:832–845.

391. Kennie DC. Health maintenance in the elderly. *J Amer Geriatr Soc.* 1984; 32:316–323.

392. Berkman LF. The assessment of social networks and social support in the elderly. *J Am Geriatr Soc.* 1983; 31:743–749.

393. Russell RM. The aging process as a modifier of metabolism. *Am J Clin Nutr.* 2000; 72(2 Suppl): 529S–532S

394. Sonn U, Rothenberg E, Steen B. Dietary intake and functional ability between 70 and 76 years of age. *Aging.* 1998; 10(4):324–331.

395. Smiciklas-Wright H, Fosmire GJ. Government nutrition programs for the aged. In: Watson RR, ed. *CRC Handbook of Nutrition in the Aged.* Boca Raton, Fla: CRC Press; 1985;323–334.

396. Fanelli MT, Kaufman M. Nutrition and older adults. In: Phillips HT, Gaylord SA, eds. *Aging and Public Health.* New York: Springer Publishing; 1985:76–100.

397. Lipschitz DA, Mitchell CO, Steele RW, Milton KY. Nutritional evaluation and supplementation of elderly subjects participating in a "Meals on Wheels" program. *J Parent Ent Nutr.* 1985; 9 343–347.

398. Mayer J. Hunger and undernutrition in the United States. *J Nutr.* 1990; 120(8):919–923.

399. Martinez-Spencer A, Westley C. Nutrition for better aging in long-term care. *Lippincotts Prim Care Pract.* 1999; 3(2):174–178.

400. Keller HH. Malnutrition in institutionalized elderly: how and why? *J Am Geriatr Soc.* 1993; 41 (11):1212–1218.

401. Finn SC. Nutrition and healthy aging. *J Womens Health Gend Based Med.* 2000; 9(7):711–716.

402. Maaravi Y, Berry EM, Ginsberg G, Cohen A, Stessman J. Nutrition and quality of life in the aged. *Aging.* 2000; 12(5):402.

403. Visser M. Nutritional state and quality of life in old age. *Aging.* 2000; 12(4):320.

404. Butler RN. Fighting frailty. Prescription for healthier aging includes exercise, nutrition, safety, and research. [editorial] *Geriatrics.* 2000; 55(2):20.

405. Villers Foundation. *On the Other Side of Easy Street: Myths and Facts about the Economics of Old Age.* Washington, DC: Villers Foundation; 1986.

406. Dwyer JT. Nutritional concerns and problems of the aged. In: Satin DG, ed. *The Clinical Care of the Aged Person: An Interdisciplinary Perspective.* Oxford University Press; 1993.

CHAPTER 8

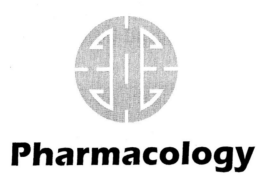

Pharmacology

Mrs. Jones, a 98-year-old woman with Parkinson's disease who recently had an amputation above the knee came to physical therapy late one day. Her therapist was busy in the gym with several other patients, but she handed Mrs. Jones a black dumbbell weight, which Mrs. Jones had frequently used to do her warm-up exercise. Instead of beginning her usual exercises, Mrs. Jones raised the dumbbell to her ear and said "Hello, Emily?" She continued to chat on what she thought was a phone. The therapist immediately went to the nurses' station and discovered that Mrs. Jones was on a new medication, which had obviously profoundly confused her. Her medication was changed, and in a few days, she was her usual coherent self. This real-life example graphically depicts one of the many complications of administering drugs to older persons.

As physical and occupational therapists, we are highly involved in our patients' care and need to be involved as part of a team in their pharmacologic management. As an individual ages, the way that a person's body handles a drug changes. Drug regimens in the elderly, particularly those who are medically compromised by illness or injury, should, therefore, be evaluated and reassessed regularly.

This chapter will explore the multiple aspects of medication management in the elderly. Drug disposition, response, and adverse reactions in the elderly patient will be discussed, as well as common drug regimens. Frequently used medications, common pathologies, and drug reactions will be explored. Monitoring techniques and compliance issues will also be examined. A discussion of the use of over-the-counter drugs and self-medication, as well as consideration of drug-induced malnutrition are included. Finally, to keep pace with the increasing popularity of the use of herbs and vitamins in the treatment of many pathological conditions, herbs, vitamins, and nutraceuticals will be presented in a concise table format for easy reference.

EPIDEMIOLOGICAL ISSUES

The number of elderly in the United States, as well as worldwide, is expanding at an ever increasing rate. Older people take more prescription and over-the-counter medications than younger people. Although those over 65 years of age and older constitute only 12% of the population, they consume 31% of all prescribed drugs.[1] Older persons tend to have more chronic problems and diseases that often involve a multisystem diagnosis. Both of these are causes for concern when managing medications for this age group. Chronicity of disease impels the prescribing physician to sample a wide array of medications for symptom relief. Physicians will, in most instances, consult a specialist for additional advice in management. Unfortunately, additional drugs usually accompany this additional management. Since chronic problem management is not curative in nature, an ongoing drug regimen use may be prescribed to alleviate symptoms. This pharmacological behavior can easily cause complications unless someone coordinates all the medications.[1,2] The multiplicity of disease that is so commonly seen in the elderly also dictates polypharmacy management and, therefore, requires careful coordination and management.

CLINICAL IMPLICATIONS

Medications are absorbed, distributed, metabolized, and excreted (pharmacokinetics) differently in the elderly, and the action of drugs (pharmocodynamics) may be exaggerated or diminished. Of special significance in the geriatric population, different drugs interact with each other either by pharmacokinetic inhibition or induction of drug metabolism or by pharmacodynamic potentiation or antagonism. Knowledge of these pharmacological pathways has a profound impact on the quality of care. The problem of polypharmacy, defined here as the use of two or more chronic medications, is often a problem in the older patient.[1,3] Medication mishaps in the elderly occur for numerous reasons. Multiple providers are often unaware of one another's new prescriptions or medication changes, especially after hospitalization. Older patients often have visual or cognitive impairments (or both) that lead to errors in self-administration. Patients may be unable to afford their medicines, so they take only some of what is prescribed based on how they are feeling, or they cut doses down to save money and extend the life of their prescription. Functional illiteracy, which is not uncommon among the elderly, makes adherence to a medical regimen difficult. Cultural diversity also changes an older individual's perspective regarding the value of taking a certain medication when a natural alternative has been used for centuries in their culture to treat the same condition.

The average rehabilitation professional is not knowledgeable about the vast number of drug interactions. It is important for therapists working with the elderly to understand the actions and interactions of drugs for several reasons. First, physical and occupational therapists design and monitor exercise programs that can adversely affect pharmacokinetics. Fat-soluble drugs, for example, may be affected by a person's decrease in fat after participation in an exercise program, and, therefore, dosages will need to be adjusted accordingly. Second, therapists see patients on a regular basis and can easily note adverse reactions, such as dizziness, confusion, and slurred speech.

If educated in pharmacology, therapists can suggest modifications of drug regimens based on patient symptoms. A good example of this is Mrs. Jones. Noting her confused state, the therapist would be able to review her medications, find the offending drug (for example, benztropine, the drug for treatment of Parkinson's), and perhaps suggest that the physician prescribe another drug for replacement or lower the present dosage of the drug.

Appropriate medication management is an interdisciplinary concern. Other health care team members, not just the physician, must take responsibility for the supervision and coordination of drug interventions.

PHARMACOKINETICS AND THE ELDERLY

Pharmacokinetics is the process by which the body handles drugs. Pharmacokinetics has four progressive stages: absorption, distribution, biotransformation, and excretion. Each stage can be affected by the aging process. Since the goal of drug administration is to reach a therapeutic level, the rate and efficiency of these stages of pharmacokinetics will be influential in achieving this goal.

Controversy exists as to whether aging or the effects of disease truly affect the absorption of drugs.[4,5] Changes in drug metabolism in the healthy elderly are often minimal and not of clinical significance. However, the clinical impact of aging changes in the gastrointestinal tract, or in older people with kidney or liver disease can be considerable. Absorption is the process by which a drug passes from the gastrointestinal tract to the bloodstream,[5] and because age-related changes occur in the gastrointestinal tract, it has been hypothesized that they are one of a number of causes for a decrease in absorption that occurs in later life. These age-related changes include decreases in the intestinal blood flow, the time needed for gastric emptying, and the mucosal cell absorbing area, which might delay or reduce absorption. In addition, there is an alteration in gastric pH that may affect ionization and drug solubility. Adverse drug reactions are two to three times more likely to occur in older individuals.[1,3] In general, drug absorption is complete in older persons, although it often occurs at a slower rate. Bioavailability, the percentage of a drug reaching the systemic circulation, depends on absorption and first-pass metabolism. Some drugs have increased bioavailability in the elderly (e.g., labetalol, levodopa, nifedipine, omeprazole), which leads to potential toxicity in an older person.

Distribution, the next phase of pharmacokinetics, determines the concentration of a drug.[2,6] The nature of drugs will cause them to have an affinity for certain body components, such as water, fat, or protein, and this will affect their action at their target site.[6] Drug distribution can change due to age-related changes in body compostion. Weight is reduced, percentage of body fat is increased, and total body water and lean mass are decreased. Hydrophilic drugs have a higher concentration, since they are distributed in a smaller volume of body water. Lipophilic drugs have a larger volume of distribution and a longer half-life, since they are distributed in a larger volume of fat. Decreased albumin and other binding proteins may or may not affect the active drug concentration.[6]

Since a drug must go through the liver, be changed to enzymes, enter the circulation, bind to protein in the blood or cells, and eventually infiltrate each of the target organs, it is easy to see that how well an organ is perfused affects the drug's distribution. The age-related changes that affect this process are decreases in lean body mass, total body water, and plasma albumin.[6,7] These changes will affect the concentration of the drug and the protein-binding ability of the drug. In addition, the increase in body fat with increased age will affect the drug's accumulation in the fatty tissue and possibly prolong its action.[7,8] The results of these changes are that the elderly are more susceptible to toxicity and are more prone to have side effects of the drug than younger patients.[9]

Biotransformation, the next phase of pharmacokinetics, is the process of metabolizing a drug to inactive or active metabolites.[8] This process determines the length of time that a drug stays in the body. Since the liver plays an integral role in biotransformation, age-related changes in liver function will affect the efficiency of this process. The age changes related to biotransformation are decreases in the size, amount of blood flow, and hepatic enzyme activity of the liver,[10] and all of these changes will result in a decreased rate of hepatic metabolism. Hepatic metabolism varies greatly among individuals based on age, sex, lifestyle, hepatic blood flow, presence of liver disease, and other factors.[1] Although enzymes are usually unchanged by aging, many drugs are metabolized more slowly in older people due to a reduction in hepatic blood flow. This decreased metabolism of the drug may cause a buildup of the drug and result in toxic effects.

The final phase of the pharmacokinetics process is excretion. Excretion is the elimination of a drug from the body. Most drugs are eliminated through the kidneys (a small portion are excreted through the skin and feces), therefore, age changes in the kidney have a significant influence on the elimination of drugs. These age changes are decreases in the renal blood flow, the glomerular filtration rate (GFR), and the rate of tubular excretion.[11] Renal excretion of drugs diminishes by 35% to 50% due to decreased GFR,[1] however, because of decreased muscle mass, measurement of serum creatinine does not reflect GFR, and many formulas to estimate creatinine clearance based on age, weight, and creatinine are inaccurate. Obtaining a 24-hour urine collection to assess creatine clearance is the most accurate way to estimate GFR. The changes in the kidney affect an overall reduction in excretion and an accumulation of drugs and drug metabolites in the body. These age-related pharmacokinetic changes result in a longer drug half-life, diminished clearance, and a longer time to reach a steady state. This is reflected in different serum levels at a given dose. Because of age-related pharmacodynamic changes, drugs have a different effect at the same serum level. For example, opioids have a greater analgesic effect, benzodiazepines have a greater sedative effect, and anticoagulants are associated with a higher risk of bleeding. Beta-blockers, in contrast, are less effective in the elderly.[12] The accumulation of drugs without clearance can lead to toxicity, and conversely, the poor absorption of a drug can lead to the need for higher doses and a greater potential for adverse drug reactions and interactions. In addition, common cardiac problems can increase the likelihood of drug toxicity because of the damaging effects of these diseases on renal functioning.

Pharmacokinetics will vary from person to person. The therapist should keep in mind the phases of this process and look for signs of drug toxicity and adverse reactions.

DRUG USE AND ADVERSE REACTIONS IN THE ELDERLY

The biggest drug users in this country are the population over the age of 65. Polypharmacy, and the potential for the excessive prescription and self-administration of medications, is an enormous problem among the elderly population.[13] In the rehabilitation setting, the use of medications is probably even more prevalent. Most rehabilitation patients have multiple problems and consequently receive multiple medications. In addition, these patients may be taking self-prescribed over-the-counter (OTC) medications to alleviate chronic symptoms associated with the diseases or inactivity due to the disease. The purpose of their behavior is to alleviate their symptoms and improve their functional status. Many times, however, adverse reactions or unwanted side effects occur. Therapists should be aware of the most commonly used OTC drugs, therefore, and any adverse effects associated with them. These will be listed later in this chapter.

When more than one drug is taken, age-related pharmacokinetic and pharmacodynamic considerations of one drug may be complicated by drug interactions. Some interactions result in less drug being available through the mechanisms of impaired absorption, induced hepatic enzymes, and inhibition of cellular uptake. Impaired absorption can be due to binding by a concurrently administered drug, such as cholestyramine-binding digoxin and thyroxine.[12] Smoking and chronic alcohol use have been found to induce similar effects.[13] Interactions that result in more drug availability can also occur and include inhibition of metabolic enzymes and inhibition of renal excretion.[12,13] Inhibition of metabolism leads to increased half-life, accumulation of the drug, and potential toxicity. Inhibition of renal excretion causes more drug availability. For example, probenecid inhibits the excretion of penicillin.[14] Pharmacodynamic interactions, those in which the actions of different drugs affect the same end point, can also occur.[14] For example, warfarin and aspirin interact by increasing the likelihood of bleeding through separate pathways. Similarly, warfarin and nonsteroidal anti-inflammatory drugs (NSAIDs) make gastrointestinal bleeding more likely. NSAIDs also raise blood pressure and may undermine the action of antihypertensive agents.[14,15] As presented in Chapter 7, Exploring Nutrition in the Aged, drug-food interactions can also complicate the picture. For example, interactions with grapefruit juice (or other acid-based substances) can potentiate the effects of buspirone or felodipine, and should be considered when adverse drug reactions occur.

The health professional must be familiar with the most common prescription drugs and be aware of all medications the elderly patient is taking, including over-the-counter drugs, vitamins, and herbal remedies. The rehabilitation professional should report any adverse reactions and investigate all complaints, as they may point to drug-drug or drug-nutrient interactions. Drug toxicity and drug interactions should be part of the differential diagnosis for altered mental status, fatigue, postural hypotenion, depression, incontinence, movement and gait disorders, and any other symptoms that are uncharacteristic of the elderly individual you are working with. Pharmacists, computer databases, and other drug interaction resources (e.g., Physician's Desk Reference), for health care professionals who have limited background education in pharmacology, are helpful for checking known drug-drug and drug-nutrient interactions.

In reviewing the most common prescription drugs and over-the-counter medications used by Medicare patients in all settings, the most frequently prescribed and non-prescribed drugs were identified.[6,15] These medications are listed in Table 8–1 according to class of drug. It is obvious from such frequent and diverse drug-taking behaviors that side effects are likely to occur, and drug-taking behavior in relation to age-related changes contributes to the occurrence of adverse reactions.

The adverse reactions or side effects of special concern to therapists are postural hypotension, fatigue

TABLE 8–1. CLASSES OF PRESCRIPTION DRUGS COMMONLY USED BY MEDICARE PATIENTS

Cardiovascular Drugs
Antianginal
Antiarrhythmic
Antihypertensive agents
  Sympatholytics
  β-Blockers
  Vasodilators
  ACE inhibitors
Antilipemic agents
Cardiac glycosides

Diuretics
Thiazide
Potassium sparing
Loop

Tranquilizers
Minor
Major

Anticoagulants
Coumadin
Heparin

Benzodiazepines
Temazepam
Triazolam
Flurazepam

Analgesics
Non-narcotic
  Acetaminophen
  Aspirin
Narcotic

Diabetic Products
Insulin preparations
Oral hypoglycemics

Antacids
Sodium bicarbonate
Aluminum hydroxide
Aluminum & magnesium
  hydroxide
Magaldrate

Cathartics
Castor oil
Psyllium

Antibiotics
Erythromycin
Amoxicillin

Anti-inflammatories
NSAIDs
  Aspirin
  Ibuprofen
  Naproxen
Cox-2 Inhibitors
Andrenal corticosteroids

Antispasmodics
Dicyclominehydrochloride

Thyroidals
Thyroidal hormones
Antithyroid agents

Vitamins & Herbs
All over-the-counter
  preparations

and weakness, depression, dehydration, confusion and dementia, movement and gait dis- orders, extrapyramidal signs, incontinence, anticholinergic actions, dizziness, and fluid volume depletion.

Postural Hypotension

Postural hypotension is defined as a drop in systolic blood pressure upon assumption of an erect posture.[15] When blood pressure drops in this manner, the person often is more susceptible to falls and fractures, as well as to cardiac and cerebral infarcts, which the older person is already at risk for because of age-related changes in the homeostatic mechanisms affecting this process.[16] Any additional impairment caused by a drug, for example, would put the person at further risk. Table 8–2 provides a list of drugs that can cause or contribute to postural hypotension.[1,2,16]

Fatigue and Weakness

Fatigue and weakness in older patients may have a pathological, pharmaceutical, or psychological cause.[15,16] The therapist can explore possible causes

TABLE 8–2. DRUGS CAUSING POSTURAL HYPOTENSION

Tricyclic Antidepressants (Depression)	Aldomet
Amitriptyline	Guanethidine
Elavil	*Esimil*
Endep	Peripheral α-blockers
Desipramine	Phenoxybenzamine
Norpramin	*Dibenzyline*
Pertofrane	Phentolamine
Doxepin	*Regitine*
Adapin	Prazosin
Sinequan	*Minipress*
Imipramine	β-Adrenoreceptor blockers
Tofranil	Atenolol
Nortriptyline	*Tenormin*
Aventyl	Pindolol
Pamelor	*Visken*
Protriptyline	Metroprolol
Vivactil	*Lopressor*
Trimipramine	Timolol
Surmontil	*Blocadren*
	ACE Inhibitors
Tranquilizers (Insomnia, psychotic behavior)	Captopril
Thiothixene	*Capoten*
Navane	Enalapril
Haloperidol	*Vasotec*
Haldol	Vasodilators
	Nifedipine
Narcotic Analgesics (pain)	*Procardia*
ALL	Calcium channel blockers
	Nicardipine
Antiparkinsonians (Parkinson's)	*Cardene*
Levodopa	Isradipine
	DynaCirc
Sedative-Hypnotics (insomnia, anxiety, behavioral)	Verapamil
	Isoptin
Benzodiazepines	*Calan*
Florazepam	
Dalmane	**Diuretics (hypertension, CHF)**
Temazepam	ALL
Restoril	
Triazolam	**Nitrates (angina)**
Halcion	Nitroglycerin
	Nitro-dur or Nitro-Bid
Antiarrhythmic Drugs (cardiovascular disease)	Erythrityl tetranitrate
ALL	*Cardilate*
	Isosorbide dinitrate
Antihypertensive Drugs (hypertension)	*(Dilatrate SR)*
Sympatholytics	
Methyldopa	

through consulting with both the physician and the patient to determine if any intervention would be successful. For psychological causes of fatigue and weakness, consult Chapter 4. For cardiovascular disease, diabetes, and arthritis, the therapist should understand the limitations posed by these pathologies and respect and progress within those limits (see Chapter 5 for pathologies of aging). Drug administration may contribute to the psychological and pathological disease component.

Several drugs deserve to be mentioned when discussing fatigue and weakness. Beta-blockers can cause fatigue because of their ability to slow down the heart and reduce blood flow. Diuretics decrease fluid volume and may cause dehydration, a decrease in cardiac output, or both, which can cause hyponatremia or hypokalemia. In addition, vasodilators, digitalis preparations, antihypertensives, and oral hypoglycemics may cause weakness and fatigue.[16]

Since fatigue and weakness are such important factors in a rehabilitation program, the therapist must work with the physician to alter the medication to fit the rehabilitation program or to alter the rehabilitation to fit the medication program.

Depression

Depression can be caused by any drug that has an adverse effect on brain function. If an individual is depressed, they lack the motivation and interest to participate in a rehabilitation program. In addition, they are unable to realistically assess their improvements. Therapists must be involved with the doctor to manage these problems. Table 8–3 lists drugs that may cause depression.

Dehydration

Many pharmacologic agents lead to dehydration, a decrease in total body water. This condition is the most common fluid and electrolyte disturbance among the elderly. Although the morbidity of hospitalized elderly with dehydration is seven times more likely than in age-matched cohorts without dehydration,[17] older persons residing in nursing homes and in the community are also at risk. Older people have an increased sensitivity to dehydration as a result of physiological changes including an increase in fat and a decrease in lean body mass, which corresponds with decreased total body water in the elderly. Other age-related changes include an increased thirst threshold, the kidneys' reduced ability to conserve water and concentrate urine, increased antidiuretic hormone secretion, and impaired renal sodium conservation. Often dehydration is iatrogenic, resulting from low-salt diets and volume-depleting drugs which include most cardiovascular medications (particularly the diuretics), many of the psychotrophic and gastrointestinal medications, in addition to many of the commonly used pain relieving drugs prescribed or purchased over the counter. Many of the drugs prescribed, such as those in the cardiovascular class, are accompanied with recommendations to decrease fluid consumption, further increasing the risk of complication from dehydration Table 8–4 provides a list of some of the drugs that may potentiate dehydration in the elderly.

Functional ramifications inherent with dehydration should alert the therapist to assess an older person for dehydration. Although an early sign of dehydration is weight loss, imminent or fulminating dehydration can present with altered mental status, agitation or lethargy, lightheadedness, confusion, and

TABLE 8–3. DRUGS ASSOCIATED WITH DEPRESSIVE SIDE EFFECTS IN THE ELDERLY

Antihypertensives
Sympatholytics
  Methyldopa
    Aldomet
  Clonidine
    Catapres
  Guanabenz
    Wytensin
Receptor Blockers / α-Blockers
  Prazosin
    Minipress
Receptor Blockers / β-Blockers
  Nadolol
    Corgard
  Propranolol
    Inderal
  Atenolol
    Tenormin
  Metaprolol
    Lopressor
  Pindolol
    Viskin
ACE Inhibitors
  Guanethidine
    Esimil
  Reserpine
    Various derivatives

Anti-inflammatories
NSAIDs
  Naproxen
    Naprosyn
  Tolmetin
    Tolectin
  Indomethacin
    Indocin
  Meclofenamate
    Meclomen
  Peroxicam
    Feldene
Steroidals
  Prednisolone
    Meticortelone

Antimycobacterial
Ethambutol
  Myambutol

Antiparkinson Drugs
Levodopa
Levodopa-Carbidopa
  Sinemet
Amantadine
  Symmetrel
Bromocriptine
  Parlodel

Diuretics
Acetazolamide
  Diamox
Methazolamide
  Neptazane
Hydrochlorothiazide and
  deserpidine
    Oreticyl

H₂ Receptor Antagonist
Cimetidine
  Tagamet

Sedative-Hypnotics
Glutethimide
  Elrodorm
Barbiturates
  Phenobarbital
    Nembutal
Benzodiazepines
  Flurazepam
    Dalmane
  Temazepam
    Restoril
  Triazolam
    Halcion
  Alcohol
    Rum, etc.

Vasodilators
Hydralazine
  Apresoline

---

should become familiar with these drugs and consider drug toxicity when observing for confusional states in their patients. See Chapter 4, Psychosocial Considerations.

Movement Disorders

Movement disorders caused by medication can be broken down into several types and causes. Drug-induced parkinsonism is characterized by bradykinesia, resting tremor and rigidity, and is relatively common in the elderly. It is usually, but not always, caused by antipsychotic medication. (See Table 8–6 for a list of drugs causing drug-induced parkinsonism).[16]

Tardive dyskinesia is a neuroleptic-induced movement disorder that usually affects the lips, jaw, and tongue and can be induced or exacerbated by medications.[16,20] This disorder may occur as a late effect of antipsychotic drug treatments, the administration of anticholinergic medications, or from withdrawal from a medication.[21] Patients with preexisting brain damage are more likely to develop tardive dyskinesia.

Akathisia, or motor restlessness, is another neuroleptic movement disorder that may result from antipsychotic drug administration.

Finally, essential tremor, which is defined as quick oscillating movements around a joint when the limb is used for active movement, can be exacerbated by lithium carbonate, tricyclic antidepressants, and adrenergic drugs.[20,21]

Incontinence

Incontinence is another severe and embarrassing problem that can be caused and exacerbated by a variety of drugs. Drugs that depress cerebral function, such as benzodiazepines and barbiturates, can exaggerate a preexisting incontinence by depressing one's ability to inhibit bladder contractions. Stress incontinence, on the other hand, is exacerbated by thioridazine and chlorpromazine, both antipsychotic phenothiazines. Anticholinergic drugs relax the muscles of the bladder and may cause urinary retention and overflow incontinence. Therapists can encourage patients to schedule the administration of these drugs so that they coordinate with activities. Further, anticholinergic effects may be evidenced in cardiac abnormalities, dryness of the mouth, difficulty in swallowing, confusion, hallucinations, fatigue, difficulty in urination, and ataxia. Table 8–7 provides a list of drugs with potent anticholinergic action.[16]

Dizziness

Drugs may be the major cause of dizziness in people over age 60.[16] The number of drugs that can cause dizziness in older persons is almost as intimidating as the list for confusion. The greatest contributors are given in Table 8–8. Since therapists work so closely

syncope. Orthostatic hypotension is also an indicator of dehydration.[18] Weakness and lethargy are often misinterpreted and attributed to other conditions prevalent in the elderly. It is important that the therapist include hydration as part of their differential diagnosis in an elderly individual.

Confusion and Dementia

Confusion and dementia are, unfortunately, caused by many drugs. Any drug that causes confusion with prolonged use can cause dementia.[19] Older adults are particularly susceptible to acute confusional states because of the higher incidence of systemic illnesses in the population and their greater vulnerability to the adverse effects of polypharmacy.[19] The drugs that most frequently cause confusion are listed in Table 8–5. This list of drugs is frighteningly long. Therapists

TABLE 8–4. DRUGS THAT CAUSE DEHYDRATION IN THE ELDERLY

Cardiovascular Drugs

Diuretics
Furosemide (Frusemide, Lasix)
Ethacrynic acid (Edecrin, Edecril)
Chlorothiazide (Diuril, Chlotride)
Hydrochlorothiazide (Esidrix, Esidrex)
Bumetanide (Bumex)

Cardiotonic glycosides
Digoxin (Lanoxin)
Digitoxin (Crystodigin, Digitox)

Calcium channel blockers
Verapamil (Isoptin)
Diltiazem (Cardizem)
Nifedipine (Procardia)

Beta-blockers
Atenolol(Tenormin)
Metoprolol (Lopressor)
Propanolol (Inderal)
Nadolol (Corgard)
Timolol (Blocadren)
Pindolol (Visken)
Dipyridamole (Cardoxine)

Vasopressors/Sympathomimetics
Dopamine (Intropin)
Dobutamine (Dobutrex)
Isoproterenol (Isuprel)

Coronary vasodilators
Nitroglycerin (Glyceryl, Trinitrate)
Isosorbide dinitrate (Sorbitrate, Iso-Bid)
Erythrityl (Cardilate)
Verapamil (Calan and Calan SR)
Penaerythritol tetranitrate (Vasodiatol)

Peripheral vasodilators
Hydralazine (Apresoline)
Diazoxide (Hyperstat)
Nitroprusside (Nipride)

Antiarrhythmic Drugs
Quinidine (Quinaglute)
Procainamide hydrochloride (Procan)
Lidocaine (Xylocaine)
Disopyramide phosphate (Norpace)
Quinidine gluconate (Duraquin)
Quinidine polygalacturonate (Cardioquin)

Pain Medications

NSAIDs
Indole acetic acids (Tolectin, Clinoril, Indocin)
Fenamic acids (Meclomen, Ponstel)

Propionic acids (Motrin, Nalfon, Naprosyn)
Phenylacetic acids (Voltaren)
Oxicams (Feldene)
Salicylates (Dolobid, Disalcid, Bufferin)

Psychotrophic Agents

Benzodiazepines
Clorazepate (Tranxene)
Alprazolam (Xanax)
Prazepam (Centrax)

Nonbenzodiazepine
Buspironic (Buspar)

Tricyclic Antidepressants
Doxepine (Sinequan)
Amitriptyline (Elavil)
Imipramine (Tofranil)
Nortriptyline (Pamelor)
Trimipramine (Surmontil)
Protriptyline (Vivactil)

MAO Inhibitors
Isocarboxazid (Marplan)
Maprotiline (Ludiomil)
Phenelzine (Nardil)

Phenothiazine derivatives
Chlorpromazine (Thorazine)
Trifluoperazine (Stelazine)
Fluphenazine (Prolixin)
Mesordazine (Serentil)
Promethazine (Phenergan)
Thioridazine (Mellaril)

Thioxanthene derivatives
Tiothixene (Navane)

Butyrophenone derivatives
Haloperidol (Haldol)

Gastrointestinal Drugs

H2 receptor blockers
Cimitedine (Tagamet)
Ranitidine (Zantac)
Famotidine (Pepcid)

Antidiarrheal absorbants
Kaolin, Pectin (Kaelin)

Hyperosmotic laxatives
Lactulose (Chronolac)
Sodium phosphate (Phosphosoda)

with patients on problems of coordination and balance, the adverse effects of these medications are important to understand. The therapist should remember that a patient will never improve on a balance program if a medication continues to make them dizzy.

Fluid Volume Depletion

Diuretics are the major cause of volume depletion in older persons. Volume depletion can cause decreased cardiac output and they may result in tiredness. Therapists should be aware of the diuretic use of their patients who are constantly tired. (See Table 8–9 for listing of diuretics.)

DRUG REGIMENS

Common drug regimens will be explored in the cardiovascular, neuromusculoskeletal, psychiatric, and gastrointestinal realms. A drug regimen is a method of administering a drug. Drug regimens must be altered for older persons. The following are brief descriptions of drug regimens.

TABLE 8-5. DRUGS THAT CAUSE CONFUSIONAL STATES IN THE ELDERLY

Cardiac Glycosides	Antiparkinsonians	Antidepressants	Anticholinergics
Digitoxin	Benztropine	Tricyclics	(See Table 8-7)
Cardigin	*Cogentin*	Amitriptyline	
Digoxin	Levodopa	*Elavil*	
Digacin	Trihexyphenidyl	*Endep*	
	Artane	Desipramine	
	Amantadine	*Norpramin*	
	Symmetrel	*Pertofrane*	
	Bromocriptine	Doxepin	
	Parlodel	*Adapin*	
		Sinequan	
		Imipramine	
		Tofranil	
		Nortriptyline	
		Aventyl	
		Pamelor	
		Protriptyline	
		Vivactil	
		Trimipramine	
		Surmontil	

Anti-inflammatories	Analgesics	Sedative-Hypnotics	H₂ Receptor Antagonists
Indomethacin	Hydromorphone	Benzodiazepine	Cimetidine
Indocin	*Dilaudid*	Flurazepam	*Tagamet*
Salicylates	Meperidine	*Dalmane*	
Bufferin	*Demerol*	Temazepam	
Anacin	Methadone	*Restoril*	
Phenylbutazone	*Fenadone*	Triazolam	
Butazolidin	Pentazocine	*Halcion*	
Oxyphenbutazone	*Talwin*	Barbiturates	
Oxalid		Phenobarbital	
		Nembutal	
		Secobarbital	
		Pramil	

Diuretics	Hypoglycemic Agents	β-Blockers	
Methyclothiazide	Tolazamide	Propranolol	
Aquatensen	*Tolinase*	*Inderal*	
Hydrochlorothiazide	Tolbutamide	Metroprolol	
Hydro-Ciuril	*Orinase*	*Lopressor*	
Furosemide		Atenolol	
Lasix		*Tenormin*	
		Acebutolol	
		Sectral	

Cardiovascular Regimens

Drug management for the cardiovascular system revolves around managing congestive heart failure (CHF), hypertension, angina pectoris, cardiac arrhythmias, and arteriosclerosis. Congestive heart failure is a condition in which the heart is unable to pump enough blood throughout the body, based on the body's metabolic needs at that time. The symptoms of CHF are tiredness, shortness of breath, edema, and an inability to take a deep breath. Frequently, CHF is a problem in the elderly.

This problem is complicated by the fact that the most commonly used drugs to treat CHF are toxic. These drugs are digoxin and digitoxin (cardiac glyco-sides) or vasodilators. Under the influence of the gly-cosides, the weakened heart is able to pump more forcefully. The glycosides, however, are not curative and do not make any permanent changes in the heart muscle and, therefore, must be given for life.[22]

Another problem with the glycosides, more so than with any other drug, is their narrow margin of safety. Even small changes, therefore, in the functioning of the body, such as an increase in an exercise program, may cause toxic effects in the older person. Another important point about this drug regimen is that it takes longer for the elimination of this drug from the system of the older person.[22] Early symptoms of toxicity from glycosides are blurred vision, slowed heart rate, and confusion. These can eventu-

TABLE 8–6. DRUGS CAUSING DRUG-INDUCED PARKINSONISM

Antipsychotics	Sympatholytics
Phenothiazines	Centrally acting
Chlorpromazine	Methyldopa
Thorazine	*Aldomet*
Fluphenazine	Presynaptic adrenergic
Permatil	inhibitors
Mesoridazine	Reserpine
Serentil	*Crystoserpine*
Perphenazine	
Trilafon, Triavil	
Prochlorperazine	
Compazine	
Thioridazine	
Mellaril	
Trifluoperazine	
Stelazine	
Triflupromazine	
Vesprin	
Butyrophenone	
Haloperidol	
Haldol	
Dihydroindolone	
Molindone	
Moban	
Dibenzoxazepine	
Loxapine	
Loxitane	

TABLE 8–7. DRUGS WITH ANTICHOLINERGIC ACTION

Drug	Trade Name
Tricyclic Antidepressants	
Amitriptyline	Elavil, Endep
Amoxapine	Asendin
Doxepin	Adapin, Sinequan
Imipramine	Tofranil
Maprotiline	Ludiomil
Nortriptyline	Pamelor, Aventil
Protriptyline	Vivactil
Trimipramine	Surmontil
Antipsychotic	
Benztropine	Cogentin
Biperiden	Akineton
Chlorpromazine	Thorazine
Molindone	Moban
Thioridazine	Mellaril
Antihistamines	
Diphenhydramine	Benadryl
Antiparkinsonians	
Orphenadrine	Disipal
Trihexyphenidyl	Artane

TABLE 8–8. DRUGS THAT MAY CAUSE DIZZINESS

Antihypertensives
Vasodilators
  Diltiazem
   Cardizem
  Nifedipine
   Procardia
  Hydralazine
   Apresoline
β-Blockers
  ALL
Sympatholytic
  Acting on CNS
   Clonidine
    Catapres
   Guanabenz
    Wytensin
   Methyldopa
    Aldomet
  Acting on PSN*
   Guanethidine
    Esimil
   Phenoxybenzamine
    Dibenzyline
  α-Receptor blockers
   Phentolamine
    Regitine
   Prazosin
    Minipress
  β-Andrenoreceptor blockers
   Atenolol
    Tenormin
   Metaprolol
    Lopressor
   Timolol
    Blocadren

ACE Inhibitors
  Enalapril
   Vasotec
  Captoril
   Capoten
  Lisinopril
   Zestril, Prinvil

Cardiovascular Antilipemic Agents
  Gemifibrozil
   Lopid
  Colestipol
   Cholestid
  Clofibrate
   Atromid-S

Sedative-Hypnotics
  Barbiturates
   ALL
  Benzodiazepines
   ALL
  Alcohol
   ALL

Analgesics
NSAIDs
  Naproxen
   Naprosyn
  Tolmetin
   Tolectin
  Indomethacin
   Indocin
  Meclofenamote
   Meclomen
  Peroxicam
   Feldene

* PSN = Postganglionic sympathetic neurons

TABLE 8–9. COMMONLY USED DIURETICS

Potassium-Sparing Diuretics	Thiazides and Combinations
Spironolactone and hydrochlorothiazide	Polythiazide
Aldactazide	*Renese*
Spironolactone	Acetazolamide
Aldactone	*Diamox*
Triamterene	Chlorthalidone
Dyazide	*Hygroton*
Dyrenium	Chlorothiazide
Amiloride	*Diuril*
Midamor	Methyclothiazide & crystenamine
Amiloride hydrochlorothiazide	*Diutensin*
Moduretic	Triamterene & hydrochlorothiazide
	Dyazide
	Hydrochlorothiazide
	Esidrix

ally lead to significant cardiac disturbances.[22] The clinician should be alert to these signs as a means of precluding more serious problems.

Vasodilators can also be used to treat CHF. They work by reducing the resistance of the vasculature. This causes the heart to work less; it pumps against less resistance and, therefore, pumps more efficiently. The vasodilators are less toxic than the glycosides, but they may also be less effective. Their toxic symptoms are similar to the ones noted for glycosides. Table 8–10 provides a list of commonly used vasodilators.

Hypertension is another common problem in the older person. Unlike CHF, hypertension is virtually symptomless until the advanced stages. Its main dangers are its possible sequelae: heart attack, stroke, and renal disease. Hypertension is difficult to define and may, therefore, be even more problematic to treat. The World Health Organization defines hypertension as diastolic blood pressure over 95 mm Hg.[23] The Framingham Study defined hypertension as diastolic over 95 mm Hg and systolic over 160 mm Hg.[24]

Before discussing the types of drugs used to treat hypertension, it should be noted that the physical therapist should realize that there is a question as to whether and when to treat patients who present with hypertension. Most physicians choose conservative methods as their first treatment course (e.g., weight control, smoking cessation, salt restriction, and exercise). If nondrug therapy is ineffective, the first reasonable step in drug therapy would be thiazide diuretics (e.g., chlorothiazide). Thiazide diuretics are slower acting (average duration of action 10 to 12 hours) and show no early peak effect. Therefore, the inconvenience (especially for the elderly patient) of an overwhelming urinary frequency produced by a faster-acting diuretic is not a factor with this drug.[6,22]

Even though thiazide diuretics are tried first, they have adverse side effects that are particularly dangerous for older persons. Thiazides are likely to produce some degree of hyperglycemia, hypokalemia, and hyperuricemia. Diuretics, because they act on the kidneys to increase excretion of water and sodium to hypothetically decrease the cardiac workload, also cause dehydration which increases

the work of the system. Because of the increased prevalence of late-onset diabetes, arrhythmias, and gout in older persons, the side effects of these drugs must be carefully monitored.[6,22]

Calcium channel blockers and β-adrenergic blockers are often the second stage of management for hypertension. Beta blockers are used for patients with hypertension, angina pectoris, and cardiac arrhythmias to decrease the effects of catecholamines (epinephrine and norepeinephrine) on the heart. Beta blockers, therefore, cause a decrease in heart rate and contractile force. Calcium channel blockers are more effective than β-blockers in the older population because of their ability to lower arterial blood pressure without increasing total peripheral resistance (TPR). In the elderly patient TPR is typically increased and cardiac reserve is restricted. Beta blockers would be counterproductive because they lower blood pressure mainly by reducing cardiac output and somewhat increasing TPR in a patient whose TPR is already high. Both, however, have the liability that an overdose can slow or even stop the heart.

Figure 8–1 is an adapted chart on the various stages for hypertension management of the elderly. Please note that the choice of drugs often depends on the other diagnoses the patient may have.

Angina pectoris requires two forms of drug management. Angina is a condition where the person suffers a sudden severe pain in the substernal area that is due to a temporary lack of oxygen to the heart. To manage this problem, the sufferer needs quick relief. Vasodilators, such as amyl nitrite and nitroglycerin, which are placed under the tongue, are absorbed quickly and travel rapidly to the heart. The other mode of drug management for angina is preventative. The drugs beneficial for this are calcium channel blocker and β-blockers.[22] Table 8–11A provides a list of the commonly used antianginal agents with route, dose, and comments.

Reduced cardiac output may result from chronic heart disease or it may occur acutely, producing symptoms such as dyspnea, dizziness, nausea, dysrhythmias, hypotension, and pale, cool, clammy skin. Many drugs are used to enhance cardiac output. For example, digoxin improves cardiac output by increasing the heart's contractility, which boosts stroke volume. It does this by disrupting the sodium-potassium pump in the cardiac cells, allowing calcium ions to move in, which produce more forceful contractions. Digoxin also has a tonic effect on the myocardium, that is, it lowers the cell membrane potential and lengthens the refractory period. This slows the heart rate to regulate atrial fibrillation. Calcium channel blockers also reduce heart rate and restore normal sinus rhythm. A calcium channel blocking drug, such as verapamil, works by inhibiting calcium influx through the slow channels of the myocardial contractile units. Table 8–11B provides a list of commonly used drugs that affect cardiac output.

TABLE 8–10. COMMONLY USED VASODILATORS*

Drug	Trade Name
Hydralazine*	Apresoline
Minoxidil*	Loniten
Calcium channel blockers	Verapamil
	Nilapamil
	Diltiazem
Diazoxide	Hyperstat
Nitroprusside	Nipride
Nitroglycerin	Glyceryl trinitrate
Isosorbide dinitrate	Sorbitrate

*Primary vasodilators used.

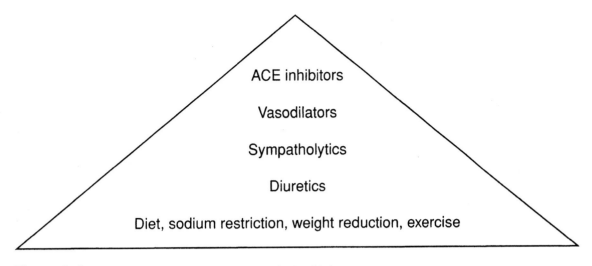

Figure 8–1. *Stages for hypertension management in the elderly.*

Management of arrhythmias is another tricky and controversial area in the older person. Often the arrhythmia, or abnormal heart beat, is a manifestation of an underlying pathology and will resolve when the pathology is treated. Nevertheless, arrhythmias should not be overlooked in the older person because of the older person's inability to maintain a normal cardiac output between 40 to 170 beats per minute as can younger persons. In the aged, there is a reduction in this range to between 45 and 120 beats per minute. The drugs of choice depend on the rhythm alteration. Table 8–12A provides a list of some commonly used antiarrhythmic agents, route, dose, and comments noted. In older persons, the rate of removal of procainamide, lidocaine, and quinidine are reduced. Disopyramide may cause voiding problems in older men.[21]

The final cardiovascular condition that is typically treated with drugs is atherosclerosis. Atherosclerosis is a buildup of plaque in the arteries, causing a thickening of the arterial walls and, therefore, diminishing the size of the lumen. Drug therapy for atherosclerosis is aimed at preventing the development of plaques by reducing the blood levels of certain lipids, especially cholesterol. The three most *common* drugs used for this problem are lovastatin, niacin, and cholestyramine.[6,22] At present lovastatin has little toxic effect. Niacin used in the high doses necessary for results may cause itching, flushing, and gastrointestinal distress. Cholestyramine is not absorbed into the body and acts by binding to cholesterol, thereby promoting its excretion in the feces. Cholestyramine may bind to fat-soluble vitamins and cause a deficiency in an undernourished older person. Finally, it may be difficult to predict the effectiveness of this drug because of the amount of laxatives that older people tend to take.[16] Table 8–12B provides a list of drugs commonly used to treat hyperlipidema and Table 8–12C provides a list of drugs used to treat overclotting problems.

Neuromusculoskeletal Regimens

This section will discuss drug management in neuromuscular and muscoloskeletal conditions such as arthritis, neuralgias, stroke, and Parkinson's disease. The latest drug regimes being utilized in osteoporosis will also be presented.

Since arthritis is so common in the older population, the chances of an older patient taking some type of medication for the management of pain and inflammation are great. Physicians prescribing drugs for the management of arthritis must understand that this is not a comprehensive program. Both environmental modifications and an appropriate physical therapy program that enhances independence must be addressed.

The most common drugs used in the management of osteoarthritis (OA) are analgesics and nonsteroidal anti-inflammatories (NSAIDs). Even though osteoarthritis is a degenerative disease, the patient may have significant inflammation, often on the initial presentation, due to overuse and irritation of the joint. The use of anti-inflammatories at this point may help in the management of the disease. In fact, NSAIDs have been the cornerstone of OA treatment because of their combined analgesic and anti-inflammatory effects. However, because appreciable inflammation is often absent and considering the risk of gastropathy, analgesics frequently suffice. Acetaminophen, in doses up to 4 g daily, has been proven efficacious, although in a survey of OA patients, 67% of the patients preferred an NSAID to acetaminophine.[25]

The most frequent NSAID prescribed for osteoarthritis is aspirin. The dosage may vary, but it should be titrated to the individual. The patient should begin with one aspirin every four hours and increase the dosage to two aspirins every four hours until the relief of symptoms is achieved and before any adverse drug reactions (e.g., gastric irritability or

TABLE 8-11A. ANTIANGINAL AGENTS

Drugs	Trade Name	Method of Action	Side Effects	Drug Interactions
Nitroglycerin	Nitro-Bid	Relax smooth muscle in arterial and venous beds	Transient headache, nausea, vomiting, dizziness, flush on face and neck, rapid pulse	Alcohol, antihypertensives, dihydroergotamine, sympathomimetics, tricyclics, antidepressants, vasodilators
	Nitro-Dur	Relax smooth muscle in arterial and venous beds	Skin rash, transient headache, tachycardia, nausea, hypotension, vomiting, rapid pulse, dizziness, flush	Antihypertensives, vasodilators, sympathomimetics
	Transderm nitro	Relax smooth muscle in arterial and venous beds	Transient headache, hypotension, flush nausea/vomiting, rapid pulse, dizziness	Antihypertensives, vasodilators, sympathomimetics
Isosorbide dinitrate	Iso-Bid	Relax smooth muscle in arterial and venous beds	Weakness, cutaneous vasodilation with flushing, hypotension	Antihypertensives, tricyclics, antidepressants, vasodilators, sympathomimetics
Erythrityl tetranitrate	Cardilate	Direct dilation of coronary conductance vessels Decreased myocardial oxygen demand (preload & afterload)	Headache, flushing, dizziness, weakness, signs of cerebral ischemia, associated hypotension (caused by overdosage)	Alcohol
Verapamil	Calan Calan SR	Blocks active and inactive calcium channels	Hypotension, peripheral edema, dizziness, headache, fatigue, constipation, nausea	Disopyramide, carbamazepine, β-blocking agents, digoxin, calcium supplements
Diltiazem hydrochloride	Cardizem	Calcium channel block	Edema, decrease in blood pressure, occasional hypotension, headache, nausea, dizziness, rash, AV block	Digoxin, calcium supplements, β-blocking agents, disopyramide
Nifedipine	Procardia	Calcium channel block	Dizziness, lightheadedness, nausea, headache, weakness, transient hypotension	β-blocking agents, cimetidine, digoxin, bentanyl, calcium supplements, long-acting nitrates
Nadolol	Corgard	Nonselective block of β-adrenergic receptors	Dizziness, fatigue, paresthesia, drowsiness, hypotension, conjunctive heart failure, peripheral vascular insufficiency	Epinephrine, lidocaine, indomethacin, oral hypoglycemic, catecholamine-depleting
Dipyridamole	Cardoxin	Selectively dilates coronary arteries resulting in increased oxygen supply to myocardium, also inhibits platelet aggregation	Dizziness, weak or syncope flushing, nausea, vomiting, skin rash, GI distress, headache	No known clinical significance
Pentaerythritol tetranitrate	Vasodiatol	Direct dilation of coronary conductive vessels	Flushing, headache, dizziness, weakness, postural hypotension	Norepinephrine, acetylcholine, histamine, alcohol

TABLE 8-11B. COMMONLY USED DRUGS AFFECTING CARDIAC OUTPUT

Drugs	Trade Name	Method of Action	Side Effects
Cardiotonic glycosides Digoxin Digitoxin	Lanoxin Crystodigin, Digitox	• Increase cardiac output (CO) by improving contractility, decreasing heart rate, and controlling dysrhythmias • Increase influx of calcium ions into myocardial cells by altering electric properties of cell membrane (sodium-potassium pump) • Decrease conduction velocity through atrioventricular node	• Nausea, vomiting, anorexia, diarrhea, headache, hypokalemia, visual disturbances, nervousness, dysrhytmias (usually conduction disturbances) • Prolonged PR interval on EKG indicates toxicity
Calcium channel blockers Verapamil Diltiazem	Isoptin Cardizem	• Increase CO by decreasing heart rate and increasing ventricular f illing time • Block influx of calcium ions, decreasing smooth muscle contract-ions and relaxing coronary arteries; in some cases, may lower CO by decreasing contractility of cardiac muscle	• Headache, hypotension, flushing, pedal edema, constipation, vertigo, atrioventricular block, dysesthesia • Severe hypotension producted when used with beta-blockers
Beta-blockers **Cardioselective** Atenolol Metoprolol **Nonselective** Propranolol Nadolol Timolol Pindolol	Tenormin Lopressor Inderal Corgard Blocadren Visken	• Cardioselective blockers inhibit beta-1 receptors in the heart, relieving hypertension angina, and dysrhythmias. • Nonselective blockers inhibit beta-1 and beta-2 receptors • Both types may decrease CO by decreasing ventricular contractility	• Lightheadedness, depression, mild paresthesia, hypotension, respiratory distress, heart failure, dysrhythmias, decreased peripheral circulation • Increased respiratory distress with COPD or asthma • Bradycardia in patients with compromised ventricular function

(continued)

TABLE 8-11B. (CONTINUED)

Drugs	Trade Name	Method of Action	Side Effects
Vasopressors/sympathomimetics Dopamine Dobutamine Isoproterenol Epinephrine Norepinephrine	Intropin Dobutrex Isuprel	• Stimulate beta-receptors in the heart • Increase CO by stimulating contractility (improving stroke volume) or increasing heart rate	• Nausea, vomiting, tachycardia, dysrhythmias, palpitation • MAO inhibitors may potentiate effects
Coronary vasodilators Nitroglycerin Isosorbide dinitrate	Glyceryl trinitrate Sorbitrate	• Relax smooth muscle of coronary arteries, increasing myocardial blood supply, but also act on all smooth muscle in vascular system • May improve cardiac output	• Headache, flushing, nausea, vomiting, hypotension, vertigo • Glaucoma patients at risk for increase in intraocular pressure
Peripheral vasodilators Hydralazine Diazoxide Nitroprusside	Apresoline Hyperstat Nipride	• Relax smooth muscle in peripheral vascular system, reducing blood pressure; also decrease preload and pulmonary capillary wedge pressure • May improve CO by decreasing afterload and allowing for more efficient ventricular function	• Nausea, vomiting, abdominal discomfort, lightheadedness, headache, anxiety, muscle twitching, skin rash, tachycardia, palpitations, angina • Hyperstat can raise blood glucose levels in diabetics
Diuretics Furosemide Ethacrynic acid Chlorothiazide Hydrochlororo- thiazide Bumetanide	Frusemide, Lasix Edecrin, Edecril Diuril, Chlotride Esidrix, Esidrex Burnex	• Inhibit renal absorption of sodium in combating chronic congestive heart failure • Relieve concomitant edema • Can increase or decrease CO by affecting preload volumes	• Fatigue, anorexia, diarrhea, skin rash, vertigo, tinnitus, loss of electrolytes, hypokalemia, weakness, muscle cramps • Severe dehydration • Severe potassium loss affecting quality and rhythmicity of heart contractions

TABLE 8–12A.   ANTIARRHYTHMIC DRUGS

Drugs	Trade Name	Method of Action	Side Effects	Drug Interactions
Quinidine	Quinaglute	Depresses pacemaker rate, depresses conduction and excitability	Nausea, vomiting, abdominal pain, diarrhea, headache, tinnitus, disturbed vision, worsening arrythmia	Amiodarone, reserpine phenothiazine, digitalis glycosides, neuromuscular blocking agents, antacids, oral anticoagulants
Procainamide hydrochloride	Procan	Supresses automaticity, decreases conduction velocity, prolongs effective refractory period	Hypotension, worsening ventricular arrhythmia, systemic lupus erythematosus symptoms, arthritis, arthralgia, fever, rash	Antiarrhythmic agents, anticholinergic agents, antihypertensive agents
Lidocaime	Xylocaine	Suppressor of abnormal cardiac activity, acting exclusively on sodium channels	Paresthesias, tremor, lightheadedness, convulsions, drowsiness	Oxytocic drugs
Propranolol	Inderal	Nonselective blockage of β-adrenergic receptors	Dizziness, fatigue, lightheadedness, nausea, vomiting, bronchospasm bradycardia, peripheral vascular insufficiency	Chlorpromazine, epinephrine, barbiturates, cimetidine, haloperidol, catecholamine-depleting, thioamines, rifampin
Verapamil	Calan	Coronary vasodilator, blocks both activated and inactivated calcium channels	Hypotension, peripheral edema, bradycardia, dizziness, headache, fatigue, constipation, nausea	Carbamazepine, β-adrenergic blocking agents, digoxin, calcium supplements, digitalis, disopyramide, antihypertensive agents, quinidine, methyldopa
Amiodarone	Cordarone, Miocard	Effective blocker of inactivated sodium channels, blocks α- and β-adrenoreceptors	Halo in peripheral vision field, yellowing of cornea, photodermatitis, grayish/ blue skin discoloration	Warfarin, theophylline, quinidine, procainamide, flecainide
Disopyramide phosphate	Norpace	Depresses pacemaker rate, depresses conduction and excitability	Dry mouth, urinary retention, constipation, blurred vision, dry nose, eyes, bloating, malaise, fatigue, weakness	Alchohol, warfarin, phenytoin, digoxin
Quinidine polygalacturonate	Cardioquin	Slows conduction time, prolongs refractory period, depresses excitability of the heart muscle	Disturbed vision, headache, diarrhea, nausea, vomiting, abdominal pain, confusion, vertigo, fever, delirium, syncope, apprehension	Digoxin, potassium supplements, phenobarbital, phenytoin, anticholinergic drugs
Quinidine gluconate	Duraquin	Prolongation of refractory period, decrease in excitability of ectopic foci of the heart	Disturbed vision, headache, diarrhea, nausea, vomiting, abdominal pain, confusion, vertigo, fever, delirium, syncope, apprehension	Potassium, coumarin, anticoagulants, thiazide diuretics, sodium bicarbonate, carbonic anhydrase inhibitors, other antiarrhythmics
Isoproterenol	Isuprel	Increases cardiac output, increases venous return to heart, lowers peripheral vascular resistance	Sweating, mild tremors, nervousness, tachycardia with palpitations	Diuretics, epinephrine, cyclopropane

TABLE 8–12B. COMMONLY USED DRUGS TO TREAT HYPERLIPIDEMIA

Drug	Trade Name	Method of Action	Side Effects
Cholestyramine	Cholybar, Questran	Decreases plasma LDL cholesteral levels	Nausea, diarrhea
Clofibrate	Abitrate, Atromid-S	Lowers plasma triclycerides by decreasing LDL and IDL levels	Nausea, diarrhea, fatigue, weakness, myalgia, myositis, arrhythmias, blood dyscrasias, angioneurotic syndrome
Gemfibrozil	Lopid	Lowers plasma triclycerides by decreasing LDL and IDL levels	Nausea, diarrhea, fatigue, weakness, myalgia, myositis, arrhythmias, blood dyscrasias, angioneurotic syndrome
Lovastatin	Mevacor	Decreases plasma LDL cholesterol levels; may decrease triglycerides and increase HDL levels	Nausea, diarrhea, fatigue, weakness, myalgia, myositis
Niacin	Niacor, Nicobid	Lowers plasma triglycerides by decreasing VLDL levels	Nausea, diarrhea, cutaneous vasodilation, sensation of warmth when administered
Pravastatin	Pravachol	Decreases plasma LDL cholesterol levels; may decrease triglycerides and increase HDL levels	Nausea, diarrhea, fatigue, weakness, myalgia, myositis
Probucol	Lorelco	Decreases LDL and HDL cholesterol; inhibits deposition of fat into arterial wall	Nausea, diarrhea, parasthesias, arrhythmias, blood dyscrasias, angioneurotic syndrome
Simvastatin	Zocor	Decreases plasma LDL cholesterol levels; may decrease triglycerides and increase HDL levels	Nausea, diarrhea, fatigue, weakness, myalgia, myositis

HDL = high-density lipoproteins; LDL = low-density lipoproteins; IDL = intermediate-density lipoproteins; VLDL = very low-density lipoproteins

tinnitus). If the older person does not tolerate aspirin, then another class of NSAID may be used. These drugs are more expensive and many different types of NSAIDs abound. Table 8–13 provides a list of the most common NSAIDs and cox-2-selective NSAIDs on the market.

Despite the fact that an estimated 70 million prescriptions are written annually, NSAIDs can have serious side effects. The major problems with NSAIDs in the older population are the adverse reactions, which include gastropathy, frontal headaches, dizziness, light-headedness, confusion, and depression.[25] In addition to these reactions, NSAIDs may also cause renal dysfunction. Risk factors for NSAID gastropathy include age greater than 60, history of ulcer, concomitant use of corticosteroids, concomitant use of warfarin, and the use of high dose and combination NSAIDs. Age-related risk is independent and linear.[26]

TABLE 8–12C. COMMONLY USED ANTICOAGULANT, ANTITHROMBOTIC, AND THROMBOLYTIC DRUGS

Drugs	Trade Name	Method of Action	Indication
Anticoagulants			
Heparin	Calciparine, Liquaemin	Inhibits synthesis and function of clotting factors	Used primarily to prevent and treat venous thromboembolism
Oral anticoagulants			
Anisindione	Miradon	Inhibits synthesis and function of clotting factors	Used primarily to prevent and treat venous thromboembolism
Dicumarol	generic		
Warfarin	Coumadin, Panwarfin		
Antithrombotics			
Aspirin	multiple brands	Inhibits platelet aggregation and platelet-induced clotting	Used primarily to prevent arterial thrombus formation
Dipyridamole	Dipridacot, Persantine		
Sulfinpyrazone	Anturane		
Thrombolytics			
Anistreplase	Eminase	Facilitates clot dissolution	Used to reopen occluded vessels in arterial and venous thrombosis
Streptokinase	Kabikinase, Streptase		
Tissue plasminogen activator	t-PA		
Urokinase	Abbokinase		

TABLE 8–13. COMMONLY USED NSAIDS

Drugs	Trade Name	Method of Action	Side Effects	Drug Interactions
Indole acetic acids				
Tolmetin	Tolectin	Inhibits cyclooxygenase resulting in biosynthesis of prostaglandin	GI symptoms, dizziness, drowsiness, depression, rash, pruritus, headache, nervousness, chest pain, hypertension, tinnitis, edema, nausea, vomiting, asthenia, heartburn	Warfarin
Sulindac	Clinoril	Inhibits cyclooxygenase resulting in biosynthesis of prostaglandin	GI symptoms, drowsiness, dizziness, headache, nausea, vomiting, pruritus, rash, diarrhea	Oral anticoagulants, salicylates, furosemide, lithium, probenecid, β-adrenergic blockers, methotrexate
Indomethacin	Indocin	Inhibits cyclooxygenase resulting in biosynthesis of prostaglandin	GI symptoms, drowsiness, dizziness, somnolence, depression, fatigue, nausea, tinnitus, headache, diarrhea, vomiting	Oral anticoagulants, salicylates, loop or thiazide, diuretics, lithium, captopril, probenecid, diflunisal, β-adrenergic blockers
Fenamic acids				
Meclofenamic acid, sodium salt, mono-hydrate	Meclomen	Inhibits cyclooxygenase resulting in biosynthesis of prostaglandin	Dizziness, tinnitus, edema, headache, nausea, vomiting, diarrhea, rash	Warfarin, salicylates
Mefenamic acid	Ponstel	Inhibits cyclooxygenase resulting in biosynthesis of prostaglandin	Diarrhea, nausea, vomiting, abdominal pain, anorexia, pyrosis, drowsiness, dizziness, nervousness, headache, blurred vision, insomnia, rash	Anticoagulants
Propionic acids				
Ibuprofen	Motrin	Inhibits cyclooxygenase resulting in biosynthesis of prostaglandin	GI symptoms (cramps, constipation), pruritus, tinnitus, dizziness, anxiety, headache, nausea, vomiting, aseptic meningitis	Coumarin-type anticoagulants, aspirin
Fenoprofen	Nalfon	Inhibits cyclooxygenase resulting in biosynthesis of prostaglandin	GI symptoms, occult blood in stool, somnolence, dizziness, rash, tremor, pruritus, headache, nervousness, dyspnea, fatigue, insomnia, decreased hearing	Salicylates, phenobarbital, coumarin-type anticoagulants
Naproxen	Naprosyn	Inhibits cyclooxygenase resulting in biosynthesis of prostaglandin	Blurred vision, edema, anorexia, shortness of breath, indigestion, tinnitus, constipation, nausea, drowsiness, dizziness, headache	Oral anticoagulants, furosemide, lithium, β-adrenergic blockers
Naproxen sodium	Anaprox	Inhibits cyclooxygenase resulting in biosynthesis of prostaglandin	Shortness of breath, indigestion, tinnitus, edema, itching, dizziness, drowsiness, headache, nausea, vomiting	Oral anticoagulants, naproxen, methotrexate, furosemide, lithium, β-blockers, salicylates, probenecid

(continued)

TABLE 8–13. (CONTINUED)

Drugs	Trade Name	Method of Action	Side Effects	Drug Interactions
Ketoprofen	Orudis	Inhibits cyclooxygenase resulting in biosynthesis of prostaglandin	GI symptoms, headache, dizziness, drowsiness, constipation, nausea, vomiting, tinnitus, visual disturbances, urinary tract infection	Antacids, aspirin, diuretics, digoxin, warfarin, probenecid, methotrexate, lithium
Pyrazoles Phenylbutazone	Butazolidin	Inhibits cyclooxygenase resulting in biosynthesis of prostaglandin	Aplastic anemia, edema, water retention, GI distress, nausea, dyspepsia, rash	Anti-inflammatory agents, phyeytoin, oral antidiabetics, sulfonamides, sodium valproate, coumarin-type anticoagulants, digitoxin hexabarbital; cortisone
Phenylacetic acids Diclofenac sodium	Voltaren	Inhibits cyclooxygenase resulting in biosynthesis of prostaglandin	Peptic ulceration, GI bleeding, abdominal cramps, headache, fluid retention, diarrhea, indigestion, constipation, dizziness, tinnitus, rash, pruritus	Aspirin, cyclosporine, methotrexate, digoxin, oral hypoglyemics
Oxicams Piroxicam	Feldene	Inhibits cyclooxygenase resulting in biosynthesis of prostaglandin	Stomatitis, anorexia, GI distress, nausea, constipation, flatulence, diarrhea, dizziness, somnolence, headache, malaise, tinnitis, anemia, leukopenia, eosinophilia, edema	Lithium, aspirin
Salicylate Diflunisal	Dolabid	Inhibits cyclooxygenase resulting in biosynthesis of prostaglandin	Abdominal cramps, diarrhea, rash, somnolence, insomnia, dizziness, nausea, vomiting, dyspepsia, fatigue, tinnitus	Aspirin, naproxen, hydrochlorothiazides, antacids, sulindac, indomethacin
Salsalate	Disalcid	Inhibits cyclooxygenase resulting in biosynthesis of prostaglandin	Tinnitus, abdominal pain, abnormal liver function, anaphylactic shock, angio-edema, vertigo, rash, bronchohepatitis, hypotension, urticaria, nephritis	Aspirin, anticoagulant drugs, penicillin, triiodothyronine, thiopental, thyroxine, naproxen, warfarin, corticosteroids, thyroid hormone, sulfinphyrazone
Aspirin	Bufferin	Inhibits cyclooxygenase resulting in biosynthesis of prostaglandin	Stomach pain, heartburn, nausea, vomiting, increased rate of GI distress	Acetazolamide, alcohol, ammonium chloride, tolbutamide, chlorpropamide, probenecid, methotrexate, NSAIDs, phenytoin, penicillin, spironolactone, heparin, corticosteroids
COX-2-Selective NSAIDS Cox-2 Inhibitors	Celecoxib, Rofecoxib	Selectively inhibit cyclooxygenase-2 sites resulting in biosynthesis of prostaglandin	Unknown	NSAIDs, corticosteroids

Combining analgesics with anti-inflammatory drugs, as well as using multiple analgesics, is relatively common in the older populations. The use of acetaminophen can be helpful for pain relief without an analgesic effect. It can also be combined with anti-inflammatories for episodes of severe pain.

Gastrointestinal ulceration is a common side effect in older adults on chronic aspirin regimes for musculoskeletal or neuromuscular pain. New drugs, called cox-2 inhibitors, relieve pain just about as well as aspirin and do not have the serious side affects. These drugs are currently referred to as the "superaspirins." The new drugs work much the same way as the old ones do. Aspirin and other NSAIDS block production of substances called protaglandins, which are among the most versatile molecules in the body. Among other things, prostaglandins trigger uterine contractions during birth; generate a layer of mucus that protects the stomach from its acids; and cause blood platelets to form clots (a mixed blessing, since the clots that help a wound heal can also lead to a heart attack or stroke). But, protaglandins trigger pain and inflammation, and when the body is injured or irritated, as it is with arthritic joints, prostaglandins are released. Aspirin reduces that pain and inflammation by lowering prostaglandin levels. It does so by blocking cyclooxygenase, or cox, which is involved in the manufacture of protaglandins. Cyclooxygenase comes in at least two versions: cox-1, ultimately responsible for protecting the stomach and making platelets sticky; and cox-2, which triggers pain and inflammation. Drugs such as aspirin and ibuprofen block both cox-1 and cox-2, reducing pain but also leading to side effects, including ulcers. The cox-2 inhibitor drugs block cox-2 only, giving pain relief without substantial side effects. The commonly used cox-2-selective NSAIDs celecoxib and rofecoxib, both used in treatment of OA, offer efficacy and an improved GI safety profile and do not interfere with platelet function. Older patients whose symptoms are not relieved with acetaminophen or who have other risk factors are candidates for cox-2-selective NSAIDs.

Of interest is that cox-2 inhibitors may not only control pain; they may also be used one day to prevent some types of cancer. Researchers have learned that malignant cells in the intestines manufacture cox-2 enzymes to accelerate their growth. That may help explain why consuming fruits and vegetables, which block cox-2 enzymes naturally, seems to protect against colon cancer. Other scientists have determined that cox-2 inhibitors could conceivably lessen some of the brain damage in Alzheimer's disease. Unfortunately, cox-2 inhibitors have little or no effect on heart disease, since it is the cox-1 enzymes that cause blood clotting. So far, no one knows how to block the cox-1 enzymes in the bloodstream without also affecting the ones that help protect the stomach.

The goal of drug intervention in rheumatoid arthritis (RA) is the control and relief of pain, to decrease joint destruction by inflammation, diminish disability, and improve quality of life and functional outcomes. The problems encountered with increasing age are multiple. The risk of toxicity from long-term drug use and the substantial increase in the risk of drug interactions and adverse reactions is problematic in the elderly patient with RA. The choice of drug therapy will depend on the progression of the disease, toxicity of the drug, and the individual's co-existing conditions.[27] Simple analgesics such as acetaminophen are ineffective in this disease. Nonsteroidal anti-inflammatory drugs are effective in the patient with mild to moderate disease, but may not be tolerated well because of gastrointestinal side effects.[25] Other potential toxicities include nephrotoxicity, hepatotoxicity, cardiovascular effects of volume overload, central nervous system effects of confusion and cognitive impairment and hematological abnormalities such as thrombocytopenia, neutropenia, and hemolytic anemia. Increasing age, history of ulcer, concomitant corticosteroid or anticoagulant use, cigarette smoking, alcohol use, and ingestion of multiple NSAIDs are risk factors for gastrointestinal complications. The new cox-2-inhibitors may provide increased protection from gastrointestinal complications, however, longitudinal studies are needed to assess the safety of these drugs over the long haul.

Hydroxychloroquine seems to be well tolerated by the elderly RA patient. The role of corticosteroids in the treatment of RA is extremely controversial because of the potential toxicities of osteoporosis, diabetes, cataracts, glaucoma, anxiety, delirium, and atherosclerosis. These drugs exert a general catabolic effect on all supportive tissue (e.g., muscle, tendon, bone).[28] Although these agents are effective in reducing inflammation, the side effects need to be cautiously weighed. Antiresorptive therapy should be initiated simultaneously to diminish potential bone loss if corticosteroids are selected as the treatment of choice.[27] Other second-line agents such as methotrexate and sulfasalazine appear to be well tolerated in the elderly and have few side effects and lower toxicity. Other agents such as cyclosporine, azathioprine, parenteral gold, and oral auranofin, and penicillamine are less popular agents in older individuals due to the extreme side effects. Of the new agents—leflunomide, an inhibitor of pyrimidine biosynthesis, has been shown to be effective in reducing disease activity. Side effects include rash, liver function abnormalities, alopecia, and gastrointestinal symptoms. Diets that are high in fish oil and certain fatty acids (e.g., gammalinolenic acid) have been advocated for patients with RA because these diets may supply precursors that enhance the biosynthesis of certain endogenous anti-inflammatory and immunosuppressant compounds.[29]

Of interest are some of the newer approaches to treatment of RA. Tumor necrosis factor (TNF) is a proinflammatory cytokine that contributes to the pathogenesis of RA. Agents have been developed to inhibit this cytokine, including etanercept, a recombinant human TNF receptor fusion protein, and infliximab, an anti-TNF alpha antibody.[30–32] Although recent studies have shown both agents to be well tolerated and effective in reducing disease activity, more data is needed to assess their long-term efficacy, safety, and toxicity in older patients.

Osteoporosis Regimens

Several drugs are being employed for the treatment of osteoporosis. Hormone replacement therapy (HRT) has been studied as a preventive measure. Estrogen replacement therapy (ERT) has been found to play a protective role against osteoporosis in postmenopausal women.[33] In addition, ERT improves cardiolipid profiles, enhances mental function, protects dentition, and improves urinary physiology. However, unopposed estrogen increases the risk of endometrial and breast cancer. Adding progestin brings the risk down slightly. Tamoxifen has been found to be a suitable substitute when an individual is at risk for estrogen-sensitive tumor development. Though tamoxifen does not increase bone mass, it has been found to at least stabilize it.[34,35]

Bisphosphonates (also called diphosphonates) have been found to inhibit osteoclast-induced bone resorption, thus decreasing bone turnover and shifting the balance toward bone formation. Alendronate (Fosamax), one 10-mg tablet daily, effectively increases bone density and reduces fracture rate.[36] There are associated side effects such as ulceration of the esophagus (secondary to espohagitis) if a specific routine is not followed. The drug needs to be taken on an empty stomach with a glass of water and the individual must wait 30 minutes, in an upright position, before eating or drinking anything.[33]

Calcitonin also increases bone density. Basically, calcitonin (Cibacalcin, Calcimar, Miacalcin) mimics the effects of endogenous calcitonin and increases bone formation in conditions such as Paget's disease and osteoporosis. However, bone density increments with calcitonin are not nearly as marked as with estrogen or the bisphosphonates. No reliable fracture prevention data is available for calcitonin, but it is reported to have significant analgesic properties, making it useful for fracture pain.

Raloxifene (Evista) is a selective estrogen receptor modulator. Its bone anabolic effects are only about 50% as effective as ERT or HRT. However, this level is sufficient for the prevention of osteoporosis. The chief advantage of raloxifene is that it does not cause any stimulation of the ovary, uterus, or breast. There is no data on the protective effect of raloxifene for heart disease or stroke or its effect on cognition, though studies are under way. The most common side effects are mild leg cramps and a minor increase in the incidence of hot flashes.

Calcium supplements (Biocal, Os-Cal, Citracal, Neo-Calglucon, etc.) are highly recommended in anyone at risk for osteoporosis or who is not getting enough calcium through diet. See Chapters 7 and 11 for further discussion of calcium and osteoporosis. The primary effect of calcium supplementation is to provide an additional source of calcium to prevent depletion and to encourage bone formation in conditions such as osteoporosis, osteomalacia, hypothyroidism, and Paget's disease. Vitamin D analogues are also often prescribed (Calderol, Rocaltrol, Drisdol, Calciferol, etc.) as a preventive measure in the battle against osteoporosis and other bone diseases. Vitamin D supplementation generally enhances bone formation by increasing the absorption and retention of calcium and phosphate in the body. Many dietary products, such as milk, have vitamin D added.

Neuralgias can be defined as sudden recurring pain that extends along the site of a nerve and affects the anatomical distribution of that nerve. The three most common types of neuralgia in older persons are postherpetic, glossopharyngeal, and trigeminal neuralgia. The pharmaceutical management of these problems revolves around pain management. For very mild cases, rest and analgesics, such as aspirin and acetaminophen, are suggested. Stronger drugs, such as carbamazepine and phenvtoin, are effective for the trigeminal and glossopharvngeal neuralgias.[37] For the management of shingles in severe cases, morphine or codeine may be necessary. In addition, systemic adrenal steroids may be recommended for most elderly patients but are contraindicated for patients with neoplasms or any underlying disease and for patients on immunosuppressive therapy.[37]

Drugs that are used in the treatment of strokes are a quickly growing area of study. The current thought, however, is to protect the area of infarct. The concern is that even a slight fall in blood pressure may aggravate a cerebral ischemia and extend the infarct area. Nevertheless, studies continue to investigate the effects of the "intracerebral steal" and the "inverse steal" effects on the poststroke brain. In the first effect, the healthier cerebral arteries may dilate and take blood from the needy arteries and the infarct. In the "inverse steal," administration of vasoactive drugs may reduce the swelling of capillary walls, which occurs after stroke.[21,37]

Despite the controversy of the previously stated effects, certain drug regimens have been used for poststroke patients for the management of cerebral edema, cerebral emboli, and blood pressure. Corticosteroids can be used to reduce cerebral edema, and glycerol can be used to improve regional blood flow. Anticoagulants are indicated for the management of cerebral emboli. (See Tables 12B and 12C.) The management of the poststroke patient's blood pressure should be aimed at maintaining pressure in the acute phases. For older patients, the use of activity or stressing the postural response is preferable to drug management for maintaining blood pressure.[21,37]

The final neuromusculoskeletal drug to be discussed in this section is a treatment for parkinsonism. Parkinsonism is a condition that reflects a deficiency of dopamine in the brain. Because dopamine does not cross the blood-brain barrier, L-dopa must be used. L-dopa is a dopamine precursor that crosses the blood-brain barrier and is converted to dopamine.[38] Unfortunately, large doses of dopamine are needed to achieve concentrations in the brain and these large doses lead to major side effects, such as involuntary movements, adverse mental changes, postural hypotension, and vomiting. Sinemet is the most widely used drug for the management of parkinsonism, and it is a combination of L-dopa and carbidopa. Carbidopa acts as an inhibitor to decarboxylase, which rapidly breaks down L-dopa thus allowing smaller doses of L-dopa to be effective. Long-term L-dopa therapy may lose its effect, and the results of this can be seen with the patient displaying end of dose "stiffness" or freezing, or swings in function.[38] The creative titration of this drug, as well as the use of dopaminergic derivatives and anticholinergic drugs, can be helpful. Table 8–14 lists the drugs commonly used to treat Parkinson's disease.[38]

Psychological Regimens

The incidence of psychological complications in the older person is a known problem, and the management of these problems has always been a challenge. The most important step in the pharmacological management is proper diagnosis. Unfortunately, it is often the case that the patient and the physician accept the psychological complication as a natural occurrence of aging. For the sake of simplicity the mental disorders to be discussed in this section are

1. Adjustment disorders
2. Affective disorders
3. Organic brain disorders
4. Anxiety disorders
5. Schizophrenic disorders
6. Personality disorders
7. Substance abuse disorders

Adjustment disorders are time-limited responses to psychosocial stressors, the most common of which is the death of a spouse. The treatment is a short-acting medication for the relief of anxiety, agitation, and sleep disturbances. Short-acting benzodiazepine-type sedative/hypnotic or antianxiety agents are appropriate versus the use of antidepressants or antipsychotic medications.[21] Table 8–15 lists the commonly used antianxiety agents.

An unresolved adjustment disorder may lead to an affective disorder. Affective disorders are composed of depressive and manic depressive disorders. The manifestations of these major depressive disorders are increased physical complaints, memory problems, guilt, hopelessness, agitation, appetite disturbances, decreased energy, helplessness, and suicidal thoughts. The first line of treatment for these problems are antidepressant medications. The next effective line of treatment, providing there are no contraindications, is electroconvulsive shock therapy, tricyclics, and monoamine oxidase inhibitors (MAOI). Because of the side effects of severe orthostatic hypotension, MAOIs may need to be avoided, as well as tricyclic antidepressants for cardiac condition defects.[21] Manic depressive illness is treated with lithium carbonate and carbamazepine. Drugs used in the treatment of affective disorders are listed in Table 8–16.

Organic brain disorders are treated symptomologically (see Chapter 3 for a full description). Cognitive agents that supposedly stop or reverse the dementia are of little or no value. The symptom most treated is agitation, and the treatment of choice is short-acting sedative/hypnotics and antianxiety agents.[21] (See Table 8–16.)

Schizophrenic disorders usually have their onset before 45 years of age and are characterized by delusions, hallucinations, social withdrawal, and an inappropriate and flattened affect. The primary treatment for schizophrenia is antipsychotic drugs, which are associated with blocking central dopamine receptors in the brain. Older persons with schizophrenic disor-

TABLE 8–14. ANTIPARKINSON DRUGS

Drug	Trade Name	Mechanism of Action
Anticholinergics		Inhibits excessive acetylcholine influence caused by dopamine deficiency
Diphenhydramine	Benadryl	
Biperiden	Akineton	
Procyclidine	Kemadrin	
Ethopropazine	Parsidol	
Trihexyphenidyl	Artane	
Orphenadrine	Disipal	
Levodopa		Resolves dopamine deficiency by being converted to dopamine after crossing blood-brain barrier
Levodopa/carbidopa	Sinemet	
Amantidine	Symmetrel	Stimulates release of remaining dopamine
Bromocriptine	Parlodel	A dopamine agent that directly stimulates dopamine receptors in the basal ganglia; a dopamine agonist
Deprenyl	Selegiline	Inhibits the enzyme that breaks down dopamine in the basal ganglia; enables dopamine to remain active for longer periods of time

TABLE 8-15. ANTIANXIETY AGENTS

Drugs	Trade Name	Method of Action	Side Effects	Drug Interactions
Benzodiazepines				
Diazepam	Valium	Facilitates neurotransmitter action of γ-aminobutyric acid (GABA), which mediates both pre- and postsynaptic inhibition in all regions of the CNS	Ataxia, drowsiness	Alcohol & other CNS depressants
Chlordiazepoxide hydrochloride	Librium	Facilitates neurotransmitter actions of γ-aminobutyric acid (GABA), which mediates both pre- and postsynaptic inhibition in all regions of the CNS	Drowsiness, ataxia, confusion	Alcohol & other CNS depressants
Clorazepate, dipotassium salt	Tranxene	Facilitates neurotransmitter actions of γ-aminobutyric acid (GABA), which mediates both pre- and postsynaptic inhibition in all regions of the CNS	Drowsiness, dizziness, nervousness, dry mouth, blurred vision, headache, confusion	Alcohol & other CNS depressants
Lorazepam	Activan	Facilitates neurotransmitter action of γ-aminobutyric acid (GABA), which mediates both pre- and postsynaptic inhibition in all regions of the CNS	Sedation, dizziness, weakness, unsteadiness, disorientation, depression	Alcohol & other CNS depressants
Oxazepam	Serax	Facilitates neurotransmitter action of γ-aminobutyric acid (GABA), which mediates both pre- and postsynaptic inhibition in all regions of the CNS	Drowsiness, dizziness, vertigo, headache	Alcohol & other CNS depressants
Alprazolam	Xanax	Facilitates neurotransmitter action of γ-aminobutyric acid (GABA), which mediates both pre- and postsynaptic inhibition in all regions of the CNS	Drowsiness, dizziness, dry mouth, hypotension	Alcohol & other CNS depressants
Prazepam	Centrax	Facilitates neurotransmitter action of γ-aminobutyric acid (GABA), which mediates both pre- and postsynaptic inhibition in all regions of the CNS	Fatigue, dizziness, drowsiness, weakness, lightheadedness, ataxia	Alcohol & other CNS depressants
Nonbenzodiasepines				
Buspirone	Buspar	Unknown	Dizziness, drowsiness, nervousness, nausea, headache, fatigue	Trazodone, haloperidol, CNS drugs, MAO inhibitors, warfarin

TABLE 8-16. DRUGS USED IN THE TREATMENT OF AFFECTIVE DISORDERS

Drugs	Trade Name	Method of Action	Side Effects	Drug Interactions
Tricyclic Antidepressants				
Desipramine hydrochloride	Norpramine	Inhibits membrane pump mechanism responsible for the reuptake of norepinephrine and seratonin at presynaptic nerve postsynaptic terminals	Tachycardia, nausea, vomiting, dizziness, headache, constipation, weight gain	Alcohol, cimetidine, CNS depressants, MAO inhibitors, sympathomimetics, anticholinergics, guanethidine
Doxepine	Sinequan	Inhibits membrane pump mechansism responsible for the reuptake of norepinephrine and serotonin at presynaptic nerve terminals, potentiating activity at postsynaptic terminals	Tachycardia, dry mouth, blurred vision, nausea, vomiting, dizziness, weakness, headache, constipation, urinary retention, weight gain	CNS depressants, anticholinergics, MAO inhibitors, clonidine, cimetidine, sympathomimetics, dicumarol, guanethidine
Amitriptyline	Elavil	Inhibits membrane pump mechansism responsible for the reuptake of norepinephrine and serotonin at presynaptic nerve terminals, potentiating activity at postsynaptic terminals	Tachycardia, dry mouth, blurred vision, nausea, weakness, headache, constipation, urinary retention, weight gain	CNS depressants, anticholinergics, MAO inhibitors, sympathomimetics, guanethidine
Imipramine	Trofanil	Blocks uptake of norepinephrine at nerve endings	Orthostatic hypotension, hypetension, tachycardia, confusional states, delusions, anxiety, numbness, tingling, incoordination, dry mouth, blurred vision, constipation, jaundice, nausea, vomiting	CNS depressants, guanethidine
Nortriptyline	Pamelor	Blocks uptake of norepinephrine at nerve endings	Orthostatic hypotension, hypetension, tachycardia, confusional states, delusions, anxiety, numbness, tingling, incoordination, dry mouth, blurred vision, constipation, nausea, vomiting	CNS depressants, thyroid medications, guanethidine & other antihypertensive drugs
Trimipramine	Surmontil	Unknown	Hypotension, hypertension, confusional states, delusions, numbness, jaundice, tingling, blurred vision, rash, nausea, vomiting	Local decongestants, catecholamine, MAO inhibitors, anticholinergics, sympathomimetics, alcohol, cimetidine
Protriptyline	Vivactil	Unknown	Myocardial infarction, stroke, heart block, hypotension, confusional states, delusions, anxiety, incoordination, seizures, tremors, dizziness, drowsiness, jaundice, urinary retention, nausea, vomiting, anorexia	Guanethidine, thyroid medication, CNS depressants, neuroleptics, sympathomimetics, cimetidine
MAO Inhibitors				
Isocarboxazid	Marplan	Potent inhibitor of amine oxidase	Orthostatic hypotension, dizziness, vertigo, disturbance in cardiac rate, headache, tremors & muscle twitches, mania, confusion, weakness, fatigue, blurred vision	Sympathomimetics, MAO inhibitors, caffeine, tryptophan, benzodiazepines, clomipramine hydrochloride, buspirone, CNS depressants

(continued)

TABLE 8–16. (CONTINUED)

Drugs	Trade Name	Method of Action	Side Effects	Drug Interactions
Maprotiline	Ludiomil	Blocks norepinephrine reuptake	Nervousness, drowsiness, dizziness, tremor, dry eyes, blurred vision, weakness, fatigue, headache, constipation	MAO inhibitors, general anesthetics, CNS depressants, sympathomimetics, guanethidine, phenothiazine, cimetidine
Tranylcypromine	Parnate	Nonhydrazine MAO inhibitors, increases concentration of norepinephrine	Hypertensive crisis, headaches, restlessness, insomnia, weakness, drowsiness, dizziness, diarrhea, abdominal pain, jerks, tinnitus, muscle spasm	MAO inhibitors, benzodiazepines, CNS depressants, caffeine, antihistamine anaesthetic drugs, buspirone, meperidine, tyramine, antiparkinson drugs, dextromethorphan, antihypertensives
Phenelzine	Nardil	MAO inhibitors	Postural hypotension, dizziness, headache, drowsiness, fatigue, constipation, GI distress	MAO inhibitors, other antidepressants, fluoxetine, thiazide, diuretics, β-blockers, benzodiazepines, buspirone, antihypertensives
Amoxepine	Ascendin	Blocks norepinephrine and serotonin reuptake	Drowsiness, blurred vision, anorexia, insomnia, nausea,	Neuroleptic MAO inhibitors, anticholinergic drugs, CNS depressants, cimetidine dizziness, headache
Alprazolam	Xanax	Increases CNS GABA effects	Drowsiness, dizziness, hypotension, dry mouth	CNS depressants
Carbamazepine	Tegretol	Unknown	Dizziness, drowsiness, nausea, vomiting, unsteadiness, bone marrow depression, urticaria, congestive heart failure, edema, aggravation of hypertension, syncope, collapse, fever, pneumonia, aplastic anemia	Phenobarbital, primidone, warfarin, doxycycline, haloperidol, phenytoin, erythromycin, cimetidine, calcium channel blockers, lithium propoxyphene, theophylline
Lithium carbonate	Carbolith	Alters sodium transport in nerve and muscle cells; it is not known how it controls mania	Blackout spells, tremor, muscle hyperirritability, ataxia, slurred speech, dizziness, vertigo, weight loss, cardiac arrhythmia, hypotension, anorexia, nausea, vomiting, blurred vision, fatigue, lethargy	Haloperidol, antipsychotic meds, neuromuscular blocking agents, indomethacin, piroxicam, NSAIDs, ACE inhibitors, enalapril, captopril

TABLE 8–17. ANTIPSYCHOTIC DRUGS

Drugs	Trade Name	Method of Action	Side Effects	Drug Interactions
Phenothiazine derivatives				
Chlorpromazine	Thorazine	Unknown, has actions at all levels of CNS, strong central adrenergic blocking activity	Tardive dyskinesia, drowsiness, jaundice, agranulocytosis, postural hypotension, tachycardia, fainting	CNS depressants (alcohol, barbiturates, etc), oral anticoagulants
Trifluoperazine	Stelazine	Unknown, has actions all all levels of CNS, strong central adrenergic blocking activity	Tardive dyskinesia, jaundice, rash, pseudoparkinsonism, dystonias, motor restlessness, drowsiness, dizziness, dry mouth, fatigue, muscle weakness	CNS depressants, oral anticoagulants, propranolol, dilantin, guanethidine, other antihypertensives, thiazide diuretics, amipaque
Fluphenazine	Prolixin	Unknown, has actions at all levels of CNS, strong central adrenergic blocking activity	Hypertension, nausea, salivation, polyuria, perspiration, headache, dry mouth, constipation, weight change	Epinephrine, alcohol, CNS depressants, anticholinergics
Mesordazine	Serentil	Acts indirectly on reticular formation; depression of hypothalamic centers	Drowsiness, hypotension, parkinsonism, dizziness, weakness, restlessness, dystonia, rigidity, dry mouth, blurred vision, nausea, slurring, fainting	CNS depressants
Promethazine	Phenergan	Unknown antitussive effect on the CNS; also has anticholinergic effects	Drowsiness, rash, nausea, vomiting, blurred vision, dry mouth, dizziness	Alcohol and other CNS depressants, anticholinergic agents, MAO inhibitors
Prochlorperazine	Compazine	Competitively blocks postsynaptic dopamine receptors in cerebral cortex, basal ganglia, hypthalamus, limbic system, medulla, and brain stem	Drowsiness, dizziness, blurred vision, hypourticaria, extrapyramidal reaction, tardive dyskinesia	Alcohol, metrizamide, CNS depressants, anticoagulants, anticholinergics, β-adrenergic blocking drugs, guanethidine
Thioridazine	Mellaril	Competitively blocks postsynaptic dopamine receptors in the cerebral cortex, basal ganglia, hypothalamus, limbic system, medulla, and brain stem	Drowsiness, dizziness, blurred vision, dry mouth, constipation, extrapyramidal reactions, tardive dyskinesia, dermatitis	CNS depressants, anticholinergics, guanethidine
Thioxanthene derivatives				
Thiothixene	Navane	Competitively blocks postsynaptic dopamine receptors in the cerebral cortex, basal ganglia, hypothalamus, limbic system, medulla, and brain stem	Drowsiness, drowsiness, tardive dyskinesia, dry mouth, urticaria, extrapyramidal symptoms, weakness, photosensitivity, diarrhea, pruritus	CNS depressants, anticholinergics,
Butyrophenone derivatives				
Haloperidol	Haldol	Blocks postsynaptic dopamine receptors in the cerebral cortex, basal ganglia, hypothalamus, limbic system, medulla, and brain stem	Hypotension, insomnia, anxiety, tachycardia, restlessness, lightheadedness, tardive dyskinesia, blurred vision, photosensitivity, nausea, vomiting, rash, pruritis	CNS depressants, guanethidine, anticonvulsants, lithium

271

ders are usually treated with lower doses of antipsychotic agents with relatively good outcomes.[21] Table 8–17 lists antipsychotic drugs used in the treatment of schizophrenia.

Anxiety disorders usually have their onset in the young to middle adult years. Interventions are usually psychological and behavioral. Psychotropic (i.e., antianxiety medications) can be used adjunctly in severe situations.[21]

Personality disorders are lifelong patterns of maladaptive ways of relating to the world. The treatment of choice is behavior modification and psychotherapy. Psychotropics may be used, but many times they are discouraged because of the potential for addiction.[21]

Substance abuse disorders are characterized by withdrawal symptoms and the inability to control the use of a substance. The primary treatment is psychotherapy and behavior modification. However psychotropics can be used in the initial stages and then tapered off.

Gastrointestinal Drugs

Understanding the types of gastrointestinal drugs is important to the rehabilitation professional because a majority of patients use them. According to Peura and Fresion, 60% to 100% of chronically ill patients suffer some type of stress-related stomach problem.[39]

The good news about gastrointestinal drugs is that they do not produce any significant side effects that may impair rehabilitation. The only potential side effect may occur with the administration of opiates for the treatment of diarrhea due to their addictive nature. The most common gastrointestinal problems are gastric ulcers, diarrhea, and constipation.

Gastric ulcers, or the hemorrhaging and ulceration of the stomach lining due to an above-normal amount of acids being produced, can be treated in a variety of ways. The main treatment is antacids. Other commonly used medications are H_2 receptor blockers, anticholinergics, and sucralfate. See Table 8–18 for dosages, side effects, and trade names.[6,39]

Antidiarrheal agents mainly take three forms: absorbants, bacterial cultures, and opiate derivatives. Absorbants, such as pectin and kaolin, have essentially no side effects and work by absorbing excess fluid. Bacterial cultures are used to replace specific active cultures that for some reason may be deficient. They do, however, have minor intestinal gas and flatulence as side effects. Finally, opiate derivatives are, perhaps, the most effective agents in the treatment of diarrhea.[16,37] They slow intestinal peristalsis, but offer such side effects as nausea, gastrointestinal disturbances, drowsiness, constipation, and fatigue.[39] Table 8–19 lists the common drugs, trade names, methods of action, and dosage for each.[6,37,39]

TABLE 8–18. DRUG TREATMENTS FOR GASTRIC ULCERS

Drugs	Trade Name	Method of Action	Dosages
Antacids			
Sodium bicarbonate	Alka-Selzer	Neutralization of gastric acid	1–2 tablets every 4 hr as needed
Aluminum carbonate	Basaljel	Relief of hyperacidity	2 capsules as often as every 2 hr, up to 12 daily
Aluminum hydroxide	Amphojel	Relief of hyperacidity	2 tablets of 0.3 g or 1 tablet of 0.6 g strength five to six times per day
Aluminum hydroxide magnesium	Maalox	Neutralizaton of acidity	1–2 tablets well chewed, or 1–2 tsp at meals and bedtime
	Mylanta	Neutralization of acidity	2–4 tablets well chewed, or 2–4 tsp after meals and at bedtime
Magaldrate	Riopan	Rapid and uniform buffering action	Chew or swallow 1–2 tablets or 1–2 tsp between meals and at bedtime
H_2 receptor blockers			
Cimitedine	Tagamet	Inhibits histamine at the H receptors on gastric cells	300 mg four times/day
Ranitidine	Zantac	Inhibits histamine at the H receptors on gastric cells	100–150 mg two times daily
Famotidine	Pepcid	Inhibits histamine at the H receptors on gastric cells	40 mg once daily at bedtime
Anticholinergics (Please see Table 8–7)			
Sucralfate	Carafate	Formation of ulcer adherent complex, which covers the ulcer site and protects it against further attack by acid, pepsin, and bile salts	1 g twice daily
Metoclopramide	Reglan	Stimulates motility in the upper GI tract	10–15 mg up to qid 30 min prior to meal or bedtime

TABLE 8–19. ANTIDIARRHEAL AGENTS

Drugs	Trade Name	Method of Action	Dosages
Absorbants			
Kaolin, Pectin	Kaelin	Absorption of excess fluid and causative agent	60–120 mL regular strength suspension after each loose bowel movement
Bacterial cultures			
Lactobacillus acidophilus	_____	Administered to reestablish flora	2 capsules, 4 tablets, or 1 packet, 2–4 times each day
Lactobacillus bulgaris	_____	Administered to reestablish flora	2 capsules, 4 tablets, or 1 packet, 2–4 times each day
Opiate derivatives			
Diphenoxylate	Lomotil	Binds to intestine opiate receptors, decreasing peristalsis	5 mg, 4 times daily
Loperamide	Imodium	Unknown	4 mg unit or 2 after each unformed stool

Laxatives, commonly used agents in the older population, are present in four different forms: bulk forming, stimulant, hyperostotic, and lubricant or stool softeners. Prior to using laxatives, the rehabilitation professional may want to encourage the patient to exercise. Decreased activity has been shown to lower gastric motility.[6] A major concern in laxative administration is the potential for abuse with long-term usage. Table 8–20 provides a list of a few of the common laxatives, their trade names, methods of action, and side effects.[6]

Diabetic Regimens

Oral diabetes medications are generally recommended when diet and exercise have failed to achieve optimal glucose control in patients with Type II diabetes. With the current knowledge regarding the relationship between hyperglycemia and chronic complications, many patients are beginning oral diabetic medications at the time of diagnosis, in combination with diet and exercise. There are currently five classes of oral diabetes medications available in the United States: sulfonylureas, meglitinides, biguanides, thiazolidinediones, and alpha-glucosidase inhibitors.[40] Individuals with Type I diabetes are not candidates for oral medications.

Sulfonylureas stimulate insulin secretion from the pancreatic β-cell. The most common side effect is hypoglycemia.[41] Meglitinides stimulate insulin secretion from the pancreatic β-cell more rapidly than sulfonylureas.[40] Meglitinides are taken prior to meals to

TABLE 8–20. LAXATIVES

Drugs	Trade Name	Method of Action	Side Effects
Bulk forming			
Psyllium	Metamucil	Polycarbophil absorbs water in the GI tract to form a gelatinous bulk that encourages a normal bowel movement	Powder may cause allergic reaction if inhaled
Perdiem	_____	Vegetable mucilages soften stool and provide painfree evacuation	Laxative dependance, excessive water and body salt loss
Stimulants			
Castor oil	Fleet-flavored castor oil	Works directly on small intestine to promote a bowel movement	Laxative dependance, excessive water and body salt loss
Bisacodyl	Ducolax	Contact laxative directly on colonic mucosa to produce peristalis through the large intestine	Abdominal cramps
Phenolphthalein	Modane	Acts on large intestine to produce semifluid stool	Excess bowel activity, abdominal discomfort, cramps, weakness, palpittion
Hyperosmotic			
Lactulose	Chronolac	Broken down in the colon to lactic acid, formic and acetic acids; causes an increase in stool water content	Intestinal cramps, nausea, vomiting, flatulence
Sodium Phosphate	Fleet Phospho-soda	Versatile in action, gentle laxative or purgative	Laxative dependence, sodium loss
Lubricants & stool softeners			
Docusate	Pericolace Disonate	Provides general peristaltic stimulation and helps keep stools soft	Nausea, abdominal cramping, rash, diarrhea
Mineral oil	Fleet mineral oil enema	Contact softens and lubricates hard stools	Abdominal pain

reduce postprandial hyperglycemia. Biguanides decrease hepatic gluconeogenesis and glycogenesis and increase insulin sensitivity.[41] Gastrointestinal problems, including abdominal discomfort, are the most common side effects of metformin, the only biguanide available in the United States.[41] An infrequent side effect of metformin is lactic acidosis. Metformin is therefore contraindicated in any condition that causes hypoperfusion, such as severe hepatic, renal, and cardiopulmonary disease. Thiazolidinediones increase insulin sensitivity.[41] Because use of thiazolidinediones has been associated with hepatic dysfunction, the manufacturers provide specific guidelines for liver function testing in patients using these drugs. Alpha-glucosidase inhibitors interfere with the ability of enzymes in the small intestinal brush boarder to break down oligosaccharides and disaccharides into monosaccharides, thus retarding glucose entry into the systemic circulation.[41] Alpha-glucosidase enzyme inhibitors are associated with a number of gastrointestinal side effects, including bloating, abdominal discomfort, diarrhea, and flatulence. These side effects can usually be minimized by slow titration of the daily dosage. Alpha-glucosidase inhibitors are contraindicated in individuals with inflammatory bowel disease, cirrhosis, or plasma creatinine greater than 2 mg/dL.

Insulin is indicated as initial therapy in patients who have Type II diabetes with a markedly elevated fasting plasma glucose level (>280 to 300 mg/dL); in patients with ketonuria or ketonemia; and in symptomatic (neuropathies, retinopathies, etc.) patients.[41] There are a number of insulin preparations currently available. These drugs are administered based on the source of the insulin (human versus animal) and the length of pharmacologic effects. Animal forms of insulin are effective in controlling glucose metabolism even though they have some structural chemical differences from their human counterparts. Human insulin is the most effective and is produced through biosynthesis using cell cultures and recombinant DNA technique. The advantage of biosynthetic products is that they are absorbed more rapidly after injection and have a lower risk of immunologic reaction.[41]

Oral diabetic medications and insulin preparations used in the treatment of diabetes mellitus are listed in Table 8–21.

Urinary Incontinence

Pharmacologic therapy of incontinence in older adults can be quite helpful, especially when combined with behavioral interventions. The type of incontinence—urge, stress or mixed incontinence—will determine the appropriate therapeutic agent. Drugs affect incontinence because they benefit either bladder storage or emptying. Table 8–22 summarizes medications used for urge and stress incontinence.[42] It is important to note that clinical trials for these

TABLE 8–21. HYPOGLYCEMIC DRUGS

Drug	Trade Name	Mechanism of Action
Oral Hypoglycemic Drugs		
Sulfonylureas	Diabeta, Diabinese, Diamicron, etc.	Stimulate the pancreas to produce more insulin
Meglitinides	———	Rapid acting. Stimulate the pancreas to produce more insulin
Biguanides	Metformin	Help the body to use glucose more efficiently
Thiazolidinediones	Actos, Avandia	Control blood glucose by making the muscle cells more sensitive to insulin
Alpha-glucosidase	———	Retard glucose entry into the systemic circulation
Acarbose	Prandase	Prolongs the absorption of carbohydrates after a meal
Therapeutic Insulin		
Rapid-acting insulin	Humulin R, Novolin R, Velsulin	Administered to complement other drugs (oral hypoglycemics) and to supplement endogenous insulin release
	Human[H] Iletin I or II, Velsulin[A]	
Prompt insulin zinc	Semilent Insulin, Semilente Iletin I[A]	Supplement endogenous insulin release
Intermediate-acting	Humulin N, Novolin	
Isophane Insulin	H, Insulatard NPH[H], NPH Inulin, NPH Iletin I, NPH Iletin II [A]	Complementary to other drugs and supplement endogenous insulin release
Insulin zinc	Humulin L, Novolin L[H], Lente Insulin, Lente Iletin I or II[A]	Supplement endogenous insulin release
Long-acting	Ultralente Insulin,	Supplement endogenous insulin release
Extended insulin zinc	Ultralente Iletin I[A]	
Protamine zinc insulin	Protamine Zinc & IletinI;[A] Protamine Zinc & Iletin II[A]	Supplement endogenous insulin release

H = lists insulin from human sources (biosynthetic; recombinant DNA)
A = lists insulin from animal sources

TABLE 8–22. MEDICATION FOR URGE AND STRESS INCONTINENCE IN OLDER ADULTS

Brand Name	Generic Name	Method of Action	Side Effects	Contraindications
Urge Incontinence				
Detrol	Tolterodine	Anticholinergic, decreases bladder contractility, increases capacity	Dry mouth, headache, constipation	Urinary retention, pyloric stenosis, uncontrolled narrow angle glaucoma
Ditropan XL, Ditropan	Oxybutynin	Anticholinergic, decreases bladder contractility	Dry mouth, constipation, somnolence	Urinary retention, pyloric stenosis, uncontrolled narrow angle glaucoma
Tofranil	Imipramine	Tricyclic antidepressant, blocks reuptake of of epinephrine and serotonin, therefore may have effect of increasing bladder capacity and increasing sphincteric closure	Dry mouth, constipation, blurred vision, dizziness	Not to be given during acute phase of myocardial infarction or with MAO inhibitors, urinary retention
Cardura	Doxazosin	Relaxes smooth muscle of urethra and prostatic capsule in men with benign prostatic hypertrophy	Postural hypotension, dizziness, dyspnea, edema	Not for use with patients with impaired liver function
Hytrin	Terazosin	Relaxes smooth muscle of urethra and prostatic capsule in men with benign prostatic hypertrophy	Postural hypotension, dizziness, nausea	Caution with other antihypertensives
Flowmax	Tamsulosin	Relaxes smooth muscle of urethra and prostatic capsule in men with benighn prostatic hypertrophy	Abnormal ejaculation, postural, dizziness, insomnia, cough	Caution with cimetidine
Stress Incontinence				
Premarin cream, Estrace	Estrogen vaginal cream	Treats atrophic vaginitis	Breast tenderness, uterine bleeding, vaginal candidiasis, headache	Endometrial cancer, impaired renal or liver function
ESTring	Estradiol	Treats atrophic vaginitis	Headache, leukorrhea, skeletal pain	Caution in patients with impaired liver function
Entex LA	Phenylpropanolamine	Increases urethral smooth muscle contraction	Nervousness, dizziness, insomnia	Uncontrolled hypertension, benign prostatic hypertrophy
Sudafed	Pseudoephedrine	Increases urethral smooth muscle contraction	Central nervous system over-stimulation, headache, elevation in blood pressure	Severe or uncontolled hypertension, benign prostatic hypertrophy, and not for use with MAO inhibitors

medications did not test the drugs on large numbers of frail elders. Therefore, the rehabiliation therapist needs to monitor a patient on these drugs for side effects such as delirium, urinary retention (which will lead to infection), blurred vision, dehydration, and other adverse reactions.

Cancer Regimens

As the second most common cause of death and a major cause of morbidity for persons aged 65 and over, it is important to discuss the implications of the chemotherapies that our patients are often undergoing. Cytotoxic chemotherapy can result in significant changes in functional capabilities. Drugs used against cancer are classified by their chemical structure, source, or mechanism of action.[6] The primary groups of antineoplastic drugs are the alkylating agents, antimetabolites, antineoplastic antibiotics, antineoplastic hormones, and several other miscellaneous drug groups and individual agents.[6] Due to the extensive list of these chemotherapy pharmaceuticals, they will not be listed in this text. For an excellent source for information on various cancer regimes and extensive discussion of the research on various agents, refer to the text, *Pharmacology in Rehabilitation,* by Dr. Charles D. Ciccone.[6]

Because aging may be associated with changes in the pharmacokinetics and pharmacodynamics of cytotoxic drugs and with increased susceptibility of normal tissues to the complications of treatment, the dosages of cytotoxic agents may need to be modified, Pharmacokinetic changes in absorption, volume distribution, metabolism, and excretion occur with age.[43] With the development of new oral drugs, changes in drug absorption may become more relevant in the use of chemotherapeuric agents. Changes in the volume concentrations of water-soluble agents occur as a result of a decline in lean body weight, a decline in albumin concentration, and anemia. Many cytotoxic agents are heavily bound to red blood cells. In the presence of anemia, the concentration of free agent in the circulation increases.[43] Changes in liver function may reduce the activation and deactivation of drugs such as the oxaphosphorines (cyclophosphamide and isfosfamide). Unfortunately, no reliable clinical tests are available to assess these reactions.[43,44]

Because the decline in GFR is one of the most consistent physiological changes in aging, the renal excretion of drugs is reduced in the majority of older adults. Many drugs, such as methotrexate, bleomycin, and carboplatin, or drugs that give origin to active and toxic metabolites, are excreted through the kidneys. Idarubicin and daunorubicin are metabolized and excreted through the kidneys. Cytarabine in high does leads to accumulation of ara-uridine, a neurotoxic metabolite, in the blood.[44] As this drug is excreted through the kid-

ney, failure to eliminate this byproduct from the body results in neurological symptoms.

Altered intracellular metabolism of drugs and a decrease in the ability to repair DNA occur in the elderly. As a result, the ability of cells to catabolize cytotoxins is diminished. With chemotherapy in the older adult, the risk and severity of myelodepression, mucositis, central and peripheral neurotoxicity, and cardiotoxicity also increase.[44]

Chronic Obstructive Pulmonary Disease: Drug Interventions

Chronic obstructive pulmonary disease (COPD), the fifth leading cause of death in the United States, peaks in prevalence between the ages of 65 to 74 years of age, a major medical disorder in the elderly.[45] Diagnoses of COPD include chronic bronchitis to emphysema. The first line of drug intervention in COPD is the use of bronchodilators, which are inhaled anticholinergics and β^2-agonists. Anticholinergic agents are the first choice for regular maintenance therapy. Ipratropium is the most commonly prescribed anticholinergic inhaler as the effects last longer than the β^2-agonists (albuterol), and ipratropium is devoid of significant side effects.

The use of theophylline in the treatment of COPD in the elderly is controversial. Theophylline and its analogues have both bronchodilator and nonbronchodilator effects. These effects include increased contractility and increased hypoxic drive to respiration. Elderly patients are vulnerable to serious toxic effects such as cardiac arrhythmia, seizures, insomnia, headache, anxiety, and tremors.

Corticosteroids clearly have a beneficial effect on airway inflammation, such as in asthma, but they are not as effective in COPD.[45] Systemic steroids in elderly COPD patients are prone to numerous side effects including hyperglycemia, osteoporosis, myopathy, cataracts, hypertension, peptic ulcer disease, adrenal insufficiency, and a range of mood and behavioral changes. Inhaled corticosteroids may produce fewer side effects than systemic steroids but are generally less effective.

As the COPD patient is apt to have frequent bouts with lower respiratory tract infections (pneumonia), empirical antibiotics are often a part of an older person's drug regime.

The only therapies that have been proven to impact the outcomes in elderly COPD patients are smoking cessation and oxygen therapy. Smoking cessation is associated with a slower rate of decline in lung function, demonstrating that it is never too late to stop smoking.[45] Oxygen therapy improves both quality of life and survival in hypoxemic patients with COPD. Supplemental oxygen is required when the PaO_2 is 55 mm Hg or less in sitting; if there are more than two hours during which the patient's SaO_2 is less than 90%; or if the PaO_2 falls to 55 mm Hg or lower during exercise.[46]

Dementia: Pharmacological Therapy

Pharmacologic therapies for cognitive impairment are gaining more attention due to the prevalence of Alzheimer's disease and other dementias as people live longer lives. Multiple pharmacotherapeutic approaches are often used, including antidepressants, anxioloytics, sedatives, and cognitive enhancers. The focus in this section is primarily on therapies for Alzheimer's disease (AD), because it is the most common form of dementia.

Drug therapies are currently being directed toward the two etiological causes of AD. It is generally thought that increases in levels of the small peptide (amyloid or β-amyloid) in the aging brains lead to neuronal dysfunction and damage. Vascular dementia is the second most common cause and felt to be a part of the progressive decline seen in AD patients.[25] Our understanding of AD was greatly enhanced by genetic findings that mutations in the β-amyloid precursor protein gene, which segregate with early-onset disease, make the accumulation of β-amyloids (what we think of as neurofibrillary plaques and tangles) central to the disease process. Although no current medications are aimed at lowering β-amyloid production, the most recent discovery of the β-secretase enzymes (see Chapter 5) ensures that there will be extensive research in this area. At this time, therapies are aimed at altering β-amyloid precursor protein metabolism.

Abnormalities in the cholinergic system, similar to those seen in Parkinson's disease, are consistently found in AD. Consideration of the role of acetylcholine in learning and memory and its potential neurotrophic effects has given rise to cholinergic therapies. Cholinergic agents include cholinesterase inhibitors, muscarinic and nicotinic receptor agonists, and direct modifiers of acetylcholine release.[47,48] Acetylcholinesterase inhibitors include tacrine, donepezil, physostigmine, rivastigmine, galantamine, ENA 713, and metrifonate. Tacrine improves cognitive performance and certain secondary psychiatric symptoms, however, hepatotoxicity and gastrointestinal side effects are a problem.[47] Donepezil (Aricept), recently approved for use in mild to moderate AD, improves cognitive performance and quality of life over the short term and is less toxic and better tolerated than tacrine. This whole family of drugs must be administered cautiously in patients with bronchospastic pulmonary disease, bradydysrhythmia, decreased cardiac contractility, or peptic ulcer disease, due to the risk of adverse reactions.[47,48]

Evidence for the role of oxidative stress in neuronal degeneration has led to the use of antioxidant therapies for the treatment of dementia. These therapies include monoamine oxidase inhibitors (MAOIs), vitamin E, vitamin C, and calcium channel blockers. Selegiline (a relatively selective MAO-B inhibitor) is believed to act as a free radical scavenger and modulator of monoaminergic neurotransmission, and has been shown to influence mood and behavioral concomitants of AD.[49] Patients with AD or vascular dementia treated with ginko biloba, a compound with putative antioxidant properties, showed modest improvements in cognition.[50-52] Other antioxidants such as vitamin E, vitamin C, melatonin, and idebenone are currently under investigation and may ultimately prove beneficial.[49]

Inflammatory dysfunction has been identified in the brains of AD patients, indicating that inflammatory and immune mechanisms accompany the neurodegenerative processes.[53] The potential role of anti-inflammatory agents in the treatment of AD was originally suggested by the unexpectedly low prevalence of the disease among patient with RA treated with NSAIDs. Case-control studies showed a slower rate of decline on several cognitive measures in AD patients using NSAIDs.[49] However, drug-related side effects such as gastrointestinal tolerance, renal toxicity, and adverse cognitive effects such as sleep disturbance and delirium may limit their use. Selective inhibition of cox-2, which is expressed in the neocortex and particularly in limbic structures such as the hippocampus, may result in reduced drug-related side effects.[49,53] Current investigations of NSAIDs, cox-2 inhibitors, and corticosteroids are ongoing and promising.

Clinical trials of other compounds with diverse therapeutic values include substances that facilitate the use of fatty acids, such as acetyl-L-carnitine, and calcium channel blockers, such as nimodipine. Drugs that protect the central nervous system from potential damage due to hypoxia, such as piracetam, oiracetam, pramiracetam, and anitacetam are currently being investigated.[48] Immunization with β-amyloid is showing significant reduction of β-amyloid plaque formation, neuritic dystrophy, and astrogliosis.[48,54] The eventual success of any pharmacological interaction requires the identification of preclinical biomarkers of disease, as AD has its origins many years before even the most mild symptoms appear.

COMPLIANCE AND MOTIVATION IN DRUG REGIMENS

The issue of compliance must be addressed when discussing pharmaceutical management of disease. The use of medications in the management of physical illness is only as useful as the patient's ability to adhere to the program. This final section will explore compliance behaviors of older patients.

Health professionals appear to believe that older persons are less compliant. In reality, older patients are no more noncompliant than younger patients.[55] However, a statistical relationship does exist between noncompliance and patients taking multiple drugs.[55] Other factors involved in noncompliance are unmanageable costs, physical weakness, and impaired vision or hearing.[55] These factors tend to be more prevalent in older persons and may be the reason health professionals see older persons in general as noncompliant. In recognizing noncompliance, the therapist should look at these factors as contributors to the problem instead of describing all older people as noncompliant.

The simplest initial step in enhancing patient compliance is giving clear, simple, and explicit instructions. Sometimes prescribing physicians omit this important information. Physical therapists can assist in ensuring compliance by researching and reiterating the correct drug procedure in concise and easily understandable terms. Devices such as pill containers, charts, and booklets may enhance compliance. A therapist may suggest these alternatives to the physician of a noncompliant patient. The supplementation of the medication regimen with clear instructions and devices, though, may still not alleviate the noncompliance problem. The literature is unclear as to what is the best answer in this case, and it appears that no program is completely effective.[55]

It does appear that the best intervention for noncompliance is to understand why the patient does or does not comply. In this regard, an interesting group to study are the self-regulators. Often this group does better than the strict compliers. This information tells the therapist to respect the patient's input into designing and monitoring the rehabilitation program in both the medication and exercise aspects. In the medication aspect, the therapist can act as an advocate for the patient.

Finally, the practitioner-patient relationship is an extremely important factor in appropriate patient compliance.[55] When a practitioner questions a patient about compliance, the most honest and useful answers are obtained when the questions are nonthreatening. In addition, explanations on the importance of compliance are also enhanced when the practitioner uses a positive tone, explains clearly, and has a close relationship with the patient.[56]

OVER-THE-COUNTER DRUGS AND SELF-MEDICATION

Age-related physiological and psychological changes, increasing prevalence of chronic disease, and the likelihood of multiple pathologies predispose older people to experience problems with medications. Medication noncompliance, polypharmacy, and the use or abuse of OTC or nonprescription drugs are common. The elderly are the major users and abusers of both OTC and prescription drugs.[57] Although older Americans spend more on prescription drugs than OTC drugs, the elderly account for 40% to 50% of all OTC drug purchases.[58] Fifty-six percent of men and 76% of women who used multiple prescribed medications also used multiple OTC drugs,[58] indicating the depth of the problem of self-medication.

Patients and even health professionals may think of OTC drugs as safe and of little pharmacological significance. All drugs, including OTC medications, carry a risk that is less easily characterized in the elderly. Polypharmacy greatly increases the occurrence of adverse reactions and interactions. In addition to "traditional" OTC drugs, self-medication may include the use of herbal medicines and complementary therapies. A number of preparations once available by prescription only are now available OTC. For example, naproxen an NSAID, was changed from prescription-only to OTC in 1994 (it still requires a prescription in the United Kingdom). Many "mild" H_2-receptor antagonists can be obtained over the counter. As the side effects of this class of drug are numerous (gastrointestinal disturbances, headache, dizziness, weakness, rash, confusion, depression, etc.) and these drugs have potentially hazardous interactions with antiarrhythmics, warfarin, tricyclic antidepressants, antidiabetics, benzodiazepines, psychotics, and beta-blockers, the unprescribed use of these substances is of great concern in an older population.[59]

Other OTC drug categories include allergy treatments, analgesia and antipyretic products, antimicrobials, bronchodilators, dermatological products, emetics, hematinics, laxatives, sedatives, stimulants, vitamin-mineral supplements, and weight-loss aids. The OTC drugs used most commonly by the elderly tend to be drugs for the treatment of pain and fever; coughs, colds, and allergy; insomnia; heartburn and acid reflux; constipation; diarrhea; and nausea and vomiting.

These OTC drugs tend to be used to treat self-described (and therefore, self-prescribed) symptoms. However, these symptoms may mask a more serious condition. A good example is an older person believing angina to be indigestion and self-medicating for heartburn or acid reflux (whichever commercial they've seen on TV that week). Although OTC drugs are usually sold with clear warnings about the need to consult a physician if symptoms persist, the elder may equate controlling the symptoms with "fixing" the problems. Late presentation for diagnosis or reduced compliance with prescribed medications can result. Over-the-counter drugs are not innocuous; they have the same potential to cause harm as prescribed drugs. Perhaps more so, as OTCs are often taken without the knowledge of the attending physician. The problem of polypharmacy and reducing the negative effects of drugs in the elderly requires a full assessment of both prescribed and OTC drugs. Careful observation by the clinician for signs of confusion, malnutrition (often occurs with the use of antacids), dehydration, and other symptoms, may lead to the discovery that the use of OTC drugs, in combination with prescribed medications, are causing adverse reactions in the older patient.

DRUG-INDUCED MALNUTRITION

Many nutritional problems may be related to the fact that often elderly people are taking various drugs or are on special diets for one or more chronic illnesses. All drugs affect the nutritional status of individuals because all drugs affect metabolism. Aside from the secondary side effects, which include depressed appetite, nausea, vomiting, and diarrhea, drugs have direct effects on the metabolism of nutrients.[57] Some drugs, such as antibiotics, can produce changes in intestinal flora which are responsible for the synthesis of certain vitamins, in particular, vitamin K and pantothenic acid. Destruction of intestinal bacteria may give rise to accelerated growth of fungi and to abnormal bacteria that require excess amounts of folic acid and vitamin B_{12} for their growth, and as a result deprive the host of these nutrients.[57,60] Some drugs and medications may interfere with nutrient absorption. For instance, iron supplements given to relieve anemia may inhibit the absorption of vitamin E. A resinous product, cholestyramine, used to reduce hypercholesterolemia by absorption of bile acids and cholesterol, absorbs other important physiological substances with structures similar to cholesterol, such as vitamin D. The chronic use of alkalizers interferes with the absorption of many nutrients, including calcium and phosphate.[57]

Antimetabolites used in cancer therapy interfere with the utilization of many nutrients. For instance, folic acid, which is required for normal as well as accelerated cell division and growth, is not absorbed. As a result, these drugs not only inhibit or prevent abnormal tissue growth of malignant tissues, they also impair the normal growth of healthy tissues. Some drugs, such as diuretics given for the control of hypertension, prevent water retention but also enhance the excretion of many essential elements, such as potassium, magnesium, chromium, zinc, and copper.

In general, drug administration results in increased vitamin requirements. Chronic aspirin users tend to have low vitamin C levels in leucocytes and synovial fluid. Alcohol ingestion inhibits the absorption of B_1, B_6, B_{12}, and folic acid, resulting in low blood levels of all of these nutrients. To prevent malnutrition, elderly individuals on drug therapies may require vitamin and mineral supplements, and special attention to increasing nutrient intake. See Chapter 7, Exploring Nutritional Needs in the Elderly.

HERBS, VITAMINS, AND NUTRACEUTICALS

More and more of our older adults are seeking alternative forms of health promotion and prevention beyond traditional pharmacologic agents. It is therefore important that we as clinicians are familiar with the effects of herbs, vitamins and nutraceutical substances. A *nutraceutical* agent is any substance that may be considered a food or part of a food which provides medical or health benefits, including the prevention and treatment of disease.[61] *Functional food* is any modified food or food ingredient that may provide a health benefit beyond the traditional nutrients it contains.[62,63] The National Institutes of Health (NIH) has also identified subcategories of pharmacologic utilization of food that include: *pharmafood* which are food or nutrients that have medical or health benefits, including the prevention and treatment of disease; and *designer food*, which are processed foods that are supplemented with food ingredients naturally rich in disease-preventing substances.[61–63]

Herbs are medicinal plants, also called *botanicals* or *phytomedicines*. Phytomedicines are medicinal products that contain plant materials as their pharmacologically active component. They are often complex mixtures of compounds that generally do not exert a strong, immediate action. Table 8–23 provides a summary of the types and kinds of herbal products contained in this pharmaceutical category. In *phytotherapy*, patients receive a specific dose based on the active ingredients in the raw plant material. The dose varies depending on: age, weight, current medical condition, and prescription medication use. Herbal products are often prescribed alone, though may be used to complement a traditional drug regime. For instance, a garlic concentration may be used in combination with other prescription agents to treat hypercholesterolemia.

Herbs are not considered "drugs" in the United States; however, they can be classified as drugs from a medical viewpoint as many provoke a pharmacologic response from a physiological perspective. In the United States, herbs and phytomedicinals are classified as nutritional supplements under the Dietary Supplement and Health Education Act (DSHEA) of 1994. According to this act, herbs, vitamins, miner-

TABLE 8–23. TYPES AND KINDS OF HERBAL PRODUCTS

- **Extracts:** Concentrated preparations of a liquid, powdered, or viscous consistency that are ordinarily made from dried plant parts (crude drug) by maceration or percolation. Fluid extracts are liquid preparations that usually contain a 1:1 ratio of fluid to dried herb. Ethanol, water, or mixtures of ethanol and water are used in the production of fluid extracts. Solid or powdered extracts are preparations made by evaporation of the solvent used in the production process (raw extract).
- **Tincture:** Alcoholic or hydroalcoholic solutions prepared from botanicals. If glycerol is used as a solvent, the preparation is known as a glycerite.
- **Plant juices:** Natural sources of nutrients formed from the freshly harvested plant parts macerated in water and pressed.
- **Teas:** All herb extracts from which potable infusions can be made.

TABLE 8–24. HERBS, DIETARY SUPPLEMENTS, AND DRUGS USED TO TREAT SLEEP DISORDERS & INSOMNIA

Active Herb, Source, Form, and Dosage	Therapeutic Effect Mechanism of Action	Side Effects; Drug Interactions; autions
Herbs for Sleep		
☐ VALERIAN ROOT		
Volatile essential oils (monoterpenes and sesquiterpenes) from dried root and rhizome.	Restlessness, sleeping disorders based on nervous conditions, muscle relaxant.	Mild headache, excitability, uneasiness.
Source: 400–900 mg capsules; 2–3 grams powdered leaf; or 3–5 ml of tincture.	Reduced sleep latency; improved perception of sleep quality.	Too much may cause severe headache, nausea, morning grogginess, blurry vision.
Dosage: 2–3 times daily and before bed.		Do not take with sedatives, anxiolytics, or alcohol. Use caution when driving or operating machinery.
Dietary Supplements for Sleep		
☐ MELATONIN		
Synthetic preparations include sublingual tablets, ordinary tablets, and capsules.	Induces sleep but does not maintain sleep.	Should not be used when person is malnourished or frail, in people taking steroids, or those with severe auto-immune diseases.
Dosage: 0.2–5 mg taken at bedtime.	May alter circadian rhythms and/or have a direct sleep inducing effect.	
Results variable: doesn't work for everyone.	Associated with a decrease in body temperature.	
Large first pass effect through liver.		
Half-life is 30–60 minutes.		
☐ 5-HYDROXYTRYPTOPHAN (5-HTP)		
Commercially produced by extraction from seeds of *Griffonia simplicifolia*.	Increased sleep compared to placebo (600 mg dose); at high doses (2,500 mg) sleep decreased.	Possible GI upset, nausea, diarrhea, and cramping. Do not use with antidepressants.
Dosage: 50 mg 3x/day with meals or 100–300 mg before bedtime.	Precursor to serotonin, a neurotransmitter associated with sleep.	Rare possibility of an eosinophilia myalgia syndrome (EMS).
Well absorbed, 70% ends up in bloodstream. Crosses blood-brain barrier without transport molecule.		
T☐ **Benzodiazepines**	Effective in short-term management of insomnia. Reduce sleep-onset latency, decrease the number and duration of nocturnal awakenings and increase total sleep time.	Used cautiously and with appropriate behavioral treatment programs.
☐ **Flurazepen** (Dalmane)	Effective in inducing and maintaining sleep for up to one month of consecutive usage.	Rapidly absorbed: half-life 48–120 hours. Accumulation with nightly use. Washout slow after termination of use.
	Decreases daytime alertness, increases daytime sedation.	Minimal tolerance for up to 3 months of use. Intermediate absorption: half-life 8–20 hours.
	Good for sleep maintenance problems.	Moderate accumulation with multiple dosing.
☐ **Temazepam** (Restoril)	Best for late-life insomnia.	Fast absorption, short half-life (2–6 hours). Minimal accumulation during multiple dosing.
☐ **Triazolam** (Halcion)	Reduces sleep-onset latency and increases total sleep. time	
	Allows maximal daytime alertness.	
☐ **Zolpidem tartrate** (Ambien)	May be associated with early morning awakening and daytime anxiety.	Rapid onset and short duration. Therapeutic gains maintained 5 wks.
	Decreases sleep-onset latency, but does not decrease number or duration of awakenings.	No next-day residual effects of rebound insomnia.
	Slow-wave sleep well preserved.	

280

TABLE 8–25. HERBS AND DRUGS USED TO TREAT DEPRESSION & ANXIETY DISORDERS

Active Herb, Source, Form, and Dosage	Therapeutic Effect Mechanism of Action	Side Effects; Drug Interactions; Cautions
Herbs for Depression and Anxiety		
❏ ST. JOHN'S WORT Anthraquinone derivatives hypercin and pseudohypercin. Also contains flavonoids, glycosides, phenols, carotenoids, organic acids, choline, pectine, tannins, and long chain alcohols. Flowers provide active constituents. Klamath weed or goatweed harvested and dried. Daily dose: 200–1000 mg alcohol abstract. Taken 2–3 times per day.	Mild to moderate depression Under investigation as a treatment for AIDS and other viruses. Exact mechanism of action unknown. Thought to exert antidepressant effects by inhibiting serotonin re-uptake by postsynaptic receptors. Some reports suggest MAO antagonism as another probable mechanism.	Side effects are rare but include: gastro-intestinal (0.6%), allergic reactions (0.5%), fatigue (0.4%), restlessness (0.3%). No known drug interactions, but not recommended to be used with other antidepressants. Effects of reserpine antagonized. Rash caused by photosensitivity rare.
❏ KAVA-KAVA Kava pryrones (kawain) found in rhizome (root). Other complex chemical components include seven kava lactones. Kava extract standardized to 55–70% kava lactones (kava alphapyrones). Dose: for anxiety 45–75 mg 3 times a day; for sedation 135–210 mg one hour before bedtime.	Sedative and sleep enhancement (CNS depressant effect). Reduced nonpsychotic-type anxiety. Masticated kava causes numbness of the mouth. Mechanism of action unknown.	May adversely affect motor reflexes and judgment for driving. Side effects include dry, flaking, discolored (yellow) skin; scaly rash; red eyes; puffy face; muscle weakness. Contraindicated if using alcohol, barbiturates, or psychoactive agents.

Drug	Side Effects; Drug Interactions; Cautions
Prescription Medications for Depression	
❏ SELECTIVE SEROTONIN RE-UPTAKE INHIBITOR (SSRI) Fluoxetine (Prozac); Sertraline (Zoloft); Paroxetine (Paxil)	May cause nausea, GI distress, anxiety, nervousness, change in appetite or weight, fatigue, drowsiness, and sexual dysfunction.
❏ TRICYCLIC ANTIDEPRESSANTS (TCAs) Tofranil (Imipramine); Anafranil (Clomipramine); Elavil (Amitriptyline)	Dry mouth, constipation, blurry vision, increased sensitivity to sunlight, increased sweating, and weight gain.
❏ BUPROPION (Wellbutrin)	Increased restlessness, agitation, anxiety, and insomnia.
❏ VENLAFAXINE (Effexor)	Nausea, headache, sweating, anxiety, and insomnia.
Prescription Medications for Anxiety	
❏ BENZODIAZEPINES Diazepam (Valium); Alprazolam (Xanax); Chlordiazepoxide (Librium)	Habit forming; withdrawal symptoms. Drowsiness, dizziness, inability to concentrate, increased salivation, constipation, weight gain, blurred vision, decreased sex drive, and impotence.
❏ BUSPIRONE (BuSpar)	Mild headache, drowsiness, nausea, and dry mouth.

See References listed

als, amino acids, and botanicals may be sold legally over the counter as long as the label does not make any therapeutic claims.

The following tables (Tables 8–24 through 8–31) are examples of commonly used complementary phytomedicines and nutrients often prescribed to manage: sleep and insomnia (Table 8–24); depression and anxiety disorders (Table 8–25); memory, Alzheimer's disease and cognitive function (Table 8–26); headache (Table 8–27); atherosclerosis, heart failure, chronic venous insufficiency, and hypertension (Table 8–28); immune and respiratory disorders (Table 8–29); skin conditions, wound healing, and oral health (Table 8–30); and gastrointestinal and liver disorders (Table 8–31).

Rubifacients have been used for many years by patients seeking relief, but only recently has scientific evidence supported the use of such agents. Though this chapter does not permit the review of each variety of treatment available, one example is particularly important in rehabilitation medicine. Capsaicin, a topical treatment has been found to be effective in OA patients for pain relief as well as maintaining joint integrity.[84] Capsaicin depletes substance P by enhancing its release from unmyelinated C fibers. Various strengths are available. Lower concentrations (.025%) need to be applied four times daily, whereas higher concentrations (.075%) can be applied twice daily. The most common side effects

TABLE 8–26. HERBS & DIETARY SUPPLEMENTS: MEMORY, ALZHEIMER'S DISEASE (AD) & COGNITIVE FUNCTION

Active Herb, Source, Form, and Dosage	Therapeutic Effect Mechanism of Action	Side Effects; Drug Interactions; Cautions
Herbs and Cognitive Function		
❑ **Ginkgo biloba**		
Standardized extract from leaves contains 24% flavone glycosides and 6% terpene lactones. Dose for dementia: 120–240 mg/day Taken in 2–3 separate doses for a minimum of 8 weeks.	Treatments for cerebrovascular insufficiency (causing anxiety, memory, concentration and mood impairment, and hearing disorders), dementia, and circulatory disorders (see Table 8–28). Antioxidant. Inhibits platelet activating factor (PAF).	Possible side effects include headache, dizziness, heart palpitation, GI and dermatologic reactions. Ginkgo seeds toxic. Contact with fruit pulp causes an allergic dermatitis. May potentiate the effects of anticoagulants.

HORMONES, VITAMINS, NUTRACEUTICALS AND DRUGS FOR COGNITIVE FUNCTION

Substance	Reported Benefits	Mechanism of Action
❑ **Estrogen (ERT)**	Associated with reduced risk of Alzheimer's disease. Enhanced response to tacrine in women with AD.	May have direct effects on neurotransmitter activity and development, enhancing growth of cholinergic neurons. May act as an antioxidant. Reduces generation of β-amyloid peptides.
❑ **Vitamin E (alpha-tocopherol)**	Slowed functional deterioration seen in moderately severe AD patients (Dose: 2,000 IUs daily for 2 years).	Antioxidant. Inhibits lipid peroxidation and reduces cell death associated with β-protein.
❑ **Selenium**	Deficiency signs include confusion	Co-factor for antioxidant enzymes.
❑ **Phosphatidylserine (PS)**	Exerted mild benefit in age-related cognitive decline and in patients with early symptom of Alzheimer's disease. Preparation used was extracted from bovine brain cortex.[48]	PS is the major phospholipid in the brain. Involved with neurotransmitter release and supports signal transduction.
❑ **Docosahexaenoic acid (DHA)**	Epidemiological correlation between low levels of serum DHA and dementia, depression, and memory loss.	DHA can make up 20–30% of the phospholipids (PE and PS) in the gray matter of the brain.
❑ **Lecithin**	Studies failed to find significant memory improvement with choline or lecithin supplementation in AD patients.[46,47]	Contains choline, the precursor to acetylcholine. Used to make phosphatidyl choline.
❑ **Vitamin B$_{12}$ and Folic acid**	Deficiency symptoms include depression and and dementia.	Methyl donors add metylmoities to monoamine neurotransmitters (dopamine and serotonin)
❑ **Acetyl-L-carnitine** (component of choline)	Improved cognitive function and memory in patients with age related dementia and slowed rate of deterioration in patients with AD.	Crosses the blood-brain barrier and produces cholinergic effects. Also increases cerebral blood flow.
❑ **Nonsteroidal anti-inflammatory drugs (NSAIDs)**	Slowed functional deterioration and cognitive impairment of AD patients. Reduced risk of developing AD.	Reduces inflammation in the brain due to the deposition of amyloid protein.

TABLE 8–27. HERBS USED TO TREAT HEADACHES

Active Herb, Source, Form, and Dosage	Therapeutic Effect Mechanism of Action	Side Effects; Drug Interactions; Cautions
❑ **Feverfew**		
Sesquiterpene lactones (parthenolide), and flavonoid glycosides. Dosage: 125 mg dried leaf preparation Containing at least 0.2% parthenolide.	Inhibits prostaglandin systhesis *in vitro*. Inhibits serotonin release from platelets; may produce an antimigraine effect in a manner similar to Sansert.	Rebound symptoms may occur after discontinuation. Side effects when chewed include mouth ulceration, inflammation of the oral mucosa and tongue, often with lip swelling and loss of taste. Long-term safety has not been established.
❑ **Peppermint oil**		
Oil obtained by steam distillation from freshly harvested, flowering sprigs (yields 0.1% to 1.0% of volatile oil composed primarily of menthol).	Applied externally for myalgia and neuralgia. Exhibits spasmolytic activity on smooth muscle.	When used topically, no known side effects or interactions with other drugs.

TABLE 8–28. HERBS USED TO TREAT CARDIOVASCULAR DISORDERS

Active Herb, Source, Form, and Dosage	Therapeutic Effect Mechanism of Action	Side Effects; Drug Interactions; Cautions
☐ **Garlic (Allium sativum)** Garlic bulbs, consisting of fresh or carefully dried bulbs, as well as its preparations in effective dosage. Garlic contains alliin, which is converted to allicin and other sulfur-containing compounds. Dose: 2–4 gm fresh garlic (1–2 cloves) or its equivalent in commercial product with daily intake of 10 mg alliin or total allicin potential of 4 mg, taken for at least 1–3 months.	Supportive to dietary measures which lower elevated levels of total and LDL cholesterol and for prevention of atherosclerosis. May help reduce systolic and diastolic blood pressure in patients with mild hypertension,* but effect is not adequate for specific antihypertensive therapy in patients with high blood pressure. Inhibits platelet aggregation by interfering with thromboxane synthesis; prolongs bleeding and clotting time; enhances fibrinolytic activity.	Side effects rare, but include GI symptoms, changes to flora of intestines, allergic reactions, and hypotensive circulatory reactions. May potentiate the effect of antihypertensive and anticoagulant medications. The odor of garlic may pervade the breath and skin.
☐ **Ginkgo biloba** Standardized extract from leaves contains24% flavone glycosides and 6% terpene lactones. Dose: 40 mg three times daily. Should be taken consistently for 12 weeks to be effective.	Supportive treatment for peripheral arterial disease. Protect against cardiac ischemia reperfusion injury, adjusts fibrinolytic activity, in combination with aspirin, treats thrombosis. Inhibits binding of platelet activating factor to membrane receptors.	Possible side effects include headache, dizziness, heart palpitations, GI and dermatologic reactions.
☐ **Guggul (Commiphora mukul)** Standardized extract known as Guggulipid contains 25 mg guggulsterones per gram. Dose: 500 mg for 12 weeks.	Appears to lower total and LDL cholesterol, and increase HDL. Stimulates thyroid-stimulating activity.	No significant adverse effects reported in clinical studies. If any symptoms: GI in nature.
☐ **Hawthorn leaf with flower** Leaf with flower, consisting of dried flowering twig tips. Main constituents are flavonoids, prodyanidins, catechins, and other compounds. Dose: 160–900 mg aqueous alcoholic extract with a designated content of flavonoids (4–30 mg) or oligomeric procyanidins (30–160 mg) per day, for at least 6 weeks.	Heart failure and coronary insufficiency, as described in functional Stage II of New York Heart Association†. Not Appropriate for more advanced stages. Improvement in cardiac performance during exercise. Peripheral vasodilator and positive inotropic agent (associated with lengthening of the refractory period) to stabilize heart rhythm.	Side effects mild, may include nausea and headache. Swelling of the lower extremities.
☐ **Digitalis (Digitalis purpurea)** Leaves and seeds of wild varieties contain at least 30 different cardiac glycosides including digoxin and digitoxin.	Used in treatment of CHF. Improves cardiac conduction, thereby improving the strength of cardiac contractility.	Narrow therapeutic margin and high potential for severe side effects.
☐ **Horse chestnut seed** Dry extract manufactured from seeds, adjusted to a content of 16–20% triterpene glycosides (calculated as anhydrous aescin) Dosage: 100 mg aescin corresponding to 250–300 mg extract 2×/day in delayed release form.	Chronic venous insufficiency (e.g., pain and a sensation of heaviness in the legs; swelling of the legs). Anti-exudative and vascular tightening effect by reducing vascular permeability.	Non-invasive treatment measures (e.g., leg compresses, support hose, or cold H_2O therapy) should be used Side effects may be pruritis, nausea, and gastric complaints.

*All of the blood pressure trials used the same dried powder preparation (Kwai), which has a standardized allicin content, in the dose range 600–900 mg daily. This is the equivalent of 1.8–2.7 gm/day fresh garlic. The median duration of therapy was 12 weeks.

†Stages I and II of NYHA refer to stages of heart disease in the New York Heart Association's 1994 Revisions to Classification of Functional Capacity and Objective Assessment of Patients with Disease of the Heart: Patients with cardiac disease but without resulting limitations of physical activity. They are comfortable at rest. Ordinary physical activity results in fatigue, palpitation, dyspnea, or anginal pain.

TABLE 8-29A.   HERBS USED TO TREAT IMMUNE AND RESPIRATORY SYSTEM DISORDERS

Active Herb, Source, Form, and Dosage	Therapeutic Effect Mechanism of Action	Side Effects; Drug Interactions; Cautions
❑ **Echinachea (E purpurea, E pallida)** Common name: cone flower 0.1R caffeic acid glycoside (echinacoside), and many other complex substances. No single compound appears to be responsible for plant's activity. Dose: 15–25 drops/day equivalent to 900 mg. Do not use for more than 8 weeks (Parenteral: no longer than 3 weeks).	Supportive treatment of recurrent infections of upper respiratory tract & lower urinary tract. Appears to shorten duration/ frequency of the common cold. Immune stimulant. Stimulates phagocytic activity, release of interleukin 1, tumor necrosis factors and interferon. Increases number of white blood cells and spleen cells. May elevate body temperature.	No known side effects. Contraindicated in patients with progressive systemic diseases, such as tuberculosis, leucosis, multiple sclerosis, collagen disorders, and other autoimmune diseases, or HIV. Metabolic condition in diabetes can decline upon parenteral application.
❑ **Ephedra (Ephedra sinica)** Common name: Ma Huang, Mormon tea, sea grape, yellow horse. Main alkaloid is ephedrine. Standard preparations have supplanted the use of the crude drug in most countries. Dosage: herb preparation corresponding to 0.5 mg total alkaloid per kg body weight. Maximum daily dosage: 300 mg total alkaloid, calculated as ephedrine. Should only be used short term (one week).	Clears up respiratory congestion, relaxes airways (bronchodilator) Stimulates the sympathomimetic and central nervous system.	Side effects: insomnia, motor restlessness, irritability, headaches, nausea, vomiting, disturbances of urination, tachycardia. In higher dosage: drastic increase in blood pressure, cardiac arrhythmia, can develop dependency. Contraindicated in anxiety and restlessness, high blood pressure, glaucoma, enlarged prostate. Do not use with cardiac glycosides, MAOIs, guanethidine.
❑ **Ginseng (Panax ginseng)** Common name: Korean ginseng Whole root used, contains triterpenoid saponin glycosides. Wide range of commercial products available. Proper dose & duration remain poorly defined. Dosage: 2–3 g standard in capsules.	Reported effective as an adaptogen: to increase physical, chemical, and biological stress, and to build up vitality.	Not usually associated with serious adverse effects. Common side effects: nervousness and excitation. Both side effects usually resolve after first few days of use. May also have hypoglycemic effect.
❑ **Eleuterococcus (Acanthopanax seticosus)** Common names: Siberian ginseng, devil's shrub, eleuthera, eleuthero, touch-me-not. Contains electherosides, glucose, sucrose, and a variety of dyestuffs. Leaves contain saponins normally found in ginseng roots. Dosage: 2–3 g/d limited to 3 months.	Immunomodulator. Increases absolute number of T cells. Used as a tonic to counteract fatigue & weakness, as a restorative for declining stamina and impaired concentration, and as an aid to convalescence.	Rare reported side effects have included slight languor or drowsiness immediately after taking. Contraindicated in hypertension.

TABLE 8–29B. HERBS USED TO TREAT IMMUNE AND RESPIRATORY SYSTEM DISORDERS: COUGH REMEDIES

Herb (Botanical Name)	Preparation
Antitussives (Cough Suppressants)	
Marshmallow root *(Althaeae officinalis)* and mallow leaf *(Malvae folium)*	• Consumed in form of tea, 1–2 tsp (5–10 g) in 150 ml water (daily dose: 6 g) Note: absorption of oral drugs taken simultaneously may be delayed
Iceland moss *(Lichen islandicus)*	• 1–2 % infusion (1–2 tsp/150 mL). Drink 1 cup 3× daily. Do not use in large quantities over extended period of time (can be toxic).
Mullein flowers *(Verbascum thapsus)*	• 3–4 tsp or 1.5–2 g used to prepare tea, drink several times/day
Plantain *(Plantago lanceolata)*	• Tea prepared from 2–3 g of herb and 150 ml water. Used also for inflammatory conditions of the oral cavity.
Slippery elm *(Ulmus rubra)*	• Lozenges most effective form
Expectorants	
Horehound *(Marrubium vulgare)*	• Tea prepared from 2 tsp cut herb steeped in one cup boiling water or hard candy used as a cough lozenge
Thyme *(Thymus vulgaris)*	• Tea prepared from 1 tsp herb per cup water, drink up to 3× daily; may be sweetened with honey, which also acts as a demulcent
Eucalyptus leaves *(Eucalyptus globulus)*	• Tea prepared from ½ tsp leaves in about 150 ml hot water, drink freshly prepared 3× daily. The volatile oil is commonly incorporated into a variety of nasal inhalers and sprays, balms and ointments for external application, and mouthwashes.
Licorice *(Glycyrrhiza glabra)*	• 1–2 g dried root taken 3× daily.
Senega snake-root *(Polygala senega)*	• Decoction prepared from 0.5 g and 1 cup water. Daily does should not exceed 3 g due to tendency to cause upset stomach, nausea, and diarrhea.

are local erythema, burning, stinging, which tends to diminish with repeated use.

Glucosamine and chondroitin sufate, two over-the-counter nutritional supplements, have become very popular. To date, there is no definitive study of glucosamine and chondroitin supplements, however, studies (especially using prescription levels) of these agents suggest efficacy in OA of the knee and hip when compared with traditional NSAID drug intervention.[85–87]

CONCLUSION

As physical and occupational therapists, we are highly involved in our patients' care and need to be involved as part of a team in their pharmacologic management. The therapist is often the first individual to identify a change in status. For example, increased confusion, complaints of fatigue, changes in muscle tone, slurred speech, and other side effects of medications, may initially be observed by the physical or occupational therapist during a period of exercise or increased exertion during training in activities of daily living. It is important for therapists to understand how a person's body handles a drug with advancing age. Drug regimens employed in the elderly will affect the older person's functional status and, in many cases, dictate their physiological responses to increased activity levels. This chapter has explored the medication management of many conditions in the elderly and discussed various areas of concern including changes in absorption, metabolism and excretion of drugs with age, polypharmacy, self-medication, and drug-induced malnutrition. It is particularly

important that rehabilitation professionals familiarize themselves with current drug regimes and gain a better understanding of how pharmacologic considerations may impact an elderly individual's functional outcomes in rehabilitation.

PEARLS

- Even though the elderly make up less than 12% of the population, they consume 30% of all prescription medications.
- The four stages of pharmacokinetics (absorption, distribution, biotransformation, and excretion) are all diminished with age, which will affect the impact of a medication when taken by an older person.
- The most common adverse reactions or side effects of drug use seen in the elderly are postural hypotension, fatigue, weakness, depression, confusion, movement disorders, incontinence, anticholinergic actions, dizziness, extrapyramidal signs, and volume depletion.
- Cardiovascular regimens revolve around controlling congestive heart failure, hypertension, angina pectoris, cardiac arrhythmias, and arteriosclerosis.
- Common neuromusculoskeletal regimens are designed to manage arthritis, osteoporosis, neuralgias, stroke, and Parkinson's disease.
- Psychological drug regimens can be used for adjustment, affective, organic brain, anxiety, schizophrenic, personality, and substance abuse disorders. The most important step in this area is proper diagnosis.

TABLE 8–30. HERBAL TREATMENTS FOR WOUNDS, SKIN, AND ORAL HEALTH

Active Constituents: Source, Form, Dosage	Therapeutic Action	Side Effects, Drug Interactions, Cautions
Echinacea (Echinacea angustifolia, E purpurea, E pallida) Common names: cone flower, black susans, comb flower, Kansas snakeroot, indian head		
Semi-solid preparation containing at least 15% pressed juice. Do not use more than 8 weeks	Used externally for poorly healing wounds and chronic ulcerations	No reported side effects or interactions
Gotu kola (Centella asiatica) Common names: hydrocotyle, Indian pennywort, talepetrako		
Contains active principle madecassol, asiatic acid, and glycoside asiaticoside	Promotes wound healing. Used in patients with surgical wounds, fistulas, and gynecological lesions. Helpful in treating psoriasis.	Contact dermatitis reported in some patients
Tea tree oil (Melaleuca alternifolia) Common names: desert essence, tea tree oil soap		
Essential oil obtained by steam distillation of leaves. Main constituent is terpin-4-ol (~ 30%)	Antimicrobial effects without irritating sensitive tissues. Effective against tinea pedia (athlete's foot) and acne Can be added to baths or vaporizers to help treat respiratory disorders	Use has resulted in allergic contact eczema and dermatitis Harmful if ingested
Aloe (Aloe vera, A. ferox) Common names: Cape, Zanzibar, Socotrine, Curacao, Barbados aloe, aloe vera		
Aloe gel is a clear, thin, gelatinous material obtained by crushing the mucilaginous cells found in inner tissue leaf. Contains the polysaccharide glucomannan	Minor burns and skin irritations Moisterizing effect, which prevents air from drying the wound Accelerates wound healing	Not associated with adverse reactions when used topically
Oil of evening primrose (Oenothera biennis) Common name: Efamol		
Rich in gamma-linolenic acid Available in capsule form. Maximum dose 4 g/day	Treats itching associated with atopic dermatitis and eczema	Mild GI upset, headache and nausea possible
Goldenseal (Hydrastis canadensis) Common names: eye balm, ground raspberry, Indian dye, jaundice root, orange root, tumeric root		
Contains hyrastine and berberine	Topically, as eye wash Astringent and weak antiseptic properties which is effective in treating oral problems	Small amounts of the plant can be ingested (as in tea) with no side effects. Large doses can be toxic Should not take during pregnancy
Myrrh (Commiphora molmol, C. abyssinica) Common names: African myrrh, myrrh, gum myrrh, bola, gal, bol, heerabol		
Oleo-gum-resin that contains from 1.5% to 17% of volatile oil. (40% commiphoric acid and 60% of gum yields a variety of sugars upon hydrolysis)	Mild astringent properties. May exert antimicrobial activity Helpful in treating canker sores Added to mouthwashes, used in fragrances, and as a food flavoring	Generally considered to be non-irritating, though several cases of dermatitis have been reported
Sage (Salvia officinalis) Common names: Garden sage, true sage, meadow sage, scarlet sage		
Contains 1–2.8% of a volatile oil	Topical use as an antiseptic and astringent Exerts antimicrobial activity against *taphySlococcus aureus*	Reports of cheilitis and stomatitis in some cases following ingestion of sage tea. Large amount may cause dry mouth or local irritation
Bloodroot (Sanguinaria cana densis) Common names: red root, red puccon, tetterwort, Indian red plant, Indian plant, sanguinaria		
Many isoquinoline derivatives, including Sanguinarine and berberine Contains a negatively charged ion that binds to dental plaque	In toothpastes and oral rinses to help reduce and limit deposition of dental plaque Effective against common oral bacteria	Should not be ingested, as it can induce CNS depression, and may also produce nausea and vomiting

TABLE 8-31. HERBAL TREATMENTS FOR GASTROINTESTINAL SYSTEM AND LIVER HEALTH

Active Constituents: Source, Form, Dosage	Therapeutic Action	Side Effects, Drug Interactions, Cautions
Gentian (Gentiana lutea) Common names: Stemless gentian, bitter root, pale gentian, gall weed Dried rhizome and roots, quickly dried. Approved for food use; usually consumes as tea prepared by gently boiling root in water	Used as bitter tonic to stimulate appetite and improve digestion May stimulate taste buds and increase flow of saliva and stomach secretions	May cause headache and gastric irritation, resulting in nausea and vomiting
Ginger (Zingiber officinale) Rhizome of plant. Contains volatile oil, which is responsible for characteristic aroma, and oleoresin Dose: 2–4 g/day	Possesses carminative, stimulant, diuretic and antiemetic properties Symptomatic relief in pregnant women suffering from hyperemesis gravidarum (250 mg, 4×/day)	No reports of toxicity Large overdoses carry potential for causing CNS depression and cardiac arrhythmias.
Chamomile (Matricaria chamomilla) Common names: German, Hungarian or genuine chamomile Flower head contains essential oil. Teas contain small amount of oil, but used over long periods of time, may have cumulative effect	Gastrointestinal antispasmodic	May cause contact dermatitis, anaphylaxis and other hypersensitivity reactions to persons allergic to ragweed, asters, and chrysanthemums May delay drug absorption from gut
Peppermint oil (Mentha x piperita) Complex chemistry; volatile oil composed primarily of menthol As a tea: cup of boiling water over 1 Tbs leaves (3–4 cups daily with meals)	Antispasmodic (carminitive) effects on smooth muscle Used in treatment of irritable bowel and abdominal pain	Persons with hiatal hernia may experience worsening of symptoms due to its relaxing effect on lower esophageal sphincter Do not use during pregnancy or in presence of gallstones
Turmeric root (Curcuma aromatica, C. domestica, C. longa) Common names: Tumeric, curcuma, Indian saffron Rhizome, contains volatile oil consisting of 60% sesquiterpene ketones known as turmerones Dosage: 1.5–3 g/day	Digestive aid Stimulated production of bile Possesses antihepatotoxic effects	No side effects reported Contradicted in obstruction of bile passages
Psyllium seen (Plantage psyllium) Common names: psyllium, Indian plantago seed, psyllium seed, flea seed, black psyllium Dried ripe seed, containing mucilages Dose: 7.5 g of seed of 1 tsp husks, mixed into 8 oz glass of water or juice (consumed quickly)	Chronic constipation; irritable bowel Acts as a bulk laxative. Mixed with water, produces a mucilaginous mass. Regulates intestinal peristalsis May lower cholesterol levels	Varying degrees of psyllium allergy including anaphylaxis, chest congestion, sneezing, and watery eyes Take with adequate fluid to avoid blockages May inhibit absorption of lithium and carbamazepine
Cascara (Rhamnus purshiana) Common names: Buckthorn, cascara sagrada, chittem bark, sacred bark Dried bark. Contains not less than 7% total hydroxyanthracene derivatives calculated as cascaroside A on a dried basis Available as ingredient in OTC laxatives. If using capsules of powdered bark, dose is 1 g.	Stimulant laxative, used for constipation Inhibits stationary and stimulating propulsive contractions in colon, resulting in accelerated intestinal passage, and reduction in liquid absorption	Reduce dosage if cramp-like discomfort Contraindicated in acute intestinal inflammation (e.g., Crohn's disease, colitis, abdominal pain of unknown origin), children under 12, and if pregnant or nursing

(continued)

TABLE 8-31. (CONTINUED)

Active Constituents: Source, Form, Dosage	Therapeutic Action	Side Effects, Drug Interactions, Cautions
Common names: senna leaf, black draught granules, Senokot Leaves contain anthraquinones and sennosides Should not be used over extended period of time (1–2 weeks) without medical advice Dose: 20–30 mg hydroanthracene derivatives daily, Calculated as sennoside B. Individually correct dosage is the smallest amount necessary to maintain a soft stool	Potent laxative effect Decreases intestinal transit time	Contradictions: same as Cascara above Aggravates loss of potassium if on diuretics. Cautions: chronic use may result in "laxative dependency syndrome" characterized by poor gastric motility in the absence of repeated axative administration.Abuse may result in diarrhea, altered electrolytes (which may enhance effectiveness of cardiac glycosides), cachexia, and reduced serum globulin levels May decrease absorption of oral medications
Aloe (Aloe vera, A ferox) Common names: Cape, Zanzibar, Socotrin, Curacao, Barbadoes aloe, aloe vera Anthraquinone glycosides aloin A and B Dose: 20–30 mg hydroanthracene derivatives daily, calculated as anhydrous aloin	Potent laxative, used for acute constipation	Contraindications and cautions: see above
Bilberry fruit (Vaccinium myrtillus) Common names: Bilberries, bog bilberries, blueberries (variety of), whortleberries Contains tannins, anthocyans, flavonoids, plant acids, inverted sugars and pectins, Must be dried to obtain tannins which come about by condensation of tannin precursors during drying process	Supportive treatment of acute nonspecific diarrhea	Effects of ingesting large doses unknown. No known side effects or interactions with other drugs
Licorice root (Glycyrrhiza glabra) Common names: licorice, Spanish or Russian licorice Dried rhizome and roots contain at least 4% triterpene glycoside. On hydrolysis, glycyrrhizin loses its sweet taste and is converted to glycyrrhetic acid	Treatment of peptic ulcers (but not as effective as cimetidine) Anti-inflammatory properties	Side effects include headache, lethargy, sodium and water retention (e.g., contraindicated in high blood pressure); excessive excretion of potassium. Potentiates toxicity to cardiac glycosides such as those in digitalis due to potassium loss in urine; should not be used with spironolactone or amiloride; or with corticoid treatment
Milk Thistle (Silybum marianum) Common names: Holy thistle, lady's thistle, marian thistle, Mary thistle, St. Mary thistle, silybum From fruits (seeds), 70% contains silymarin, a mixture of 4 isomers, including main constituent silybin (silibinin) Doses: 12-15 g; formulations equivalent to 200–400 mg silymarin, calculated as silybinin Poorly soluble in water, so aqueous preparations (e.g., teas) ineffective. Best administered parenterally or as a capsule containing concentrated extract due to poor absorption from GI tract	Dyspeptic complaints For supportive treatment in chronic inflammatory liver disease and hepatic cirrhosis. Also used in *Amanita phalloides* poisoning Alters structure of outer cell membrane of hepatocytes to prevent penetration of liver toxin into interior of cell and/or stimulates regenerative ability of the liver and formation of new hepatocytes Acts as an antioxidant	No known side effects or contraindications

- Gastrointestinal drugs are commonly used by the elderly; they have minimal side effects that may impair rehabilitation.
- Insulin is indicated as initial therapy in patients who have Type II diabetes with a markedly elevated fasting plasma glucose level (>280 to 300 mg/dL); in patients with ketonuria or ketonemia; and in symptomatic (neuropathies, retinopathies, etc.) patients.
- Pharmacologic therapy of incontinence in older adults can be quite helpful, especially when combined with behavioral interventions.
- Drugs used against cancer are classified by their chemical structure, source, or mechanism of action.
- The first line of drug intervention in COPD is the use of bronchodilators, which are inhaled anticholinergics and β₂-agonists.
- Multiple pharmacotherapeutic approaches are used in the treatment of dementias including antidepressants, anxiolytics, sedatives, and cognitive enhancers.
- Compliance and motivation for using drugs appropriately by the aged can be enhanced by initially assessing the economic and physical decrements of the person and then providing clear and simple instructions.
- The elderly are the major users and abusers of both OTC and prescription drugs.
- Aside from secondary side effects of drugs that include depressed appetite, nausea, vomiting, and diarrhea, drugs have direct effects on the metabolism of nutrients, thereby placing older persons at risk for malnutrition.
- A *nutraceutical* agent is any substance that may be considered a food or part of a food which provides medical or health benefits, including the prevention and treatment of disease.
- Phytomedicines are medicinal products that contain plant materials as their pharmacologically active component.
- Herbs are not considered "drugs" in the United States; however, they can be classified as drugs from a medical perspective as many provoke a pharmacologic response from a physiological perspective.

REFERENCES

1. Hanlon JT, Schmader KE, Koronkowski MJ, Weingerger M, Landsman PB, Samsa GP, Lewis, IK. Adverse drug events in high risk older populations. *J Amer Geriatr Soc.* 1997; 45(8):945–958.
2. Yee B, Williams B, O'Hara N. Medication management and appropriate substance use for elderly persons. In Lewis, ed. *Aging: Health Care's Challenge,* 2nd edition. Philadelphia: F.A. Davis; 1990: 298–330.
3. Gupta S, Rappaport HM, Bennett LT. Polypharmacy among nursing home geriatric Medicaid recipients. *Ann Pharmacother.* 1996; 30(8):946–950.
4. Krammer P. Influences of aging in drug disposition and response. *Top Geriatr Rehabil.* 1987; 2(3): 12–23.
5. White D, Lewis C. The older patient and the effects of drugs on rehabilitation. In: Malone T, ed. *Physical and Occupational Therapy: Drug Implications of Practice.* Philadelphia: JB Lippincott; 1989: 144–182.
6. Ciccone CD. *Pharmacology in Rehabilitation.* 2nd edition. Philadelphia, PA: F.A. Davis; 1996: 15–31.
7. Myers-Robfogel MW, Bosmann HB. Clinical pharmacology in the aged—aspects of pharmacokinetics and drug sensitivity. In: Williams TF, ed. *Rehabilitation in the Aging.* New York: Raven Press; 1984: 23–40.
8. Robertson D. Drug handling in old age. In: Brocklehurst JC, ed. *Geriatric Pharmacology and Therapeutics.* Boston: Blackwell Scientific Publications; 1984:41–59.
9. Woo E. Drug treatment of the elderly. In: Walshe TM, ed. *Manual of Clinical Problems in Geriatric Medicine.* Boston: Little, Brown; 1985:21–26.
10. Stevenson IH. Pharmacokinetics in advancing age. In: Barbagallo-Sangiorgi G, Exton-Smith AN, eds. *Aging and Drug Therapy.* New York: Plenum Press; 1984:1–9.
11. Lamy PP: Comparative pharmacokinetics changes and drug therapy in an older population. *J Am Geriatr Soc.* 1982; 30:S11–S19.
12. Swanger AK, Burbank PM. *Drug Therapy and the Elderly.* Boston: Jones & Bartlett Pubs. 1995.
13. Stewart RB, Cooper JW. Polypharmacy in the aged. Practical solutions. *Drugs & Aging.* 1994; 4(6):449–461.
14. Rizack M, Gardner D. The Medical Letter drug interaction program. *Med Letter.* 1998; 40(9):1–4.
15. Atkin PA, Shenfield GM. Medications-related adverse reactions and the elderly: a literature review. *Adverse Drug React Toxicol Rev.* 1995; 14(2): 175–191.
16. Chapron D, Besdine RW. Drugs as an obstacle to rehabilitation of the elderly: A primer for therapists. *Top Geriatr Rehabil.* 1987; 2(3): 63–81.
17. Davis KM, Minaker KL. Disorders of fluid balance: Dehydration and hyponatremia. In: Hazzard WR, Blass JP, Ettinger WH, Halter JB, Ouslander JG, eds. *Principles of Geriatric Medicine and Gerontology.* 4th edition. New York: McGraw-Hill. 1999; 1429–1441.
18. Mentes J, Adkins J, Culp K, et al. *Hydration Management Research-Based Protocol.* Iowa City, IA: University of Iowa Gerontological Nursing Interventions Research Center; 1998.
19. American Psychiatric Association. Practice guidelines for the treatment of patients with Alzheimer's disease and other dementias of late life. *Amer J Psychiatry.* 1997; 154(suppl 5):1–39.
20. Catterson ML, Preskorn SH, Martin RL. Pharmacodynamic and pharmacokinetic considerations in geriatric psychopharmacology. *Psychiatr Clin North Am.* 1997; 20(2):205–218.

21. Chapron DJ. Clinical pharmacology in the elderly: Recognizing and preventing of adverse drug effects during rehabilitation. In: Jackson O ed. *Physical Therapy of the Geriatric Patient,* 2nd ed. New York: Churchill Livingston; 1989:145–173.

22. Ciccone CD. Current trends in cardiovascular pharmacology. *Phys Ther.* 1996; 76(3):481–497.

23. WHO Expert Committee. Arterial hypertension. Technical Report, Series 628. Geneva: World Health Organization; 1978.

24. Kannel W, Gordon T. *The Framingham Study: An Epidemiological Investigation of Cardiovascular Disease,* Washington, D.C.: U.S. Government Printing Office; 1970.

25. Wolfe F, Zhao S, Lane N. Preference for nonsteroidal antiinflammatory drugs over acetminophen by rheumatic disease patients: A survey of 1,799 patients with osteoarthritis, rheumatoid arthritis, and fibromyalgia. *Arthritis & Rheumatism.* 2000; 43(2): 378–385.

26. Singh G, Triadafilopoulos G. Epidemiology of NSAID induced gastrointestinal complications. Review. *J Rheumatol.* 1999; 26(56) [suppl]:18–24.

27. Glennas A, Kvien RK, Andrup O, Clarke-Jenssen O, Karstensen B, Brodin U. Auranofin is safe and superior to placebo in elderly-onset rheumatoid arthritis. *Br J Rheumatol.* 1997; 36:870–877.

28. Porter DR, Sturrock RD. Fortnightly review: Medical management of rheumatic arthritis. *B MJ.* 1993; 307(4):425–429.

29. Leventhal LJ, Boyce EG, Zurier RB. Treatment of rheumatoid arthritis with gammalinolenic acid. *Ann Intern Med.* 1993; 119:867–869.

30. Girolomoni G, Abeni D. Anti-tumor necrosis factor alpha therapy in psoriatic arthritis and psoriasis. *Arch Dermatol.* 2001; 137(6):784–785.

31. Kassiotis G, Kollias G. TNF and receptors in organ-specific autoimmune disease: multi-layered functioning mirrored in animal models. *J Clin Invest.* 2001; 107(12):1507–1508.

32. Smith JR, Levinson RD, Holland GN, et al. Differential efficacy of tumor necrosis factor inhibition in the management of inflammatory eye disease and associated rheumatic disease. *Arthritis Rheum.* 2001; 45(3):252–257.

33. Schussheim DH, Siris ES. Osteoporosis: Update on prevention and treatment. *Women's Health in Primary Care.* 1998; 1(2):133–140.

34. Demissie S, Silliman RA, Lash TL. Adjuvant tamoxifen: predictors of use, side effects, and discontinuation in older women. *J Clin Oncol.* 2001; 19(2): 322–328.

35. Rubin CD. Treatment considerations in the management of age-related osteoporosis. *Am J Med Sci.* 1999; 318(3):158–170.

36. Piper BA, Galsworthy TD, Bockman RS. Diagnosis and management of osteoporosis. *Contemp Int Med.* 1995; 7(7):61–68.

37. Chapron DJ. Drug-drug interactions in the elderly: A potential consequence of polypharmacy. *Top Geriatr Rehab.* 1987; 2(3):5–12.

38. Aminoff MJ. Pharmacologic management of parkinsonism and other movement disorders. In: Katzung BG, ed. *Basic and Clinical Parmacology*, 5th edition. Norwalk, CT: Appleton & Lange Publishers; 1992.

39. Peura D, Freston J. Introduction evolving perspectives on parenteral H$_2$ receptor antagonist therapy. *Am J Med.* 1987; 18:1–2(suppl 6a).

40. American Diabetes Association. Report of the expert committee on the diagnosis and the classification of diabetes mellitus. *Diabetes Care.* 1998; 21(suppl 1):S5-S19.

41. DeFranzo RA. Pharmacology therapy for type 2 diabetes mellitus. *Ann Int Med.* 1999; 131(4): 281–303.

42. Smith DA, Ouslander JG. Pharmacologic management of urinary incontinence in older adults. *Top Geriatr Rehabil.* 2000; 16(1):54–60.

43. Redmond K, Aapro MS. *Cancer in the Elderly: A Nursing and Medical Perspective.* Oxford, England: Elsevier Science Ltd.; 1997.

44. Cova D, Beretta G, Balducci L. Cancer chemotherapy in the older patient. In: Balducci L, Lyman GH, Ershler W, eds. *Comprehensive Geriatric Oncology.* Harwood Academic Publishers. 1998:429–442.

45. Adair N. Chronic airflow and respiratory failure. In: Hazzard WR, Blass JP, Ettinger RL, Halter JB, Ouslander JG (eds). *Principles of Geriatric Medicine and Gerontology.* 4th edition. New York: McGraw-Hill; 1999:745–755.

46. Dow JA, Mest CG. Psychosocial interventions for patients with chronic obstructive pulmonary disease. *Home Healthcare Nurse.* 1997; 15(6): 414–420.

47. Francis PT, Palmer AM, Snape M, Wilcock GK. The cholinergic hypothesis of Alzheimer's disease: A review of progress. *J Neurol, Neurosurg & Psych.* 1999; 66(2):137–147.

48. Wheatley D, Smith D. *Psychopharmacology of Cognitive and Psychiatric Disorders in the Elderly.* London: Chapman and Hall. 1998.

49. Felician O, Sandson TA. The neurobiology and pharmacotherapy of Alzheimer's disease. *J Neuropsych & Clin Neurosciences.* 1999; 11(1): 19–31.

50. Kleijnen J, Knipschild P. Ginkgo biloba for cerebral insufficiency. *Br J Clin Pharmacol.* 1992; 34: 352–358.

51. Reuter HD. Ginkgo biloba—botany, constituents, pharmacology, and clinical trials. *Br J Phycother.* 1997; 4:3–20.

52. LeBars PL. A placebo-controlled, double-blind, randomized trail of an extract of gingko for dementia. *JAMA.* 1997; 278:1327–1332.

53. Paris D, Town T, Parker TA, Tan J, Humphrey J, Crawford F, Mullan M. Inhibition of Alzheimer's beta-amyloid induced vasoactivity and proinflammatory response in microglia by a cGMP-dependent mechanism. *Experimental Neurol.* 1999; 157(1): 211–221.

54. Kato A, Fukunari A, Sakai Y, Nakajima T. Prevention of amyloid-like deposition by a selective prolyl endopeptidase inhibitor, Y-29794, in senescence-accelerated mouse. *J Pharmacol & Experimental Therapeutics.* 1997; 283(1): 328–335.

55. Fuchinetti N. Adherence by patients to prescribed therapies: A social psychotic perspective. *Top Geriatr Rehabil.* 1987; 2(3):33–45.

56. Becker MH. Patient adherence to prescribed therapies. *Med Care.* 1985; 23:539–555.

57. Roe DA: Therapeutic effects of drug-nutrient interactions in the elderly. *J Amer Diet Assoc.* 1985; 85: 174–178.

58. Simons LA, Tett S, Simons J. Multiple medication use in the elderly: Use of prescription and nonprescription drugs in a community setting. *Med J of Australia.* 1992; 157:242–246.

59. Parkes AJ, Cooper LC. Inappropriate use of medications in the veteran community: How do doctors and pharmacists contribute? *Australian & New Zealand J Pub Health.* 1997; 21(5):469–476.

60. Smith CH, Bidlack WR: Dietary concerns associated with the use of medications. *J Amer Diet Assoc.* 1984; 84:901–908.

61. Kratz AM. Nutraceuticals: new opportunities for pharmacists. *JAMA.* 1998; 1:27–28.

62. Hasler C. Functional foods for health: the nation's first academic nutraceutical research program. *JANA.* 1998; 1:29.

63. Hasler C. Functional foods: the western perspective. *Nutr Rev.* 1996; 54: S33–37.

64. Bartels CL, Miller SJ. Herbal and related remedies. *Nutr in Clin Pract.* 1998; 12:5–19.

65. Vann A. The herbal boon: understanding what patients are taking. *Cleveland Clin J Med.* 1998; 65: 129–132,

66. Garfinkel D. Improvement of sleep quality in elderly people by controlled release of melatonin. *Lancet.* 1995; 346:541–544.

67. Lamberg L. Melatonin potentially useful but safety, efficacy remain uncertain. *JAMA.* 1996; 276: 1011–1014.

68. Wyatt RJ. Effects of 5-hydroxytryptophan on the sleep of normal human subjects. *Electroencep and Clin Neurop.* 1971; 30:505–509.

69. 5-Hydroxytryptophan. *Monograph.* www.thorne. com, 1999. www.thorne.com/altmedrev/monograph. html

70. Heiligenstein E, Guenther G. Over-the-counter psychotropics: a review of melatonin, St. John's wort, valerian, and kava-kava. *J Am Coll Health.* 1998; 46:271–276.

71. Miller AL. St. John's wort (Hypericum perforatum): clinical effects on depression and other conditions. *Alt Med Rev.* 1998; 3:18–26.

72. NIH News Release. St. John's wort study launched. http://www.nih.gov, 1999. http:/nccam.nih.gov/fcp /stjohnswort

73. Clay A, Reichert R. Kava-kava in modern drug research: portrait of a medicinal plant. *Quart Rev Nat Med.* 1996; 4:259–274.

74. King AC. Effects of differing intensities and formats of 12 months of exercise training on psychological outcomes in older adults. *Health Psychol.* 1993; 12:292–300.

75. Birge SJ. Hormones and the aging brain. *Geriatrics.* 1998; 53:S28–S30.

76. Knopman DS. Current pharmacotherapies for Alzheimer's disease. *Geriatrics.* 1998; 53:S31–34.

77. Foster NL. An enriched-population double-blind, placebo controlled, crossover study of tacrine and lecithine in Alzheimer's disease. *Dementia.* 1996; 7:260–266.

78. Kidd PM. Phosphatidylserine: membrane nutrient for memory: A clinical and mechanistic assessment. *Alt Med Rev.* 1996; 1:70–84.

79. Koppal T. Vitamin E protects against Alzheimer's amyloid peptide (25–35)-induced changes in neocortical synaptosomal membrane lipid structure and composition. *Brain Res.* 1998; 786:270–273.

80. Meydani SN. Assessment of the safety of supplementation with different amounts of vitamin E in healthy older adults. *Am J Cln Nutr.* 1998; 68: 311–318.

81. Perrig WJ. The relation between antioxidants and memory performance in the old and very old. *J Am Geriatr Soc.* 1997; 45:718–724.

82. Merikangas KR. Tyramine conjugation deficit in migraine, tension-type headache and depression. *Biol Psych.* 1995; 38:730–736,

83. Sun AY, Cirigliano MD. Internist's guide to herbal treatments. *Int Med.* 1998; 19:43–54.

84. Berman BM, Singh BB, Lao L, et al. A randomized trial of acupuncture as an adjunctive therapy in osteoarthritis of the knee. *Rheumatology.* 1999; 38(4): 346–354.

85. McAlindon TE, LaValley MP, Gulin JP, et al. Glucosamine and chondroitin for treatment of osteoarthritis: a systematic quality assessment and meta-analysis. *JAMA.* 2000; 283(11):1469–1475

86. Deal CL, Moskowitz RW. Nutraceuticals as therapeutic agents in osteoarthritis. The role of glucosamine, chondroitin sulfate, and collagen hydrolysate. *Rheum Dis Clin North Am.* 1999; 25(2): 379–395.

87. Kelly GS. The role of glucosamine sulfate and chondroitin sulfates in the treatment of degenerative joint disease. *Alt Med Rev.* 1998; 3(1):27–39.

CHAPTER 9

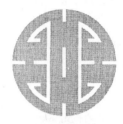

Principles and Practice
of Geriatric Rehabilitation

Normal aging is not necessarily burdened with disability; however, almost all conditions that cause disability are more frequently seen in the older population. As a result, the aged are more likely to require assessment for rehabilitative services. The mutual exclusion of geriatrics and rehabilitation is unjustified and functional assessment for needed rehabilitative services should be an essential part of routine evaluation by all health care disciplines working with the aged population. Geriatrics teaches that maximal functional capabilities be attained; therefore, it can be argued that rehabilitation is the foundation of geriatric care. The purpose of this chapter is to provide clinicians with knowledge of rehabilitation principles and practices in working with the aged individual and to help them apply interventions to provide high quality care.

The basis of geriatric rehabilitation is to assist the disabled aged in recovering lost physical, psychological, or social skills so that they may become more independent, live in personally satisfying environments, and maintain meaningful social interactions. This may be done in any number of settings including acute and subacute care settings, rehabilitation centers, home and office settings, or in long-term care facilities such as nursing homes.

Because of the complexity of the interventions needed in dealing with the aged, an interdisciplinary team approach is required. The rehabilitation process also requires that patients and their families be educated. Finally, rehabilitation is more than a medical intervention: it is a philosophical approach that recognizes that diagnoses and chronological age are poor predictors of functional abilities, that interventions directed at enhancing function are important, and that the "team" should always include patients and their families.

DISABILITY: A DEFINITION

The meaning of disability is key to an understanding of rehabilitation. When referring to alterations in an individual's function, three terms are often used interchangeably: impairment, disability, and handicap. A more distinct understanding of these concepts is useful in geriatric rehabilitation, and a "systems approach" is most useful. In the systems approach, a problem at the organ level (e.g., an infarct in the right hemisphere) must be viewed not only in terms of its effects on the brain, but also its effects on the person, the family, the society, and, ultimately, the nation. It goes beyond the pure "medical model," in which only the current medical problem is assessed to determine rehabilitative goals. From this perspective "impairment" refers to a loss of physical or physiologic function at the organ level. This could include alterations in heart function, nerve conduction velocity or muscle strength. Impairments usually do not affect the ability to function. However, if impairment is so severe that it inhibits the ability to function "normally," then it becomes a "disability." Rehabilitation interventions are most often oriented toward adaptation to or recovery from disabilities. Given the proper training or adaptive equipment, people with disabilities can pursue independent lives. Obstructions in the pursuit of independence can arise, however, when people with disabilities confront inaccessible buildings or situations that limit rehabilitation interventions, such as low toilet seats, buttons on an elevator that are too high, or signs that are not legible. In these cases a disability becomes a "handicap." Society's environment creates the handicap.

In this chapter we will be primarily concerned with rehabilitative approaches employed to reduce disabilities.

DEMOGRAPHICS OF DISABILITY IN THE ELDERLY

The elderly are disproportionately affected by disabling conditions when compared with younger cohorts. According to Wedgewood,[1] the old-old age group (85 plus years of age) comprises the highest percentage of disabled persons; indeed, 40% of all disabled persons are over the age of 65. Three-fourths of all cerebrovascular accidents occur in persons over the age of 65;[2,3,4] the highest incidence of amputations has been reported in the aged;[5,6] and hip fractures occur most frequently between the ages of 70 to 78, on average.[6,7] The Federal Council on Aging has reported that, of all those persons studied over the age of 65, 86% have at least one chronic condition, and 52% have limitations in their activities of daily living (ADLs).[8] It is the impact of these disabilities on the level of independence that needs to be considered, rather than the presence of an impairment or disability.

Disabilities in old age are associated with a higher mortality rate, a decreased life span, greater chronic health problems (e.g., cardiovascular, musculoskeletal, or neurological) and an increased expenditure for health care. Disabilities resulting in an inability to ambulate, feed oneself, or manage basic ADLs, such as toileting or self-hygiene (e.g., bathing), are very strong predictors of loss of functional independence and an increased burden on caregivers.[9] The greater the disability, the greater the risk of institutionalization. Rehabilitative measures can be cost-effective when they enhance the patient's functional ability and help him or her attain greater levels of independence. Higher functional capabilities and greater levels of independence have been associated with fewer hospitalizations and a lower mortality rate among the aged.[10,11,12]

Geriatric rehabilitation includes both institutional and noninstitutional services for aged with chronic medical conditions that are marked by deviation from the normal state of health and manifested in physical impairment. Unless treated, these conditions have the potential for causing substantial, and frequently cumulative, disability. The aged with disabilities need assistance with such daily functions as bathing, dressing, and walking. This increased need for help is often compounded when there is no spouse, nearby family, or friends able to assist the patient. With this social isolation, which is common in the elderly, continuing professional medical care is required to ward off the debilitating effects of inactivity and depression.

It is difficult for 32% of people over the age of 75 who live at home to climb ten steps; 40% have difficulty walking a mile; and 22% are unable to lift ten pounds. These percentages translate into millions of older people with some limitation in ADLs.[12,13] While dramatic gains have been made; we need to seek ways to prevent frailty and to help the frail elderly cope with ADLs. The impact of frailty is enormous in terms of costs of care in long-term care settings. Disability in the elderly is not inevitable. In fact, disability rates fell during the 1980s, according to the National Institute on Aging's National Long-Term Care Survey.[13] While the general population of people aged 65 and older grew by 14.7% between 1982 and 1989, the number of people with chronic disabilities or in nursing homes increased by 9.2%. This means that the proportion of people with disabilities fell, and there were hundreds of thousands fewer people with disabilities than expected.[14] Figure 9–1 provides a graphic representation of the number of projected and the number of actual chronically disabled persons aged 65 and over.

FRAILTY: MEDICALLY COMPLEX ELDERLY

Though it is difficult to concisely define the term frailty, the concept of frailty is well understood in geriatric rehabilitation. The use of the word "frail" conjures up a clear mental image for most clinicians. Compromises in cognition, sensorimotor input and integration,[15] polypharmacy, dehydration, and malnutrition are components of frailty. Decline in muscle strength and mass,[16] respiratory reserve and cardiovascular functioning, kyphotic postural changes, poorer eyesight, poor hydration and marginal nutritional intake, and many other physiological and physical changes associated with inactivity and aging, lead to frailty. Any of these conditions, in isolation or in combination, can create frailty. The presence of multidiagnostic situations in the elderly leads to multiple drug and nutrient interactions and complex medical management with the resulting side effects of progressive loss in functional reserve and

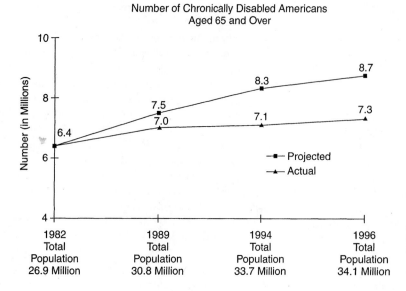

Figure 9–1. *Number of Chronically Disabled Older Americans. (Created from data: Manton KG, Corder L, Stallard E. Chronic disability trends in elderly United States populations: 1982–1994. Proc Natl Acad Sci USA. 1997; 94:2593–2598.)*

physiological homeostasis. Concomitant diseases such as congestive heart failure, renal disease, osteoporosis, diabetes, chronic lung disease, and arthritis (to name a few), add to the level of frailty.

Impaired physical functioning has been documented in one-third of older hospitalized patients.[17] With any admission for acute illnesses or injury in an older person, there is significant short-term deterioration in mobility and other functional domains.[18] Decline in physical function, while a negative outcome in itself, has also been associated with a number of adverse consequences such as falls, disability, and mortality.[12,18,19]

Functional dependence develops in approximately 10% of nondisabled community-dwelling persons over the age of 75 each year.[12] Increasing levels of disability are associated with substantial mortality leading to the adverse outcomes of hospitalization, nursing home placement, and greater use of home care services.[19] It is estimated that it costs $9,600 for each disabled, community-living older person annually and at least 15 billion dollars is spent each year on long-term care.[14,20] Functional dependence leads to increasing levels of frailty, especially in the medically complex, multisystem-involved elder. With each medical insult and hospitalization, there is a decreasing level of physiologic capacity associated with difficulty in recovery to premorbid functional abilities.[20,21] Movement of frail older people through the health care system is relevant for clinicians. Cost-containment strategies that encourage providers to substitute less costly care in the community for the more expensive care in hospitals and nursing homes may have implications for the patient's functioning, ability to remain at home, or other treatment outcomes.[19,21] An understanding of this issue is essential to assure that frail older patients receive the services they need and are treated appropriately.

Mrs. K, 78 years of age, who lived alone and independently, became frail because of the complacency of preventive and medical interventions and because of the limitations in the reimbursement system. Diagnosed with worsening arthritis and osteoporosis, she fell and broke her hip. Following surgery, rehabilitation was only partially successful when she was discharged from this service due to lack of insurance coverage, and sent home. After a second fall, she entered a nursing home and became depressed. Antidepressant drugs made her lightheaded and dizzy. She fell again, breaking her other hip. She was unable to participate in rehabilitation due to confusion and medical complications, and she became bedridden. Unfortunately, this is not an atypical rehabilitation scenario. Mrs. K's progressive frailty might have been prevented or reversed at several points. One such point might have been from a preventive perspective, before she developed osteoporosis, which can be prevented or at least alleviated through exercise, nutrition, and in some cases, hormone replacement therapy. Mrs. K's first fall could have been prevented with simple and practical measures, such as muscle-strengthening exercises, balance training, protective ambulatory devices, and environmental assessment and modification for safety.

FUNCTIONAL ASSESSMENT OF THE ELDERLY

The assessment of functional capabilities is the cornerstone of geriatric rehabilitation. The ability to walk, to transfer (e.g., from bed to chair or chair to toilet), and manage basic ADLs independently is often the determinant of whether hospitalized aged patients will be discharged home or to an extended-care facility. Functional assessment tools, which are practical, reliable, and valid, are necessary to assist all interdisciplinary team members in determining the need for rehabilitation or long-term care services. In the home care setting, precise assessment of a patient's function can detect early deterioration and allow for immediate intervention.

In response to the growing importance of chronic diseases and need for long-term care, the Commission on Chronic Illness was established in 1949.[22] The Commission highlighted the importance of function and disability, and concluded that there was a need for a means of classifying functional ADLs.[23]

Since that time functional assessment tools have gone through many evolutional stages. Early in this evolution, scales included such variables as locomotion and traveling, dressing, toileting, eating, and hand activities such as managing coins or knitting.[24] Some assessment tools addressed bowel and bladder function,[25] while others had measures for muscle strength, overall functional capacity, communication and behavior.

From these early efforts, a series of more sophisticated methodological scales were developed under the direction and sponsorship of the National Institute on Aging, the Administration on Aging, and the National Center for Health Services Research. These studies were concerned with reliability, validity, and usefulness of the various tools proposed. Among those who helped to clarify the theoretical framework for functional assessment, Lawton proposed a behavioral model in which function is viewed within a hierarchy of domains.[27] Each domain includes a set of functions that can be ordered along a continuum from simple to complex activities. For example, the simple task might be picking up the telephone receiver, while the more complex task would be picking up the telephone receiver, and dialing a number. This model revealed the component ADLs covering more than one domain of self-maintenance functions within a broader set of functions. For instance, Lawton included mobility and ambulation (or locomotion) as basic self-maintenance functions that enabled an aged individual to adjust and adapt within their environment. For example, the ability to ambulate one block and ascend and descend stairs four stairs would enable the aged person to walk to the bus stop and board a bus.

Lawton's conception of functional capacity defined three levels of ADLs: (1) basic ADLs, including such self-care activities as bathing, dressing, toileting, continence, and feeding; (2) instrumental activities of daily living (IADL), such as using the telephone, driving, shopping, housekeeping, cooking, laundry, managing money, and managing medications; (3) mobility, described as a more complicated combination of IADL activities, such as leaving one's residence and moving from one location to another by using public transportation. Mobility and IADL are more complex and are concerned with people's ability to cope with their environments.[26,27] This classification of ADL, IADL, and mobility has become standard in most functional assessment tools.

As a clinical tool, functional assessment scales are invaluable. Initial assessment identifies areas of functional deficit and can assist clinicians in developing treatment regimens that address specific needs. Subsequent assessments measure progress towards rehabilitation goals. On a broad scale, functional assessment can assist public policy makers in the provision of health care services by determining the levels of need in a population. Demographically, it is apparent that Americans are living longer; the question is, are these added years of life years of vigor and independence or years of frailty and dependence?

By design, functional assessment scales are meant to determine specific outcomes. Outcomes of interest to those working with the aged include mortality, hospitalization, institutionalization, special interventions, and declining physical function, to name a few. Numerous functional assessment tools are available to determine physical, emotional, cognitive, and social functioning in various care settings. Table 6–5 summarizes a number of ADL and IADL scales and indexes, including those summarized by Branch and Meyers.[28] Though this table of functional assessment tools is not exhaustive, it represents a relatively comprehensive reference list of currently used scales. In reviewing this list, the reader will notice some tools include only basic ADL skills (more useful in the institutional setting), while others are comprehensive and include all three levels of functioning defined by Lawton (more useful in discharge planning and the home care setting).

FUNCTIONAL ABILITIES OF THE CAREGIVER: A REHABILITATIVE CONSIDERATION

Aged patients, given a choice, would prefer to stay at home rather than recuperate and rehabilitate in an institutional setting. The elderly have strong ties to their homes, and the help of their spouses, other relatives, and friends is a crucial component in making rehabilitation in their homes possible. Home care by professionals can protect the health of informal caregivers and maximize the patient's ability to perform ADLs by including a systematic assessment of the living environment as a key part of care planning. Provision of such assistance openly acknowledges that caregivers (often aged themselves) have some decrease in physical ability which needs to be considered as it relates to caring for disabled relatives. It has been demonstrated that more than 90% of persons 75 to 84 years of age can manage, without help, to perform such tasks as grooming, bathing, dressing, and eating.[29] The more complicated skills of transferring and ambulation are more compromised, with more than 50% of persons aged 75 to 84 years of age presenting with limitations in their capabilities of performing these activities without assistance. These ADLs require greater assistive skills on the part of the caregiver. Assessment of the home environment needs to incorporate the abilities (or disabilities) of the individual(s) providing care. Adaptive equipment, such as a sliding board for transfers or a rolling walker for ambulation, are available to assist the caregiver in caring for his or her spouse, relative, or friend. Attention to the abilities of the caregiver can facilitate the ease of care and decrease the burden placed on the caregiver. The provision of home health care services may be necessitated when safety is an issue. Thorough evaluation of the functional capabilities of the aged individual and the caregiver, in addition to assessment of the environmental obstacles that may be encountered, will increase the likelihood of a positive outcome.

PRINCIPLES OF GERIATRIC REHABILITATION

Three major principles are important in the rehabilitation of the aged. First, the variability of the aged must be considered. Variability of capabilities within an aged group is much more pronounced than within younger cohorts. What one 80-year-old can do physically, cognitively, or motivationally, another may not be able to accomplish. Second, the concept of activity is key in rehabilitation of the aged. Many of the changes over time are attributable to disuse. Finally, optimum health is directly related to optimum functional ability. In acute situations, rehabilitation must be directed toward (1) stabilizing the primary problem(s); (2) preventing secondary complications such as bedsores, pneumonias, and contractures; and (3) restoring lost functions. In chronic situations, rehabilitation is directed primarily toward restoring lost functions. This can best be accomplished by promoting maximum health so that the aged are best able to adapt to their care environment and to their disabilities. Each of these principles—variability, inactivity, and optimum health—will be discussed in greater detail in the following sections.

Variability of the Elderly

Unlike any other age group, the aged are more variable in their level of functional capabilities. In the clinic, we often see 65-year-old individuals who are severely physically disabled, yet, sitting right alongside of that individual is a 65-year-old who is still building houses and felling trees. Even in the old-old, variability in physical and cognitive functioning is

remarkable. For example, at one end of the spectrum is John Kelly who, at the age of 87, was still running the Boston Marathon, while at the other end of the spectrum is a frail bedridden 87-year-old person in a nursing home who is not responsive to his or her environment. The differences can also be identified cognitively, and are just as remarkable. The spectrum moves from the demented, institutionalized aged to those aged who are presidents and Supreme Court justices. Chronological age is a poor indicator of physical or cognitive function.

The impact of this variability is an important consideration in defining rehabilitation principles and practices of the aged. A wide range of rehabilitative services must be provided to address the varying needs of the aged population in different care settings. Awareness of this heterogeneity helps to combat the myths and stereotypes of aging and presents a foundation for developing creative rehabilitation programs for the aged. Older persons tend to be more different from themselves (as a collective group) than other segments of the population. Given this fact, interdisciplinary team members, policy makers, and planners in rehabilitation settings need to be prepared to design a wide range of services and treatment interventions. This becomes more difficult as the number of aged increase and the budget decreases, however, creating new and innovative rehabilitation programs could ultimately improve the functional capabilities and the resulting quality of life for many aged individuals.

Examples of Variability in Aging

Reaction time is one concept of variability to be considered in the aged patient. In general, reaction time tends to slow with age,[30] but this is not necessarily a decline in functioning of the nervous system. Such an assumption may result in inaccuracies such as decreasing the amount and intensity of exercise and rehabilitative measures that older persons require. Research indicates that those aged who are more physically active are capable of performing as well as, and in some cases better than, younger subjects on reaction time performance tasks.[31] Reaction time is a complex variable that may be affected by disease or social stigma. For example, an aged individual with arthritis may react slower as a result of stiff and painful joints. Their discomfort may lead to a sense of physical instability and inadequate physical adaptability, and result in a fear of falling. When evaluating functional capabilities, underlying pathologies or a sense of a social parameter (fear or discomfort) that may have an impact on a person's functioning may be discovered. Seeing variability in the older person in the area of reaction time may help to determine causes for functional declines in other areas.

There is a marked range of visual capabilities in the aged that also impacts an aged person's reaction time and the ability to function safely in a given environment. Several changes normally occur within the aging eye:

1. The lens begins to thicken and becomes yellowed.
2. The muscles that control dilation of the pupil weaken.
3. The older eye needs three times the amount of light to function adequately.
4. The thickening of the lens and delayed pupil dilation means that the glare and reflections often encountered in the environment cannot be tolerated.[32]
5. The older person has difficulty with depth perception and color differentiation, which can interfere with ambulation, ADLs, and driving an automobile.

The combination of these changes presents many ramifications and creates many obstacles for the aged person. A decline in visual acuity may ultimately result in a decrease in function. Even when errors of aged refraction are corrected, a loss of visual receptors in the aging retina or macula will result in a decrease of acuity. Fortunately, with modern technology, the majority of older people are able to maintain a high degree of visual function and independence. Research indicates that visual capabilities do not normally decline as part of aging. Instead, like so many other systems, the eyes are affected by nutritional deficits and environmental hazards, such as intense sunlight, poor lighting, and air-borne contaminants, all of which are preventable causes of visual loss.[33,34]

Strength is another variable, which directly affects an aged individual's ability to function at their maximum capability. Strength measures in a group of 70 plus year olds compared to a group of 40- to 50-year-olds (both male and female subjects) showed a greater range in strength values in the 70 plus year group.[35] Part of the variability results from the difficulty in separating age-dependent muscle changes from other factors that influence muscle strength, such as physical activity, disease, cardiovascular condition, and hormonal and neural influences. The younger group had fewer confounding factors. This variability in strength leads to different levels of functioning within an aged population and will be discussed further in the subsequent section of this chapter.

Mental ability is another area that varies greatly within an aged population and directly affects the rehabilitation potential of an aged individual. The presence of pathology, such as Alzheimer's disease, can severely influence an aged individual's ability to safely function within their environment. In the absence of pathology, however, an individual's cognitive abilities have been shown to undergo little or no change.[36]

What happens to intelligence and cognition with age? The answers are many, complex, and controversial. Some researchers say that cognition enters a process of irreversible decline in the adult years, because the brain becomes less and less efficient, just as do the heart, lungs, and other physical organs.[37] Other investigators say that intelligence and cognition are relatively stable through the adult years, with the brain providing more than enough capacity for any brain functioning necessary until serious disease sets in late in life.[38] Yet, other researchers indicate that cognition declines in some respects (in mental quickness, for example) and increases in others (in knowledge about life, for example).[39]

The decline of intelligence and cognition over the age of 65 or 70 is variable and subject to several interpretations. In addition to notions of inevitable biological decrement, intellectual and cognitive decline due to inactivity, social isolation, decreasing motivation to perform irrelevant tasks, disease, or a combination of such factors.

All in all, many researchers have begun to believe that the search for the curve of normal deterioration in mental abilities is a fruitless task.[40] In this view, there is too much variability in age trends to postulate one as normal or basic. Some people decline in intellectual ability, others increase. Some abilities seem to be increasing with each new generation; others seem to be decreasing. An environmental event (the development of television, for example) can change age trends for some people and have little effect on others. Thus the search goes on, but it is a search now for the determinants of change or stability and much less for inevitable and irreversible decrements.

The principle of variability in geriatric rehabilitation is key in providing therapeutic interventions that address the range of mental capabilities in aged individuals. Though we're bound to see cognitive decline in the rehabilitative setting, it's possible that healthy aged individuals who maintain an active intellectual life will show little or no loss of intellectual abilities even into their 80s and beyond.

Activity Versus Inactivity

The most common reason for losses in functional capabilities in the aged is inactivity or immobility. There are numerous reasons for immobilizing the aged. "Acute immobilization" is often considered to be accidental immobilization. Acute catastrophic illnesses include severe blood loss, trauma, head injury, cerebral vascular accidents, burns, and hip fractures to name only a few. The patient's activity level is often severely curtailed until acute illnesses become medically stable. "Chronic immobilization" may result from long-standing problems that are undertreated or left untreated. Examples of chronic problems include cerebral vascular accidents (strokes), amputations, arthritis, Parkinson's disease, cardiac disease, pulmonary disease, and low back pain. Environmental barriers are a major cause of "accidental immobilization" in both the acute and chronic care settings. These include bedrails, the height of the bed, physical restraints, an inappropriate chair, no physical assistance available, fall precautions imposed by medical staff, no orders in the chart for mobilization, social isolation, and environmental obstacles (stairs or doorway thresholds are examples). Cognitive impairments, central nervous system (CNS) disorders (such as cerebral vascular accidents, Parkinson's disease, and multiple sclerosis), peripheral neuropathies resulting from diabetes, and pain with movement can also severely reduce mobility. Affective disorders such as depression, anxiety, or fear of falling, may also lead to accidental immobilization. In addition, sensory changes, terminal illnesses (such as cancer or cirrhosis of the liver), acute episodes of illness like pneumonia or cellulitis, or an attitude of "I'm too sick to get up" can negatively affect mobility.

The process of deconditioning involves changes in multiple organ systems, including the neurological, cardiovascular, and musculoskeletal systems to varying degrees. Deconditioning is probably best defined as the multiple changes in organ system physiology that are induced by inactivity and reversed by activity (e.g., exercise).[16,41] The degree of deconditioning depends on the degree of superimposed inactivity and the prior level of physical fitness. The term "hypokinetics" has been coined to describe the physiology of inactivity.[42] Deconditioning can occur at many levels of inactivity. For simplicity and clarity, two major categories of inactivity or hypokinetics will be examined: the acute hypokinetic effects of bed rest, and the chronic inactivity induced by a sedentary lifestyle or chronic disease.

Looking at the aging process with one eye on the adverse effects of bed rest or hypokinetics as a possible concomitant of deconditioning and disability can lead to discovering more about the potential use of exercise as one of our primary rehabilitation modalities. The phrase "use it or lose it" is a concept with tremendous ramifications for aging, especially in geriatric rehabilitation. Exercise has not been viewed as an important factor in health until recently. Until the 1950s the rate-of-living theory was promoted. According to this theory, the body would be worn out faster and life shortened by expending energy during exercise.[43] Conversely, studies in the past decade have shown that regular exercise does not shorten life span, and may in fact increase it.[44] Exercise is increasingly viewed as beneficial for both the primary and secondary prevention of disease.[45]

There are several challenges to understanding the interaction between inactivity and health in older persons. The first is that the process of aging itself causes some changes that parallel the consequences of hypokinetics or inactivity. Several studies have provided strong evidence, which separates the aging process from the sedentary lifestyle.[46–61] It has been found that older individuals can improve their flexibility, strength, and aerobic capacity to the same extent as younger individuals. The second challenge in studying inactivity is separating the effects of inactivity from those of disease.[54,55] It is obvious that some effects of aging can be directly related to inactivity. Many aged individuals who are deconditioned may also have superimposition of acute or chronic disease. Studies on younger subjects have helped to clarify some of the effects of inactivity alone (e.g., bed rest on physiological changes and functional performance).

Another challenge exists: the challenge of understanding the relationship between physiologic decline and functional loss. Is the inability to climb stairs in an 85-year-old primarily from cardiovascular deconditioning, muscle weakness, impaired balance secondary to sensory losses, or a sedentary lifestyle? Is there a new disease process beginning? Is this normal aging? An important concept in geriatric rehabilitation is that threshold values of physiologic functioning may exist.[45,49] An aged person, who is below these thresholds, may suddenly lose an essential functional skill. An understanding of the consequences of inactivity is particularly important in addressing rehabilitation needs of the aged individual. Table 9–1 summarizes the complications of bed rest.

Inactivity's effect on the nervous system has not been studied as intensely as other organ systems. Perhaps this is related to the complexity of the nervous system and the lack of assessment techniques. In younger individuals changes in the nervous system with inactivity are minimal. In the aged, however—especially those individuals with concurrent acute or chronic illnesses - the consequences of inactivity on the nervous system may be particularly extreme.[47,50,53,59]

Bed rest has been compared to the experience of sensory deprivation. In a study of prolonged immobilization (immobilized during the day followed by bed rest at night), showed that occipital lobe frequencies on EEG were substantially decreased in awake subjects.[61] Exercise prevented some of these changes.[60,61] In addition to physical changes, performance on several intellectual tests deteriorated, including verbal fluency, color discrimination, and reversible figures.

Changes in affect, cognition, and perception are well described within a variety of settings of sensory deprivation including bed rest. Affective changes include anxiety, fear, depression, and rapid mood changes. Perceptual distortions ranging from daydreaming to hallucinations, difficulty concentrating, loss of sense of time, somatic complaints, and noncompliant behavior are well recognized with sensory deprivation.[61]

In a study on sensory deprivation, young subjects were put on bed rest and periodically stimulated by audiotapes of disjointed conversations.[53] Within a three-hour test period, the subject's perception of time intervals became distorted, and several subjects described hallucinatory-like experiences. Social isolation was also very disconcerting to the subjects and made them feel uncomfortable. Frequent complaints

TABLE 9–1.   SYSTEMIC COMPLICATIONS OF BED REST

Neurosensory	Sensory deprivation ↓ EEG activity ↓ thermoregulation ↓ cognition ↓ in reaction time ↓ balance ↑ postural sway	**Musculoskeletal**	Muscle atrophy ↓ muscle strength ↓ muscle oxidative capacity ↓ aerobic capacity Bone loss (osteoporosis) ↓ hyaluronic acid ↓ glycoproteins Joint contractures Osteoarthritis
Cardiovascular	↓ cardiac output ↑ resting heart rate (HR) ↓ oxygen uptake ↓ total blood volume ↓ aerobic capacity ↑ HR & BP with activity Delayed postactivity recovery time Orthostatic hypotension Venous thrombophlebitis	**Gastrointestinal**	Constipation
		Genitourinary	Urinary tract infection Urinary incontinence Renal calculi
		Skin	Pressure sores
		Functional	Impaired ambulation ↓ Activities of daily living ↑ Risk of falls
Respiratory	Atelectasis Relative hypoxemia ↑ risk of pneumonia ↓ chest wall compliance ↓ intercostal muscle strength ↓ vital capacity Impaired gas exchange ↓ resting arterial oxygen tension ↑ alveolar-artial oxygen gradient ↓ peripheral perfusion	**Psychological**	Sensory deprivation Anxiety, fear, depression Mood changes Hallucinations Perceptual disturbances Sleep disturbances

included feelings of loneliness and longing for some sign of recognition from the investigator. In young subjects, other emotions occur during prolonged bed rest such as anxiety, irritability, and a depressed mood.[60,61] These dramatic feelings occurred in healthy young persons during a three-hour bed rest period; reactions were more intense in subjects who were not allowed to exercise compared with those allowed to exercise three times a day.[61]

It has been found that bed rest also affects the EEG pattern of sleep. A longer period of time is spent in the deep stages of sleep, stages 3 and 4, in subjects on bed rest.[61] This was even more pronounced in individuals who were not allowed to perform light supine exercise. Rapid eye movement (REM) sleep periods also increased in subjects on bed rest. In addition, there was a noted increase in mental lethargy observed during waking hours. In conditioned subjects the onset of stage 3 sleep was sooner and the time spent in this deep, slow-wave sleep was longer than in subjects who were deconditioned.[46] These findings may have significant clinical implications in the aged person, especially one who is hypokinetic. Less time spent in deep sleep can lead to a feeling of tiredness, depression, anxiety, and lack of motivation. All of these sequelae could have a significant impact on an aged individual's level of functioning and rehabilitation potential.

Thermoregulation is also altered by bed rest.[46] Both oral and skin temperatures show a decline, which may have great clinical implications for the aged individual who already has decreased thermoregulatory responses.

Several neurological changes occur which affect motor performance. Balance decrements are significant after two to three weeks of bed rest.[47] Muscle-strengthening exercises during bed rest did not reverse this deterioration, but recovery of the balance losses was accomplished within three to five days following cessation of bed rest. Testing included assessment with the patient's eyes shut and open. Allowing visual cues greatly improved the relearning rate and overall performance scores.

Coordination was also found to decline with bed rest.[48] Pattern tracing skill tests were used to test coordination. Performance of these activities decreased in accuracy by 10% after three weeks of bed rest and resolved within four days of the resumption of activity.

Each of these changes will have significant clinical implications for aged individuals on acute or chronic bed rest or severely restricted levels of activity. The neuropsychologic consequences of a chronic level of inactivity, as in a sedentary lifestyle, are not easy to determine. Shepard[49] found that a moderate level of physical activity makes a person feel better, leading to better intellectual and psychomotor development. The underlying mechanism may include increased arousal, improved self-esteem and body image, and a decreased level of anxiety, stress, and depression.

Chronic inactivity also negatively affects balance. Postural sway is known to increase with aging, and inactivity may contribute to the progression of this decline. Research indicates that balance is better in active, as compared to inactive, older women.[50] Results were similar for different types of exercise (e.g., golf, walking, range-of-motion exercise). In a study by Emes,[51] standing balance on one foot was improved following a twelve-week exercise program.

A sedentary lifestyle is also associated with prolonged reaction times.[50,52] A comparison between young versus older persons revealed an 8% decline in reaction and movement times when age was considered alone. A 22% decrement was present when nonactive young and old groups were compared. Spirduso[53] has proposed that "exercise prevents the cycle in which disuse increases brain metabolism leading to decreased blood flow and neuronal loss."

The summary of the effects of inactivity on the nervous system is of great significance in geriatric rehabilitation. Acute bed rest induces some cognitive changes including distortion of time perception and decrements in some intellectual tests. Mood changes occur as well. Consequences on cognitive and emotional function of chronic inactivity may include a poorer sense of well-being. Balance is impaired after both acute and chronic inactivity. Prolonged reaction times are associated with chronic inactivity. Realizing the consequences of inactivity superimposed on the normal changes with aging should alert the rehabilitation team to the importance of maintaining activity and maximal functional capabilities in the aged person.

Changes in the cardiovascular system have been studied most in relation to inactivity versus activity. An aged individual in good physical condition responds to submaximal exercise levels without significant increases in heart rate or blood pressure. In contrast, a deconditioned person encountering minimal to moderate activity level experiences a marked increase in these vital signs. Maximal workloads elicit similar increases in heart rate and blood pressure in both deconditioned and conditioned individuals, however, the recovery rate (i.e., the return to resting vital sign values) is slower in deconditioned individuals. Table 9–2 summarizes the hemodynamic changes on standing in older individuals on acute (brief) and chronic (prolonged for a week or more) bed rest.

Within the first week of bed rest there is a noted increase in resting heart rate.[49,54,55] In other words, the work of the heart is increased in spite of the fact that the body remains at rest. In very early studies on the effects of bed rest on cardiovascular function it was found that by the end of the third week of bed rest the morning heart rate increased by as much as 21% and the evening heart rate by 33%. This is an average increase in resting heart rate of approximately one beat for every two bed rest days.[48] Other investigations showed approximately a four-beat increase, documenting lesser increases in resting heart rate over a one week period.[55] In each of these studies, six weeks of submaximal exercise was necessary before the resting heart rate returned to its baseline value.

Total blood volume has been found to decrease after several weeks of bed rest.[56] These findings were based on studies of astronauts in the aerospace program, a presumably healthy group of individuals. It was determined that plasma volume decrements were greater than red cell mass decrements. Such a change could have significant import for older persons. There is a strong possibility that a decrease in total blood volume could be correlated with orthostatic hypotension in the aged, though this has not been studied in an elderly population to date.

Orthostatic hypotension occurs within the first week of inactivity in young subjects. This, and other cardiovascular signs of deconditioning, occurs even with armchair rest.[57] Orthostasis resolves very slowly, even when the recovery period includes maximal exercise levels.

In addition to the deterioration of the cardiovascular system at rest, any level of activity above the resting level becomes more strenuous. At submaximal levels of exercise, heart rate increases of ten to twenty beats are common in the deconditioned individual. In addition to an increase in the heart rate, the stroke volume tends to decrease, making the heart less efficient in delivering blood to the working muscles.[45,49] Delayed recovery rates also indicate an increased cardiac and metabolic stress. Before bed rest, the return to baseline heart rate in the conditioned individuals occurs in less than two minutes and the systolic blood pressure returns to a resting level within four minutes. After six weeks of bed rest imposed on a healthy individual, it takes three to six minutes for the heart rate and five to seven minutes for the systolic blood pressure to return to pre-exercise resting levels.[45]

Normal aging is accompanied by a 1% per year decline in oxygen uptake starting at the age of 30,[45,49] although it has been shown that oxygen uptake is improved with activity. There is less of a decrease in oxygen uptake in armchair rest versus bed rest. In one of the few studies of older men, maximal oxygen uptake decreased 15% after ten days of bed rest.[58] Oxygen uptake at submaximal levels of activity was approximately 10% less after bed rest despite a increase in heart rate. These oxygen uptake levels returned to their baseline within one month following resumption of daily activities. Interestingly, recovery

TABLE 9–2.   HEMODYNAMIC CHANGES WITH STANDING FOLLOWING BED REST

Cardiac Parameter	After Acute (brief) Bed rest	After Chronic (prolonged) Bed rest
Cardiac output	↓	↓↓
Heart rate	↑ or No change	↑↑
Stroke volume	↓	↓↓
Peripheral vascular resistance	↑	↑↑
Blood pressure	No change	↓↓

rates were similar for subjects who participated in an aerobic exercise program as well as for those who just returned to their usual activities.

The cardiovascular system undergoes significant changes with bed rest. The alterations are noted even without activity by an increase in resting heart rate. Mere standing can be accompanied by orthostasis. Any level of activity stresses the heart eliciting a greater heart rate and a diminished stroke volume. These factors contribute to the overall decrease in maximal oxygen uptake resulting in decreased physical capabilities, decreased endurance, and lost function.

The cardiovascular consequences of chronic inactivity are similar to those seen in acute bed rest. Resting heart rates are higher. At submaximal activity levels, heart rate and blood pressure are greater than in physically fit individuals performing at the same intensity of exercise. Maximal oxygen uptake is lower than in individuals who exercise aerobically. The well-documented decline in maximal oxygen uptake with age is 50% less in physically active individuals compared to inactive persons and the latter's recovery rate is prolonged. The biggest difference in acute versus chronic inactivity's effects on the cardiovascular system are the cumulative effects of long-term inactivity. In other words, the longer an individual remains inactive, the more pronounced the above mentioned cardiovascular changes are and the longer it takes to return to a healthy, predeconditioned baseline.

The skeletal muscle system of the body is the largest organ system by mass, and its physiological capabilities are closely related to levels of activity. Alterations in skeletal muscle with aging and with inactivity resemble those observed with denervation. The classic cross-innervation studies of Buller and associates[59] established the importance of the trophic influence on skeletal muscle function and demonstrated that the metabolic and physiologic profile of a muscle fiber (i.e., the fiber type) was primarily determined by the type of neural innervation (phasic or tonic firing pattern and other trophic factors) it received. Adult skeletal muscle is composed of three distinct fiber types: type IIA (fast twitch, high oxidative fiber), type IIB (fast twitch, low oxidative fiber) and type I (slow twitch, high oxidative fiber). This heterogeneous fiber pattern is lost with aging and fibers become more homogeneous in respect to their physiological and metabolic profile.

It is well known that decreases in muscle mass occur with old age—with proximal muscles of the lower extremity particularly affected. This decrease in muscle mass is due to a decrease in both fiber number and diameter. No change in the number of motor neural fibers has been found, but the size of the motor unit decreases due to the loss of muscle fibers. The reported decrease in fiber number primarily affects the red oxidative fiber, the preponderance of evidence based on enzyme histochemistry and physiological properties suggest a greater loss in the fast type II fiber. The decrease occurs in both type IIA and IIB fibers such that the type IIB/IIA fiber ratio is unaltered with increasing age. As a result of this selective loss of type II fibers, the percentage of type I fibers increases from about 40% in 20- to 30-year-old persons to 55% in 60- to 65-year-old individuals.[45,49]

With aging and with inactivity, then, we see a loss of lean body mass. The same changes are also observed in younger subjects on bed rest and in astronauts in a gravity-free environment.[60,61] Exercise positively affects body composition. Bed rest imposes inactivity in a nonuniform way in muscle groups. Functionally, neck extensors and the antigravity muscles of the legs are the least exercised. Arm, back, and abdominal muscles may be used more frequently during positional changes and basic activities of care. During several weeks of bed rest in young men, grip strength, abdominal, and back muscle strength did not show any discernible change.[45] A decrease of 6% in shoulder and arm flexor muscles was observed. The tibialis anterior (the muscle that pulls the foot up) decreased in strength by 13%, and the gastrocsoleus (the muscle group that pulls the foot into a ballerina position and assists in flexion of the knee) lost 20% of its strength. Muller reported a loss of approximately 1.5% per day during a two-week period of bed rest.[62]

Most of the studies of bed rest effects on skeletal muscle have been done on younger subjects; therefore, the amount of strength lost by aged persons during bed rest has not been extensively studied. Inactivity superimposed on the normal aging process previously mentioned, however, is likely to have significant disabling consequences. The decrement in strength with aging is likely to be due partially to inactivity. Exercise programs have been found to improve strength in all age groups.[49]

The skeletal system functions to support, protect, and shape the body. Additionally, bone has the metabolic functions of blood cell production, the storage of calcium and a role in acid-base balance.

Cortical thickening starts to decline at approximately age 35 and becomes 20% less in men and 30% less in women in the 8th and 9th decades. Bed rest or a lack of weight-bearing activities produces bone loss. Astronauts lose four grams calcium during an 84-day space flight simulation.[60]

The most commonly known age-related change involving bone is calcium-related loss of mass and density. This loss ultimately causes the pathological condition of osteoporosis. Bone density is lost from within by a process termed reabsorption. As the body ages, an imbalance occurs between osteoblast activity (bone buildup) and osteoclast activity (breaks down bone). Osteoclast activity proves to be the stronger. As one ages, a decline in circulating levels of activated vitamin D_3 occurs,[63] and this causes less calcium to be absorbed from the gut and more calcium to be absorbed from the bones to meet body needs. In postmenopausal women, decreased estrogen levels influence parathormone and calcitonin to increase bone reabsorption, which decreases bone mass. Certain factors such as immobility, decreased estrogens, steroid therapy, and hyperthyroidism are known to accelerate bone erosion to pathological levels. Easily occurring fractures are the most common result.[64,65]

Bone mass and strength decline with age. Osteoporosis is a major bone mineral disorder in the older adult. A decreased bone mineral composition, an enlarged medullary cavity, a normal mineral composition, and biochemical normalities in plasma and urine have characterized this bone loss. The rate of bone loss is about 1% per year for women starting at age 30 to 35 and for men at age 50 to 55. In elderly subjects, regions of devitalized tissue with osteocyte lacunae and haversian canals containing amorphous mineral deposits have been described indicating a change in the bone mass/mineral ratio. These have been identified as micropetrotic regions and are noted to increase in frequency in the skeleton with age. Thus, it is clear that the mineral content of bone qualitatively changes with age.

Qualitatively, osteoporotic bone exhibits a reduction in bone mass with a resulting decrease in bone strength. There is some evidence, however, that alterations occur in the composition and structure of bone in the aged. Evans[66] observed that the tensile strength of bone in man is related to the number and size of osteons. It has been found that bone from older humans has smaller osteons and fragments and more cement lines than younger bone. This would account for some of the reduced bone strength of the older bone specimens. The remaining difference in strength results from the geometric structure of the bone in its distribution per unit area as a response to environmental stress placed upon the bone. According to Wolff's law, bone is laid down in the direction of stresses it must withstand. In the absence of stress (i.e., bed rest or varying levels of inactivity), the composition of bone becomes diffuse rather than uniform, and losses it's tensile strength.

Throughout life, red blood cells continue to be replaced after a life span of about 120 days. Some morphological changes do occur with aging. Red cells are slightly smaller and more fragile. Blood volume, however, is maintained until approximately 80 years of age. In the absence of pathology, few changes are seen in the white blood cells and in the platelet count. What is lost with aging is the functional reserve to quickly accelerate the production of red blood cells when needed,[64] and this inability is further accentuated by inactivity.

In the pulmonary system, age changes and changes associated with inactivity can be organized according to mechanical properties, changes in flow, changes in volume, alteration in gas exchange and impairments of lung defense. Decreases in chest wall compliance and lung elastic recoil tendency are two mechanical properties, which are altered with age.

Increased calcification of the ribs, a decline in intercostal muscle strength, and changes in the spinal curvature (resulting from osteoporotic collapse of the thoracic vertebrae) all result in a lower compliance and increased work of breathing.

At normal lung volume, airway resistance is not increased, however, normal aging results in a reduction of maximum voluntary ventilation, maximum expiratory flow and forced expiratory volume in one second (alone and in relation to forced vital capacity). Though tidal volume remains fairly constant throughout life, vital capacity decreases while residual volume increases. Bed rest has a relatively small effect on pulmonary function in healthy subjects,[55] however, chronic inactivity may cause some reversible decrement in vital capacity, and exercise training leads to a more efficient respiratory function.[49]

Ventilation, diffusion and pulmonary circulation are the three major components of the respiratory system that lose efficiency with age. There is an increased thickening of the supporting membranes between the alveoli and the capillaries, a decline in total lung capacity, an increase in residual volume, a reduced vital capacity and a decrease in the resiliency of the lungs. It is difficult to completely separate pulmonary changes resulting with age from those associated with the pathology of emphysema or chronic bronchitis. Throughout a lifetime, exposure to occupational and environmental inhalants as well as cigarette smoke may result in chronic pulmonary changes and lung pathologies. These disease states closely parallel those of the aging process and also increase in incidence with advancing age.[67] Normal pulmonary aging includes a loss of elastic tissue leading to expiratory collapse of the larger airways, difficulty with expiration, and dilitation of the terminal air passages.[68]

Aging and inactivity also affect the diffusion efficiency of peripheral vascular system. Starting with the pulmonary system, impairment of gas exchange is illustrated by a reduced diffusing capacity of carbon monoxide, a lower resting arterial oxygen tension and an increased alveolar-arterial oxygen gradient. Alveolar surface area and pulmonary capillary blood volume diminish with age. As a result, the oxygen dissociation curve shifts to the left, which makes oxygen less available at the tissue level.

The ability to provide oxygen to working tissues diminishes with inactivity. Normal aging affects the cardiopulmonary system in a variety of ways, however, in the absence of pathology, the heart and lungs can generally meet the body's needs. The most evident change in the cardiovascular and cardiopulmonary functioning with bed rest is that the reserve capacities are diminished. In other words, with any challenge, the body's demand for oxygen and perfusion may exceed available supply.

Of importance clinically in an older person is an impairment of pulmonary defenses resulting from normal aging changes and a decreased level of mobility. Cilia are reduced in number, and those, which remain, become less strong. The "mucus escalator" and alveolar macrophages (the germ killers) become less effective in removing inhaled particulate matter. In the absence of physiological challenges, the system maintains fairly adequate defenses; however, an older individual who is chronically exposed to particle-laden air in addition to inactivity, which in essence diminishes the efficiency of the lungs, will become at risk for pulmonary dysfunction.[64,69]

As previously mentioned, the postexercise recovery period following effort is prolonged. Among other factors, this reflects a greater relative work rate, an increase proportion of anaerobic metabolism, a slower heat elimination, and a lower level of physical fitness.

Extremes of immobilization can lead to a decrease in joint range of motion secondary to connective tissue changes. There are many types of connective tissue in the body (loose, adipose, fibrous, etc.), but it is loose connective tissue which functions to bind organs together while holding tissue fluids and permitting cellular-molecular diffusion. Loose connective tissue is located beneath most layers of epithelium and fills spaces between muscles (fascia). The most common type of cell in loose connective tissue is called a fibroblast. Fibroblasts work to produce protein fibers called collagen and elastin.[70]

In youth, collagen fibers are strong and flexible and are arranged in bundles, which criss-cross to form structure in the body. As a person ages, there is an increased criss-crossing or cross-linkage of the fibers resulting in denser extracellular matrices. The collagen structure becomes stiffer as it becomes denser. This increased density also impairs molecular movement of nutrients and wastes at the cellular level.[71]

Structurally, elastin fibers also develop increased cross-linkage with age. Water and elasticity are lost. The elastin fibers become more rigid, may tend to fray and, in some cases, are replaced by collagen completely.[64]

The clinical significance of this increased cross-linking is seen in resultant collagenous contractures. Bonds between adjacent collagen strands can produce shortening and distortion of the collagen fibers. This shortening may result in contractures with a progressive restriction in tissue mobility.[72] Collagen fiber contractures are tough and inelastic, and their bonds can not be broken by mechanical stretching forces.

Fibrinous adhesions have great clinical implications in working with the elderly. Fibrinogen, a soluble plasma protein is a normal molecular exudate within the capillary. When this substance passes through the capillary wall into the surrounding tissues, it is converted to strands of insoluble fibrin.[73] Fibrin strands can adhere to tissue structures and restrict movement of these structures. Normally, fibrin is removed as debris, but with age, the exudation of fibrinogen into the surrounding tissues is increased,[74] and with reduced activity levels, complete breakdown of fibrin may not occur. This leads to the accumulation of fibrin, which restricts movement and may result in adhesions.

Fibrinogen also accumulates at the site of tissue damage following an injury (traumatic or surgically induced). If activity is limited, these strands can consolidate and create an adhesion.[75] Some decrements in flexibility can be reversed by exercise,[49] but, the most effective means of maintaining mobility is early intervention using bed exercises. What is not lost does not need to be regained, therefore, the prevention of contractures is of extreme importance in geriatric rehabilitation, and the only way to accomplish this is to maintain activity (even if an aged person is on bed rest).

Other connective tissue also affected by aging and inactivity includes hyaline cartilage, elastic cartilage, and articular cartilage. Hyaline cartilage is found in the nose and the rings of the respiratory passages as well as in the joints. Elastic cartilage is found in parts of the larynx and the outer ear. Articular cartilage is found between the intervertebral discs, between the bones of the pelvic girdle, and at most articular joint surfaces.[76] With aging, cartilage tends to dehydrate, becomes more stiff, and thins in weight-bearing areas.

Cartilage is formed when its cells are subjected to compressive forces (weight bearing) in an environment of low oxygen concentration. Cartilage is a unique connective tissue in that it has no direct blood supply. Blood flow in adjacent bones and synovial fluid provides nutrients to the cartilage. A strong osmotic force attracts water with dissolved gases, inorganic salts, and organic materials into the cartilage providing materials necessary for normal metabolism. The concentration of glycoproteins in the matrix of the cartilage determines the amount of fluid drawn into the cartilage. Normal aging is accompanied by a reduction in the amount of glycoproteins produced,[77] resulting in a decrease in osmotic attraction forces and impairment in the ability of the cartilage to attract and retain fluids.

Nutrients enter the matrix of the cartilage only when compressive forces are absent.[49] In a loaded or compressed state, fluid and nutrient substances are squeezed out. To provide regular movement of substances in and out of the cartilage, it is necessary that alternating application and release of compressive forces occur. Metabolites remain in the cartilage in the absence of compression, and the presence of metabolites reduces the oxygen content, resulting in a reduction of the secretion of glycoproteins.[49] The destruction of the joint becomes a viscous cycle in the absence of activity.

In synovial joints, the articular surfaces are covered by hyaline cartilage. The secretion of hyaluronic acid provides lubrication at the interface of the hyaline cartilage. Hyaluronic acid molecules form a viscous layer covering the hyaline cartilage. Compression facilitates production of hyaluronic acid ensuring continual lubrication of the joint during movement.[78] The secretion of hyaluronic acid decreases with age, and in the absence of weight-bearing activity, the efficiency of the lubrication system of the joint is reduced.[79] Degenerative changes of the cartilage are not reversible and rehabilitation efforts need to be directed towards regular (but not excessive) compression and release of compression in the aging joint. Normal weight-bearing exercises are recommended to maintain cartilagenous health.

The cartilage, which normally covers body joints, thins and deteriorates with aging. This especially occurs in the weight-bearing areas. Because cartilage has no blood supply or nerves, erosion within the joint is often advanced before symptoms of pain, crepitation, and limitation of movement are perceived. Decreased hydration, reduced elasticity, and increased fibrous growth around bony prominences all contribute to increased stiffness and decreased functioning. Advanced stages of cartilage-joint deterioration are commonly known as osteoarthritis.[70,64,80]

Since some types of connective tissue exist almost everywhere in the body, the effects of aging superimposed on inactivity are widespread. Increased rigidity of collagenous and elastin fibers results in a greater amount of energy being needed to produce a given stretch. Skin becomes less elastic and more wrinkled. Lungs lose some recoil tendency, arteries become more rigid, and the heart becomes less distensible. Joints become stiffer while decreased hydration in the intervertebral discs results in vertebral compaction and shrinkage of height. Cellular repair, nutrition, and waste removal are impaired.[64] All of these consequences of inactivity and aging have been shown to be preventable with regular exercise.[49]

The changes in bowel and bladder function with aging have been discussed in Chapter 3, and lack of activity or deconditioning per se do not appear to directly impair these functions. Of note in considering inactivity on an acute basis, however, is the increased incidence of constipation, urinary incontinence, and urinary tract infections.[81] The effect of chronic inactivity is less clear. It is difficult to sort out effects solely related to inactivity from dietary and functional problems.

Constipation and fecal impaction are frequent complications of bed rest. Hospitalized elderly with limited mobility have longer gastrointestinal transit times than nonhospitalized, ambulatory elderly.[82] Mass propulsion by the colon correlates with physical activity.[83] Movement of radioactive markers through the colon varies with somatic activity. With inactivity, there is slowed movement of feces into the descending colon and sigmoid.[83] Environmental factors associated with bed rest in the elderly also predispose to constipation. Bedpans, delay in assistance, and lack of privacy can lead to constipation. Weakness, confusion, and drugs prescribed for conditions requiring bed rest may make constipation worse.

Urinary incontinence is common in patients on bed rest. It is more difficult to void in a supine position. The irritability of the bladder may be reduced with immobilization leading to incomplete emptying of the bladder. As a result, incontinence may occur, or residual urine can create an environment for bacterial infection and urinary tract complications. Conditions that require bed rest such as strokes, and complications of conditions such as delirium and weakness, may limit access to toileting, predisposing the patient to urinary incontinence. The hypercalciuria that occurs with bed rest predisposes to renal calculi. Calcium renal stones have been reported in immobilized older adults.

The effects of bed rest on metabolic function include an increased excretion of calcium within the first two days of bed rest[61] (perhaps indicative of skeletal changes), peaking in the fourth week of immobilization.[54] Calcium losses stabilize by the fifth week of activity resumption. Negative nitrogen balance can start by the fifth day of bed rest. This is indicative of protein degradation, primarily in the skeletal muscle. Following a return to activity, a return to normal occurs by the 6th week of exercise. Accelerated loss of calcium and nitrogen induced by bed rest has important implications with regard to the high incidence of osteoporosis and loss of lean muscle tissue with aging.

Decubitus ulcers or pressure sores are widely recognized complications of bed rest. Sustained pressure from immobilization is the most important cause of skin breakdown. Pressure is transmitted to skin, subcutaneous tissue, and muscle, particularly over bony prominences, and can result in ischemia and necrosis. Constant pressure of 70 mmHg for more than two hours produces irreversible skin damage as discussed in Chapter 14. In addition to the effects of pressure with bed rest, bedding frequently occludes the skin. When occluded, skin is softened by sweat and other body fluids, the skin is predisposed to maceration and breakdown. Shearing forces and friction to which the bedbound elder is often subjected may cause direct injury to the skin.

It seems obvious from these body systems that the evaluation and treatment of hypokinetics is crucial in the total care of the elderly. Passive range of motion (PROM) or active-assistive range of motion (A-AROM) is appropriate even in the most immobilized patients to prevent the consequences of immobilization. Aging and inactivity are both associated with loss of lean body mass and a gain in body fat.[49,52] Some degree of changes associated with aging are directly related to inactivity. Active aged individuals show lesser degrees of these changes, and exercise programs in sedentary aged persons have been shown to positively modify those changes associated with aging. Exercise has been shown to reverse the physiological changes of inactivity including a return of cardiovascular and cardiopulmonary response to pre-bed rest base lines, and a return of muscle strength and flexibility.[45] A mnemonic representation of the effects of bed rest is helpful in remembering the overall effects of inactivity on functional capabilities:

B— Bladder and bowel incontinence and retention; bedsores

E— Emotional trauma; electrolyte imbalances

D— Deconditioning of muscles and nerves; depression; demineralization of bones

R— ROM loss and contractures; restlessness; renal dysfunction

E— Energy depletion; EEG activity decreases

S— Sensory deprivation; sleep disorders; skin problems

T— Trouble

The elderly are especially susceptible to the complications of bed rest. Aging changes and common chronic diseases result in a decrease in physiologic reserve and a decreased ability to tolerate the changes which occur with bed rest. The physiology of aging and bed rest have many features in common and may be additive in their effects. The changes that commonly occur with aging and prolonged bed rest independently lead to osteoporosis, decreased endurance and impaired mobility, and increase the predisposition to falls, deep venous thrombosis, sensory deprivation, and pressure sores.

With the numerous adverse effects of bed rest discussed above, clearly bed rest should be prescribed judiciously and with full awareness of its potential complications and the need for preventive exercise prescription. Any elderly patient on bed rest should be on a physical or occupational therapy program. When full activity is not possible, limited activity such as movement in bed, activities of daily living, intermittent sitting and standing will reduce the frequency of some complications of bed rest. Prolonged bed rest causes significant cardiovascular, respiratory, musculoskeletal, and neuropsychological changes. Complications are often irreversible. Complete bed rest should be avoided at all costs.

Optimal Health

The last principle in geriatric rehabilitation is the principle of "optimal health." The great English statesman, Benjamin Disraeli said, "The health of people is really the foundation upon which all their happiness and their powers as a state depend." The World Health Organization defines health as a state of complete physical, mental, and social well-being, not merely the absence of disease or infirmity.[84] The existence of complete physical health refers to the absence of pathology, impairment, or disability. Physical health is quite achievable. Mental and social well-being are closely related, and possibly less obtainable in this day and age. Mental health as defined by the World Health Organization would include cognitive and intellectual intactness as well as emotional well-being. The social components of health would in-

clude living situation, social roles (i.e., mother, daughter, vocation etc), and economic status.

As seen in Chapter 3, there are some cumulative effects—biological, physiological, and anatomical—that may eventually lead to clinical symptoms. It has also been noted in the chapter that some of these changes are associated with inactivity and not purely a result of progressive aging effects. In light of this, a preventive approach to physical health needs to be in the foreground when addressing the needs of the aged.

Preventing impairment and disability is a key principle in geriatric rehabilitation. It is reasonable to assume that the health status of individuals in their 70s and subsequent decades of life are in a suboptimal range. Thus, the scope of health status for the aged should be focused toward preventing the complications that could result from suboptimal health. When considering suboptimal health then, the goal of geriatric rehabilitation should be to strive for relative optimal health (i.e., the maximal functional and physical capabilities of the aged individual considering their current health status).

In reviewing the importance of promoting relative optimal health in terms of the musculoskeletal, sensory, or cardiopulmonary systems, an example of an aged woman with a hip fracture may help.

The patient may be in suboptimal health and suffering from osteoporosis; however, she is not treated until she fractures her hip. The resulting complications could include pneumonia, decubiti from bed rest, all of the changes previously noted in relation to inactivity, and possibility of death. Intervention at the suboptimal level was needed here rather than waiting for an illness or disability to occur. This intervention could include weight-bearing exercises to enhance the strength of the bone, strengthening exercises of the lower extremities to provide adequate stability and endurance, balance and postural exercises to facilitate effective balance reactions and safety, education in nutrition, and modification of her living environment to ensure added safety in hopes of avoiding the kind of fall that results in a hip fracture.

Another excellent example of preventive intervention to maintain optimal health would be in the case of the diabetic aged individual. It is known that sensory loss in the lower extremities resulting from diabetes mellitus often predisposes diabetic individuals to ulceration of the foot. An ill-fitting shoe or a wrinkle in the sock may go unnoticed and lead to friction, skin breakdown and a resulting foot ulcer. If undetected, even the smallest ulcer may lead to amputation of a lower extremity. Screening of the foot during evaluation can prevent this devastating loss. Intervention could include education of the aged individual in foot inspection (or education of a family member or friend if the diabetic aged individual's eyesight is compromised), proper shoe fitting, and techniques for dealing with their sensory loss (e.g., as temperature sensation diminishes, the individual needs to test bath water temperature with a thermometer, or have their spouse test the water before they put their insensitive feet into a steamy bath). With proper skin care and professional (podiatric) care of the nails and calluses, there is less likelihood that injury will occur. The cost of a therapeutic diabetic shoe (the P.W. Minor Thermold shoe for example) is $130 to $160 per pair and provides protection and ample room for the forefoot. Compare this to the cost of ulcer care, which averages $6,000, and the cost of hospitalization and rehabilitation for amputation, which averages $30,000.[85]

The principle of obtaining relative optimal health in geriatric rehabilitation is not only cost- effective, but clearly would lead to an overall improvement in the quality of life. Encouraging healthy behaviors, such as decreasing obesity, stress, and smoking, and increasing activity, could be the elements necessary in maintaining health and striving for optimal health as defined by the World Health Organization.[84]

Health care professionals involved in geriatric rehabilitation need to be good *evaluators* and *screeners*. Good investigative skills could detect a minor problem with the potential of developing into a major problem. Thorough assessment of physical, cognitive, social needs could help us to modify rehabilitation programs accordingly to truly improve the health and functional ability of our aged clients.

Rehabilitative Measures

Rehabilitation should be directed at preventing premature disability. A deconditioned aged individual is less capable of performing activities than a conditioned aged individual. For example, the speed of walking is positively correlated to the level of physical fitness in an aged person.[86] When cardiovascular capabilities are diminished (i.e., maximum aerobic capacity), walking speeds are adjusted by the aged person to levels of comfort. Himann[86] found that exercise programs geared for improving cardiovascular fitness improved the speed of walking. The more conditioned the individual, the faster the walking pace. The faster the walking pace, the smoother the momentum decreasing the likelihood of falling. The better-conditioned elder is also more agile and has improved reaction times to balance perturbation when compared to an unfit older individual.

If disease and physical disability are superimposed on a hypokinetic sequelae, the functional consequences can be disastrous, because pain often prevents mobility. For instance, the pain experienced by an aged individual with an acute exacerbation of osteoarthritic knee pain accompanied by inflammation of the knee capsule may reflexively inhibit quadriceps contraction. While strength of the quadriceps may have been poor in the first place due to inactivity, the absence of pain still permitted this individual to rise from a chair or ascend shallow steps. Now, with the presence of acute pain, these activities cause

severe discomfort and threaten the capability of maintaining an independent lifestyle. In this situation, rehabilitation efforts should focus medically on

- Reducing the inflammation through drugs or ice (physician, nurse);
- Maintaining joint mobility during the acute phases by joint mobilization techniques of oscillation and low grade passive range in addition to modalities, such as interferential current, to assist in reducing the edema, and decreasing the discomfort (physical therapy);
- Joint protection techniques and prescription of adaptive equipment such as a walker to protect the joint (occupational and physical therapy);
- Provision for proper nutrition in light of medications/nutrient (pharmacist/dietician) effects and evidence that vitamin C is a crucial component in health of the synovium;[79]
- Social and psychological support (social worker, psychologist, religious personnel) to provide emotional and motivational support.

These interventions to prevent the debilitating effects of bed rest highlight the need for an interdisciplinary approach when addressing geriatric rehabilitation.

Rehabilitation of the aged individual should emphasize functional activity to maintain functional mobility and capability, improvement of balance through exercise and functional activity programs (e.g., weight shifting exercises, ambulation with direction and elevation changes, reaching activities), good nutrition and good general care (including hygiene, hydration, bowel and bladder considerations, appropriate rest and sleep) as well as social and emotional support.

It is important to optimize overall health status by implementing the concept of independence. The more an individual does for his- or herself, the more they are capable of doing independently. The more that is done for an aged individual, the less capable they become of functioning on an optimal independent level and the more likely the progression of a disability.

The advancing stages of disabilities increase an individual's vulnerability to illness, emotional stress, and injury. An older person's subjective appraisal of her or his health status influences how they react to their symptoms, their perception of their vulnerability, and their perception of their abilities to perform a given activity. Often an aged person's self-appraisal of their health is a good predictor to the rehabilitation clinician's evaluation of health and functional status, but such assessments may also differ in many ways. In older persons, perceptions of one's health may be determined in large part by one's level of psychological well-being and by whether or not one continues in rewarding roles and activities.[87]

Because an aged individual's perception of their health status is an important motivator in compliance with a rehabilitation program, it is important to discuss this further. One interesting study showed that even when age, sex, and health status (as evaluated by physicians) were controlled for, perceived health and mortality from heart disease were strongly related.[88] Those who rated their health as poor were two to three times as likely to die as those who rated their health as excellent. A Canadian longitudinal study of persons over 65 produced similar results.[89] Over three years, the mortality of those who described their health as poor at the beginning of the study was about three times that of those who initially described their health as good.

Yet, despite this apparent awareness among older persons of their actual state of health, the elderly are known to fail to report serious symptoms and wait longer than younger persons to seek help. Rehabilitation professionals need to listen carefully to their aged clients with this in mind. It appears that, contrary to the popular view that older individuals are somewhat hypochondriacal, aged persons generally deserve serious attention when they bring complaints to their caregivers.

The perceived level of health will greatly impact the outcomes of functional goals in the geriatric rehabilitation setting, whether it is acute, rehabilitative, home, or chronic care. Rosillo and Fagel[90] found that improvement in rehabilitation tasks correlated well with patients' appraisal of their potential for recovery, but not very well with others' appraisal. Stoedefalke[91] reports that positive reinforcement (frequent positive feedback) for older persons in rehabilitation greatly improved their performance and feelings of success. This indicates that aged persons can improve in their physical functioning when modifications in therapeutic interventions provide feedback more often. Some research indicates that older persons with chronic illness have low initial aspirations with regard to their ability to perform various tasks.[92] As situations in which they succeeded or failed occurred, their aspirations changed to more closely reflect their abilities.

Older persons may have different beliefs about their abilities compared to younger persons.[93] When subjects were given an unsolvable problem, younger subjects ascribed their failure to not trying hard enough, while older subjects ascribed their failure to inability. On subsequent tests, younger individuals tried harder and older subjects gave up. This holds extreme importance in the rehabilitation potential of an aged person. If the person sees the cause of failure as an immutable characteristic, then little effort in the future can be expected.

Aged individuals may have a higher anxiety level in rehabilitation situations because they fear failure or are afraid of "looking bad" to their family or therapist.[94] Eisdorfer[94] found that if anxiety is high enough, then the behavior is redirected toward reducing the anxiety rather than accomplishing the task.

Weinberg[95] found that subjects set their own goals for task achievement, even if they are directed to adopt the therapist's goals. In another study, Mento, Steel, and Karren[96] found that the best performance at difficult tasks, as many rehabilitation tasks are, occurs when the aged person sets a very specific goal, such as walking ten feet with a walker. If the person simply tries to "do better," then performance is not improved as much. These are important motivational components to keep in mind when working with an aged client. Perhaps the therapeutic approach of the clinician may have the greatest impact on the successful functional outcomes in a geriatric rehabilitation setting.

Exercise programs have potential for improving physical fitness, agility, and speed of response.[49] They also serve to improve muscle strength, flexibility, bone health, cardiovascular and respiratory response, and tolerance to activity.[97] Evidence suggests that reaction time is better in elders who engage in physical exercise than in those who are sedentary.[98] Stelmach and Worringham[98] showed a positive correlation between individuals' ability to maintain their balance when stressed and their level of fitness. Initial test scores on reaction time were significantly improved following a six-week stretching and calisthenics program in individuals 65 years of age and older. This has great clinical significance when considering the increasing incidence of falls with age (an area to be discussed in more detail in a subsequent section of this chapter).

In addition, exercise has been shown to provide social and psychological benefits affecting the quality of life and the sense of well-being in the elderly.[99] Intuitively, it would appear plausible that an aged individual who is in better physical condition will experience less functional decline and maintain a higher level of independence and a resulting improvement in their perceived quality of life. The risks of encouraging physical activity are small and can be minimized through careful evaluation. While all the exercise and activity programs that constitute therapeutic exercise cannot be described in detail in this chapter, Table 9–3 summarizes therapies for various conditions seen most frequently in geriatric rehabilitation settings.

Specialized exercise techniques, such as proprioceptive neuromuscular facilitation (PNF), Bobath, and sensory integration techniques are very useful in regaining and maintaining functional mobility and strength and improving sensory awareness in elderly individuals.[100] Though these therapeutic exercises vary in application techniques, the concept of integrating sensory and motor function is consistent in each.

These exercise techniques are methods of placing specific demands on the sensory motor system in order to obtain a desired response. Facilitation, by definition, implies the promotion or hastening of any natural process—the reverse of inhibition; specifically, the ef-

TABLE 9–3.   REHABILITATION THERAPIES FOR COMMON CONDITIONS

Cerebral Vascular Accident (Stroke)

Physical Therapy
- Pre-gait activities (if individual is not ambulatory)
- Gait/Balance training (if individual is ambulatory)
- Provision of assistive ambulatory devices (quad cane, hemi-walker)
- Ambulation on different types of surfaces (stairs, ramps)
- Provision of appropriate shoe gear and orthotics
- Education and provision of appropriate bracing
- Range-of-motion, strengthening, coordination exercises
- Proprioceptive neuromuscular facilitation
- Bobath techniques to modify tone
- Sensory integration
- Joint mobilization techniques (when appropriate)
- Functional electrical stimulation (when appropriate)
- Positioning and posturing (chair, feeding needs)
- Family and patient education for home management
- Alternative interventions—Qi Gong, T'ai Chi, Yoga, Feldenkrais

Occupational Therapy
- Training in activities of daily living (grooming, dressing, cooking, etc)
- Transfer training (toilet, bathtub, car, etc)
- Activities and exercise to enhance function of upper extremities
- Training to compensate for visual-perceptual problems
- Provision of adaptive devices (reachers, special eating utensils)

Speech Therapy
- Language production work
- Reading, writing, and math retraining
- Functional skills practive (checkbook balancing, making change)
- Therapy for swallowing disorders
- Oral muscular strengthening

Parkinson's Disease

Physical Therapy
- Gait training
- Provision for appropriate shoe gear and orthotics
- Training in position changes
- General conditioning, strengthening, coordination, and range of motion exercises
- Breathing exercises
- Training in functional instrumental activities of daily living
- Proprioceptive neuromuscular facilitation/Sensory integration
- Alternative interventions—T'ai Chi, aquatic therapy, Qi Gong, Feldenkrais

Occupational Therapy
- Fine/gross motor coordination of upper extremities
- Provision of adaptive equipment
- Basic self-care activity training
- Transfer training

Speech Therapy
- Improving respiratory control
- Improving coordination between speech and respiration
- Improving control of rate of speech
- Use of voice amplifiers and/or alternate communication devices

Arthritis

Physical Therapy
- Joint protection techniques
- Joint mobilization for pain control and mobility
- Conditioning, strengthening, and range-of-motion exercises
- Gait training
- Provision of proper shoe gear and orthotics
- Modalities to decrease pain and edema, and break up adhesions
- Provision of assistive ambulatory devices (when appropriate)
- Alternative interventions—T'ai Chi, Qi Gong, Feldenkrais, Yoga, aquatics

(*continued*)

TABLE 9–3.   (Continued)

- Refer for nutritional counseling

Occupational Therapy
- Range-of-motion and strengthening exercise of upper extremities
- Splinting to protect involved joints, devrease inflammation, and prevent deformity
- Joint protection techniques
- Provision of adaptive devices to promote independence and avoid undue stress on involved joints

Amputees

Physical Therapy
- Fitting and provision of temporary and permanent prosthetic devices
- Teaching donning and doffing of prostheses
- Progressive ambulation
- Provision of assistive ambulatory devices
- Training in stump care
- Wound care (when appropriate)
- Provision of shoe gear and protective orthotic for uninvolved extremity
- Instruction in range-of-motion, strengthening, and endurance activites for both involved and uninvolved extremi ties
- Balance activities
- Transfer training
- Patient education in skin care and monitoring
- Alternative therapies—Qi Gong, Yoga, Feldenkrais
- Refer for nutritional counseling

Occupational Therapy
- Teaching donning and doffing of prostheses
- Training in stump care
- Transfer training
- Training in activities of daily living

Cardiac Disease

Physical Therapy
- Patient education
- Conditioning and endurance exercises (walking, biking, etc)
- Breathing and relaxation exercises
- Strengthening and flexibility exercises
- Monitoring of patients' vital signs during exercise
- Stress management techniques
- Alternative interventions—Qi Gong, T'ai Chi, Yoga
- Refer for nutritional counseling

Occupational Therapy
- Labor-saving techniques
- Improving overall endurance for participation in activities of daily living
- Monitoring patients' participation in activities of daily living

Pulmonary Disease

Physical Therapy
- Patient education
- Breathing control exercises
- Chest physical therapy
- Conditioning exercises
- Joint mobilization of rib cage
- Relaxation and stress management techniques
- Alternative interventions that incorporate controlled breathing patterns—Yoga, Qi Gong, T'ai Chi, Feldenkrais

Occupational Therapy
- Training in labor-saving techniques
- Monitoring of participation in activities of daily living
- Improving endurance of upper extremities

Low Back Pain

Physical Therapy
- Joint mobilization/stabilization
- Modalities to decrease pain and improve tissue mobility

(continued)

TABLE 9–3.   (Continued)

- Strengthening and flexibility exercises
- Instruction in proper body mechanics for lifting, sitting, and sleeping
- Provision of proper shoe gear and shock-absorbing orthotics
- Correction of leg length discrepancy (when appropriate)
- Postural training for positioning
- Relaxation and stress management techniques
- Alternative approaches to encourage posture—Qi Gong, T'ai Chi, Yoga, Feldenkrais

Occupational Therapy
- Training in ergonomic techniques
- Training in energy conservation and positioning at rest

Alzheimer's Disease

Physical Therapy
- Sensory integration techniques
- Gait training (when appropriate)
- Balance activities
- Provision of proper shoe gear and orthotics
- General conditioning exercises
- Reality orientation activities/validation techniques
- Alternative interventions—dancing, hammock, T'ai Chi, Qi Gong

Occupational Therapy
- Sensory integration techniques
- Activities of daily living (grooming, feeding, etc)
- Reality orientation activities/validation techniques

Hip Fractures

Physical Therapy
- Range-of-motion, strengthening and conditioning exercises
- Positioning
- Progressive weight bearing and gait training
- Provision of assistive ambulation devices
- Provision of proper shoe gear, life on the involved side and orthotics for shock absorption
- Balance activities
- Transfer training
- Referral to nutritionist if presence of osteoporosis

fect produced in nerve cells by the introduction of an impulse. Thus, these techniques, though highly complex and requiring specialized training to employ, may simply be defined as methods of promoting or hastening the response of the neuromuscular mechanism through stimulation of the proprioceptors.[101]

The normal neuromuscular mechanism is capable of a wide range of motor activities within the limits of the anatomical structure, the developmental level, and inherent and previously learned neuromuscular responses. The normal neuromuscular mechanism becomes integrated and efficient without awareness of individual muscle action, reflex activity, and a multitude of other neurophysiological reactions. Variations occur in relation to coordination, strength, rate of movement, and endurance, but these variations do not prevent adequate response to the ordinary demands of life.

The deficient neuromuscular mechanism is inadequate to meet the demands of life in proportion to the degree of the deficiency. Responses may be limited in aged persons by the faulty neuromuscular response previously discussed as sequelae of the aging process, inactivity, trauma, or disease of the nervous or the musculoskeletal system.

Deficiencies present themselves in terms of limitation of movement as evidenced by weakness, incoordination, adaptive muscle or connective tissue shortening, or immobility of joints, muscle spasm, or spasticity. It is the deficient neuromuscular mechanism that becomes the concern of the rehabilitation team in a geriatric setting. These techniques are very useful in successfully retraining the neuromuscular system in the aged person. Specific demands placed on the patient by a physical or occupational therapist have a facilitating effect upon the individual's neuromuscular mechanism. The facilitating effects of these therapeutic exercises are the means used in physical and occupational therapy to reverse limitations of the aged person.[101]

A general measure to ensure the highest functional capacity should encourage early resumption of daily activities following trauma or acute illness. Safety measures to prevent falls and avoid accidents should include reinforcing the use of properly fitted shoes with good soles, low broad heels, and heel cups or orthotics to stabilize the foot during ambulation. The importance of wearing prescription eyeglasses needs to be stressed, and the staff and family should be educated in reducing potential hazards within the patient's living environment (decreasing the amount of furniture, securing all loose rugs and carpeting, obtaining a commode, installing handrails around the toilet and tub areas and railings in the hallways as needed). These are just a few examples of safety proofing the environment in which the elder lives so that individuals may function at their maximum level. Adaptive equipment to enhance the ease of activities of daily living is often a useful adjunct for gaining independence. Adapting the environment to improve safety is essential in geriatric rehabilitation and will be discussed more thoroughly in a subsequent section of this chapter.

Pain management is a very important factor in geriatric rehabilitation, but it is one of the most difficult pathophysiologic phenomena to define. Pain is human perception or recognition of a noxious stimulus. In geriatric rehabilitation two basic types of pain—acute and chronic—are dealt with. Chronic pain can be broken down even further into two subcategories—acute-chronic and chronic-chronic.

Treatment of acute pain may include medications to reduce inflammation, ice, heat, or compression (also to reduce edema when warranted), rest, and gentle mobility exercises (low-grade oscillation techniques of joint mobilization are very helpful in pain relief and maintenance of joint mobility). Rarely are modalities such as ultrasound or electrical currents (high galvanic current reduces edema, interferential current neutralizes the tissue and assists in fluid removal) used in the acute pain situation in the aged individual, although they are widely used in acute sports-related injuries in younger populations. The reasons for this are not documented, though the authors of this book clinical experience teaches that the more conservative approaches of rest, ice, compression or elevation, and gentle exercise in combination with nonnarcotic analgesics seem to be quite effective in treating acute pain in the older person.

Chronic pain is more frequently observed in the aged and is more difficult to control. Chronic pain may not always correspond with objective findings. It is well recognized that emotional and socioeconomic factors play a role in chronic pain. Tension and anxiety often lead to muscle tension and decreased activity, and this can be a viscious cycle. Situational depression may exacerbate this type of pain. In management of acute-chronic pain, such as the example of an acute osteoarthritic condition, treatment is similar to the acute pain management with the exception of the inclusion of various modalities. For instance, ultrasound may be used to break up a tissue adhesion, interferential or high galvanic electrical stimulation may be used to break up adhesions, reduce swelling, and enhance circulation to the painful area. Joint mobilization techniques are often employed to improve and maintain

mobility. Nonnarcotic analgesics can be prescribed, but the aged are more susceptible to the cumulative effects, as well as side effects, of the long-term use of these drugs.

Foot pain and/or discomfort from bony changes, such as those induced by lifelong use of ill-fitting shoes, arthritic changes, or age-related shifting of the fat pads under the heel and the metatarsal heads, can severely curtail the ambulatory abilities of the aged. Proper shoe gear and shock absorbing orthotics that place the foot in a neutral position have been clinically observed to facilitate ambulation and prevent disability.

Though few studies have documented this effect of reducing plantar foot pressures or altering the weight-bearing pattern of the foot during gait in aged individuals, this author has completed one study (currently unpublished) that clearly demonstrates a decrease in discomfort as a result of reduced pressure and alteration in the weight-bearing pattern and an increase in walking distance and functional capabilities. This has important ramifications in the area of geriatric rehabilitation.

Assistive devices, such as a cane, a quad cane (a more stable, four-legged cane), or a walker can also be prescribed to improve stability during ambulation and reduce the stresses on painful joint.

Wheelchair prescription may be necessary for longer distances (usually recommended for use outside the home) or when ambulation is no longer possible (e.g., in the case of a bilateral amputation or severe diabetic neuropathy). Wheelchairs should be prescribed to meet the specific needs of the aged individual. For instance, removable arms may be needed to enhance the ease of transfers, or elevating leg rests may be prescribed for lower extremity elevation when severe cardiac disease results in lower extremity edema.

Likewise, if advanced rheumatoid arthritis or quadriplegia limits upper extremity capabilities, an electric wheelchair will greatly improve an individual's capabilities of locomotion. Other considerations may be a one-arm manual drive chair for a hemiplegic or a "weighted" chair to shift the center of gravity and improve the stability of the chair in transfers for the bilateral amputee. This author often prescribes the use of golf-like carts or other motorized carts for community-dwelling elders to enhance their ability to move around town or long corridors in assisted living or senior housing environments. Though the older individual may be an independent ambulator within their home, the use of such a cart is a means of energy conservation when longer distances of locomotion are required. All of these considerations necessitate team approach in obtaining the equipment that best suits the individual's needs.

Proper positioning and seating for the aged individual who must sit for extended periods is required to decrease discomfort and keep pressures off of bony prominences, provide adequate postural support, facilitate feeding, and prevent progression of joint contractures and deformities. Many specialized chairs and adaptive positioning pads are on the market and address specific positioning needs. Armchairs which assist in rising from a seated position include higher chairs that decrease the work of the lower extremities for standing, or electric "ejection" chairs that actually extend to bring the individual to a near standing position. Functional assessment of the aged person is vital in the prescription of these specialized devices.

SPECIAL GERIATRIC REHABILITATION CONSIDERATIONS

While the present design of active rehabilitation programs, which involves learning and problem solving on the part of the aged individual, may not be realistic in severe dementias, such as that encountered in Alzheimer's disease, because of impaired cognition, inability to learn new tasks, and difficulty in cooperating or participating in a regimented physical exercise program, functional capabilities can be maintained. Refer to Chapter 12, Neurological Treatment Considerations, for a review of interventions in Alzheimer's disease and other dementias. Until the end stages of Alzheimer's, physical functioning remain relatively intact. It is the integration of movement, the motor planning (for instance, putting the sock on before the shoe), and the judgment required for safe functioning that becomes distorted.

The body communicates through its nervous system, which relays information and initiates motor activity. A breakdown in the system can lead to less-efficient communication and a slowing of the body's responses. Thus, it is important to consider the degenerative effects on the body of an aging nervous system. Neuromuscular changes with aging include deficits in coordination, strength, and speed of motion.

Changes in the sensory system with age provide less information to the CNS, which results from decrease in sensory perception. With loss of sensory input in combination with dementia of any degree, the aged individual is less able to assess their environment accurately, and this leads to incorrect choices. Diminished hearing can also lead to incorrect choices due to inaccurately received and perceived communications. As a result of normal aging, we will all experience changes in our ability to hear. For example, older individuals experience a decreased ability to separate one sound or voice from background noises. Specific effects of aging on the auditory system include a decrease in auditory acuity and poorer speech discrimination skills based on their pure tonal losses.[102] In other words, as the ear ages, there is a greater distortion of auditory signals. In the aged person with dementia, these changes can add to confusion. Sensory losses and cognitive impairments, in addition to physical changes associated with aging, need to be given special consideration in

geriatric rehabilitation (specific interventions will be discussed in the subsequent section on adapting the environment).

With aging there is a loss of neurons. Neurons are postmitotic cells and do not duplicate themselves.[103] This cell loss results in the narrowing of the convolutions and widening of the sulci in the aging brain. In fact, brain mass itself decreases by 10% to 20% by 90 years of age.[104] The areas of the brain that show the greatest loss of neurons with normal aging are the frontal lobe (which is the area of cognition), the superior area of the temporal lobe (the main auditory area), the occipital area (the visual area), and the prefrontal gyrus (the major sensorimotor area of the brain).[105] A loss of neurons can be equated with a decrease in function if the losses are significant in any one area of the brain, and the rehabilitation of an elderly individual is directly affected by these changes. In the special case of Alzheimer's patients, the transcortical pathways are affected by the disease process and result in an inability to integrate activity. For instance, normally aging individuals know instinctively to alternate feet when walking. This may not be an automatic response of an individual with Alzheimer's disease, especially in the later stages of the disease. (See Chapter 12.) Compensation for cognitive, hearing and visual decrements should be incorporated into rehabilitation programs (these changes will be readdressed in the subsequent section on adapting the environment).

Diminished tactile sense often accompanies aging. Although vision and hearing are the predominant means of communication, touch is an important physical sensoricommunicator and should be considered when designing a rehabilitation program for aged patients. Information from receptors in muscles, joints, and the inner ear aid in movement and positioning. Decreased kinesthetic sensitivity owing to a general slowing and loss of receptor sensitivity with aging results in postural instability and difficulty in reacting to bodily changes in space.

Muscle strength determined by neurological function is defined by the rate of motor unit firing, the number and frequency of motor unit recruitment, and the cross-sectional diameter of the muscle.[42] The effects of the aging process on the neuromuscular system are seen clinically in deterioration of strength, speed, motor coordination, and gait. Muscular atrophy may be attributed to a decrease in the number of muscle fibers as previously described.[106] Other changes include a decrease in the clear differentiation of fiber type functioning.[107,108] It has been suggested that muscle weakness in aging is a result of the replacement of skeletal muscle by fibrous tissue rather than free fat,[109] however, there is great variability in loss of strength. Despite the obvious relationship between neuromuscular changes and loss of strength, disuse appears to play a very important role.[42] Changes in lifestyle as one ages apparently contribute to disuse of the muscles. As a result, aging changes of the muscle system closely parallel those discussed in the section on activity versus inactivity.[110]

Activity not only decreases but slows with aging and with disuse, and the elderly exhibit slower reaction times. Nerve conduction velocity decreases at approximately 0.4% per year starting at 20 years of age,[104] but reaction time is a complex response pattern to measure. The pathways involved include CNS processing, afferent nerve pathways, and the effector organ (muscles). Sensory stimuli and cognitive functioning are intimately involved in reaction time, and these factors must be considered when developing a rehabilitation program for the aged.

There are significant differences between the young and the old on tests measuring coordination and fine motor skills.[111] An increase in "sway" as a normal balance correction that diminishes the ability to maintain balance is observed in the aged population. As a result, gait changes are observed. To compensate for the loss of balance, a wide base of support (a greater distance between feet) is frequently employed. Declines in sensory input due to inactivity also lead to sensorimotor deficits, which alter gait in other ways.

Neurologic assessment must include psychologic factors and physiologic pathologies. The changes seen in the aging nervous system compound disabilities resulting from physiologic or cognitive decline. (Refer to Chapter 12.)

Musculoskeletal changes that occur with aging influence flexibility, strength, posture, and gait. Functional changes in lifestyle and activity add to these age-related changes. (See Chapter 11.)

Collagen, the supportive protein in skin, tendon, bone, cartilage, and connective tissue changes with aging.[97] The collagen fibers become irregular in shape as a result of increased cross-linking, and this decreases the elasticity of the collagen fibers, decreasing the mobility of all the body tissues.

Inactivity, too, has been shown to decrease muscle and tendon flexibility. Full immobilization in bed results in loss of approximately 3% per day of strength.[104] Increased time spent in sitting significantly affects the body's flexor muscles, as adhesions are more likely to develop if the flexors of the body are maintained in a shortened position for extended periods of time. This has been observed in studies of astronauts, which demonstrate the relationship between what we know to result from aging, and the effects of "disuse."[49]

A decrease in lean muscle mass and changes in muscular function result from a variety of factors, including a decrease in efficiency of the cardiovascular system to deliver nutrients and oxygen to the working muscles and changes in the chemical composition of the muscle. Glycoproteins, which produce an osmotic force important in maintaining the fluid content of muscle tissues, are reduced in aging.[112] The inability of the muscle tissues to retain fluid, causes the

hypotrophic changes observed in aging muscles, and there is a decrease in the permeability of the muscle cell membrane, which makes the cell less efficient. At rest, high concentrations of potassium, magnesium, and phosphate ions are found in the sarcoplasm, while sodium, chloride, and bicarbonate ions are prevented from entering the cell. In the senescent muscle there is a shift in this resting balance with a decrease in potassium. Lack of potassium in the aging muscle reduces the maximum force of contractions generated by the muscle.[108] Clinically, tiredness and lethargy result from a depletion of potassium stores.

A decrease in total bone mass is a characteristic change with age. Osteoporosis is the result of progression of this loss past the threshold of what is considered normal (see Chapter 11 for bone mass density measurements). Four times more women than men, including 30% of women over the age of 65 years, are osteoporotic.[104] The older the person and the poorer the nutritional history, the greater the risk for this condition. Hormonal changes (as seen with menopause in women and andropause in men) and circulatory changes (as seen with decreased activity) also play a role. Though often asymptomatic, osteoporosis can be a major cause of pain, fractures, and postural changes in the musculoskeletal system.[42]

Balance, flexibility, and strength provide the posture necessary to ensure efficient ambulation. In aging, poor posture results from a decline in flexibility and strength and from bony changes in the vertebral spine, resulting in less safe gait patterns. Gait is the functional application of motion. Changes in the gait cycle seen in the elderly include (1) mild rigidity (greater proximally than distally), producing less body movement; (2) fewer automatic movements with a decreased amplitude and speed (such as arm swing); (3) less accuracy of foot placement and speed of cadence (step rate per minute); (4) shorter steps due to changes in kinesthetic sense and slower rate of motor unit firing; (5) wider stride width (broad-based gait) in an attempt to enhance safety; (6) decrease in swing-to-stance ratio, which improves safety by allowing more time in the double support phase (i.e., both feet in contact with the ground at the same time); (7) decrease in vertical displacement which is the up and down movement created by pushing off from the toes for forward propulsion and the alternate heel strike, usually secondary to stiffness (a distinct push-off and heel strike are not observed in the aged); (8) decrease in toe-to-floor clearance; (9) decrease in excursion of the leg during swing phase; (10) decrease in the heel-to-floor angle (usually due to the lack of flexibility of the plantar flexor muscles and weakness of dorsiflexors); (11) slower cadence (another safety mechanism); and (12) decrease in velocity of limb motions during gait.[42]

Exercise is a physical stimulus, which produces a metabolic increase above the resting levels of vital signs. In a healthy, young individual, the cardiovascular system responds quickly to increase the metabolic rate by increasing heart rate, stroke volume (the amount of blood delivered to the system with each heartbeat), and peripheral blood flow to deliver oxygen to the working muscles. In the aged, response time of the cardiovascular system is delayed in restoring homeostasis when the level of physical activity has been increased.[49] The aged have a lower resting cardiac output and basal metabolic rate primarily due to age-related loss of lean body mass[97] and inactivity.[49] Heart rate and stroke volume decrease 0.7% per year after 30 years of age, decreasing from approximately 5L/min at 30 years to 3.5L/min at 75 years. As exercise levels increase, this is manifest as reduced oxygen uptake.[110] In respiration there is a 50% decrease in the maximum volume of ventilation and 40% decrease in the vital capacity by the age of 85.[104] These limitations in oxygen transport capability translate directly into a reduced physical work capacity.

Understanding and managing the patient's sensation of fatigue is essential in any exercise program. Fatigue, a word understood by everyone, lacks precise definition. Darling[113] likened the concept of fatigue to the concept of pain. Both must be considered from physiologic and psychologic points of view. Physiologic types of fatigue include "muscle" fatigue from prolonged use of a muscle group, "circulatory" fatigue associated with elevated blood lactate levels during prolonged activity, and "metabolic" fatigue in which exercise depletes glycogen (energy) stores. General fatigue is related to more subtle factors like interest, reward, and motivation.

Given these definitions, it is easy to understand why a deconditioned person can experience fatigue. From a treatment perspective it is essential to determine what sensation the aged individual is describing as fatigue. Elevated vital signs and progressively weak muscle contractions suggest that rest is needed. A vaguer complaint of fatigue in the absence of these changes would not necessarily be a basis for reducing exercise. In fact, poor aerobic fitness may be related to an otherwise healthy aged person's complaint of fatigue.[114]

One therapeutic principle we often use successfully in motivating elderly individuals is to not give them instructions that include specific times or numbers of repetitions. For instance, "do this exercise for as long as you feel comfortable and then stop and rest." Or, "lift this weight as many times as you feel comfortable lifting it and then stop and rest." This omits the potential for failing by not making it to the prescribed time or number of repetitions. The authors of this book find that once a specific "number" is not looming in front of the older exerciser, fatigue does not set in as readily. They no longer have markers (i.e., "I'm halfway there.") by which to measure, so the task becomes less ominous and never results in failure.

Another principle that works well with the older adult exerciser is the communication rule of exercise.

Rather than having the patient focus on vital sign monitoring (which the clinician can do during assessment and evaluation), the level of exercise is based on the ability to speak. Mild exercise that is not aerobic results in the individual's ability to carry on a fluid conversation without shortness of breath. Moderate exercise, or exercise in the submaximal aerobic range, results in more staccato sentences with frequent pauses for breath. In other words, the individual can speak but would rather not. The maximal exercise range, which you rarely want to take an individual into, results in the inability to speak. This is the range that mountain climbers in low oxygen environments find themselves in. In the maximal range, all air inhaled is needed for the provision of oxygen to the working muscles.

What should be the prescribed level of exercise in an older adult? This will be based on the elder's overall physical, physiological, emotional, and cognitive condition. However, a good rule of thumb in activity and exercise in the elderly is *anything above rest works.*

In providing activity and exercise programs for the aged, normal aging changes in the musculoskeletal, neuromuscular, cardiovascular and pulmonary systems will affect functional capacity. In addition, confusion, decreased sensory awareness, postural changes, cardiovascular limitations resulting from deconditioning, motivation, and perceived level of fatigue all affect the potential for rehabilitation and need to be assessed prior to implementing activity or exercise programs. Specific exercise recommendations are included in the chapters specific to each system (e.g., Chapters 11 through 14).

NUTRITIONAL CONSIDERATIONS

Nutrition in the aged has been covered extensively in Chapter 7. Nutrition is reviewed here only as it impacts functional capabilities.

A car needs gas in order to run; a human being needs adequate energy sources in order to function on an optimal level. Nutritional levels need close monitoring in relation to energy needs and functional activity levels. Increased feeding difficulties may be secondary to decreased appetite, poor oral status, visual or sensorimotor agnosia, cognitive declines (decreasing attentiveness), and physical limitations. Environmental cues and adaptive eating equipment can often be employed to facilitate feeding. Postural considerations need to be addressed as well. A poor sitting posture can further decrease the ease of feeding by preventing upper extremity movement or making chewing and swallowing difficult as a result of head position. For example, an elderly woman with severe osteoporosis and resulting kyphosis is at a postural disadvantage for feeding. Seated in an upright chair, her entire upper trunk will be forced forward and her face directed downward. Gravity only serves to allow the food to drop out of her mouth, especially if dentures are loose, she is edentulous, or oral motor skills are compromised.

Specialized feeding programs may be necessitated if there is neuromuscular involvement. For instance, an aged person sustaining a cerebral vascular accident may have difficulty swallowing or closing the mouth due to weakness in the muscles needed for these activities. In these cases, specialized muscle facilitation techniques can be employed to promote swallowing and facilitate mouth closure. What is commonly termed a "dysphasia team," made up of nursing, dietary, speech, physical, and occupational therapy, can comprehensively address the feeding needs of a neurologically involved individual. In the geriatric rehabilitation setting, this team is a vital component in obtaining maximal functional capabilities. They function to promote adequate nutrition through neuromuscular facilitation techniques, proper posturing and supportive seating, and adaptive eating utensils. Ultimately the goal of this team is to permit independent feeding by the aged person.

RESTRAINTS

The use of physical restraints, in an attempt to keep patients safe, continues to be practiced despite evidence that restraints often increase the incidence of falls.[115] Decreasing the use of physical restraints continues to be a challenge for the health care team. It is important to understand the law regarding restraints as well as the risks, benefits, and implications for their use. This section of the chapter addresses regulations, types of restraints, documentation, and alternatives to the use of restraints.

The Omnibus Budget Reconciliation Act (OBRA) states that "a patient has the right to be free from any physical or chemical restraints imposed for purposes of discipline or convenience, and not required to treat the resident's medical symptoms."[116] By this statement, OBRA did not mandate an environment free of restraints but placed restrictions on the use of physical or mechanical devices that are not medically necessary. Despite OBRA guidelines, restraints still rank in the top 10 of the Center for Medicare and Medicaid's Service's (CMS—formerly Health Care Finance Administration [HCFA]) list of most commonly cited deficiencies in long-term care facilities.

The reasons given by long-term care team members for the use of physical restraints are numerous: to prevent injury to self and other residents; control of agitated or restless behavior; management of a resident's cognitive deficit and poor judgment; mobility impairments placing the resident at risk for falls; and resistance to medical treatment. Although these may seem to be noble support statements, there are a number of risks associated with physical restraints. A list of benefits and risks associated with the use of restraints is provided in Table 9–4.

TABLE 9–4. BENEFITS AND RISKS OF PHYSICAL RESTRAINTS

Benefits of Restraints

- Prevention/protection from falls and other accidents or injuries
- Allows medical treatment to proceed without patient interference
- Maintenance of body alignment
- Increases patient's feeling of security and safety
- Protects other patients and staff from physical harm

Risks of Restraints

- Injury from falls
- Accidental death by strangulation
- Skin abrasions and breakdown
- Immobilization sequelae (deconditioning, muscle atrophy, contractures, osteoporosis, orthostatic hypotention, deep vein thrombosis, pneumonia, incontinence)
- Decline in ADLs, functional mobility
- Cardiac stress
- Increased mortality
- Dehydration, reduced appetite
- Disorganized behavior
- Social/emotional isolation

Physical restraints affect a number of aspects of the elderly person's life in the institutional setting. A great deal of research has investigated the association of restraint use with other parameters such as falls, cognition, and activities of daily living impairment. Phillips[117] found that residents in long-term care facilities with the poorest ADL function were more likely to be restrained. A balance problem further increased this likelihood. Ejaz and colleagues[115] compared a restrained group who underwent restraint reduction to a nonrestrained group. They found that serious falls, resulting in hematoma, fracture, or loss of consciousness, did not increase in the restraint reduction group although non-serious falls did (i.e., those requiring first aid, cuts, bruises). Rate of falls in the experimental group, however, matched but did not exceed the rate of falls in the control group. This provides some evidence to dispel the myth that untying the elderly would increase serious falls.

In order for the long-term care team to reduce restraints, it is important to understand which devices are considered restraints and the implications of their use. CMS interpretive guidelines define a physical restraint as "any manual method or physical or mechanical device, material or equipment attached to or adjacent to the resident's body, which the individual cannot remove easily, that restricts freedom of movement or normal access to one's body."[118] Further, the guidelines state that physical restraints include leg, arm and vest restraints, hand mitts, soft ties, binding a resident who is bedbound by tucking sheets in tightly, bedrails, and chairs that prevent rising.

"Devices on clothing that trigger electronic alarms to warn staff that a resident is leaving a room"[118] are not necessarily considered restraints, according to the guidelines. This definition, although helpful, often leaves the long-term care team with questions regarding the proper use of restraints. The following is information and recommended practice for a number of physical restraints.

Side rails are often utilized to keep an individual from falling out of bed and to deter attempts to get out of the bed. A number of deleterious effects have been cited due to the use of side rails. These negative consequences include increasing the distance one falls from the bed, obstruction of vision, creating noise, trauma if the body strikes the side rails, creating a sense of being trapped, and dislodging/pulling tubes during raising and lowering.[119] Donius and Radar[119] recommend a thorough risk level assessment to determine necessity of side rail use. Table 9–5 is an example of a risk level assessment for the use of side rails.

Vest, waist, pelvic and extremity tie-on devices are generally considered to be restraints. These types of restraints should rarely be used and only if alternatives have failed. Further, they should be used for only brief periods of time.

Position change and body alarm devices in and of themselves are not considered restraints, however, if the staff responds to the sound of the alarm by restricting the resident's mobility (i.e., making the resident sit back down when attempting to stand up rather than addressing needs), then the facility's response would be considered restrictive.

Reclining wheelchairs and geri chairs are considered restraints when they restrict a resident's normal mobility and require a physician's order for use. Lap

cushions or trays, wheelchair bars, and seatbelts can be restraints if the resident is unable to remove these devices independently. Lap cushions and trays particularly are not restraints if they are used to provide support for residents who do not attempt to stand or lean forward. Wedge cushions that raise residents' feet off the floor if they propel a wheelchair or that limit their ability to stand would be considered a restraint.

A number of restraint alternatives have been proposed for various resident impairments. Cohen[120] found the most common restraint-reducing alternatives to include wedge cushions, wheelchair modifications (e.g., lowering seats, footrests, etc.), and physical and occupational therapy consultation to improve functional mobility and safety through exercise and activity. This author has successfully employed a seated hammock in cognitively compromised patients who are at risk for falls because of sundowning, pacing, or both. Placed in a calming environment (e.g., paying attention to noise, activity, and colors) the hammock serves to soothe the typically confused and anxious patient. Hung so that the front edge of the hammock is 18 inches from the floor, an elderly individual with fair or better quadriceps strength can easily arise from the hammock. The seated hammock has been used on Alzheimer's units for well over a decade, and anecdotal experience reveals a high level of success in calming and protecting these patients from falls without restraining them.

Regardless of whether a device considered a restraint is used or a restraint alternative is found, appropriate documentation is necessary. The Food and Drug Administration (FDA) recommends that each facility define and communicate an institutional policy for restraints and that restraints are removed at least every two hours for ADLs. Further, documentation in the chart for use of restraints should include the medical reason for the restraint; the type of restraint selected; and the time frame for use.[121] When a restraint is used, a physician's order is necessary.

A responsible party should sign a consent form that explains the benefits and risks of the restraint. Restraints and restraint alternatives can be determined and documented in the context of a team restraint committee consisting of social services, physical and occupational therapy, appropriate nursing staff, the administrator, and the physician if available. Consultants to the team may include the pharmacist and nutritionist.

The use of physical restraints has become a concern for nursing home caregivers due to the OBRA guidelines and accusations of elderly abuse. The most common definition of a physical restraint is "any device placed on or near one's body to limit freedom of voluntary movement or normal access to one's own purpose." It is easy to say, "no restraints"; however, there are circumstances for use and emergency procedures. A fundamental ethical dilemma occurs as well as a caregiver's responsibility to pro-

TABLE 9–5.   RISK LEVEL ASSESSMENT FOR USE OF SIDE RAILS ON BED

Level I: Low Risk

Side rails are not necessary for residents in this group. They may be used because of the person's preference but are not considered restraints. Residents at this level are able to get into and out of bed without assistance and safely, or do not move without staff assistance.

Level II: Moderate Risk

These residents have the desire to get into and out of bed unassisted but lack the ability to do so safely. These residents need side rails or an alternative if side rails are not used. Side rails are then considered restraints and need a physician's order.

Level III: High Risk

Side rails are used to restrict movement of these residents because there are no alternatives, alternatives have failed, or the benefit of using side rails outweighs the burden. Side rails are then considered restraints and need a physician's order.

Donius and Radar (see ref 119)

tect the patient. Initiation of a restraint should be a team effort, and the removal of restraints should also be a team process to give the resident the least restrictive device. Finding appropriate options to maintain safety and mobility for the residents of long-term care institutions continues to be a challenge. Only through a coordinated team approach can we decrease the use of restraints in the institutional setting. A guiding principle is to "use restraint before using restraints" and to be creative in finding alternatives.

FALLS IN THE ELDERLY

Falls are not part of the normal aging process, but are due to an interaction of underlying physical dysfunction, medications, and environmental hazards.[122] Poor health status, impaired mobility from inactivity or chronic illness, postural instability, and a history of previous falls are observable risk factors. The ultimate goals of rehabilitation are to combat the inactivity and loss of mobility that predisposes to falls.

Some of the ad hoc measures currently used to prevent falls, such as physical restraints and medications to reduce activity, are now suspected of increasing the risk of falling.[122]

Medical conditions are often a cause of falling. A pathological fracture secondary to severe osteoporosis may result in a fall (rather than the fracture resulting from the fall), or an arrhythmia may induce dizziness. Certain drugs, such as digoxin used in treating an arrhythmia, may also induce dizziness or fatigued (see Chapter 8 for tables listing drugs that cause adverse side effects that may result in falls in the elderly).

The fear of falling is often a cause for inactivity and is commonly seen in an individual who has sustained a previous fall. It must be noted here that older individuals may not have experienced a fall themselves, but may limit their activity because their neighbor fell. Their observation of the sequelae of events experienced by their neighbor makes them fearful of having the same thing happen in their life. As a result, they limit their activities and the activities they do are guarded. The guarding patterns that aged individuals use as a result of this fear (e.g., grabbing furniture that may not be stable or supportive) may in fact lead to further danger. Intervention by a psychiatrist or psychologist is often necessitated to diminish this fear.

Functionally, limitations of range of motion, decreased muscle strength and joint mobility, coordination problems, or gait deviations can predispose an elderly individual to falling. Specific strengthening and gait training programs assist in preventing falls by improving overall strength and coordination, balance responses and reaction time, and awareness of safe ambulation practices (for example, freeing one hand for use of a handrail when carrying packages up the stairs). Some individuals will have inadequate

strength and balance to ambulate without an assistive device, or assistive ambulatory devices may also provide a safer mode for locomotion. Walking aids, such as canes and walkers, are beneficial for prevention of falls in some cases,[123] whereas, in other cases, they actually contribute to the cause of the fall.[124] Assess the appropriateness of the assistive device, and ensure that the aged individual is using it properly. With proper instruction, patients can usually function safely within their environment without falling.

Gait evaluation is one of the most important components in fall prevention. The "get up and go" test is a method used often to test functional strength, balance, coordination, and safety during gait. The aged individual is asked to get up out of the chair without using their hands, walk approximately twenty feet down the hall, turn around, come back to the chair, and then stand still. While the patient is standing still with the eyes closed, the rehabilitation therapist can give a gentle push on the sternum to test the patient's righting reflexes. Finally, the individual is directed to sit down without the use of their hands. Each component of the test is analyzed. For instance, the inability to arise from the chair without the assistance of the hands is indicative of hip extensor, quadriceps weakness, or both. If step symmetry is absent (i.e., if the individual is taking irregular steps), the cause can often be pinpointed just by observation. A leg length discrepancy may be present or the hip abductors may be weak. These alterations in anatomical structure or muscle status can easily be determined by close evaluation of the gait pattern. Lower extremity pain may also result in nonrhythmical steps as the individual attempts to avoid the painful extremity. Tendencies to veer, lose balance, or hold on to surrounding objects may be indicative of dizziness, muscle weakness or poor vision. A loss of balance while turning or a stiff, disjointed turn may alert the clinician to the possibility of neurological disorders, such as Parkinson's disease or drug-induced muscle rigidity (often seen in aged individuals on haloperidol or other psychotropic medications).

With good basic education for the patient and the family and modification of the environment to reduce hazards, it is possible to prevent falls through methods that do not undermine mobility or autonomy. It is important to identify and treat reversible medical conditions, as well as physical impairments in gait and balance. Many falls can be prevented through: proper exercise to maintain strength; sensory integration techniques to promote all functional activities by improving balance and coordination; good shoes and orthotics to provide a proper base of support and gait training activities; and modifications to safety proof the living environment.

Rehabilitation specialists have an important role in recommending interventions to prevent falls. When disease states and medications responses are stable, an individualized program of safety education, environmental adaptations, lower extremity strengthening exercises, balance exercises, and gait training should be implemented.

Safety education is an important first step in the prevention of falls. Many older individuals are not aware that they are at risk for falling. Often, simple instructions about environmental adaptations and encouraging a person to allow plenty of time for functional activities are all that is needed to facilitate their safety. Many aged people feel the need to rush to answer a phone or doorbell. They should be discouraged from rushing, because that could result in a fall. Caregivers and visitors should also be a part of the safety education process. They are often able to remind the person who is at risk for falling of the need for added precaution.

Aged persons who complain of dizziness during changes of position should be evaluated for postural hypotension. These individuals should be taught to change positions slowly and to wait before moving to another position in order to allow the blood pressure to accommodate to the change.

Any individual who has fallen is at risk for falling again. In fact, clustering of falls has been seen in some older individuals during the months preceding death.[125] Inability to rise or lack of assistance after a fall can produce devastating consequences. In one study, half of the aged persons who lay on the floor for longer than six hours after a fall died within six months.[126] Having a phone in every room or obtaining a cellular phone may be a necessity for aged persons who live alone. A "buddy system" in which older persons call each other regularly during the day is a means of "checking up" and early detection of a fall. In a community program that this author is involved in (described in Chapter 15 on Screening and Prevention Programs), firemen from each township have been enlisted to call elders living alone (in their respective communities) twice each day. As firemen, who hopefully are cooking at the station rather than fighting fires, generally have the time to attend to this task (in addition to being skilled at responding to an emergency when one occurs), this program has been extremely successful in early detection and response to falls in the elderly. Individuals at risk can also be provided with a device such as the "life-line," that summons emergency personnel by pushing a button.

Eighty-five percent of all falls occur at home,[127] most commonly on stairs,[128] on the way to and from the bathroom,[129,130] and in the bedroom.[131] Environmental evaluation and adaptation is needed for those aged individuals who have fallen or are at risk for falling. Table 9–6 presents a safety check list for use in the home.[127]

Safety evaluation should address such questions as, "Are the carpets tacked down?" "Is the pathway from the bed to the bathroom obstacle free?" and "Is there night time lighting?" Additional environmental suggestions include adaptive equipment for the shower or bathtub (i.e., using a tub seat and a hand held showerhead can improve safety and independence while bathing). Adaptations may also be necessary in order to avoid falls in route to the bathroom. Individuals with urinary urgency, evening fatigue, or disorientation in the middle of the night should be encouraged to use a bedside commode.

The purpose of strengthening exercises to prevent falls is to provide adequate force production of the lower extremities and trunk muscles for support of posture and control of balance. Some aged individuals will tolerate a progressive resistive exercise program. Others will derive greater benefit from a more functional approach to strengthening exercises. For example, practicing sit-to-stand movements and the reverse is a functional means of strengthening extensors and flexors of the lower extremity. Going up and down stairs one stair at a time requires less strength, range of motion, and balance than walking step over step. A functional way to progress this activity, then, is to begin with one stair at a time and progress to step over step. Marching in place while standing can also be a lower extremity flexor strengthening activity. It can be progressed by asking the individual to hold the leg in flexion for a count of three or for as long as they feel comfortable. During this activity, isometric strengthening also occurs in the extensors, abductors, and adductors of the stance leg. Aged individuals should hold on to the back of a chair or the rim of the kitchen counter during this exercise for safety.

No matter which approach is selected for strengthening, the following precautions are recommended:

- Many aged individuals suffer from osteoporosis. Resistance and unilateral weight bearing may be excessive for them. It is possible to fracture an osteoporotic bone during strengthening exercises.
- Many aged individuals have osteoarthritis. Isometric exercise may be less painful for them. Prolonging the amount of time that the contraction is held is an effective way to increase strength without adding external resistance.[132]
- It is especially important for aged individuals to avoid holding their breath (Valsalva maneuver) during exercise. Counting out loud helps to avoid this problem.
- The aged individual should be taught to monitor their heart rate during exercise.

Therapeutic exercises designed to improve balance are an important part of fall prevention. Balance exercises address three areas of posture control: response to perturbation, weight shifting, and anticipatory adjustments to limb movements.[133] Individuals must be able to respond to an external perturbation, such as a push to the shoulder or sternum, with a postural adjustment that brings the center of gravity back over the base of support. The usual response to a lateral perturbation will be extension of the weight-bearing leg along with elongation of the trunk on the weight-

TABLE 9–6. HOME ASSESSMENT CHECKLIST - PREVENTION OF FALLS

Exterior

Are step surfaces nonslip?

Are step edges visibly marked to avoid tripping?

Are stairway handrails present? Are handrails secure?

Are walkways covered with a nonslip surface and free of objects that could be tripped over?

Is there sufficient outdoor lighting to provide safe ambulation at night?

Interior

Are lights bright enough to compensate for limited vision?

Are light switches accessible before entering a room?

Are lights glare free?

Are handrails present on both sides of staircases?

Are stairways adequately lit?

Are handrails securely fastened to walls?

Are step edges outlined with colored adhesive tape and nonslip?

Are throw rugs secured with nonslip backing?

Are carpet edges taped or tacked down?

Are rooms uncluttered to permit unobstructed mobility?

Are chairs throughout home strong enough to provide support during transfers? Are armrests present?

Are tables (dining room, kitchen) strong enough to lean on?

Do low-lying objects (coffee tables, stools) present a hazard?

Are telephones accessible?

Kitchen

Are storage areas easily reached without standing on tiptoes or a chair?

Are linoleum floor slippery?

Is there a nonslip mat in front of sink to soak up spilled water?

Are chairs wheelfree, armrest equipped, and of the proper height to allow for safe transfers?

If the pilot light goes out, is odor strong enough to alert the person?

Are step stools strong enough to provide support?

Are stool treads strong, in good repair, and slip resistant?

Bathroom

Are doors wide enough to accommodate assistive devices?

Do door thresholds present tripping hazards?

Are floor slippery, especially when wet?

Are skid-proof strips or mats in place in tub or shower?

Are tub and toilet bars available? Are they well secured?

Are toilets low in height? Is an elevated toilet seat available?

Is there sufficient, accessible, and glare-free light available?

Bedroom

Is there adequate, accessible lighting? Are there nightlights and/or bedside lamps available?

Is the pathway from the bed to the bathroom unobstructed?

Are beds of appropriate height for safe transfers on and off?

Are floors covered with a nonslip surface and obstacle free?

Can individual reach objects on closet shelves without standing on tiptoes or a chair?

Adapted from Tideiksaar, R (1987) Tideiksaar F. Fall prevention in the home. *Top Geriatr Rehabil.* 1987; 3:57.

bearing side. Flexion and abduction of the nonweight-bearing leg will also be seen.[134] A small backward force should stimulate the reaction of the dorsiflexors at the ankles and flexion at the hips, whereas a small forward push should be followed by plantarflexion at the ankles and extension at the hips.[135]

Weight shifting of the entire body during standing involves muscular activity similar to that used in response to a perturbation; however, during weight shifting, the muscle activation occurs voluntarily. Balance must also be controlled when a limb movement occurs, such as reaching with the upper extremity or swinging with the lower extremity. In this case, the postural adjustment actually occurs in anticipation of the limb movement, in order to prevent the center of gravity from moving outside of the base of support. For example, a forward movement of the arm should be preceded by ankle plantar flexion and hip extension. In this way, a small backward movement of the center of gravity counteracts the forward displacement caused by the moving arm. Practicing each of these activities, that is, response to perturbation, voluntary weight shifting, and postural adjustments in anticipation of limb movement in standing, will help prepare the aged individual to use postural adjustment effectively during functional standing activities, such as cooking, transfers, and ambulation. These activities are directed toward improvement of the motor component of balance.

Altering the sensory conditions during balance activities encourages the aged person to attend to support surface or visual information selectively. Balancing in bare feet with eyes open or closed helps maximize the amount of somatosensory information that is available from the soles of the feet. On the other hand, balancing while standing on a piece of foam[136] disrupts information from the sole of the foot and from stretch receptors in the ankle muscles and forces the individual to practice using visual input to stabilize posture. Maintaining balance while turning the head from side to side or nodding the head is also important. Many aged people report falling during head movements,[137] while looking up to hang curtains, while getting the cereal off the second shelf in the cabinet, or while changing a lightbulb. Aged individuals should be instructed to use caution during upward head movements.

When an individual is unable to control standing balance and is about to fall, the normal response is protective extension of the arms or legs. Protective reactions, such as arm extension and the stepping response, should also be practiced. Upper extremity protective extension can be practiced both forward and sideways against the wall in the standing position.[138] Lower extremity protective reactions should be practiced in standing in forward, sideways, and backward directions. Brisk and accurately directed limb extension is the goal.

Balance exercises can be incorporated into functional activities for the aged. Moving from sit-to-stand

and from stand-to-sit are examples of controlled voluntary weight shifting. Shifting the trunk forward and back and from side to side while sitting are also examples of voluntary weight shifting. Voluntary weight shifting while standing with the back to a wall is a safe way to facilitate control of balance. Dancing has also been recommended as a functional activity to improve balance for prevention of falls.[139] T'ai Chi and Qi Gong exercise, because of the slow, controlled movements beyond the center of gravity, have also been shown to substantially improve balance and postural stability in the elderly.[140,141] Postural adjustments in anticipation of arm movements can be practiced during functional activities by standing and reaching for objects on the kitchen or closet shelves. Reaching should be practiced in a variety of directions.

Ambulation requires weight shifting. Manual guidance during ambulation helps organize the time and direction of weight shifting.[49,138] Functional ambulation requires interaction with a variety of different support surfaces, therefore, it should be practiced on smooth as well as uneven surfaces and on level as well as inclines, curbs, and stairs. Varying the amount of available light and background noise also stimulates realistic environmental conditions. If step lengths are irregular, footprints on the floor make good targets for foot placement.[142]

Manual guidance is also useful for improving ambulation speed. A variety ambulation speeds is necessary for function. Challenging activities, like crossing a busy street, can be made less threatening if the aged individual practices with the therapist or caregiver.

An area of intervention which is commonly overlooked (or avoided) in working on balance and falls in the elderly, is teaching an elder *how* to fall, and more importantly, *how* to get back up from the floor. It is helpful to use the thick track and field mats used for the high bar and pole vault jumps. These mats are at least 18 inches thick and provide sufficient protection during a fall. Aquatic falling is also helpful. In both instances, the elderly individual can practice falling knowing they will land on a soft and forgiving medium. The key to falling is *relaxation*. As many readers have learned in ski school, if an individual tries to stop a fall, she or he is more likely to be rigid when meeting the ground, and much more likely to sustain an injury. Conversely, it the individual relaxes into the fall, they will more likely roll with impact and sustain the least amount of injury.

Difficulty rising from the floor after a fall is common in older adults and is associated with substantial morbidity.[143] This tends to be an underappreciated problem, one which is rarely addressed when working with the elderly. In a study by Tinetti and colleagues[143] only 49% of community-dwelling fallers were able to get up after a fall without assistance. Interestingly, most of the falls associated with the inability to get up without help (85%) were not associated with serious injury.[143] Thus, the inability to get up after a fall is common and not simply a conse-

quence of a fall-related injury. Up to 20% of fallers remain on the floor for one hour or more,[144] and dehydration, pressure sores, muscle injury, and renal failure may be associated with long periods of time spent on the floor following a fall. Fear of falling appears to be increased in previous fallers, particularly those with a history of difficulty rising alone after a fall.[145] Despite the high risk of difficulty in rising from the floor after a fall, few therapists teach older adults how to rise from the floor.[146]

Some researchers have analyzed the motions used to rise from a supine position on the floor to a standing position,[147,148] finding that movement patterns differ somewhat as age increases[149] and when comparing sedentary to physically active adults.[150] Few studies have included healthy or frail older adults, however, Alexander and associates[144] investigated the ability of older adults in rising from the floor and explored how rising ability might differ based on initial body position and with or without the use of an assistive device. The findings from this study were that older adults (in their sixth and seventh decades of life) have more difficulty rising from the floor regardless of initial body position compared to younger adults, and it takes two to three times longer to accomplish this task with or without support (e.g., assistance using furniture). There were no significant advantages to using support to assist with rising. Data from this study and others may serve as the foundation for future interventions to improve the ability to rise from the floor. The Section on Geriatrics of the American Physical Therapy Association has developed a poster that provides a nine-step protocol for getting up from the floor. This is a helpful tool for teaching an older adult a step-by-step way of rising after a fall. Figure 9–2 provides this poster as an example for how to teach this strategy to older adults.

Risk factors for falling among the aged suggest that falling should not be considered a normal concomitant of aging; rather, it should alert the health care professional to the possibility of underlying disease or accelerated sensory or neuromuscular degeneration secondary to disuse. Secondary or multiple diagnoses, use of multiple medications, especially diuretics and barbiturates, decreased vision and lower extremity somatosensation, and decreased lower extremity strength all appear to contribute to balance and gait deficits, which in turn result in falling. Prevention of falls depends on addressing the specific problem area for each individual at risk. A team approach will be the most effective means to prevent falling by the aged.

ADAPTING THE ENVIRONMENT

The process of adapting to the environment, or of adapting the environment to the aged person, is especially important in geriatric rehabilitation. With de-

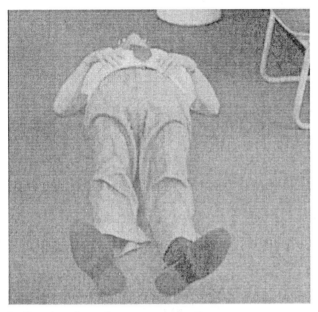

1. Remain calm and assess your situation.

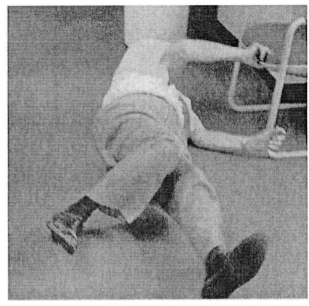

2. Roll over slowly. Locate the nearest sturdy chair.

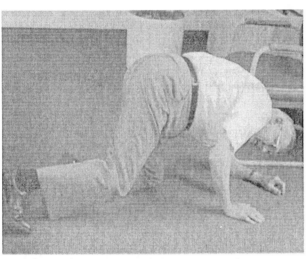

3. Crawl or shuffle to the chair.

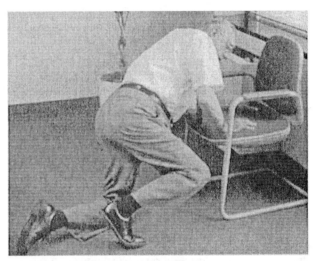

4. Kneel, then stand up using the chair.

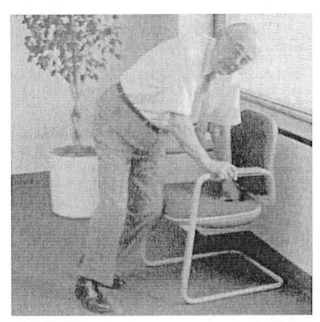

5. Then turn and sit down.

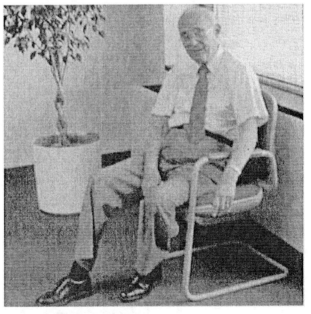

6. Call or wait for help.

Figure 9–2. Falls: What to do if you fall at home.

creased physiologic reserves, the aged person may not be able to continue an activity that is extremely demanding. For instance, an older person with a stroke and underlying cardiac insufficiency may need to learn wheelchair mobility skills. Therefore, the environment will need significant modification. Doors may need to be widened, ramps installed, and counters lowered. Financial concerns and personal preferences may restrict opportunities for obtaining new housing or adapting the present home.

The interaction between the aged person and his or her environment becomes potentially precarious as one ages. These interactions are affected by the aged person's underlying physical status, their living surroundings, and their social support systems. Of course, all persons interact with their environment. As one ages, however, the physiologic reserves, underlying medical problems, affective states, and a host of other factors complicate the relationship between the aged individual and their environment.

The purpose of rehabilitation providers is to manipulate the environment to make it safer. Assistive walking devices or modifications of the home may be recommended. But even these interventions are subject to differences when dealing with aging persons. The aged person with a disability may view such aids as unattractive or demeaning. The individual has a choice in selecting eyeglasses, which may enhance their appearance, but walkers or chrome-plated grab bars seem to project an image of illness and disability, which the aged person may try to avoid. The older person may have difficulty finding someone who can install home modifications. Some retired senior volunteer programs (RSVPs) have carpenters available for this purpose, but many communities are without such support services. As a result, often needed modifications are not affordable for the older individual.

Tasks are carried out within a physical and social context, which has the potential for facilitating or hindering the use of functional capabilities. Push-button controls placed at the front of a range assist aged individuals with low vision, whereas dials situated at the back of the range handicap them. Similarly, caregivers can enhance functional independence by providing aged individuals with adaptive equipment, such as plate guards, bath brushes with elongated handles, and sock aids, or they can promote dependence by feeding, bathing, and dressing the individual.

Evaluation of the environment is more difficult than task analysis because the environment of concern is the one in which the individual actually lives and has to function, rather than a hospital or nursing home. Evaluation of physical space aims at ascertaining architectural barriers, safety and functional features, and the extent to which available equipment can be operated by the aged individual. Evaluation of the social context probes the availability of caregivers, their skills in rendering care and their need for training, their attitudes toward functional independence, and their experience of caregiver burden.

Those with disabilities or physiological or anatomical changes resulting from inactivity and aging may experience memory loss, disorientation, decreased ability to perform normal physical activity, a deteriorating ability to remember details, difficulty in verbal expression, and impairment in judgment. Each of these factors is important when modifying the physical and social environment to meet the rehabilitation needs of the aged. Recent US government hearings and reports suggest that social and organizational characteristics of institutions and the home setting could postpone the time when aged people become bedridden and require skilled nursing care.[151,152]

It is reasonable for the direct caregiver to seek advice about practical strategies that could reduce confusion or injury on the part of the disabled aged to prolong care at home. Environmental designs for aged patients have been studied, and several factors are consistently identified as environmental hazards: poor illumination; inadequate color differentiation; cluttered furnishings; confusing layout, such as a table in a dimly lit hallway; bland, nondistinct textiles; architectural features, such as split level rooms; and climate control.[153] Certain environmental features are a threat to safety, can produce anxiety, and amplify cognitive deficits.[154] Cohen[155] found that behavioral approaches, (i.e., using environmental cues like color coding or labeling objects) had advantages over drugs in the treatment of cognitive impairments. Additional studies emphasized that encouragement of independence, self-sufficiency, and social interaction is critical to prolonging cognitive functions.[156]

The aged individual's environment may have some negative effects on their communication. Older people living alone are often isolated in home or community settings; that is, an environment in which few opportunities for successful, meaningful communication are available.[157] This can result in impairment in their communication skills. An aged person needs an environment that stimulates and reinforces communication. Geriatric rehabilitation should encourage participation in a variety of activities that can serve as a basis for conversation and interaction. Providing socially stimulating environments within a hospital, rehabilitation, or long-term care setting can be provided by organized recreational and social therapies. This becomes more difficult in the home setting; although often resources, such as church, community groups, or senior centers, can facilitate social interaction. Meaningful conversation is a crucial component in enhancing and reinforcing cognitive functioning and a sense of well-being for the aged individual.[156,157]

Visual limitations, such as farsightedness, decreased ability to adapt to changes in lighting conditions requiring increased illumination to see, and an increased sensitivity to glare, are not uncommon in the elderly patient.

Several changes normally occur within the aging eye that affect safety and need to be considered when adapting an older person's environment. The lens of the eye begins to thicken and yellow, and the muscles that control dilation of the pupil weaken. The thickening of the lens and delayed pupil dilation means that the glare and reflections often encountered in the environment cannot be tolerated.[32] In fact, the older eye needs approximately three times the amount of light to function adequately. The older person also has difficulty with depth perception and color differentiation that can interfere with ambulation (poor judgement in distance), ADLs, and driving an automobile. Color vision deficiencies in the aged have been described by Andreasen.[32] He found that the aged individual has difficulty distinguishing between shades of blue-green, blue, and violet and is unable to distinguish between two shades of a similar color. The elderly maintains their ability to differentiate between brighter colors, such as orange and red.[32] Several authors suggest the need for large pattern designs or solid bright colors in upholstery and textiles to enhance visibility, interest, and appeal (reducing the likelihood of bumping into or falling over furniture). Small patterns can produce blurring of vision, eye fatigue, and dizziness.[158]

Independence can be facilitated by bright and sharply contrasting colors. Considering the poorer differentiation of similar colors, if an aged individual is in a poorly lit living room with a blue carpet, light blue walls and lavender and blue flowered furniture and draperies, it could be trouble. Contrasting colors or better lighting, which even is economically more feasible, could positively facilitate safety in that room. Color coding of walls and corridors in hospitals and nursing homes using bright colors can help aged persons find their own rooms, bathrooms, sitting rooms, and so on. Contrasting colors are extremely important, because they can eliminate the difficulty of independently managing a stairwell or a poorly lit hall where shadows can be hazards. Often this contrast can be accomplished through the use of fluorescent colors of tape (orange, lime green, or red).

Different colors have differing effects on an individual's emotional state.[158] The colors red, yellow, and orange have been associated with excitement, stimulation, and aggression.[158] Red increases muscular tension and increases blood pressure. It could be used as a visual stimulant with the elderly to alert them of environmental changes or hazards, such as stairs or level changes. It must be noted, however, that individuals with cataracts lose the shorter frequencies in the spectrum. This includes red, orange, and in extreme cases, yellow.

Although elderly persons often need to be stimulated, the aged individual with dementia requires soothing and warm colors, such as light oranges and blues in their living quarters to enhance relaxation and comfort.

Higher, reasonably firm, supportive, comfortable chairs with high backs allow rising from a sitting position with minimal assistance. Wide armrests, either wooden or metal, allow identification by touch when eyesight is poor or trunk rotation is limited. An aged individual should always be instructed to feel the chair seat with the back of their legs before attempting to sit down.

Human beings have a great propensity for adapting to less than ideal conditions. The aged, particularly those with a severe disability, have much more difficulty. Sensory stimulation should be incorporated into every aspect of rehabilitation. Repetitive visual cues using graphics, color, and lighting encourage independence, thereby increasing pride and self-esteem.

Hellbrandt[159] proposes a focus on the maintenance of good health and residual mental function, the latter through socialization, physical, and recreational activities. The relationship between physical condition and behavior is particularly important in patients with dementia.[160] Changes in environmental design can accommodate the normal physiological changes of aging and prevent the effects of disuse. If the older person cannot manage the environment safely, her or his independence, socialization and ADLs are hindered.

CONCLUSION

Rehabilitation of the aged patient is one of the most challenging tasks for health care professionals. It is often difficult to separate the physiological aspect of aging and disability from cognitive changes when designing a rehabilitation treatment program. With increased knowledge, the natural history of normal aging may eventually be altered. Until then, rehabilitation of aged individuals needs to focus on obtaining the maximal functional capacity within the care environment by simplifying that environment and providing activity to ensure that disabilities do not result from disuse. To maintain the highest level of functional ability for the longest amount of time, decline in all sensory integration and physical functioning capabilities must be considered when providing rehabilitative care. One of the most salient aspects of geriatric rehabilitation is the simultaneous management of multiple conditions and the concept of frailty. For the rehabilitation specialist, these multiple diagnoses translate into multiple, and often multidimensional, impairments that complicate the management of ADLs and hinder maximal functional capabilities.

Rehabilitation is a process that is not determined by a specific diagnosis or the care setting in which services are provided but by multidiagnostic circumstances and the aged individual's level of motivation. The primary goal of rehabilitation is to promote independent living, as defined by the aged themselves. When working with aged people, rehabilitation specialists need to be aware of the number of factors that make caring for them more complex, more challenging, and more fulfilling.

PEARLS

- The purpose of geriatric rehabilitation is to assist the disabled aged in recovering lost physical, psychological, or social skills so that they may become more independent.
- Forty percent of all disabled persons are over age 65; the oldest-old (over 85) compose the highest percentage of disabled persons.
- The decline in muscle strength and mass, respiratory reserve and cardiovascular functioning, kyphotic postural changes, poorer eyesight, poor hydration and marginal nutritional intake, and many other physiological and physical changes associated with inactivity and aging, lead to frailty.
- Lawton[27,160] defines three levels of ADLs as: (1) basic ADLs, such as self-care activities; (2) instrumental ADLs, such as cooking and cleaning; (3) mobility, a more complicated form (combining basic and instrumental ADLs) of ADLs, such as using public transportation.
- Attention to the abilities of the caregiver can facilitate the ease of care and decrease the burden placed on the caregiver.
- Three major principles influence geriatric rehabilitation. These are variability, hypokinetics, and optimal health. The influence of these can be seen in the systems of the body and should be differentiated from normal versus pathological aging.
- Rehabilitation of the aged should emphasize maintenance of functional mobility, improvement of balance, good nutrition, and general care, as well as social and emotional support.
- Special geriatric rehabilitation considerations must be implemented for patients with cognitive, sensory, and generalized physical decline.
- Increased feeding difficulties may be secondary to decreased appetite, poor oral status, visual or sensorimotor agnosia, cognitive declines (decreasing attentiveness), and physical limitations.
- CMS (previously HCFA) interpretive guidelines define a physical restraint as "any manual method or physical or mechanical device, material or equipment attached to or adjacent to the resident's body, which the individual cannot remove easily, that restricts freedom of movement or normal access to one's body."
- Managing falls in the aged requires recognizing that falls are not a normal part of aging and may be due to medication, fear of falling, inactivity, chronic illness, postural instability, the use of restraints or a combination of these.
- The goals for adapting an environment for the older person are to ensure safety, increase mobility, and enhance comfort and communication.

REFERENCES

1. Wedgewood J. The place of rehabilitation in geriatric medicine: an overview. *Int Rehabil Med.* 1985; 7(1);107.
2. Warshaw GA, Moore JT, Friedman SW, et al. Functional disability in the hospitalized elderly. *JAMA.* 1982; 248(7):847–850.
3. National Center for Health Statistics. *Health, United States, 1999, with Health and Aging Chartbook.* Hyattsville, MD: National Center for Health Statistics, 1999; 36–37.
4. National Center for Health Statistics. *Health, United States, 1999, with Health and Aging Chartbook.* Hyattsville, MD: National Center for Health Statistics, 1999; 34–35.
5. Clark G, Blue B, and Bearer J. Rehabilitation of the elderly amputee. *J Am Geriatr Soc.* 1983; 31:439.
6. Centers for Disease Control and Prevention. *Unrealized Prevention Opportunities: Reducing the Health and Economic Burden of Chronic Disease.* Atlanta, GA: Centers for Disease Control and Prevention, National Center for Chronic Disease Prevention and Health Promotion. 1997.
7. Kumar VN, Redford JB. Rehabilitation of hip fractures in the elderly. *Am Fam Physician.* 1984; 29:173.
8. Federal Council on the Aging. *The Need for Long-Term Care. A Chartbook of the Federal Council on Aging.* Washington, DC: US Government Printing Office; 2000. US Department of Health and Human Services publication No. (OHDS) 81-20704, 29.
9. Enright RB, Friss L. Employed care-givers of brain-damaged adults: an assessment of the dual role. Unpublished thesis, University of Arizona. 1997.
10. Lehman JF, Guy AW, Stonebridge JB, et al. Stroke: does rehabilitation affect outcome? *Arch Phys Med Rehabil.* 1975; 56;375.
11. Rubenstein LZ, Josephson KR, Guriand B. Effectiveness of a geriatric evaluation unit: a randomized trial. *N Engl J Med.* 1984; 311:1664.
12. Fried LP, Guralnik JM. Disability in older adults: evidence regarding significance, etiology, and risk. *J Am Geriatr Soc.* 1997; 45(1):92–100.
13. Ferrucci L, Gauralnik JM, Pahor M, Corti MC, Havlik RJ. Hospital diagnoses, Medicare charges, and nursing home admissions in the year when older persons become severely disabled. *JAMA.* 1997; 277:728–734.
14. Manton KG, Corder L, Stallard E. Chronic disability trends in elderly United States populations: 1982–1994. *Proc Natl Acad Sci USA.* 1997; 94: 2593–2598.
15. Lundin-Olsson L, Nyberg L, Gustafson Y. Attention, frailty, and falls: The effect of a manual task on basic mobility. *J Am Geriatr Soc.* 1998; 46(6): 758–761.
16. Fiatarone MA, O'Neill EF, Ryan ND, Clements KM, Solares GR, Nelson ME, Roberts SB, Kehayias JJ, Lipsitz LA, Evans WJ. Exercise training and nutritional supplementation for physical frailty in very elderly people. *N Engl J Med.* 1994; 330(25): 1769–1775.

17. Inouye SK, Wagner DR, Acampora D. A predictive index for functional decline in hospitalized elderly medical patients. *J Intern Med.* 1993; 8(7): 645–652.

18. Winograd CH, Lindenberger EC, Chavez CM, Mauricio MP, Shi H, Bloch DA. Identifying hospitalized older patients at varying risk for physical performance decline: a new approach. *J Am Geriatr Soc.* 1997; 45(5):604–609.

19. Fried TR, Mor V. Frailty and hospitalization of long-term stay nursing home residents. *J Am Geriatr Soc.* 1997; 45(3):265–269.

20. Buchner DM, Wagner EH. Preventing frail health. *Clin Geriatr Med.* 1992; 8(1):1–17.

21. Pearlman DN, Branch LG, Ozminkowski RJ, Experton B, Li Z. Transitions in health care use and expenditures among frail older adults by payor/provider type. *J Am Geriatr Soc.* 1997; 45(5): 550–557.

22. Commission on Chronic Illness. *Chronic Illness in the United States: Prevention of Chronic Illness.* Cambridge, Mass: Harvard University Press; 1957: 1; 285–311.

23. Trussel RD, Elinson J. *Chronic Illness in the United States: Chronic Illness in a Rural Area.* Cambridge, Mass: Harvard University Press; 1959:3.

24. Dinken H. Physical treatment of the hemiplegic patient in general practice. In: Krusen FH, ed. *Physical Medicine and Rehabilitation for the Clinician.* Philadelphia: Saunders; 1951; 205.

25. Heather AJ. *Manual of Care for the Disabled Patient.* New York: Macmillan; 1960; 12–15.

26. Rusk H. *Rehabilitation Medicine.* St Louis; Mosby Co.; 1958; 40–44.

27. Lawton MP, Brody EM. Assessment of older people: self-maintaining and instrumental activities of daily living. *Gerontologist.* 1969; 9:179–186.

28. Branch LG, Meyers AR. Assessing physical function in the elderly. *Clin Ger Med.* 1987; 3(1): 29–51.

29. Branch LG, Jette A. The Framingham Disability Study: social disability among the aging. *Am J Public Health.* 1981;71:1202.

30. Woollacott MJ. Changes in posture and voluntary control in the elderly: research findings and rehabilitation. *Top Geriatr Rehabil.* 1990; 5(2):1–11.

31. Woollacott MJ. Response preparation and posture control: neuromuscular changes in the older adult. *Ann NY Acad Sci.* 1988; 515:42–53.

32. Andreasen MK. Making a safe environment by design. *J Gerontol Nurs.* 1985; 11(6):18–22.

33. Boyer GG. Vision problems. In: Carnevali P, Patrick B, eds. *Nursing Management for the Elderly.* Philadelphia: Lippincott; 1989: 482–484.

34. Kasper RL. Eye problems of the aged. In: Reichel W, ed. *Clinical Aspects of Aging.* Baltimore, Md: Williams and Wilkins Co.; 1988: 393–395.

35. Fitts RH. Aging and skeletal muscle. In: Smith EL, Serfass RC, eds. *Exercise and Aging: The Scientific Basis.* Hillside, NJ: Enslow Publishers; 1980.

36. Schaie KW. Historical time and cohort effects. In: McCuskey KA, Reese HW, eds. *Lifespan Developmental Psychology: Historical and Generational Effects.* New York; Academic Press; 1984.

37. Wechsler D. "Hold" and "Don't hold" tests. In: Chown SM, ed. *Human Aging.* New York; Penguin Press; 1972.

38. Siegler IC. Psychological aspects of the Duke longitudinal studies. In: Schaie KW, ed. *Longitudinal Studies of Adult Psychological Development.* New York; Guilford Press: 1983.

39. Botwinick J. *Aging and Behavior.* 2nd ed, New York; Springer Publishing Co., 1987.

40. Baltes PB, Schaie KW. On the plasticity of intelligence in adulthood, and old age. *Am Psychol.* 1986;31: 720–725.

41. Siebens AW, Schmedt JF, Eckberg DL, et al. Homodynamic consequences of cardiovascular deconditioning—functional effects. *Circulation.* 1990; 82(4):694.

42. Lewis CB. *Aging: The Health Care Challenge.* Philadelphia: Davis; 1990.

43. Holloszy JO. Exercise, health, and aging: a need for more information. *Med Sci Sports Exerc.* 1983; 15:1.

44. Schneider El, Reed JD. Modulations of aging processes. In: Finch Ce, Schneider EL, eds. *Handbook of the Biology of Aging.* New York; Academic Press; 1985.

45. Astrand PO. Exercise physiology and its role in disease prevention and in rehabilitation. *Arch Phys Med Rehabil.* 1987; 68:305.

46. Greenleaf JE, Reese RD. Exercise thermoregulation after 14 days of bed rest. *J Appl Physiol.* 1980; 48:72–77.

47. Haines RF. Effect of bed rest and exercise on body balance. *J Appl Physiol.* 1974; 36:323.

48. Taylor HL, Henschel JB, Keys A. Effects of bed rest on cardiovascular function and work performance. *J Am Physiol.* 1949; 2:223.

49. Shepard RJ. *Physical Activity and Aging.* 2nd ed. Rockland, Md: Aspen Publishers, Inc.; 1987.

50. Rikli R, Busch S. Motor performance of women as a function of age and physical activity level. *J Gerontol.* 1986; 41:645.

51. Ernes CG. The effects of a regular program of light exercise on seniors. *J Sports Med.* 1979; 19:185.

52. Buskirk ER. Health maintenance and longevity; exercise. In: Finch CE, Schneider EL, eds. *Handbook of the Biology of Aging.* New York; Academic Press, 1985.

53. Spiraduso WW. Physical fitness, aging, and psychomotor speed: a review. *J Gerontol.* 1980; 35: 850.

54. Dietrick JE, Whedon GD, Shorr E. Effects of immobilization upon various metabolic and physiologic functions of normal men. *Am J Med.* 1948; 4:3–9.

55. Saltin B, Astrand PO, Grover RF, et al. Response to exercise after bed rest and after training. *Circulation.* 1968; 38(suppl 7):I.

56. Miller PB, Johnson RL, Lamb LE. Effects of four weeks of absolute bed rest on circulatory functions in man. *Aerospace Med.* 1964; 35:1194.

57. Lamb LE, Stevens PM, Johnson RL. Hypokinesia secondary to chair rest from 4 to 10 days. *Aerospace Med.* 1965; 36, 755.

58. DeBusk RF, Convertino VA, Hung J, Goldwater D. Exercise conditioning in middle-aged men after 10 days of bed rest. *Circulation.* 1983; 68:245.

59. Buller AJ, Eccles JC, Eccles RM. Interaction between motor neurons and muscles in respect of the characteristic speeds of their responses. *J Physiol.* 1960; 150:417–419.

60. Ryback RS, Lewis OF, Sewab RS, Blum K. Psychobiologic effects of prolonged weightlessness (bed rest) in young healthy volunteers. *Aerospace Med.* 1971; 42:408–411.

61. Ryback RS, Lewis OF, Lessard CS. Psychobiologic effects of prolonged bed rest (weightless) in young, healthy volunteers (study II). *Aerospace Med.* 1971; 42:529–534.

62. Muller EA. Influence of training and of inactivity on muscle strength. *Arch Phys Med Rehabil.* 1970; 51:449.

63. Fugiswawa Y, Kida K, Matsuda H. Role of change in vitamin D metabolism with age in calcium and phosphorus metabolism in normal subjects. *J Clin Endocrinol Metab.* 1984; 59:719–726.

64. Kenney RA. *Physiology of Aging: A Synopsis.* Chicago: Year Book Medical Publishers, Inc.; 1982.

65. Ham RJ, Marcy ML. Normal aging: a review of systems/the maintenance of health. In: Wright J, ed. *Primary Care Geriatrics.* Boston: PSG, Inc.; 1983.

66. Evans CE, Galasko CS, Ward, C. Effect of donor age on the growth of in vitro cells obtained from human trabecular bone. *J Orthop Res.* 1990; 8(2): 234–237.

67. Zadai CC. Cardiopulmonary issues in the geriatric population: implications for rehabilitation. *Top Geriatr Rehabil.* 1986; 2(1):1–9.

68. Cummings G, Semple SG. *Disorders of the Respiratory System.* Oxford, England; Blackwell; 1973.

69. Wynne JW. Pulmonary disease in the elderly. In: Rossman I, ed. *Clinical Geriatrics.* 2nd ed. Philadelphia: Lippincott; 1979.

70. Goldman R. Decline in organ function with age. In: Rossman I, ed. *Clinical Geriatrics.* 2nd ed. Philadelphia: Lippincott; 1979.

71. Ham RJ, Marcy ML, Holtzman JM. The aging process: biological and social aspects. In: Wright J, ed. *Primary Care Geriatrics.* Boston: PSG, Inc.; 1983.

72. Hamlin CR, Luschin JH, Kohn RR. Aging of collagen: comparative rates in four mammalian species. *Exp Gerontol.* 1980; 15:393–398.

73. Astrand PO, Rodahl K. *Textbook of Work Physiology.* San Francisco, London: McGraw–Hill Book Co.; 1970.

74. Meyer K, Hoffman P, Linker A. Mucopolysaccharides of costal cartilage. *Science.* 1958; 128:896.

75. Pickles LW. Effects of aging on connective tissues. *Geriatrics.* 1983; 38(1):71–78.

76. Hole JW. *Human Anatomy and Physiology.* Iowa: WC Brown Co.; 1978.

77. Kaplan D, Mayer K. Distribution of alkaline phosphatase. *Nature.* 1959; 183:1262–1263.

78. Calliet R. Mechanisms of joints. In: Licht S, ed. *Arthritis and Physical Medicine.* Baltimore: Waverly Press; 1969.

79. Palmoski Mj, Colyer RA, Brandt KD. Joint motion in the absence of normal loading does not maintain normal articular cartilage. *Arthritis Rheum.* 1985; 23:325.

80. Gardner DL. Aging of articular cartilage. In: Brockehurst JC, ed. *Textbook of Geriatric Medicine and Gerontology.* New York: Longman Group Ltd., 1978.

81. Larson EB, Bruce RA. Health benefits of exercise in an aging society. *Arch Intern Med.* 1987; 147:353.

82. Klein H. Constipation and fecal impaction. *Med Clin North Am.* 1992; 186:1135–1144.

83. Holdstein DJ, Misiewicz JJ, Smith T. Propulsion (mass movements) in the human colon and its relationship to meals and somatic activity. *Gut.* 1999; 251(1):91–103.

84. World Health Organization. *Constitution of the World Health Organization.* Geneva; World Health Organization; 1964.

85. American Diabetes Association. *Direct and Indirect Costs of Diabetes in the United States in 1997.* Alexandria, Va: American Diabetes Association Report; 1998.

86. Himann JE. Age-related changes in speed of walking. *Med Sci Sports Exerc.* 1998; 44: 161–165.

87. Siegler IC, Costa PT, Jr. Health behavior relationships. In: Birren JE, Schaie KW, eds. *Handbook of the Psychology of Aging.* 2nd ed. New York: Van Nostrand Reinhold; 1985.

88. Kaplan E. Psychological factors and ischemic heart disease mortality: a focal role for perceived health. Paper presented at the annual meeting of the American Psychological Association, Washington, DC; 1999.

89. Mossey JM, Shapiro E. Self-rated health: a predictor of mortality among the elderly. *Am J Public Health.* 1982; 72:800–808.

90. Rosillo RA, Fagel ML. Correlation of psychologic variables and progress in physical therapy: I. degree of disability and denial of illness. *Arch Phys Med Rehabil.* 1970; 51:227.

91. Stoedefalke KG. Motivating and sustaining the older adult in an exercise program. *Top Geriatr Rehabil.* 1985; 1;78.

92. Nader IM, et al. Level of aspiration and performance of chronic psychiatric patients on a simple motor task. *Percept Mot Skills.* 1985; 60:767.

93. Prohaska T, Pontiam IA, Teitleman J. Age differences in attributions to causality: implications for intellection assessment. *Exp Aging Res.* 1984; 10:1–11.

94. Eisdorder L. Arousal and performance: experiments in verbal learning and a tentative theory. In: Talland GA, ed. *Human Aging and Behavior.* New York: Academic Press; 1968.

95. Weinberg R, Bruya L, Jackson A. The effects of goal proximity and goal specificity on endurance performance. *J Soc Psychol.* 1985; 7:296.

96. Mento A, Steele RP, Karren RJ. A metaanalytic study of the effects of goal setting on task performance: 1966-1984. *Organ Behav Hum Decis Process.* 1987; 39:52.

97. Smith E, Serfass R. *Exercise and Aging: The Scientific Basis.* Hillside, NJ; Enslow Publishers; 1981.

98. Stelmach CE, Worringham CJ. Sensorimotor deficits related to postural stability: implications for falling in the elderly. In: Radebaugh TS, et al., eds. *Clinics of Geriatric Medicine*. Philadelphia: Saunders; 1985:1(3).

99. McPherson BD, ed. *Sport and Aging: The 1984 Olympic Scientific Congress Proceedings*. Champaign, III: Human Kinetics Publishers, Inc.; 1986:5.

100. Seltzer B, Rheaume Y, Volicer L, et al. The short-term effects of in-hospital respite on the patient with Alzheimer's disease. *Gerontologist*. 1988; 28(1):121–124.

101. Knott M, Voss DE. *Proprioceptive Neuromuscular Facilitation: Patterns of Techniques*. 2nd ed. New York: Harper and Row Publishers; 1968.

102. Marshall L. Auditory processing in aging listeners. *J Speech Hear Disord*. 1981; 46: 226–238.

103. Gutman E. *Age Changes in the Neuromuscular System*. Great Britain; Bristol, Ltd.; 1972.

104. Payton OD, Poland JL. Aging process: implications for clinical practice. *Phys Ther*. 1983; 63(1):41–48.

105. Brody H. Kliemer lecture, Gerontological Society Meeting. *Gerontology News*. Washington, DC: Gerontological Society of America. November, 1979.

106. McCarter R. Effects of age on contraction of mammalian skeletal muscle. In: Kalkor G, DiBattista J, eds. *Aging in Muscle*. New York; Raven; 1978; 1–22.

107. Moritani T. Training adaptations in the muscles of older men. In: Smith EL, Serfass RC. *Exercise and Aging: The Scientific Basis*. Hillside, NJ; Enslow Publishers: 1981; 149–166.

108. Gutman E, Hanzlikova V. Fast and slow motor units in aging. *Gerontology*. 1976; 22:280–300.

109. MacLennan WJ, Hall MRP, Timothy JI. Postural hypotension in old age: is it a disorder of the nervous system or of blood vessels? *Age Aging*. 1980; 9:25–32.

110. Ragen PB, Mitchell J. The effects of aging on the cardiovascular response to dynamic and static exercise. In: Weisfelt ML, ed. *The Aging Heart*. New York: Raven; 1980; 269–296.

111. Murray MP. Normal postural stability and steadiness: quantitative assessment. *J Bone Joint Surg (Am)*. June, 1975; 57(A):510.

112. Carlson KE, Alston W, Feldman DJ. Electromyographic study of aging skeletal muscle. *Am J Phys Med*. 1964; 43:141–152.

113. Darling RC. Fatigue. In: Downey JA, Darling RC, eds. *Physiological Basis of Rehabilitation Medicine*. Philadelphia: Saunders; 1971.

114. Kohl HW, Moorefield DL, Blair SN. Is cardiorespiratory fitness associated with general chronic fatigue in apparently healthy men and women? *Med Sci Sports Exerc*. 1987; 19(S6).

115. Ejaz F, Jones J, Rose M. Falls among nursing home residents: An examination of incident reports before and after restraint reduction programs. *J Am Geriatr Soc*. 42(7):960–964.

116. OBRA '87. Omnibus Budget Reconciliation Act of 1987, Public Law 100-203. Washington DC: US Government Printing Office. 1987:172.

117. Phillips C. Use of physical restraints. *Med Care*. 1996; 34(11).

118. HCFA. *State Operations Manual, Part II: Guidance to Surveyors for Long Term Care Facilities, Interpretive Guidelines*. 483.13(a); 2000.

119. Donius M, Rader J. Use of side rails: Rethinking a standard of practice. *J Gerontol Nursing*. 1994; 20 (11):23–27.

120. Cohen C. Old problem, different approach: Alternatives to physical restraints. *J Gerontol Nursing*. 1996; 22(2):23–29.

121. Stolley JM. Freeing your patients from restraints. *Am J Nursing*. 1995; 43(2):27–31.

122. Christiansen J, Juhl E, eds. The prevention of falls in later life. *Danish Med Bull*. 1987; 34(Suppl) (4):1–24.

123. Kalchthaler T, Bascon RA, Quintos V. Falls in the institutionalized elderly. *J Am Geriatr Soc*. 1978; 26:424.

124. Tinetti ME. Factors associated with serious injury during falls by ambulatory nursing home residents. *J Am Geriatr Soc*. 1987; 35:644.

125. Gryfe CI, Amies A, Ashley MJ. A longitudinal study of falls in an elderly population: I. incidence and morbidity. *Age Ageing*. 1977; 6:201.

126. Wild D, Nayak US, Isaacs B. How dangerous are falls in old people at home? *Br Med J*. 1981; 282:266.

127. Tideiksaar R. Fall prevention in the home. *Top Geriatr Rehabil*. 1987; 3(1):57–64.

128. Droller H. Falls among elderly people living at home. *Geriatrics*. 1955; 10:239–244.

129. Archea JC. Environmental factors associated with stair accidents by the elderly. *Clin Geriatr Med*. 1985; 1:555.

130. Ashley MJ, Gryfe CT, Aimes A. A longitudinal study of falls in an elderly population. II. Some circumstances of falling. *Age Ageing*. 1997; 30: 211–217.

131. Louis M. Falls and their causes. *J Gerontol Nurs*. 1993; 33:142–148.

132. Lawrence MS. Strengthening the quadriceps: progressively prolonged isometric tension method. *Phys Ther Rev*. 1956; 36:658.

133. Horak FB. Clinical measurement of posture control in adults. *Phys Ther*. 1987; 67(12):1881.

134. Bobath B. *Adult Hemiplegia: Evaluation and Treatment*. 2nd ed. London: Heineman Medical Books; 1978.

135. Woollacott MJ, Shumway-Cook A, Nashner L. Aging and posture control. *Int J Aging Hum Devel*. 1986; 23:97.

136. Shumway-Cook A, Horak FB. Assessing the influence of sensory interaction on balance. *Phys Ther*. 1986; 66(10):1548.

137. Stout RW. Falls and disorders of postural balance. *Age Ageing*. 1978; 7:134.

138. Carr JH, Shepard RB. *A Motor Relearning Program for Stroke*. 2nd ed. Rockville, MD: Aspen Publishers; 1987.

139. Gabell A. Falls in the elderly: will dance reduce their incidence? *Human Movement Studies*. 1986; 12:119.

140. Bottomley JM. The use of T'ai Chi as a movement modality in orthopaedics. *Ortho Phys Ther Clinics North Am*. 2000; 9(3):361–373

141. Wolf SL, Coogler C, Xu T. Exploring the basis for Tai Chi Chuan as a therapeutic exercise approach. *Arch Phys Med Rehabil.* 1997; 79: 886–892.

142. Bottomley JM. Gait in later life. *Ortho Phys Ther Clinics North Am.* 2001; 10(1):131–149.

143. Tinetti ME, Liu WL, Claus EB. Predictors and prognosis of inability to get up after falls among elderly persons. *JAMA.* 1993; 269(1):65–70.

144. Alexander NB, Ulbrich J, Raheja A, Channer D. Rising from the floor in older adults. *J Am Geriatr Soc.* 1997; 45(5):564–569.

145. Tinetti ME, Richman D, Powell L. Falls efficacy as a measure of fear of falling. *J Gerontol.* 1993; 45 (3):P239–P243.

146. Simpson JM, Salkin S. Are elderly people at risk of falling taught how to get up again? *Age Ageing.* 1993; 22(3):294–296.

147. Van Sant AF. Rising from a supine to erect stance: description of adult movement and a developmental hypothesis. *Phys Ther.* 1988; 68(2): 185–192.

148. Unrau K, Hanrahan SM, Pitetti KH. An exploratory study of righting reactions from a supine to standing position in adults with Down syndrome. *Phys Ther.* 1994; 74(12):1116–1124.

149. Ford-Smith CD, Van Sant AF. Age differences in movement patterns used to rise from a bed in subjects in the third through fifth decades of age. *Phys Ther.* 1993; 73(5):300–309.

150. Green L, Williams K. Differences in developmental movement patterns used by active versus sedentary middle-aged adults coming from a supine position to erect stance. *Phys Ther.* 1992; 72(8): 560–568.

151. Government Document. *Alzheimer's Disease: Report of the Secretaries Task Force on Alzheimer's Disease.* Washington, DC; US Government Printing Office; 1999. Rockville, Md; US Department of Health and Human Services, Public Health Service, Alcohol, Drug Abuse, and Mental Health Administration. DHHS pub. no. (ADM) 84–1323.

152. Government Document. *Alzheimer's Disease.* Washington, DC: US Government Printing Office; 1999. Joint hearing before the Subcommittee on Health and Long-Term Care of the Select Committee on Aging and the Subcommittee on Energy and Commerce. House of Representatives, 105th Congress, first session.

153. Liebowitz B, Lawton MP, Waldman A. Evaluation: designing for confused elderly people. *AIA Journal.* 1979; 2:59–61.

154. Weldon S, Yesavage JA. Behavioral improvement with relaxation training in senile dementia. *Clinical Gerontologist.* 1982; 1(1):45–49.

155. Cohen GD. The mental health professional and Alzheimer's patient. *Hosp Community Psychiatry.* 1984; 35(2):115–116, 122.

156. Reifler BV, Wu S. Managing families of the demented elderly. *J Fam Pract.* 1982; 14(6): 1051–1056.

157. Lubinski R. Speech, language, and audiology programs in home health care agencies and nursing homes. In: Beasley DS, Davis GA, eds. *Aging: Communication Processes and Disorders.* New York: Grune and Stratton; 1981.

158. Sharpe DT. *The Psychology of Color and Design.* Chicago: Nelson-Hall Co.; 1974.

159. Hellebrandt FA. The senile dement in our midst: a look at the other side of the coin. *Gerontologist.* 1978; 18:67–70.

160. Lawton MP. Assessing the competence of older people. In: Kent D, Kastenbaum R, Sherwood S, eds. *Research Planning and Action for the Elderly.* New York: Behavioral Publications; 1972.

CHAPTER 10

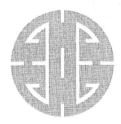

Patient Evaluation

Preparation	Pain Assessment
Setting	Physical Assessment—How To
Tools	**Environmental Assessment**
Timing	**Psychosocial Assessment**
Expectations	**Conclusion**
Interview	**Appendices**
Physical Assessment	

Of all the elements of patient care, evaluation is the most crucial. A comprehensive evaluation provides the practitioner with all the necessary information for designing an appropriate program. Since older patients often present with complex problems because of multiple pathologies and the effects of aging, a thorough evaluation may be more difficult. Nevertheless, it is even more important to determine the exact nature of the problem. This chapter divides evaluation into six main components: preparation, expectations, the interview, physical assessment, environmental assessment, and psychosocial assessment. Assessment will be covered briefly here in terms of the initial evaluation. For a more detailed account, please refer to Chapter 6.

PREPARATION

Setting

What background is essential for a good evaluation of older patients? A quiet noncompeting environment is important because there is a high probability that the patient will have some hearing loss,[1] and background noise will make it difficult for the patient to hear questions. In addition, many older persons suffer from vision loss. Therefore, examination areas should be well lit and nonglare. Therapists should provide enough room for movement, and doorways and room space should be large enough to be wheelchair accessible.

The room should have a comfortable, sturdy, 18-inch (or higher) chair available.[1] Optimally, the bed or treatment table should be automatically adjustable for height. The floor should have a low pile carpet or a low gloss nonslippery floor. Finally, the colors in the room should be those that make the older person most at ease, such as reds, oranges, gold, and beige. These colors should also be contrasted to avoid visual misinterpretation.[2] This scenario is for a clinical setting; however, many evaluations are done in the home. In the home setting try to imitate this background as closely as possible.

Tools

Any general evaluation form can be sufficient for the initial evaluation visit; however, specific forms for functional, physical (orthopedic, neurological, and cardiopulmonary), environmental, and psychosocial assessment are helpful and often cue the clinician to ask appropriate questions. It should be noted that many of the functional evaluation forms listed in Chapter 6 can be given to the patient prior to the evaluation. Forms for different diagnoses can be used by the clinician to look for specific problems. (See Appendix A for orthopedic, neurological, and cardiopulmonary forms.)

Timing

When is the best time to do an evaluation? There are times during the day when people perform better. It would be impossible to schedule evaluations to fit each patient's peak performance; however, a thorough clinician should ask the patient when he or she performs the best and note it. Only one time is contraindicated for an initial evaluation, and that is immediately following a large meal.[3] This is due to the decrease in blood flow to the brain for one hour after a large meal, which is most apparent in older patients.[3] Therefore, it is not good to overtax the system by doing an evaluation immediately after a large meal.

EXPECTATIONS

A clinician unfamiliar with treating geriatric patients can expect different levels of performance from an older person in an initial evaluation as compared to a younger person. Clinical experience shows that the older patient cannot tolerate a similar history taking session as younger patients. Initial evaluation may need some modification, especially in the physical performance area. Robin McKenzie, for example, requests that his patients both extend and flex the trunk approximately ten times.[4] This type of repetition is too rigorous for most older persons. Physically, most older persons can tolerate one or two repetitions of a movement, and can tolerate rolling into different positions one to two times. For these reasons, a clinician may need to anticipate two sessions to complete a thorough evaluation.

INTERVIEW

Though a great deal of information can be collected from the interview process, much of it is not useful. Limiting responses and directing questions is the key to a successful interview.

A good way to start an interview is to ask the patient, "Why are you here to see me?" A good follow-up to this question is, "What do you expect from physical therapy?" These two questions give the interviewer the main problem (usually in functional terms) and the patient's goals (again, in functional terms).

The next important piece of information is the relevant history. One way to get this information is to ask, "How did this happen?" Follow-up questions along this line are, "Have you had anything similar to this before?" or, "What do you think contributed to this?" To obtain additional medical history information that could impact the rehabilitation progress ask, "What other medical problems do you have that I need to know about?" or, "What other medical problems do you have that may affect your progress?"

Other important information that can easily be gathered in the initial interview is the patient's social support system, for example, a question like, "Do you

live alone?" followed by, "Who is the main person that helps you when you are ill or having difficulties with any of your daily activities?" will give the clinician important insight into the patient's social support. Age, weight, and medication usage can all be asked in the initial interview.

The initial interview session can also be used to gather information on subjective areas. Pain assessments are the major subjective tests used by the geriatric therapist. When assessing pain in the elderly person the clinician should be aware of two different presentations of symptoms in the older patient from the younger. First, older people tend to under report pain, and second, they are less sensitive to pain.[5,6] There are several pain ratings available for assessing pain in the elderly; some are better than others.

PHYSICAL ASSESSMENT

Physical assessment is probably the most important aspect of the physical therapist's time with a patient. Physical assessment will provide the therapist with both subjective and objective data from which to develop and monitor a treatment program. Appendix A contains sample forms for the orthopedic, neurological, and cardiopulmonary assessment. Chapter 6 provides specific information on aging changes that will affect some of the outcome measures in the tools listed in Appendix A.

The application of physical assessment tools in the geriatric patient is similar to younger patients except for the variables listed in the beginning of the chapter as well as the following:

1. The therapist should relate physical findings to function. For example, what is the patient unable to do with shoulder flexion limited to 90°?
2. An entire assessment may need to be broken up and conducted in several sessions. The older person may not have the endurance to complete an entire physical assessment.
3. Psychosocial components must be considered along with physical parameters (see subsequent section).
4. Pain can be a major component and should be assessed thoroughly in an older person (see next section).

Pain Assessment

Pain evaluation tools can be divided into four categories. The first includes general pain evaluation tools. (For example, asking a patient to rate his or her pain as severe, moderate, or mild.) Pain diagrams are the second type of pain evaluation tools. An example of a pain diagram is the visual analog scale, which is simply a 100 mm line with a label at top and bottom.[7] Figure 10–1 is an example of a visual analog scale. To use this scale, the older person simply marks the place that cor-

No Pain

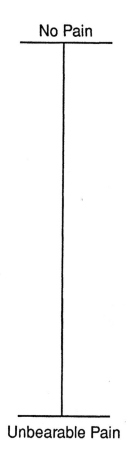

Unbearable Pain

Figure 10–1. *Visual analog scale.*

responds to their pain. The clinician then measures the distance from no pain to the mark. For example, on an initial evaluation a patient may have 67 mm of pain on the visual analog scale and two weeks later they mark their pain as 23 mm. However, pain diagrams pose potential problems for older patients. The tests require abstract thinking, and older persons do not tend to perform as well on tests of this nature.[6]

The third group of pain assessment tools are pain language tools. A good example of a pain language tool is the McGill-Melzak Pain Questionnaire.[8] This one-page questionnaire uses different pain descriptors to rank the person's pain. This particular test has been used with older populations; however, specific reliability and validity for this test and the older population has not been demonstrated.

The final type of pain tool is a pain diary, which is a running record of the person's pain. There are pros and cons for this tool. A pain diary can be useful, because it helps the patient focus and become aware of how pain affects their life.[9] A major drawback of it is that the patient often becomes too focused on his or her pain as a result.[10]

The interview process can provide a wealth of information for the clinician. According to Rothstein and associates the information synthesizing process begins in the interview process, even before the clinician lays hands on the patient.[11]

Physical Assessment—How To

Once the interview session is over, the physical process begins. If a treatment session could be extended to four hours, it would be possible to evaluate every aspect of the person during the physical assessment session. In reality, though, treatment sessions often last less than an hour, and it becomes crucial that the clinician choose to assess the areas that may affect the problem. The other reason for focusing on the major problem area is that the older person may have limited stamina.[12]

Appendix A contains many different types of evaluation forms. The first group of forms are orthopedic forms that can be used for the different body parts. For example, if a patient complains of neck pain, the therapist should evaluate the pain using a neck evaluation form. The forms included in Appendix A were specifically developed in a geriatric clinic.[13] The neurological forms look at various functional problems related to mobility. Appendix A contains forms to evaluate problems with bed mobility, sitting, standing, gait, and balance. In addition, stroke and Parkinson's evaluation forms are included.

The final area for evaluation is the cardiopulmonary system. A specific cardiopulmonary evaluation form is provided in Appendix A. Even though the physical assessment forms are divided into specific areas, it is often necessary to assess the patient's cardiopulmonary status, even if treating the patient for neck pain. Therefore, the wise clinician will use different pieces of various forms depending on individual patients needs.

Table 10–1 lists the more common problems among older people that a clinician should be aware of during an initial evaluation.[14]

ENVIRONMENTAL ASSESSMENT

Because there are so many changes that are common among the older population, environmental assessments may be necessary for the institution or the home. Appendix B contains an environmental assessment form for the home and the institution. These forms can be used by the clinician, family, or patient.

Assessing the environment should not be taken lightly. Lawton's "environmental docility hypothesis" states that the proportion of the behavior attributable to the environment increases as the person's competence decreases.[15] In addition, the older person has diminished senses and, therefore, reacts less to the environment. This results in a cascade of internalization and a decrease in reality and function.[16] Some evidence shows that enriched environments can favorably affect older persons.[17,18]

The assessment of color and lighting is an extremely important aspect of the environmental evaluation. The use of appropriate color can minimize the adverse effects of sensory deprivation, enhance

TABLE 10–1. PROBLEMS MORE COMMON OR SEVERE IN THE ELDERLY

1. Falls
2. Syncope
3. Hip fracture
4. Urinary incontinence
5. Fecal incontinence
6. Fecal impaction
7. Pressure sores
8. Hearing and vision impairment
9. Stroke
10. Dementia syndrome
11. Parkinsonism
12. Normal pressure hydrocephalus
13. Polymyalgia rheumatica/giant cell arteritis
14. Osteoporosis
15. Osteoarthritis
16. Paget's disease
17. Carpal tunnel syndrome
18. Spinal stenosis
19. Diabetic hyperosmolar nonketotic coma
20. Inappropriate antidiuretic hormone secretion
21. Accidental hypothermia
22. Chronic lymphatic leukemia
23. Basal cell carcinoma
24. Angioimmunoblastic lymphadenopathy with dysproteinemia
25. Solid tumors
26. Tuberculosis
27. Herpes zoster
28. Arteriosclerosis
29. Amyloidosis
30. Colonic angiodysplasia
31. Isolated systolic hypertension
32. Postural hypotension

Reprinted with permission from Besdine RW. Clinical approach to the elderly. In: Rowe JW, Besdine RW. Geriatric Medicine. ed 2. Boston: Little Brown & Co.; 1988: Table 3–5:30.

mood, and improve function.[19] Color usage follows several simple rules:

1. Increase lighting as much as possible (up to three times as much as for younger persons).[20]
2. Use matte surfaces. Avoid glare on any surface.
3. Use contrasting colors as much as possible (that is, light and dark, different hues, cold and warm colors).
4. Use cues; however, make sure they are of adequate size and are clear and visible.
6. Use daylight fluorescent light. This light offers a broader distribution of light.[21]

PSYCHOSOCIAL ASSESSMENT

Specific psychosocial assessment forms are described in Chapters 4 and 6, therefore, this section will discuss when a psychosocial assessment is appropriate. The areas most important to the outcome of rehabilitation are depression and dementia. Depression is important because it will affect the participant's assessment and expectation of the rehabilitation program.

The depressed client will have lower expectations and tend to underassess progress. In addition, depression can cause lethargy, which may discourage the client from participating in an exercise program.[22] Therefore, if the astute clinician senses depression from the global signs (e.g., pessimism, low self-esteem, loss of interest, and preoccupation with body aches), administering a depression test may be beneficial. The Geriatric Depression Scale is a good tool for assessing the older population. (See Chapters 4 and 6 for further discussion.) Once the clinician has determined that depression is a major problem, he or she should be aware that complaints of lethargy may only be a manifestation of depression. In addition, the clinician can also be on guard for subjective ratings of improvement or lack thereof.

Dementia, or brain syndromes, may also require special considerations in the rehabilitation program. If the clinician notices that the client has difficulty remembering during the initial questioning, then dementia may be the cause. Any of the brain syndrome screening tools may be administered at this time. If a patient does have a dementia, then the clinician must modify and simplify the treatment program so that the patient will derive the most benefit. Making the program more familiar, shorter, simpler, and more dependent on automatic responses will assist the patient with dementia. In addition, providing instruction to the care giver is crucial.

The final aspect of applying a psychological assessment is implementation. Many patients will resent being asked psychosocial questions in a physical therapy setting. A good approach is to say, "I am going to ask you a few questions that will measure mental processes. The questions may seem silly, but if we begin an exercise program that is too stressful for you, one of the first areas to show a change is your mental processing. Therefore, I need to get an initial assessment." Finally, as stated above, psychological assessments can be used to measure exercise tolerance.

CONCLUSION

Patient evaluation provides some of the most valuable time a therapist spends with a patient. The initial evaluation provides the clinician with information that will enable him or her to design the most appropriate rehabilitation program. Once a thorough evaluation has been done, the rehabilitation program can begin. The next step is to conduct periodic reevaluations.

PEARLS

- The essential setting for evaluating an older person is a noncompeting environment that is well lit, has nonglare surfaces, is wheelchair accessible, and is

- color contrasted with low pile carpet or nonslip floors.
- The initial interview should focus on functional decrements and include questions on history, social support, and subjective findings.
- When physically assessing the aged, consider breaking up the initial evaluation into several visits.
- When assessing pain in the elderly, use additional pain tools, such as pain diagram, pain diaries, pain language tools, and general pain evaluations.
- The environment should be assessed for safety and optimal functioning because as the older person becomes frailer, they become more dependent on the environment.
- Psychosocial aspects of an older person may be awkward for the physical therapist to assess; however, using the straightforward approach will be easiest.

REFERENCES

1. Cooper BA. Model of implementing color contrast in the environment of the elderly. *Am J Occup Ther.* 1985; 39:253–258.
2. Cristarella M. Visual functions of the elderly. *Am J Occup Ther.* 1977; 31:432–440.
3. Lipsitz L, Fullerton R. Post prandial blood pressure reduction in healthy elderly. *J Am Ger Soc.* 1986; 34(4):267–270.
4. McKenzie R. *The Lumbar Spine: Mechanical Diagnosis and Therapy.* Waikanee, New Zealand: Spinal Public; 1981.
5. Harkins S, Kiventis J, Price D. Pain and the elderly. In: Benedette C, et al., eds. *Advances in Pain Management in the Elderly.* New York: Raven; 1984.
6. Ferrel B. Pain management in the elderly. *J Am Ger Soc.* 1991; 36:64–73.
7. Lewis C. *Documentation: Physical Therapists Course in Successful Reimbursement.* Bethesda, Md: Professional Health Educators; 1987.
8. Melzak R. *The Puzzle of Pain.* New York: Basic Books; 1973.
9. Mannheimer J. *Clinical Transculaneous Nerve Stimulation.* Philadelphia: Davis; 1984.
10. Woodruff L. Pain and Aging. Paper presented at APTA June Conference; 1990.
11. Echternach J, Rothstein J. Hypothesis-oriented algorithms. *Phys Ther.* 1989; 69:559–564.
12. Haines RF. Effect of bed rest and exercise on body balance. *J Appl Physiol.* 1974; 36:323.
13. Lewis C. Forms from physical therapy services of Washington, DC, Inc., 1990.
14. Besdine RW. Clinical approach to the elderly. In: Rowe JW, Besdine RW. *Geriatric Medicine.* 2nd ed. Boston: Little Brown & Co.; 1988.
15. Lawton MP. Assessment, integration and environments for older people. *Gerontologist.* 1970; 10: 38–46.
16. Kraus A, Spasoff R, Beattie E. Elderly applicants to long-term care institutions: their characteristics, health problems and state of mind. *J Am Ger Soc.* 1976; 24(3):117–125.
17. Birren F. Human response to color and light. *Hospitals.* 1979; 53(14):93–96.
18. Whelihan W. Geriatric centers environment fosters interaction. *Hosp Prog.* 1980; 61:50–55.
19. Hiatt L. Care and design for color and use of color in environments for older persons. *Nursing Homes.* 1981; 30:18–22.
20. Corso J. Sensory processes and age effects in normal adults. *J Gerontol.* 1971; 26:90–105.
21. Sylvania GTE. Engineering Bulletin 0-341. Fluorescent Lamps. Montreal, Canada.
22. Zarit S. Aging and mental disorders. In: *A Psychological Approach to Assessment and Treatment.* New York: The Free Press; 1980.

Appendix A   Orthopedic, Neurological, and Cardiopulmonary Evaluation Forms

Orthopedic Evaluation Forms
  Hip Pain Evaluation
  Hip Fractures
  Knee Evaluation
  Foot Assessment
  Shoulder Evaluation
  Neck Evaluation
  Back Evaluation
Neurological Evaluation Forms
  Hemiplegic Evaluation
  Coordination Evaluation

  Mobility Assessments
  Transfer Evaluation
  Balance and Falls Assessment
Cardiopulmonary Evaluation Forms
  Cardiopulmonary Evaluation
  Step Test
  Medical History Form
  Physical Activity Questionnaire
  Exercise Data Sheet

ORTHOPEDIC EVALUATION FORMS

Hip Pain Evaluation

Name _____ Age: _____ Sex: _____

Diagnosis _____

History _____

Precautions _____

Function _____

Pain
    Character _____

       When _____

       Where _____

       What increases _____

       What decreases _____

       Position of comfort _____

Low back check
    History _____

    ROM _____

    Pain _____

    Movement _____

Range of motion and strength

	ROM		STRENGTH	
	L	R	L	R
Hip Flexion				
Extension				
Adduction				
Abduction				
IR				
ER				
Knee Flexion				
Knee Extension				
Unilateral Stance				

Tenderness or Spasm _____

    Hip _____

    Thigh _____

    Knee _____

Posture _____

Gait _____

Sensation _____

Other _____

Figure 10A–1. (© Carole B Lewis, Geriatric Orthopedics Handout.)

Physical Therapy Evaluation and Treatment Report for Patients with Hip Fracture in Extended Care Settings

Name _____ Date _____ Record # _____

Age _____ Sex _____ Referring Physician _____

Description of fracture _____

Onset _____ Fixation used _____

Surgery date _____ Additional diagnoses _____

_____

Medications potentially impacting rehab performance _____

Other significant medications _____

Current weight bearing orders _____

Preinjury living arrangements _____

Preinjury functional/ADL status _____

Social support available _____

Bowel and bladder control _____

HOSPITAL DISCHARGE PHYSICAL THERAPY STATUS
Exercise program _____

Assistive devices used _____

Distance ambulating _____

Equipment brought to facility _____

SKIN EVALUATION
At risk bony prominences (heel of affected leg, sacrum, trochanters) _____

_____

General skin condition; other bony prominences _____

_____

Suture line _____

PHYSICAL AND FUNCTIONAL EVALUATION
Ability to go sitting to supine _____

Ability to relieve pressure from affected heel _____

Ability to roll to either side _____

Range of Motion

Affected Limb:

Hip _____

Knee _____ Ankle _____

Other Extremities and Trunk _____

_____

Leg length comparison _____

Ability to go supine to sitting _____

Manual Muscle Testing

	(R) arm	(L) arm		Unaffected Leg	Affected Leg
Shoulder flexors	_____	_____	Hip flexors	_____	Not tested
Serratus Anterior	_____	_____	Hip extensors	_____	Not tested
Biceps	_____	_____	Hip abductors	_____	Not tested
Triceps	_____	_____	Knee extensors	_____	_____
Wrist extensors	_____	_____	Knee flexors	_____	_____
			Ankle dorsiflexors	_____	_____
			Ankle plantarflexors	_____	_____

Continued

Continued from previous page

Tool for Physical Therapy Evaluation

Transfer ability: to horizontal surface _____
_____ to toilet _____
_____
Ability to come to standing _____
Gait Analysis (Address device, distance, ability to maintain weight bearing orders, posture, gait deviations, endurance, balance, etc.)

Discomfort in the affected limb _____
Other pain/discomfort _____
Wheelchair safety _____
Wheelchair mobility _____
Ability to stair climb _____

SENSORY AND EMOTIONAL EVALUATION
Vision _____ Hearing _____
Emotional state _____
Motivation _____
Ability to follow instructions _____

OTHER SIGNIFICANT FINDINGS

ASSESSMENT/REHABILITATION POTENTIAL
Short-range Goals:

Long-range Goals:

Treatment Plan:

_____
Physician's Comments: Therapist's Signature

Physician's Certification/Recertification

I certify _____ re-certify _____ that I have examined the patient and physical therapy is necessary and that service will be furthered while the patient is under my care, and that the plan is established and will be reviewed every 30 days or more often if the patient's condition requires. I estimate that these services will be needed for about _____ (specify no. of days, weeks, or months)
Physician's name	Physician's Signature	Date	Telephone

Figure 10A–2. *(Reprinted with permission from Hielema F, Mitchell R, Dyster R. A tool for the physical therapy evaluation of patients with hip fractures in the extended care setting. Top Geriatr Rehabil. 1989; 4(2):56–57.)*

Knee Evaluation

Date _____

Name _____ Age and Sex _____

Diagnosis _____

History _____

Pain _____

Functional activities _____

   Sitting to Standing _____

   Ambulation (device & assistance needed) _____

   Approximate distance ambulates before resting _____

   Elevations (stairs, curbs, & ramps) _____

Range of motion—muscle strength

	(R) - ROM - (L)	(R) - MS - (L)
Hip Flexion _____		
Abduction _____		
External Rotation _____		
Internal Rotation _____		
Straight Leg Raise _____		
Knee Flexion _____		
Extension/Extension lag _____		
Ankle Plantarflexion _____		
Dorsiflexion _____		

Crepitations _____

Patellar Tracking _____

Leg length (ASIS —Med. Malleolus) (R) _____ (L) _____

Gait and posture

   Summary gait analysis _____

   Standing Time _____ Bilateral _____ Left _____ Right _____ 8 Steps _____

   Genu valgus or varus _____

   Sensation _____

Girth

	Left	Right
0 cm		
5 cm		
10 cm		
15 cm		
15 cm		

Swelling _____

Skin _____

Medication _____

Mentation _____

Goals _____

Treatment plan _____

Additional comments _____

Figure 10A–3. *(© Carole B Lewis, Geriatric Orthopedics Handout.)*

Assessment of the Foot

Name _____ Age _____ Assistive Device _____

Past Medical History _____

Current Medications _____

Complaints of Pain   Type _____   Location _____

                               At rest _____ Incessant _____ On movement _____

Light Touch Sensation: L4 _____   L5 _____   S1 _____

Vibratory Sensation _____

Inspection   Swelling? Volumetric measurements skin (ulcers? bunion? color, temp, nails, dryness, calluses?)

_____   R.A. Nodules? _____

Circulatory Status   Pulses: Posterior Tibialis _____   Dorsal Pedalis _____

Posture of Foot   Hallux Valgus/Varus _____   Foot Pronation _____

                               Forefoot Splaying _____   Lesser Toe Deformities _____

                               Calcaneal Valgus _____   Other _____

		Active	Passive	Resistive	(Pain) (Strength)
Ankle ROM	Dorsiflexion				
	Plantarflexion				
Subtalar Motion	Supination				
	Pronation				
Midtarsal Motion	Inversion/Eversion				
	ABduction/ADDuction				

Abductor Halluxes   Strength: _____

                               ROM: _____

Hallux Extension/Flexion   Strength: _____

                               ROM: _____

Digit Extension/Flexion   Strength: _____

                               ROM: _____

Digit Addubction   Strength: _____

Strength/ROM Deficits in   Hip _____

Figure 10A–4.   *(© Carole B Lewis, Geriatric Orthopedics Handout.)*

Shoulder Evaluation

Name: _____   Date: _____

Age: _____   Diagnosis:_____

_____

History:

1. Where is your pain?

_____

2. Was there an injury?

_____

3. How long have you had your problem?

_____

4. Have any other joints been affected?

_____

5. Has your pain spread?

_____

6. When does your pain occur?

_____

Observation: (check symmetry, atrophy or subluxation)

1. A-C Joint: _____   2. Superior border
                                                   of scapula: _____

3. Inferior angle of   4. Other areas: _____
   Scapula: _____   _____

Palpation:

1. A-C joint (place arm in abduction past 90°, then horizontally adduct in forward flexion)
   Pain _____   No Pain _____

2. Rotator Cuff Insertion (Place arm in internal rotation, extension and adduction)
   Pain _____   No Pain _____

3. Crepitus
   Yes _____   No _____

(FR = Full Range; LR = Limited Range; P = Pain; NP = No Pain)

―――――*Continued* ―――――

─────────────── *Continued from previous page* ───────────────

4. Temperature (state whether hot, warm, cool; compare to other side) _____

	Active Movements	Passive Movements	Resisted Movements
Forward Flexion			
Abduction			
External Rotation			
Internal Rotation			
Extension			

Special Tests

Drop Arm Test: (Abduct arm to 90°, patient should be able to lower arm slowly down; if test is positive, patient unable to control arm)

Positive: _____   Negative: _____

Arthrogram Results: _____

_____

X-Ray Findings: _____

_____

Figure 10A–5. *(© Carole B Lewis, Geriatric Orthopedics Handout.)*

Neck Evaluation

Date: _____ Age: _____ Sex: _____

Name: _____

Diagnosis: _____

Precautions: _____

History: _____

Function: _____

Range of Motion	Strength		Passive		Normal	Active		Comments
	Left	Right	Left	Right		Left	Right	
Flexion					0–30			
Extension					0–35			
Lat Flexion					0–40			
Rotation					0–130			

Shoulder ROM _____

Description of pain:

_____ Localized   _____ Sharp   _____VAS

_____ Diffuse   _____ Prolonged; Intense

_____ Other   _____ Burning   Posture:

          Forward Head _____

          Scoliosis _____

          Kyphosis _____

Shoulder Radiation _____

Related Pain _____

    When pain occurs _____

    Frequency and duration _____

    Position of comfort _____

Abnormal Sensation _____

Spasms (indicate position tested, area and degree) _____

Medication _____

Vocation or Avocation _____

Sleep position _____

Goals _____

Treatment _____

Additional Comments _____

Figure 10A–6. (© *Carole B Lewis, Geriatric Orthopedics Handout.*)

Low Back Evaluation

Patient: _____   Date:_____

Diagnosis:_____

HX: _____

I. Pain Description

A. Where: _____

B. How long:_____

C. At rest: _____

    Sitting: _____

    Standing: _____

    Lying: _____

    Other: _____

D. With activity: _____

    Walking: _____

    Lifting: _____

    Bending: _____

    Other: _____

E. Character: _____

    Sharp: _____

    Dull: _____

    Radiating: _____

F. Spinal Tenderness: _____

    Locale: _____

G. Muscle Spasm: _____

    Locale: _____

II. Muscle Strength & ROM

	ROM		STRENGTH	
	L	R	L	R
Lumbar Flexion				
Lumbar Extension				
Hip Flexors				
Hip Extensors				
Int. Rotators				
Ext. Rotators				
Knee Flexors				
Knee Extensors				
Ankle Dorsiflexors				
Ankle Plantar Flexors				
Ankle Invertors				
Ankle Extensors				
Toe Flexors				
Toe Extensors				

—Continued —

Continued from previous page

Postural Examination

HEAD
Forward _____
Level _____
Other _____

HIPS
High _____
Low _____
Other _____

ABNORMALITIES
SPINAL
Kyphosis _____
Lordosis _____
Scoliosis _____

SHOULDERS
High _____
Low _____
Other _____

LEG LENGTH
Supine _____
Upright _____

LOWER EXTREMITIES
Normal _____
Genu Valgum _____
Genu Varum _____
Genu Recurvatum _____
Tibial Torsion _____

Functional Evaluation

How is the patient's pain affecting his activities of daily living?

What makes you feel better?

_____ PT

Figure 10A–7. *(© Carole B Lewis, Geriatric Orthopedics Handout.)*

NEUROLOGIC EVALUATION FORMS

Hemiplegic Evaluation

General Observations

1. Sitting (symmetry)_____ Leg position _____ Arm _____

2. Up from sit

3. Standing (with cane) _____ (without) _____

   Wiggle bottom _____ Leg (Wt) _____ Shoulder _____

4. Gait   Control _____ 2 Gaits? _____

   Turns _____ Backward _____

   Side Step _____ Push-faster
   Spontaneous _____

   Push pull _____ Spontaneous _____

   Wiggle bottom _____

5. Standing

   Bend strong side _____

   Shoulder with elbow extension _____

   Tone   hand wrist _____

   Shoulder abduction _____

6. Undress

   Arm _____

   Leg _____

7. Sitting—left arm _____

   left leg _____

   tickle foot _____

   arm clasp _____

   cross leg _____

   uncross _____

   cross leg & clasp _____

Figure 10A–8.   *(© Carole B Lewis, Geriatric Orthopedics Handout.)*

Coordination Evaluation

By each item, briefly describe deficits, abnormal posturing, etc. Put "N" beside each item that is normal. Put "—" in those categories not tested.

ITEM	DESCRIPTION

I. LOW LEVEL COORDINATION

A. Shoulder and UE

1. Weight shifting in prone on elbows (forward and backward, side to side)_____

2. Weight shifting sitting propped on hands (side to side)_____

B. Pelvis and LE

1. Weight shifting in bridging (forward and backward, side to side)_____

2. Pelvic tilt (anterior and posterior) in supine_____

3. Hip abduction and adduction in supine_____

4. Alternate knee to chest in supine_____

5. Weight shifting in kneeling (forward and back, side to side, diagonals)_____

6. Weight shifting in 1/2 kneeling (forward and back, side to side, diagonals)_____

7. Weight shifting in standing (forward and back, side to side, diagonals)_____

C. Combined UE and LE

1. Weight shifting in quadruped (forward and back, side to side, diagonals)_____

2. Jumping jack motion in supine_____

II. MIDDLE LEVEL COORDINATION

A. Shoulder and UE

1. Reaching in prone on elbows (forward and sideways)_____

2. Chopping and lifting patterns in kneeling_____

3. Alternate UE lifts in quadruped_____

————————Continued ———

Continued from previous page

ITEM	DESCRIPTION

B. Pelvis and LE

1. Unilateral bridging with other LE extended _____

2. Alternate LE lifts in quadruped _____

3. Kneel-walking (forward and back, sideways) _____

4. Heel slides opposite knee to ankle along tibial crest _____

5. Making circles with extended LE _____

6. Walking (forward, backward, sideways) _____

C. Combined UE and LE

1. Creeping _____

2. Alternate UE and LE lifts in quadruped (opposite sides, same sides) _____

III. HIGH LEVEL COORDINATION

A. UE

1. Bouncing ball (same hand, alternate hands) _____

2. Catching and throwing a ball _____

3. Finger to nose _____

4. Alternate forearm pronation/supination (same direction, opposite direction) _____

B. LE (upright)

1. One limb balance (right and left) _____

2. Two-foot hop _____

3. Jogging in place _____

4. One-foot hop (right and left) _____

5. Crossover walking (right and left) _____

6. Balance beam walking (forward, backward, sideways) _____

7. Foot tapping (right and left) _____

8. Tracing shapes with feet (right and left) _____

C. Combined UE and LE

1. Jumping rope _____

2. Jumping jacks _____

3. Crab walking _____

Figure 10A–9. *(Reprinted with permission from Cruz, V. Evaluation of coordination—a clinical model. Clin Management. 1986; 6(3): 6–10. Reprinted with permission of the American Physical Therapy Association.)*

Mobility Assessment

Name _____ Date _____

Functional Problem _____

Goals _____

History _____
_____

Physical Evaluation _____

        Skin _____

            Cardiopulmonary BP _____ HR _____

            Pathology _____

        Musculoskeletal

            ROM _____

            STR _____

            FEET _____

        Neurological

            Reflexes _____ Proprioception _____

            Vibration _____ Sway _____

            Tremor _____ Tone_____

Psychological

            Motivation _____ Depression _____

            Dementia _____ Falling Fear _____

Drugs _____

            Prescribed _____ OTC _____

Environment _____

Mobility Grade

            Bed _____ Sitting _____

            Transfer _____ Wheelchair _____

            Standing _____

            Gait _____

Support System _____

MISC _____

Figure 10A–10. *(© Carole B Lewis, Geriatric Neurology Handout.)*

Transfer Evaluation

Cardiopulmonary Status
    HR _____
    BP _____
    Sit to Stand _____
Neuromusculoskeletal
    Tone _____
    Strength _____
    Flexibility _____
    Phsychosocial _____
    Personal _____
    Support System _____
Transfer Position

	Initial	Mid	Ending
Head			
Neck			
Trunk			
Hips			
Pelvis			
Knees			
Feet			

Figure 10A–11. *(© Carole B Lewis, Geriatric Neurology Handout.)*

Balance and Falls Assessment

1. Current medical problems _____
_____
2. Medications _____
_____
3. History of Falls _____
_____
    Frequency _____
    Time of day _____
    Position _____
    Activity _____
    Circumstances _____
4. Balance with eyes open _____
_____
    Balance with eyes closed _____
5. Push balance recovery _____
_____
6. Balance actuator _____
_____
7. VAS _____
_____
8. Lying to sit _____
_____
9. Sit to stand _____
_____
10. Flexibility _____
_____

Figure 10A–12. *(© Carole B Lewis, Geriatric Neurology Handout.)*

Cardiopulmonary Evaluation

Name _____

Date _____

RHR _____

RBP _____

RR _____

Current Activity Level _____

Posture

       C-Spine _____

       T-Spine _____

       Shoulders _____

Meds _____

Mental Status _____

History _____

      _____

Pain   _____

      _____

Stress Level _____

Chair Step Test

		HR	BP
6"	2 min.		
	5 min.		
12"	2 min.		
	5 min.		
18"	2 min.		
	5 min.		
18" &	2 min.		
arms	5 min.		

Comments _____

Figure 10A–13. *(© Carole B Lewis.)*

Step Test Data Sheet

Name _____

Age/DOB_____   Date _____

Weight _____   Examiner _____

Target Heart Rate Range (circle appropriate level)

Age	Target HR
61–70	114–132
71–80	108–125
81–90	102–118

Workload			HR	BP	Comments (symptoms)
Rest					
Step Test					
Step height	Steps/min	Met level			
0"	13	2			
8"	10	3			
8"	15	4			
8"	20	5			
8"	26	6			
Recovery					
3 minutes					
6 minutes					

Figure 10A–14.

Medical History Form

Have you ever had any indications of, or been treated for, any of the following? (underline applicable item)

		YES	NO
1.	High blood pressure? (If "yes", list drugs prescribed and dates taken)	____	____
2.	Disorders of the heart or blood vessels, such as rheumatic fever, heart murmur or irregular pulse?	____	____
3.	Disorders of the lungs, such as asthma, tuberculosis, bronchitis or emphysema?	____	____
4.	Cancer, tumor, cyst, or any disorder of the thyroid, skin or lymph glands?	____	____
5.	Diabetes or anemia, or other blood disorder?	____	____
6.	Sugar, albumin, blood or pus in the urine, or venereal disease?	____	____
7.	Any disorder of the kidney, bladder, prostate, breast or reproductive organs?	____	____
8.	Ulcer, intestinal bleeding, hepatitis, colitis or other disorder of the stomach, intestine, spleen, pancreas, liver or gall bladder?	____	____
9.	Fainting, convulsions, migraine headache, paralysis, epilepsy or any mental or nervous disorder?	____	____
10.	Arthritis, gout, amputation, sciatica, back pain or other disorder of the muscles, bones, or joints?	____	____
11.	Disorder of the eyes, ears, nose, throat or sinuses?	____	____
12.	Varicose veins, hemorrhoids, hernia or rectal disorder?	____	____
13.	Alcoholism or drug habit?	____	____

HAVE YOU:

14.	Had, or been advised to have, an x-ray, cardiogram, blood or other diagnostic test in the past 5 years?	____	____
15.	Been a patient in a hospital, clinic, or other medical facility in the past 5 years?	____	____
16.	Ever had a surgical operation performed or advised?	____	____
17.	Had any oral or respiratory infections in the past week?	____	____

Give details of "yes" answers on reverse, including number of attacks and dates.

Figure 10A–15.

Physical Activity Questionnaire

1. How often do you take walks?
   a. 4 or more times per week
   b. about 3 times per week
   c. very infrequently or never (Do not answer question 2 if your answer is c)
2. Of the walks you take at least three times per week, how far do you walk?
   a. less than 1/2 mile
   b. 1/2 mile or more, but less than 1 mile
   c. 1 mile or more, but less than 2 miles
   d. 2 miles or more
3. How many hours a day are you on your feet working in your apartment?
   a. 0–1 hour
   b. 1–2 hours
   c. 2–3 hours
   d. more than 3 hours
4. Do you do your own grocery shopping and carry your groceries? (May use wheeled cart to bring them home)
   a. frequently
   b. sometimes
   c. very infrequently or never
5. Do you do your own laundry?
   a. frequently
   b. sometimes
   c. very infrequently or never
6. Do you do any volunteer work or physical activity outside the building?
   a. frequently
   b. sometimes
   c. very infrequently or never
7. Do you go out of your apartment to socialize?
   a. frequently
   b. sometimes
   c. very infrequently or never
8. Do you invite friends and relatives over to socialize?
   a. frequently
   b. sometimes
   c. very infrequently or never

Continued

Continued from previous page

Indicate how often you do each activity on the list below using the following scores:

0 = never or almost never
1 = once a month or every other month
2 = 2 or 3 times a month
3 = 1 to 5 times a week
4 = about every day
5 = more than once a day

_____ Play cards, bingo, other games	_____ Cook
_____ Watch television	_____ Sleep
_____ Sing	_____ Iron, do laundry
_____ Socialize	_____ Listen to radio or music
_____ Play billiards	_____ Work in apartment
_____ Ride stationary bike	_____ Sit
_____ Read	_____ Walk
_____ Take care of plants	_____ Watch sports
_____ Shop	_____ Write letters
_____ Do needle work, art, crafts	_____ Exercise
_____ Eat	_____ Babysit
_____ Do crossword puzzles	_____ Participate in organizations, committees
_____ Travel	_____ Dance
_____ Go to church	

Figure 10A–16.

Exercise Data Sheet

MD_____ Date_____

Admission Date _____ Age _____ Sex_____

Diagnosis _____ Marital Status _____ # of Children_____

Apt. or House_____ # of Stairs _____ Family Assess._____

Significant PMH: _____

Risk Factors _____

Complications: _____

Present Hx _____

Telemetry _____ CPK _____ MB _____ E.F. _____

Medications _____

Psych. Status _____

Date	Pre-Exercise BP & HR	Distance	Post Exercise BP & HR	Initials	Comments

Assessment:

Discharge:

Figure 10A–17.

Appendix B Environmental Evaluation Forms

Institutional Environmental Evaluation
General Sensory Evaluation

Home Asessment Checklist for Fall Hazards
General Environmental Evaluation

Institutional Environmental Evaluation

Instructions: evaluate the resident's environment, checking either yes, no, or D/A (does not apply). Then check if the area needs work (NW). At the end, list all areas for correction.

	YES	NO	D/A	N/W
Resident's Room				
Colors				
1. Are the colors contrasted?				
2. Are reds predominant and blues and greens pale?				
Objects				
1. Are rugs and/or carpets secured safely?				
2. Are chairs or tables secure enough to support weight if needed?				
3. Is there any clutter or unsafe objects (i.e. low furniture)?				
4. Is ADT equipment (i.e. telephone, etc) easily accessible?				
5. Are grab bars or rails secure and accessible?				
Lighting				
1. Is lighting bright enough and from multiple sources?				
2. Are lights glare free and properly situated?				
3. Are glare situations minimized (i.e. mirrors)?				
Dangerous areas				
1. Are objects easily seen and reached without excessive reaching, stooping?				
2. Are doorways wide enough and trip-proof?				
3. Are bathtubs or showers furnished with skid proof surfaces?				
4. Is a night light used?				
Miscellaneous				
1. Is the room adequately sound-proofed?				
Exterior				
1. Are steps and edges clearly marked?				
2. Are color-contrasted handrails present in hallways and stairs?				
3. Are rooms, signs, etc. marked with sufficiently large and well spaced letters and written on a color contrasted background?				
4. Are social areas far from outside noise areas?				
5. Is background noise in general low-level?				
6. Are walkways and steps in good repair and free of cracks or bulges?				
7. Is adequate diffuse lighting available in all public areas?				
8. If music is playing, is it in the lower tones?				
9. Are foods presented on color contrasting plates and mats?				

Areas for improvement:

_____

_____

_____

_____

Figure 10B–1.

General Sensory Evaluation

Name _____

Place _____

Date _____

Vision

Color Contrasting _____

Food _____ Table _____ Plates _____

Pills _____

Rugs, Floors, Chairs _____

Stairs _____ Doorways _____

Glare

Windows _____

Floors _____

Furniture _____

Night Lighting _____

Reading Material _____

Lighting _____

Aids _____

Hearing

The Person

Aids _____ Motivation _____

Vision _____ Stress _____

Skills _____ Social Activities _____

_____

Figure 10B–2.

Home Assessment Checklist for Fall Hazards

Exterior
- Are step surfaces nonslip?
- Are step edges visually marked to avoid tripping?
- Are steps in good repair?
- Are stairway handrails present? Are handrails securely fastened to fittings?
- Are walkways covered with a nonslip surface and free of objects that could be tripped over?
- Is there sufficient outdoor lighting to provide safe ambulation at night?

Interior
- Are lights bright enough to compensate for limited vision? Are light switches accessible to the patient before entering rooms?
- Are lights glare free?
- Are stairways adequately lighted?
- Are handrails present on both sides of staircases?
- Are handrails securely fastened to walls?
- Are step edges outlined with colored adhesive tape and slip resistant?
- Are throw rugs secured with nonslip backing?
- Are carpet edges taped or tacked down?
- Are rooms uncluttered to permit unobstructed mobility?
- Are chairs throughout home strong enough to provide support during transfers? Are armrests present on chairs to provide assistance while transferring?
- Are tables (dining room, kitchen, etc) secure enough to provide support if leaned on?
- Do low-lying objects (coffee tables, step stools, etc) present a tripping hazard?
- Are telephones accessible?

Kitchen
- Are storage areas easily reached without having to stand on tiptoe or a chair?
- Are linoleum floors slippery?
- Is there a nonslip mat in the sink area to soak up spilled water?
- Are chairs wheelfree, armrest equipped, and of the proper height to allow for safe transfers?
- If the pilot light goes out on the gas stove, is the gas odor strong enough to alert the patient?
- Are step stools strong enough to provide support? Are stool treads in good repair and slip resistant?

Bathroom
- Are doors wide enough to provide unobstructed entering with or without a device?
- Do door thresholds present tripping hazards?
- Are floors slippery, especially when wet?
- Are skid-proof strips or mats in place in the tub or shower?
- Are tub and toilet grab bars available? Are grab bars securely fastened to the walls?
- Are toilets low in height? Is an elevated toilet seat available to assist in toilet transfers?
- Is there sufficient, accessible, and glare-free light available?

Bedroom
- Is there adequate and accessible lighting available? Are night-lights and/or bedside lamps available for nighttime bathroom trips?
- Is the pathway from the bed to the bathroom clear to provide unobstructed mobility (especially at night)?
- Are beds of appropriate height to allow for safe on and off transfers?
- Are floors covered with a nonslip surface and free of objects that could be tripped over?
- Can patient reach objects from closet shelves without standing on tiptoe or a chair?

Figure 10B–3. *(Reprinted with permission from Tideiksaar R. Fall prevention in the home. Top Geriatr Rehabil. 1987;3(1):59. Permission from Aspen Publishers, Inc.)*

General Environmental Evaluation

	Yes	No	D/A
Lighting:			
Does each room have multiple sources of light?			
Is the lighting diffuse?			
Is the lighting sufficiently bright?			
Are there blinds, drapes, sheer curtains across windows through which bright light shines?			
Are mirrors placed so that they do not reflect blinding amounts of light?			
Are older people seated so that bright sources of light are to the side of them?			
Colors:			
Do wall colors contrast with the colors of floors and rugs?			
Are the predominant colors red, orange, pink, and yellow?			
Are the blues and greens intense rather than pale?			
Are colors used to mark the edges of steps, curbs?			
Do small rugs contrast sharply in color with their floors?			
Is the paper used in making announcements, pamphlets, etc., a beige, off-white, yellow, or other warm color?			
Lettering:			
Are rooms, offices, signs, elevators, mailboxes, menus, notices, schedules, and so on, marked with sufficiently large and well spaced lettering?			
Are letters and numbers in sharp contrast to their background?			
Is the print easy to read for the older person?			
Are the markings on appliances easily discerned, such as OFF/ON, or HOT/COLD?			
Are personal letters to older people written in large, legible script or in large type?			
Hearing Environment:			
Is background noise reduced as much as possible?			
Are frequent interruptions by phones, people, or noises minimized?			
Are rooms adequately sound-proofed to facilitate conversation?			
Are conversational areas separated from areas containing noise-generating equipment?			
Communication:			
Are your voice tones moderate?			
Do you avoid shouting?			
Is your speech moderate in pace?			
Do you enunciate your words?			
Do you directly face older people and catch their attention?			
Do you inform the hard-of-hearing person of changes in conversation?			
Are you seated within three to five feet of the older person?			
Are children instructed about ways of interacting with older people?			
Are phone amplifiers available?			

Continued

—— *Continued from previous page* ——

Are receivers available in public halls, churches, etc.?

Is adequate lighting available for the older person to see lips and facial expressions?

Touch:

Does the environment contain a rich variety of textures that are easily accessible for the older person to feel?

Does the environment contain a rich variety of objects that are interesting to touch?

Do you and others shake hands warmly with older persons being welcomed into your setting?

Do you know what forms of touch are appreciated by older persons with whom you interact?

Dangerous Areas:

Are the edges of individual steps marked with a bright, contrasting color?

Are protrusions on walls or floors carefully marked?

Are curbs and driveways clearly marked?

Are kitchen appliances, showers, baths, and so on, clearly marked as to on/off or hot/cold positions?

Figure 10B–4. *(Reprinted with permission and adapted from The Sixth Sense. The National Council on Aging. Washington, DC; 1985.)*

CHAPTER 11

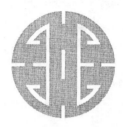

Orthopaedic Treatment Considerations

The principles of geriatric rehabilitation, posed in *Archives of Physical Medicine and Rehabilitation*, state that approximately 30% of all geriatric patients consult their physicians because of musculoskeletal problems.[1] Therefore, it appears that orthopaedics are a primary concern to therapists working with the elderly. This chapter will explore the changes with age in the musculoskeletal system. Pathologies specific to an older population will be discussed. Then a joint by joint approach will be taken that will examine evaluation and treatment of orthopaedic conditions in the elderly.

STRENGTH

Numerous studies cite the loss of strength with age.[2,3,4] The greatest loss of strength appears to be related to the selective loss of type II muscle fibers, which is thoroughly discussed in Chapter 3 of this text. Other variables can lead to strength loss. Lower levels of physical activity certainly heads the top of this list. A decrease in cardiovascular endurance results in less stamina even during activities of daily living. This sets the stage for progressive loss in overall strength. Poor nutrition can change the metabolic efficiency of energy exchange at the level of the sarcolema. A decrease in activity also leads to a diminished neuromuscular connection whereby transmission of nerve impulses to the muscle is slowed and the strength of the impulse lessened. Inhibition of muscle contraction is the consequence of the presence of edema, often seen in older adults with arthritic changes in the joints.[5] All of these variables will lead to a loss in overall muscular contraction strength. The clinical implications of these changes are that increasing activity could potentially reverse these strength changes. Some hypothetical examples might be:

1. If the decrease in strength is due to cardiovascular inefficiency leading to poor nutrient exchange, then an increase in activity level above rest would increase blood flow to the muscle and positively affect the health of the muscle tissue.
2. If the loss of strength is due to a decrease in the efficiency of the neuromuscular junction contact, exercise has been shown to improve nerve conduction velocities, reaction times, and strength of muscle contraction.[4]
3. If the decrease in strength is due to swelling (i.e., reflex inhibition due to joint distention), then the swelling and subsequent strength loss can be alleviated by using modalities and anti-inflammatory medication prior to joint strength training.[5]

Other major reasons for the decline in strength with age are pathological in nature, all of which appear to be more prevalent in the elderly. An example of this is polymyalgia rheumatica, a systemic inflammatory disease of multiple joints that causes swelling, pain and weakness.[6] Systemic rheumatological problems such as rheumatoid arthritis and lupus, like polymyalgia rheumatica, will diminish activities level secondary to pain and inflexibility and lead to a progressive loss in muscular strength. Parkinson's disease and cerebral vascular accidents, as well as other neurological pathologies, can result in strength loss owing to tone changes and the quality of muscle contraction. The presence of underlying pathology in addition to normal changes in muscle strength with age should be considered in the evaluation and intervention of elderly individuals.

FLEXIBILITY

Another major area of function change with age is flexibility. As a person ages, the muscles become more rigid and tend to become less flexible. There is a higher proportion of type I muscle fibers, making the muscle a stabilizer instead of the fast-reacting muscle.[7] There is also a decrease in elastin and an increase in collagen of the muscle tissue, further affecting the flexibility of muscle tissue (see Chapter 3).

In addition to these changes in muscle tissue, all connective tissues are affected by changes in elastin

and collagen as described in detail in Chapter 3. The cartilage breaks down restricting joint mobility. Tendons and ligaments become more rigid and less resilient to length changes often resulting in injury. Flexibility into extension is most often lost in the elderly.[8,9] Postural changes from kyphosis of the thoracic spine lead to flexed positions of all of the lower extremity joints which may result in irreversible soft tissue contractures if not attended to by the therapist. The presence of contractures requires special consideration in older persons. To get the best results, prolonged static stretching—preceded by a heat modality—is often needed to restore flexibility of collagenous tissue. Functional activities that incorporate elongated muscle positions are also helpful in regaining flexibility.[9]

It must be recognized that once a contracture occurs in older adults, it takes longer to achieve the benefits of a stretching program. Prevention of contractures in the first place is the best mode of intervention. Encouraging extension-strengthening exercises, positioning to facilitate extension, postural and balance exercises, proper nutrition and hydration will help to establish healthy and flexible muscle tissue in the older adult. The key phrase here is *"Extension Equals Function."*[8]

POSTURE

The third area of orthopaedic functional change is posture. The classic "senile posture," which is flexed, is certainly not an inevitable consequence of aging. However, in the presence of osteoporosis, compression wedge fractures of the thoracic vertebrae and compression fractures in the lumbar vertebrae result in characteristic postural changes.

As noted in Figure 11–1, normal posture, absected with a plumb line running from the ear to the ankle, should fall through:

1. The middle of the earlobe.
2. The middle of the acromion process.
3. The middle of the greater trochanter.
4. Posterior to the patella but anterior to the center of the knee joint.
5. Slightly anterior to the lateral malleolus.

The most common posture changes with age, as depicted in Figure 11–2 (see also Figure 10–3), include a forward head, rounded shoulders, decreased lumbar lordosis, and increased flexion in the hips and knees.[9] There are some variations in the way in which posture is evaluated, as discussed in Chapter 10 with progressive postual changes, modification of postual status is often more easily assessed using the middle of the latoral malleolus as the starting point and going up the kinetic chain. Treatment for postural changes in the elderly is to concentrate on extension throughout the kinetic chain. Stretching and flexibility exercises should be employed for any of the body parts that have deviated from the norm.

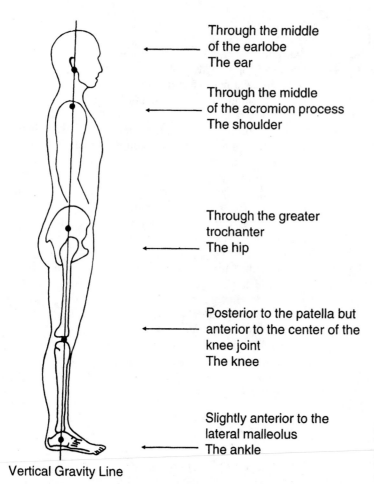

Through the middle
of the earlobe
The ear

Through the middle
of the acromion process
The shoulder

Through the greater
trochanter
The hip

Posterior to the patella but
anterior to the center of the
knee joint
The knee

Slightly anterior to the
lateral malleolus
The ankle

Vertical Gravity Line

Figure 11–1. Proper posture shown with a vertical gravity line. *(Reprinted with permission from Lewis CB, Bottomley JM. Musculoskeletal changes with age. In: Lewis CB, ed.* Aging: The Health Care Challenge. *Philadelphia, PA: FA. Davis; 1990.)*

Strengthening of extensors and work on balance activities are very important components to a postural intervention program. The key to maintaining posture is prevention, prevention, prevention. The key to any exercise program is extension, extension, extension.[8,9,10]

After reviewing strength, flexibility, and posture changes with age, it is important to note that there are several musculoskeletal orthopaedic pathologies that are extremely prevalent in the elderly.

OSTEOPOROSIS: A SPECIAL CONSIDERATION OF A PREVALENT PATHOLOGY

Distinguishing "Normal" Aging of Bone from Osteoporosis

Osteoporosis is no longer considered an inevitable consequence of aging. Many of the sequalae associated with the development of osteoporosis can be prevented by development of a healthy peak bone mineral density during childhood with a maximum density at the time of physiological maturity and by utilizing sound nutritional and exercise practices throughout the lifetime to maintain mineralization of the bone.[10]

Understanding the controlling mechanisms of bone cell response to nutritional and biochemical interventions and mechanical loading is important in preventing the development of osteoporosis (see also Chapter 3).

Two types of bone or osseous tissue have been identified: compact bone, which is dense bone characterized by the arrangement of minerals and cells into haversian systems; and cancellous or spongy bone, also called *trabecular bone,* which has no haversian system. Compact bone makes up approximately 80% of the skeletal mass and is located in the cortices and in the shafts of long bones.[11] Cancellous bone, which comprises the other 20%, is found primarily in the metaphyseal and epiphyseal regions of long bones, areas of the bone exposed to maximal stress, and in the middle layer of flat bones. Although cancellous bone makes up a smaller proportion of overall bone mass, it contributes approximately 70% of the skeletal bone volume, and because of its trabecular arrangement, allows for marrow and fat storage and provides the microstructure that gives bone strength.[12] Loss of trabeculae and cancellous bone mass severely compromises bone strength, increasing the risk for fracture. Figure 11–3 demonstrates the differences in the structure and location of compact and cancellous bone.

Changes in posture (more forward head and kyphosis)

Demineralization of the bone (especially dangerous in the spine—may lead to fractures)

Decreased flexibility (especially in hips and knees)

Loss of strength; greater difficulty in doing functional activities

Changes in gait patterns; less motion and strength, causing less toe off and floor clearance

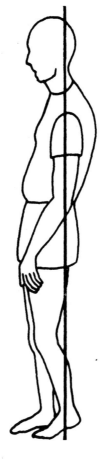

Figure 11–2. *Postural changes with age. (Reprinted with permission from Lewis CB. What's so different about rehabilitating the older person? Clinical Management. May-June 1984; 4(3):12.)*

Compact bone is a highly organized structure as seen in Figure 11–4. Bone cells (called *osteocytes*), nerves, and blood and lymph vessels together form the structural units. Each unit is called a *haversian system* or *osteon*. Haversian systems include concentric *lamellae* surrounding longitudinal channels containing neurovascular bundles, the *haversian* canals. The osteocytes deposit matrix in layers around and between the haversian canals. Between each channel is a matrix of bone mineral, and the circles formed by the bone mineral and osteocyte channels are called lamellae. This lamellar arrangement characterizes mature or lamellar bone.

Cancellous bone is less complex than compact bone, and not as dense. Cancellous bone is composed of thin trabeculae of bone connected to each other in a three-dimensional pattern that looks like a honeycomb from a bee hive as seen in Figure 11–4.

Normal bone contains an abundance of viable cells which are metabolically active. The part of the bone having the most functional significance to the living organism is composed of proteinaceous secretions of these cells in which a large amount of inorganic matter has been deposited. Thus the noncellular components of the skeleton are responsible for the strength and rigidity of the bones, and also serve as the body's largest mineral reserve.[13] The skeleton is the product of cells, and since it remains under the influence of these cells and is consistently being renewed, the nature and function of the living component of bone is important in distinguishing "normal" aging of bone from osteoporotic bone.

Changes in Bone Remodeling During the Life Cycle

Bone growth and bone remodeling are two processes that occur in the formation and maintenance of the axial and appendicular components of the human skeleton.

Bone is formed in a succession of layers by a process called osteogenesis or ossification. These layers, or lamellae, are formed sequentially by osteoblasts. As they are formed, a number of osteoblasts remain within each layer, become entrapped within the bone, and are transformed into osteocytes, the metabolically active cells of bone. Each set of lamellae is arranged so that the living cells remain in contact with a blood supply. In spongy, cancellous bone such as that found in vertebral bodies, or at the diaphysis of long bones such as the femur, these lamellae form spicules which remain in direct contact with the marrow cavity. In compact or cortical bone, lamellae are laid down concentrically around a central arteriole, forming a haversian system. Each set of lamellae (or each haversian system) forms a meta-

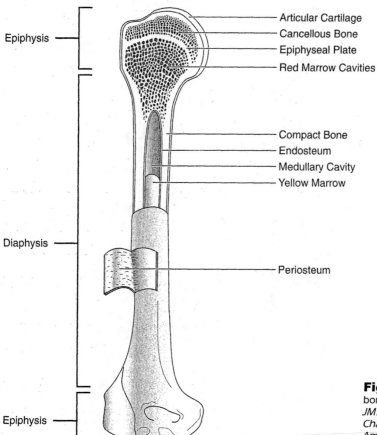

Epiphysis

Diaphysis

Epiphysis

Articular Cartilage
Cancellous Bone
Epiphyseal Plate
Red Marrow Cavities

Compact Bone
Endosteum
Medullary Cavity
Yellow Marrow

Periosteum

Figure 11–3. Cancellous and compact bone. *(Reprinted with permission from Bottomley JM. Orthopedic Interventions with Seniors: Bone Changes in Seniors. Orthopaedic Section of the American Physical Therapy Association. 1999 Home Study Course 9.2.2. Artist: JM Bottomley.)*

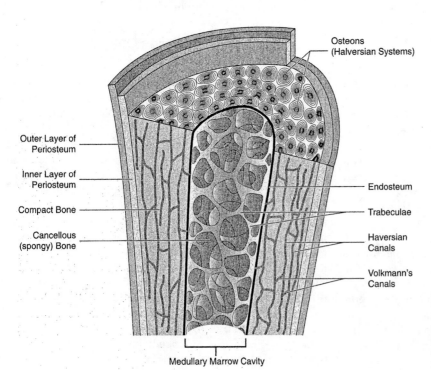

Osteons
(Halversian Systems)

Outer Layer of
Periosteum

Inner Layer of
Periosteum

Compact Bone

Cancellous
(spongy) Bone

Endosteum

Trabeculae

Haversian
Canals

Volkmann's
Canals

Medullary Marrow Cavity

Figure 11–4. Microscopic structure of compact bone. *(Reprinted with permission from Bottomley JM. Orthopedic Interventions with Seniors: Bone Changes in Seniors. Orthopaedic Section of the American Physical Therapy Association. 1999 Home Study Course 9.2.2. Artist: JM Bottomley.)*

bolic unit called the basic multicellular unit. The cells that are embedded within the bone maintain contact with each other by means of fine extensive cellular processes. This web-like system of cellular filaments accounts for the ability of bone to react as a metabolic unit.

The organic phase of bone formation results in the development of the matrix by osteoblasts. The matrix contains a variety of glycoproteins and mucopolysaccharides but is primarily composed of collagen. Collagen is the basis for much of the bone's strength and is the framework on which the minerals are deposited. Of all proteins, it is unique in that it contains the amino acids hydroxyproline and hydroxylysine in high concentrations. Collagen is secreted by the osteoblasts as three peptide chains, which are twisted together (procollagen). A small fragment from one end of the procollagen helix separates from the unit after the peptide triad is secreted and tropocollagen units are formed. These units then polymerize. This continued process leads to the maturation of bone.[13,14]

Prostaglandins, growth factors, and cyctokines have been shown to be important in the control of bone homeostasis and will be discussed further in subsequent sections of this chapter as they are related to hormones such as parathyroid hormone and growth hormones and in response to mechanical loading of the bone.

The mineralization of the matrix is a complex process which is influenced by several factors. Calcium is deposited in bone both as amorphous calcium phosphate and as crystalline hydroxapatite. Much of the initial mineralization occurs in relation to the collagen and the crystals are located between the individual collagen units, within the "gaps" formed by the staggered arrangement and also in the interstices of the fibrils. In the later phases of mineralization, crystals are formed in the matrix between the collagen fibrils. The mineralization is responsible for the rigidity of the bone.

Osteoblast and Osteoclast Activity

The osteocytes play an active role in mineralization. The mitochondria of the osteocyte transfers calcium and phosphates into the matrix of bone.

Bone remodeling, which occurs throughout life, involves the continual breakdown, repair, and replacement of osteocytes and bone mineral. Through the action of multinucleated cells (osteoclasts), both organic and mineral phases of the bone are reabsorbed in localized areas and then replaced by osteoblasts, with a new metabolic unit. Bone deposition occurs at the sites of injury or stress. Bone resorption occurs when bones are unstressed, or when an imbalance exists in the regulatory processes of bone mineral content.

The balance of bone mineral results from the activity of the osteoblasts and osteoclasts. Together they function as parts of a basic multicellular unit (BMU) that responds to regulatory conditions (Figure 11–5). An increase in conditions favoring bone resorption increases osteoclast activity relative to osteoblast activity. Bone resorption occurs when catalytic enzymes are secreted by the osteoclasts. Osteoclasts also have a phygocytic action. The mineral salts released during reabsorption diffuse into the interstitial fluid, where they are removed by the circulation. During conditions of bone resorption, a negative bone mineral balance occurs. Conversely, stimuli that favor bone deposition increase osteoblast activity relative to osteoclast activity, and a net positive bone mineral balance is attained. Estimates indicate that most bone mineral BMUs are in a state of quiescence,[15] with approximately 20% active in cancellous bone and less than 5% active in compact bone. Hormonal components will directly influence

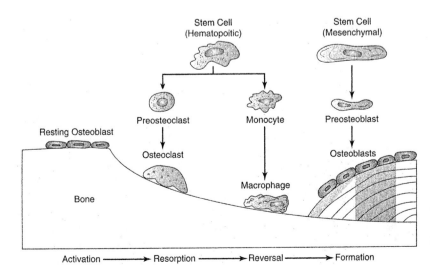

Figure 11–5. *Basic multicellular unit (BMU) which responds to hormonal and physical stress during bone remodeling and is affected by exercise, calcium and estrogen. (Reprinted with permission from Bottomley JM. Age-related bone health and pathophysiology of osteoporosis. Ortho Phys Ther Clinics of No. Amer. 1998; 7(2): 117–132. Artist: JM Bottomley.)*

the transient accelerated bone loss associated with menopause and impact the absorption of nutrients ingested.

Hormonal Influence

Bone remodeling occurs by means of a multiple-hormone regulation system (see Table 11–1.) and in response to physical stress, calcium intake, and other dietary factors (e.g. magnesium, phosphorus, zinc, etc.) (see Figure 11–6).

Estrogen acts on the thyroid gland to produce calcitonin. Calcitonin protects the bones by acting on the parathyroid gland and inhibiting the production of parathyroid hormone, which in excess has a negative impact on bone density. The loss of estrogen at menopause means that there is less available calcitonin and therefore the PTH serum level is left unchecked resulting in more bone activity. Additionally, estrogen acts to decrease osteoclastic activity. The lower levels of estrogen associated with menopause result in increased osteoclastic activity and subsequent acceleration in bone loss. Testosterone also plays a role in decreasing bone resorption by acting to decrease the systems sensitivity to PTH. As is evident in Table 11–1 most of the growth hormones and the morphogenetic proteins can initiate and perpetuate the entire cascade of events that convert stem cells to osteoblasts and appear to be powerful factors in stimulating bone formation locally. Stress on the bone, as will be discussed in an ensuing part of this chapter, is also a significant factor in facilitating osteoblast activity.

Homeostatic Mechanisms: Controlling Plasma Calcium & Skeletal Minerals

The hormonal regulation of bone remodeling is sensitive to blood calcium concentrations. Normal total blood calcium concentrations range between 85 and 105 mg/L. When blood calcium decreases, the parathyroid gland releases parathyroid hormone (PTH), which increases the activity of the osteoclasts, thereby increasing bone resorption. Conversely, when blood calcium concentrations are above normal, the thyroid gland releases calcitonin, which inhibits osteoclast activity, favoring osteoblast activity and bone deposition. In this hormonal system the primary element is blood calcium, because bone resorption will continue until a severely low bone mineral content develops if blood calcium concentrations remain low. This priority is understandable because blood calcium concentrations influence the membrane potential of excitable cells (e.g., nerves, myocardium, smooth muscle, and skeletal muscle), and optimal functioning of many of these tissues is essential for life. Also, excess blood calcium can be deposited in organs (e.g., kidneys and blood vessels), impairing their function.

Estrogen is an important hormone regulator of bone remodeling. Estrogen reduces both the number of active BMUs and their sensitivity to PTH. This results in reduced osteoclast activity and bone resorption,[14,15] favoring the retention of bone mineral. Testosterone has similar mechanisms in men. Other hormones also are known to influence bone mineral content through permissive and minor direct effects. These hormones are thyroxine (T_4), growth hormone (GH), somatomedin C (SM-C), Vitamin D, corticosteroids, protaglandins, interleukin-1 (IL-1), and endothelial growth factors.[14–16]

Mechanical Stress

Physical stress on bone stimulates increased bone deposition. Exercise can apply compressive and tensile stress, and in addition, simply overcoming the forces of gravity on the musculoskeletal system, or resisting impact, can stimulate bone deposition. Because of the large number of muscles (more than 600) that originate and insert on the numerous bones of the skeletal system (around 206), muscle contraction, especially against resistance (gravity or external loads), can place large forces on the muscle tendon-bone joints, and these forces are relayed to the bone matrix. These facts are being revealed in tests with astronauts in the US space shuttle program; in addition, efforts are being made to use exercise in zero gravity as a means to retard increased bone resorption during space flights.

TABLE 11–1. HORMONAL AND STRESS-RELATED FUNCTION ON BONE AND MECHANISM OF ACTION

HORMONE	FUNCTION	MECHANISM
Calcitonin	↑ Bone Deposition	↑ Osteoblast activity
	↓ Bone Resorption	↓ Osteoclast activity
Parathyroid Hormone (PTH)	↑ Bone Resorption	↑ Osteoclast activity
Estadiol-β 17	↓ Bone Resorption	↓ Sensitivity to PTH
Testosterone	↓ Bone Resorption	↓ Sensitivity to PTH
Growth Hormones (GH):		
Insulin-like GH	↑ Bone Deposition	↑ Osteoblast activity
Transforming GH	↑ Bone Deposition	↑ Osteoblast activity
Platelet-derived GH	↑ Bone Deposition	Unknown mechanism
Fibroblast GH	↑ Bone Deposition	↑ Osteoblast activity
Interleukins	↓ Bone Deposition	↑ Osteoclast activity
Morphogenetic Proteins	↑ Bone Deposition	↑ Osteoblast activity
Bone Stress	↑ Bone Deposition	↑ Osteoblast activity

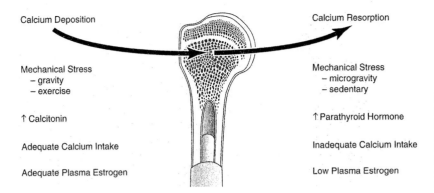

Calcium Deposition

Mechanical Stress
– gravity
– exercise

↑ Calcitonin

Adequate Calcium Intake

Adequate Plasma Estrogen

Calcium Resorption

Mechanical Stress
– microgravity
– sedentary

↑ Parathyroid Hormone

Inadequate Calcium Intake

Low Plasma Estrogen

Figure 11–6. *Factors that influence and regulate bone remodeling. (Reprinted with permission from Bottomley JM. Orthopedic Interventions with Seniors: Bone Changes in Seniors. Orthopaedic Section of the American Physical Therapy Association. 1999 Home Study Course 9.2.2. Artist: JM Bottomley.)*

There is a clear age-related loss in bone mineral content. This loss occurs first in cancellous bone, which begins to decline before the third decade of life. Compact bone is retained for another decade before resorption increases[17,18,19] (Figure 11–7). The decline in trabecular bone mineral content is greater for women than men and greater again for postmenopausal women.[11,15,20–22] After menopause, the rate of trabecular bone mineral loss in women can increase to 7% per year, with the greatest loss in the first five years. This rate of loss is large compared with the average loss before menopause of less than 1% per year.[11]

Pathophysiological Mechanism of Osteoporosis

Since no specific defect in the cellular elements, the matrix, the mineral components, or the structural arrangement of bone has ever been demonstrated, osteoporosis is presumed to result from an imbalance between bone remodeling, resorption, and formation. Many factors influence bone remodeling including age, hormones, dietary factors, and a variety of environmental and constitutional factors.

Osteoporosis may result from the uncoupling of bone resorption and formation with resorption of bone exceeding formation to such an extent that the structural integrity of bone is compromised.

Postmenopausal Osteoporosis

This form of osteoporosis characteristically affects women within fifteen to twenty years after menopause, with the most rapid loss occurring around 5 to 7 years following menopause. During this accelerated phase, trabecular-plate perforation with loss of structural trabeculae weakens the vertebrae and predisposes them to acute collapse.[23] The turnover of bone is decreased and osteoporosis is caused by factors closely related to or exacerbated by menopause. This leads to the following cascade: accelerated bone loss, decreased secretion of PTH and increased secretion of calcitonin.[15,18] In addition, a functional impairment in 25-OH-D 1-α-hydroxylase activity (responsible for converting vitamin D to its active form) with a decreased production of $1,25(OH)_2D$ (active vitamin D metabolite) results in a decrease in calcium absorption.[24] This decrease in calcium absorption into the bone may further aggravate bone loss.

All women are estrogen deficient after menopause and serum levels of hormones are similar in postmenopausal women with and without osteoporosis. Thus, other factors must interact with estrogen deficiency to determine individual susceptibility to the development of postmenopausal osteoporosis.

Primary Osteoporosis

This syndrome occurs equally in men and women who are 70 years of age or older. It is manifested mainly by hip and vertebral fractures, although fractures of the proximal humerus, proximal tibia, pelvis, and metatarsal bones are common. Trabecular thinning associated with the slow phase of bone loss is responsible for gradual loss of bone integrity.[23] In pri-

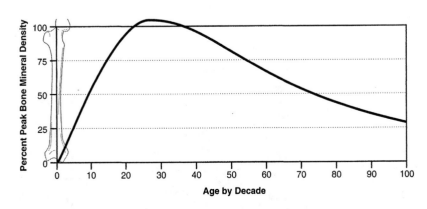

Figure 11–7. *Life-cycle changes in bone mineral content. Peaking at maturity and showing a gradual decline throughout the remainder of the life cycle. (Reprinted with permission from Bottomley JM. Age-related bone health and pathophysiology of osteoporosis. Ortho Phys Ther Clinics of No. Amer. 1998; 7(2):117–132. Artist: JM Bottomley.)*

mary osteoporosis there is a proportionate loss of cortical and trabecular bone and a rate of loss that is higher than in age-matched peers.[25] The two most important age-related factors are decreased osteoblast function and impaired production of 1,25(OH)$_2$D, leading to decreased calcium absorption and secondary hyperthyroidism. The effects of all risk factors for bone loss occurring over a lifetime are cumulative.

Table 11–2 compares the differences between postmenopausal and primary osteoporosis.

Conditions That Influence *Age-Related* Decrease in Bone Mineral Content

With aging there is a loss of bone mineral content as depicted in Figure 11–7. Several conditions can exaggerate this loss including nutrition, endocrinologic factors, and exercise-related factors. The two main determinants in the development and severity of osteoporosis are peak bone mineral content and the rate of bone mineral loss.[26] Thus it is important to understand the factors that increase peak bone mineral content, as well as how to retard bone mineral loss.

Effects of Nutrition on Bone Remodeling

Because bone is the storage site for calcium, and endocrine regulation of serum calcium involves modifying bone resorption and deposition, it is reasonable to hypothesize that an inadequate intake of calcium would favor increased bone resorption. Nutritional intake of calcium is critical to bone mineral content and adolescence is the most important time during the life cycle for building bones. This is the period when the growth spurt in body mass and skeletal mineral mass occurs and approximately 60% of the peak skeletal mineral mass is deposited.[11] Nutritional

data indicates that the calcium intake of girls before pubescence is inadequate,[11] which may limit skeletal mineral mass development in adolescent girls, placing them at higher risk for the development of osteoporosis later on in life.

Dietary intake and/or supplementation of calcium, regardless of age or gender, is an important factor in establishing a healthy bone mass. This is especially true given that calcium absorption by the small intestine is compromised by protein and caffeine ingestion. Getting enough calcium in the diet does not automatically ensure that this amount is available to the body. It is currently recommended that men and premenopausal women consume 1200 mg of calcium a day and that postmenopausal women increase this amount to 1500 mg/day.[11,22,27]

The parathyroid hormone secretion rate is directly related to the serum calcium level as discussed in the subsequent section of this chapter.

Vitamin D, phosphate, protein, caloric content, sodium, magnesium, fluoride, ascorbic acid, zinc, copper, and manganese have all been found to play a fundamental role in bone metabolism and have been demonstrated to play a role in modulating bone mass and bone strength.[28]

Effects of Endocrine Status on Bone Remodeling

Despite media attention on calcium intake for individuals over 50 years of age, research indicates that nutritional influences on bone mineral status are more likely affected by endocrinologic influences. The most important determinant of bone mineral content in women is the circulating concentration of estrogen. Consequently, any condition that reduces estrogen concentrations affects bone remodeling. The most prevalent conditions that influence estrogen concentrations in women are the normal menstrual cycle; menstrual cycle abnormalities, with complete lack of menses (amenorrhea) being the most influential; and menopause.

The changes in serum estrogen and progesterone concentrations during the menstrual cycle are large, especially during the estrogen surge portions of the follicular and luteal phases when menstrual function is normal. Drinkwater and colleagues[29] were the first to document the reduced bone mineral content (14%) in the vertebrae of amenorrheic women compared with eumenorrheic women. Subsequent research of amenorrheic female athletes verified this finding, with relative reductions in bone mineral density reported to be as great as 25% compared with sedentary controls.[22,27] These differences have been reported only for vertebral bone. The bone mineral content of bones from the appendicular skeleton (femoral neck, radius, trochanter) have shown no differences between eumenorrheic and amenorrheic women.

The influence of menopause on bone mineral content has revealed a negative correlation. The greatest

TABLE 11–2. COMPARING PRIMARY OSTEOPOROSIS TO POSTMENOPAUSAL OSTEOPOROSIS

Characteristic/ Variable	Primary	Postmenopausal
Age	> 70	51–75
Sex Ratio (F:M)	2:1	6:1
Type of Bone Loss	Trabecular, cortical	Mainly trabecular
Rate of Bone Loss	Not accelerated	Accelerated
Fracture Sites	Vertebrae, hip	Vertebrae, hip, wrist
Parathyroid Function	↑	↓
Calcium Absorption	↓	↓
Metabolism 25-OH-D to 1,25(OH)$_2$D	Primary ↓	Secondary ↓
Main Cause	Age-related factors	Menopausal factors

bone mineral loss in postmenopausal women occurs during the first 5 years after menopause.[11,22] Interestingly, evidence from amenorrheic women who resume menstrual function and normal circulating estrogen indicates that the increased estrogen has the potential not only to retard bone resorption but also to slightly increase bone mineral content.[30] Estrogen supplementation in menopausal women significantly attenuates or reverses bone resorption.[20]

Parathyroid hormone stimulates both osteoblastic activity (bone formation) and osteoclastic activity (resorption), but its primary effect is on resorption. Slight elevations in PTH levels result in a change in the metabolic activity of the "resting" bone units to supply amounts of calcium for fine regulation of mineral homeostasis, whereas greater elevations of PTH activate mechanisms for supplying larger amounts of calcium to the system.[20,25,30] Hypocalcemia tends to stimulate the secretion of PTH, whereas hypercalcemia inhibits the stimulation of PTH.

Effects of Exercise on Bone Remodeling

Exercise was reported to influence bone mineral content in a 1991 study that used a cross-sectional design.[31] Bone density was higher in athletes compared with sedentary controls, and athletes involved in weight-bearing activities had the highest bone mineral content. The finding of increased bone mineral density in individuals involved in weight-bearing activities has been shown repeatedly in similar cross-sectional studies.[27,31] Furthermore, it is believed that the amount of muscle mass is proportional to bone mineral content.[26,32] In other words: the stronger the muscle, the stronger the bone.

Exercise can affect the retention of bone mineral even in amenorrheic athletes involved in weight-bearing activities. Exercise involving weight-bearing retains more bone mineral than nonweight-bearing. For individuals who have been involved in exercise throughout their lives, there is evidence that they maintain a higher bone mineral density (decreased resorption) compared to sedentary controls.[33] The effects of exercise on the bone are discussed more extensively in a subsequent section of this chapter.

Risk Factors for Osteoporosis

Risk factors are not the cause, but they are contributing factors to the development of osteoporosis. The number of risk factors that predispose an individual to osteoporosis are not cumulative. That is to say, if you have three risk factors you are not three times more likely to develop osteoporosis. Rather, the more risk factors identified, the greater the predisposition towards the development of osteoporosis. Factors such as age, gender, genetic makeup, race, body type and complexion may initiate the process. Other factors such as poor nutrition, inactivity, and smoking may serve to accelerate bony loss.

Age is by far the most important empirical determinant of bone mass. From the fourth decade on, less bone is formed than is resorbed at individual remodeling foci, and this imbalance increases with advancing age.[34] Although this imbalance in bone remodeling could be caused by osteoblast senescence, the observation that healing of fractures in the elderly is not delayed suggests that aging does not impair the response of osteoblasts to appropriate stimuli. Serum levels of both growth hormone and insulin-like growth factor 1, (which mediates the effect of growth hormone on bone and cartilage) have been shown to decrease with aging.[35]

There may be impaired regulation of osteoblast activity caused by abnormalities in either systemic or local growth factors which are *genetically* influenced. Therefore, genetic factors may predispose an individual to the development of osteoporosis. At least twelve local regulators of growth produced by bone, cartilage, or marrow cells, have been identified.[36] Either age-related or genetic defects in the synthesis of one or more of these regulators may explain the uncoupling of bone formation from resorption that allows age-related bone loss. These factors include: skeletal growth factor, bone-derived growth factor, macrophage-derived growth factor, a factor resembling β-transforming growth factor, and prostaglandin E_2.

Table 11–3 summarizes the relative risk factors in the development of osteoporosis.

Gender clearly influences the development of osteoporosis. Females have a higher incidence of osteoporosis related to lower levels of estrogen.

Race also appears to have an impact on the development of osteoporosis. White women, particularly of northwestern European background and Asians are more at risk than black women, in whom osteoporosis is actually very rare.[13] *Family history* also plays a part in the development of osteoporosis. Slight build, fair complexioned individuals with freckles and blond hair, all of which are genetically regulated, have a higher incidence of osteoporosis. Environmental factors, such as customary dietary habits developed within family structures, could play a role in increasing the risk for osteoporosis.

The Calcium Connection: Effects of Calcium Intake

Mechanism for Calcium Absorption Calcium absorption decreases with advancing age both in males and in females.[37,38] Serum levels of $1,25(OH)_2D$, the physiologically active vitamin D metabolite, decrease by as much as 50%[39,40] and this decrease is the probable cause of decreased calcium absorption. A primary impairment of 25-hydroxyvitamin D_3 (25-OH-D 1-α-hydroxylase), the renal enzyme responsible for the conversion of 25-OH-D to $1,25(OH)_2D$ (also called calcitriol), has been demonstrated to blunt the serum $1,25(OH)_2D$ response to infusion of PTH in normal el-

TABLE 11–3. RISK FACTORS FOR OSTEOPOROSIS

Age (postmenopausal)

Genetic Factors
Genders (females at risk)
Race (Caucasians, Asians more at risk)
Family history
Body build / small frame
Fair complexion

Nutritional Factors
Low body weight
Low dietary calcium intake
High alcohol consumption
Eating disorders (anorexic, bulimic, chronic crash dieting patterns)
High caffeine consumption (leaches calcium)
High vitamin A, D intake
High protein intake
High soft drink consumption (phosphorus binding with calcium)

Lifestyle Factors
Inactive/sedentary lifestyle (immobilization, bedrest, no gravity)
Cigarette smoking

Medical Factors
Early menopause (natural or surgically induced)
■ Bilateral oophorectomy
Medication use: corticosteroids, anticoagulants, anticonvulsants, antacids
Menstrual cycle disorders (amenorrhea, dysmenorrhea)
No pregnancies
Contraceptive use

Safety Issues and Falls

Diseases causing secondary osteoporosis
Endocrine diseases (hyperparathyroidism)
Gastrointestinal diseases (IBS, malabsorption syndromes)
Bone marrow disorders (myeloma, carcinoma)
Connective tissue disorders (Marfan's, osteogenesis)

---

derly subjects and in elderly subjects with osteoporosis.[39,40] Parathyroid hormone serum levels increase with aging, perhaps in response to decreased calcium absorption.

Menopause marks the onset of an acute change in calcium balance and rapid bone loss in women.[41,42] In addition to its direct effect on bone metabolic processes, estrogen affects calcium homeostasis, enhancing calcium absorption and improving renal conservation of calcium.[41] Therefore, when this hormone is decreased at menopause, not only will less calcium be absorbed but more of it will be excreted. This overall decrease in the availability and utilization of dietary calcium contributes to the rapid postmenopausal acceleration of bone loss.[41] Other factors which may contribute to this bone loss include low intake of dietary calcium, a high protein diet, and inactivity.[41]

As reviewed by Heaney and colleagues,[43] elderly persons have consistently been shown to require a calcium intake of 1200 mg and higher to achieve a calcium balance and decrease the risk of fractures. The recommended daily allowance for postmenopausal women and elderly in general is 1500 mg per day.

Intestinal calcium absorption is less, and there is inadequate conversion of vitamin D to calcitrol, the metabolite necessary for calcium absorption. Vitamin D deficiencies are prevalent in the elderly due to the lack of exposure to sunlight and low dietary intakes. It is also believed that the requirements for vitamin D actually go up with age from the RDA of 400 IU to 600 to 800 IU/day.[44]

Additionally, several diseases common to the elderly, such as diabetes, chronic renal failure, and malabsorption syndromes either directly or indirectly impact the intestinal absorption of calcium and vitamin D.[42] Nutritional components that adversely affect calcium absorption include coffee, oxalates and phytates, protein, sodium, vitamins A and D, and alcohol. Coffee and other caffeinated beverages act as diuretics, flushing the system of many essential nutrients. Oxalates and phytates, produced with overconsumption of fatty substances, work in opposition to antioxidants, such as vitamins C, E, and A, all responsible for interferring with the oxidative process of free radicals which may bind to calcium, prevent their absorption. Protein ingestion in excess increases the urinary excretion of calcium; overingestion and absorption of foods rich in vitamins A or D have a negative impact on utilization of calcium; and alcohol tends to flush the system of all nutrients, including calcium, and may be used as a substitute for nutrient-rich food sources. Attention has also focused on the high consumption of phosphorus, contained in processed foods and soft drinks. Phosphorus binds with calcium and is never absorbed in the system.[45] Several studies have shown that dietary fiber reduces the bioavailability of calcium if ingested in high quantities.[41,42]

Figure 11–8 provides an overview of the effects of aging on calcium metabolism.

Both calcium intake and calcium absorption diminish with advancing age. With advancing age, there is a decrease in vitamin D synthesis in the skin and a decrease in the 1α-hydroxylase in the kidney. As depicted in Figure 11–8, older individuals have a decrease in $25(OH)D_3$ and its active metabolite, $1,23(OH)_2D_3$. As noted, lower vitamin D levels are particularly prevalent in institutionalized and home-bound elderly people.

A decrease in the secretion of growth hormone, especially of the insulin-like growth factor 1 (IGF I), somatomedin C, increases the activity of osteoclasts. In combination with a decrease in physical activity, the osteoblast activity is suppressed.

These changes can lead to a decrease in ionized calcium which, in turn, results in a compensatory increase in PTH levels. Calcitonin levels may decline with advancing age as well. As already discussed, the age-related declines in IGF 1 and testosterone also impede calcium metabolism. All of these changes in combination result in an exacerbation of bone loss and osteopenia.

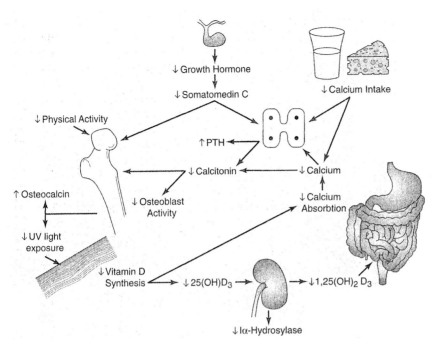

Figure 11–8. An overview of the effects of aging on calcium metabolism. (*Reprinted with permission from Bottomley JM. Orthopedic Interventions with Seniors: Bone Changes in Seniors. Orthopaedic Section of the American Physical Therapy Association. 1999 Home Study Course 9.2.2. Artist: JM Bottomley.*)

Mechanisms of the Benefits of Exercise

The effects of gravity and mechanical stress on the bone have been associated with functional adaptation of the bone.[45] In other words, there is a continual remodeling of bone in response to functional demands placed on the bone. According to Wolff's law, the internal architecture of the bone responds to stress by laying down more bone wherever the muscles are exerting their greatest force. Additionally, stress on the bone creates a negative potential within the bone according to the piezoelectric effect, thereby attracting positive ions, such as calcium.[45]

When force is applied to bone, bone bends and there is an inherent moment of inertia applied to the bone. These mechanical stresses or loads are crucial in keeping bone healthy. Mechanical loads stimulate bone cells within the loaded region to deform and increase their synthesis of prostacyclin (PGI_2), prostaglandin E_2 (PGE_2), and other growth hormones, and increase their synthesis of RNA. This causes the cascade of events described in a previous section of this chapter within the osteoblasts and osteoclasts in response to changes in bone strain, reflecting an adaptation to the imposed loading environment.[45] A minimum amount of strain is required to be effective for increased bone remodeling.

The major impact of activity on bone mass is localized. Bone mineral density is increased only in the areas that are stressed.[46,47,48] Weight-bearing and bone-site-specific forces are the key factors in the relationship of bone development and muscle pull.[47,48]

Muscle mass and strength bears an interesting relationship to bone mass. There is a positive correlation between muscle strength and muscle mass with the bone mineral density.[49,50] It appears that overall strength is the key factor as strength in one area typi-

cally reflects strength in other regions of the body. To effect change in bone mass, the training stimulus must exceed the normal loading of the muscle.

The type of exercise is very important. Sinaki's landmark studies[51,52] clearly demonstrated that in postmenopausal women who had sustained osteoporotic vertebral fractures, extension exercises significantly reduced the incidence of fracture reoccurrence, whereas flexion exercises increased the risk of fracture.

Based on current research it is important to consider the following factors when prescribing exercise to enhance bone mass: 1. Weight-bearing physical activity is essential for the normal development and maintenance of a healthy bone mass. 2. Sedentary elderly individuals may increase bone mass by becoming more active, but the primary benefit of the increased activity may be in avoiding the further loss of bone that occurs with inactivity. 3. The optimal program for older adults would include activities that improve strength, flexibility, and coordination that may indirectly, but effectively, decrease the incidence of osteoporotic fractures by lessening the likelihood of falling.[45–50]

Problems in Studying Exercise Effects on Bone

There are many unanswered questions in osteoporosis research. Many of the problems inherent in the research done to date is that most research looks at specific age or activity groups (e.g., immediately postmenopausal women and athletes, respectively). This information can not be easily generalized to women aging as a whole. Future research needs to focus on the development and maintenance of bone as a tissue across the life cycle. At the same time, there is a great need for clinical and epidemiological research that explores and extends further the current potential for practical prevention and treatment of osteoporosis. A deeper knowledge of factors controlling bone cell activity and regulation of bone mineral and matrix formation and remodeling would contribute ultimately to our understanding of how to intervene earlier in life to prevent the devastating sequalae associated with osteoporosis. This understanding would permit a more rational choice and evaluation of therapies related to exercise, nutrition, and hormone replacement therapies.

Research in the area of osteoporosis needs to be sensitive to differing requirements for various phases of skeletal development, different racial groups, and the needs of special populations such as those with lifelong disabilities, and stroke or spinal cord injury patients. These studies should be designed and conducted with the same scientific rigor that is demanded of other intervention and outcome studies.

Figure 11–9 shows the devastating effects of progressive end-stage osteoporosis. We have the means of preventing this outcome. Osteoporosis is a preventable disease entity.

Table 11–4 shows the World Health Organization's (WHO) recommended classification of osteo-

porosis based on bone mass measurements. Categories are defined by comparing an individual's bone mass to that of the average young adult. By WHO's definitions, *osteopenia* is described as a state of low bone mass. Individuals in this range are at a increased risk for fracture, and steps need to be taken to address diet modification and weight-bearing exercise to prevent further bone loss. Individuals with greater loss in bone mass with no history of fracture are defined as having *osteoporosis*. These individuals are at an increased risk for fracture with minimal or no trauma. The most severe category are those people with marked loss in bone mass in addition to a history of fracture. These individuals are defined as having *severe osteoporosis*.[53]

OSTEOPENIA

Osteopenia refers to metabolic bone diseases that are characterized by x-ray findings of a subnormal amount of mineralized bone mass. The most common osteopenia is osteoporosis, generally defined as a decrease in the quantity of bone, with an increased incidence of fractures from minimal trauma. One of the first signs of osteoporosis is alveolar bone loss, called *dental osteopenia,* followed by bone loss in vertebrae and long bones. Indeed there appears to be a strong correlation between skeletal osteopenia and density of alveolar bone.[54] Dental osteopenia leads to an inadequate amount of bone mass in the mandible, loss or mobility of teeth, edentulousness, and inability to wear dentures.[55]

It has been found that calcium deficiencies and calcium-phosphorus imbalances contribute to the development of osteopenia and the subsequent pathogenesis of osteoporosis.[56] Prevention and management include not only increased calcium intake, but also estrogen therapy, dietary vitamin D, and exercise.

Osteopenia commonly is present in hyperthyroidism, and the development of hyperthyroidism aggravates normal age-related bone loss. Mild hypercalcemia is commonly seen in hyperthyroidism due to the endocrine imbalance of the thyroid hormone. Estrogen acts on the thyroid gland to produce calcitonin. In a condition in which there is too much thyroid hormone and too little estrogen, calcium absorption is decreased and calcium excretion is increased. In hypothyroidism, there is a mild decrease in the rate of calcium deposition in bone related to the imbalance between the decrease amount of thyroid hormone and a surplus of PTH.

OSTEOMALACIA

Osteomalacia is a bone disorder caused by a failure of normal calcification of the bone matrix. The most common causes of osteomalacia are vitamin D defi-

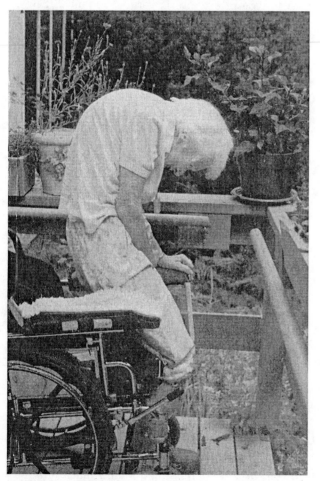

Figure 11–9. Progressive end-stage thoracic kyphosis secondary to progressive osteoporosis. *(Photo by: JM Bottomley.)*

TABLE 11–4. WORLD HEALTH ORGANIZATION CLASSIFICATION OF OSTEOPOROSIS

Normal	Bone mineral density that is not more than one standard deviation below the young adult mean value
Osteopenia or low bone mass	Bone mineral density that lies between 1.0 and 2.5 standard deviations below the young adult mean value
Osteoporosis	Bone mineral density that is more than 2.5 standard deviations below the young adult mean value without a history of fracture
Severe osteoporosis	Bone mineral density more than 2.5 standard deviations below the young adult mean value with history of one or more fractures

World Health Organization as per Kanis JA, Melton LF III, Christiansen C, Johnson CC, Khalten N. The Diagnosis of osteoporosis. *J. Bone Mirer Res* 1994; 9: 1137–1141.

ciency, a calcium deficiency, abnormal metabolism of vitamin D, and low serum calcium-phosporus levels. In contrast to osteoporosis, where there is a loss of bone mass and resulting brittleness of the bones, osteomalacia causes the bones to soften due to poor mineralization and an inability to absorb vitamin D, calcium, and phosphate.[57]

The primary etiology is a vitamin D deficiency, which results in poor absorption of calcium in the intestines and increased excretion of phosphate from the kidneys. Vitamin D is obtained from the diet (D_2 and D_3) and from biosynthesis following exposure to sunlight (D_3). Its metabolite, $1,25(OH)_2D$, enhances the gastrointestinal absorption of calcium and phosphate, and thus has a direct effect on the bone calcification process. Vitamin D deficiency may result from dietary restriction of food (e.g., too little fish, whole grain flour, and dairy products), malabsorption of vitamin D, or insufficient exposure to ultraviolet radiation.[57,58]

Vitamin D from the diet is absorbed in the upper small bowel via fat-dependent absorption. Derangement in upper intestinal function or fat malabsorption can result in vitamin D deficiency. Diagnoses such as pancreatic insufficiency, irritable bowel syndrome, biliary obstruction, or sprue can lead to poor absorption of this essential nutrient.

Once absorbed, vitamin D_2 and D_3 are hydroxylated in the liver to 25-hydroxyvitamin D; and subsequently in the kidneys to $1,25(OH)_2D$. Interference with the metabolism of vitamin D may contribute to the development of osteomalacia. Liver disease, particularly cirrhosis of any etiology, may interfere with hepatic 25-hydroxylation of vitamin D. In renal failure, the deficiency of renal 25-OH-D 1-α-hydroxylase activity is the primary cause of osteomalacia, because it produces a deficiency of $1,25(OH)_2D$.

Certain drugs may also impede the absorption of vitamin D by causing an increase in vitamin D excre-

tion or catabolism. Drugs that increase the hepatic degradation of 25-hydroxyvitamin D, such as phenytoin and phenobarbital, are known to predispose individuals to osteomalacia. In nephrotic pathologies, there may be an increase in vitamin D clearance and excretion, which results in a deficiency of vitamin D.[57,58]

Phosphorus is also essential for the calcification of bone. Hypophosphatemia may result from gastrointestinal or renal loss of phosphate, which is independent of parathyroid or vitamin D metabolism. Malabsorption and subsequent gastric and intestinal tract wasting of phosphates may be compounded by vitamin D deficiency and hyperparathyroidism. This malabsorption also may be exacerbated by phosphate-binding antacids. Renal wasting of phosphorus is a prominent feature of proximal renal tubular disorders. These disorders range from defects that limit phosphate absorption and increase phosphate clearance to renal failure which results in defects involving absorption of phosphorus, glucose, amino acid, uric acid, and vitamin K. In renal tubular acidosis, the acidotic state will repel positive ions, such as calcium and phosphorus, and contribute to the development of osteomalacia.[58]

The classic symptom of osteomalacia is generalized or localized bone pain. The pain is often exaggerated by movement, and bony tenderness is common. A complaint of general fatigue and achiness is often heard. Proximal myopathy and sensory polyneuropathy may accompany these complaints. Initially the progression of osteomalacia is insidious and deformity is unusual, though pathologic fractures ultimately may occur as bone strength declines and result in vertebral wedge fractures, bowing of the femur and tibia, and postural changes similar to those seen in osteoporosis. Gait and functional declines are associated with the overall loss in muscle strength.[57]

Treatment must address the nutritional-malabsorption component of this metabolic disorder. Dietary supplementation of vitamin D may be required to restore positive calcium balance and normal bone mineralization. The gastrointestinal, hepatic, or renal disorder underlying osteomalacia must be treated. Research indicates that exercise has a positive effect on osteomalacia only when adequate dietary vitamin D is provided and the metabolic disorder corrected. Then exercise has a positive effect on bone mass, similar to that described in osteoporosis.[57,58]

AVASCULAR NECROSIS

Death of bone and the cellular components of bone in the absence of infection is referred to as *osteonecrosis* or *avascular necrosis*. Avascular necrosis is the result of a disrupted arterial supply and most commonly affects the femoral head following an intracapsular or femoral neck fracture in which the circumflex arteries are injured as a result of the fracture. Avascular necrosis also can be the end result of a thrombosis of an artery supplying bone. The bone tissue becomes ischemic and permanent loss of bone occurs.[59]

Osteonecrosis, a process of "creeping substitution" where there is resorption of "dead" trabeculae and woven bone is laid down on dead trabeculae, results in the collapse of bone. Osteonecrosis can result from a number of etiologies, but most commonly it is associated with fracture, alcoholism, pancreatitis, diabetes mellitus, obesity, or gout. Other conditions that may lead to avascular necrosis include systemic lupus erythematosus, Cushing's disease, caisson disease, Gaucher's disease, idiopathic Chandlers disease, sickle cell anemia, and long-term corticosteroid use.[60]

Although the talus, scaphoid, and proximal humerus are susceptible to osteonecrosis, the femoral head is the most common site associated with this pathology. The femoral head and neck receive their circulatory supply from the medial and lateral femoral circumflex artery which travel in a distal to proximal direction in the femoral neck and head. Fracture or displacement secondary to fracture of the neck of the femur can compromise the circulation to the head of the femur and lead to death of the bone. Following trauma or with insidious conditions, pain is reported in the groin, medial thigh, and knee, which is intermittent and associated with weight-bearing activities. Internal rotation, flexion, and adduction of the hip exacerbate the pain, and the patient will present with an antalgic gait. Radiographic examination will show the source of arterial disruption; if a fracture is present but not for conditions like thrombosis. A more sensitive evaluation of bony status—a bone scan, magnetic resonance imaging (MRI), or CT scans—is required to detect earlier and subclinical stages of bone loss.

In the elderly, the treatment of choice is a total joint replacement.

PAGET'S DISEASE

Also known as osteitis deformans, Paget's disease of bone is an example of an imbalance in which bone formation overtakes bone resorption. Paget's disease is a progressive disorder associated with a marked increase in osteoblastic activity. At first there is a softening, and later, an overgrowth and hardening of bone. The disease progresses in three distinct stages: (1) osteoclastic, (2) osteoblastic, and (3) sclerotic. In the early stages, blood flow increases to the affected bone: primarily the skull, vertebrae, pelvis, and the bones of the lower extremities. There is an initial osteoclastic, resorptive stage where abnormal proliferation of osteoclasts occurs. During this period of softening, characteristic deformities develop. The skull thickens and the forehead becomes prominent, the lower extremities bow, and the individual experiences the development of kyphosis in the thoracic vertebrae and a loss of the lumbar curve in the lumbar area with posterior prominence of the vertebrae. The initial resorption is followed by abnormal regeneration of bone through an overactive osteoblastic phase followed by sclerosis. The serum alkaline phosphatase levels are extremely high (over 100 units), indicating overactivity of the osteoblasts. The normal cancellous architecture is replaced by coarse, thickened layers of trabecular bone, and the cortical bone becomes thickened, irregular, eroded, and uneven. One would think that with the increased calcification of bone that the bone would be stronger, however, the converse is true: the bone is enlarged, eroded, and weakened by irregular alignment of trabeculae.[58,61]

The postural deformities seen in Paget's disease result in a progressively increased thoracic kyphosis and bowing of the femur and tibia. If the femoral neck softens to the point of collapse, a reduced femoral neck angle (coxa vara) results in a waddling gait pattern. These postural changes increase local mechanical stress and are associated with increasing fatigue and bone pain.[58]

On radiographs the vertebrae appear to be flattened and broadened. The cortical bone and end plates become exaggerated and the cancellous bone develops a coarse yet almost transparent appearance. Primarily affecting the axial skeleton, the progressive stages of Paget's disease weaken the bony structures resulting in significant postural deformities. If the femur and tibia are involved, they, in addition to the vertebrae, are common sites of pathological or stress fractures in individuals with Paget's disease.[58]

Symptoms are initially nonexistent and the disease begins insidiously and progresses slowly. Often the disease is first detected by an abnormal radiograph or an incidentally elevated serum alkaline phosphatate level. Pain that develops is deep, aching bone pain often associated with stress fractures, hypervascularity, and mechanical stress of the excessively weakened bones. If the skull is involved, headaches, tinnitus, vertigo, and hearing loss are frequent complaints. Hearing loss is associated with the involvement of the ossicles of the inner ear or foraminal collapse and encroachment of the eighth cranial nerve. As the disease progresses, individuals usually complain of extreme fatigue, lightheadedness, and overall "stiffness." If pain occurs acutely, it is usually indicative of a pathological fracture.

Cardiovascular involvement is often associated with Paget's disease as well. Due to vasodilatation of blood vessels in the bones, skin, and subcutaneous tissues overlying the affected bones, the individual may present with peripheral vascular involvement and an increase in cardiac output severe enough to result in congestive heart failure. In fact, it is the cardiac involvement that is the most common cause of death in the Paget's disease patient.[61]

Other clinical manifestations of Paget's disease include nerve palsy syndromes and dementia. Nerve palsy syndromes occur as a result of entrapment of the nerves due to bony collapse. With bony impingement on the structures at the base of the skull, slurred speech, incontinence, diplopia, and impaired swallowing can occur.

Osteosarcoma is reported in fewer than 1% of individuals with pagetic bone and may be heralded by a rapid enlargement of bone, increased bone mass, or an elevation in serum alkaline phosphate levels.

Two classes of drugs are approved by the FDA for the treatment of Paget's disease. Both classes of drugs suppress the abnormal bone remodeling that is associated with this disease. (1) Bisphosphonates (such as alendronate sodium (Fosamax), etidronate disodium (Didronel), and pamidronate disodium (Aredia) are drugs that inhibit abnormal bone resorption. (2) Calcitonin is a hormone secreted by the thyroid gland that also inhibits abnormal bone resorption (e.g., Calcimar, Miacalcin, and Osteocalcin). Other forms of treatment may include: chemotherapy in the presence of osteosarcoma, limb sparing resection, total joint replacement, or amputation.[61]

OSTEOARTHRITIS

The most prevalent orthopaedic joint pathology is osteoarthritis. It occurs in 50% of individuals aged 65 to 75 years old, and 70% of people over the age of 75.[61] Osteoarthritis is termed the wear-and-tear arthritis. The cause of primary osteoarthritis is unknown. It is defined as a noninflammatory progressive pathology of a movable articulation, especially weight-bearing joint, and is characterized by deterioration of articular cartilage and formation of new bone at joint margins and remodeling of subchondral bone.[62] Osteoarthritis most commonly occurs in the carpometacarpal joint, the knees, and the hips. Patients will complain of pain during weight bearing in the joints, and the pain tends to be relieved by rest.

Classic treatment consists of nonsteroidal anti-inflammatory drugs (NSAIDs). However, NSAIDs for older persons have received a somewhat negative review in the medical literature due to side effects associated with long-term use.[63] Laing and Fortin[63] have encouraged physicians to use more local and specific approach modalities, such as exercises that are specific to improve a person's functioning in the osteoarthritic joints. It has been demonstrated that strengthening around an osteoarthritic joint can alleviate some of the pain, as well as increase the strength and improve the functional mobility of arthritic patients.[64,65] The clinical implication of these studies is that therapists should work with these patients on stretching and strengthening exercises, frequently throughout the day. Specific techniques for the various joints of the body will be given in subsequent sections of this chapter.

In addition to pharmacological agents and exercise, typical interventions for osteoarthritis include education, rest, and possibly surgery. Patients should be instructed in joint protection and energy-conserva-

tion techniques that can help prevent acute flare-ups and help to minimize joint stress and pain.

Rehabilitation should include appropriate weight-bearing and nonweight-bearing exercises. An individually designed program of strengthening, range-of-motion, and cardiovascular fitness exercises should be implemented. The design of the strengthening program should include low weight and much repetition so as to minimize stress on the joints. Exercise that produces pain indicates that the joint is being overstressed through too much resistance or incorrect performance of the exercise. Exercises incorporating low-load, prolonged stretching performed several times a day will help to gain a more appropriate, length-tension relationship for the muscles surrounding the affected joint and may lead to decreased stress in the intra-articular and periarticular joint structures. Heat modalities may assist in decreasing pain and stiffness, and cold modalities may decrease pain and inflammation. Splints, braces, and walking aides may also be warranted to decrease the joint stresses.

Surgical interventions such as arthroscopy, arthroplasty, and osteotomy are often employed to provide symptomatic relief, improved joint mobility, and improved joint mechanics. More than 70% of hip and knee joint replacements are performed in older adults with osteoarthritis.[66] Rehabilitation following total hip or total knee replacement will be discussed in a subsequent section of this chapter.

RHEUMATOID ARTHRITIS

Rheumatoid arthritis (RA), a chronic, systemic inflammatory autoimmune disease, is the second major orthopaedic pathology affecting the joints in the elderly. Over 10% of people over the age of 65 are affected by rheumatoid arthritis and the prevalence of this disease increases with advancing age.[67] Rheumatoid arthritis classically affects younger women three times more than men, although this predominance is less evident beyond the age of 60.[67] The major differences between late onset RA and early onset are that the exacerbations tend to be severe and the remissions tend to be much better. Therefore, the therapist must be cautious during the exacerbation phases and limit therapy to active assistive and active exercises. During the remission phases, the therapist can be much more aggressive when designing a strengthening and stretching program for an older patient than one for a younger person.

The characteristic feature of RA is chronic inflammation of the synovium, peripheral articular cartilage, and subchondral marrow spaces. Due to chronic inflammatory states, granulation tissue called *pannus* is laid down and the resulting friction erodes the articular cartilage.[67] Inflammation of the tendon sheaths also occurs, resulting in the fraying and eventual rupture of the tendons. The resultant deformities of the hands, with dislocation and lateral migration of the fingers, and the same deformities of the toes, are examples of the typical extremity deformities seen in patients with RA. Knee valgus is another example of deformities seen in this pathology.

Though the cause of RA is not specifically known, recent literature suggests that there is evidence of a genetic predisposition for the disease that is triggered by bacteria or viral infection. A definitive diagnosis is based on a combination of clinical manifestations and laboratory results. An individual with RA will often have a decreased red blood cell count, increased erythocyte sedimentation rates, and a positive rheumatoid factor (RF).

Clinically, RA manifests itself bilaterally, primarily affecting the small joints of the hands and feet, ankles, knees, hips, shoulders, elbows, and wrists. Table 11–5 describes the typical joint deformities seen in RA. The other area commonly involved is the cervical spine. Tenosynovitis of the transverse ligament of the first and second cervical vertebra and erosion of the facet joints may lead to cervical instability with the risk of neurological damage from compression.[67]

THE AGING SPINE

Pain in the neck and back is not uncommon in the older population. Although there is a higher preva-

TABLE 11–5. COMMON JOINT DEFORMITIES OF EXTREMITIES IN RHEUMATOID ARTHRITIS

Joint	Typical Deformity or Contracture
Hands (MCP/PIP/DIP)	MCP ulnar drift, swan-neck deformity, boutonnière deformity, mallet deformity, rheumatoid thumb deformity
Wrist (Carpal joints)	Volar subluxation, radial deviation
Elbow	Nodular enlargement, flexion and pronation contracture and/or deformity
Shoulder	Adduction and internal rotation contracture and/or deformity, may have subluxation
Toes (MTP/PIP/DIP)	Hallux valgus, hallux rigidus, hammer toes, claw toes, mallet toes, overlapping toes, lateral subluxation with lateral deviation
Subtalar/Midtarsal	Pronation, pes planus, instability
Ankle	Plantar equinus contracture and/or deformity
Knee	Genu valgus or genu varus, flexion contractures and/or deformity, subluxation of patella
Hip	Leg length discrepancy, flexion and adduction contractures and/or deformity

Key: MCP-Metacarpal phalangeal joint
PIP-Proximal interphalangeal joint
DIP-Distal interphalangeal joint
MTP-Metatarsal phalangeal joint

lence of this problem in the population aged 35 to 55, older persons do have a relatively high incidence of back and neck dysfunction.[68,69] Some of the major changes that are considered to be part of the normal aging process affect the cervical spine and back.

Muscles are less flexible, resilient, and strong.[68,69] Nevertheless, Rider and Daly found that older adults respond well to flexibility and strength training.[70] In their study, a group of older women whose average age was 72 were put on a spinal mobility program consisting of strengthening and stretching activities. The finding of this study was that functional mobility improved significantly.[70] The loss of flexibility of all soft tissues will affect mobility of the spine. For a comprehensive review of aging changes of cartilage, tendon, ligament, and muscle refer to Chapter 3 in this text.

The bone tends to become less dense or be affected by osteoporosis, and as a result the older person will tend to lose height. Approximately 20% of height is lost by the thinning of the intervertebral discs, but the majority of the height loss is caused by the collapse of the cartilaginous end plates secondary to a decrease in bone density and ballooning in the disc area.[71]

Joints are more prone to osteophytes. Twomey[71] states that the layer of fat pads in older joints acts as cushions against osteophytes, and that these vascular systems are more highly innervated, which may cause more pain and sensitivity. If joint congruity is not maintained by the tone of the multifidus, there is a chance that torn portions of the cartilage would be displaced, particularly with sudden rotatory movement. Manipulative techniques, therefore, would be particularly successful in freeing the torn pieces of cartilage; however, if the techniques are too aggressive, they may gap the joints and conceivably exacerbate the damage due to shearing of articular cartilage in the joint capsules.[72] Aging changes in the cervical spine mean that older patients suffer from osteophyte formations and decreased range of motion with age. This was shown in an excellent study by Hayashi and associates.[69] In addition, older patients experience a higher incidence of vertebral anterolisthesis and retrolisthesis, and a slight decrease in the diameter of the spinal cord, which may or may not cause neurological symptomology.[71]

The implication of these changes is that the therapist needs to work on strengthening, flexibility, and the appropriate manual therapy techniques to alleviate the elderly patient's symptoms. Alternative exercise forms such as T'ai Chi and Qi Gong have also been shown to be effective in enhancing spinal mobility.[73]

SPINAL PATHOLOGY OF THE ELDERLY

Lumbar Stenosis

There are many pathologies that can affect the spine of an older person. The first spinal pathology to be discussed is *lumbar stenosis,* which is a multilevel impingement on structures in the lumbar spine ligaments, usually by osteophytes.[72] Pain may be in the back, hips, or lower extremities, and worsens when the person walks or extends their lumbar spine.[72] It is usually partially or completely relieved with flexion. Lumbar stenosis rarely affects anyone under the age of 60.[74] Treatment for lumbar stenosis consists of:

- Rest for one to two hours in the afternoon with knees higher than the hips.
- Flexion exercises of the trunk.
- Heat and massage to decrease muscle spasm.
- Teaching and enforcing posterior pelvic tilting in all positions and activities.

Vertebral Compression Fractures

Vertebral compression fractures usually affect the spinal areas of the thoracic and upper lumbar spine. Fractures can occur during any kind of routine activity, such as bending, lifting, or rising from a chair. The patient often complains of immediate, severe local back pain. The pain may subside in several months, but in some cases, may continue for years. Other vertebral compression fractures, however, may cause no pain at all. The fracture may be gradual and asymptomatic, and only diagnosed by radiographs.[75] Multiple vertebral compression fractures will cause shortening of the spine and leads to the classic kyphotic position described earlier in this chapter. Progression of thoracic kyphosis can result in alveolar hyperventilation and retention of bronchial secretions with poor respiratory reserve. Eventually, the person may develop repeated episodes of pneumonia. Because all of the organs are compressed into a smaller space, often there are additional problems with abdominal symptoms, bloating, and constipation.[75]

Treatment for acute compression fractures is bed rest, but the patient must get out of bed every hour for ten minutes to work on stabilization of the back.[75] Pain relief modalities may be helpful, such as heat, ice, TENS, or electrical stimulation, to relieve some of the symptoms.[76] The authors of this book has found that the use of a six-inch ace wrap or the binders used with rib fracture is very helpful in providing support and comfort in the area of the compression fracture. Once the person can tolerate exercise, extension exercises should be used extensively.[76] Any type of extension exercises to the thoracolumbar spine is helpful.[51,76]

Cervical Spondylosis

One of the pathologies affecting the neck of an older person is cervical spondylosis, which is defined as degenerative changes in the cervical spine. Symptoms of this are pain in the cervical spine with possible radiculitis into the shoulder, arms, or fingers.[77] The treatment for cervical spondylosis includes anti-inflammatories, keeping the neck in neutral or a slightly flexed position, manual traction, heat, active range of motion, and progressive resistive exercises that the patient can tolerate.[78]

Vertebral Artery Syndrome

A second pathology of the cervical spine is vertebral artery syndrome (VAS). An encroachment on the vertebral foramina results in VAS, and this can be caused by a multitude of things. The most likely cause is the combination of a narrowing of the disc, osteophyte formation from osteoarthritis, and a forward head positon.[79] The symptoms of VAS are dizziness, tinnitus, and blurred vision that occur in conjunction with a combination neck rotation and extension. The treatment for VAS is wearing a cervical collar to prevent extension, axial extension exercises, and cervical isometric exercises.[79]

The standard test for VAS is to rotate and fully extend the cervical spine while evaluating for dizziness, nausea, and nystagmus of the eyes. Caution when evaluating an elderly individual with suspected vertebral artery syndrome needs to be applied. Utilizing the standard vertebral artery test is not advisable and could actually be dangerous.[80–85] Performing the vertebral artery test may decrease blood flow in the vertebrobasilar circulation enough to result in infarction.[84,85] Arterial diagnostic testing would confirm the therapist's suspicions of the presence of VAS. The Dix-Hallpike maneuver[86] is the typical test performed in 45° of cervical rotation and 30° of extension to diagnose benign paroxysmal positional vertigo (BPPV). This maneuver does not place the older adult in as much risk as the vertebral artery test because the patient is not placed in end-range rotation or extension. Often nystagmus can be seen in older adults by placing them in supine with their head turned, although the supine position may not be comfortable for the severely kyphotic individual. An alternative is to perform the Dix-Hallpike test on the person with kyphosis using a tilt table with pillows to support their spine and head. By lowering the person's entire body, the person's alignment remains the same, yet there is stimulation to the semicircular canal. If the patient becomes vertiginous in the Trendelenburg position and complains of vertigo with head rotation and extension, this is indicative of the possibility that the individual has VAS.[87,88]

Rheumatoid Arthritis

A third pathology causing problems in the neck in the elderly is rheumatoid arthritis. Patients/clients with RA with subsequent neck pain will tend to experience the pain in the middle area and the posterior aspect of the cervical spine. Therapists should check the x-rays for atlanto-occipital subluxation. If present, the therapist should not use any manual techniques that could further exacerbate dislocation (e.g., mobilization, traction, or occipital release).[79] Proper treatment includes supporting the neck with a cervical collar, heat, ultrasound, gentle massage, range of motion, and progressive resistive exercises.[79]

Ossification of the Posterior Longitudinal Ligament

The fourth pathology of the neck is ossification of the posterior longitudinal ligament (OPLL). In OPLL, the ligament tends to ossify, usually over several segments of the cervical spine. This causes limitation in neck flexion and radiculopathy.[89] The treatment for OPLL consists of heat, cervical traction, and rest from sedentary static activities such as knitting, reading, computer, or desk work. In addition, stretching and range of motion or progressive resistive exercises are helpful.

In all of these pathologies, the therapist must first check the person's environment. Frequently, adding pillows between the knees while the person sleeps in the side lying position can provide relief for low back pain. Putting a lumbar pillow in the wheelchair or changing the level of the footrests can provide relief for the entire spine. Since older patients spend so much time sitting, and wheelchair patients are so often bound to their chairs, the therapist must check their environments to make sure they are not exacerbating any spinal symptoms. Often a simple modification of the environment can provide tremendous relief from spinal pain.

THE UPPER EXTREMITY

The Shoulder

As noted in Chapter 3, range of motion in the shoulder does decline with age. Despite the fact that studies have documented age changes,[90,91] clinically there is evidence to show that if a person uses the shoulder more frequently, the range of motion decrease will be less. The aging shoulder is more prone to certain pathologies, such as the ones discussed here: osteoarthritis, bursitis, and rotator cuff tears.

Osteoarthritis The first pathology, osteoarthritis, is very rare and may be over diagnosed. Only 2% of shoulder problems in the elderly are truly osteoarthritis.[92] The symptoms of true osteoarthritis are a constant ache, crepitus, difficulty sleeping, and weakness. When the therapist moves the shoulder, there is a hard-end felt with joint movement. In addition, there will be a grinding and a dryness with shoulder movement.[93,94]

Treatment of osteoarthritis, when the patient has severe joint pain, is rest, gentle pain-free range of motion exercises and anti-inflammatories.[93] Once the patient can move through range with less pain, however, heat or ice, functional adaptation, joint mobility, gentle weight bearing isometrics, and range of

motion exercises can be helpful. In addition, thermal modalities, such as ultrasound and ice, can be very helpful in alleviating pain.

Bursitis The second shoulder problem, which is more commonly seen than osteoarthritis in the elderly population, is bursitis. The symptoms of bursitis are:

1. A palpable tenderness in the area of the inflamed bursa;
2. Pain with movement of the muscle affected by the temporary bursa;
3. Symptom relief with rest.[94]

The patient will usually have a recent history of overuse of the shoulder prior to the initial onset of symptoms.[95]

Treatment for bursitis is heat or ice, ultrasound, and energy conservation. Painful movements should be avoided, and the patient should begin pain-free isometrics when he or she can tolerate them. No exercise should be done that exacerbates the pain, but having the patient exercise below and above a painful arc will be useful.

Rotator Cuff The third shoulder pathology, and the one most commonly seen in the elderly, is rotator cuff problems. The rotator cuff is composed of the infraspinous, the supraspinatus, subscapularis, and teres minor. X-ray of the subacromical space of less than 5 mm is diagnostic of a rotator cuff tear.[95]

With the rotator cuff, the patient will complain of pain when sleeping on the shoulder. He or she will be positive on the impingement sign when the arm is brought to full passive flexion, and pain will be present for the last 10 to 20 degrees. Crepitus and catching sensations due to fibrosis and scarring may also be present. If the problem progresses, the patient/client may even have atrophy of the rotator cuff muscles and definite weakness in the shoulder abductors and flexors.[96]

Treatment for impingement, tears, and tendonitis of the rotator cuff is symptomological management. If the person has pain throughout an arc, the therapist should avoid range-of-motion exercises that use the arc and irritate the rotator cuff. The patient can be instructed to passively move the shoulder through that range and to do some end-range stretching and strengthening exercises. Heat, ultrasound, and electric stimulation may help decrease the inflammation. Passive-active assistive stretching exercises can also be helpful, as will isometrics that do not encourage tightness in the shoulder musculature. The person must exercise the arm at least twice a day to see significant improvement.

Adhesive Capsulitis Rotator cuff dysfunctions can become more irritating problems if the person develops a frozen shoulder. Although frozen shoulders are not always preceded by rotator cuff problems, it is a common occurrence in the aged. With frozen shoulders or adhesive capsulitis a person may or may not experience pain. A capsular pattern, where external rotation is most limited and abduction, flexion and internal rotation of the shoulder are also limited, is a symptom of adhesive capsulitis. The person may display a protracted scapula and atrophy of the deltoid, rotator cuff,[95] biceps, and triceps. Tenderness of the anterior joint may also be present.

Treatment for a frozen shoulder is heat or ice, depending on how painful the joint is and how well the person tolerates ice. Extremely painful joints may need the numbing effect of ice. Ultrasound can also be used to relieve some inflammation. Joint mobilization must be done in all limited directions, followed by active assistive or passive range of motion and contract-relaxed stretching. Posture work and scapular retraction exercises are also helpful.

Humeral Fracture Humeral fractures are the final pathology to be discussed here. Classically, they will either be displaced or nondisplaced. Slightly more nondisplaced fractures occur, and they usually require pinning or wires. A fractured humerus usually requires that the patient use a sling for one week. After that time, the patient can remove the sling to work on general pendulum exercises, shoulder shrugs and circles, protraction and retraction, and any active motion exercises for the hand or wrist. At this point, the person should be doing no passive range of motion. For the first week, the patient should also learn ways of writing, eating, and performing daily ADLs without stressing the shoulder.[94]

By the third week the patient can begin gentle isometrics, either against the wall or using Theraband™. Active range of motion in the pain-free ranges can begin at this point as well, and the person should begin doing scapular humeral rhythm motion in front of the mirror, that is elevating the arms without raising the shoulder. This type of activity can also be used for all the previously noted shoulder pathologies. One of the most prevalent problems is that patients with shoulder pathologies have poor scapular humeral rhythm. Normally, they do not achieve full range of motion, because they are never taught how to properly move the shoulder. Simply working with patients in front of a mirror and encouraging them not to lift the shoulders as the arm is lifted is adequate for attaining the desired results.

By the sixth or eighth week, if the patient is healed, joint mobilization can begin. Passive range of motion can also begin, but scapular humeral rhythm should be stressed.

THE LOWER JOINTS OF THE UPPER EXTREMITY

The joints of the upper extremity (the elbows, wrists, and hands) show minimal changes in the range of motion with age. However, as seen in Chapter 6, grip strength does decline.[97,98] The practitioner should be careful when looking at grip strength measures in the elderly, because studies have shown that the older patient's grip and pinch strength may be influenced by extraneous variables. These variables range from mental status to gait and balance problems. Therefore, grip strength may not be a true indicator of strength in the older population.[99,100]

The Elbow

Almost one quarter of all elbow traumas and one third of elbow fractures are fractures of the radial head,[101] which usually are stabilized with an internal fixation device. For the first three weeks, the patient is immobilized in a hinged splint with the forearm held neutral. The patient can do range-of-motion exercises with the hand and shoulder, and to control swelling, cold packs can be applied for ten minutes every hour. At day twenty-one, active range of motion exercises can be started and passive range and progressive resistive exercises (PRE) can be increased gently as the patient/client tolerates. This regimen is followed slowly until twelve to fifteen weeks.[101]

It is important to note that since this is such a painful fracture, practice and skill acquisition on a visual level may be beneficial. According to Maring,[102] the experimental group who visualized a forearm activity did much better than the control group who did not.

The Wrist

The most common pathology of the wrist is Colles' fracture, which is a fracture of the distal radius as a result of a fall on the hand. It can be treated by closed reduction, or it can be reduced by screws.[103] The therapist will usually see the patient once while the extremity is in a cast for instruction in edema control and for range of motion exercises for the uncasted upper extremity joints. After four weeks, the cast is usually removed, and at that time the therapist can use modalities as needed, such as heat, ice, and electrical stimulation to control swelling and increase circulation. Gentle joint mobilizations to the carpal joints, active range of motion, and gentle passive and resistive exercises can be started at this time. By six weeks, when the person is completely healed, the therapist can begin work on more vigorous passive resistive, contract-relax stretching exercises, or both. The therapist should be sure to reinforce the exercises with daily, functional activities at home.

Rheumatoid arthritis or osteoarthritis often affect the wrist. Marked limitation in joint mobility can severely impede functional capabilities. Often splints are advised to protect the wrist during activity. Joint protection techniques should be a part of therapy intervention. Teaching an individual how to manage activities of daily living without stressing the joints of the wrist will decrease the amount of pain and inflammation.

The Hand

The most common pathologies in the aging hand are (1) rheumatoid arthritis (2) osteoarthritis and (3) Dupuytren's contracture. In rheumatoid arthritis, the synovial fluid in the joints of the hand become particularly painful, and the person may develop ulnar drifting and significant deformities of the hand. The patient may undergo surgery or arthroplasty for severe deformities; nevertheless, the therapist can work on light exercises and splinting to help alleviate pain symptoms, as well as focusing on range-of-motion deficits.[104]

Arthritis Osteoarthritis of the hand is more common than RA. It most commonly involves the interphalangeal joints and the carpometacarpal joint of the thumb. Since the thumb is so important for functioning, this particular problem can be devastating. The patient will present with pain, swelling, and weakness, possibly due to overuse of the hand. The treatment involves joint protection, splinting to stabilize the thumb, joint mobilization and strengthening exercises. Heat, ice, paraffin, and ultrasound can also give relief from pain and inflammation.[104,105]

Dupuytren's Contracture The final pathology involving the hand is Dupuytren's contracture, which is relatively uncommon in people under 50. It is caused by excessive collagen formation around tendons, nerves, and blood vessels in the palm of the hand, and it can cause minimal or permanent flexion of the fingers, usually of the proximal interphalangeal joints. Figure 11–10 demonstrates a typical Dupuytren's contracture. It is usually not painful, and, therefore, people often delay treatment. However, treating the problem early can be extremely effective. Heat and ultrasound to the fascia of the hand followed by unidirectional transverse friction massage, stretching, and splinting in a stretched position can be extremely helpful. Patients are encouraged to continue the friction massage, range-of-motion exercises and heating at home to enhance the benefits of the therapeutic regimen.[104]

THE LOWER EXTREMITY

The Hip

The hip shows a decrease in range of motion similar to the other joints of the body, as demonstrated in the work of James and Parker[106] (see also Chapter 6). In addition, Kramer and coworkers[107] found that older women have 61% less force in their hip abductors than younger women.

The normal changes with age of decreased range of motion and strength will have a significant impact on an older person's gait, stability, and balance and may lead to a downward spiral for some of the pathologies that are commonly seen by therapists. The three major pathologies to be discussed in this section are hip fractures, osteoarthritis, and total hip replacements.

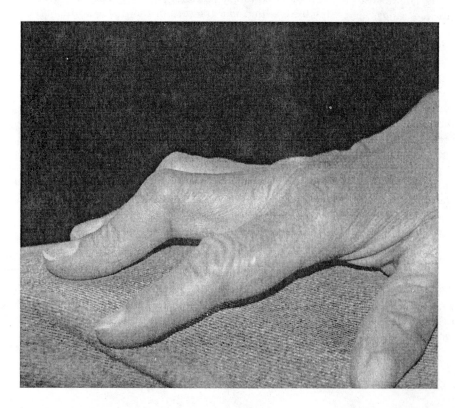

Figure 11–10. Typical Dupuytren's contracture in an elderly homeless male. (*Photo by: JM Bottomley.*)

Hip Osteoarthritis

Patients with hip osteoarthritis may constantly complain of pain around or over the hip area. Even if a patient has radiographic evidence of hip osteoarthritis, the patient may also have an inflamed bursa or tensor fascia lata tendinitis that relates pain to the hip.[64] It is imperative that the therapist assess this to treat it appropriately. If the patient's hip abductors are weak, they may be carrying the body's weight differently and irritating the bursas or the tendons around the hip area.[108] A thorough examination of these areas will help achieve an appropriate targeted treatment plan.

In arthritis of the hip, the patient will complain of an aching sensation, especially with weight bearing by the hip, and there will be corresponding radiographic evidence. The treatment for hip osteoarthritis includes alleviating stress, through the use of a cane, to decrease weight bearing until a person increases his or her strength. This can be followed by strengthening exercises to the areas around the hip, especially for the abductors and extensors, to increase the shock-absorbing system of the hip joint.[79]

Proper range of motion, stretching to the joint capsule, and ergonometric modifications may also be helpful, as can biomechanical alterations. According to Neumann and associates,[108] a patient can decrease the hip force by carrying loads on the same side or with both hands. If a patient is carrying a purse on the uninvolved side, it may actually increase the pain felt by the patient.[108] Strengthening and range-of-motion exercises have also been shown to be very beneficial for patients with osteoarthritis.[70]

Hip Fracture

Hip fracture is the most common acute orthopedic condition of the elderly. Tinetti et al[109] found that active elderly persons fell less frequently than inactive, but when they did fall, it was more serious. Kampa[110] said, "Every 10 minutes someone dies from a hip fracture, and one out of every 20 women over 65 will suffer hip fracture.[110] In the United States, there are 267,000 fractures per year, and 97% of these involve persons 65 years or older, and two-thirds are women.[111]

A study by Cummings and Nevitt[111] raised some interesting points about the relationship of osteoporosis to falls. They found that osteoporosis alone does not explain the exponential increase in the incidence of falls among the elderly. They proposed that four conditions cause elderly people to fall and fracture their hips:

1. The faller is positioned so that impact occurs near the hip.
2. The faller's protective responses fail.
3. Local soft tissue absorbs less shock than necessary to prevent the fracture.
4. The residual energy of the fall exceeds the strength of the femur.

Frequently, a fracture in older people occurs in the neck and intertrochanteric area of the femur where there is less of a blood supply and the bone is of the cancellous rather than the cortical type. Due to the distal arterial supply from the circumflex artery to this area, often these fractures result in nonunion. Subtrochanteric fractures occur with very high velocity falls and thus are rarely seen in the elderly population. The orthopedic surgeon has a multitude of choices in the types of fixation used, ranging from screws, to pins, to rods and plates. Table 11-6 lists some of these devices and the method of weight-bearing progression that can be used by therapists.[112] It is imperative that the therapist gets the older patient to bear weight on the limb as soon as possible so as to enhance normal walking patterns, proprioception, and the integrity of the bone.[113]

Hip fractures are usually treated on a protocol basis. A total hip fracture protocol that is commonly used in departments around the United States is provided in Appendix A. In addition, Baker and coworkers[114] showed that treadmill gait retraining following a fracture of the neck of the femur can significantly increase gait strength in patients.[114]

Total Hip Replacement

The third hip pathology of the elderly is total hip replacement. Total hip replacements may be used for hip fractures, as well as for patients who have very severe rheumatoid arthritis, osteoarthritis, or carcinomas. Patients receiving total hip replacements tend to do well. They are usually put on a specific protocol procedure. For an example of this protocol, please see Appendix A (Figure 11A–1). Depending on the approach used by the surgeon, various simultaneous motions need to be avoided by the patient so as not to cause dislocation. Unfortunately, there is no definitive time frame for dislocation, and some orthopedic surgeons may put patients on precaution protocols for anywhere from 3 months to the rest of their lives.

Some of the best predictors of outcomes for both hip fractures and total hip replacement's are the number of visits that the patient makes to physical therapy.[115,116,117] It is imperative that patients who have had hip replacements or hip fractures receive adequate instruction in both exercise, activities of daily living, and proper precautions and methods of improving their weight bearing status. See Appendix A Figure 11A–2 for a total hip protocol and Figure 11A–3 for general patient home instructions.

THE KNEE

The knee, similar to the hip, has been shown to lose strength with age.[118] According to Borges,[118] older patients showed a significant decrease in torque values likely to be generated at the knee. The knee, however,

TABLE 11–6.   MOST FREQUENTLY USED HIP FIXATION DEVICES

Device	Characteristics	Weight Bearing Precautions	Comments
Rods Enders	Three rods stablize hip fracture. Rods are inserted into femoral condyle to knee joint.	PWB – PO day 2 FWB – as tolerated	Can cause toe-out posture. Rehab of hip and knee crucial.
Nails Jewett Smith-Peterson	Long stainless steel rods are used to stablize intertrochanteric fracture.	TDWB–PO 2-5 days FWB – when totally healed	Strict weight bearing secondary to fixation possibly piercing femoral head.
Pins Knowles	Sharp stainless stell rod used to reduce non-comminuted intracapsular fracture.	TDWB-PO 2-5 days FWB - 6th –7th week	Strict weight bearing secondary to fixation, possibly piercing femoral head.
Screws & Plates Richard's Compression	Most commonly chosen device for intertrochanteric fixation.	PWB – PO day 2 FWB – 6th – 7th week	The screwing mechanism enhances healing.

PWB = Partial weight bearing; FWB = Full weight bearing; TDWB = Touch down weight bearing; PO = Postoperative. (Modified and reproduced with permission from *Zimmer Product Encyclopedia. Warsaw IN: Zimmer USA; December 1999.*[112])

shows only a very slight decrease in range of motion with age.[106]

Osteoarthritis

Osteoarthritis of the knee is defined as a wearing away of the articular cartilage of the knee.[119] The articular cartilage softens, fissures occur, ostephytes form, and the synovium becomes fibrous. The capsule also thickens.[119] Barrett[120] found that older patients tend to have a slight decrease of proprioception in the knee; however, there was a significant decrease in patients who had osteoarthritis of the knee in this study. This study also found that when patients received a joint replacement, they have an improvement in proprioception in the knee, but it is still not at the same level as normal.[120]

The important points to consider in osteoarthritis of the knee are the pain and other difficulties encountered by the patient. Frequently, the pain will occur with weight bearing, and the patient will have difficulty with gait activities and simple weight bearing. Therapists, again, need to work on decreasing forces on the knee joint until the patient is strong enough for daily activities.

According to the work of Radin,[121] the major shock-absorbing mechanism of the joint is not the cartilage but is in fact the muscle, which absorbs 80% of the shock. Therefore, a very comprehensive exercise program to improve the strength around the joint will be helpful. According to the work of Fisher and associates[64] and Kriendler and Lewis,[65] strengthening around the joint can improve range of motion and strength. Therefore, a nonweight-bearing strengthening program should be initiated early.

An article by Steinlan and coworkers[122] showed that infrared therapy helps to decrease pain in patients with osteoarthritis of the knee. In this study,

patients used home infrared units for twenty minutes every eight hours with significant pain relief.[122]

According to Liang and Fortin,[63] when therapists evaluate osteoarthritis problems of the knee, they must consider other causes for the pain, such as patellar-femoral problems, bursitis, as well as tendonitis and inflammation of the ligament around the knee. If it is a patellar-femoral problem, the patient needs to work on patella-femoral tracking exercises to stimulate the vastus medialis.[123] The simplest exercise to facilitate this is a combination hip abduction with quadricep setting (Fig. 11–11).

Prior to starting any strengthening program, however, the therapist must consider decreasing the swelling of the knee joint. This treatment is based on reflex inhibition due to joint extension that may cause difficulty initiating a proper contraction.[5] This can be achieved with ice or electrical modalities. In addition, the patient may complain of stiffness after sitting for long periods of time. This may be caused by an inflammatory response in the knee joint, causing cross-linking of the collagen or synovial thickening. Simply having the person roll the foot back and forth on a soda bottle or something similar can help to increase extensibility of this tissue.

Total Knee Replacement

The next pathology to be discussed here is the total knee replacements, which have been extremely successful in the United States.[124] In Appendix A (Figure 11A–4) are intervention protocols for total knee replacements. These protocols are specific and work with patients on active, range-of-motion exercises, various passive exercises, as well as strengthening exercises to improve the range of motion.

For the older patients, it is extremely important to encourage frequent but limited bouts of exercise

Total Hip Arthroplasty Protocol

Purpose

To guide patients through the pre- and postoperative phases of rehabilitation following total hip arthroplasty to assist the patient in becoming functionally independent following surgery.

Indications

Patients who have been admitted for or who have acutely undergone total hip arthroplasty.

Contraindications

Any surgical or postoperative complications as stated by the attending orthopedic surgeon.

Physical Therapy Goals

1. Increase range of motion of the operative hip with progression towards full anatomical range of motion and limited only by the prosthetic design and the patient's potential.
2. Muscle strengthening primarily of the hip abductor muscle groups. These exercises are not to be instituted until approximately 2–6 weeks after surgery and without the use of ankle weights.
3. Gait training. Assistive devices are used to enable the patient to achieve the proper weight bearing status on the operative extremity and to assist with balance. These devices are ultimately discontinued at the discretion of the attending orthopaedic surgeon.

Physical Therapy Program Shall Consist of

1. Preoperative instruction via "Total Hip Information" class.
2. Preoperative evaluation and teaching.
3. Postoperative rehabilitation.
4. Home instructions prior to discharge.
5. Home/outpatient physical therapy follow-up.
6. Progression in outpatient therapy per and with the attending orthopedic surgeon in the orthopedic clinic on follow-up clinic visits.

Preoperative Physical Therapy Evaluation

History

Mentation

Range of motion of both lower extremities

Muscle function and strength

Pain

Sensation

Skin, including edema, erythema, increased heat or cold

Posture

Continued

Continued from previous page

Leg length measurements. Taken with the patient supine, measure from ASIS to the medial malleolus

Gait analysis

Functional abilities of the patient

Equipment used by the patient

Other medical problems

Statement of physical therapy goals. Long- and short-term goals are set and reviewed with the patient

Prognosis, duration, and frequency of physical therapy.

Physical Therapy Preoperative Teaching

1. Explanation of the role of physical therapy in total hip arthroplasty rehabilitation.

2. Statement of physical therapy goals for total hip arthroplasty.

3. Step-by-step explanation, instruction, and demonstration of postoperative physical therapy treatments.

4. Answering of general questions regarding the actual surgical procedure and rehabilitation following total hip arthroplasty.

Generally Precautions in Hip Arthroplasty

1. No combination movements of the operative lower extremity. Patients are allowed to flex, extend, rotate, and so forth their operative hip to tolerance (i.e., no limitations on range of motion), but are not to combine any of these motions. All range of motion exercises are done in single planes of movement.

2. No straight leg raises.

3. No use of ankle weights with any of the prescribed exercises.

4. No sleeping on the operative hip for 6 weeks.

5. Low, soft, contour-type furniture (i.e., sofas, chairs) is to be avoided.

6. Patient may resume driving at 10 weeks from the date of surgery.

7. Patient may return to work at the discretion of the surgeon.

8. Sexual activity may be resumed when comfortable. Specific literature on this subject is available from the nursing staff upon request.

9. Ambulation guidelines.

   a. **Cemented Protheses:** WBAT ambulation. Patients will be required to ambulate using a walker/crutches for a total of 6 weeks following their surgery. At that time, they are begun on ambulation programs using a cane with emphasis on strengthening their hip abductor muscle groups. At the time they are able to ambulate without a Trendelenburg limp, the cane may be discontinued, and they are encouraged to ambulate without any assistive device.

Continued

— *Continued from the previous page* —

b. Uncemented Prosthesis: TDWB ambulation. Patients are to ambulate using walker/crutches with TDWB status for a total of 6 weeks. At 6 weeks postop, the patient is begun on a progressive weight bearing program using the walker/crutches. Patients begin by bearing 1/3 of their body weight on the operative extremity; in 2 weeks, they progress to 2/3 body weight on the operative extremity (continuing to use their assistive device); in 2 weeks, they are allowed full weight bearing on the operative extremity for a total of 2 more weeks. At the end of these 2 weeks, 12 weeks from the date of surgery, walker/crutches are discontinued and cane ambulation is begun. Patients are to continue ambulating using a cane until they are able to ambulate without a Trendelenburg limp. At this time, the cane may be discontinued, and patients are encouraged to ambulate without any assistive device.

Physical Therapy Treatment Protocol for Total Hip Arthroplasty

Preoperative: 1 Month Prior to Hospitalization

1. Attend total joint class on hip arthroplasty. Material covered in the class includes discussions on anatomy of normal and abnormal hip joint components and types of hip prosthesis, admission procedures for VUH, inpatient preoperative care, intraoperative sequence of events, identification of postoperative complications and preventative measures, inpatient/home rehabilitation via physical therapy, and occupational therapy and postdischarge needs. Class personnel includes nursing, PT, OT, and SW.

Prepoerative: Day of Admission

1. Preoperative evaluation of range of motion, strength, limb length discrepancy, pain, gait, etc.

2. Review basic precautions and instruct in immediate postoperative exercises.

3. Fit walker/crutches and instruct in appropriate gait pattern. Three-point gait if one extremity is involved, four-point gait if both lower extremities are involved: WBAT if cemented prosthesis is to be used, TDWB if noncemented prosthesis is used.

Postop Day 1

1. Begin lower extremity isometrics and ankle pumping exercises.

2. Initiate bilateral upper extremity and contralateral limb strengthening exercises.

3. Begin bed-to-chair transfers with assistance to a chair of appropriate height. Patients are not required to "slouch" sit and may sit in an upright position if comfortable.

Postop Day 2

1. Review lower extremity isometrics and ankle pumping exercises.

2. Begin active-assisted lower extremity range of motion exercises to the operative extremity in bed. Operative limb motions should be to the patients tolerance and the limb should be kept in a single plane of motion.

3. Begin assisted walker/crutch ambulation with weight bearing status dependent on prosthesis design and implantation.

— *Continued* —

Continued from previous page

Postop Day 3–5

1. Continue supine exercises.

2. Instruct patient in sitting exercises.

3. Instruct in bathroom transfers. Patients are to use an over-the-commode chair that the nursing staff will secure for their use while hospitalized.

4. Continue gait training on level surfaces.

Postop Day 6–Discharge

1. Review and reinforce supine and sitting exercises.

2. Reinforce postopeative precautions.

3. Further gait refinement to achieve maximum, safe, energy-efficient gait pattern with appropriate weight bearing status.

4. Instruct in stair climbing.

5. Begin and complete discharge plans and arrangements for follow-up home/outpatient physical therapy (follow-up physical therapy services arranged for 6 weeks with three sessions per week).

6. Review home instructions and exercise program with patient and family members.

After Discharge

First clinic follow-up visit. Approximately 2 to 3 weeks from hospital discharge; seen in orthepedic clinic with surgeon.

1. Review home instructions and exercise program.

2. Instruct in hip abduction exercises—standing only, and instruct in supine IT band stretches.

3. Continue walker/crutch ambulation with appropriate weight bearing status.

Second clinic follow-up visit. Approximately 6 weeks postop.

1. Review complete exercise program.

2. Instruct in hip abduction exercises, side-lying and instruct in supine IT band stretches.

3. Instruct in increased activity schedule.

4. If cemented prosthesis, can begin ambulation. Continue to use the cane until patient is able to ambulate without a Trendelenburg limp.

5. If noncemented prosthesis, begin on progressive weight bearing program using walker/crutches.

Third clinic follow-up visit. Approximately 12 weeks postop.

1. Review complete exercise and activity program.

2. Noncemented prothesis, begin can ambulation. Continue to use cane until patient able to ambulate without a Trendelenburg limp.

All other clinic follow-up visits.

1. Continue to review and reinforce exercises and activity regimens.

389 ORTHOPAEDIC TREATMENT CONSIDERATIONS

Hip Arthroplasty General Instructions

1. The exercise program should be carried out two to three times per day building up to 20 repetitions of each exercise.

2. You may sit for up to 30 minutes at one time, as often as desired, as long as you walk or lie flat on your back or stomach for a few minutes between sitting periods.

3. It is very common to note swelling of the lower leg when first home; do not be concerned as long as the swelling is down in the morning.

4. Do not sleep on your operative side until approved by your surgeon.

5. Sexual activity may be resumed when comfortable.

6. Try to keep your operative leg positioned in bed so that the toes and kneecap point upwards toward the ceiling when you are backlying.

7. When advised by your surgeon, you may take a shower (tub baths are not advised). You may wish to put a chair in your shower to sit on while bathing (mesh lawn chairs work well).

8. Low, soft contour-type chairs should be avoided.

9. Dining out: Do not sit in booths or low chairs.

10. Walk in short sessions as tolerated to gradually improve your physical endurance. You may walk out of doors when stamina and strength are adequate.

11. You may return to work at the discretion of your surgeon.

12. Walking

    a. Keep erect posture at all times with buttocks tucked under shoulders.

    b. Look straight ahead.

    c. Walk in a heel-to-toe sequence, with toes pointed straight ahead.

    d. Tighten your buttocks and the knee of the supporting leg until the heel of the moving leg hits the ground.

    e. Never lean on your crutches. Distribute your weight on the hand grips.

13. Stairs

    UP: Step up with your_____leg first. Lean slightly forward and push down on your crutches. Raise your other leg. After both feet are firmly on the stair above, raise your crutches.

    DOWN: Come to the edge; lower your crutches to the stair below as you bend your knees. Lower your———————leg, then lower your other leg.

Additional Comments:

and to emphasize range of motion. Therapists need to be aware that total knee replacements are very painful operations and are more prone to infection than total hip replacements.[124] Therefore, the therapist needs to not only work on range of motion and strength, but also to check for infection and utilize pain management techniques. Frequently, the use of ice and various weight-bearing protocols have been shown to be effective.[123]

THE FOOT AND ANKLE

The foot requires a special introduction from Arthur Helfand:

"Have you ever imagined the difficulties you might encounter if your feet were in such condition that you could not walk or stand without chronic pain? The foot has received less attention than any other

Total Knee Replacement Home Instructions and Exercise Program

General Instructions

1. It is very common to note swelling of the lower leg when first home. Do not be concerned as long as the swelling is down in the morning.

2. Do contact your physician if you have any evidence of infection in any part of your body (i.e., redness, edema, or increased heat in a joint).

3. Sit or stand with the operative leg out in front of the other leg.

4. Never pivot or twist on your operative leg when turning; take small steps to turn.

5. Wear your knee splint at night unless your surgeon discontinues its use.

6. You may sit for 30 minutes with your knee bent, but then you must stretch your knee muscles by walking approximately 5 minutes or by practicing your exercises.

7. Avoid low chairs! A straight back chair (kitchen type) is best for getting up and down comfortably.

8. As tolerated, walk in short sessions to gradually improve your physical endurance. Continue to use your walker or crutches until your surgeon specifies otherwise.

9. Stairs: when ascending stairs, the nonoperative leg goes up first, followed by the operative leg and your crutches. When descending stairs, the crutches and operative leg go first, then the nonoperative leg.

Exercise Program

- Exercises are to be performed two to three times per day building up to 20 repetitions of each exercise.

- Do not place any resistance on your ankle or foot when doing your exercises (i.e., remove heavy shoes, use no ankle weights).

1. **Supine:** Lying on your back on a firm, flat surface; exercise both legs!

   a. Tighten the muscles on the top of the thighs pushing the back of the knees down into the bed. Hold 5 seconds. Relax; repeat.

   b. Tighten buttock muscles. Hold 5 seconds. Relax.

   c. Slowly make circles with your ankles moving your feet in clockwise and counterclockwise directions. Only your foot should move, not the entire leg.

   d. Tighten your knee and bend your ankle so that your toes point toward your face. Lift your leg straight up in the air. Tighten the knee again before slowly lowering your leg to the bed, making the back of your knee hit the bed first.

   e. With one leg straight, bring the opposite knee to your chest allowing your knee to bend as much as possible. Hold your thigh up with your hands or a towel as you kick your foot in the air to straighten your knee. Lower your leg to the bed with the knee straight.

   f. Place a large towel roll (12 inches in diameter) under your thigh. Straighten your knee by lifting your foot up toward the ceiling and by tightening your knee cap. Do not lift your thigh or upper leg off the roll. Hold 5 seconds. Relax.

— Continued —

─── *Continued from previous page* ───

2. **Long Sitting:** Sit in the bed with our back straight. Stretch your legs out in front of you. Push the back of your knees down into the bed and bend your ankle by pulling your toes toward your face. Keeping knees tight, reach forward toward your toes in order to feel stretching in the back of your knees. Hold 5 seconds. Relax.

3. **Sitting:** Sit on a firm surface with a small towel under your knee. Straighten the operative leg, using the foot of the nonoperative leg for support if necessary. Let your operative leg drop by gravity slowly, then force it to bend using the other foot to exert pressure on top of the ankle within limits of pain tolerance.

4. **Prone:**

   a. Roll over your operative knee to get on your stomach. Lie on your stomach, feet hanging over the edge of the bed, and thigh rolls in place. Assume this position for 15 minutes twice each day. You may wear your shoes to give an added stretch to the muscles behind the knee.

   b. After resting, bend your operative knee as much as is possible. Hold 5 seconds. Relax *Discontinue this exercise if it is too painful.

5. **Biking:** Gradually increase your bike riding endurance to two 15 minute sessions per day. Initially adjust the seat to the height determined in the hospital.* Once riding the bike comfortably at that seat height, lower the seat 1/4 inch each week.

*Seat height at discharge:_____. Measure from the tip of the seat to the top of the pedal at its lowest point.

Note—NO RESISTANCE IN BIKING!!!

If you have any questions or problems with your exercises, please contact your therapist.

───────────────────PT

part of the human anatomy, possibly because injuries, disorders of the foot are seldom causes of mortality."[125]

White and Mulley found that 30% of community-dwelling elderly complain of pain in their feet.[126] Common foot disorders and deformities can cause a great deal of pain and severely curtail ambulation activities.[127] Ill-fitting or worn-out shoes can also lead to ulceration and discomfort during weight-bearing activities. Many simple and inexpensive modifications of shoes, and fabrication of shock absorbing, total contact orthotics to redistribute weight evenly on the plantar surface, can greatly enhance mobility for an older adult.[128]

When evaluating feet, therapists must first check the skin for dryness and calluses. If they note that they are dry, rough, or callused, the therapist should encourage patients to use creams, unless there are open lesions. The therapist should also check the skin for the integrity of vibratory, temperature, and protective sensations; and hair growth and color to determine diminished circulation or changes consistent with metabolic disorders such as diabetes.[129]

The skin on the feet should be checked for corns and calluses. These are layers of compacted skin that have built up over irritated areas. Calluses are usually found on the soles of the feet or heels. Corns are cone-shaped areas that occur on the toes and are caused by friction and pressure from the skin rubbing against bony areas, such as when the patient wears ill-fitting shoes. The person should be encouraged to wear shoes that fit properly.[128]

The bony alignment of the foot also needs to be checked. The therapist should check for lesser toe deformities such as clawlike, hammer toes, mallet toes, dislocated and/or overlapping toes. These lesser toe deformities are usually the result of weakness in the soft tissue surrounding metatarsal heads, which can lead to tendonitis or capsulitis. Treatment is aimed at relieving pressure. Interventions, such as metatarsal bars or "cookies" (pads) to splay the metatarsal heads, intrinsic exercises to strengthen the foot, such as toe spreads and stretches, as well as anti-inflammatory medication can be very helpful.[128,130] Hallux valgus, another bone deformity, is an inward deviation of the first metatarsal, coupled with an outward deviation and rotational deformity of the great toe.[127] A person

Sit or lie on a flat surface with your legs straight out. With a rolled towel between your knees, push knees together. Then, still keeping your knees together, tighten the muscles in the front of your thigh by forcing your knee straight. Hold for 10 seconds. Do _____ times. Count out loud and breathe while holding.

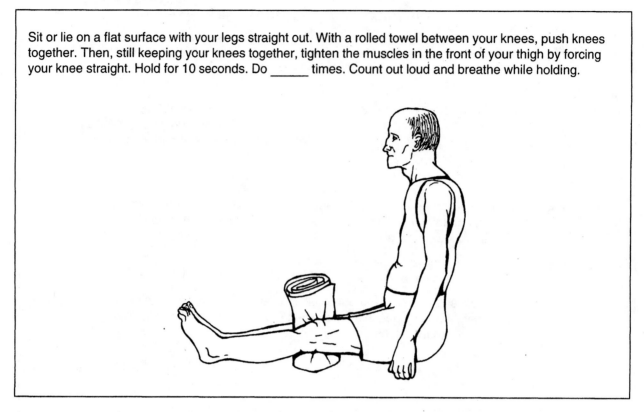

Figure 11–11.   *Exercise for facilitating a combination of hip abduction with quadricep setting.*

can develop osseous enlargements and joint pain. Treatments include: ultrasound, whirlpool, iontophoresis, joint mobilization and exercise to the great toe. Orthotics are extremely important for redistributing the forces under the second metatarsal head and for assisting these patients in pressure and pain relief.[128]

Circulation and sensation should be checked in the foot. Patients complaining of cramping and fatigue should receive special attention. For these patients, it is important that they inspect their feet, keep them warm and dry, and that they do not wear circular garters that cut off the blood supply to the feet. Patients also need to be careful about any type of medication used on their feet, so as to not cause skin damage. Buerger-Allen exercises may be helpful in improving circulation in the aging foot. Chapter 13 of this text provides a comprehensive description of Buerger-Allen exercises for improving circulation. Chapter 13 provides evaluation forms and flow sheets developed by Dr. Bottomley for the assessment of circulatory and sensory changes in the lower extremity.

There are strength and joint mobility changes in the foot, as noted in Chapter 6. Vandervoort and Hayes[131] showed a slowing and a decrease in torque generation applied to foot and ankle flexors in old persons of 71%, when compared with younger persons.[131] This means that older people will be significantly weaker in their plantarflexion strength, which may be a very important factor in balance. (See also Chapter 3.) In addition, ankle and foot range of mo-

tion decrease with age, limiting adaptability of the foot to changing walking surfaces.[106]

The approach for foot problems is a thorough evaluation, and then treatment of the appropriate problem with modalities and exercises as needed. The importance of properly fitting shoes cannot be stressed enough. Frequently, older persons have been purchasing inappropriately sized shoes for many years, and it will be difficult to convince them they need different sized shoes. To instruct an older person in the proper shoe fit, the following criteria should be used: When a person stands, a thumb (rule-of-thumb) should fit between the end of the longest toe to the end of the shoe. When the therapist squeezes the person's shoe (while they are standing) at the metatarsal head, a slight give should be felt prior to feeling the metatarsal heads. The metatarsal heads should never be in contact with the lateral borders of the toe box of the shoe.[132] In approximately 99% of cases, patients have poor-fitting shoes. In addition, the shoes should have a strong, supportive sole made of rubber or crepe, so that they do not slip. The sole should have a wide base, and high heels should be strongly discouraged.[132]

CONCLUSION

Even though this chapter has divided orthopedic treatment into various conditions and joints, any thorough examination, evaluation and intervention needs to look at the person as a whole. This chapter provides information on specific musculoskeletal changes that occur with age, as well as orthopedic pathologies that occur more predominately in an older adult population. General treatment suggestions have been provided (see Chapter 10 for further details on evaluation of orthopedic conditions).

PEARLS

- Thirty percent of all geriatric patients/clients consult their physicians because of musculoskeletal problems.
- Therapists need to assess the cause of strength declines (e.g., neuromuscular, cardiovascular, joint swelling or joint changes) and treat the strength decrease accordingly.
- Treatment suggestions for flexibility decrements in the aged are to heat the muscle, gently stretch the muscle, reinforce the stretch by doing functional activities, and cool the muscle down in the lengthened position.
- Normal changes of the spine include less flexibility in the soft tissues, decreased mineralization of bones, osteophyte formation, and disc space narrowing.
- Osteoporosis is no longer considered an inevitable consequence of aging.
- Osteopenia refers to metabolic bone diseases that are characterized by x-ray findings of a subnormal amount of mineralized bone mass.
- Osteomalacia is a bone disorder caused by a failure of normal calcification of the bone matrix.
- Death of bone and the cellular components of bone in the absence of infection is referred to as *osteonecrosis* or *avascular necrosis*.
- Paget's disease is a progressive disorder associated with a marked increase in osteoblastic activity.
- Lumbar stenosis can be treated with flexion exercises and environmental modifications, whereas vertebral compression fractures are treated with extension exercises.
- Pathologies of old age seen in the shoulder include rotator cuff problems, adhesive capsulitis, fractures, and osteoarthritis.
- Aging causes a decrease in motion of almost all of the body joints. Nevertheless, the older person can maintain independence. Osteoporosis, arthritis, fractures, as well as many other pathologies, respond favorably to exercise and rehabilitation programs.

REFERENCES

1. Steinberg FU. Principles of geriatric rehabilitation. *Arch Phys Med Rehabil.* 1989; 70(1):67–68.
2. Eva P, Lyyra AL, Viitasalo JT, et al. Determinants of isometric muscle strength in men of different ages. *Eur J Appl Physiol.* 1992; 64(1):84–91.
3. Frontera W, Hughes VA, Lutz KS, et al. A cross-sectional study of muscle strength and mass in 45- to 78-year-old men and women. *J Appl Physiol.* 1992; 72(2):644–650.
4. Hakkinen K, Hakkinen A. Muscle cross-sectional area, force production and relaxation characteristics in women at different ages. *Eur J Appl Physiol.* 1991; 62(4):410–414.
5. De Andrade J, Grant C, Dixon, et al. Joint distension and reflex muscle inhibition in the knee. *J Bone Joint Surg.* 1965; 47-A(2):312–322.
6. Healy L. Late-onset rheumatoid arthritis vs. polymyalgia rheumatica in blacks may be an artifact. *J Am Ger Soc.* 1990; 38(9):824–826.
7. Thompson LV. Physiological Changes Associated with Aging. In: Guccione AA. *Geriatric Physical Therapy.* 2nd Edition. St. Louis, MO: Mosby, Inc; 2000: 28–55.
8. Bottomley JM. Extension equals function. *Geri-Notes.* September 2000; 7(5):1–4.
9. Lewis CB, Bottomley JM. Musculoskeletal changes with age: clinical implications. In: Lewis CB, ed. *Aging: Health Care's Challenge.* 2nd Ed. Philadelphia: FA Davis; 1990:135–160.
10. Bottomley JM. Age-related bone health and pathophysiology of osteoporosis. *Ortho Phys Ther Clinics of No Amer.* 1998; 7(2):117–132.
11. Snow-Harter C, Marcus R. Exercise, bone mineral density, and osteoporosis. *Exercise Sport Sci Rev.* 1991; 19:351–388.
12. Marieb EN. *Human Anatomy and Physiology.* 3rd ed. Redwood City, Calif: Benjamin Cummings; 1995.
13. Wheeler M. Osteoporosis. *Medical Clinics of North America.* 1996; 80(6):1213–1224.
14. Robergs RA, Roberts SO. Bone function and adaptation to exercise. In: Robergs RA, Roberts SO. eds. *Exercise Physiology: Exercise Performance and Clinical Applications.* St. Louis Missouri: Mosby Year Book, Inc; 1997:380–393.
15. Dalsky GP. Effect of exercise on bone: permissive influence of estrogen and calcium. *Med Sci Sports Exercise.* 1990; 22(3):281–285.
16. Raisz LG, Smith J. Pathogenesis, prevention, and treatment of osteoporosis. *Ann Rev Med.* 1989; 40:251–267.
17. Geusens P, Dequeker J, Verstraeten A, Nijs J. Age, sex-, and menopause-related changes of vertebral and peripheral bone: population study using dual- and single-photon absorptiometry and radiogrammetry. *J Nucl Med.* 1986; 27:1540–1549.
18. Riggs BL, Wahner HW, Dann WL. Differential changes in bone mineral density of the appendicular and axial skeleton with aging. *J Clin Invest.* 1981; 67:328–335.
19. Riggs BL, Wahner HW, Melton LJ III. Rates of bone loss in the appendicular and axial skeletons of women. *J Clin Invest.* 1986; 77:1487–1491.
20. Buchanan JR, Myers C, Lloyd T. Determinants of trabecular bone density in women: the role of androgens, estrogen, and exercise. *J Bone Mineral Research.* 1988; 3:673–680.

21. Grove KA, Londeree BR. Bone density in post-menopausal women: high-impact versus low-impact exercise. *Med Sci Sports Exercise.* 1992; 24 (11):1190–1194.

22. Suominen H. Bone mineral density and long-term exercise. *Sports Med.* 1993; 16(5):316–330.

23. Parfitt AM, Mathews CHE, Villaneuva AR, Kleerekoper M, Frame B, Rao DS. Relationships between surface, volume, and thickness of trabecular bone in aging and in osteoporosis. *J Clin Invest.* 1993; 82:1396–1409.

24. Gallagher JC, Riggs BL, Eisman J, Hamstra A, Arnaud SB, DeLuca HF. Intestinal calcium absorption and serum vitamin D metabolites in normal subjects and osteoporotic patients: effect of age and dietary calcium. *J Clin Invest.* 1979; 64: 729–736.

25. Riggs BL, Wahner HW, Seeman E. Changes in bone mineral density of the proximal femur and spine with aging: differences between the postmenopausal and senile osteoporosis syndromes. *J Clin Invest.* 1982; 70:716–723.

26. Sanborn CF. Exercise, calcium, and bone density. *Gatorade Sports Science Exchange.* 1990; 2(24): 1–5.

27. Dalsky GP, Stocke KS, Ehsani AA. Weight-bearing exercise training and lumbar bone mineral content in postmenopausal women. *Ann Intern Med.* 1988; 108:824–828.

28. Parfitt AM. Dietary risk factors for age-related bone loss and fractures. *Lancet.* 1993; 2: 1181–1185.

29. Drinkwater BL, Nilson K, Chesnut CH III. Bone content of amenorrheic and eumenorrheic athletes. *N Engl J Med.* 1984; 311(5):277–281.

30. Drinkwater BL, Nilson K, Chesnut CH III. Bone mineral density after resumption of mensus in amenorrheic athletes. *JAMA.* 1986; 256: 380–382.

31. Nilsson BE, Westline NE. Bone density in athletes. *Clin Orthop.* 1991;97:179–182.

32. Block JE, Friedlander AL, Brooks GA. Determinants of bone density among athletes engaged in weight-bearing and non-weight-bearing activity. *J Appl Physiol.* 1989; 67(3):1100–1105.

33. Aisenbrey JA. Exercise in the prevention and management of osteoporosis. *Phys Ther.* 1987; 67(1): 100–104.

34. Lips P, Courpron P, Meunier PJ. Mean wall thickness of trabecular bone: changes with age. *Calcif Tissue Res.* 1988; 26:13–17.

35. Rudman D, Kutner MH, Rogers CM, Lubin MF, Fleming GA, Bain RP. Impaired growth hormone secretion in the adult population: relation to age and adiposity. *J Clin Invest.* 1991; 77:1361–1369.

36. Centrella M, Canalis E. Local regulators of skeletal growth: a genetic perspective. *Endocr Rev.* 1985; 6:544–551.

37. Ivey JL, Baylink DJ. Postmenopausal osteoporosis: proposed roles of defective coupling and estrogen deficiency. *Metab Bone Dis Relat Res.* 1981; 3:3–7.

38. Bullamore JR, Gallagher JC, Wilkinson R, Nordin BEC, Marshall DH. Effect of age on calcium absorption. *Lancet.* 1990; 2:535–537.

39. Manolagas SC, Culler FL, Howard JE, Brickman AS, Deftos LJ. The cytoreceptor assay for 1,25–dihydroxyvitamin D and its application to clinical studies. *J Clin Endocrinol Metab.* 1993; 56: 751–760.

40. Tsai KS, Health H III, Kumar R, Riggs BL. Impaired vitamin D metabolism with aging in women: possible role in pathogenesis of senile osteoporosis. *J Clin Invest.* 1994; 83:1668–1672.

41. Heaney RP, Gallagher JC, Johnston CC, Neer R, Parfitt AM, Whedon GD. Calcium nutrition and bone health in the elderly. *Am J Clin Nutr.* 1982; 36(suppl):986–1013.

42. Allen LH. Calcium bioavailability and absorption: a review. *Am J Clin Nutr.* 1982; 35:783–808.

43. Heaney RP, Recker RR, Saville PD. Menopausal changes in calcium balance performance. *J Lab Clin Med.* 1988; 102:953–963.

44. Parfitt AM, Gallagher RP, Heaney PR, Johnston CC, Neer R, Wheldon GD. Vitamin D and bone health in the elderly. *Am J Clin Nutr.* 1992; 46 (suppl): 1014–1031.

45. Greger K, Krystofiak M. Phosphorus intake of Americans. *Food Technol.* 1992; 46:78–84.

46. Frost HM. Structural adaptations to mechanical usage. Redefining Wolff's Law. *Anat Rec.* 1990; 226:403–422.

47. Heinrich Ch, Going RW, Parmenter CD, Perry T, Boyden W, Lohman TG. Bone mineral content of cyclically menstruating female resistance and endurance trained athletes. *Med Sci Sports Exerc.* 1990; 22:558–563.

48. Jacobsoen PC, Beaver W, Grubb SA, Taft TN, Talmadge RV. Bone density in women: college athletes and older athletic women. *J Orthop Res.* 1994; 2:328–332.

49. Pocock N, Eisman JA, Gwinn T. Muscle Strength, physical fitness and weight but not age, predict femoral neck bone mass. *J Bone Miner Res.* 1989; 4:441–446.

50. Snow-Harter C, Bouxsein M, Lewis BT, Charette S, Weinstein S, Marcus R. Muscle strength as a predictor of bone mineral density in women. *J Bone Miner Res.* 1990; 5:589–595.

51. Sinaki M, Mikkelson BA. Postmenopausal spinal osteoporosis. Flexion versus extension exercises. *Arch Phys Med Rehabil.* 1984; 65:593–596.

52. Sinaki M. Musculoskeletal challenges of osteoporosis. *Aging.* 1998; 10(3):249–262.

53. Kanis JA, Melton LF III, Christiansen C, Johnson CC, Khaltev N. The diagnosis of osteoporosis. *J Bone Miner Res.* 1994; 9:1137–1141.

54. Kribbs PJ, Smith DE, Chestnutt CH III. Oral findings in osteoporosis. Part II: relationship between residual ridge and alveolar bone resorption and generalized skeletal osteopenia. *J Prosthet Dent.* 1983; 50(5):719–724.

55. Shapiro S, Bomberg TJ, Benson BW, et al. Postmenopausal osteoporosis: dental patients at risk. *Gerodontics.* 1985; 1(5):220–225.

56. Wical EE, Swoope CC. Studies of residual ridge resorption. Part II: The relationship of dietary calcium and phosphorus to residual ridge resorption. *J Prosthet Dent.* 1974; 32(1):13–22.

57. Gunta KE. Alterations in skeletal function: congenital disorders, metabolic bone disease, and neoplasms. In: Porth C, ed. *Pathophysiology: Concepts of Altered Health States.* 4th ed. Philadelphia, Pa: JB Lippincott; 1994: 1230–1235.

58. Hahn BH. Osteopenic bone diseases. In: McCarty DJ, Koopman WJ, eds. *Arthritis and Allied Conditions.* Vol 2, 12th ed. Philadelphia, Pa; Lea & Febiger; 1994: 1935–1938.

59. James J, Steijn-Myagkaya GL. Death of osteocytes. Electron microscopy after in vitro ischemia. *J Bone Joint Surg.* 1986; 68:620–624.

60. Jones JP. Osteonecrosis. In: McCarthy DJ, Koopman WJ, eds. *Arthritis and Allied Conditions.* Vol 1 12th ed. Philadelphia, Pa: Lea & Febiger; 1993; 1677–1696.

61. Schiller AL. Bones and joints. In: Rubin E, Farber JL (eds): *Pathology,* 2nd Ed. Philadelphia, PA: JB Lippincott, 1994; 1273–1347.

62. Pigg JS, Bancroft DA. Alterations in skeletal function: rheumatic disorders. In: Mattson-Porth C (ed): *Pathophysiology,* 4th Ed. Philadelphia, PA: JB Lippincott, 1994; 1267–1268.

63. Liang MH, Fortin P. Management of osteoarthritis of the hip and knee. *N Eng J Med.* July 11, 1991; 325(2):125–126.

64. Fisher N, Pendergast DR, Calkins EC, et al. Maximal isometric torque of the knee extension as a function of muscle length in subjects of advancing age. *Arch Phys Med Rehabil.* 1990; 71(9): 729–734.

65. Kreindler H, Lewis CB. The effects of three exercise protocols on osteoarthritis of the knees. *Top Geriatr Rehabil.* 1989; 4(3):389–409.

66. Felson DT. Weight and osteoarthritis. *Am J Clin Nutr.* 1996; 63(5):430–432.

67. Schumacher RH, ed. *Primer on the Rheumatic Diseases.* 10th ed. Atlanta, GA: Arthritis Foundation; 1993.

68. Gandy S, Payne R. Back pain in the elderly: updated diagnosis and management. *Geriatrics.* 1986; 41(12):59–72.

69. Hayashi K, Okada K, Hamada M. Etiological factors of mylopathy: a radiographic evaluation of the aging changes in the cervical spine. *Clin Ortho.* 1987; 214(1):200–209.

70. Rider R, Daly J. Effects of flexibility training of enhancing spinal mobility in older women. *J Sports Med and Phys Fit.* 1991; 3(2):213–217.

71. Twomey LT, Taylor JR. *Physical Therapy of the Low Back.* New York, NY: Churchill Livingston; 1987.

72. Fast A. Low back disorders conservative management. *Arch Phys Med Rehabil.* 1988; 69(10): 880–891.

73. Bottomley JM. The use of T'ai chi as a movement modality in orthopedics. *Ortho Phys Ther Clin No Amer.* 2000; 9(3):361–374.

74. Frost H. Clinical management of the symptomatic osteoporotic patient. *Ortho Clin No Amer.* 1981; 12(3):671–681.

75. Turner P. Osteoporotic back pain—its prevention and treatment. *Physiotherapy.* 1991; 77(9): 642–646.

76. Sinaki M, McPhee MC, Hodgson SF. Relationship between bone mineral density of spine and strength of back extensors in health postmenopausal women. *Mayo Clin Proc.* 1986; 61(2): 116–122.

77. Payne R. Neck pain in the elderly: a management review, part I. *Geriatrics.* 1987; 42(1):59–65.

78. Payne R. Neck pain in the elderly: a management review, part II. *Geriatrics.* 1987; 42(2):71–73.

79. Lewis CB, McNerney T. Neck pain and the elderly. *Phys Ther Practice.* 1992; 1(1):43–53.

80. Furman JM, Whitney SL. Central causes of dizziness. *Phys Ther.* 2000; 80(2):179–187.

81. Cote P, Kreitz BG, Cassidy JD, Thiel H. The validity of the extension-rotation test as a clinical screening procedure before neck manipulation: a secondary analysis. *J Manipulative Physiol Ther.* 1996; 19:159–164.

82. McGregor M, Haldeman S, Kohlbeck FJ. Vertebrobasilar compromise associated with cervical manipulation. *Top Clin Chiro.* 1995; 2:63–73.

83. Terrett AG. *Vertebrobasilar Stroke Following Manipulation.* Nat Chiro Mutual Co: West Des Moines, IA; 1996.

84. Di Fabio RP. Manipulation of the cervical spine: risks and benefits. *Phys Ther.* 1999; 79(1):50–65.

85. Bolton PS, Stick PE, Lord RS. Failure of clinical tests to predict cerebral ischemia before neck manipulation. *J Manipulative Physiol Ther.* 1989; 12:304–307.

86. Dix M, Hallpike C. The pathology, symptomatology and diagnosis of certain common disorders of the vestibular system. *Ann Otol Rhinol Laryngol.* 1952; 61:341–354.

87. Whitney SL. Treatment of the older adult with vestibular dysfunction. In: Herdman SJ, ed. *Vestibular Rehabilitation.* 2nd edition. FA Davis: Philadelphia, PA; 1999: 512–543.

88. Borello-France DF, Whitney SL, Herdman SJ. Assessment of vestibular hypofunction. In: Herdman SJ, ed. *Vestibular Rehabilitation.* FA Davis: Philadelphia, PA; 1994:247–286.

89. Harsh G, Sypert GW, Weinstein PR. Cervical spine stenosis secondary to ossification of the posterior longitudinal ligament. *J Neurosurg.* 1987; 67(3): 349–357.

90. Bassey E, Morgan K, Calloso HM, et al. Flexibility of the shoulder joint measured at range of abduction in a large representative sample of men and women over 65 years of age. *Eur J Appl Physiol.* 1989; 58:353–360.

91. Faulkner C, Jensen RH, Nosse L. The aging rotator cuff: internal/external rotation torques for youth vs. senior citizen. *Phys Ther.* June 1991; 71(6): (suppl S75).

92. Sundstrom W. Painful shoulders: diagnosis and management. *Geriatrics.* March 1983; 38(3): 77–96.

93. Warren R, O'Brien S. Shoulder pain in the geriatric patient, part 11: treatment options. *Ortho Rev.* 1989; 18(2):248–263.

94. Warren R, O'Brien S. Shoulder pain in the geriatric patient, part 1: evaluation and pathophysiology. *Ortho Rev.* 1989; 18(1):129–135.

95. Simon E, Hill J. Rotator cuff injuries. *Orthop Sport Ther*. April 1989; 10(10):394–399.

96. Harrell L, Massey E. Hand weakness in the elderly. *J Am Ger Soc*. 1983; 31(4):223–227.

97. Imrhan S. Trends in finger pinch strength in children, adults and elderly. *Human Factors*. 1989; 31(6):689–701.

98. Kallman D, Plato CC, Tobin JD, et al. The role of muscle loss in the aging related decline of grip strength cross-sectional and longitudinal perspectives. *J Gerontol*. 1990; 45(3):M82–M88.

99. Denham M, Modkinson MH, Furesh KN, et al. Loss of grip in the elderly. *Gerontol Clin*. 1973; 15: 286–271.

100. Balogun J, Akinloye AH, Adeneola SA, et al. Grip strength as a function of height, body weight and quetelet index. *Physiotherapy Theory and Practice*. 1991; 7:111–119.

101. Sobel JS. Elbow injuries: a rehabilitation perspective. In: Lewis CB, Knortz K, eds. *Orthopedic Asssessment and Treatment of the Geriatric Patient*. St. Louis: Mosby Year Book; 1993: 133–144.

102. Maring J. Effects of mental practice on rate of skill acquisition. *Phys Ther*. March 1990; 70(3): 165–172.

103. Villar R, Marsh D, Rushton N, et al. Three years after Colles' fracture. *J Bone Joint Surg*. 1987; 69-B(4):635–638.

104. Douvall S. Hand injuries: a rehabilitation perspective. In: Lewis CB, Knortz K, eds. *Geriatriczithopedics: Surgical and Rehabilitative Management*. St. Louis: Mosby Year Book; 1992.

105. Maddali-Bongi S, Giuidi G, Cencett A, et al. Treatment of carpo-metacarpal joint osteoarthritis by means of a personalized splint. *Pain Clinic*. 1991; 4(2):119–123.

106. James B, Parker A. Active and passive mobility of lower limb joints in elderly men and women. *Am J Phys Med Rehabil*. August 1989; 68(4):165.

107. Kramer J, Vaz MD, Vandervoort AA, et al. Reliability of isometric hip abductor torques during examiner and belt-resisted tests. *J Gerontol*. 1991; 46(2): M47–M51.

108. Neumann D, Cook TM, Sholty RL, et al. An electromyographic analysis of hip abductor muscle activity when subjects are carrying loads in one or both hands. *Phys Ther*. March 1992;72(3):207–217.

109. Tinetti ME, Williams TF, Mayewski R. Fall risk index for elderly patients based on number of chronic disabilities. *Am J Med*. 1986; 80(3):429–434.

110. Kampa K. Mortality of hip fracture patients within one year of fracture . . . an overview. *Geritopics*. April 1989; 14(1):10–11.

111. Cummings S, Nevitt M. A hypothesis: the causes of hip fractures. *J Gerontol Med Sciences*. 1989; 44(4):MI07–Mlll.

112. *Zimmer Product Encyclopedia*. Warsaw, IN: Zimmer USA; December 1999.

113. Zuckerman JD, Zetterber C, Kummer FJ, Frankel VH. Weight bearing following hip fractures in geriatric patients. *Top Geriatr Rehabil*. December 1990; 6(2):34–50.

114. Baker P, Evans OM, Lee C, et al. Treadmill gait training following fractured neck-of-femur. *Arch Phys Med Rehabil*. 1991; 72(8):649–652.

115. Bohannon RW, Kloter KS, Cooper JA. Outcome of patients with hip fracture treated by physical therapy in an acute care hospital. *Top Geriatr Rehabil*. 1990; 6(2):51–58.

116. Barnes B, Dunovan K. Functional outcomes after hip fracture. *Phys Ther*. 1987; 67(11):1675–1679.

117. Bonar S, Tinnetti ME, Speechley M, et al. Factors associated with short versus long-term skilled nursing facility placement among community living hip fracture patients. *J Am Ger Soc*. 1990; 38 (10):1139–1144.

118. Borges O. Isometric and isokinetic knee extension and flexion torque in men and women aged 20–70. *Scand J Rehab Med*. 1989; 21(1):45–53.

119. Altman R. Development of criteria for the classification and reporting of osteoarthritis of the knee. *Arthritis and Rheumatism*. 1986; 29(8): 1039–1049.

120. Barrett D. Joint proprioception in normal osteoarthritis and replaced knees. *J Bone Joint Surg*. 1991; 73-B(1):53–56.

121. Radin E. Mechanical aspects of osteoarthritis. *Bull Rheumatic Dis*. 1975–1976; 26(7):862–865.

122. Steinlan J, Gil I, Habot B, et al. Improvement of pain and disability in elderly patients with degenerative osteoarthritis of the knee treated with narrow-band light therapy. *J Am Ger Soc*. 1992; 40(1): 23–26.

123. Knortz K. Knee injuries: a rehabilitative perspective. In: Lewis CB, Knortz K, eds. *Orthopedic Assessment and Treatment of the Geriatric Patient*. St. Louis: Mosby Year Book; 1993. 301–322.

124. Berry G. Assessment and treatment of knee injuries with particular attention to the hamstring muscles and joint swelling. *Physiotherapy*. 1989; 75(8):690–693.

125. Helfand A. Podiatry in a total geriatric health program: common foot problems of the aged. *J Am Ger Soc*. 1967; 15(6):593–599.

126. White EG, Mulley GP. Foot care for very elderly people: a community survey. *Age and Aging*. 1989; 18(4):275–279.

127. Herman H, Bottomley JM. Anatomical and biomechanical considerations of the elder foot. *Top Geriatr Rehabil*. 1992; 7(3):1–13.

128. Bottomley JM, Herman H. Making simple, inexpensive changes for the management of foot problems in the aged. *Top Geriatr Rehabil*. 1992; 7(3): 62–77.

129. Evans S, Nixon BP, Lee I, et al. The prevalence and nature of podiatric problems in elderly diabetic patients. *J Am Ger Soc*. 1991; 39(3): 241–245.

130. Helfand A. The aging foot. *Focus on Ger Care and Rehab*. April 1989; 2(10).

131. Vandervoort A. Hayes K. Plantarflexor muscle function in young and elderly women. *Eur J of Appl Physiol*. 1989; 58(4):389–394.

132. Bottomley JM. Footwear: foundation for lower extremity orthotics. In: Lusardi MM, Nielson CC. *Orthotics and Prosthetics in Rehabilitation*. Boston, MA: Butterworth-Heinemann; 2000.

PART II

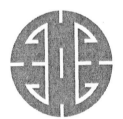

Patient Care Concepts

CHAPTER 12

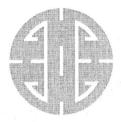

Neurological Treatment Considerations

This chapter will build upon the discussion of specific biological changes that occur with age or pathology, as developed in Chapters 3 and 5. This section will discuss a model for looking at neurological dysfunction, followed by sections on mobility, balance and coordination, weakness, and tremor. The major pathologies that will be discussed are cerebral vascular accidents (CVA) and Parkinson's disease, which will be discussed in terms of prevalence, efficacy of treatment interventions, evaluation, and treatment strategies. This will be followed by a discussion of evaluation and treatment of the common neurological pathology—Alzheimer's disease—which requires special consideration. The last section of this chapter will focus on balance and falls, evaluation of the numerous causes of dizziness and physical changes that increase the risk of falling, and treatment interventions aimed at decreasing the incidence of falls.

The model for neurological dysfunction used is that of Schenkman and Butler.[1] Figure 12–1 illustrates the progression of the stages that result in ultimate disability. This model is best explained using an example; therefore, a patient with a CVA in which the neuroanatomic pathology is a parietal lobe lesion will be discussed. The impairment's direct effects might include a motor loss from the parietal lesion resulting in hypotonicity of the shoulder. An indirect pathological effect could be a rotator cuff tear, and the resulting impairment would be a subluxed shoulder. The impairment's composite effects would be de- creased use of the upper extremity and pain on movement, as well as movement dysfunction in the upper and lower extremities. The resultant functional disability is the patient's inability to dress or walk independently, or sleep without discomfort,

The therapist can then use this model to examine where physical or occupational therapy can benefit the patient. In this example, the therapist may have little effect on the insult or neuroanatomic pathology, but the therapist could positively affect the other areas. Using this information, the therapist can choose the most effective intervention for the problem. This problem-solving model should be kept in mind when reviewing the subsequent dysfunctions.

PARKINSON'S DISEASE

Parkinson's disease is the primary neurological disease of the elderly.[2] It affects 1% of people over 50 years of age, and 50,000 new cases are diagnosed annually.[2] The description of Parkinson's disease and its causes have been covered in detail in Chapter 5. The most common symptoms in Parkinson's disease are:

- Slowness in ambulation and dressing.
- Difficulty in getting out of a chair and in turning in bed.
- Shuffling.

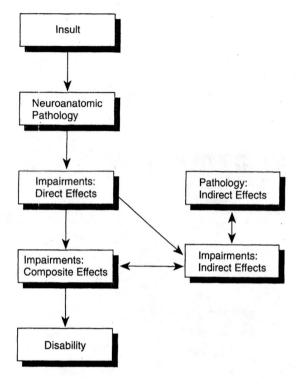

Figure 12–1. Outline of model for evaluating, interpreting, and treating individuals with neurologic dysfuntion. *(Reprinted with permission from Schenkman M, Butler RB. A model for multisystem evaluation, interpretation and treatment of individuals with neurologic dysfuntion. Physical Therapy. July 1989; 69(7):538–547.)*

- Stooping when walking or falling to one side when sitting.
- Difficulty with speech.
- Tremor and handwriting changes.
- Difficulty initiating movements.[3]

Medical management of Parkinson's disease revolves mainly around the use of drugs such as L-dopa. (Information is available on the use of L-dopa in Chapter 8, Pharmacology.) It is important to note that the side effects associated with L-dopa's use are less virulent in the elderly and, therefore, it can be prescribed at the onset.[4] The literature is filled with controversy as to dosage and side effects of anti-Parkinson medications (again see Chapter 8 for the side effects). The most noteworthy and deleterious side effects in the elderly are mental side effects, such as disorientation and confusion.[5]

The medical management of Parkinson's disease depends on the stage of disability. The Hoehn and Yahr[6] stages are as follows:

Stage I: Is characterized by minimal or no functional impairment and unilateral involvement only.
Stage II: Is characterized by bilateral involvement without any type of balance impairment.
Stage III: Is characterized by mild to moderate disability; here, the patient may lose righting reflexes as evidenced by unsteadiness on turns.
Stage IV: Is characterized by moderate to severe disability. The patient can still walk and stand unassisted, but is not stable.
Stage V: Is severe disability and here the patient is confined to bed or a wheelchair.[6]

The medical literature has shown that medication alone is not adequate treatment for this disease and that rehabilitation therapy is an important adjunct to medical treatment.[4–8]

Physical therapy has been shown to be efficacious for these patients.[8] In a study by Banks, Parkinson's patients with all degrees of impairment and duration of the disease improved in walking and other mobility skills after physical therapy.[8]

Evaluation

Schenkman and Butler have developed a model for the evaluation of patients with Parkinson's disease (Fig. 12–2).[9]

This model can be used as a guideline for evaluating Parkinson patients. The therapist can begin by assessing the direct effects of the nervous system, such as tremor rigidity, hypokinesis, and autonomic nervous system effects. While it is important to note these, it is also important to recognize that these impairments will respond less dramatically to physical therapy procedures than the indirect effect impairments.[9] The indirect effect impairments are changes in the musculoskeletal system, such as flexibility, strength, and vital capacity. The combined changes of these two areas make up the major impairments listed in composite effects.

Evaluation Form Figure 12–3 is an evaluation form that highlights and expands on the relevant impairments. This form affords the therapist the ability to differentiate between the various types of impairment.

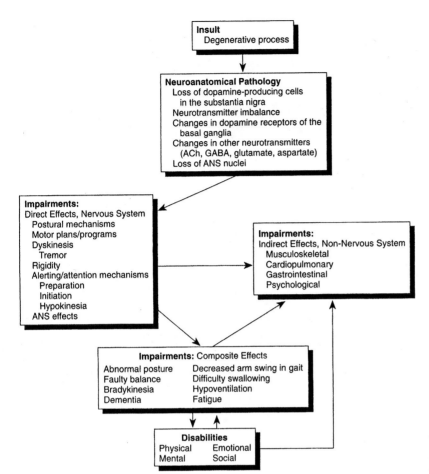

Figure 12–2. Overview of model for evaluation and treatment of patients with Parkinson's disease. ACh, acetylcholine, GABA, gamma-aminobutyric acid; ANS, autonomic nervous system. (Reprinted with permission from Schenkman M, Butler R. A model for multisystem evaluation treatment for individuals with Parkinson's disease. Physical Therapy. 1989; 69(11):932–943.

Under the impairment categories the therapist looks for the following:

1. **Musculoskeletal impairments**

   Trunk mobility—unilateral and then bilateral trunk limitation. Increased kyphosis, decreased lumbar extension.

   Pelvic mobility—decreased rotation, decreased ability to tilt the pelvis.

   a. Range-of-motion limitations: Decreased motion in the plantar flexors, hip flexors, and neck rotators.

   b. Strength limitation: Weak hip extensors, dorsi/plantar flexors, and trunk extensors.

   c. Postural limitations: Forward head, rounded shoulders, kyphosis, increased hip and knee flexion.

2. **Cardiopulmonary impairments:** Decreased chest expansion and increased heart rate and blood pressure.

   a. Slowed movements and difficulty breathing.

   b. Increased fatigue and orthostatic hypotension.

3. **Neurological impairments:** Increased rigidity, resting tremor, slowness of movement, difficulty

initiating movement, and increased drooling and flushing.

   a. Balance impairment: Increased loss of balance.

   b. Gait impairment: Shuffling, festination, retropulsion, no arm swing, slow pace.

   c. Swallowing impairments: Increased difficulty swallowing.

Even with an extremely comprehensive form such as Figure 12–3, there are still areas that require special mention. Tremor, for example, may be overlooked because it is only present intermittently, minimally, or in one joint. Because tremor may be difficult to assess, the therapist should have the patient sit with arms resting on legs. The patient is then instructed to count backward by 2 from 100. This activity stresses the patient and brings out the resting tremor, which the therapist can then observe. Once the therapist has observed the tremor, placing the hands over the moving part will elicit the four-to-seven second tremor and confirm the resting tremor.[10]

A good test for bradykinesia is to have the patient sit with both hands in his or her lap. The patient then supinates and pronates the forearms as rapidly as

Name _____

History _____

FUNCTIONAL

Complaint _____

_____

MUSCULOSKELETAL IMPAIRMENTS

Trunk mobility _____

_____

Pelvic mobility _____

_____

Range of Motion Limitations _____

_____

Strength Limitations _____

_____

Limitations _____

_____

CARDIOPULMONARY IMPAIRMENTS

Chest Expansion _____

Pulmonary Limitations _____

_____

Heart rate, Blood Pressure _____

NEUROLOGICAL IMPAIRMENTS

Rigidity _____

Tremor _____

Motor Planning _____

ANS

Function _____

COMPOSITE IMPAIRMENTS

Balance _____

Gait _____

Swallowing _____

Bradykinesia _____

_____

Hypoventilation _____

_____

Fatigue _____

_____

Goals _____

_____

_____

_____

_____

Treatment Plan _____

_____

_____

_____

_____

_____

_____

_____

Figure 12–3. *Parkinson Evaluation Form. (© Carole B. Lewis)*

possible on one side and then the other. If the symptoms are unilateral the therapist should start with the uninvolved side. The patient must do this activity for at least 20 seconds with the therapist observing for quality of movement. There may be no noticeable impairment at first; however, after three to four seconds, the patient will begin to substitute by shortening the arc, or will fail to flip hands over completely, and movement will generally slow. If this is noted, bradykinesia is confirmed.[10]

Hand posture can be checked by standing above and behind the patient, grasping both wrists, and shaking both hands up and down. The therapist observes for looseness and thumb position. If the patient fails to show general looseness or opposition of the thumb while shaking this may be a sign of early stage involvement. As the disease progresses, the patient will display finger adduction and flexion of the metacarpals, interphalangeal extension, and ulnar deviation. In the very advanced stages, the wrist may be drawn into flexion and pronation.[10]

Rigidity should be assessed in the neck, trunk, and all the extremities. Assessment for rigidity simply involves moving the part through the range of motion, making sure the patient is relaxed and not tensing the muscles. The therapist then notes any resistance or tension. All normal muscle movements should float.[10]

Weindrich and associates[11] noted that limitations in the wrist and head in axial rotation related to the improvement of symptoms of Parkinson's disease. Therefore, this measure may be an important tool in assessment.

Gait Evaluation   Gait changes in Parkinson patients deserve special mention. According to the works of Murray and co-authors[12] there are significant changes in the Parkinson's gait as compared to the normal gait. These changes are

1. Decreased step length.
2. Wider stride width.
3. Increased knee flexion in the standing position. (Normally, 3° of hyperextension at the knee is observed in standing. Parkinson patients tend to stand in 3°, 6°, and 12° of flexion for mild, moderate, and severely disabled groups, respectively.
4. Decreased mean total amplitude for flexion-extension used during free walking (degrees respectively in disabled Parkinson patients).[12]
5. Simultaneous thoracic and pelvic rotation in free speed walking.
6. Decreased heel floor angle at heel strike (norms 21° to 16°, 11° to 6° for Parkinson patients).[12]

Functional Assessment   A final area of evaluation of the Parkinson patient is functional assessment. In a study by Henderson and associates,[13] functional or activities of daily living (ADL) assessments were shown to be good for assessing functional deficits. The study did find, however, that if a description of the disease was sought, then an assessment of the actual signs of the disease would be better.[13]

Two ratings scales that incorporate both signs and ADL assessment are found in Table 12–1 and Figure 12–4.[10,14]

Once the therapist has conducted a thorough evaluation then the treatment can be initiated.

Treatment Considerations

When designing a treatment program for patients with Parkinson's disease, the model of Schenkman and co-authors[15] can be useful. The therapist must keep in mind which deficits can be corrected and which respond minimally to physical therapy. Rigidity, for example, may be temporarily relaxed in order to facilitate muscle stretching. However, the permanent effects of relaxation training on muscle rigidity will be minimal.[16] Therefore, prior to initiating a program the therapist must prioritize the problems and interpret the goals in terms of what is efficacious. Table 12–2 is an example of this process.[15]

Schenkman's Approach   Schenkman suggests the following treatment progression:

■ Relaxation.
■ Breathing exercises.
■ Passive muscle stretching and positioning.
■ Active range of motion and postural alignment.
■ Weight shifting.
■ Balance responses.
■ Gait activities.
■ Patient home exercises.[15]

As mentioned previously, relaxation can be used to temporarily decrease rigidity and increase flexibility. Relaxation of the muscles can be induced by slow rhythmic rotating movements beginning with very small motions and progressing to larger ones. Other techniques, such as biofeedback, contract-relax stretch, and deep breathing, can be helpful. The relaxation will be more effective if the approach begins supine and progresses to sitting and standing, and the more supported the individual is, the better will be their ability to relax. In addition, relaxation is better if it is begun passively and is progressed to active. Finally, the relaxation is more effective if the patient is taught to relax individual functional segments (for example, the head on the thorax, the shoulder on the thorax, and the lower extremity on the pelvis).

Breathing or breathing control should be encouraged throughout the various stages of treatment. The patient is taught to take deep relaxed breaths while doing the relaxation exercises. Once the patient has achieved some degree of relaxation in the thoracic area then deeper breathing combined with trunk stretching can help to increase chest expansion.

TABLE 12–1. *PARKINSON'S DISEASE RATING SCALE*

Directions: Apply a gross clinical rating to each of the ten listed items, assigning value ratings of 0–3 for each item, where (0) = no involvement and (1), (2), and (3) are equated to early, moderate, and severe disease, respectively. Refer to the discussion in the text for details of the examination and the ratings.

Bradykinesia of Hands—Including Handwriting
(0) No involvement.
(1) Detectable slowing of the supination–pronation rate evidenced by beginning difficulty in handling tools, buttoning clothes, and handwriting.
(2) Moderate slowing of supination—pronation rate, one or both sides, evidenced by moderate impairment of hand function. Handwriting is greatly impaired, microphagia present.
(3) Severe slowing of supination—pronation rate. Unable to write or button clothes. Marked difficulty in handling utensils.

Rigidity
(0) Nondetectable
(1) Detectable rigidity in neck and shoulders. Activation phenomenon is present. One or both arms show mild, negative, resting rigidity.
(2) Moderate rigidity in neck and shoulders. Resting rigidity is positive when patient is not on medication.
(3) Severe rigidity in neck and shoulders. Resting rigidity cannot be reversed by medication.

Posture
(0) Normal posture. Head flexed forward less than 4 inches.
(1) Beginning poker spine. Head flexed forward up to 5 inches.
(2) Beginning arm flexion. Head flexed forward 6 inches. One or both arms raised but still below waist.
(3) Onset of simian posture. Head flexed forward more than 6 inches. One or both hands elevated above waist. Sharp flexion of hand, beginning interphalangeal extension. Beginning flexion of knees.

Upper Extremity Swing
(1) One arm definitely decreased in amount of swing.
(2) One arm fails to swing.
(3) Both arms fail to swing.

Gait
(0) Steps out well with 18–30 inch stride. Turns about effortlessly.
(1) Gait shortened to 12–18 inch stride. Beginning to strike one heel. Turn around time slowing. Requires several steps.
(2) Stride moderately shortened—now 6–12 inches. Both heels beginning to strike floor forcefully.
(3) Onset of shuffling gait, steps less than 3 inches. Occasional stuttering-type or blocking gait. Walks on toes—turns around very slowly.

Tremor
(0) No detectable tremor found.
(1) Less than one inch of peak-to-peak tremor movement observed in limbs or head at rest or in either hand while walking or during finger to nose testing.
(2) Maximum tremor envelope fails to exceed 4 inches. Tremor is severe but not constant and patient retains some control of hands.
(3) Tremor envelope exceeds 4 inches. Tremor is constant and severe. Patient cannot get free of tremor while awake unless it is a pure cerebellar type. Writing and feeding are impossible.

Facies
(1) Detectable immobility. Mouth remains closed. Beginning features of anxiety or depression.
(2) Moderate immobility. Emotion breaks through at markedly increased threshold. Lips parted some of the time. Moderate appearance of anxiety or depression. Drooling may be present.
(3) Frozen facies. Mouth open 1/4 inch or more. Drooling may be severe.

Seborrhea
(0) None.
(1) Increased perspiration, secretion remaining thin.
(2) Obvious oiliness present. Secretion much thicker.
(3) Marked seborrhea, entire face and head covered by thick secretion.

Speech
(0) Clear, loud, resonant, easily understood.
(1) Beginning of hoarseness with loss of inflection and resonance. Good volume and still easily understood.
(2) Moderate hoarseness and weakness. Constant monotone, unvaried pitch. Beginning of dysarthria, hesitancy, stuttering, difficulty to understand.
(3) Marked harshness and weakness. Very difficult to hear and understand.

Self Care
(0) No impairment.
(1) Still provides full self-care but rate of dressing definitely impeded. Able to live alone and often still employable.
(2) Requires help in certain critical areas, such as turning in bed, rising from chairs, etc. Very slow in performing most activities but manages by taking much time.
(3) Continuously disabled. Unable to dress, feed him- or herself, or walk alone.

Reprinted with permission from Webster D. Critical analysis of the disability in Parkinson's disease. *Mod Treat.* 1969;5:257–282.

Parkinson Patient Disability Rating

PATIENT
  Name:
  Sex:
  Age:
  Ward:
Total score:

Note:
Use 0–4 for rating:

None	Never
Mild	Occasional % time
Moderate or	Moderate % time
Severe	Considerable % time
Complete	Constant

Use 0.5 for readings that are not clearly categorized.

HEAD

1. *Ocular Movements* (consider rapidity of conjugate gaze in all directions, and the ability to open eyes after closure).
   Limitation of voluntary control.

   complete . . . .
   severe . . . .
   moderate . . . .
   mild . . . .
   none . . . .

2. *Blinking*
   (inability to blink)
   (1 min and over)
   (30–60 sec)
   (10–30 sec)
   (free)

   complete . . . .
   severe . . . .
   moderate . . . .
   mild . . . .
   none . . . .

3. *Emotional facial control*
   (Check degree of flattening of facial lines.
   Note facial expression with smiling.)

   Upper (forehead, eyes, nose)
   (absence of facial expression)

   complete . . . .
   severe . . . .
   moderate . . . .
   mild . . . .
   none . . . .

   Lower (mouth)
   (absence of facial expression)

   complete . . . .
   severe . . . .
   moderate . . . .
   mild . . . .
   none . . . .

Continued

Continued from previous page

4. *Voluntary facial control*
   (Ask patient to frown upward, inward; wrinkle nose; close eyes)

   Upper (forehead, eyes, nose)
   (absence of control)

complete	. . . . . .
severe	. . . . . .
moderate	. . . . . .
mild	. . . . . .
none	. . . . . .

   Lower (mouth). Ask patient to grimace and purse lips.
   (absence of control)

complete	. . . . . .
severe	. . . . . .
moderate	. . . . . .
mild	. . . . . .
none	. . . . . .

Note: If there is considerable difference between the two sides of the face, please rate.

5. *Swallowing*
   (inability to swallow)
   (not voluntary and chokes reflexly)
   (slowed)
   (drooling, occasional choking)

complete	. . . . . .
severe	. . . . . .
moderate	. . . . . .
mild	. . . . . .
none	. . . . . .

6. *Motor speech*—degree to which speech is inaudible and unintelligible (inability to talk)

complete	. . . . . .
severe	. . . . . .
moderate	. . . . . .
mild	. . . . . .
none	. . . . . .

7. *Tongue movement*
   (inability to move)
   (can protrude tongue to lip margin)
   (can protrude tongue beyond lips but not full forward or in other directions)
   (full movement, but slowed)

complete	. . . . . .
severe	. . . . . .
moderate	. . . . . .
mild	. . . . . .
none	. . . . . .

NECK AND UPPER EXTREMITIES

8. *Head rotation* (sitting)
   (Best rating taken when patient decreases range with repetition—100% equivalent of 90°)

	Right		**Left**	
(inability to rotate)	complete	. . . . . .	complete	. . . . . .
(25–0%)	severe	. . . . . .	severe	. . . . . .
(50–25%)	moderate	. . . . . .	moderate	. . . . . .
(75–50%)	mild	. . . . . .	mild	. . . . . .
(100–75%)	none	. . . . . .	none	. . . . . .

Note: The head may be in an asymmetrical starting position, but where this is of a considerable degree, marked limitation of head movement to right and left has been found and it has not interfered with rating.

Continued

Continued from previous page

9. *Shoulder elevation* (sitting)
   (Best rating taken when patient decreases range with repetition)

	Right		Left	
(inability to rotate)	complete	. . . . . .	complete	. . . . . .
(25–0%)	severe	. . . . . .	severe	. . . . . .
(50–25%)	moderate	. . . . . .	moderate	. . . . . .
(75–50%)	mild	. . . . . .	mild	. . . . . .
(100–75%)	none	. . . . . .	none	. . . . . .

10. *Lowering head to plinth* (supine position)

(inability)			complete	. . . . . .
(can lower head to some extent)			severe	. . . . . .
(can lower head to plinth but slowly)			moderate	. . . . . .
(can lower head to plinth—moderate speed)			mild	. . . . . .
			none	. . . . . .

11. *Elevation of arms* (sitting)

	Right		Left	
(inability)	complete	. . . . . .	complete	. . . . . .
(below shoulder)	severe	. . . . . .	severe	. . . . . .
(shoulder level)	moderate	. . . . . .	moderate	. . . . . .
(partial hyperabduction)	mild	. . . . . .	mild	. . . . . .
(full hyperabduction)	none	. . . . . .	none	. . . . . .

12. *Handwriting* (depending on handedness—one score)

(inability)			complete	. . . . . .
			severe	. . . . . .
			moderate	. . . . . .
			mild	. . . . . .
			none	. . . . . .

TRUNK AND LOWER EXTREMITIES

13. *Arising from standard chair with sidearms*

(inability)			complete	. . . . . .
(can arise with examiner's support)			severe	. . . . . .
(can arise with maximal arm support by self)			moderate	. . . . . .
(can arise with moderate arm support by self)			mild	. . . . . .
(can arise with arms folded)			none	. . . . . .

14. *Walking*

(cannot walk)			complete	. . . . . .
(can walk with observer's assistance)			severe	. . . . . .
(can walk with arm support by self)			moderate	. . . . . .
(can walk independently but slowly)			mild	. . . . . .
(can walk well)			none	. . . . . .

15. *Walking*

	Right		Left	
(cannot walk on heels and toes)	complete	. . . . . .	complete	. . . . . .
Can walk:				
(on heels or toes with maximal support)	severe	. . . . . .	severe	. . . . . .
(on heels or toes with moderate support)	moderate	. . . . . .	moderate	. . . . . .
(on heels and toes with moderate support)	mild	. . . . . .	mild	. . . . . .
(on heels and toes with no support)	none	. . . . . .	none	. . . . . .

16. *Climbing*

	Right		Left	
(cannot lift foot in walking and climbing)	complete	. . . . . .	complete	. . . . . .
(can lift foot in walking with observer's support but cannot climb)	severe	. . . . . .	severe	. . . . . .
(can lift foot in walking and climb with observer's support)	moderate	. . . . . .	moderate	. . . . . .

Continued

Continued from previous page

	Right		**Left**	
(can lift foot in walking and climb with own support)	mild	. . . . . .	mild	. . . .
(can lift foot in walking and climb 8 in. step without support)	none	. . . . . .	none	. . . .

17. *Trunk raising* (supine position)

(cannot lift head and shoulders off table)	complete	. . . . . .
Can lift head and shoulders:		
(off table with hands on side of plinth)	severe	. . . . . .
(off table with hands on abdomen or chest)	moderate	. . . . . .
(off table with hands on head)	mild	. . . . . .
(can arise to sitting position with hands on head)	none	. . . . . .

18. *Trunk turning* (supine position)

(cannot turn to right or left)	complete	. . . . . .
(can make some attempt to turn using arms)	severe	. . . . . .
(can turn to one side using one arm but not other)	moderate	. . . . . .
(can turn to both sides using arms)	mild	. . . . . .
(can turn to both sides without using arms)	none	. . . . . .

19. *Straight leg raising*

	Right		**Left**	
(cannot flex thigh)	complete	. . . . . .	complete	. . . .
Can flex thigh:				
(with heel remaining on bed)	severe	. . . . . .	severe	. . . .
(30° lifting partially extended lower extremity)	moderate	. . . . . .	moderate	. . . .
(60° lifting partially extended lower extremity)	mild	. . . . . .	mild	. . . .
(60° lifting fully extended lower extremity)	none	. . . . . .	none	. . . .

20. *Movement of ankles and toes*

	Right		**Left**	
(no spontaneous movement)	complete	. . . . . .	complete	. . . .
(slight movement)	severe	. . . . . .	severe	. . . .
(moderate movement)	moderate	. . . . . .	moderate	. . . .
(good, but slowed movement)	mild	. . . . . .	mild	. . . .
(free movement)	none	. . . . . .	none	. . . .

GENERAL

21. *General mobility*

(complete immobility at rest)	complete	. . . .
(mobility limited to head and neck)	severe	. . . .
(slight mobility in trunk and extremities)	moderate	. . . .
(moderate mobility in trunk and extremities)	mild	. . . .
(freely mobile)	none	. . . .

22. *Abnormal tone* (rigidity)

	Neck	**Back**
complete	. . . . . .	. . . . . .
severe	. . . . . .	. . . . . .
moderate	. . . . . .	. . . . . .
mild	. . . . . .	. . . . . .
none	. . . . . .	. . . . . .

RUE

	Shoulder	**Elbow**	**Wrist & Fingers**
complete	. . . . . .	. . . . . .	. . . . . .
severe	. . . . . .	. . . . . .	. . . . . .
moderate	. . . . . .	. . . . . .	. . . . . .
mild	. . . . . .	. . . . . .	. . . . . .
none	. . . . . .	. . . . . .	. . . . . .

Continued

Continued from previous page

LUE

	Shoulder	Elbow	Wrist & Fingers
complete	. . . . . .	. . . . .	. . . . . .
severe	. . . . . .	. . . . .	. . . . . .
moderate	. . . . . .	. . . . .	. . . . . .
mild	. . . . . .	. . . . .	. . . . . .
none	. . . . . .	. . . . .	. . . . . .

RLE

	Hip	Knee	Ankle & Toes
complete	. . . . . .	. . . . .	. . . . . .
severe	. . . . . .	. . . . .	. . . . . .
moderate	. . . . . .	. . . . .	. . . . . .
mild	. . . . . .	. . . . .	. . . . . .
none	. . . . . .	. . . . .	. . . . . .

LLE

	Hip	Knee	Ankle & Toes
complete	. . . . . .	. . . . .	. . . . . .
severe	. . . . . .	. . . . .	. . . . . .
moderate	. . . . . .	. . . . .	. . . . . .
mild	. . . . . .	. . . . .	. . . . . .
none	. . . . . .	. . . . .	. . . . . .

Use finger or toe rating where wrist or ankle are immobile from fusion or contractures.

23. *Contractures and deformities*

	Neck	Back
complete	. . . . .	. . . . . .
severe	. . . . .	. . . . . .
moderate	. . . . .	. . . . . .
mild	. . . . .	. . . . . .
none	. . . . . .	. . . . . .

RUE

	Shoulder	Elbow	Wrist & Fingers
complete	. . . . . .	. . . . .	. . . . . .
severe	. . . .	. . . . .	. . . . . .
moderate	. . . . . .	. . . . .	. . . . . .
mild	. . . . . .	. . . . .	. . . . . .
none	. . . . . .	. . . . .	. . . . . .

LUE

	Shoulder	Elbow	Wrist & Fingers
complete	. . . . . .	. . . . .	. . . . . .
severe	. . . . . .	. . . . .	. . . . . .
moderate	. . . . . .	. . . . .	. . . . . .
mild	. . . . . .	. . . . .	. . . . . .
none	. . . . . .	. . . . .	. . . . . .

Continued

Continued from previous page

RLE

	Hip	Knee	Ankle & Toes
complete	. . . .	. . . .	. . . . . .
severe	. . . .	. . . .	. . . . . .
moderate	. . . .	. . . .	. . . . . .
mild	. . . .	. . . .	. . . . . .
none	. . . .	. . . .	. . . . . .

LLE

	Hip	Knee	Ankle & Toes
complete	. . . .	. . . .	. . . . . .
severe	. . . .	. . . .	. . . . . .
moderate	. . . .	. . . .	. . . . . .
mild	. . . .	. . . .	. . . . . .
none	. . . .	. . . .	. . . . . .

24. *Tremor*

	Eyelids	Face	Jaw
constant	. . . .	. . . .	. . . .
considerable % time	. . . .	. . . .	. . . .
moderate % time	. . . .	. . . .	. . . .
occasional % time	. . . .	. . . .	. . . .
never	. . . .	. . . .	. . . .

	Tongue	Neck	RUE
constant	. . . .	. . . .	. . . .
considerable % time	. . . .	. . . .	. . . .
moderate % time	. . . .	. . . .	. . . .
occasional % time	. . . .	. . . .	. . . .
never	. . . .	. . . .	. . . .

	LUE	RLE	LLE
constant	. . . .	. . . .	. . . .
considerable % time	. . . .	. . . .	. . . .
moderate % time	. . . .	. . . .	. . . .
occasional % time	. . . .	. . . .	. . . .
never	. . . .	. . . .	. . . .

Figure 12–4. *(Reprinted with permission from Alba A, et al. A clinical disability rating for Parkinson's disease. Chron Dis 1968;21:507–522.)*

Passive muscle stretching is another commonly used modality for physical therapy. What is different for the patient with Parkinson's disease is the mode and area of application. As with relaxation, the most effective stretch will be with the body in the most supported position due to the patient's decreased protective responses; therefore, begin with stretching in the supine or side-lying position. Areas requiring special stretching are:

■ Lumbopelvic extensions are important for balance.
■ Rotation and lateral flexion of the pelvis.
■ Hamstring and plantar flexion.
■ Cervical and thoracic extension rotation, and lateral flexion
■ Hip extension, external rotation, and abduction
■ Elbow extension and supination
■ Finger flexion and extension

To achieve passive stretching, contract-relax stretching and passive stretching using Gustaffson's principle of fifteen to thirty second stretches gives the best results.[17] Stretching is followed by active range of motion and postural alignment.

The key to achieving the best results in active range of motion and postural alignment is repetition. According to Nelson,[18] for a movement to become assimilated by the nervous system it needs millions of repetitions, which equates to hundreds to thousands of repetitions a day. Therefore, the patient should do the activity for five to ten minutes instead of five to ten times. Some of the most useful active motion activities

TABLE 12-2. EXAMPLES OF PROBLEMS, INTERPRETATIONS, AND GOALS FOR PATIENTS WITH PARKINSON'S DISEASE

Problem[a]	Quantitative	Descriptive	Interpretation	Goal
Gait	Ambulates 25 ft[b] in 18 sec (18 steps)	Small steps; decreased left heel-strike; decreased trunk rotation; left knee in flexion from weight acceptance to push-off; no left arm swing	Problems attributable to limitations in left knee and ankle range of motion and decreased available trunk rotation combined with trunk and limb rigidity with motor programming and planning deficits	Ambulate 25 ft in 10 sec (12 steps); improved heel-strike, pushoff, trunk rotation, and arm swing
Bed mobility (supine to sitting)	7 sec to complete task	Lacks trunk rotation and dissociation of pelvic complex from shoulder complex; appears fearful of losing balance	Problems attributable to combination of limited available trunk ROM, rigidity, and impaired balance	2 sec to complete task; improved trunk rotation with dissociation of shoulder complex from pelvic complex
Transfers (sitting to standing from low treatment table)	Sitting to standing from mat takes 10 sec	Lack of anterior pelvic tilt and of scooting forward on mat; excessive use of arms for push-off from mat	Problems attributable to lack of lumbo-pelvic mobility, rigidity, and difficulty motor planning and programming	Patient will accomplish task in 5 sec, use anterior tilt, scoot forward, and decrease need for use of arms
Decreased hip ROM	Straight leg raise (left leg: 0°–50°; right leg: 0°–45°; internal rotation (left leg: 0°–25°; right leg: 0°–30°)		Problems result from rigidity and improper posturing	Hip ROM within normal limits
Rigidity[c]		Moderate[d]	Attributable to primary impairments of disease	Patient will self-relax rigidity for increasing ROM

[a]Patient problems may relate to disabilities or impairments.
[b]1 ft = 0.3048 m.
[c]Rigidity is listed as a problem because of its causal role in most impairments of Parkinson's disease; however, objective measures of rigidity do not exist, and physical therapy does not appear to affect long-term changes.
[d]Feldman R, Lannon M. Parkinson's disease and related disturbances. In: Feldman R, ed. Neurology: The Physician's Guide. New York: Thieme Medical Publishers, 1984; 147–162.

Reprinted with permission from Schenkman M, et al. Management of individuals with Parkinson's disease: rationale and case studies. *Phys Ther*, November 1989;69(11)944–955.

for these areas are (1) pelvic clocks to enhance pelvic and lumbar motion, (2) isolated lateral and anterior pelvic tilts, and (3) clocks around any joint in the body. If the patient has limitation in the lumbar spine, the patient may substitute for lumbopelvic motion with pelvic-femoral motion. Therefore, evaluate and treat any loss of mobility in the lumbar spine.

Once the patient is able to actively move the various body parts in a supine and then a standing position following stretching, then weight shifting in a standing position with the pelvis in a balanced position is practiced. Weight shifting, like the previous sequences, can be practiced from the supine to the standing positions.

Finally, balance activities and responses must be stressed. Here the patient's balance can be challenged intrinsically and extrinsically. Methods of challenging the patient's intrinsic balance include having the patient reach overhead, from side to side, and backward in a rotational direction when sitting and standing. For extrinsic balance challenges, the therapist can apply an outside stress, such as a gentle shove, to disturb the patient's balance. Both are needed for everyday activity and should be practiced when sitting and standing.

Function is the final area of treatment and must always be kept in mind when designing the exercise program, because exercises are most effective if they relate to function. For example, trunk rotation should be followed by rolling in bed as an active functional activity that the patient can do on his or her own at home. Anterior pelvic tilting when standing is another useful home exercise employing a needed functional activity. When designing a home exercise program, be sure to stress the functional carry-over. This way when the patient does daily activities, he or she is constantly doing the exercise program.

Flewitt-Handford Exercises Another well-known program for Parkinson patients are the Flewitt-Handford exercises. These exercises were developed to help improve the gait of Parkinson patients. The developers of the exercises believe that the gait seen is a result of adaption to gain control of forward progression and balance. Parkinson patients have plenty of propulsion, but they lack a braking mechanism. Flewitt-Handford exercises are directed to reteach heel strike, improve weight transference, increase motion of the hip and knee, and prevent stiffness of the lower extremity (Table 12–3).[19]

Patient education is an important component for the treatment of the Parkinson patient. The Parkinson's Disease Foundation is an excellent resource for information and assistance for the patient and the families. They have developed an exercise videotape for Parkinson patients called "Get up and Go," which is a useful tool for helping patients maintain the benefits of a rehabilitation program in a fun and interesting way.

Group Rehabilitation Another treatment con-sideration is group rehabilitation.[20] Table 12–4 is a sample group evaluation and exercise progression.

TABLE 12–3.   THE FLEWITT-HANDFORD EXERCISES

1. **Long sitting.** Alternate flexion/extension of toes, feet, and knees.
2. **Crook lying.** Rolling knees from side to side.
3. **Lying.** Alternate hip and knee flexion/extension, lift each foot off the plinth.
4. **Stand** facing and holding onto either parallel bars in a gym, or a heavy chair, table, or mantelpiece at home.
   a. High stepping.
   b. With straight knees and not leaning backward alternate feet dorsiflexion.
   c. Cross the left leg in front of the right and vice versa each time trying to touch the floor heel first.
   d. If in the gym, the patient should practice weight transference by walking sideways up and down the parallel bars.Then the same again, but crossing the legs over each other.
5. **Standing** at right angles to the parallel bars or chair, practice taking strides from toe off to heel-strike of first one leg, then the other. Pay attention to hip extension and proper heel-strike.
   When walking, patients must learn to put their heels down first with every step. Many patients become "stuck" while walking. They can easily unstick themselves by rocking backwards so their weight is going through their heels. Though taking a step backwards or sideways, they will find themselves able to move forwards again.

Reprinted with permission from Handford F. *The Flewitt-Handford exercises for Parkinson's gait.* Physiotherapy. August 1986; 72(8) 382.

STROKE

Even though stroke is not the major neurological problem of old age, it is significant because it is such a functionally devastating disease. In the United States alone between 250,000 and 300,000 persons have CVAs a year.[21,22] Most strokes occur late in life; 43% of stroke patients are over the age of 74.[22,23]

In absolute numbers, women and men over age 75 are almost equally afflicted with CVAs; however, because the ratio of women to men is so much greater (3:2), statistically men have a greater likelihood of developing stroke.[24] Blacks and Japanese Americans are more likely to have strokes than whites, and the geographic area with the highest percentage of strokes is the southern United States.[22,25]

Besides causing tremendous morbidity (it is estimated that 20% to 40% of stroke patients die within 30 days,[26] nearly 40% of people with this disease report limitations in their activities. Cerebral vascular disease results in an average of 36 days of restricted activity for stroke victims.[27]

There are three major types of strokes. The cerebral thrombosis occurs when an artery that supplies blood to the brain becomes narrowed by plaque and deposits. The blood may coagulate and form a clot that does not allow sufficient blood through to the area. A cerebral emboli is caused by a blockage of some foreign object in the bloodstream, such as a clot, that can become wedged where it obstructs blood flow to the brain. The final type of stroke is a cerebral hemorrhage, where the artery is not blocked but bursts and blood seeps into the surrounding brain tissue. Depending on the extent of the damage, a cerebral hemorrhage is usually the most severe type of stroke, followed by thrombosis, then emboli. The severity of the stroke also depends on what area of the brain is affected and the extent and duration of the blockage of blood. Table 12–5 shows the clinical symptoms of vascular lesions and neurovascular disease.[28]

Risk factors associated with stroke are similar for young and old. Spriggs and co-workers[29] noted such factors as previous cerebral vascular disease, taking certain prescribed medicines, and regular cigarette smoking as high risk factors. Family history was also a factor but was not found to be significant in the older population.[22,29]

Perceptual deficits occur in varying degrees with a stroke. Table 12–6 is a chart of these deficits.

A central problem in tone occurs in approximately 10% of stroke patients. This condition, which severely affects gait and balance in the hemiplegic, has been termed the Pusher syndrome.[30] This problem is one of postural imbalance due to ipsilateral pushing or lateropulsion. The patient pushes strongly away from the unaffected side towards the hemiplegic side. Ipsilateral pushing varies in severity from mild to severe and may be transient or pronounced and prolonged.[31] If severe, pushing occurs in all posi-

TABLE 12–4. PARKINSONISM EVALUATION

Occupational Therapy

Upper Extremity Function	Activities of Daily Living

1. Drawing concentric circles
   a. number in 30 sec
   b. size of circles
   c. line quality
2. Alternating finger flexion/extension: number
   of complete repetitions in 10 sec
3. Grasp strength
4. Signature: time, legibility
	1. Dressing (in seconds)
	   a. put on shirt
	   b. fasten three buttons
	   c. put one shoe
	   d. tie one shoelace
	2. Transfers (in seconds)
	   a. standing to supine
	   b. supine to standing
	   c. standing to sitting
	   d. sitting to standing
	3. Mobility (in seconds)
	   a. rolling supine to prone
	   b. standing 360° turn
	   c. opening/entering doors
	   d. ascending/descending stairs

Physical Therapy

Muscle Tightness	Balance
1. Pectorals—active range 2. Hamstrings—passive range 3. Hip flexors—passive range 4. Hip adductors—passive range	1. Quadruped-balance on opposite arm and leg, 5 sec 2. Standing on one foot, 5 sec 3. Propulsion (push patient forward) 4. Retropulsion (push patient backward)

Reciprocation (repetitions in 30 sec)
1. Supine
2. Gait
3. Stop start walk: sec/15 m
	Posture
	1. Standing
	   a. anterior—posterior
	   b. lateral
	2. Walking
	3. Supine

Phase I:
Warm-up exercises for range of motion, reciprocality, and mobility.
Mat exercises: bridging, trunk rotation, side leg raises, and reciprocal movements
Parallel bars: knee bends, side leg raises, balancing.
Bicycle/pulleys.

Phase II:
Activities for mobility and equilibrium.
Range of motion exercises for all major joints.
Facial exercises.
Static and dynamic balance: *Hokey Pokey, Alley Cat*

Phase III:
Activities for coordination and socialization:

Week 1: Special exercises for breathing
   Alley Cat
   Shuffleboard
   Frisbee
	Special exercises for face, lips
	Marching
	Hot potato
	Instrument playing
	Tic-Tac-Toe

Week 2: *Hokey Pokey*
   Ball: reciprocal bouncing, tossing, kicking,
     pass and reverse, beach ball
	Subgroup *a*: *Alley Cat*
	   cotton ball blow
	   hand-clapping patterns
	Subgroup *b*: individual tasks:
	   perceptual tasks, dexterity
	   boards, tracing

Week 3: Bean bag toss Sitting relay: overhead, sideways	Horseshoes Hot potato
Week 4: *Hokey Pokey* Bowling	Special exercises for arms, hands Wang passing Basketball

Reprinted with permission from Davis J. Team management of Parkinson's disease. Am J Occup Ther. May–June 1977;31(5)300–308.

TABLE 12–5. CLINICAL SYMPTOMS OF CEREBRAL VASCULAR LESIONS AND NEUROVASCULAR DISEASE

Vessel	Clinical Symptoms	Structures Involved
Cerebral Vascular Lesions		
Middle cerebral artery	Contralateral paralysis and sensory deficit	Somatic motor area
	Motor speech impairment	Broca's area (dominant hemisphere)
	"Central" asphasia, anomia, jargon speech	Parietoccipital cortex (dominant hemisphere)
	Unilateral neglect, apraxia, impaired ability to judge distance	Parietal lobe (nondominant hemisphere)
	Homonymous hemianopsia	Optic radiation deep to second temporal convolution
	Loss of conjugate gaze to opposite side	Frontal controversive field
	Avoidance reaction of opposite limbs	Parietal lobe
	Pure motor hemiplegia	Upper protion of posterior limb of internal
	Limb-kinetic apraxia capsule	Premotor or parietal cortex
Anterior cerebral artery	Paralysis—lower extremity	Motor area—leg
	Paresis in opposite arm	Arm area of cortex
	Cortical sensory loss	Sensory area
	Urinary incontinence	Posteromedial aspect of superior frontal gyrus
	Contralateral grasp reflex, sucking reflex	Medial surface of posterior frontal lobe
	Lack of spontaneity motor inaction, echolalia	Uncertain
	Perseveration and amnesia	Uncertain
Posterior cerebral	Homonymous hemianopsia	Calcarine cortex or optic radiation
	Bilateral homonymous hemianopsia, cortical blindness, inability to perceive objects not centrally located, ocular apraxia	Bilateral occipital lobe Inferomedial portions of temporal lobe Nondominant calcarine and lingual gyri
	Memory defect	
	Topographic disorientation	
Central area	Thalamic syndrome	Posteroventral nucleus ophthalmus
	Weber's syndrome	Cranial nerve III and cerebral peduncle
	Contralateral hemiplegia	Cerebral peduncle
	Paresis of vertical eye movements, sluggish pupillary response to light	Supranuclear fibers to cranial nerve III Uncertain
	Contralateral ataxia or postural tremor	
Internal carotid artery	Variable signs according to degree and site of occlusion—middle cerebral, anterior cerebral, posterior cerebral territory	
Basilar artery		
Superior cerebellar	Ataxia	Middle and superior cerebellar peduncles
	Dizziness, nausea, vomiting, horizontal nystagmus	Vestibular nucleus
	Horner's syndrome on opposite side, decreased pain and thermal sensation	Decending sympathetic fibers Spinal thalamic tract
	Decreased touch, vibration, position sense of lower extremity greater than upper extremity	Medial lemniscus
Anterior inferior cerebellar artery	Nystagmus, vertigo, nausea, vomiting	Vestibular nerve
	Facial paralysis on same side	Cranial nerve VII
	Tinnitus	Auditory nerve, lower coclear nucleus
	Ataxis	Middle cerebral peduncle
	Impaired facial sensation on same side	Fifth cranial nerve nucleus
	Decreased pain and thermal sensation on opposite side	Spinal thalamic tract
Hemorrhage		
Hypertensive hemorrhage	Severe heacache	CT scan can detect hemorrhages greater than 1.5 cm in cerebral and cerebellar hemispheres; they are diagnostically superior to arteriography; they are especially helpful in diagnosing small hemorrhages that do not spill blood into cerebrospinal fluid; with massive hemorrhage and increased pressure, cerebrospinal fluid is grossly bloody; lumbar puncture in necessary when CT scan is not available; radiographs occasionally show midline shift (this is not true with infarction); EEG shows no typical pattern, but high volt to age and slow waves are most common with hemorrhage; urinary changes may reflect renal disease
	Vomiting at onset	
	Blood pressure > 170/90; usually "essential" hypertension but can be from other types	
	Abrupt onset, usually during day, not in sleep	
	Gradually evolves over hours or days according to speed of bleeding	
	No recurrence of bleeding	
	Frequency of blacks with hypertensive hemmorage is greater than frequency of whites	
	Hemorrhaged blood absorbs slowly—rapid improvement of symptoms is not usual	
	If massive hemorrhage occurs, client survive a few hours or days, secondary brainstem compression	

(continued)

TABLE 12–5.   (Continued)

Vessel	Clinical Symptoms	Structures Involved
Ruptured saccular aneurysm	Asymptomatic before rupture With rupture, blood spills under high pressure into subarachnoid space: Excruciating headache with loss of consciousness Sudden loss of consciousness Decerebrate rigidity with coma If severe—persistent deep coma with respiratory arrest, circulatory collapse leading to death; death can occur within 5 minutes If mild—consciousness regained within hours then confusion, amnesia, headache, stiff neck, drowsiness Hemiplegia, paresis, homonymous hemianopsia, or aphasis usually absent	CT scan detects localized blood in hydrocephalus if present; cerebrospinal fluid is extremely bloody; radiographs are usually negative; carotid and vertebral arteriography are performed only if certain of diagnosis
Basilar artery Complete basilar syndrome	Bilateral long tract signs with cerebellar and cranial nerve abnormalities Coma Quadriplegia Pseudobulbar palsy Cranial nerve abnormalities	_____ _____ _____ _____
Vertebral artery	Decreased pain and temperature on opposite side Sensory loss from a tactile and proprioceptive Hemiparesis of arm and leg Facial pain and numbness on same side Horner's syndrome, ptosis, decreased sweating Ataxia Spinal cerebellar tract Paralysis of tongue Weakness of vocal cord, decreased gag Hiccups	Spinal thalamic tract Medial lemniscus Pyramidal tract Descending tract and fifth cranial nucleus Descending sympathetic tract Cranial nerve XII Cranial nerves IX and X Uncertain
Neurovascular Disease		
Thrombosis	*Extremely variable* Preceded by a prodromal episode Uneven progression Onset develops within minutes, hours, or over days ("thrombus in evolution") 60% occur during sleep—awaken unaware of problem, rise, and fall to floor Usually no headache but may occur in mild form Hypertension, diabetes, or vascular disease elsewhere in body	Cerebrospinal fluid pressure is normal Cerebrospinnal fluid is clear EEG: limited differential diagnostic value Skull radiographs are not helpful Arteriography is the diffinitive procedure, it demonstrates site of collateral flow CT scanning is helpful in chronic state when cavitation has occurred Usually none
TIAs	Linked to atherosclerotic thrombosis Proceeded or accompanied by stroke Occur by themselves Last 2–30 minutes Experience a few attacks or hundreds Normal neurological examination between attacks If transient symptoms are present on awakening, may indicate future stroke	
Embolism Cardiac	*Extremely variable* Occurs extremely rapidly—seconds or minutes	Generally same as thrombosis except for following:

Noncardiac
  Atherosclerosis
  Pulmonary thrombosis
    Fat, tumor, air
	There are no warnings
	
	Branches of middle cerebral artery are involved most frequently, large embolus will block internal carotid artery or stem of middle cerebral artery
	If in basilar system, deep coma and total paralysis may result
	Often a manifestation of heart disease, including atrial fibrillation and myocardial infarction
	As embolis passes through artery, client may have neurological deficits that resolve as embolis breaks and passes into small artery supplying small or silent brain area
		If embolism causes a large hemorrhagic infarct, cerebrospinal fluid will be bloody
		30% of embolic strokes produced small hemorrhagic infarct without bloody cerebrospinal fluid

Reprinted with permission and adapted from Ryerson S. Hemiplegia resulting from vascular insult or disease. In: Umphred D, ed. Neurological Rehabilitation. St. Louis: Mosby: 1985: 476.

TABLE 12–6. PERCEPTUAL DEFICITS IN CNS DYSFUNCTION

LEFT HEMIPARESIS: right hemisphere--general spatial-global deficits
Visual-perceptual deficits
  Hand-eye coordination
  Figure-ground discrimination
  Spatial relationships
  Position in space
  Form constancy
Behavioral and intellectual deficits
  Poor judgment, unrealistic behavior
  Denial of disability
  Inability to abstract
  Rigidity of thought
  Disturbances in body image and body scheme
  Impairment of ability to self-correct
  Difficulty retaining information
  Distortion of time concepts
  Tendency to see the whole and not individual steps
  Affect lability
  Feelings of persecution
  Irritability, confusion
  Distraction by verbalization
  Short attention span
  Appearance of lethargy
  Fluctuation in performance
  Disturbances in relative size and distance of objects
Right Hemiparesis: left hemisphere—general language and temporal ordering deficits
Apraxia
  Motor
  Ideational
Behavioral and intellectual deficits
  Difficulty initiating tasks
  Sequencing deficits
  Processing delays
  Directionality deficits
  Low frustration levels
  Verbal and manual perseveration
  Rapid performance of movement or activity
  Compulsive behavior
  Extreme distractibility

Reprinted with permission from Ryerson S. Hemiplegia resulting from vascular insult or disease. In: Umphred D, ed. *Neurological Rehabilitation.* St. Louis: Mosby; 1985, 476.

tions, supine, sitting, and standing, and during remission or resolution pushing typically disappears first in the supine position, then in the sitting position, and finally in the standing position. Pushing increases in intensity with the difficulty of the postural challenge.[32] The most apparent problem of this syndrome is that is represents a threat to safety during standing and transfers, as the hemi side cannot effectively support body weight.

It has been suggested that the damage from the stroke lesion occurs in the subcortical sensory pathways.[31,32] Pusher syndrome affects sensory feedback in relationship to posture and gravity leading to a misperception of the individual's position in space. In other words, the patient reflexively compensates for a false feeling of leaning toward the unaffected side by leaning in the opposite direction.[30]

Before a therapist can begin evaluating and treating a stroke patient, a thorough understanding of the various stages of recovery of limb tone is essential. In the majority of cases, the predominant abnormality on admission in both upper and lower extremity is flaccidity.[33] The recovery of tone goes through stages of progression occurring mainly in the first seven to fourteen days. By day 28, a total of 20% of the patients had normal upper limb tone and 28% of the patients had normal lower limb tone.[34]

Table 12–7 shows the recovery of limb tone at 28 days.[33]

Many of the following evaluative techniques are for assessing tone. It is imperative to realize that the greatest recovery occurs within the first seven days, and many patients do regain spontaneous motor recovery within that time. Studies as of yet have not shown a difference in this early recovery stage between young and old.[33]

The efficacy of rehabilitation techniques for stroke patients has been questioned by legislature as well as administrative personnel. Nevertheless, there are several references that point to the efficacy of physical therapy.[34–36] Lehman, in the *Archives of Physical Medicine Rehabilitation,* showed that there are excellent improvements for stroke patients over the age of 80 who are discharged to the home for up to 2 years.[37] Longitudinal studies are needed to determine the long term effects of rehabilitation. Older patients can improve on a stroke rehabilitation program if it is properly applied. Evaluation and treatment techniques for the older patient will be described next.

Evaluation

Several models for evaluating stroke patients can be used. As mentioned in the Parkinson's disease section, Schenkman focuses on impairments and direct and indirect effects of the disease as well as on functional disability.[38] This model stresses that there are certain areas where physical therapy will be more beneficial.

Other authors have developed extensive forms and methods of evaluating stroke patients, and one interesting model developed by Tripp divides assessment into the following areas[39]:

1. Motor neuron response: Evaluates tone in terms of spasticity and ability to activate and relax muscle, with associated reactions.
2. Fractionated movement: Evaluates the ability of the patient to move individual limb segments.
3. Movement consistency: Evaluates whether or not the patient's ability to perform gross motor activities is consistent with his or her ability to form isolated movements.
4. Mental status: Looks at ability to follow commands and ability to learn safety and judgment.
5. Functional assessment: Includes mobility and gross upper extremity function.[39]

TABLE 12–7. RECOVERY OF LIMB TONE AT 28 DAYS

Admission limb tone	Limb tone at 28 days					
	No.	Normal	Flexor	Extensor	Flaccid	Dead
Upper limb						
Normal	19	16	0	0	0	3
Flexor	43	10	14	1	4	14
Extensor	8	4	1	1	0	2
Flaccid	87	17	20	3	17	30
Lower limb						
Normal	47	38	0	2	0	7
Flexor	11	4	1	0	1	5
Extensor	45	15	5	9	3	13
Flaccid	54	15	4	4	7	24

Reprinted with permission from Gray C, French J, Bates D. Motor recovery following acute stroke. *Age Ageing, 1900;*19:179–184.

Bobath Evaluation Bobath,[40] one of the leaders in the area of stroke rehabilitation, provides one of the most in-depth assessments of stroke patients. The Bobath evaluation tool looks not only at range of motion and sensory deficits, but also tests various movement patterns. The first test (Fig. 12–5) is for postural reactions in response to being moved. In addition, Bobath looks at tests for voluntary movements on request (Fig. 12–6) and at tests for balance and other automatic protective reactions (Fig. 12–7).

These tests are defined in detail in Bobath's text.[40] Looking at these assessment forms, a therapist can get an idea of some of the various movements and reactions being analyzed in the treatment setting. One of the strengths of Bobath's evaluative techniques is that they can be used not only to evaluate the patient, but the actual tests can also be used as treatment techniques.[40]

Brunnstrom Evaluation Brunnstrom[41] looks at the motor behavior of adults in terms of synergies. Brunnstrorn discusses the flexor synergy of the various limbs of the body, describes them in detail, then asks the therapist to evaluate these synergy levels throughout the entire evaluation and treatment progression of the patient. The flexor synergy of the upper limb is:

■ Flexion of the elbow to an acute angle;
■ Full range supination of the forearm;
■ Abduction of the shoulder to 90°;
■ External rotation of the shoulder;
■ Retraction or elevation of the shoulder girdle.

The extensor synergy of the upper limb shows:

■ Extension of the elbow, complete range;
■ Full range of pronation-supination;
■ Abduction of the forearm in front of the body;
■ Internal rotation of the arm;
■ Fixation of the shoulder girdle in a somewhat protracted position.

The flexor synergy for the lower limb is:

■ Dorsiflexion of the toe;
■ Dorsiflexion and inversion of the ankle;
■ Flexion of the knee to 90°;
■ Flexion of the hip;
■ Abduction and external rotation of the hip.

Finally, extensor synergy of the lower limb is:

■ Plantarflexion of the toes (inconsistent);
■ Plantarflexion and inversion of the ankle;
■ Extension of the knee;
■ Extension of the hip;
■ Abduction and internal rotation of the hip.

Brunnstrom[41] suggests looking for the various synergies and patterns in patients who have sustained a stroke.

Figure 12–8 is the form used by Brunnstrom[41] for classification and recording of motion. The various synergies are noted as numbers in the chart. The synergy levels for flaccidity progressing to normal tone would be noted as:

■ No movement initiated or elicited;
■ Synergies or components first appearing;
■ Synergies or components initiated voluntarily;
■ Movements deviating from basic synergies;
■ Relative independence;
■ Coordinated movements.

The remainder of the forms are self-explanatory and can be found in Brunnstrom's *Movement Therapy in Hemiplegia.*[41]

Carr and Shepherd Evaluation Carr and Shepherd,[42] physical therapists from Australia, have a different way of analyzing patients who have sustained strokes. These therapists have developed an entire strategy based on motor relearning. Their strategy is to eliminate unnecessary movements and to better organize the movement patterns. It is important to understand

Tests for Postural Reactions in Response to Being Moved

Patterns to be tested:

Tests for shoulder girdle, arm, and hand to be tested separately in supine, sitting, and standing as results are different.

At the end of each test, and at any one stage of each movement performed by the therapist, the normal reaction would be that the person tested should be able to maintain the position unaided when left unsupported.

	Abnormal resistance?	Abnormal assistance?	Uncontrolled full weight?

Grade 1

a. Elevation of the extended arm in external rotation with supination. Wrist and fingers extended and fingers abducted. The arm is lifted forward-upward.

b. Horizontal abduction, the arm and hand in the position described above.

c. Placing the arm by the side of the patient's body, position of the arm and hand as above.

Grade 2

d. From any one of the above three positions the patient's arm is moved forward across body and palm placed on the opposite shoulder

This is followed by lifting elbow so that forearm touches face, the hand remaining on the shoulder, with wrist extended.

e. From the elevated extended position, the patient's elbow is flexed, while upper arm is kept in elevation; palm is placed on the top of head.

Then palm is placed to the back of head, while arm is abducted, and wrist extended.

Supine Tests for Pelvis, Leg, and Foot

	Abnormal resistance?	Abnormal assistance?	Uncontrolled full weight?

Grade 1

a. The patient's leg is fully flexed at all joints, so that the foot is off support.

This is tested first with the sound leg fully flexed and held actively by the patient.

Then with the sound leg extended on support.

b. From the above flexed position the patient's foot is placed on the support; the leg remains flexed. Ankle and toes are dorsiflexed, foot everted, so that the heel only touches the support.

c. From this position (b) the patient's foot is slowly and in stages moved downward so that leg extends gradually. Dorsiflexion of the ankle and toes is maintained and tested at each stage, as well as testing for extensor thrust of the leg.

Continued

this principle when looking at their evaluation strategies. In evaluating upper limb function, for instance, instead of grading the function in terms of synergies or range of motion deficits, this approach outlines common problems and compensatory strategies. For example, in the arm, common problems are (1) poor scapular movement and persistent depression of the shoulder girdle; (2) poor muscular control of the glenohumeral joint caused by a lack of abduction, flexion, and inability to sustain position; and (3) excessive and unnecessary elbow flexion, internal rotation, shoulder, and forearm supination.

Continued from previous page

Grade 2

d. From the fully flexed position (a) the patient's leg is moved across the sound leg, and foot placed on the support on the opposite side. (Resistance to adduction of the leg and to rotation forward of the pelvis is tested.)

e. The patient lies near the edge of the plinth, the affected leg over the edge. Keeping hip extended the therapist bends knee, the foot and toes in dorsiflexion and eversion. (Resistance to flexion and to extensor thrust when extending the knee are tested.)

Abnormal resistance?	Abnormal assistance?	Uncontrolled full weight?

Prone Tests for the Leg and Hip

Grade 1

a. The patient supports him- or herself on both forearms. The affected leg is externally rotated, foot dorsiflexed and everted and then bent at the knee to a right angle without hip being flexed. (Resistance to the movement is tested and whether there is extensor thrust when it is gradually extended.)

b. The patient's legs are extended with external rotation, feet dorsiflexed and everted so that heels touch each other. (Resistance is tested and whether the position can be kept.)

Grade 2

c. Test (b) is followed by the patient's knees being bent, heels kept together and feet dorsiflexed and everted. (Resistance to this movement is tested as above (a) and whether there is extensor thrust when the affected leg is extended.)

Abnormal resistance?	Abnormal assistance?	Uncontrolled full weight?

Sitting Tests for the Legs
(The patient is sitting on a chair, feet on the ground)

Grade 2

a. Toes and ankles are dorsiflexed and foot placed backwards behind the sound one, knee being bent and heel kept on the ground. (Resistance to flexion of knee, ankle and to dorsiflexion of toes is being tested and whether there is downward pressure of the foot.)

b. The patient's leg is lifted, foot in dorsiflexion, and heel is placed on the edge of the chair, and from there it is placed on the knee of the sound leg. (Resistance to flexion is tested and whether patient can keep foot on the chair or on the sound knee.) The leg is then slowly lowered again until the foot reaches the ground. (Undue assistance to extension is tested when the leg is moved downward.)

Abnormal resistance?	Abnormal assistance?	Uncontrolled full weight?

Continued

──────── *Continued from previous page* ────────

Grade 2 (continued)

c. The patient sits with knees adducted in midline. The therapist moves both knees as far as possible to either side, and feet remain in the original position. (Resistance to adduction of the affected leg and to rotation of the pelvis forward is tested when moving knees toward the sound side.)

Abnormal resistance?	Abnormal assistance?	Uncontrolled full weight?

Standing Tests for the Legs
Grade 2

a. The patient's affected leg is lifted, flexed at all joints and then slowly lowered into a step forward, toes and ankle held dorsiflexed and foot everted. (Resistance to flexion is tested and whether there is downward pressure of the leg and foot on lowering foot to the ground.)

b. The patient stands in step position, the affected leg behind. Knee is then bent, the foot supported in dorsiflexion and eversion, the hip to remain extended. (Resistance to flexion of knee and extension of hip is tested.)

c. The foot is then slowly lowered again to the initial position behind the sound leg, foot everted and dorsiflexed and the heel placed to the ground. (Undue assistance to lowering the foot with stiffening of the knee is tested.)

Abnormal resistance?	Abnormal assistance?	Uncontrolled full weight?

Figure 12–5. *(Reprinted with permission from Bobath B. Adult Hemiplegia: Evaluational Treatment. London: William Heineman Medical Books, 1970; 18–71.)*

In looking at the hand, this approach would consider the following dysfunctional movement patterns:

1. Difficulty in grasping;
2. Difficulty in extending and flexing metacarpal phalangeal joints;
3. Difficulty with abduction and rotation of the thumb;
4. Difficulty cupping the hand;
5. Inability to hold different objects while moving the arm;
6. Tendency to pronate the forearm;
7. Excessive extension of the fingers and thumbs;
8. Inability to release objects;
9. Difficulty with abduction and rotation with the thumb in order to grasp.

During assessment the therapist would look at these deficits, identify them, and treat them.

Carr and Shepherd's method[42] of assessing lower extremity and trunk deficits is to describe them in terms of functional tasks, such as walking, balance, standing, standing from sitting, and sitting over the edge of the bed. In an analysis of sitting over the side of the bed, Carr and Shepherd identified two common problems: (1) flexion of the hip and knee on the affected side; and (2) flexion of the shoulder and protraction of the shoulder girdle, which results in the patient's inability to use the appropriate body mechanics to get out of bed.

This analysis can then be easily transferred to the appropriate treatment strategies for working with these patients. More specific evaluative and treatment information is available in Carr and Shepherd's *A Motor Re-Learning Programme for Stroke.*[42] In a subsequent section of this chapter, a specific form developed by Carr and Shepherd will be examined that goes over some of these points.[42]

In evaluating strength deficits, several studies have made a comparison between extension and torque in the knees, as well as various other joints of the body, and it can be a reliable and valid measure in stroke patients. Therefore, therapists can use manual muscle tests or dynamometry readings to assess strength in their elderly patients with a stroke.[43–45]

Olney and Colbourne's Gait Assessment Another consideration that is extremely important in the area of stroke is the analysis of gait. In a particularly valu-

TESTS FOR VOLUNTARY MOVEMENTS ON REQUEST
Patterns to be tested
Tests for Arm and Shoulder girdle
To be tested separately in supine, sitting, and standing, so each will be different.

	Supine Yes	No	Sitting Yes	No	Standing Yes	No

Grade 1

a. Can patient hold extended arm in elevation
   after having it placed there?
     With internal rotation?
     With external rotation?
b. Can patient lower the extended arm from the
   position of elevation to the horizontal plane
   and back again to elevation?
     Forward-downward?
     Sideways-downward?
     With internal rotation?
     With external rotation?
c. Can patient move the extended abducted arm
   from the horizontal plane to the side of body
   and back again to the horizontal plane?
     With internal rotation?
     With external rotation?

Grade 2
a. Can the patient lift arm to touch the opposite
   shoulder?
     With palm of hand?
     With back of hand?
b. Can patient bend elbow with upper arm in elevation to touch the top of head?
     With pronation?
     With supination?
c. Can patient fold hands behind head with both
   elbows in horizontal abduction?
     With wrist flexed?
     With wrist extended?

Grade 3
a. Can patient supinate forearm and wrist?
     Without side-flexion of trunk on the
     affected side?
     With flexed elbow and flexed fingers?
     With extended elbow and flexed fingers?
b. Can patient pronate forearm without adduction
   of arm at shoulder?
c. Can patient externally rotate the extended arm?
     (i) in a horizontal abduction?
     (ii) by the side of his body?
     (iii) in elevation?
d. Can patient bend and extend elbow in supination
   to touch the shoulder of the same? starting with:
     (i) arm by side of body?
     (ii) horizontal abduction of the arm?

Continued

Continued from previous page

Tests for Wrist and Fingers

Grade 1

	Yes?	No?
a. Can patient place the flat hand forward down on table in front?		
Can patient do this sideways when sitting on plinth?		
With fingers and thumb adducted?		
With fingers and thumb abducted?		

Grade 2

a. Can patient open hand to grasp?		
With flexed wrist?		
With extended wrist?		
With pronation?		
With supination?		
With adducted fingers and thumb?		
With abducted fingers and thumb?		

Grade 3

a. Can patient grasp and open fingers again?		
With flexed elbow?		
With extended elbow?		
With pronation?		
With supination		
b. Can patient move individual fingers?		
Thumb?		
Index finger?		
Little finger?		
Second and third finger?		
c. Can patient oppose fingers and thumb?		
Thumb and index finger?		
Thumb and second finger?		
Thumb and little finger		

Tests for Pelvis, Leg, and Foot: Prone Tests

Grade 1

	Yes?	No?
Can patient bend knee without bending hip?		
With foot in dorsiflexion?		
With foot in plantiflexion?		
Foot inverted?		
Foot everted?		

Grade 2

Can patient lie with both legs externally rotated and extended, feet dorsiflexed and everted, heels touching?		
Hold position when placed?		
Turn affected leg out again to touch heel of sound leg after it has been internally rotated by therapist?		
Perform internal and external rotation unaided?		

Grade 3

a. Can patient keep heels together and touching while bending both knees to right angle?		
Affected foot inverted?		
Affected foot everted?		
b. Can patient hold knee of affected leg flexed at right angle and alternately dorsiflex and plantiflex ankle?		
Foot inverted?		
Foot everted?		
Without moving knee?		

Continued

— Continued from previous page —

Tests for Pelvis, Leg, and Foot: Supine

	Yes?	No?

Grade 1

a. Can patient bend affected leg?
   With sound leg flexed, foot off support?
   With sound leg extended?
   Without bending affected arm?
b. Can patient bend hip and knee with foot remaining on the support from the beginning of extension until the foot is near pelvis?
   Can patient extend leg by degrees, with foot remaining on the support?

Grade 2

Can patient lift pelvis without extending affected leg, both feet on the support?
Can patient keep pelvis up and lift sound leg?
Without dropping pelvis on the affected side?
Can patient keep pelvis up and adduct and abduct knees?

Grade 3

a. Can patient dorsiflex ankle?
   Dorsiflex toes?
   With flexed leg, foot on the support?
   With extended leg?
   With foot inverted?
   With foot everted?
b. Can patient bend knee while lying near the edge of plinth, the leg over side of plinth?

Sitting Tests on Chair

	Yes?	No?

Grade 1

a. Can patient adduct and abduct affected leg, foot on ground?
b. Can patient adduct and abduct affected leg, foot placed on seat of chair?

Grade 2

a. Can patient lift affected leg and place foot on sound knee? (without use of hand to lift leg.)
b. Can patient draw affected foot back under chair, heel on the floor?
c. Can patient stand up with sound foot in front of affected one? (without use of hand?)

Standing Tests

	Yes?	No?

Grade 1

Can patient stand with parallel feet, both feet touching?

Grade 2

a. Can patient stand on affected leg, lifting sound one?
b. Can patient stand on affected leg, sound one lifted and bend and extend standing leg?
c. Can patient stand in step position, weight forward on affected leg, sound leg behind on toes?
d. Can patient stand in step position, sound leg forward with weight on it, affected leg behind and bend knee of affected leg without taking toes off ground?

Grade 3

a. Can patient stand in step postion, weight forward on sound leg, affected leg behind and lift foot without bending hip of affected leg?
   Foot in inversion?
   Foot in eversion?

— Continued —

—————————— Continued from previous page ——————————

Tests for Pelvis, Leg, and Foot: Supine (continued)
Standing Tests (continued)
Grade 3 (continued)

	Yes?	No?
b. Can patient stand on affected leg and transfer weight over it to make step with sound leg?		
Forward?		
Backward?		
c. Can patient stand on sound leg and make step forward with affected leg without hitching pelvis up?		
d. Can patient stand on sound leg and make step backward with affected leg without hitching pelvis up?		
e. Can patient stand on affected leg and lift toes?		

Figure 12–6. *(Reprinted with permission from Bobath B. Adult Hemiplegia: Evaluational Treatment. London: William Heineman Medical Books, 1970;18–27.)*

able journal article, Olney and Colboume describe some of the deficits in gait and discuss methods of treating the gait problem. They also divide the gait pattern into phases. The first phase, "late swing to foot flat," identifies three problems for stroke patients: (1) inability to attain full hip flexion during swing, (2) inability to extend the knee fully, and (3) inability to activate ankle dorsiflexor muscles. In addition, stroke patients may hyperextend the knee to avoid the problem of instability.

The next phase of gait that presents problems is "foot flat to heel off." Problems noted here are the decreased use of hip extensor muscles, limited hip extension motion, and that ankle plantar flexors contract inappropriately.

The next phase, "push off, pull off in early swing," causes residual weakness of ankle plantar flexors and hip flexors. It also results in the stance phase of the affected side being longer than normal, and the body's weight being transferred to the lower limb through push off.[46]

Rancho Los Amigos Gait Evaluation Another interesting analysis of hemiplegic gait comes from Rancho Los Amigos medical center in California. This method is called the Upright Control Evaluation. Its purpose is to assess the patient's static ability to flex and then accept weight on the involved lower extremity. It is an intricate method of testing upright control and the criteria for this are given in specific detail in Table 12–8.[47]

Pusher Syndrome Assessment Common findings of sensory deficits on the hemi side of a patient with Pusher syndrome are hemianopsia, problems with proprioception, and somatosensory deficits which contribute to postural inattention and difficulties with postural adjustments.[48] Perceptual dysfunction includes unilateral neglect and agnosia. Cognitive function is usually decreased with significant memory

impairments, impulsivity with decreased attention (typical of left hemiplegia), lack of insight or understanding of problems, and apraxia.

Motor function in Pusher syndrome includes overuse of extension on the sound side with ipsilateral pushing and predominance of a flexion synergy pattern in the affected lower extremity.[30,31,48] Posturally, the head and trunk are held toward the hemi side with increased weightbearing on the involved side and shifting of the trunk away from the sound side. The patient's balance is severely disturbed with an inability to find a midline orientation. In fact, the patient resists all attempts to assist in centering of the center of motion within the base of support. The patient pushes back strongly when weight transfer is attempted.

Typically, the individual shows no concern or fear of falling and does not automatically compensate for loss of balance with adjustments to support body weight. During the stance phase of gait, the patient demonstrates inadequate extension of the involved leg. During stepping, the patient is unable to transfer the weight efficiently onto the sound limb and the hemi leg typically adducts strongly during swing (sissors).[30–32,48] Functional assessment reveals profound difficulties with sit-to-stand and transfers. The patient is often unable to stand without assistance.

Motor Assessment Scale Specific compacted tests for the assessment of stroke patients are somewhat difficult to find, but they do exist. Carr and Shepherd have developed the Motor Assessment Scale in Figure 12–9A. All items on the form are constructed so that a score of six indicates optimal motor behavior. The criteria for scoring is listed in Figure 12–9B. These particular criteria are self-explanatory and give the examiner a six-point scale from which to assess the patient and show improvement in a very simple form.[49]

When evaluating a stroke patient, it is important to choose the tools that will appropriately reflect the patient's status and the methods to be used in the

TESTS FOR BALANCE AND OTHER AUTOMATIC PROTECTIVE REACTIONS

(N.B.) In order to test these reactions the patient must be able to assume and hold the test position. The patient should react with specific movements in order to regain balance or protect self against falling when being moved or pushed unexpectedly.

Balance Reactions

Yes? No?

1. *Patient in prone lying, supporting body on forearms. State reaction.*
a. Patient's shoulder girdle is pushed toward affected side. Does patient remain supported on affected forearm? ☐ ☐
b. Sound arm is lifted forward and up, as when reaching out with one hand. Does patient immediately transfer weight toward the affected arm? ☐ ☐
c. Sound arm is lifted and moved backward and patient is turned to side, support on affected arm. Does patient remain supported on affected arm? ☐ ☐

These three tests can be done in slight cases with patient supporting self on extended arm instead of on forearm.

2. *Patient sitting on the plinth, feet unsupported. State reaction.*

Yes? No?

a. If patient is pushed toward the affected side, does he or she stay upright? ☐ ☐
   Does patient laterally flex head toward the sound side? ☐ ☐
   Abduct sound leg? ☐ ☐
   Use the affected forearm for support? ☐ ☐
   Use the affected hand for support? ☐ ☐
b. If patient is pushed forward, does he or she bend affected hip and knee? ☐ ☐
   Extend spine? ☐ ☐
   Lift head? ☐ ☐
c. Both legs are lifted up by the therapist, knees flexed. Does patient stay upright? ☐ ☐
   Move affected arm forward? ☐ ☐
   Support body backward with affected arm? ☐ ☐

3. *Patient in four-foot kneeling. State reaction.*
a. Body is pushed toward the affected side
   Does patient abduct the sound leg? ☐ ☐
   Remain on all fours? ☐ ☐
b. Patient's sound arm is lifted and held up by the therapist
   Does patient keep affected arm extended? ☐ ☐
c. Sound leg is lifted.
   Does patient keep affected leg flexed and transfer weight on to it? ☐ ☐
d. Sound arm and affected leg are lifted
   Does patient keep affected arm extended? ☐ ☐
e. Affected arm and sound leg are lifted
   Does patient remain on affected flexed leg? ☐ ☐
f. Sound arm and leg are lifted
   Does patient transfer weight toward the affected side and maintain position? ☐ ☐

4. *Patient in kneel-standing. State reaction.*
a. Patient is pushed toward the affected side
   Does patient abduct the sound leg? ☐ ☐
   Bend head laterally toward the sound side? ☐ ☐
   Use affected hand for support? ☐ ☐
b. Patient is pushed toward the sound side
   Does patient abduct the affected leg? ☐ ☐
   Extend the affected arm sideways? ☐ ☐

Continued

Continued from previous page

	Yes?	No?
c. Patient is pushed backward and asked not to sit down		
Does patient extend the affected arm forward?	☐	☐
d. Patient is pushed gently forward, sound arm held backward by therapist		
Does patient use affected arm and hand for support on the ground?	☐	☐
Lift affected foot off the ground?	☐	☐

5. *Patient half-kneeling, sound foot forward. (Patient should not use sound hand for support.) State reaction.*

	Yes?	No?
a. Sound foot is lifted up by the therapist		
Does patient remain upright?	☐	☐
Keep affected hip extended?	☐	☐
b. Sound foot is lifted by the therapist and placed sideways		
Does patient remain upright?	☐	☐
Show balance movements with affected arm?	☐	☐
c. Sound foot is placed from the above position back to kneel-standing		
Does patient keep upright?	☐	☐
Keep affected hip extended?	☐	☐

6. *Patient standing, feet parallel, standing base narrow. State reaction.*

	Yes?	No?
a. Patient is tipped backward and not allowed to make step backward with sound leg. (Therapist puts foot on patient's sound one to prevent step.)		
Does patient step backward with affected leg?	☐	☐
b. Patient is tipped backward and not allowed to make steps with either leg.		
Does patient dorsiflex toes of affected leg?	☐	☐
Big toe only?	☐	☐
Dorsiflex ankle and toes of affected leg?	☐	☐
Move affected arm forward?	☐	☐
c. Patient is tipped toward sound side.		
Does patient abduct affected leg?	☐	☐
Abduct and extend affected arm?	☐	☐
Make steps to follow with affected leg across sound leg?	☐	☐
d. Patient is tipped toward the affected side		
Does patient abduct the sound leg?	☐	☐
Bend head laterally toward the sound side?	☐	☐

7. *Patient standing on affected leg only. (Patient is not allowed to use sound hand for support.) State reactions.*

	Yes?	No?
a. Sound foot is lifted by the therapist and moved forward as in making a step, extending knee.		
Does patient keep the heel of affected leg on the ground?	☐	☐
Keep the knee of the affected leg extended?	☐	☐
Assist weight transfer forward over affected leg with extended hip?	☐	☐
b. Sound foot is lifted by the therapist and moved backward as in making a step backward		
Does patient keep the hip of affected leg extended?	☐	☐
Assist weight transfer backward over affected leg?	☐	☐
c. Sound foot is lifted by the therapist and held up while patient is pushed gently sideways toward the affected side.		
Does patient follow and adjust balance, moving the foot of the affected leg sideways by inverting and everting foot alternately?	☐	☐
The same maneuver is done pulling with patient toward the affected side.		
Does patient follow and adjust balance by moving foot as above?	☐	☐

Continued

Continued from previous page

	Yes?	No?

Tests for Protective Extension and Support of the Arm

1. When testing these reactions the patient's sound arm should be held by hand, so that patient cannot use it. It is advisable to hold the sound arm in extension and external rotation because this facilitates the extension of the affected arm and hand. State reaction.

a. The patient stands in front of a table or plinth. Sound arm is held backward and patient is pushed forward toward the table.

Does patient extend affected arm forward? ☐ ☐
Support self on fist? ☐ ☐
On the palm of hand? ☐ ☐
Thumb adducted? ☐ ☐
Thumb abducted? ☐ ☐

b. The patient stands facing a wall, at a distance that allows patient to reach it with hand. Patient is pushed forward against the wall, sound arm held backward.

Does patient lift affected arm and stretch it out against the wall? ☐ ☐
Place hand against the wall, fingers flexed, thumb adducted? ☐ ☐
Fingers open, thumb abducted? ☐ ☐

2. *State reaction.*

c. The patient is sitting on the plinth, with sound arm held sideways by the therapist. Patient is pushed toward the affected side.

Does patient abduct the affected arm and support self on forearm? ☐ ☐
On extended arm? ☐ ☐
Support self on fist? ☐ ☐
On open palm? ☐ ☐
Thumb and fingers adducted? ☐ ☐
Thumb and fingers abducted? ☐ ☐

d. The patient stands sideways to a wall, at a distance that allows patient to reach it with affected hand.

Does patient abduct and lift the affected arm? ☐ ☐
With flexed elbow? ☐ ☐
Reach out for the wall with extended elbow? ☐ ☐
Support self with fist against the wall? ☐ ☐
With open hand? ☐ ☐
With adducted thumb and fingers? ☐ ☐
With abducted thumb and fingers? ☐ ☐

3. *State reaction.*

e. The patient lies on the floor on back with sound hand placed under hip so that patient cannot use it. The therapist takes a pillow and pretends to throw it toward patient's head.

Does patient move affected arm to protect face? ☐ ☐
With flexed elbow? ☐ ☐
With extended elbow? ☐ ☐
With internal rotation? ☐ ☐
With external rotation? ☐ ☐
With fisted hand? ☐ ☐
With open hand? ☐ ☐
Can patient catch the pillow? ☐ ☐

Figure 12–7. *(Reprinted with permission from Bobath B:* Adult Hemiplegia: Evaluational Treatment. *London: William Heineman Medical Books; 1970; 18–71)*

HEMIPLEGIA—CLASSIFICATION AND PROGRESS RECORD (p. 1)
Upper Limb—Test Sitting

Name _____ Age _____ Date of onset _____ Side affected _____

Date

_____ Passive motion sense, shoulder _____ elbow _____

_____ pron.-supin. _____ wrist flex.-ext. _____

_____ 1. NO MOVEMENT INITIATED OR ELICITED _____

_____ 2. SYNERGIES OR COMPONENTS FIRST APPEARING. Spasticity developing _____

_____ Flexor synergy _____

_____ Extensor synergy _____

_____ 3. SYNERGIES OR COMPONENTS INITIATED VOLUNTARILY. Spasticity marked _____

FLEXOR SYNERGY

		Active Joint Range		Remarks
_____ Shoulder girdle	Elevation			
_____	Retraction			
	Hyperextension			
_____ Shoulder joint	Abduction			
	Ext. rotation			
_____ Elbow	Flexion			
_____ Forearm	Supination			

EXTENSOR SYNERGY

_____ Shoulder	Pectoralis major			
_____ Elbow	Extension			
_____ Forearm	Pronation			
4. MOVEMENTS DEVIATING FROM BASIC SYNERGIES Spasticity decreasing	Hand to sacral region			
	Raise arm forw.-horiz.			
	Pron.-supin. elbow at 90°			
5. RELATIVE IN-DEPENDENCE OF BASIC SYNERGIES Spasticity waning	Raise arm side-horiz.			
	Raise arm over head			
	Pron.-supin. elbow extended			

6. MOVEMENT COORDINATION NEAR NORMAL. Spasticity minimal

Continued

Continued from previous page

Name _____
Date

_____ SPEED TESTS for classes 4, 5, 6   Strokes per 5 sec.

Hand from	Normal		
_____ lap to chin	Affected		
Hand from lap	Normal		
_____ to opposite knee	Affected		

_____ Passive motion sense, digits _____

_____ Fingertip recognition _____

_____ Wrist stabilization   1. Elbow extended _____
for grasp   2. Elbow flexed _____

_____ Wrist flexion   1. Elbow extended _____
and extension

_____ Fist closed   2. Elbow flexed _____

_____ Wrist circumduction _____

DIGITS

_____ Mass grasp _____ Dynamometer test   Normal _____ lb.
                                                        Affected _____ lb.

_____ Mass extension _____

_____ Hook grasp (handbag, 2 lb.) _____

_____ Lateral prehension (card) _____

_____ Palmar prehension (pencil) _____

_____ Cylindrical grasp (small jar) _____

_____ Spherical grasp (ball) _____ catch _____ throw _____

_____ Indiv. thumb movements   1. Vertical movements _____
hands in lap ulnar side down   2. Horizontal movements _____

_____ Individual finger movements _____

_____ Button and unbutton shirt   Using both hands _____
                                        Using affected hand only _____

_____ Other skilled activities _____

Figure 12–8. *(Reprinted with permission from Brunnstrom S. Movement Therapy in Hemiplegia. New York: Harpewr & Row; 1970;8–12;38–41.)*

evaluation treatment progression. Several different types of tools have been provided and will be considered next.

Treatment Interventions

There are a number of treatment techniques commonly used by physical therapists ranging from the classic therapeutic exercise to the proprioceptive neuromuscular facilitation (PNF) to the Bobath and Brunnstrom techniques. A brief discussion of Bobath's, Brunnstrom's, and Carr and Shepherd's work will follow in the next section. Treatment considerations for gait will also be discussed, as will research on various types of ancillary modalities that can be used for the treatment of stroke deficits.

Boboth's Treatments Bobath's principles for treating stroke patients with deficits revolve around the idea that their problem is not their lack of power; rather it is that they cannot perform normal movements. Therefore, her beliefs are in sharp contrast to strengthening techniques such as PNF, therapeutic exercise, and even Brunnstrom's techniques.[40] The aim of Bobath's approach is to change the abnormal movement patterns of the stroke patient into normal movement patterns. Bobath's theory revolves around reflex-inhibiting movement patterns as a means of fa-

TABLE 12–8. UPRIGHT CONTROL (UC)

Criteria for UC Evaluation (Flexion and Extension)
1. Patient requires no more than one person to assist double or single limb stance.
2. Patient can understand instructions adequately to perform test

FLEXION

Number of Examiners

Two examiners required for testing; assisting examiner provides hand support, testing examiner demonstrates test to patient and determines grade.

Position for Test

Standing with use of assisting examiner's hand for support (balance only). Support should be sufficient for patient to maintain standing balance.

Technique for Administering Flexion Test for Each Segment
1. One demonstration by examiner.
2. One practice trail by patient (or two trials if needed to help patient understand test).
3. One test trial to determine grade.
4. If patient has bilateral lower extremity involvement, provide opposite lower extremity stabilization (manually, with Ankle-Foot Orthotic, Knee-Ankle-Foot Orthosis) as needed to provide standing stability.

Pretest for Hip Flexion Test

Prior to the test for each segment:
1. Position the patient's limb that is to be tested in neutral or maximum available hip and knee extension.
2. The assisting examiner provides hand support in line with the greater trochanter of the femur on the side opposite the leg being tested.

Range of Motion

Measure and record the freely available range; do not stretch part through spasticity or soft tissue restriction. For the lower extremities, use standard range of motion evaluation and recording procedure (including beginning and ending range of motion), except evaluate dorsiflexion range with the knee extended using only two-finger pressure. For the trunk and upper extremities record Within Normal Limits if range is within normal limits, record IF if limited range interferes with function.

Tone

Determine if muscle tone is normal or abnormal for the neck, trunk, and extremities by moving the part through a fast range of motion. Prior to evaluating muscle tone determine the available slow range of motion. If pain is present with passive movement of the part, defer fast motion assessment and note in comment section.

If spasticity (an exaggerated response to stretch) is present, evaluate its effect on the patient's overall function and record the grade based on the following key:

Slight (SL): Present but has no influence on patient's function.

Severe (SEV): Present to the degree that it interferes with or prevents function.

PROPRIOCEPTION

Evaluate proprioception of the upper extremity with the patient sitting; evaluate the lower extremity with the patient supine. Demonstrate the procedure to the patient before testing. Use either of the following methods.
1. Ask patient to close eyes or occlude vision. Move the part to any normal, pain-free position without putting the muscles on stretch, and ask patient to copy the position with uninvolved extremity.
2. Occlude patient's vision and move part. Ask patient to indicate if part is up, down, in, or out.

Use the following grading key:

Normal (N): Intact proprioception; characterized by rapid, correct response.

Impaired (I): Responses are slow but correct the majority of the time.

Absent (O): Unable to duplicate or identify position of body part.

Instructions to Patient for Hip Flexion Test
1. "Stand as straight as you can."
2. "Bring your knee up toward your chest three times as high and as fast as you can."

Grading Hip Flexion

When observed range is borderline between Weak and Moderate, or Moderate and Strong give the lesser grade. If patient is unable to complete the three flexion efforts within 10 seconds, give Weak grade.

Weak (W): No motion or actively flexes less than 30°.

Moderate (M): Actively accomplishes an arc of hip flexion between 30° and 60°.

Strong (S): Actively accomplishes an arc of hip flexion more than 60°.

Base grade on true hip motion and not on substitutions, such as backward trunk lean or pelvic tilt.

Instructions to Patient for Knee Flexion Test
1. "Stand as straight as you can.
2. "Bring your knee up toward your chest three times as high and as fast as you can."

Grading Knee Flexion

When observed range is borderline between Weak and Moderate, or Moderate and Strong give lesser grade. If the patient is unable to complete the three flexion efforts within 10 seconds, give the Weak grade.

Weak (W): No motion or knee-flexes less than 30°.

Moderate (M): Knee flexes between 30° and 60°.

Strong (S): Knee flexes more than 60°.

Instructions to Patient for Ankle Flexion Test
1. "Stand as straight as you can."
2. "Bring you knee and your foot up toward your chest three times as high and as fast as you can."

Grading Ankle Flexion

When observed range is borderline between Weak and Strong give the lesser grade. If the patient is unable to complete the three flexion efforts within 10 seconds, give Weak grade.

(continued)

TABLE 12–8.   (CONTINUED)

Weak (W): No motion or actively dorsiflexes to less than a right angle at the ankle joint.

Strong (S): Actively dorsiflexes to a right angle or greater at the ankle joint.

Extension

Number of Examiners

Two examiners required for testing; testing examiner determines grade, assisting examiner assists in stabilizing or providing hand support as indicated under "Pretest Position and Stabilization."

Position for Test

Standing with the use of the examiner's hand for support (balance support adequate to maintain single limb stance).

Technique for Administering Test for Each Segment

1. One demonstration by examiner.
2. One practice trial by patient (or two trials if needed to help patient understand test).
3. One test trial to determine grade.
4. If patient has bilateral lower extremity involvement, assist opposite lower extremity flexion as needed to determine extension control of the stance limb.

Pretest Positioning and Stabilization for Hip Extension Test

1. Testing examiner positioned beside patient to provde hand support and to assure that patient begins from a position of neutral or maximum hip extension range.
2. Assisting examiner provides manual stabilization as demonstrated in diagram to maintain neutral knee extension and a stable ankle.
3. If there is a fixed equinus contracture greater than neutral, accommodate for the contracture by placing a 30° wedge under the patient's heel.
4. If unable to maintain a stable plantigrade platform for single limb stance either manually or with an AFO, record UT (Unable to test) for hip and knee extension. See "Grading Ankle Extension" for testinng and recording an appropriate ankle grade.

Instructions to Patient for Hip Extension Test

1. "Stand on both legs as straight as you can."
2. "Now stand as straight as you can on just your (R) (weaker) leg."--"Lift this leg up."--"Keep standing as straight as you can."

Grading Hip Extension

When patient is balanced on weaker leg, testing examiner gradually decreases amount of hand support to determine hip control.

Weak (W): Uncontrolled trunk flexion on hip (testing examiner must prevent continued forward motion of the trunk by providing additional hand support).

Moderate (M): Unable to maintain trunk completely erect or at end of available hip extension range but patient stops own forward trunk motion or trunk wobbles back and forth or patient hyperextends trunk on hip.

Strong (S): Maintains trunk erect on hip or at end of available hip extension range.

Pretest Positioning and Stabilization for Knee Extension Test

1. Assisting examiner positioned behind patient. Assisting examiner provides hand support and maintains trunk erect on hip.
2. Testing examiner positions patient's knees in 30° of flexion bilaterally.
3. If unable to maintain feet flat with approximately 30° knee flexion, use a 30° wedge.

Instructions to Patient for Knee Extension Test

1. "Stand on both feet with your knees bent" (approximately 20° to 30°; use a wedge to accommodate for limited ankle dorsiflexion range if necessary).
2. "Keep your knees bent and lift your (L) (R) (stronger) leg."

Demonstrate and give instruction number 3 only if patient can support body weight on a flexed knee during single limb support without further collapse into flexion.

3. "Now, straighten your knee as much as you can."

Grading Knee Extension Control

If knee flexion contracture present, grade cannot exceed "moderate."

Weak (W): Unable to maintain body weight on a flexed knee (knee continues to collapse into flexion or heel rises).

Moderate (M): Supports body weight on a flexed knee without further collapse into flexion or without heel rise.

Strong (S): Supports body weight on a lfexed kknee and, on request, straightens knee to end of available knee extension range (hyperextension allowed).

Excessive (E): Unable to position knee in flexion secondary to severe extensor thrust or extensor tone.

Pretest Positioning and Stabilization for Ankle Extension Test

If patient has knee flexion contracture, record UT (unable to test) for ankle extension control.

1. Assisting examiner positioned behind patient to maintain trunk erect on hip.
2. Testing examiner positioned to prevent knee hyperextension (i.e., plantar flexion of ankle).
3. Assess passive ankle range with knee extended and accommodate for neutral or less than neutral ankle range with a 30° wedge.

Instructions to Patient for Ankle Extension Test

1. "Stand on both legs as straight as you can."
2. "Lift and hold up your (L) (R) (stronger) leg."

Demonstrate and give instructions for number 3 only if patient can control the knee at neutral.

3. "Keep your knee straight and go up on your toes as high as you can."

Grading Ankle Extension

Weak (W): Unable to maintain knee at neutral (knee collapses into flexion or wobbles back and forth between flexion and extension or hyperextenssion/extensor thrust cannot be controlled by examiner).

Moderate (M): Maintains knee at neutral.

Strong (S): Maintains knee at neutral and lifts heel off floor on command (any degree of heel lift while maintainng neutral knee).

Excessive (E): Equinus or varus so severe patient is unable to maintain stable plantigrade platform

---

Reprinted with permission from Parker K, Zablotny C, Jordan C. Analysis and management of hemiplegic gait dysfunction. Stroke Rehabiliation State of the Art. Downey, Calif: 1984. Rancho Los Amigos Medical Center.

MOTOR ASSESSMENT SCALE

NAME _____

MOVEMENT SCORING SHEET

DATE _____	0	1	2	3	4	5	6
1. Supine to side lying	____	____	____	____	____	____	____
2. Supine to sitting over side of bed	____	____	____	____	____	____	____
3. Balanced sitting	____	____	____	____	____	____	____
4. Sitting to standing	____	____	____	____	____	____	____
5. Walking	____	____	____	____	____	____	____
6. Upper-arm function	____	____	____	____	____	____	____
7. Hand movements	____	____	____	____	____	____	____
8. Advanced hand activities	____	____	____	____	____	____	____
9. General tonus	____	____	____	____	____	____	____

Figure 12–9A. *(Reprinted with permission from Carr J, Shepherd R, et al. Investigation of a new motor assessment scale for stroke patients. Phys Ther. February 1985;65(2).)*

cilitating more normal movement patterns. The patients in the program learn to know what normal movement feels like. Using this assessment tool, the therapist develops a treatment plan based on the following:

1. Whether the patient needs to increase or decrease body tone;
2. What type of movement patterns should be taught and which patterns should be facilitated and which inhibited;
3. What functional skills the patient needs to work on.

With this in mind, Bobath pursues various stages of recovery and designs a treatment program.

The first stage is the initial flaccid stage, during which the treatment must be coordinated with the nursing staff and with family members. The patient's sleeping and sitting positions must be designed to facilitate proper tone. For example, when the patient is supine, the extensor tone will be accentuated and, therefore, the patient must be positioned with some flexion in the lower extremity, possibly on the side or on the back, with pillows to accentuate that flexion.

An example of movement patterns would be having the patient lie on his or her side with knees bent and the involved extremity on top. The therapist provides active and passive movement to the shoulder girdle with the arm in extension and external rotation while extending and abducting the thumb. This can be followed by providing resistance and distraction to stimulate active movement in the upper extremity. The patient can also be encouraged to have the arm placed in a outward position by a family member while he or she is lying on the side in bed and holding on to the headboard while reaching overhead. Bo-

bath does a lot of work with mobilizing the shoulder, and when the patient is able to sit, she also stresses the importance of weight bearing on the arm in a sitting position.

The next stage of recovery is spasticity. It is extremely important for the therapist to work on decreasing the spastic patterning and on facilitating the person's use of the arm in functional positions. The patient is encouraged to move the arm in the supine position. For example, with the elbow pointing toward the ceiling, the patient is encouraged to straighten the elbow and touch the head, or the patient is told to bring the arm across the body toward the mouth, which encourages a functional position. In the lower extremity, the patient may be asked to lie prone and bend the knee. Bobath also uses quite a bit of quadruped and biped training, which encourages weight transfer onto the affected side to encourage more normal tone and weight bearing.[40]

The final stage of relative recovery focuses on placing the patient in the proper positions and challenging proper movement. An example of a technique used in this stage is patterning to break up some of the associated reactions. For example, to facilitate ankle dorsiflexion-plantar flexion while walking, the therapist may push the patient unexpectedly backward to facilitate the ankle dorsiflexion reaction. Bobath's techniques are extremely practical and a detailed analysis of these are given in her book.[40]

Brunnstrom's Treatment Brunnstrom's approach to the treatment of hemiplegic patients is first to facilitate the stages of the spasticity development and then to eventually facilitate the patient's ability to overcome the tone. For example, in the flaccid first stage, the therapist attempts to stimulate muscle activity

Criteria for Scoring Figure 12–9A.

I. Supine to Side Lying onto Intact Side

1. Pulls self into side lying. (Starting position must be supine lying, not knees flexed. Patient pulls self into side lying with intact arm, moves affected leg with intact leg.)
2. Moves leg across actively and the lower half of the body follows. (Starting position as above. Arm is left behind.)
3. Arm is lifted across body with other arm. Leg is moved actively and body follows in a block. (Starting position as above.)
4. Moves arm across body actively and the rest of the body follows in a block. (Starting position as above.)
5. Moves arm and leg and rolls to side but overbalances. (Starting position as above. Shoulder protracts and arm flexes forward.)
6. Rolls to side in 3 seconds. (Starting position as above. Must not use hands.)

II. Supine to Sitting over Side of Bed

1. Side lying, lifts head sideways but cannot sit up. (Patient assisted to side lying.)
2. Side lying to sitting over side of bed. (Therapist assists patient with movement. Patient controls head position throughout.)
3. Side lying to sitting over side of bed. (Therapist gives stand-by-help by assisting legs over side of bed.)
4. Side lying to sitting over side of bed. (With no stand-by help.)
5. Supine to sitting over side of bed. (With no stand-by help.)
6. Supine to sitting over side of bed within 10 seconds. (With no stand-by help.)

III. Balanced Sitting

1. Sits only with support. (Therapist should assist patient into sitting.)
2. Sits unsupported for 10 seconds. (Without holding on, knees and feet together, feet can be supported on floor.)
3. Sits unsupported with weight well forward and evenly distributed. (Weight should be well forward at the hips, head and thoracic spine extended, weight evenly distributed on both sides.)
4. Sits unsupported, turns head and trunk to look behind. (Feet supported and together on floor. Do not allow legs to abduct or feet to move. Have hands resting on thighs, do not allow hands to move onto plinth.)
5. Sits unsupported, reaches forward to touch floor, and returns to starting position. (Feet supported on floor. Do not allow patient to hold on. Do not allow legs and feet to move, support affected arm if necessary. Hand must touch floor at least 10 cm [4 in] in front of feet.)
6. Sits on stool unsupported, reaches sideways to touch floor, and returns to starting position. (Feet supported on floor. Do not allow patient to hold on. Do not allow legs and feet to move, support affected arm if necessary. Patient must reach sideways not forward.)

IV. Sitting to Standing

1. Gets to standing with help from therapist. (Any method.)
2. Gets to standing with stand-by help. (Weight unevenly distributed, uses hands for support.)
3. Gets to standing. (Do not allow uneven weight distribution or help from hands.)
4. Gets to standing and stands for 5 seconds with hips and knees extended. (Do not allow uneven weight distribution.)
5. Sitting to standing to sitting with no stand-by help. (Do not allow uneven weight distribution. Full extension of hips and knees.)
6. Sitting to standing to sitting with no stand-by help three times in 10 seconds. (Do not allow uneven weight distribution.)

V. Walking

1. Stands on affected leg and steps forward with other leg. (Weight-bearing hip must be extended. Therapist may give stand-by help.)
2. Walks with stand-by help from one person.
3. Walks 3 m (10 ft) alone or uses any aid but no stand-by help.
4. Walks 5 m (16 ft) with no aid in 15 seconds.
5. Walks 10 m (33 ft) with no aid, turns around, picks up a small sandbag from floor, and walks back in 25 seconds. (May use either hand.)
6. Walks up and down four steps with or without an aid but without holding on to the rail three times in 35 seconds.

Continued

Continued from previous page

VI. Upper-Arm Function

1. Lying, protract shoulder girdle with arm in elevation. (Therapist places arm in position and supports it with elbow in extension.)
2. Lying, hold extended arm in elevation for 2 seconds. (Physical therapist should place arm in position and patient must maintain position with some external rotation. Elbow must be held within 20° of full extension.)
3. Flexion and extension of elbow to take palm to forehead with arm as in step 2. (Therapist may assist supination of forearm.)
4. Sitting, hold extended arm in forward flexion at 90° to body for 2 seconds. (Therapist should place arm in position, and patient must maintain position with some external rotation and elbow extension. Do not allow excess shoulder elevation.)
5. Sitting, patient lifts arm to above position, holds it there for 10 seconds, and then lowers it. (Patient must maintain position with some external rotation. Do not allow pronation.)
6. Standing, hand against wall. Maintain arm position while turning body toward wall. (Have arm abducted to 90° with palm flat against the wall.)

VII. Hand Movements

1. Sitting, extension of wrist. (Therapist should have patient sitting at a table with forearm resting on the table. Therapist places cylindrical object in palm of patient's hand. Patient is asked to lift object off the table by extending the wrist. Do not allow elbow flexion.)
2. Sitting, radial deviation of wrist. (Therapist should place forearm in midpronation-supination, that is, resting on ulnar side, thumb in line with forearm and wrist in extension, fingers around a cylindrical object. Patient is asked to lift hand off table. Do not allow elbow flexion or pronation.)
3. Sitting, elbow into side, pronation and supination. (Elbow unsupported and at a right angle. Three-quarter range is acceptable.)
4. Reach forward, pick up large ball 14 cm (5 in.) in diameter with both hands and put it down. (Ball should be on table so far in front of patient that he or she has to extend arms fully to reach it. Shoulders must be protracted, elbows extended, wrist neutral or extended. Palms should be kept in contact with the ball.)
5. Pick up a polystyrene cup from table and put it on table across other side of body. (Do not allow alteration in shape of cup.)
6. Continuous opposition of thumb and each finger more than 14 times in 10 seconds. (Each finger in turn taps the thumb, starting with index finger. Do not allow thumb to slide from one finger to the other or to go backwards.)

VIII. Advanced Hand Activities

1. Picking up the top of a pen and putting it down again. (Patient stretches arm forward, picks up pen top, releases it on table close to body.)
2. Picking up one jellybean from a cup and placing it in another cup. (Teacup contains eight jellybeans. Both cups must be at arms' length. Left hand takes jellybean from cup on right and releases it in cup on left.)
3. Drawing horizontal lines to stop at a vertical line 10 times in 20 seconds. (At least five lines must touch and stop at the vertical line.)
4. Holding a pencil, making rapid consecutive dots on a sheet of paper. (Patient must do at least two dots a second for 5 seconds. Patient picks pencil up and positions it without assistance. Patient must hold pen as for writing. Patient must make a dot not a stroke.)
5. Taking a dessert spoon of liquid to the mouth. (Do not allow head to lower toward spoon. Do not allow liquid to spill.)
6. Holding a comb and combing hair at back of head.

IX. General Tonus

1. Flaccid, limp, no resistance when body parts are handled.
2. Some response felt as body parts are moved.
3. Variable, sometimes flaccid, sometimes good tone, sometimes hypertonic.
4. Consistently normal response.
5. Hypertonic 50% of the time.
6. Hypertonic at all times.

Figure 12-9B.

and to elicit movement. Brunnstrom uses primitive reflexes to stimulate increased tone at this point. The therapist can get the asymmetrical tonic neck reflex by having the patient turn the head, which elicits associated movements in the upper extremity.[41]

In the second stage, when the synergies first appear, the therapist should attempt to strengthen the synergies by working with the patient on associated reactions and on muscle strengthening programs using repetition.[41]

The third stage of recovery is synergy, and isolated muscle components are initiated voluntarily. During this phase, the therapist is attempting to decrease the spastic pattern by using techniques that can break this pattern. The person then progresses to the next phase, and becomes relatively independent. In this phase, the therapist begins to work with normal strengthening patterns. The last phase involves the area of coordination and normal movement, and the therapist works with coordination exercises to facilitate normal movement.[41]

Carr and Shepherd's Approach Other well-accepted physical therapy interventions are the Carr and Shepherd techniques.[49] Their treatment revolves around five principles:

1. Elimination of unnecessary muscle activity.
2. Any human activity becomes better organized and more effective when it is practiced.
3. A muscle response depends on the condition of the muscle at the moment with the following perimeters: length, velocity, temperature, and joint ankle.
4. The body must have the ability to adjust to gravity and change segmental alignment for all motor activities. Therefore, the person must be trained to preserve balance.
5. A learned task is not just doing the task in front of a therapist. A learned task is when a person can do it in a situation without actually thinking.

In their treatment approach, Carr and Shepherd go through four steps: (1) analyze the task, (2) practice the missing component, (3) practice the task as a whole, and (4) transference of training.

An example of this would be a patient who has difficulty standing. First, analyze the difficulty (e.g., hip position). Second, practice the missing component. For instance, the difficulty in standing comes from the patient's hip position (i.e., work with the hip). Third, practice this task (i.e., standing with proper hip position). Fourth, transfer to another activity with the same problem (i.e., standing in the proper position with a slight bend on a stool or a wedge under the foot).[49]

During treatment, motor tasks are practiced in their entirety. There is no "technique," the person is just instructed and manually guided through various deficits. The patient may first be passively placed in the proper position, and then the patient takes over active control. As the patient develops more control, the therapist does less.

The most important component of Carr and Shepherd's approach is the patient's contribution to the effort. Patients are encouraged to do the exercises as often as possible and to keep a notebook of their efforts and responses. In the notebook, the patient is encouraged to write down their actual program progression.[49]

Shoulder Problems in Hemiplegic Shoulder pain in hemiplegia has always been a concern and several clinicians have suggested that excessive distraction on the shoulder may lead to pain.[28,40,49]

In an article by Kumar and associates,[50] the use of overhead pulleys is described as the highest risk of developing shoulder pain for patients with hemiplegia, and it was suggested that this should be strongly discouraged with these patients.[50] In training upper extremity problems, it is preferred to provide increased weight training through the upper extremity, as well as facilitating proper positioning.[40,49]

Bohannon and associates[51] found that it is not necessarily the position that explained the "synergistic" increased force of the elbow strength, but possibly the length of the muscle in various positions. Therefore, in working with the upper extremity, it is important not only to look at the neurological factors, such as tone, but also at the length-to-tension relationship of the muscles. Therapists should facilitate range of motion and proper posture, as well as encourage weight bearing through the upper extremity in the proper position.

Gait Treatment Suggestions The upright control evaluation mentioned earlier differentiated different gait variations. In addition, in the same study from Rancho Los Amigos, the authors outlined a specific program for lower extremity problems.[47] Their treatment techniques revolve around the use of ankle-foot orthotics with various types of dorsiflexion stops, as well as electrical stimulation to the weak areas. For example, if a therapist notices stance deviation of inadequate hip and knee extension, he or she can suggest ankle-foot orthotics with dorsiflexion stops and electrical stimulation to the quadriceps or gluteus maximus for strengthening and facilitation. Inhibitive casting is used for excessive plantar flexion or with increased tone. Prolonged icing is suggested to inhibit tone. The treatment approach is to divide the various phases of gait and treat each separately according to deficit.

Treatment of gait disturbances in the patient with Pusher syndrome requires intact cognition and active patient participation. The focus needs to be on early resumption of upright postures (sitting and standing), transitional movements (supine-to-sit and sit-to-stand), and a concentration on active movements (guided or assisted). The goal is basically to "recalibrate" the patient's perception of upright posture by providing them with feedback about movement outcomes and positional correctness. Maximizing tactile and proprioceptive inputs facilitates correct muscle contraction. Emphasizing stability during early standing with biofeedback for regaining a symmetrical and stable midline position can be accomplished through physical and verbal cues.[52]

In the area of gait, it appears that weight shifting is one of the biggest problems. Patients must be taught the concept of proper weight shifting, which can be done using bicycle ergonometry or EMG for proper muscle use.[51,53]

Despite the various techniques suggested for stroke intervention (ranging from therapeutic exercise to biofeedback), the therapist must be careful to check the efficacy of the various treatment programs.[54] For example, Sackley[55] showed that symmetry and weight shifting strongly correlated with motor function. These components appear to be very important and should be treated vigorously with weight-shifting exercises. In contrast, Trueblood and co-workers[56] showed that pelvic positioning exercises were helpful while the patient did the exercise. However, after the exercise session, stroke patients did not carry the pelvic position into daily activities.[56]

Finally, Logigian and associates[57] showed that both facilitation and traditional exercise improved functional and motor performances and that there was no difference between the two exercises.[57] This study provides food for thought, especially for those working with the geriatric patient. Finding the most appropriate program, working within the patient's tolerance, and reviewing the results that accompany the treatment progression are extremely important for achieving the optimal outcomes.

ALZHEIMER'S DISEASE

A concise discussion of the incidence and etiology of Alzheimer's disease (AD) is provided in chapter 5. This discussion focuses on evaluation, staging, and intervention in patients with AD. The challenge for the geriatric rehabilitation therapist working with AD patients is to apply creative solutions to the problem of finding activities that maintain physical health. Keeping these individuals active enough to generate fitness benefits should be the primary goal of intervention in this population. Avoiding restraints is crucial. While this patient population may appear physically healthy, they are susceptible to falls and other accidents resulting in orthopedic and other types of injuries.

The clinical features of patients with AD are a gradual but relentless onset of symptoms including impairment of recent memory, disorientation, confabulations, and retrogressive loss of remote memories.[58] Over time, reasoning ability, concentration, speech, and handwriting degenerate. In the early phases of the disease motor function is well maintained, however, as the disease progresses neurological involve-

ment often renders the AD patient bedridden. In late stages, patients can deteriorate to a nonfunctional, vegetative state.

Alzheimer's disease is generally staged based on the progression of the disease. Various staging strategies are used, employing as few as three stages and as many as twelve stages, depending on the setting.[59] This therapist uses a four-stage progression scale which is provided in Table 12–9. This staging breaks the disease into early, middle, late, and terminal stages based on symptomatology. Staging allows the health care team to quantify changes in functional and cognitive abilities over time, which helps in establishing a patient's treatment plan. It must be noted, however, that from an outcomes viewpoint, it is unclear whether AD patients do in fact pass through a specific sequence of deterioration. It is unlikely that the "staging" of a patient has any prognostic implications in terms of speed of decline. Staging basically captures a moment in time, that is, the point at which the initial and subsequent evaluations occurred. Nevertheless, there is considerable practical utility in developing some form- ulation of the patient's current functional status since this directly influences decisions for management.

Six different, although overlapping, functional spheres are affected and need to be evaluated in the AD patient. (1) Cognitive or intellectual disturbance is the clinical hallmark of Alzheimer's dementia. This includes symptoms of memory impairment, language disorder, apraxia, visuoconstructive difficulty, and problems with abstract thinking. Common symptoms such as getting lost, failure to recognize familiar faces, and certain types of hallucinations are also manifestations of cognitive disturbance. Tools for testing cognition are presented in Chapter 6. (2) Another important functional domain to assess is the noncognitive function. Changes in affect, personality, and behavior are extremely common, though this aspect of the syndrome is rarely evaluated in any formal manner. There are scales, such as the Blessed Performance of Everyday Activities,[60] and the Alzheimer's Disease Assessment Scale,[61] which do measure features such as irritability, apathy, hyperactivity, and bothersomeness. Depression, anxiety, and delusions may be apparent on psychiatric assessment, however, noncognitive symptoms occur sporadically and do not necessarily coincide with the time of the examination. (3) Neurologic function is usually preserved through the early and middle stages of AD, although seizures, gait disorders, and tremors may occur at any time. In the later stages of the disease, neurologic signs include hyperactive reflexes, increasing primitive tone (gegenhalten), flexion contractures and primitive reflexes. These are tested just as they are tested in neurologically impaired pediatric patients. (4) Activities of daily living (ADL) are affected by cognitive, noncognitive, and elementary neurologic changes. This is another important functional domain to explore in assessing the status of the patient with AD. Tools for assessing

TABLE 12–9. STAGES OF ALZHEIMER'S DISEASE

STAGES	SIGNS AND SYMPTOMS
Early Stage (I)	Forgetfulness Mild memory deficit Difficulty with novel or complex tasks Apathy and social withdrawal
Middle Stage (II)	Moderate to severe objective memory deficit Disorientation to time and place Language disturbance Visuoconstructive difficulty Apraxia Personality and behavioral changes Requires supervision
Late Stage (III)	Intellectual functions virtually untestable Verbal communication severely limited Incapable of self-care Incontinence of bladder and bowel
Terminal Stage (IV)	Unaware of environment Mute Bedridden Joint contractures Pathological reflexes Myoclonus
Associated Coexisting Neurological Disorders	Increased Tone Seizures Movement disorders Gait disorders

function are discussed in Chapter 6. (5) As patients gradually loose the ability to perform many ADL, there is a corresponding increase in their need for assistance. In addition to determining the availability of family members to assist with personal care, one must also probe caregivers understanding of their patient's deficits and their physical and emotional capability to cope satisfactorily with them. (See chapter 9.) (6) Finally, all diseases occur in a psychosocial context, and this aspect assumes special importance in Alzheimer's disease (see Chapter 4). Psychosocial evaluation provides objective data on the patient's social circumstances, as well as an impression of the patient's family; its structure, sociocultural beliefs, attitudes to health and disease, myths, patterns of communication, and degree of psychopathology, if any. Through assessment one can identify the situation and psychosocial stressors that impact on the patient and family and define the coping strategies that they use to meet them, including their ability to seek out appropriate community resources.[62]

Evaluation of the AD patient is challenging from a rehabilitation perspective. Determination of baseline levels in the functional spheres discussed above is important. Physical capabilities, mobility, balance, muscle strength, flexibility, safety, and other physical realms of functioning are important in maintenance of maximal functional capabilities. During the early stages of the disease, the individual is able to follow simple one-step instructions. As the disease progresses, verbal cueing along with physical guidance of movement for testing may be necessary, though often the AD patient becomes anxious and is confused by physical assistance. The AD patient may mimic an activity or perform a task that they are familiar with (such as folding laundry). Using a recognizable activity may be a useful means of evaluating posture, strength, flexibility, endurance, balance, and the like, simply by watching. In fact, the best way to evaluate an AD patient is through observation of functional activities. For instance, the ability to rise from a chair without the use of hands would place the quadriceps strength somewhere in the 3+ (Fair +) grade for Manual muscle test (MMT). Ten different attempts of testing the quadriceps strength in the standardized manner would result in ten different muscle grades. Therefore, the functional activity of rising unassisted from the chair objectively measures functional strength for this activity. The ability to get up from the chair and move immediately away from the chair smoothly without staggering or balance loss would indicate that orthostatic hypotension is not a problem, and at least during that activity, balance is not a problem. Watching an individual don a pair of socks and shoes can give the examiner information about sitting balance, hip and knee flexibility, motor planning, eye-hand coordination, attention span, and numerous other parameters.

In the evaluation of individuals with advancing stages of AD, it is of importance to recognize the neurological signs unique to the AD patient.[63] The primitive reflexes that were encephalized shortly after birth in the human return in virtually the opposite order in which they disappeared in the AD patient. The return of these reflexes is called the "release" phenomena.[63] This represents a reversal of the encephalization process of childhood and gives the only true validity to the aphorism—"once a man, twice a child." In the child, primitive infantile reflexes fade as higher cortical areas develop and exert their control over lower subcortical centers. With Alzheimer's there is a release from this higher control, allowing the re-emergence of these primitive relexes.[64] As the reflexes become more primitive, the clinician can determine the severity of neurological and motor involvement. For instance, in the middle-to-late stages of this disease, the muscle tone termed *gegenhalten tone* (paratonia or "motor negativisim") reappears.[63] It may appear that the patient is tense or unable to relax and is often mistaken for spasticity, or more frequently, parkinsonism. There is nonvolitional resistance to passive motion and the greater the attempt of movement the greater the resistance. This tone is present during fetal life. When there is pressure on a body part in the womb, reflexively the fetus moves (pushes) in that direction (e.g., if a fetus' arm is against the uterine wall, he or she will push in that direction with the arm). This tone returns in the mid-to-late stages of Alzheimer's and becomes severe in the terminal stage. Therefore, a therapist who is attempting to move an extremity with the hands improperly placed may elicit gegenhalten tone rather than the desired movement. This is often interpreted as "patient resistance," when in fact the therapist is facilitating reflexive tone with her hand position. With proper hand placement the extremity can be moved in the intended direction. For example, the therapist can trick this resistance by attempting to move in the opposite direction desired (e.g., if you want extension, try to passively move the extremity into flexion and you'll get extension).

Release signs such as primitive grasp and sucking reflexes occur in most patients in the latter stages of the disease.[63,64] The gabellar tap reflex (Myerson's sign) reappears within days of death.[64] This reflex is stimulated by tapping between the eyebrows. Each tap elicits eye closure, constant pressure will result in maintenance of eye closure. It is thought that this reflex has the purpose of keeping the eyes shut during normal delivery through the birth canal. The palmomental response can be elicited by stroking the thenar eminence and observing contraction of the ipsilateral mentalis muscle (chin on the same side). Primitive oral responses such as the patient puckering their lips in response to percussion of the maxilla just above the lips, or other infantile sucking and rooting reflexes may be noted. An AD patient may reflexively open or clamp their mouth shut as an object is visualized approaching the oral zone. In the terminal stage of AD, the therapist will observe the return of the atonic neck reflex (ATNR), the Morrow and Labyrinth reflexes. These are all very primitive responses and indicative of eminent death.

Seizures and myoclonus also occur in the latter stages of the disease. Myoclonic jerks, whereby an extremity moves spontaneously without apparent stimulus (even when the patient is asleep), are not uncommon in the end phases of AD.

Another neurological sign is abnormality of both saccadic (volitional) and smooth pursuit eye movements. Pursuit movements are slowed and have superimposed compensatory saccades.[63,64] Saccadic disturbances include hypometria in response to predictable targets, prolonged latencies and reduced velocities with unpredicted targets, gaze impersistence, and a visual grasp reflex.[63] Visual field is also affected in the AD patient. There is a decrease in the visual field in patients with dementia of the Alzheimer's type which makes them more susceptible to bumping into door jams, and other objects in their periphery.[65] Steffes and Thralow[65] found that patients with AD have visual field losses significantly greater than other demented patients. Clinically this restriction in visual field appears to be progressive and become more severe as the disease advances. This visual loss is unique to the AD population and has significant ramification in environmental design and safety.[65]

Motor impersistence is also a classic sign. This is an apractic phenomenon resulting in an inability to carry out purposeful, usually spontaneous movements such as walking. The patient will be doing a task, such as walking, and all of a sudden he or she will freeze. In the absence of paralysis or other apparent sensory or motor impairment, the AD patient fails to persist in an action (e.g., doesn't maintain grasp around a cup and nonvolitionally drops the cup). In the latter stages, because of the deterioration of the transcortical spinal track, integration of movement is affected. An ataxic, shuffling, scissoring-type gait pattern coupled with balance and coordination problems are frequently observed. Motor planning deficits including apraxia and agnosia are also seen in AD. Perceptual-motor deficits impede judgment, which may lead to falls.

Extrapyramidal signs, including diminished arm swing, mild rigidity, and loss of facial expression occur in relation to the use of psychotrophic drugs. Generally, if an AD patient showing these signs is taken off a drug, such as Haldol, these extrapyramidal symptoms will disappear.

Treatment in the AD patient is focused on maintaining the highest level of function. Although physical and occupational therapists don't treat the disease itself, when caring for an elderly patient who has Alzheimer's, caregivers can call on their knowledge, compassion, and understanding to help patients achieve rehabilitation goals, despite the challenges associated with this difficult disease. It is rarely indicated in the literature that physical therapy has a direct impact on the course of Alzheimer's, however, therapists can play a primary role in mitigating the disease's impact as a complicating factor throughout the rehabilitation process.

In the early stages of the disease, maintaining physical fitness and providing as much neurosensory stimulus as possible, assists in improving functional capabilities and enhancing overall well-being. In addition to exercise, focus should be placed on good nutrition and minimizing the use of drugs, both prescribed and over-the-counter medications. Providing a structured, protected environment with warmth and emotional support is crucial. Maintenance of a familiar environment is helpful. For instance, if the AD patient is admitted to a nursing home, having their own furniture moved into the facility often helps to improve patient responsiveness and connectedness with their surroundings (see Chapter 4).

Exercise should consist of functionally oriented activities. Walking, performing ADL, dancing, gardening, and the like can be activities that translate into physical fitness. This therapist has found that the use of T'ai Chi, which is similar to dance, is a wonderful means of stimulating a cardiovascular response and has the added benefits of promoting calm and relaxation. Though the use of calisthenic exercises may be employed, the exercise sessions need to be set in a calm environment (paying attention to noise and color—see Chapter 9) and instructions should be kept simple and accompanied by demonstration. Music (classical or new age) is often helpful in the background as it has a calming effect.

The use of a rocking chair also facilitates muscle contraction through reflexive activity. However, Bottomley has observed (and recorded using EMG monitoring) that the primary muscle contractions occur in flexor groups while the extensor groups remain relatively inactive. (Remember: Extension equals Function). A wonderful substitute that Bottomley has discovered is the seated hammock. When the AD patient is in the hammock it can be swung backwards, forwards, sideways, and twisted to set it into a rotational pattern. All trunk muscles, in addition to extremity rotators, flexors, and extensors, have been observed to contract using this modality. This therapist is currently working with a group of students to collect data related to the use of this modality for strengthening, flexibility, and overall neurosensory stimulation. An added advantage to the seated hammock has been the discovery that it appears to be an effective tool in managing *sundowning*. Sundowning, which is a phenomenon unique to the AD patient, is a syndrome characterized by restlessness, excitement, increased confusion, hallucinations, and agitation seen in the late afternoon or early evening in patients in the middle and late stages of Alzheimer's disease.[62]

A primary emphasis in treating the AD patient must be the prevention of falls. As with any aging patient, falls in people with AD are often precipitated by a number of intrinsic risk factors. Additionally, AD is associated with specific cognitive and systemic effects that place individuals at increased fall risk. Any significant loss of cognitive function can result in:

- Lack of understanding and awareness of their potential for falls;
- Need for assistance;
- Judgmental errors, inability to recognize dangers; and misperception of environmental hazards;
- Overestimation of capacity for safe mobility resulting in attempts to do things without assistance;
- Failing to remember limitations in ADL;
- Insistence on performing activities, such as getting out of bed or going to the bathroom without assistance because of forgetfulness or failure to understand the intervention (such as the use of bed rails);
- Inability to ask for assistance with mobility because of communication problems, such as word finding or aphasia;
- Refusing or forgetting to use assistive devices (canes, walkers, grab rails) when indicated;
- Inability to understand the correct use of assistive devices (Note: the authors of this book avoid using assistive devices whenever possible due to the inherent dangers);

- Behavioral manifestation such as wandering, pacing agitation, restlessness, disorientation, hallucinations, delusions, irritability, and anxiety, which can result in attention deficits and worsening cognition;
- Sundowning—disruptive behaviors that appear during the late afternoon or evening (associated with dusk and darkness).

With respect to visual performance, AD is associated with an excess of dysfunction that is beyond what would be expected on the basis of age or underlying disease as discussed above. Significant visual problems that may lead to falls in the AD patient include:

- Restriction of visual fields (loss of peripheral vision; homonymous hemianopia);
- Decrease in visuospatial function (ability to match and integrate the position of self and objects in the environment);
- Decline in depth perception (ability to judge distances and relationship among objects in the visual field);
- Loss of contrast sensitivity (ability to perceive colors and dark from light);
- Agnosia (decreased recognition of familiar objects and places).

Last, numerous gait and balance abnormalities are associated with AD and include:

- Apraxia (inability to perform routine motor tasks);
- Loss of proprioception (awareness of posture, movement, and changes in equilibrium)—
  - Decreased stride length;
  - Decreased step height, shuffling;
  - Decreased speed of walking with bradykinesia and latent balance reactions;
  - Cautious gait. Alzheimer's patients have a classic gait pattern generally characterized by a wide base of support, flexed posture, and short, shuffling steps that are especially prominent when turning. They can be uncertain of their step or foot placement, and may hold arms tightly to their sides or crossed in front of them without arm swing. (Appears in early stages of AD.)
- Frontal lobe gait disorder characterized by a wide base of support, slightly flexed posture, and small, shuffling, hesitant steps. (Appears in late stages of AD.)
- Gait initiation failure characterized by a delay during the first few steps of walking; as a result, the body sometimes moves forward before the feet start to move, placing individuals at risk for balance loss;
- Motor impersistence in which normally automatic motions (e.g., left foot-right foot alternating foot pattern) are frozen or abruptly stopped;
- Motor incoordination in which normally automatic motions such as alternating foot pattern are disrupted, so that patient takes two or three steps with the right foot without moving the left (may be completely thrown off center of gravity);

■ Disequilibrium failure—characterized by an inability to maintain stability during postural challenges, such as standing on one foot or stepping over obstacles in the path.

While these factors by themselves increase fall susceptibility, their relationship to the likelihood of falling is more accurately reflected by their effects on mobility—the ability of the AD person to ambulate and transfer independently and safely in their living environment.

The risk of fall-related injury in AD is dependent on several intrinsic and extrinsic factors operating simultaneously. For example, the risk of sustaining a hip fracture is enhanced by the presence of poor vision, neuromuscular diseases resulting in a loss of protective reflexes, difficulty rising from a chair, osteoporosis, decreased adipose tissue surrounding the hip, the height from which the fall occurs (e.g., elevated beds, climbing over side rails, falling down stairs), and falls against harder surfaces (e.g., nonabsorptive linoleum, concrete, or wooden floors).

The management approach advocated for all older persons who fall, or are at risk, is appropriate for AD patients. These strategies are discussed in the subsequent section of this chapter.

The accumulated effects of medical diseases, altered cognition, medications, and resulting functional abilities, combined with extrinsic factors, predispose many AD patients to falls, and subsequently cause them. However, the degree of individual fall risk and the etiology, or causes, of falls among persons with AD varies considerably. Because of interindividual variability, both assessment and intervention should be customized to meet each AD patient's needs.

Patients with chronic neuromuscular disorders affecting gait and balance may respond to a number of rehabilitative strategies. These include exercise, proper footwear, hip-protective pads (this therapist uses ice hockey shorts), and limited use of ambulation devices to assist with mobility when warranted.

In AD patients, a daily program of walking can offset altered gait and balance problems that usually result from inactivity (e.g., strength, coordination, postural control). Also, habitual exercise may improve cognitive functioning (see Chapter 5) and reduce falls that result from poor judgment. Low intensity strengthening, stretching, and range-of-motion exercises can improve muscle strength and joint flexibility, and help to maintain or restore cardiovascular conditioning and endurance, and improve functional capabilities (e.g., ambulation, transfers) and safety.

BALANCE AND FALLS

In the elderly, falls often precipitate a series of events with catastrophic potential. The fear of falling is a major concern for many elderly persons. This fear is restrictive and constraining and often results in functional losses and substantially increases the risk of falls. It results in withdrawal, a progressive decrease in activity, and a steady decline in the quality of life and mental well-being.[66]

The maintenance of posture and the ability to move about the environment depend on orientation and balance.[67] Orientation, the awareness of the relationship of the body and body parts to each other and to the environment in a dynamic and reciprocal interaction, is a complex function that relies on multiple sensory input and central nervous system integrity. Likewise, balance is the process by which individuals maintain and move their bodies in relationship to the environment, and requires an automatic and unconscious process to resist the destabilizing effect of gravity. Balance is essential for purposeful movement and effective function. Many central nervous system disorders affect both.

The complexity of the integrated neurosensory system, as the following discussion reveals, translates to balance problems in the elderly. Dysfunction in any one of the components of balance will affect motor control. An older person may have postural changes affecting her or his center of gravity, mobility of the neck, thoracic, and lumbar spines may be limited. Elders frequently have poor neck rotation and extension capabilities. Muscles may be weak and inflexible. Joints may be restricted or contracted. Vision may be diminished. The vestibular system may not be working correctly due to dehydration, either due to self-restriction of fluids (to prevent incontinence), medical restriction of fluids (often related to the use of diuretic drugs), or drugs that cause dehydration. Gait patterns may be slow, with poor foot clearance or inaccurate foot placement. The older adult may be confused and misinterpret neurosensory and neuromuscular cues. Numerous pathologies can lead to a higher likelihood of falling.

To achieve balance, the body's center of gravity (COG) must be perpendicular to the center of support. This is accomplished through the integration by the central nervous system of information received from sensory organs and through the execution of coordinated and synchronized movements.[68] A loss of balance occurs when the sensory information about the position of the COG is inaccurate, when the execution of automatic right movements is inadequate, or when both are present. The postural control system receives information from receptors in the proprioceptive, visual, and vestibular systems. All of these systems, in addition to appropriate motor function, need to be intact for ultimate balance control.

Somatosensory inputs provide information about the position of the body and body parts relative to each other and to the support surface. The somatosensory input the brain receives from muscles and joints stems from sensory receptors called proprioceptors. These proprioceptors are sensitive to pressure and the stretching motion in the tissues that surrounds them. For instance, the impulses that come from the mechanoreceptor in the neck, which indicate head position and movement, and impulses that come from the ankles and the bottom of the feet, which indicate the movement of the body over the base of support are important in maintaining balance. Somatosensory inputs are the dominant sensory information for balance when the body is standing still on a fixed, firm surface, or moving through the environment. Conditions that alter sensory input, such as cerebral vascular accidents, peripheral neuropathies or nutritional deficits (see Chapter 7) may affect input and subsequent interpretation of somatosensory information.[48]

Vision informs the individual about the physical environment and the relation of the body relative to the surroundings. Visual input is the primary back-up when the somatosensory system is deficient.[69] It is not uncommon for an older adult to have visual changes or pathologies (see Chapters 3 and 5), which can play a major role in balance loss when the support system is precarious. Balance also involves the ability to stabilize gaze.

The vestibular system originates in the inner ear from five balance receptor sites. These sites are located in three semicircular canals (anterior, horizontal, and posterior) and two sacs (the saccule and the utricle). Each semicircular canal lies roughly perpendicular to the other two. When a person rotates her or his head in the plane of a particular canal, the endolymphatic fluid within the canal lags behind the movement of the canal. The fluid pushes against sensory receptors (hair cells) in the canal and temporarily bends them. This bending of the hair cells in the inner ear sends impulses to the brain via the nervous system. This mechanism varies slightly when people change their head position or move their head in a straight line. Calcium carbonate crystals produced naturally by the body make the hair cells of the saccule and utricle react to the pull of gravity or to translational movement of the head. The hair cells in the saccule and utricle send messages to the CNS. When both inner ears are functioning properly, the vestibular system sends symmetrical messages to the brain.

The vestibular system has both a sensory and a motor function, and measures the head's angular velocity and linear acceleration and detects head position relative to the gravitational axis. This is a sensory function. Head angular velocity is measured by the cristae of semicircular canals, while the maculae of the statolabyrinth (utricle and saccule) register linear acceleration and changes in gravitational force. Because the vestibular system senses head motion, it is less sensitive to body sway than is the visual or the somatosensory system.[70] When somatosensory and visual information are adequate, the vestibular system plays a minor role in the control of the COG position. Its role is dominant when there is a conflict between visual and somatosensory information and during ambulation.[67,71]

The component of motor function controlled by the vestibular system input is muscular activity. During erect posture, it initiates transitory muscular contractions and controls muscle tone. In addition, it assists in stabilizing gaze during head and body movements by generating conjugate, smooth eye movements opposite in direction and approximately of equal velocity to head movements.[72] The vestibulo-ocular reflex stabilizes gaze during target fixation and unsuspected perturbation of head and body position. Gaze stabilization is essential for clear vision; it results from the combined effect of the vestibulo-ocular reflex on the nuclei of the extraocular muscles, neck proprioception, and the position of images on the retina.[67]

The vestibulospinal reflex initiates the compensatory body movements necessary to maintain posture and to stablize the head over the trunk.[68] There are positional, acceleratory, and righting vestibulospinal reflexes.[72] The positional reflexes are initiated by a change in the support surface. The acceleratory reflexes, attributed to the semicircular canals, assist in tilt detection and sway displacement. Righting reflexes tend to keep the head in an upright position and facilitate contraction of the neck receptors and the axial musculature.[73]

The central neurological component, termed the vestibular-nuclear complex, is located in the pons and consists of four major nuclei and seven minor ones. It processes information from the peripheral vestibular system and the visual, proprioceptive, tactile, and auditory system. The vestibular nuclei are extensively connected to the cerebellum, to the nuclei of the extraocular muscles, and to the reticular formation in the brainstem.[73]

The cerebellum plays a prominent role in regulating the output of the vestibulospinal system through extensive reciprocal connections with the vestibular nuclei. Cerebellar lesions can result in severe postural disturbance.[74]

Located beneath the skin, pressure sensors measure the intensity of contact made by the different parts of the body with the environment. These sensors play a dominant role in the maintenance of balance as they relay information about the base of support.[70]

The inertial-gravitational reference provided by the vestibular system is critical to the resolution of sensory conflicts between visual and vestibular inputs and between spinal and vestibular inputs. The vestibular inputs are critical to the selection of appropriate postural movement strategies. The cerebellum and basal ganglia help to mediate visual, vestibular, and proprioceptive interactions and coordinate the proprioceptive reflexes subserving balance.[72] Information from proprioceptive, visual, vestibular, auditory, tactile, and stretch receptors in various organs is integrated to create a picture of the position and movements of the body parts relative to each other and to the environment. This picture is stored and constantly upgraded. It is the essence for all body movement and the determinant for sudden and rapid corrective motor activity.

Impaired balance, often seen in older patients, is the result of inaccurate information about the position of the COG, inadequately executed movements to bring the COG to a balanced position, or a combination of both. Vestibular information for body orientation is particularly important for an elderly individual who lacks good somatosensory or visual cues for orientation. Equilibrium is maintained through a flexible postural synergy.[75] When deterioration in the function of one or more systems subserving the balance function is progressive, as frequently seen in aging, balance remains unaffected as long as the central nervous system is able to adapt and to compensate for these functional changes. Disequilibrium is the consequence of inadequate balance function.[76] Imbalance will not manifest as long as compensation is adequate for the tasks at hand. Whenever the demands on the system exceed the function capabilities, however, instability becomes evident. As functional competence continues to deteriorate, imbalance becomes more prevalent. Chronic instability occurs when the compensating strategies can no longer offset the functional decline.

Falls occur whenever the righting reflexes are either insufficient or too slow to counter the force of attraction exerted by the earth's gravity on an individual. In the elderly, falls are usually the result of the accumulation of multiple chronic disabilities. Falling is a clinical entity in its own right in the practice of geriatrics. Falls are potentially preventable if the causative factors can be recognized and addressed.[77] Diminished alertness, poor concentration, general fatigue, drug-induced sedation or dizziness, and impaired situational judgment increase the likelihood of falls.

Age-related morphologic changes occur in all body systems, including those essential for the maintenance of posture. As discussed in Chapter 3, aging has been shown to be associated with a significant loss of hair cells in the vestibular sensors, a decrease of primary vestibular neurons, a diminution in the neuronal cell density of the cerebral cortex, and a decrease in the number of Purkinje's cells in the cerebellum. In addition, there are degenerative changes in the sensory and motor systems, in the tendon receptors of the lower extremities, and in the musculoskeletal system.

The vestibulo-ocular reflex gain and dominant time constant decrease with age.[78] This is probably the result of a combination of age-related changes in the hair cells at the center of the cristae,[79] a relatively selective loss of large-diameter primary vestibular afferents, and neuronal loss in the superior vestibular nuclei.[79,80] The superior vestibular nucleus is a major relay for the canal-ocular reflex.

Changes in the vestibulospinal reflex are difficult to assess because of functional overlap with sensory and motor functions. Distinction among vestibulospinal, visual, and somatosensory dysfunction is difficult in the elderly.[81] The increased body sway seen after the age of 60 is the consequence of cumulative degenerative changes in the vestibular, proprioceptive, sensory, and musculoskeletal systems.[82] Increased body sway shrinks the limits of stability. As the COG moves rapidly, the momentum of the body acts as an additional destabilizing force.

The visual system is of most importance in the control of balance, especially in the aged.[80] Degenerative ocular changes, such as macular degeneration and cataract, decrease the visual acuity and contribute to instability. Because vision operates slowly, when an older person loses balance, the visually guided postural reflexes do not react quickly enough to prevent a fall.

The elderly have a tendency to walk flexed forward, with the head fixed to the trunk or flexed at the neck and the eyes fixating on the ground in front of them. Such a stance places the COG in a forward position—that is, close to the anterior periphery of the limits of stability. In addition, this impairs orientation by limiting the visual field. The forward position of the head also alters the position of the statolabyrinth relative to the gravitational axis.

Instability manifests as an exaggeration of the COG sway and is the expression of the difficulty encountered in resisting the destabilizing effects of gravity. It is the consequence of the interaction between normally functioning and abnormally functioning components that result in functionally inappropriate and/or ineffective balance response.[72] As the destabilizing forces increase or the corrective measures become inadequate, or both, sway oscillations increase.

The amplitude of the COG sway, therefore, is representative of an individual's difficulty in achieving balance, and the amplitude and velocity of the sway are proportional to the difficulty experienced counteracting gravity.

The COG sway can be measured by computer analysis of information received from a force plate on which the individual stands, or can be assessed using the Romberg's test or the Functional Reach Test described in Chapter 6. Computerized dynamic posturography (Senory Organization Test) was introduced as a means to assess the vestibular, visual, and proprioceptive contributions to posture and the ability of the central nervous system to integrate sensory information.[83] Romberg's test measures the central neurological involvement of proprioceptive loss, though it is insensitive to the detection of labyrinthine impairment.[84] The functional reach test measures the extent of movement within the cone of stability to determine the distance from the COG prior to balance loss forward and sideways.[85] In each of these evaluations, the clinician is looking for appropriate motor responses to balance perturbation. Measurements in the computerized sensory organization test are taken with the individuals eyes opened and closed and after introducing conflicting visual and proprioceptive information. This tool assesses balance, but does not provide localizing or lateralizing information in the neurologic sense. It does not directly assess peripheral or central vestibular function, though it is a objective technique for the appraisal of a patient's functional ability[86] and a predictor of falls.[87]

The evaluation of an elderly patient with a vestibular disorder can be a most challenging task. The great overlap that exists between the different systems that subserve the balance function renders the interpretation of measurements of the vestibulo-ocular and the vestibulospinal reflexes difficult. Because of the effects of adaptation and habituation, these measurements do not reflect an organic loss but rather functional loss that remains uncompensated for at the time the measurements are made.

In the evaluation of vestibular disorders in the elderly, there is no gold standard, rather, experienced clinicians make use of the history, physical examination, assessment of drug regimes and diet, and a medley of laboratory tests, as well as their own best judgment regarding a particular individual. For instance, clinical experience has taught that subtle differences in testing outcomes occur. When testing for vestibular involvement, head movements are used to elicit nystagmus of the eyes, a positive finding. Vertebral artery impingement testing, as well as central nervous system involvement, also results in nystagmus of the eyes as a positive indicator of involvement. How do you differentiate? When the nystagmic movements are jerky, it is usually vestibular involvement. When the nystagmic movements are smooth and rhythmical, the patient generally has central nervous system or circulatory involvement. It is important to thoroughly question the older adult relative to the circumstances that cause dizziness. Table 12–10 provides a summary of some of the complaints older persons may relay to their therapist regarding episodes of dizziness; determining what those symptoms "feel like" may assist the clinician in pinpointing the causes of dizziness.

In the elderly, the causes of unsteadiness and falls are multifactoral and overlapping. The approach to the management of an elderly individual with unsteadiness encompasses more than the diagnosis of the disease entity or entities that are causing the problem. Often, there is no consistent relationship between anatomic abnormalities and physical signs, nor between physical signs and resulting function. The presence of fear of falling can greatly confound any evaluative tests. Nonetheless, comprehensive assessment and evaluation of an elderly patient with balance problems should include:

■ Measurement of the functional competence of the vestibular, visual, proprioceptive, sensory, auditory, and musculoskeletal systems;

TABLE 12–10. ELDER'S DESCRIPTION OF DIZZINESS: PINPOINTING THE CAUSE

Patient Complaint	Possible Cause
Dizziness "Feels Like" Vertigo	
❑ Certain head positions trigger it.	Benign paroxysmal positional vertigo (BPPV), in which small calcium stones in the inner ear's otolith (gravity detectors) become dislodged and start floating.
❑ Ringing in the ears or hearing loss.	Ménière's syndrome, a result of fluid buildup in the inner ear (with pain, pressure, or fullness). In rare cases, could be a slow-growing tumor pressing on the auditory nerve.
❑ Dizziness provoked by loud noises.	The result of head trauma or, in rare cases, thinning of the bony cover of the inner ear, which can lead to a fistula, or abnormal opening through which fluids can pass.
❑ Difficulty swallowing or speaking, or feel weakness or numbness in face or limbs.	Stroke or a tumor.
❑ Recent cold or flu.	A viral infection in the inner ear (labyrinthitis).
❑ Taking medications.	Drug side effects. Long-term use or high doses of many drugs (sleeping pills, alcohol, tranquilizers, antidepressants, blood pressure medications) can cause dizziness, and sometimes vertigo.
Dizziness "Feels Like" Physical Loss of Balance	
❑ Neurological or neuroendocrine disease.	Neuropathy.
❑ Age-related changes.	Multisensory deficit, a blunting of neurosensory input, such as vision, hearing, proprioception, kinesthetic sense. Decrease in muscle strength, endurance, flexibility. Poor posture. Cardiovascular changes.
Dizziness "Feels Like" Lightheadedness or Near Fainting	
❑ Sweating, racing heart, fast tilation, tachycardia.	Anxiety, which can cause dizziness as blood pressure drops, hypervenbreathing.
❑ High blood pressure, heart or vascular disease.	Insufficient blood to brain due to poor circulation.
❑ Dizzy when standing.	Orthostatic hypotension, hypothyroidism, anemia, B12 deficiency, or diabetes.
❑ Sweating, trembling, feel shaky and hungry.	Low blood sugar from poor food ingestion or diabetes.
❑ Taking medications.	Side effects of drugs. Polypharmacy--drug interactions.

- Evaluation of gait and movement patterns;[88]
- Evaluation of cognitive function and psychological characteristics;
- Determination of the impact of the functional loss (physiologic, functional, social, and societal) on the particular individual.

The goal of a treatment program in rehabilitation is to prevent impairments by optimizing function. The authors strongly believe that many of the balance and fall problems seen in an older adult population are related to inactivity. In other words, patients fall when they are attempting to perform activities that they have not practiced in a long while. Therefore balance reorganization strategies are the cornerstone of the management of balance disorders, especially in the elderly. Intervention should promote orientation, gaze stabilization, postural realignment, muscle strength, and joint mobility. Practicing activities, such as standing of one foot or varying the walking surfaces, enhance the integration of the input or affect the way the brain responds to a deficit in one or more of the three sensory systems (e.g., somatosensory, visual, vestibular). The improvement to be expected depends on accurate assessment of the multisystem causes of the imbalance, functional conceptualization of the exercises, severity of the impairments, the general physical and mental health of the patient, patient motivation, and family support.

Patients should be encouraged to incorporate exercises that challenge their COG into their daily routines and to use new strategies in their everyday activities. The home environment should be made safe as discussed in Chapter 9. Despite all efforts, when the COG can no longer be maintained over the base of support provided by the two feet, the base of support may need to be extended with the use of a cane, walker, or other assistive devices.

Too many elderly individuals with imbalance and dizziness receive inappropriate and ineffectual care, simply because of the bias that they are falling because they are old. Falls are not an inevitable consequence of aging changes, although age-related changes may predispose an older individual to falls. In many cases, falls can be prevented. Table 12–11 provides a list of age-related changes that increase the risk of falls. Strengthening, flexibility, postural, and balance-challenging activities can actually decrease the risk of falling. Home modifications with a focus on safety can be made, especially for activities such as walking to the bathroom at night (providing night lighting, a clear path), going up or down stairs (providing railings and sufficient lighting on nonskid stairs), cooking activities (placing most commonly used utensils in easily accessible location, improving kitchen lighting, providing a stool for counter activities). Counseling and balance reorganization strategies have proven successful in the management of balance dysfunction in the elderly.

TABLE 12–11. AGE-RELATED CHANGES THAT INCREASE THE RISK OF FALLS

Gait Changes
❏ Decreased step height, poor foot clearance
❏ Narrow-based waddling gait pattern
❏ Shorter step, wider base
❏ Slower movement (stop/start gait pattern)
❏ Shuffling (no heel strike or push off)
❏ Decreased ankle dorsiflexion

Postural Instability
❏ Increase in body sway, both lateral and anterior-posterior
❏ Decreased responsiveness of sensory receptors that alert muscle to contract when movement is away from the center of gravity
❏ Co-contraction of antagonists and agonists upon balance perturbation
❏ Weakening of muscles (anterior tibialis, knee extensors and flexors, hip extensors and abductors, trunk and neck extensors)
❏ Forward flexed posture shifting center of gravity beyond toes

Vision Diminished
❏ Decrease light entering eye secondary to opacities
❏ Cataracts
❏ Presbyopia (far sightedness)—increased time required for near/far adaptation
❏ Increase in interocular pressure (black "floaters" in field of vision) secondary to dehydration or hypertension
❏ Diminished color perception, especially blue-green perception (cataracts—can't see red, orange)
❏ Increased time required for light/dark adaptation
❏ Increased glare (especially with macular degeneration)

Hearing Reduced
❏ Reduced ability to hear high frequency sounds
❏ Reduced tendency to notice approaching car, bicycle on sidewalk, bus, siren, etc.
❏ Startles easily

Sense of Touch Diminished
❏ Somatosensory loss
❏ Unable to detect change in support surface

Cognitive Changes
❏ Confused by environment
❏ Inattentive
❏ Decreased level of alertness
❏ Poor judgement

Orthostatic Hypotension
❏ Drop of 20 mm Hg in systolic blood pressure when assuming upright position
❏ Decrease blood supply to brain with lightheadedness upon standing
❏ Decreased efficiency of baroreceptors

Nocturia
❏ Decreased bladder capacity
❏ Delay in signal to void
❏ Post mictoration syncope
❏ Urgency to reach bathroom
❏ Frequency during the night—half asleep or with poor lighting

Intervention does not necessarily need to be a formal exercise program. Simply increasing daily activities may be the trick to practicing movement. Many times elderly people fall because they are so inactive. Because inactivity reduces muscle function, flexibility, and strength, as exercise program which focuses on the involved muscle groups can greatly help an elderly person. A study by Tinetti and associates[89] confirmed the importance of activity. This study found that community-dwelling people at least 75 years old with low mobility test scores were nearly twice as likely to fall as those who had high mobility scores. Staying in shape can prevent the "trip and fall" syndrome commonly caused by the deteriorating sensory system associated with inactivity. Exercise/activity prevents this deterioration and keeps the fine motor sensory system finely tuned and increases overall muscle strength and endurance.

Intervention should be directed toward sensory and motor, peripheral, and central impairments specific to the individual. It is important to identify those impairments which can be rehabilitated and those which will require compensation strategies. Cognition as well as perceptual problems may affect the ability to relearn skills or acquire new ones. Optimal learning for motor control, skilled movements, and balance requires:

- Patient's knowledge of abilities and limitations;
- Patient's knowledge of the environmental risks and advantages;
- Knowledge of the critical components of the task to be performed;
- Problem-solving abilities, using the knowledge sets listed above;
- The ability to modify and adapt movements as the task and environment changes.

With older individuals, using practice and feedback to teach motor skills requires repetition of the activity, as well as modifying lighting, surfaces, background distractions, and other environmental conditions that challenge their concen- tration as well as their balance. Treatment should be multi-impairment oriented with tasks and environments selected to stimulate involved systems.

The less sensory information available, the more difficult the task of balancing. Initially, treatment might start by providing adequate sensory inputs (somatosensory, visual, vestibular) with augmented feedback if sensory channels are deficient. Progression of the treatment would then add the challenge of manipulating visual, somatosensory, or vestibular inputs so that equilibrium is taxed in varying conditions.

To stimulate the somatosensory system, a stable surface for standing can be provided and the other senses modified (eyes open, eyes closed, practicing in low lighting). Eyes closed with weight shifting during standing can further challenge the somatosensory system.

To stimulate the use of visual inputs, treatments that disrupt the somatosensory system (destabilize) are helpful. For instance, the use of rocker boards, BAPS boards, Fitters™, and foam pads will provide differing stimuli to the somatosensory system and en- courage the visual system to assume a dominant role in determining where the individual is in relation to their environment. Varying the surface for walking with different levels of light can also challenge this system.

The vestibular system can be stimulated by practicing activity on unstable or compliant surfaces with vision either absent (eyes closed), destabilized (eye movements or head movements), or confused (background movements, activity). Adding head movements to any activity will place the vestibular organ at different angles in relationship to gravity. Gaze stabilization (keeping a stationary object in focus) while moving the head or body is also a helpful approach in the elderly. Starting slow and gradually increasing the rate of head or body movement is a excellent stimulus to the vestibular system. Gaze stabilization with head movement while standing or walking on uneven surfaces increases the challenge. Head movements should be practiced in whatever direction provokes dizziness. Though it is beyond the scope of this chapter to discuss all the possible exercise protocols for treating vestibular disorders, in general, quick movements of the head, head tilts, or forward/backward and side-to-side will progressively challenge and improve the vestibular response to movement.[90] It is also important to keep in mind the importance of proper hydration.

Challenging the center of gravity should be done in sitting, sit-to-stand and stand-to-sit, standing balance, strategy training (e.g., stimulating the ankle, hip, and stepping responses with sternal nudges or decentralizing activities), and during gait (e.g., obstacle courses).

Another treatment consideration should be footwear. An older person should be fitted with supportive, flat-soled, non-slip and non-stick soles, with a good heel counter and adequate room in the shoe for the foot. Elderly individuals often fall because of poor foot gear.

Many balance exercises can be incorporated into home activities. The older persons should be instructed to do things, such as standing tasks, in a corner or near a counter to initially enhance their stability. The community setting is a natural challenge for gaining postural control. Grocery or library aisles, public transport systems, elevators, escalators, lawns, beaches, ramps, trails, hills, and varied environmental conditions can provide a challenge to the balance with significant functional relevance.

CONCLUSION

This chapter has built upon the discussion of specific biological changes that occur with age or pathology. Neurological dysfunction seen in the aging process as well as the common major pathologies of Parkinson's disease and cerebral vascular accidents (CVA) were discussed in terms of prevalence, efficacy of treatment interventions, evaluation, and treatment strategies. Evaluation and treatment of Alzheimer's disease was presented and a discussion focusing on balance and falls, evaluation of the numerous causes of dizziness and physical changes that increase the risk of falling and treatment interventions aimed at decreasing the incidence of falls was provided.

PEARLS

- *Parkinson's disease is the number one neurological disease in the elderly.*
- *The most common symptoms of Parkinson's disease are slowness with ADLs, shuffling, tremor, difficulty with speech, and erratic movements.*
- *When assessing and treating Parkinson patients, it is imperative to thoroughly assess and discriminate between direct, indirect, and composite impairments when designing treatment interventions.*
- *Parkinson patients may respond to a specific evaluation and treatment progression as outlined by Schenkman, the well-known Flewitt-Handford exercises, or group classes.*
- *Numerous methods exist for assessing older stroke patients. Schenkman, Bobath, Brunnstrom, Olney and Coulbourne, Rancho Los Amigos, and Carr and Shepherd have the greatest functional emphasis and applicability to geriatric rehabilitation.*
- *Pusher syndrome is a central neurological problem in 10% of patients following stroke and results in postural imbalance due to ipsilateral pushing or lateropulsion.*
- *Treatment strategies for stroke range from those devised by Bobath to Brunnstrom to Carr and Shepherd; when modified for the aged, the most functional aspects of each are stressed.*
- *The hemiplegic shoulder can respond to modalities, proper sling use, and appropriate exercise.*
- *Exercise and rehabilitation can help the older patient to improve in function. To date, no specific technique has been statistically shown to have superior results, however.*
- *The primitive reflexes that were encephalized shortly after birth in the human return in virtually the opposite order in which they disappeared, as Alzheimer's disease progresses.*
- *Exercise should consist of functionally oriented activities in the Alzheimer's population.*
- *The maintenance of posture and the ability to move about the environment depend on orientation and balance.*
- *The postural control system receives information from receptors in the proprioceptive, visual, and vestibular systems.*

REFERENCES

1. Schenkman M, Butler R. A model for multisystem evaluation, interpretation and treatment of individuals with neurologic dysfunction. *Phys Ther.* 1989; 69(7):538–547.
2. Topp B. Towards a better understanding of Parkinson's disease. *Ger Nurs.* July/August 1987; 180–182.
3. Mutch W, Strudwick A, Sisare R, et al. Parkinson's disease: disability, review and management. *Br Med J.* 1986; 293(9):675–677.
4. Wilson J, Smith R. The prevalence and aeitology of long-term L dopa side effects in elderly Parkinson's patients. *Age Ageing.* 1989; 18:11–16.
5. Amenoff MJ. Parkinson's disease in the elderly: current management strategies. *Geriatrics.* 1987; 42(7): 31–37.
6. Hoehn M, Yahr M. Parkinsonism: onset, progression and mortality. *Neurology.* 1967; 17(5): 427–442.
7. Greer M. Recent developments in the treatment of Parkinson's disease. *Geriatrics.* 1985; 40(2):34–41.
8. Banks M. Physiotherapy benefits patients with Parkinson's disease. *Clin Rehab.* 1989; 3:11–16.
9. Schenkman M, Butler R. A model for multisystem evaluation treatment for individuals with Parkinson's disease. *Phys Ther.* 1989; 69(11):932–943.
10. Webster D. Critical analysis of the disability in Parkinson's disease. *Mod Treat.* 1968; 5:257–282.
11. Weinrich M, Koch K, Garcia F, et al. Axial versus distal motor impairment in Parkinson's disease. *Neurology.* 1988; 38(4):540-,545.
12. Murray MP, Sepic S, Gardner G, et al. Walking patterns of men with parkinsonism. *Am J Phys Med.* 1978; 57(6):278–294.
13. Henderson C, Kennard C, Crawford S, et al. Scales for rating motor impairment in Parkinson's disease: studies of reliability and convergent validity. *J Neur Psych.* 1991; 54(1):18–24.
14. Alba A, Trainor F, Ritter W, et al. A clinical disability rating for Parkinson's disease. *J Chron Dis.* 1968; 21:507–522.
15. Schenkman M, Donovan J, Tsubota J. Management of individuals with Parkinson's disease: rationale and case studies. *Phys Ther.* 1989; 69(11):944–955.
16. Hallet M. Physiology and pathophysiology of voluntary movement. In: Tyler K, Dawson D, eds. *Current Neurology.* Boston: Houghton-Mifflin; 1979: 351–376.
17. Saal JS, ed. *Flexibility Training and Rehabilitation of Sports Training.* Philadelphia: Hardey & Belfus; 1987.
18. Nelson A. Lecture Notes. New York: Hospital for Special Surgery; September 1988.
19. Handford F. The Flewitt-Handford exercises for Parkinson's gait. *Physiotherapy.* 1986; 72(8):382.
20. Davis J. Team management of Parkinson's disease. *Am J Occup Ther.* 1977; 31(5):300–308.
21. Rusin M. Stroke rehabilitation: a geropsychological perspective. *Arch Phys Med Rehab.* October 1990; 71:914–920.
22. Centers for Disease Control and Prevention. *Unrealized Prevention Opportunities: Reducing the Health and Economic Burden of Chronic Disease.* Atlanta, GA: Centers for Disease Control and Prevention, National Center for Chronic Disease Prevention and Health Promotion; 1997.
23. Robins M, Baum H. Incidents. *Stroke.* 1981; 12 (suppl 1):45–57.

24. Kelley R. Cerebral vascular disease. In: Weiner W, Goetz C, eds. *Neurology for the NonNeurologists.* 2nd ed. Philadelphia: Lippincott; 1989:52–66.

25. Gillum R. Stroke in blacks. *Stroke.* 1988; 19:1–9.

26. Baxter D. Clinical syndromes associated with stroke. In: Brandstater M, Basmajian JV, eds. *Stroke Rehabilitation.* Baltimore: Williams and Wilkins; 1987: 36–54.

27. Dawson D Adams P. Current estimates from the National Health Interview Survey. United States 1986 National Center for Health Statistics. *Vital Health Statistics* 1987; 10:164.

28. Ryerson S. Hemiplegia resulting from vascular insult or disease. In Umphred D, ed. *Neurological Rehabilitation.* 4th edition St Louis: Mosby; 2001.

29. Spriggs D, French J, Murdy J, et al. Historical risk factors for stroke—a case controlled study. *Age Ageing.* 1990; 19:280–287.

30. Ashburn D, Ward C. Asymmetrical trunk posture, unilateral neglect and motor performance following stroke. *Clinical Rehab.* 1994; 8(1):48–53.

31. Bohannon R. Correction of recalcitrant lateropulsion through motor relearning. *Phys Ther Case Reports.* 1998; 1:157–159.

32. Gottlieb D, Levine D. Unilateral neglect influences the postural adjustments after stroke. *J Neuro Rehab.* 1992; 6(1):25–41.

33. Gray C, French J, Bates D. Motor recovery following acute stroke. *Age Ageing. 1990;* 19:179–194.

34. Feigenson JS. Stroke rehabilitation: effectiveness, benefits, and costs. Some practical considerations. *Stroke.* January/February 1979; 10(l):1–4.

35. Anderson TP, McClure WJ, Athelstan G, et al. Stroke rehabilitation: evaluation of its quality by assessing patient outcomes. *Arch Phys Med Rehab.* 1978; 79(4):170–175.

36. Anderson TP, Baldridge M, Ettinger MG. Quality of care for completed stroke without rehabilitation: evaluation by assessing patient outcomes. *Arch Phys Med Rehab.* 1979; 60(3):103–107.

37. Lehman JF, Delateur BJ, Fowler RS, et al. Stroke: does rehabilitation affect outcome? *Arch Phys Med Rehab.* 1975; 56(9):375–382.

38. Schenkman M, Butler RB. A model for multisystem evaluation interpretation and treatment of individuals with neurologic dysfunction. *Phys Ther.* 1989; 69:538–547.

39. Tripp N, Boudoures K, Dalum A, et al. Initiation of a systemic evaluation to categorize the hemiplegic patient. *Phys Ther.* 1991; 71(suppl 6):57.

40. Bobath B. *Adult Hemiplegia: Evaluational Treatment.* London: William Heinemann Medical Books; 1970:18–71.

41. Brunnstrom S. *Movement Therapy in Hemiplegia.* New York: Harper & Row; 1970:8–12, 34–41.

42. Carr J, Shepherd R. *A Motor Re-Learning Programme for Stroke.* Rockville, Md: Aspen; 1986.

43. Bohannon R. Knee extension torque in stroke patients: comparison of measurements obtained with a hand-held and a Cybex Dynamometer. *Physiotherapy Canada.* November/December 1990; 42(6).

44. Bohannon R. Consistency of muscle strength measurements in patient with stroke: examination from a different perspective. *J Phys Ther Sci.* 1990; 2:1–7.

45. Bohannon R. Is the measurement of muscle strength appropriate in patients with brain lesions? A special communication. *Phys Ther.* March 1989; 69(3). 189–191.

46. Olney S, Colbourne GR. Assessment and treatment of gait dysfunction in the geriatric stroke patient. *Top Geriatr Rehabil.* 1991; 7(1):70–78.

47. Parker K, Zablotny C, Jordan C. Analysis and management of hemiplegic gait dysfunction. In: *Stroke Rehabilitation State of the Art.* Rancho Los Amigos Medical Center, Downey Medical Center, Downey, CA; 1984.

48. Shumway-Cook A, Horak F. Assessing the influence of sensory interaction on balance: Suggestions from the field. *Phys Ther.* 1986; 66(10): 1548–1550.

49. Carr J, Shepherd R, Nordholm L, Lynne D. Investigation of a new motor assessment scale for stroke patients. *Phys Ther.* 1985; 65(2).

50. Kumar R, Metter EJ, Mehta AJ, et al. Shoulder pain in hemiplegia. *Am J Phys Med.* August 1990; 69(4): 205–208.

51. Bohannon R, Warren M, Cogman K. Influence of shoulder position on maximum voluntary elbow flexion force in stroke patients. *Occup Ther J of Research.* March/April 1991; 11(2):73–79.

52. Davies P. *Steps to Follow.* 2nd edition. New York, NY: Springer-Verlag. 2000; 403–428.

53. Brown DA, DeBacher GA. Bicycle ergometer and electromyographic feedback for treatment of muscle imbalance in patients with spastic hemiparesis. *Phys Ther.* 1987; 67(11):1715–1719.

54. Wissel J, Ebersbach G, Gutjahr PDL, et al. Treating chronic hemiparesis with modified biofeedback. *Arch Phys Med Rehab.* August 1989; 70: 612–617.

55. Sackley CM. The relationship between weight-bearing asymmetry after stroke, motor function and activities of daily living. *Physiotherapy Theory and Practice.*1990; 6:179–185.

56. Trueblood PR, Walker JM, Perry J, et al. Pelvic exercise and gait in herniplegia. *Phys Ther.* 1989; 69(l): 18–26.

57. Logigian MK, Samuels MA, Falconer J. Clinical exercise trial for stroke patients. *Arch Phys Med Rehab.* August 1983; 64:364–367.

58. Glenner GG. Alzheimer's disease (senile dementia): A research update and critique with recommendations. *J Am Geriatr Soc.* 1982; 30(1):59–62.

59. Forsyth E, Ritzline PD. An overview of the etiology, diagnosis, and treatment of Alzheimer's disease. *Phys Ther.* 1998; 78(12):1325–1331.

60. Blessed G, Tomlinson BE, Roth M. The association between quantitative measures of dementia and of senile changes in the cerebral grey matter of elderly patients. *Br J Psychiatry.* 1968; 114:797–911.

61. Rosen WB, Mohs RC, Davis KL. A new rating scale for Alzheimer's disease. *Am J Psychiatry.* 1984; 141: 1256–1364.

62. Boller F, Huff FJ, Querriera R, Kelsey S, Beyer J. Recording neurological symptoms and signs in Alzheimer's disease. *Am J Alzheimer's Care and Res.* May/June 1987; 19–29.

63. Alzheimer A. A unique illness involving the cerebral cortex. Originally published 1907. In: Hochberg

CN, Hochberg FH, translation. *Neurologic Classics in Modern Translation.* New York: Hafner Press; 1977:41–43.

64. Huff FJ, Boller F, Lucchelli F, Querriera R, Beyer J, Belle S. The neurologic examination in patients with probable Alzheimer's disease. *Arch Neurol.* 1987; 44:929–932.

65. Steffes R, Thralow J. Visual field limitation in the patient with dementia of the Alzheimer's type. *J Am Geriatr Soc.* 1987; 35:198–204.

66. Bhala RP, O'Connell J, Thoppil E. Ptophobia: Phobic fear of falling and its clinical management. *Phys Ther.* 1982; 62(2):187–190.

67. Hobeika CP. Equilibrium and balance in the elderly. *Ear, Nose & Throat J.* 1999; 78(8):558–566.

68. Horak FB. Clinical measurement of postural control in adults. *Phys Ther.* 1987; 67(12): 1881–1885.

69. Dornan J, Fernie GR, Holliday PJ. Visual input: Its importance in the control of postural sway. *Arch Phys Med Rehabil.* 1978; 59(5):586–591.

70. Keshner E, Peterson B. Frequency and velocity characteristics of head, neck, and trunk during normal locomotion. *Soc Neurosci Abst.* 1999; 15(12):1200–1204.

71. Begbie GH. Some problems of postural sway. In: de Reuck AVS, Knight J, eds. *Myotatic, Kinesthetic, and Vestibular Mechanisms.* Boston: Little, Brown & Co; 1967:80–92.

72. Horak FB, Shupert CL. Role of the vestibular system in postural control. In: Herdman SJ, ed. *Vestibular Rehabilitation.* 2nd ed. Philadelphia: F.A. Davis Co; 2000:22–46.

73. Hain CH. *Vestibular Rehabilitation.* Philadelphia: F.A. Davis Co. 1994.

74. Shimazu H, Smith CM. Cerebellar and labyrinthine influences on singular vestibular neurons identified by natural stimuli. *J Neurophysiol.* 1971; 34(5):493–508.

75. Mergner T, Becker W. Perception of horizontal self-rotation: Multisensory and cognitive aspects. In: Warren R, Wertheim AH, eds. *Perception and Control of Self-motion.* Mahwah, NJ: Lawrence Erlbaum. 1990:219–224.

76. Weber PC, Cass SP. Clinical assessment of postural instability. *Am J Otol.* 1993; 14(5):566–569.

77. Tinetti ME, Williams CS. Falls, injuries due to falls, and the risk of admission to a nursing home. *N Engl J Med.* 1997; 337:1279–1284.

78. Wall C, Black FO, Hunt AE. Effects of age, sex and stimulus parameters upon vestibulo-ocular responses to sinusoidal rotation. *Acta Otolaryngol.* 1984; 98:270–278.

79. Rosenhall U. Degenerative patterns in the aging human vestibular neuro-epithelia. *Acta Otolaryngol.* 1973; 76:208–220.

80. Paige GD. Senescense of human visual-vestibular interactions: Smooth pursuit, optokinetic, and vestibular control of eye movements with aging. *Exp Brain Res.* 1994; 98(3):355–372.

81. Keshner EA, Allum JH. Plasticity in pitch sway stabilization: Normal habituation and compensation for peripheral vestibular deficits. In: Bles W, Brandt T, eds. *Disorders of Posture and Gait.* Amsterdam: Elsevier; 1986:289–298.

82. Allum JH, Keshner EA, Honegger F, Pfaltz CR. Indicators of the influence a peripheral vestibular deficit has on vestibulo-spinal reflex responses controlling postural stability. *Acta Otolaryngol.* 1988; 106:252–263.

83. Black FO, Wall C, O'Leary DP. Computerized screening of the human vestibulospinal system. *Ann Otol Rhinol Laryngol.* 1978; 87:853–860.

84. Romberg MH. *Manual of Nervous Diseases of Man.* London: Sydenham Society; 1853:395–401.

85. Duncan P. Functional reach: A new clinical measure of balance. *J Gerontol.* 85(5):529–531.

86. Furman JM. Role of posturography in the management of vestibular patients. *Ortolaryngol Head Neck Surg.* 1995; 112(1):8–15.

87. Miller K, Hobeika CP, Sick S. Platform posturography as a predictor or falls. Proceedings of the Association for Research in Otolaryngology. St. Petersburg, FL. 1997.

88. Bottomley JM. Gait in later life. *Ortho Phys Ther Clinics North Am.* 2001; 10(1):131–149.

89. Tinetti ME, Speechly M, Ginter SF. Risk factors for falls among elderly persons living in the community. *N Engl J Med.* 1988; 319(26):1701–1707.

90. Furman JM, Cass SP. Benign paroxysmal positional vertigo. *N Engl J Med.* 1999; 341:1590–1596.

CHAPTER 13

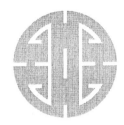

Cardiopulmonary and Cardiovascular Treatment

Cardiopulmonary considerations are particularly important in treating the elderly population in geriatric rehabilitation settings. Diseases of the heart, lungs, and blood vessels are by far the most prominent causes of morbidity and mortality among elderly individuals, rising logarithmically with age.[1,2] As the number of older individuals at risk for cardiovascular disease continues to rise, and as successful medical treatments for ischemic and hypertensive diseases in the middle-aged population drive up the number of people with known diseases surviving into older age, health care providers will be managing increasing numbers of elderly individuals with cardiopulmonary and cardiovascular disease. Eventually, the process of aging and inactivity takes its toll on the cardiovascular and cardiopulmonary systems and compromise each individual's ability to meet the oxygen demands of activity beyond the resting state.[3]

This chapter covers the cardiopulmonary and cardiovascular changes associated with aging and the physiological aspects of exercise associated with improving cardiopulmonary and cardiovascular health. Evaluation techniques specific to a frailer elderly population are covered and special considerations when prescribing exercises for people with diseases, including obesity, medications, diabetes mellitus, and osteoporosis, are presented.

INCIDENCE OF CARDIOPULMONARY AND CARDIOVASCULAR DISEASE

The projected shift in the age distribution of the population, as described in Chapter 1 of this text, indicates that older individuals comprise an increasing proportion until the middle of the next century, when they will constitute about one fifth of the total. Currently there are over 33.9 million people in the United States who are 65 years of age and older.[4] Of these, 50% of them have some form of cardiopulmonary or cardiovascular disorders. Indeed, cardiovascular disease is the major cause of death after the age of 65, accounting for more than 40% of deaths in this age group.[1] Figure 13–1 demonstrates the rates for leading causes of death among persons aged 65 or older. In 1997, though showing a slight decline in heart disease since 1980, the leading cause of death among persons age 65 or older continues to be heart disease (1,832 deaths per 100,000 persons).[2] Elderly people, who contribute 68% of all deaths in the United States annually, account for 78% of deaths attributed to cardiovascular disease.[5] In the most rapidly growing segment of the US population, those 85 years of age and older, cardiovascular and cardiopulmonary diseases account for greater than 76% of all deaths.[5,6] Morbidity is similarly prevalent in the population over the age of 65. Twenty-eight percent reported significant health impairments related to heart, lung, and vascular conditions, including angina, congestive heart failure, rhythm disturbances, chronic obstructive and restrictive lung diseases, and peripheral vascular disease.[1,2]

The majority of US residents receiving cardiovascular services are believed to be Medicare beneficiaries, and the age-associated increase in prevalence and incidence is true for all forms of cardiovascular and cardiopulmonary disease (except congenital). Although women are often thought to be at lower risk for cardiovascular disease, this relative immunity represents only a 7- to 10-year delay in onset. In fact, as age

increases, prevalence rates become more equal with those of men, and ultimately cardiovascular mortality rates in women and men are equivalent.[7] More people in the US population, as a whole, die of cardiovascular disease than the combined total of other leading causes of death (Figure 13–2). As Figure 13–2 depicts, cardiovascular disease tops the list of the 10 leading causes of death in the United States and annually kills more Americans than all the other diseases combined, including cancer, diabetes, AIDS and suicide. One in four Americans, nearly 59 million, suffers from cardiovascular disease. The American Heart Association estimates that the cost per year in health care and lost productivity is approximately $138 billion, which represents about one-seventh of the total health bill. As cardiovascular disease doesn't start in old age (i.e., after the age of 65), preventive measures must be addressed throughout the life cycle.

Implications

The most frequently occurring problem is atherosclerotic heart disease. It is common to find hypertension coexisting with atherosclerotic heart disease. Congestive heart failure, arrhythmias, and electrocardiographic abnormalities have an increased incidence with aging.[8] Cardiac disease in the elderly is complicated by the fact that it rarely occurs in isolation. Pulmonary problems, such as chronic obstructive pulmonary disease (COPD) and emphysema, usually result in death from the cardiac complications they impose and vascular diseases generally accompany cardiac disease or predispose an individual to the development of cardiovascular and cardiopulmonary pathologies (see Chapter 5). Chronic inactivity, resulting from musculoskeletal, neuromuscular causes, or systemic diseases, further exacerbates the effects of aging on the cardiovascular system. Deaths from cardiovascular disease are only part of the story. The debilitating effects on individuals who survive a stroke or a heart attack lead to a loss in functional capabili-

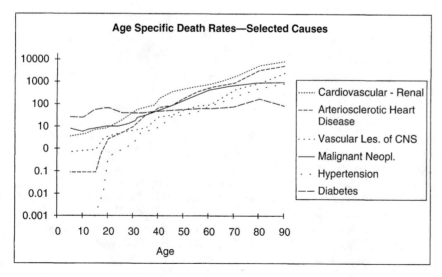

Figure 13–1. *Age-Specific Death Rates Indicate that Cardiovascular Causes of Death Occur Most Frequently with Advancing Age. (Source: National Center for Health Statistics. Health, United States, 1999 with Health and Aging Chartbook. 1999 Hyattsville, MD: National Center for Health Statistics.)*

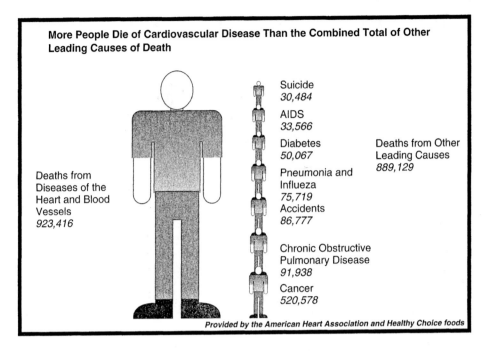

More People Die of Cardiovascular Disease Than the Combined Total of Other Leading Causes of Death

Deaths from Diseases of the Heart and Blood Vessels
923,416

Suicide
30,484

AIDS
33,566

Diabetes
50,067

Pneumonia and Influeza
75,719

Accidents
86,777

Chronic Obstructive Pulmonary Disease
91,938

Cancer
520,578

Deaths from Other Leading Causes
889,129

Provided by the American Heart Association and Healthy Choice foods

Figure 13–2. Comparison of Deaths from Cardiovascular Disease to Other Leading Causes of Death. (*Source: American Heart Association and Healthy Choice Foods, 1998.*)

ties and severely impact the individual's ability to maintain independence as depicted in Figure 13–3.

Cardiac rehabilitation is a means of improving the cardiopulmonary response to increased oxygen demands during increased activity through endurance and conditioning exercises. The progression of the aging process eventually evolves into diseases in the cardiovascular and cardiopulmonary systems. Any of the pathologies mentioned above will lead to an inhibition of the cardiopulmonary responses to increased

oxygen demands. Functional level of activity decreases as a result of a vicious cycle of inactivity and deconditioning, imposed by a variety of medical problems in the musculoskeletal, neuromuscular, and sensory systems, that can cause cardiovascular disability or may exacerbate underlying cardiac disease.

Prolonged inactivity and bed rest quickly and markedly impair cardiovascular functional capacity.[9–11] All too often, deconditioning of the cardiopulmonary system is potentiated by excessive bed rest

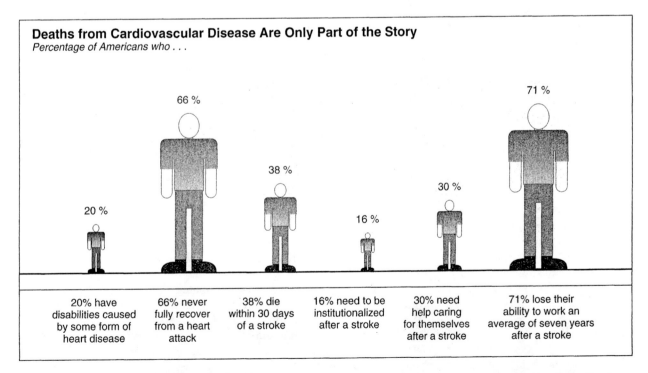

Deaths from Cardiovascular Disease Are Only Part of the Story
Percentage of Americans who . . .

20 %

66 %

38 %

16 %

30 %

71 %

| 20% have disabilities caused by some form of heart disease | 66% never fully recover from a heart attack | 38% die within 30 days of a stroke | 16% need to be institutionalized after a stroke | 30% need help caring for themselves after a stroke | 71% lose their ability to work an average of seven years after a stroke |

Figure 13–3. Debilitating Effects of Cardiovascular Disease. (*Source: American Heart Association and Healthy Choice Foods, 1998.*)

and overmedication for the elderly cardiac patient. Even prior to illness, many elderly patients decrease their activity level due to a varied combination of musculoskeletal and neuromuscular problems. Additionally, because of the decreased aerobic capacity with aging, any submaximal task is perceived as requiring increased work because of its increased relative energy cost and resulting fatigue. Relative inactivity thus potentiates the decreased physical work capacity in the elderly, often threatening the possibility of an independent lifestyle. This can be avoided, and indeed, functional capacity can be improved with conditioning and endurance exercises, and the reinstitution of the older person's participation in functional activities of daily living (ADL).

There has been increased interest in research about the effects of exercise on the aged cardiac patient.[9-11] Perhaps this is a result of the growing numbers of the elderly and changing demographic and sociologic patterns.[6] Individuals are living relatively healthy lives well beyond the socially imposed demarcation line that defines old age.[12,13] The expectations of acceptable levels of function for the elderly segment of the population have changed. Research studies have demonstrated that exercise is not only beneficial for maintaining functional baseline condition in the unimpaired elderly individual, but it is also therapeutic for reversing the effects of impairment and improving baselines in individuals who have become deconditioned as a result of symptom limitations (e.g., angina and dyspnea).[11,14]

American society's increased focus on exercise and a corresponding broadening of the expectations among the elderly for an active life-style, have increased their participation in physical activity programs. As a result, it is important that physical therapists be involved with the development of clinical procedures that are safe and effective in exercise assessment and prescription for the elderly. Therapeutic evaluation and program planning have now reached the point where the elderly individual, who was once confined to bed because of angina and dyspnea resulting from cardiopulmonary disease, can be evaluated and treated with a total rehabilitation program. This should include an individualized exercise prescription that considers the severity of disease, attempts symptom reversal, and has functional improvement as its primary goal. Cardiopulmonary considerations are important in the geriatric population for the prescription of any activity, as cardiopulmonary pathological manifestations are most likely to accompany increasing age in close to 100% of the elderly population we see in the clinic.

PHYSIOLOGICAL ASPECTS OF EXERCISE

Human performance is a remarkable integration of all of the systems of the body. Practically no tissue or organ escapes involvement in increasing activity lev-els. While the muscles perform the work, the heart and peripheral vascular systems deliver the nutrients, and with the assistance of the pulmonary system, provide O_2 to and remove CO_2 from the working tissues. The nervous and endocrine systems integrate all of this activity into meaningful performance. At the cellular level, the mitochondria and numerous enzymes are activated and energy generated to enable the muscle to contract. Skin acts as the heating and cooling system as activity is prolonged, and the kidneys assist in maintaining a homeostatic fluid balance. It is apparent that any pathological manifestation involving any of the body systems will negatively influence the physiologic response to exercise.[9]

The heart is an amazing organ. Despite its decreased power and ability to contract, slower rate of recovery, diminished cardiac reserve, and the other changes of aging and disease, the human heart continues to function well as long as it is not overwhelmed by disease. By the time a person is eighty to ninety years of age, the heart has long outperformed the best mechanical pumps devised by man. By the age of one hundred, the human heart has beat more than 3.6 billion times and pumped more than 288 billion cubic centimeters of blood. The ability of the cardiovascular and cardiopulmonary systems to respond to stress admittedly decreases with advancing age, but many elderly people, even with heart disease, can continue their normal routine activities well into older age.

During the normal life span, the cardiovascular and cardiopulmonary systems are subject to a variety of normal physiologic stimuli and processes that may create pathological consequences. In addition, the biologic changes of aging, beginning after the process of growth and development, the evolution of maturity and adulthood, and proceeding into the phases of senescence and old age, modify the anatomic, physiologic, and functional capabilities of the heart, lungs, and vascular systems.

CARDIOPULMONARY CHANGES WITH AGING AND DISEASE

The changes in the cardiopulmonary system related to aging and disease have been discussed in Chapters 3 and 5 respectively, and will only be summarized in this chapter as a foundation for cardiopulmonary treatment considerations in the elderly.

There is some controversy over the degree of physiologic change that is expressly age related as opposed to disease related. Most investigators agree, however, that certain changes in muscle strength, and in cardiac and pulmonary function are so common that they may be thought of as universal. Because rehabilitation exercise programs increase the level of activity above resting states, these changes are likely to affect the older person. Aerobic capacity (VO_2 max) decreases with advancing age,[14] and declines in aerobic capacity are probably greater in the patient who has become deconditioned during a recent hospital stay or who had poor exercise habits prior to developing a disability. Exercise capacity may be further affected by decreases in vital capacity and minute volume.[15] Additional cardiopulmonary changes related to aging include increased blood pressure and decreased maximum cardiac output.[11,14] Maximal obtainable heart rate and stroke volume decline in relation to the decrease in maximal oxygen consumption (VO_2 max).[15] With age, lean muscle mass decreases as does muscle strength[16] and will be discussed in this chapter as it relates to the cardiopulmonary systems need to meet working muscles energy demands. Orthostatic hypotension is frequently seen, particularly in those recently bedridden. Peripheral vascular resistance rises with age, increasing the risk of developing hypertensive episodes with exercise programs.

The heart demonstrates little change in the size of its chambers, but the left ventricular wall thickens and becomes less compliant.[17] There is a thickening of or a development of nodular ridges along the attachments of the aortic cusps.[18] The conduction system displays relatively little change in the atrioventricular (AV) node or the bundle of His, though the number of proximal bundle fascicles connecting the left to the main bundle may be reduced.[19]

Coronary artery or ischemic heart disease is the most prevalent disease in individuals over the age of 60.[13] In 90% to 95% of the cases, the reduction of blood flow to the heart is the result of atherosclerotic narrowing of the coronary lumen.[17] This reduction in flow creates the manifestations of angina, myocardial infarction, and sudden death. Angina and infarction impair function by decreasing the maximum cardiac output and maximum oxygen consumption. Infarction or necrosis of the heart muscle limits the distensibility of the heart and reduces the stroke volume. Collectively, these pathologic changes produce a self-limiting impediment to cardiac function. Increased systemic demands for oxygen necessitate an increase in cardiac output or myocardial work. Increased work requires an increase supply of O_2 to the myocardial muscle. The restricted coronary blood flow results in ischemia which increases the left end-diastolic pressure, prolongs systole as the heart is unable to relax, and stiffens the ventricle wall. A distructive cycle is instituted as these physiological changes reduce perfusion of the myocardium and increase the degree of ischemia further damaging cardiac tissue.[14] The result of this vicious circle is progressive deconditioning of the heart as angina and dyspnea self-limit and impair functional activity and exercise capacity.

Lung changes are characterized by an increase in residual volume accompanied by a decrease in vital capacity. Declines are seen in maximal voluntary ventilation, the surface area for gas exchange, the rate of diffusion, and the arteriovenous oxygen differential.[20] Both the lung tissue and chest wall lose elasticity. Cardiopulmonary demands usually can be met, but when disease or deconditioning are present, the demands may exceed the available reserve. All of these changes result in reduced tolerance for physical activity and are important to consider with regard to rate and intensity of activities for the older person. Due to the wide variety in lifestyles, the rate and magnitude of changes cannot be predicted and may not be apparent until they impact on ADL.

The anatomic and functional changes seen in COPD mimic those seen in aging. Both are characterized by microtraumas that occur over time, which do not interfere with resting or low-level ventilatory function.[21,22] The pathological tissue changes seen with emphysema and chronic bronchitis are also similar to the tissue changes of advancing age. The degree of impairment is the distinguishing factor between what is considered "normal" aging and the degree of impairment and compromise that is considered pathological. In emphysema there is an abnormal enlargement of the terminal airspaces as a result of a loss in tissue elasticity of the lung. This results is expiratory collapse of the larger airways. Expiration is difficult for the patient with emphysema. Chronic bronchitis is accompanied by a persistant productive cough on a daily basis. The result of these respiratory conditions is an increase in the work of breathing and an inability to meet the energy demands required for functional activities of living, exercise, or both.

Maximal Oxygen Consumption (VO_2 max)

The major function of the cardiovascular and cardiopulmonary systems during exercise is to deliver blood to the active tissues, supplying O_2 and nutrients, and removing metabolic waste products. If exercise is prolonged, the cardiovascular system also assists in maintaining body temperature.

The cardiac and pulmonary systems integrate a number of component functions in order to adequately acquire and distribute O_2 to the working muscles. The muscles of the thorax contract to initiate an increase in thoracic volume and to lower the intrathoracic pressure. A decrease in the intrathoracic pressure creates gas flow from the higher-pressured atmosphere into the conducting tubules where the gas is warmed, filtered, humidified, and mixed with existing gases to produce an alveolar oxygen tension of 90–100 mmHg.[9] Alveolar oxygen is diffused across the 70-square meter blood gas interface into pulmonary capillaries via an approximate 40 mmHg pressure gradient where it combines with hemoglobin and then enters the left atrium. The heart, through rhythmic contraction, delivers the oxygenated blood to the myocardial muscle first, and then to the peripheral tissues. The pressure created by the contraction of the heart (systolic) overcomes systemic pressure and generates blood flow through the arterial vascular system.

Maximal oxygen consumption (VO_2 max) is the best measure of cardiopulmonary fitness. It can be derived by a simple equation: $VO_2 = Q \times (aO_2 - vO_2)$. VO_2 is the amount of oxygen the system absorbs and is equal to cardiac output (Q) multiplied by the arterial oxygen content (aO_2) minus the central venous oxygen content (vO_2). Each link of this multistaged process needs to be adequately functioning in order for the system to efficiently acquire, transport, and deliver O_2. An impairment at any phase as a result of disease, age, or deconditioning limits the amount of O_2 uptake and competent delivery to the working tissues.

Heart Rate

The resting heart rate is influenced by age, body position, the level of cardiopulmonary fitness, and various environmental factors (e.g., temperature, humidity, altitude). Resting heart rate remains relatively constant with age though in advanced age may show a decline. Better cardiopulmonary fitness results in a decrease in resting heart rate, whereas, the resting heart rate will increase in higher environmental temperatures or at an increase in altitude.[23]

Before exercise the heart rate may be increased by an anticipatory response, a reflection of a sympathetic neurohumoral effect. As exercise begins, the heart rate increases, but during low levels of exercise at a constant workload, the heart rate will attain a plateau or steady state. As workload increases, the heart rate increases in a roughly linear manner. At higher workloads, the heart rate takes longer to plateau. For the same workload, the more fit individual will have a lower steady-state value.

The older individual shows a lower response given the same workload, but at progressively higher workloads, will eventually reach a level that is totally exhausting. Prior to this, however, the heart rate will have reached a plateau at its maximum.

The maximum heart rate declines with age. Each individual has a definable maximum heart rate. The equation for maximum achievable heart rate is 220 minus the person's age. Figure 13–4 provides a worksheet for calculating aerobic and anaerobic training ranges. This provides an approximation of the mean maximal heart rate for any one age category with a standard deviation of 10, so this equation should be used cautiously. The decline in maximum heart rate with age has been attributed mainly to changes in the myocardial oxygen supply, but additional factors include pathological impairment of blood flow to the sinus node, producing a lower heart rate during maximal exercise (the "sick sinus" syndrome), and greater stiffness (reduced compliance) of the heart wall which increases the time required for filling of the ventricles and interfers with the "feedback" of information on venous filling to the cardioregulatory center.[23]

Heart rate responses will vary at rest and submaximal exercise levels according to the degree of cardiovascular impairment, whereas, the maximum achievable heart rate shows a progressive decline with age.[9,23] Heart rate responses to physiologic stimuli such as postural change and cough have also been shown to decrease with age.[18] In an older, frailer population, it is not necessary to reach aerobic heart rate levels to gain improvements in cardiovascular health. Any activity above rest works! The importance of activity beyond the resting level can not be emphasized enough in an elderly population.

Stroke Volume

The difference between the end-diastolic and end-systolic blood volumes is the stroke volume. The stroke volume response is highly dependent on hydrostatic pressure effects. When sitting or standing,

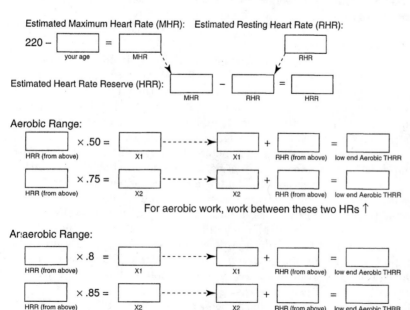

Figure 13–4. Worksheet for Calculating Aerobic and Anaerobic Training Heart Rate Ranges. *Aerobic Example: Using 70 years of age with a resting heart rate (RHR) of 80. Maximum Heart Rate (MHR) = 220−80 = 140. Subtracting RHR from MHR you get 140−80 = 60 for Heart Rate Reserve (HRR). Aerobic training heart rate range (THRR) will lie between 50% and 75% of the HRR added to the RHR: 50% of 60 = 30; 75% of 60 = 45. Adding these figures to the RHR gives: 80 + 30 = 110 and 80 + 45 = 125. Thus the THRR would be 110 to 125.*

Anaerobic Example: To calculate anaerobic heart rate range take 80% of 60 = 48 and 85% if 60 = 51. Adding these figures to RHR gives: 80 + 48 = 128 and 80 + 51 = 131. Thus the anaerobic threshold THRR is 128 to 131 beats per minute.

without exercise, the stroke volume is reduced relative to the supine position due to blood pooling in the extremities. The maximum stroke volume attained during exercise in supine or sitting is only slightly higher. The increase is sufficient to overcome the effect of venous pooling. Stroke volume at rest in the erect position varies between 50 ml to 80 ml. In a highly trained athlete, this volume can be as high as 200 ml. The stroke volume increases linearly with the workload until it reaches its maximum at approximately 50% of the individual's capacity for exercise.[9]

There is some controversy as to whether there is a change in stroke volume with age or if the changes are a result of a decline in VO_2 max, a slower maximum heart rate response, and increased peripheral resistance which diminishes the ejection fraction.[24] Understanding the significance of stroke volume changes has been hampered to some extent by the inability to accurately measure absolute left ventricular dimensions (i.e., end-diastolic and end-systolic volumes).[25] Studies have suggested that there is no age-related change in stroke volume at rest[26] and that the ejection fraction remains unchanged with age at rest.[27] During exercise, end-diastolic volume and end-systolic volume showed marked age-related increases as higher levels of exercise were achieved according to a study by Rodeheffer and associates.[28] Elderly subjects showed an increase in end-diastolic volume at low levels of exercise and continued to show progressive increases with increasing exercise intensity. End-systolic volume in elderly subjects also increased with exercise, though less dramatically. Younger subjects at high levels of exercise showed no change in the end-diastolic volume from resting levels while end-systolic volume decreased significantly. The implication of these volume changes is that the young population maintains cardiac output by achieving a high heart rate and that healthy older individuals maintain cardiac output by dilating the ventricle and utilizing the Frank-Starling mechanism to increase stroke volume.[28]

Cardiac Output

The cardiac output (CO) at rest is 4 to 6 liters per minute (L/min). It increases linearly with workload. At exercise levels of 40 to 60%, the increase in CO is accomplished through an increase in both the heart rate and the stroke volume. At higher levels of exercise, the increase in CO results solely from the continued increase in heart rate. Maximal values of cardiac output during exercise are dependent on many factors. Body size and the degree of physical fitness appear to have the most prominent influence on CO. For instance, in a small, deconditioned individual the maximum CO during exercise could be as little as 20 L/min, whereas, in a large, well-conditioned individual the CO can reach 40 L/min.[14,23]

Physiologic changes in the cardiovascular system primarily involve the determinants of CO. Cardiac output is affected by preload and afterload conditions, which are altered by aging. Early diastolic filling is decreased as a result of mitral valve thickening and/or the decrease in the compliance of the left ventricle.[19] There is an increase in afterload with aging as well. This is possibly produced by an increase in the rigidity of the ascending aorta and a general decrease in the diameter of the peripheral vascular system. This combination of factors increases the overall load on the myocardium and is responsible for the age-associated decrease in cardiac output.

Blood Pressure

The normal response of the blood pressure is a linear increase in systolic pressure with increasing work (200 Hg or higher). Blood pressure changes in aged individuals are dependent on many factors, including extracellular fluid volume, vascular tone and reactivity, the autonomic nervous system, and the arterial baroreceptor reflexes. Each component factor can affect responsiveness in the aged individual somewhat differently. Resting systolic and diastolic blood pressures tend to rise with age, however, the range is quite variable.[19,23] Diastolic blood pressure changes little in healthy elderly individuals. An increase in systemic blood pressure with age is related to the loss of elasticity in the walls of the larger arteries, which raises systolic and depresses diastolic pressures. There is also the increased liability of vasopressor control which tends to raise both systolic and diastolic pressures. As a result, the systolic arterial blood pressure rises progressively up to the age of 75 years; and the diastolic pressure rises slightly to the age of 60 and then gradually declines.[29]

Arteriovenous Oxygen Differential

The arteriovenous oxygen difference is the difference between the O_2 in the arteries compared to the O_2 content in the veins. It reflects the amount of O_2 that the peripheral tissues extract. The maximum arteriovenous oxygen difference tends to decrease with age.[30] Shepard[14] suggests that factors contributing to this decline with age include: lower levels of physical fitness; a reduction of arterial oxygen saturation; a decreased hemoglobin level; poor peripheral blood distribution; a loss of activity in tissue enzyme systems; and a greater relative blood flow to the skin.

The arteriovenous oxygen difference tends to be larger in the elderly compared to young adults both at rest and at submaximal exercise levels, indicating that there is a decrease in the amount of O_2 extracted in older subjects.[31] Some increase in the stroke volume in combination with a decrease in mechanical efficiency of the cardiopulmonary and cardiovascular systems could explain this. Horvath and Borgia[32] report that there is no reduction in the amount of O_2 saturation/transport capacity of arterial blood. The metabolic potential of skeletal muscle does not decline;[33] however, there is a decrease in the capillary/

fiber ratio in the aged muscle[34] and a reduction in the amount of blood that flows to the periphery.[35]

Peripheral Vascular Resistance

Blood flow from the heart varies with tissue needs. During exercise, blood is shunted from areas of little or no metabolic activity (e.g., the gut) to those tissues that are involved in the exercise. Blood to the heart increases proportionally to the increase in metabolic activity.[9] Blood to the skin and muscles is increased, and blood to the stomach and intestines is decreased. The effective blood volume decreases from maximal levels with prolonged work and in a hot and humid environment, because of the increased blood flow to the periphery that promotes both metabolic and environmental heat loss.[14]

Vascular changes of age affect each tissue layer differently. The cells of the intima become irregularly aligned instead of orienting themselves along the longitudinal axis of the vessel.[19] The subendothelial layer becomes thickened due to lipid deposition, calcification, and increased cross-linking of the connective tissue. The media demonstrates increased calcification and fraying of the elastic fibers. These changes all lead to regional differences in vessel diameter and increase in the resistance to blood flow.

The peripheral vascular resistance may be increased by atheromatous plaques in the lumina and, with a loss in vessel elasticity, and a failure to vasodilate in response to increasing activity. Regular exercise can reduce the resting systemic pressure by about 5 mmHg, but it has little influence on the peripheral pressure during maximum effort.[36]

Neurohumoral Factors

There is a decline in the neurohumoral controls with aging which reduces the ability to adjust to external and internal stresses.[14] The body hormones contribute to the regulation of circulating fluid volumes and cardiovascular performance. They also mobilize blood glucose, liberate fat, and break down protein to provide energy for increasing activity levels. Neurohumeral factors are important in tissue repair because they are involved with the synthesis of new protein (anabolism), which is important in the healing process at the cellular level.

Fluid loss in prolonged exercise results in a decrease in plasma volume, hemoconcentration of red blood cells (RBCs) and plasma proteins. This hemoconcentration results in an increase in RBCs by 20 to 25%, and there is a shift of fluid from the plasma to the interstitial fluid.[14]

The blood pH shows little change up to approximately 50% intensity of exercise. Past 50%, the pH decreases and the blood becomes more acidic. This decrease in pH is primarily the result of an increase in anaerobic muscle metabolism and corresponds to an increase in blood lactate.

Neurohumeral regulatory changes affect the physiologic response of the elderly individual. Catecholamines function to maintain the systemic pressure, mobilize muscle glycogen to sustain plasma glucose, liberate fatty acids, stimulate gluconeogenesis in the liver, stimulate glucagon secretion, and inhibit insulin secretion.[14] Although there may be an increase in the plasma-catecholamine levels with advancing age,[37] there is a decrease in the end-organ responsiveness to β-adrenergic stimulation.[19] This variation in circulating catecholamines or decrease in neuroresponsiveness may partially account for the decreased heart rate and blood pressure response to activities such as a cough or Valsalva's maneuver. This attenuated responsiveness is also partly attributed to decreased baroreceptor sensitivity.[37]

PULMONARY RESPONSE TO EXERCISE

Pulmonary ventilation or minute volume increases from approximately 6 L/min at rest to above 100 L/min during maximal exercise, and in a well-conditioned individual, this can exceed 200 L/min. This is accomplished by an increase in both the tidal volume and respiratory frequency. Tidal volume at rest is about 0.5 L/min and can increase to 2.5 to 3.0 L/min during maximal exercise efforts. Resting respiratory frequency ranges from 12 to 16 breaths/min and increases to 40 to 50 breaths/min during maximal exercise.[9]

The respiratory system is responsible for ventilation through the coordinated contraction of the diaphragm and associated ventilatory muscles, the displacement of the rib cage, and the expansion of the lungs by the negative pressure created by the contraction of these muscles. The resting length and strength of the ventilatory muscles, the thoracic cage compliance and the compliance of the lungs are important factors in generating adequate gas flow. Aging produces a progressive decrease in the thoracic wall and bronchiolar compliance.[38] Because of structural changes in bone, cartilage, and elastic structures with age, the chest wall becomes stiff. There is an increase in cross-linking of collagen fibers, a decrease in the resiliancy of elastic and cartilaginous tissue, and a decrease in collagen and the annulus fibrosis.[14,36] The elastic fibers within the lung change so that there is an increase in compliance of the lung, but a decrease in its elastic recoil.[39] Superimposed on a decreased compliance of the thoracic wall, this results in a decrease in total lung compliance with age. There is an increase in the size and number of alveolar fenestrae[40] that, in combination with the change in elastic features at the alveolar levels and the loss of tissue from the alveolar walls and septa, result in a decrease in the surface area available for gas exchange. The conducting tubules become more rigid, decreasing their radius and increasing resistance to gas flow.[36] The result is an increased mechanical workload for breathing and a decrease in the efficiency of gas exchange.

The pulmonary systemic changes produced by pathological lung changes as those seen in COPD, emphysema, and chronic bronchitis increase the work of breathing and decrease the energy supply available to working muscles. There is a reduction in vital capacity due to an increased residual volume, decreased forced expiratory volume, and a reduced arterial oxygen tension with an increase in the carbon dioxide tension.[3,14] In combination with a decrease in thoracic compliance and progressive narrowing of the airways, the force required for the ventilatory muscles to create air flow severely stresses the cardiopulmonary system and compromises the ability to efficiently supply O_2 to peripheral tissues.[41]

BENEFITS OF EXERCISE TRAINING IN THE ELDERLY

Cardiac, vascular, and pulmonary diseases need not be a barrier to better fitness. Too many health care professionals working with the elderly have set their sights low by accepting as normal the reduced ability of aging people who are inactive, sedentary, or incapacitated by subclinical or clinical disease. For instance, a decline in cardiac output is considered a normal process in aging, however, according to noninvasive studies with radioactive thallium nuclear and echocardiographic studies, the decline in cardiac output is absent in physically fit older people without occult coronary artery disease.[28] Most studies dealing with changes in cardiopulmonary response to exercise are done on more sedentary and less physically fit elderly individuals who may very likely have subclinical cardiopulmonary or cardiovascular disease.

There are limited studies on the role of exercise in the prevention of coronary and pulmonary problems in the elderly population. However, epidemiological studies suggest the clear role that increased activities (exercise, occupational, recreational, and leisure) play in decreasing the risk of developing cardiovascular and cardiopulmonary diseases.[9,10,23,42,43] Lack of exercise progressively becomes a more important risk factor in the development of cardiopulmonary and cardiovascular pathologies.[10,11,42-44] The relative body weight has less influence on the chances of developing a fatal heart attack.[45] Shepard[14] suggests that this may reflect the confounding influence of an increasing loss of lean tissue.

Regularly performed aerobic exercise results in an increase in VO_2 max in young adults. The magnitude of the change is determined by the intensity, frequency, and duration of exercise.[14] Sidney and Shepard[46] have reported that elderly men and women respond to endurance-exercise training with similar relative increases in VO_2 max as young people. They demonstrated that the frequency, intensity, and duration of the exercise also impacted the beneficial exercise outcomes in older subjects. Cross-sectional studies have shown that older endurance athletes have a higher VO_2

max than age-matched sedentary controls.[47,48] This difference ranges between 44% and 62% when VO_2 max is expressed in L/min and between 62% to 100% when corrected for body weight (mL/kg/min). In master athletes (65 plus years of age), the VO_2 max was only 9% lower compared to younger runners with whom they were matched in terms of performance, training, body weight, and body composition.[49] This means that regular exercise could positively influence the integrated response to an external (e.g., environmental) or internal stress (e.g., pneumonia), and could play a role in putting up a barrier to those internal accentuations.

Endurance exercise results in a significant increase in VO_2 max in older men and women.[10,11,43,47] Verg and associates[47] observed a 25% increase in VO_2 max after one year of training in a group of subjects aged 60 to 66 years of age. With low-intensity training, male and female subjects aged 61 to 65 years increased their VO_2 max by 12%.[50] An additional six months of high-intensity training produced a further substantial effect increasing the VO_2 max gains to 18%. Thomas et al[51] found that the best predictor of what an elderly subject's VO_2 max will be after one year of training is the initial VO_2 max. These findings support the hypothesis that the age-related decline in aerobic capacity is in part due to modifiable factors such as inactivity.

Cross-sectional comparisons of master athletes between the ages of 61 and 65 years and similarly aged sedentary subjects suggest that endurance-exercise training protects against the decline in ventilatory function with age.[47] When the minute volume was compared to controls at the same absolute submaximal exercise intensity, it was 12% lower in the study group of exercising individuals, which indicates a decrease in the actual work of breathing in the trained elderly. The master athletes also had a higher maximum voluntary ventilation and used a significantly higher percentage of their maximum voluntary ventilation capacities at maximal exercise than sedentary controls. Frontera and Evans[52] evaluated sedentary, healthy men and women aged 61 to 65 and found that endurance training for one year increased their VO_2 max by 25%. There were no significant changes in the maximum voluntary ventilation, however, at the same submaximal VO_2, the minute volume was 9% lower after training—a reflection of a more efficient ventilation. In addition, the maximal minute ventilation and the percentage of the maximum voluntary ventilation used at maximal exercise increased significantly. This study made it apparent that the older sedentary individual can expect to achieve the same efficient level of ventilation during submaximal exercise and utilize the same percentage of maximum voluntary ventilation during maximal effort as the master athlete. The age-related changes in the ventilatory apparatus do not preclude improvements in function with endurance-exercise training.

Prolonged endurance-exercise training results in significant adaptations in cardiovascular function.

Heath and coworkers[48] compared endurance athletes aged 53 to 65 to a group of 20- to 24-year-old athletes of similar body weight and training habits. All of the athletes were compared with similarly age-matched, healthy, untrained men. Both young and master athletes in the study groups had significantly greater left ventricular volume and mass when compared to the untrained group, and all of the athletes in both age groups had higher values for posterior wall thickness and septal thickness when normalized for body surface area. The master athletes had a significantly larger end-diastolic volume index compared to the younger athletes. The difference in ventricular mass was not statistically significant in either athletic group. Also of significance in this study was that no differences among the three groups were noted in indicators of myocardial contractile function measured by echocardiography (i.e., percentage of fiber shortening and mean velocity of fiber shortening at rest). Both groups of athletes had significantly slower heart rates at rest and during three levels of submaximal exercise than did the group of untrained subjects. This suggests that regular exercise, for men, is likely to maintain cardiovascular function above that of deconditioned younger men.

According to Seals and associates,[53] endurance training for one year resulted in a significant increase in functional aerobic capacity. There was a small but significant rise in maximal stroke volume though changes in maximal cardiac output were not significant. An increase in the arteriovenous oxygen difference suggests that there is a more efficient O_2 extraction at the muscular level suggesting that peripheral adaptations are more important than central changes.

Skeletal muscle increases its oxidative capacities with endurance training. Endurance exercise increases the muscle mitochondrial-protein content and improves its oxidative capacity even if it does not reduce the skeletal-muscle atrophy associated with aging in rats.[54] Beyer and associates[55] substantiated that finding and concluded that the capacity to oxidize fats and carbohydrates can be maintained in aging animals with increased physical activity.

Endurance training for eight weeks also has a positive effect on skeletal muscle metabolism in sedentary men aged 56 to 70.[56] Souminen and associates[56] found that there was an increased level of the activity of the enzymes with endurance training, which represents aerobic muscle metabolism. These metabolic alterations in skeletal muscle are associated with lower blood lactate levels during submaximal exercise.[10,53,56] This suggests that the lower blood levels are due to a decrease lactate production and a greater aerobic contribution to energy production.

Regular exercise helps the body to fight off the buildup of low-density lipoprotein (LDL) cholesterol. Long-term exercise has been found to keep LDL from turning into deposits that eventually result in reduced blood flow or artery-blocking clots. Exercise changes the way in which the body handles free radicals, highly reactive oxygen molecules that encourage LDL particles to form deposits.[50]

The amino acid called homocysteine is closely linked to heart disease. Homocysteine is used by the body to help manufacture proteins and carry out cellular metabolism. Too much of it appears to cause blood platelets to clump and vascular walls to break down.[57,58,59] Evidence points to a shortage of vitamin B_6, vitamin B_{12}, and folic acid, all of which work to convert the amino acid into a molecular form the body can use. Eating nutrients rich in these nutritional components helps to break homocysteine down.[57] Exercise appears to enhance the absorption and utilization of these nutrients.[58,59] A large multicenter European trial found that among men and women younger than age 60, the overall risk of coronary and other vascular disease was 2.2 times higher in those with plasma total homocysteine levels in the top fifth of the normal range compared with those in the bottom four-fifths.[58] This risk was independent of other risk factors, but was notably higher in smokers and persons with high blood pressure.[58] A Norwegian study found that among 587 patients with coronary artery disease, the risk of death after four to five years was proportional to plasma total homocysteine levels.[59]

Extremes in cardiovascular fitness in the elderly exist, especially in aging athletes. John A. Kelley of East Dennis, Massachusetts, who ran the Boston Marathon for his 58th time in 1992 at the age of 84, is clearly a good example. Hazel Wolf, who died in the year 2000 at the age of 101 years kayaked extensively when she was in her mid 90s, even portaging her own kayak and camping gear. Wolf, a Seattle resident, founded most of Washington State's Audubon Society chapters. Hilda, who climbs Mount Everest (not always to the top) each year on her birthday, climbed again in 1999 at the age of 100. These are clearly exceptions to the rule. These are individuals whose self-discipline and ability to achieve and perform great physical activity has been a way of life since very early in their lives. By contrast, most individuals who reach the age of 65 years have slowed down considerably, and inactivity is one of the major predisposers to cardiovascular and cardiopulmonary pathologies.

BENEFITS OF EXERCISE FOR PERIPHERAL VASCULAR CIRCULATION

Peripheral vascular disease results in increased peripheral vascular resistance due to narrowing and loss of elasticity in the vessel walls. Peripheral arterial insufficiency is present in most elderly individuals in varying degrees.

Indications of poor circulation in the feet include the absence of the dorsal pedal and posterior tibialis pulses, muscle fatigue, cramps in the foot and leg, intermittent claudication, pain, burning, coldness, pallor, paresthesias, atrophy of soft tissues, nail bed alterations, and trophic dermal changes such as dryness and loss of hair on the lower extremities. Prime significance should not be placed upon the absence or presence of pedal pulses as the pulses may not be palpable at pressures between 70 and 100 mmHg and are usually absent below 70 mmHg. The ankle/brachial index may be lower in some patients with palpable pulses due to hypertension compared to normotensive patients with lower ankle pressures and nonpalpable pulses.

Decreased vascularization increases the likelihood of injury due to fragility of the tissues. Delayed and inadequate healing results because there is a decrease in oxygen supply to the peripheral tissues. Assessment of the two separate vascular beds in the lower extremity should include the major arterial system as well as the small arteries, arterioles, capillaries, and venules which nourish the skin. In most cases the small vessels are dependent on the flow of the major vessels. However, in chronic occlusive vascular disease in which partial or complete occlusion of the major vessels occurs, the blood supply to the tissues may be adequate due to extensive collateral arterial circulation developed by the body as a defense to the slowly progressing ischemia.

The physiological basis for the use of Buerger-Allen exercises is hypothetical and the authors of this book present this theoretical explanation based on clinical experience. The importance of treating individuals with arterial insufficiency is threefold: to enhance peripheral circulation, to prevent limb loss, and to permit healing of wounds. The aim of Buerger-Allen exercises in the treatment of occlusive arterial disease is to improve circulation in a noninvasive therapeutic way.

Buerger-Allen exercises are postural exercises that hypothetically increase local collateral circulation and stimulate circulatory flow through postural changes thereby enhancing tissue nourishment and blood supply.[60] The addition of active muscle contraction during each positional change also appears to improve circulation by stimulating blood flow to the working muscles to increase oxygenation and by the "milking" of the contracting muscles around the vascular structures. Buerger-Allen exercises are based on the theory that the alternating emptying and filling of blood vessels increases the efficiency of transporting blood by stimulating the peripheral vascular system.[61] Research currently underway clearly indicates that there are physiological improvements observed that enhance circulation, facilitate wound healing, and decrease hypersensitivity and pain in the lower extremities of elderly patients with peripheral vascular involvement.[62] Additionally, preliminary results indicate that Buerger-Allen exercises employed in the diabetic population are effective in enhancing circulation in the lower extremities and diminishing, if not eliminating, paresthetic pain in diabetics, in addition to improving muscle function through active foot and ankle pumping.[62]

Buerger-Allen exercises are performed according to the protocol displayed in Figures 13–5 through 13–7. The starting position is with the legs horizontal in supine, as depicted in Figure 13–5. The individual elevates the lower extremities at an angle of 45° until blanching occurs or for a maximum time of 3 minutes (Fig. 13–6). Active pumping and circling of the feet and isometric quadriceps and gluteal contractions are performed for one minute or more (not necessarily a consecutive minute) in the elevated position. Once the blanching has occurred in the elevated position, the subject returns to the horizontal position for three minutes, pumping and circling the feet for one minute of that time. The feet should go from a blanched color to a warm, rosy pink color. The subject then sits up and hangs the legs over the edge of the bed (Fig. 13–7). While in this position, again the individual is encouraged to actively plantarflex, dorsiflex, and circle the feet. This position is maintained for a minimum of three minutes or until rubor has occurred. Lastly, the individual returns to the horizontal position with the lower extremities flat for another three minutes (Fig. 13–5). Again, active muscle contraction of the leg muscles is performed for at least one minute in this position. One note of caution: in the elderly Bottomley recommends assuming the flat/supine position between the elevation and dependent phases to prevent the consequences of orthostatic hypotension. Buerger's original protocol goes from the elevated position directly to the dependent position. The entire sequence is repeated three times in each exercise session (for a total of thirty-six minutes of exercise). Buerger-Allen exercises should be performed once each day for maximum benefit. If the patient is not able to actively contract the muscles in the lower extremities (e.g., peripheral neuropathy is present and active muscle contraction is not possible, patient has a flaccid lower extremity due to hemiplegia) the clinician can passively plantarflex and dorsiflex the foot in each of the respective positions to increase blood flow and facilitate the pumping action of the surrounding musculature. The authors of this book have successfully employed high frequency

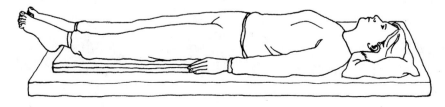

Figure 13–5. Buerger-Allen Protocol – Horizontal Position. Lying flat on back in rest position, pump and circle feet to facilitate circulation. Position maintained for at least 3 minutes. (Bottomley, JM (artist).)

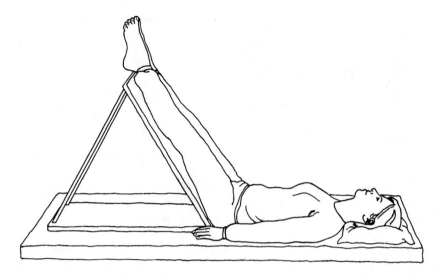

Figure 13–6. Buerger-Allen Protocol—Legs Elevated. *Lie on back with legs elevated at least 12 inches higher than the chest and ideally at 45 degrees. Pump and circle feet to enhance circulation. Maintain this position for 3 minutes.*

electrical stimulation to elicit threshold muscle contractions in the lower extremities of the elderly patient with peripheral neuropathy as well.

If the individual is in congestive heart failure (CHF), the Buerger-Allen protocol is modified by omitting the elevated position or having the patient seated upright (in cases of extreme CHF) and moving the lower extremities from a horizontal to a dependent position only. An absolute contraindication in the use of Buerger-Allen exercises is cellulitis.

EXAMINATION, EVALUATION, AND MODIFIED EXERCISE TESTING

In an elderly person's routine cardiopulmonary and vascular physical evaluation, particular attention must be paid to the neuromuscular, musculoskeletal, and sensory examination, because results of these tests will yield valuable information on residual abilities and potential for improvement. Goals of the examination include observation of deviations from normal structure or function, evidence of secondary complications from cardiopulmonary and cardiovascular diseases, and assessment of residual strengths.

Skin should be closely inspected, particularly over bony prominences, for evidence of excessive pressure, friction, or maceration that may lead to breakdown. With the high prevalence of diabetic and arteriosclerotic peripheral vascular disease in the elderly, it is also prudent to inspect the skin of the feet, particularly between the toes.

A musculoskeletal exam should include an evaluation for posture, joint range of motion, flexibility, and tenderness, and muscle strength with an emphasis on existing imbalances or asymmetry. An assessment for any complaints of pain should also be incorporated. Ambulatory status and gait pattern assessment is crucial in developing a reconditioning program.

In a neurological examination, mental status should be routinely evaluated. A routine check on appearance, affect, orientation, and communication is helpful in determining an elderly individual's level of functioning and safety. Other areas of importance in the neurologic examination include testing of sensation (particularly vibration, protective sensation, and proprioception), deep tendon reflexes, balance (sitting and standing), and coordination.

In the cardiopulmonary examination, a check for orthostatic hypotension may prove valuable, particularly in an older person who is complaining of light-headedness, dizziness, or episodes of blacking out with falling. This is particularly important in patients on hypertensive medications with orthostatic side effects. Checking the resting heart rate with comparison to a postactivity heart rate may yield valuable clues as to a person's level of endurance and tolerance of exercise. Identifying arrhythmias, murmurs, rales, or evidence of COPD may help explain exercise intolerance with easy fatiguability or dyspnea. Evaluating the respiratory pattern, posture, strength of cough, segmental lung expansion, and diaphragmatic excursion should be a routine part of evaluation, especially in an individual with known pulmonary disease. Cardiopulmonary patients often present with chronic musculoskeletal problems or peripheral adaptations such as clubbing of the fingers and toes, discoloration of the nail beds, or edema in the feet and ankles.

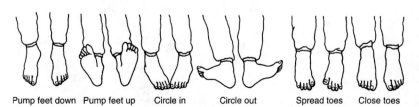

Pump feet down Pump feet up Circle in Circle out Spread toes Close toes

Figure 13–7. Buerger-Allen Protocol—Legs Dependent. *Sit with legs hanging over side of bed. In this position pump and circle feet, spread toes, then pinch toes together. Maintain the dependent position for 3 minutes.*

Checking extremity pulses is important, especially if the patient presents with complaints of claudication or peripheral sensory changes. The amount of activity needed to induce claudicant pain should be determined. As objective measures, local blood pressures and the time it takes for claudication to occur are helpful measures for establishing a baseline with which treatment effects can be compared. For instance, in a normal individual, treadmill or walking exercise tends to increase the systolic pressure at the ankle, but in the claudicant individual, the ankle pressure falls to a very low level and is slow to recover.[63]

Stress testing to determine an elderly individual's cardiopulmonary response to exercise is a crucial component of evaluation. There are several means of acquiring a baseline exercise level, which will be discussed in the subsequent section of this chapter. The appropriate stress test protocol and method for exercise testing employed will be determined by the older person's ambulatory and functional status, level of physical fitness, medical status, motivation, mentation, and safety of the test chosen. Many elderly individuals will not tolerate maximal test levels, and submaximal testing should be utilized to determine the level that is safe for prescribing and starting endurance training protocols. The importance of stress testing can not be overstated.

Another important consideration in determining the protocol that best tests an individual's exercise capacity is the method of exercise that will be used in the endurance training.

Step Tests

Steps are among the least expensive devices available for the administration of an exercise stress test. The most commonly employed step test is the *Master's 2-step exercise*. It requires a platform of two steps each nine inches high. The individual walks up and down the steps at a given rate determined by age and sex using a metronome to keep pace. This diagnostic test lasting only three minutes. Step testing is usually inadequate for measurement of aerobic work capacity and has its limitations in the elderly, especially with advanced aging. Quadriceps strength and endurance may not be adequate to maintain stepping for the full three minute period. The test is too strenuous for some cardiac patients, yet does not induce enough stress to adequately determine exercise capacity in elderly without occult cardiopulmonary problems.

Another step test uses a *single platform,* which can be raised vertically to increase the external workload is used to determine cardiovascular reponse to progressive exercise. This graduated multilevel step test parallels the principles used in the design of treadmill tests.[64] A stepping rate of 24 steps/minute is maintained while the platform is raised verically at periodic intervals (generally 2 cm each minute). The second phase of the step test increases the cadence to 30 steps/minute, again gradually increasing the height of the platform at the same time.

Modified Chair-Step Test for the Elderly

A particularly helpful modification of the step test is employed more commonly in the nursing home setting or with the frail elderly who can not maintain their balance during a step, bicycle, or treadmill testing.[65] This test is done in sitting using a bar or a platform of adjustable height placed in front of the seated individual. The feet are alternately lifted and placed on the bar or platform as in stepping at a cadence of twenty four to thirty steps/minute. The height of the bar or platform is gradually increased, dependent on physical capabilities of the elder, in three to six inch increments every one to three minutes up to the height of eighteen inches. In frail elderly, this author often modifies the increases the platform height to increments of one to two inches to a maximum of twelve inches and decreases the stepping pace to eighteen to twenty four steps/minute. If the person is able to reach the twelve or eighteen inch height, he or she can continue with the final phase of the testing protocol, which employs upper extremity reaching over the head each time a foot is raised. This has been found to be an effective means of evaluating cardiovascular and cardiopulmonary response to gradually increasing levels of work in the deconditioned elderly.

Walking Tests

A test that is applicable to the elderly without balance problems or ambulatory deficits is the walking test. A *twelve-minute walk*[66] or a *six-minute walk*[67] is employed in the elderly with cardiac or respiratory problems. Once again, this author modifies the length of this test based on the individual's capabilities. For instance, if the elder can only ambulate for three minutes, the length of the walk is decreased accordingly. The walk is accomplished on a level surface at a pace as brisk as the individual can manage and the distance recorded at the end of the timed period. This test is particularly useful in establishing a baseline walking level for those elderly who cannot accomplish either treadmill walking or bicycle riding because of angina or dyspnea.

For the more physically fit elderly, the use of a one-mile walk is a good measure of cardiopulmonary capabilities. The *one-mile walk test*[68] is on a level surface. A brisk pace is established by the individual and the amount of time it takes the individual to cover the last quarter mile is recorded. The VO_2 max is determined by a formula that incorporates the heart rate during the last quarter mile, the distance covered in the last quarter mile, and the age, sex, and weight of the individual exercise regressed against a constant (see Kline and associates[68] for details).

A *low level functional walking test* employs a ECG chest strap (e.g., Polaris™) to monitor cardiopulmonary responses during functional activities. The individual is evaluated during activities of daily living. For instance, ambulating from bedroom to bathroom, toileting activities, or dressing activities are monitored for cardiovascular response to those tasks that the elderly individual are required to perform for self maintenance on a daily basis. Often this assessment can be coordinated with the Cardiologist when a *Holter monitor* is utilized to evaluate cardiac response to daily activities over a 24 hour period.[69]

Treadmill Tests

The most commonly used treadmill test for the determination of maximal oxygen intake is the *Bruce or modified Bruce protocol*.[70] The modified test, which incorporates a much more gradual increase in the speed and incline of the treadmill, is most frequently employed for elderly individuals. Initially the speed is set at 1.7 mph at a grade of 10% (though in some protocols, the initial grade is set at 5% and increased to 10% during the first three minutes of the test for the more impaired elderly). Every three minutes the speed and the percent of incline is increased in a specified manner until a speed of 5 mph at a grade of 18% is reached. This stress test protocol can be used with relatively fit elderly individuals to accurately measure the cardiopulmonary response to exercise.

The *modified Balke test* is an alternative to treadmill stress testing. The rationale of the test is the same, but the speed of the treadmill is held constant (as determined by the individual's perceived capabilities) and every two minutes the grade is increased from 0% by 3.5% increments.[69]

In both of these protocols, assessment parameters include: expired air analysis, ECG, heart rate, blood pressure, and respiratory rate monitoring. The test is terminated using the following criteria: a decrease in blood pressure; ischemic drop of the ST segment or arrhythmias on the ECG, tachycardia; bradycardia; severe shortness of breath; angina; dizziness; or leg pain. Often the elderly individual's perceived limit of exersion will be the ending point of the stress test.

A *low level functional treadmill walking test* is an intermittent walking test used with patients with moderate to severe cardiac or respiratory involvement. It is divided into three stages and monitors ECG, blood pressure, respiratory rate, heart rate, O_2 saturation, and pulmonary function tests. Stage I is a six-minute walk on a level surface at a pace of approximately 1.5 to 2.0 mph. The objective of this phase of the assessment is to determine the cardiopulmonary response at this intensity of walking. At the end of six minutes, the patient is allowed to return to baseline heart rate, respiratory rate, and O_2 saturation.

Stage II is a functional ambulation assessment. The treadmill is set at a speed and incline equal to the functional work capacity based on the individual's physiologic and symptomatic response during stage I. This phase is also six minutes long and the

patient is allowed to return to baseline before proceeding to stage III.

Stage III is the maximum exercise tolerance component of the test, and it is also six minutes. The treadmill is set to produce a heart rate of 70% to 85% max or a pre-established ventilatory maximum. Termination of the test is based on the following criteria: (1) reaching 85% of the predicted heart rate maximum; (2) O_2 saturation of 85% or below; (3) reaching the predicted ventilatory maximum; (4) development of significant cardiac arrhythmias; or (5) the development of significant symptoms. This modified stress test elicits a safe exercise response that produces an actual exercise limit and enables accurate measurement of maximal levels in elderly individuals with severe pulmonary, coronary, or both impairment. It also allows flexibility in establishing the workload to be accomplished by modification according to the person's physiological and symptomatic response, and establishes an accurate baseline for exercise prescription.

Cycle Erogometer Test

The bicycle ergometer provides another alternative to exercise testing. The advantage is that individual are supported by the bike, and can maintain their balance using the handlebars. The use of a tractor seat in place of a regular bike seat to further facilitate the patient's stability and comfort while on the bike is helpful. For screening an older person for exercise prescription, a continuous test of six to nine minutes of cycling with gradual incremental increases in intensity and speed is employed.[65] The individual should work up to 70% to 85% of their predicted maximum heart rate. The same parameters are monitored during the bike stress test as in the treadmill tests.

Buerger-Allen Test for Peripheral Circulation

An objective means of measuring peripheral circulation is to time the emptying and filling times of the lower extremities. This is best accomplished using the *Buerger-Allen Testing Protocol* for peripheral circulation. In this test, the initial position is in supine with the legs resting in a horizontal plane (see Figure 13–5). Allow the individual to rest in this position for at least 3 minutes. Note the color of the feet (particularly the color of the nail beds). Ideally, the nail beds will be a healthy pink color. In the presence of peripheral vascular disease, however, the nail beds and skin color of the feet will be progressively deeper shades of pink to red based on the severity of the disease. One objective means of documenting skin color is through the use of photography, using instamatic film and taking care to keep the light source and distance of the camera from the lower extremities constant, so that subsequent photo documentation will be consistent. Other measures, such as skin temperature, circumference measures and grading of pitting edema if present, palpate for resting pulse rate and grade the pulse intensity (e.g., 0, 1+, 2+, 3+), sensory testing for protective sensation and vibratory sensation are valuable baseline measures to obtain during initial and subsequent examination. An evaluation form and flow sheet for managing Buerger-Allen exercise protocol, developed by Jennifer M. Bottomley for a recent research project, is provided as an example in APPENDICES 13A–1 (evaluation form) and 13A–2 (flow sheet).

The next part of the examination is to time the amount of time in takes the lower extremities to drain when placed in an elevated position. This is accomplished by raising the lower extremities to 45° as seen in Figure 13–6. The time needed for the nail beds and feet to blanch (whiten) is measured using a stop watch. Normal emptying time is around 20 to 30 seconds. With increasing severity of peripheral vascular disease, the length of time it takes for the lower extremities to drain will increase. Severe involvement of the vascular system may result in drainage times of three minutes and beyond. On initial evaluation, the skin temperature and objective pulse grading should be documented in the elevated position as well. When severe edema exists, it is also helpful to measure circumference of the lower extremities following a minimum of three minutes in an elevated position. This is relatively simple to do using the figure-8 circumferential measurement techniques described in Chapter 6 of this text.

In the original testing protocol using the Buerger-Allen evaluation technique, Buerger described changing the position of the lower extremities in relationship to gravity, by lowering the legs from the elevated to the fully dependent position as depicted in Figure 13–7. Once again, the time it takes for the lower extremities to fill is established using a stop watch, and the therapist will be looking for the deep pink coloration of the feet and nail beds. Normal filling time is twenty to thirty seconds. Filling time will increase exponentially in relationship to the severity of the disease. In severest cases, the filling time will take three minutes or more. With peripheral vascular involvement, the color of the feet will range from a deep, reddish pink to a deep, dusky, purple coloration. Pulses should be graded and skin temperature recorded in the dependent position.

In the case of the frailer older adult, a modified testing protocol is recommended by this author. Especially if the patient has problems with orthostatic hypotension, testing may require that the horizontal position be assumed between the elevated and dependent positions. In this case, the time it takes for the lower extremities to return to the original horizontal coloration will be timed and recorded. Then the change in position from horizontal the dependent position described above will be timed and recorded. This will allow more time for the individual to accommodate physiologically to postural changes and avoid orthostatic complications.

Other Evaluations of Circulatory Status

Vascular evaluation should include the palpation and grading of the femoral, popliteal, dorsalis pedis, and posterior tibial pulses, as previously mentioned, and the observation of other clinical signs and symptoms indicating vascular compromise to the lower extremities. These include intermittent claudication, foot temperature (e.g., cold feet), nocturnal pain, rest pain, nocturnal and rest pain relieved by dependency, blanching on elevation, atrophic skin, absence of hair growth, and presence of wounds or gangrene. Any lesions, areas of hyperkeratosis or discoloration should be observed and documented.[71]

Palpating for the pedal pulses can yield a qualitative measure of the dorsalis pedis or posterior tibial circulation, but the examiner must realize that there can be a substantial decrease in flow to the extremity even though arterial ankle pulses are good. To differentiate an organic disorder, such as blockage of the lumen of the vessel, from a vasospastic condition, temporary dilation of the vessel in question is a useful vascular test. This approach is accomplished by using an arterial tourniquet for one minute and then releasing it. The perfusion distal to the tourniquet should increase if the condition is due to vasospasm.

The evaluation of skin temperatures and circumferential measures are other means of assessing circulatory insufficiency and determining the presence of infection.

Skin temperature measurements are useful if the circulatory problem is asymmetrical though test results may be variable because of ambient temperature. In an individual with peripheral vascular disease, the extremities are often cool to touch and in the presence of infection, there may be "hot spots." The use of a skin temperature monitoring device to obtain precise temperature measures is helpful, however, the therapist can also objectively evaluate skin temperature by touch and grading cold, cool, warm, and hot accordingly.

Circumferential measurements of the lower leg and foot also aid in the assessment of the individual with peripheral vascular involvement. Edema is often present when the peripheral vascular system is involved, due to an inability of the involved vessels to efficiently remove waste materials from the interstitial tissues. This edema will increase in the dependent position owing to gravity. Measurement of circumference can be accomplished using Jobst measurement tapes (which are free from your local vendor). Measure around the metatarsal heads, midfoot, figure-8 around the ankle and incrementally every three inches up the lower leg from the malleolar level to the subpatellar level. Another means of determining the level of edema is volume displacement using a bucket of water with a ruler taped to the inside and measuring the amount of water that is displaced upward when the lower extremity is submerged (in inches or centimeters). This method will give an objective and reproducible means for assessing edema in the lower extremity.

The evaluation of wound status is also very important, and is discussed in detail in Chapter 14.

The neurological examination requires a reflex hammer, tuning fork (128 cycles per second, i.e., the musical key of C), and Semmes-Weinstein monofilaments. Testing for vibratory, proprioceptive, temperature, and protective sensation should be done with the patient's eyes closed. Distinguish the boundaries of any hyper- or hypo-esthesias and determine if these patterns are symmetrical or asymmetrical. The absence or presence of sweating should be noted. Reflexes to be tested include the patellar reflex and the ankle jerk. As the ankle jerk becomes more difficult to elicit with increasing age, it may appear to be absent. To aid this reflex, gently pronate and dorsiflex the foot to put tension on the Achilles and gently tap the tendon. Test for the Babinski reflex to determine if there is a superficial plantar response. To determine if there is clonus, forcibly dorsiflex the foot at the ankle. To test for loss of balance, have the individual stand with eyes closed and feet close together and compare this to the same stance with the eyes open (Romberg's sign). See Chapter 6 for greater detail on these testing procedures and examples of evaluation forms.

Muscle strength should be tested in all lower extremity muscles using a graded manual muscle test. Again, symmetry should be noted. Gait evaluation is a helpful adjunct to muscular evaluation to determine unsteady gait patterns, foot drops, or the presence of a "steppage" gait. Range-of-motion and joint mobility should be evaluated and any deformities (e.g., Charcot joints, hammer, claw, or mallet toes, hallux abductus valgus) should be noted as these abnormalities are usually indicative of intrinsic foot muscle weakness. Trophic nail changes should also be evaluated.

Vibratory and temperature sense are diminished very early in the peripheral vascular disease process compromising proprioception, kinesthesia, and awareness of temperature gradients.

Protective sensation defined by Nawcozenski and Birke[72] is 5.07 grams of pressure using the Semmes-Weinstein monofilaments. Specific evaluation of the entire plantar surface of the foot will determine areas of sensory loss vulnerable to breakdown.[73,74]

The Semmes-Weinstein monofilaments have been found to be a reproducible and accurate mode for testing sensation, and reliable in predicting those individuals at risk for ulceration due to loss of protective sensation.[73,74] The Carville group[73] measured protective sensation using the Semmes-Weinstein monofilaments and found that those individuals who could not feel the 5.07 mono filament were at greater risk for skin breakdown than those who could feel this level of stimulation. They demonstrated that 5.07 grams was the protective sensation threshold. Standardizing of sensory testing is crucial in the evaluation, so that adequate protective measures can be taken to prevent feet at risk from developing ulcers.

EXERCISE PRESCRIPTION

Intensity, duration, and frequency are the three major components of exercise prescription. These three elements are used in formulating an appropriate exercise level based on the results of exercise stress testing. Evidence suggests that the best prescription to improve cardiovascular training effects should incorporate an intensity of 60% or greater of the maximum heart rate, be done for a duration of twenty minutes or more with a frequency of three or more times per week.[10,15,52] In the absence of cardiopulmonary impairment, the elderly can achieve a cardiovascular training effect with aerobic exercise. As a result of the decline in maximum heart rate with age, a training effect occurs at lower relative heart rate increases compared with younger subjects.[14] Several alternative exercise forms have also been shown to provide substantial cardiovascular benefits as will be described in greater detail in a subsequent portion of this chapter.

Elderly individuals with cardiopulmonary impairment may be restricted in the amount of aerobic activity they can do because of dyspnea or angina. Individuals with comorbidities, such as chronic obstructive lung disease, superimposed on cardiac pathology, may not experience the same training effects as a person with cardiac disease alone. As Irwin and Zadai[21] so aptly put it:

> At the present time, the question remains of whether patients with COPD ever achieve the hallmark "anaerobic threshold" even at the higher heart rates they demonstrate with lower levels of exercise. The improvements seen in COPD patients after exercise training are not consistent with the changes demonstrated by exercising normals (central cardiovascular training effect).

Intensity of exercise is a significant factor in determining the success of improving aerobic capacity with exercise.[15,47] In healthy elderly, usually the heart rate is utilized as a reliable indicator of exercise intensity. Heart rate can be a useful indicator for those people who can palpate their own pulse (or have access to a wrist monitoring device). In prescribing exercise for the elderly, it is important to establish a target heart rate that is 60% plus that achieved during exercise testing in order to obtain the desirable VO_2 max. Once an exercise prescription has been determined that provides the time and the distance necessary to improve endurance at a safe heart rate (usually between 60% to 70% max initially), patients are instructed to maintain that heart rate level throughout their exercise session.

In the elderly individual with cardiopulmonary disease, however, heart rate may be an inadequate reflection of oxygen consumption as the oxygen cost of an ineffective breathing pattern and inefficient cardiac pump can shift the amount of O_2 supply away from the working peripheral muscles. In addition, heart rates are often modified by the medications prescribed for cardiac conditions. It is important to instruct the individual in heart rate monitoring, as the heart rate is correlated with the oxygen demand that produced significant symptoms during the patient's stress test. The elderly individual is instructed, therefore, not to exceed that heart rate during an exercise session. Given the unreliability of the heart rate as an indicator of O_2 consumption during exercise, rather than having these individuals rely on heart rate as an indicator of exercise intensity, the intensity is prescribed by recommending a certain amount of work be accomplished over a given period of time. For instance, a person who was able to walk 0.5 miles in the twelve minute walking test can continue to walk for endurance with the goal of one mile in thirty minutes. Gradually the distance can be extended as determined by the patient's cardiopulmonary tolerance, self-perceived endurance, and motivation. In endurance terms, the intensity of the exercise is determined by the distance covered in a specific amount of time.

If exercise stress tests are not available, establishing the intensity of exercise in an older adult may be accomplished by using the "communication rule." In this measure, if an individual who is exercising is able to carry on a conversation without shortness of breath, they are exercising at a level well within their physiological capabilities. An individual who is exercising at a submaximal level (40% to 60%) can carry on a conversation, but has apparent shortness of breath and is talking between periods of breaths. When aerobic levels of exercise are reached (60% to 80%), the individual can communicate, but, would prefer not to. Anerobic levels of exercise result in the inability to communicate at all.

The primary goal of endurance training is to increase the elderly individual's functional activity level by improving their exercise capacity. In order to improve endurance, the duration of exercise should also to be a part of the prescription. If an elderly individual is only able to accomplish Stage I (six minutes) of the low level functional test, intermittent exercise periods would be a way to incorporate the principle of duration. The initial prescription has a duration time (e.g., twenty minutes) that equals the eventual goal, however, the exercise is performed in 4- to 5-minute segments with 2- to 3-minute rest periods in between. As the exercise progresses, the rest periods are gradually decreased until the individual is able to walk the entire twenty minute period continuously. In the nursing home environment, it is not uncommon to exercise an elderly patient two to three short sessions a day at first, before progressing to one long session. The same principle is applicable for those elderly exercising in the community on their own. Gradually the time of the exercise session can be increased as endurance improves.

Frequency is another consideration in exercise prescription. Initially, especially with the intermit-

tent exercise program, it is recommended that the exercise session be done daily unless the individual is limited by symptoms or the weather. Once the person is able to exercise for twenty to thirty consecutive minutes, four to five times per week is beneficial in maintaining and improving the training effects of exercise.

As previously discussed, recovery times are frequently longer in the elderly due to the increased O_2 demands. Warm-up and cool-down sessions are essential as part of the exercise prescription. Individualized warm-up and cool-down sessions can address muscle imbalances, postural problems, flexibility, and overall strength. Stretching and flexibility exercises can also incorporate breathing exercises to facilitate the mobilization of the thorax and improve ventilation. Balance and coordination are often facilitated with rhythmic aerobic exercises as well.[75]

The importance of *activity* cannot be overemphasized. Daily activities are also beneficial in maintaining and improving cardiac and pulmonary function. Though reaching target heart rates established during stress tests is the most effective means of improving aerobic fitness, the truth of the matter is that *Anything Above Rest Works!* Appendix 13B provides the metabolic equivalence of various activities of daily living. The heart responds to activity like any other muscle. Moderate amounts of regular work can help strengthen the heart and improve circulation. Aerobic activities include raking, gardening, pushing a lawn mower, dancing, walking, and many other activities that are done on a daily routine, as you will see in Appendix 13B.

Figure 13–8 provides a pictorial representation (just like the food triangle) of activities and exercises based on a weekly recommendation for increasing fitness and improving health.

SPECIAL CONSIDERATIONS IN PRESCRIBING EXERCISE

Pacemakers and Intracardiac Defibrillators

Pacemakers and intracardiac defibrillators (ICDs) are frequently used in an elderly population to treat abnormally slow heart rhythms and the resulting symptoms of lightheadedness and fatigue. Pacemakers and ICDs are also used in patients with heart failure and those with atrial fibrillation.

Exercise testing can act as a diagnostic and a therapeutic tool in the adjustment of rate-responsive pacemakers. Once a permanent pacemaker with rate-responsive pacing capacity has been implanted, exercise testing is useful in the evaluation of pacemaker behavior, as well as optimizing the pacemaker response. Since most patients with pacemakers are the elderly, the exercise protocol should use gradual increments in workload, such as modified Bruce, Balke, or Naughton protocol. It is important to remember

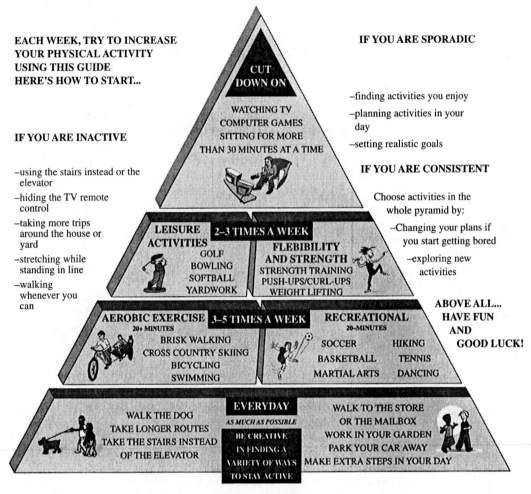

Figure 13–8. Activity Triangle: Recommended Weekly Allowance for Activity and Exercise. (Distributed by: Park Nicollet Health Source (1–800–372–7776). *Copyright ©1996 Institute for Research and Education Health-System, Minnesota.*)

that in patients with pacemaker dependence, ST segment changes do not reflect ischemic changes, and thus other diagnostic tests are required (e.g., thallium scan).[76]

Recent technologic advances have dramatically improved pacemaker function to the point at which they can nearly mimic normal cardiac function at rest and during exercise. Nevertheless, it is important that the exercise training upper heart rate limit be set below the patient's ischemic threshold.

When developing an exercise program for pacemaker patients, basic information about the pacemaker must be understood. Atrial, ventricular, and dual-chamber devices can produce varying exercise responses and impact the exercise prescription. The type of rate adaptive sensor the pacemaker has will affect the nature of heart response, and therefore, must be taken into account when prescribing exercise.[77]

Patients with ICDs are at risk of receiving inappropriate shocks during exercise. This can occur if the sinus heart rate exceeds the programmed threshold rate or if the patient develops and exercise-induced supraventricular tachycardia. For this reason,

patients with ICDs should be closely monitored during exercise to ensure that their heart rate does not approach the activation rate for the device. At least a 10% safety margin between exercise heart rate and rate cut-off for the device is advised.[77]

The elderly patient with an ICD or a pacemaker can benefit from exercise training. In addition to improvements in functional capacity, exercise training can also reduce cardiac risk factors (e.g., cholesterol, high blood pressure) and improve psychosocial outcomes.

Obesity

Obesity is related to increased risk for cardiovascular disease in the elderly. In fact, Jarret[78] found an increased risk for the development of cardiovascular problems at both extremes of the weight distribution curve. The evidence suggests that obesity heightens other atherogenic risk factors (e.g., smoking, coexisting disease) and thereby contributes to increased risk.[79] Data from the Framingham study at 30-year follow-up demonstrates a continuous relationship between obesity and coronary morbidity and mortality (stronger in men than in women). Obesity is associated with both increased blood pressure and increased serum lipoprotein levels.[80] In the Framingham study,[81] correlation between relative weight and either systolic or diastolic pressure declined steadily over adult life. Using the body mass index (BMI) Body mass index (BMI) is the body weight expressed in relation to height; BMI = weight (kg) ÷ height^2 (m).) and blood pressure, Havlik and associates,[82] reported similar declines in men over the age range 30 to 70 years. Harlan and co-workers[83] showed a reduction in association between BMI and systolic blood pressure in older women. The weaker association at older ages remains significant for men, but not for women.

In the Framingham study, the correlation between relative body weight and total plasma cholesterol is not significant over age 50 years for men; for women, it is significant only among 35- to 39-year olds.[84] Further analyses showed that, over age 50 years, BMI is no longer significantly associated with low-density lipoprotein (LDL) cholesterol in either sex. However, the strong inverse relationship between high-density lipoprotein (HDL) cholesterol and BMI remains statistically significant, even among subjects aged 70 to 79 years.[84,85] Therefore, the benefits of maintaining optimal weight for height are associated with a positive effect on HDL cholesterol levels.[86]

The effects of weight change on blood lipid profiles are considerable. In the Framingham study, the investigators found that a 10-unit change in weight relative to height was associated with a change in serum total cholesterol of 11 mg/dL in men and 6.3 mg/dL in women. There was no diminution in these relationships among older age groups.[81] Both Wolf and Grundy[87] and Zimmerman and associates[88] found modest increases in HDL cholesterol with weight reduction.

Both blood lipids and blood pressure are sensitive to the degree of obesity.[86] A significant drop in age-specific blood pressure indicates that effective control of obesity, especially the prevention of weight gain in middle adult life, is of potentially great value in reducing cardiovascular mortality.[89] Few studies compare the relative risks associated with weight fluctuation and sustained obesity. In the Framingham study, weight at younger ages has been found to be an important predictor of cardiovascular disease.[90,91] Weight reduction through exercise and diet has been shown to confer substantial improvement in the cardiovascular risk profile. Therefore, it is recommended for elderly individuals who are 20% or more above desireable weight as defined by BMIs of 27.2 for men and 26.9 for women.[92] In individuals with diabetes, hypertension, dyslipidemia and gout, lesser degrees of overweight should be reversed.[93]

Epidemiologic studies have generally shown that the transition from a normal state to overt non-insulin-dependent diabetes mellitus (NIDDM) with increasing age is characterized by a gradual increase in glucose in-tolerance.[94–96] There is evidence, however, that deterioration in glucose tolerance over the course of a lifetime may not be solely a consequence of aging.[96] In fact, the contribution of aging may be relatively modest. Data from several studies[97–99] suggest that although there is some decline in glucose tolerance with age, the degree to which this occurs is modulated by other factors, namely body fat and level of physical activity.

Excess abdominal adiposity is an important correlate of NIDDM[100] and a primary condition for loss of insulin sensitivity and glucose tolerance in aging.[101] Physical activity performed regularly is associated inversely with both prevalence and incidence of NIDDM. Regular exercise appears to protect from the development of insulin resistance and glucose intolerance. The effects of exercise training on fat distribution and glucose regulation has been shown to eliminate the occurrance of NIDDM and moderate-intensity aerobic training can help to normalize glucose responses, especially in older people with glucose intolerance.[96] These training-related improvements in glucose regulation have been found to be regulated by free fatty acids (FFA) concentrations. Thus, even in successful aging, regular moderate-intensity exercise has been shown to have a beneficial effect on glucose regulation, and an even greater significance in older people with established hyperglycemia and insulin resistance.[96]

Diabetes Mellitus

Cross-sectional studies have shown that the impaired glucose tolerance of aging is significantly related to the level of physical fitness or activity.[102] Few studies have been done specifically on those 60 years of age and older. One prospective trial of the effects of exercise on glucose tolerance was carried out on men 60 years of age and older. It was found that, while glucose levels did not change, both insulin and C peptide levels were lower.[50] In addition, high-density lipoprotein cholesterol levels increased and triglyceride levels decreased. Exercise trials in patients with type II diabetes mellitus have failed to show a major advantage of short-term exercise programs over diet alone.[45] However, trials that last five or more months did find improvements in glucose tolerance.[103–105]

Besides the possible beneficial effects of exercise on glucose tolerance, exercise training may also improve cardiovascular fitness, lipid profiles, hypertension, osteopenia, and psychologic function in diabetic patients. Risks of exercise in diabetics include hypoglycemia, ketosis, dehydration, myocardial ischemia, arrhythmias, acceleration of proliferative retinopathy, increased proteinuria, and trauma (particularly in patients with neuropathy). The National Institutes of Health (NIH) consensus panel concluded that the effects of exercise on metabolic control in non-insulin-dependent diabetes mellitus is often variable and of small magnitude.[106] Pacini and associates[107] demonstrated that normal weight, physically active older subjects have normal insulin-binding capacity, insulin sensitivity, and insulin secretory capacity in response to glucose stimulus. Helmrich and coworkers[105] showed that increased activity levels actually decreased the incidence of diabetes mellitus. Studies of long-term exercise programs need to be undertaken before a formal recommendation for an exercise prescription can be given, however, the benefits of exercise for cardiovascular conditioning and the potential for modifying glucose intolerance in the diabetic clearly outweigh the risks.

Medications

Almost all elderly patients who have cardiac problems are on medications such as β-blockers or calcium channel blockers. Beta-blockers are cardioselective adrenoreceptor blocking agents which usually result in a reduction in both the resting and exercise heart rate and cardiac output. Calcium channel blockers inhibit the influx of calcium thereby reducing the heart rate and blood pressure for any given load. In other words, these medications reduce the cardiac responsiveness to increasing activity levels, and, therefore, heart rate is not a good measure of exercise stress.

Recovery rates appear to be a good practical indicator of stress levels in these individuals. If a return to the resting heart rate occurs within two minutes following cessation of exercise, it is considered a safe level of activity. If the individual returns to a resting heart rate within one minute or less, they may increase their exercise level. A period of recovery three minutes or greater is considered to be an indication that the individual is exercising at a level that is too stressful to the cardiopulmonary system, and the intensity of exercise needs to be decreased.

Medications used for patients with pulmonary diseases include: oxygen, systemic and inhaled bronchodilators, steroids, and antibiotics. Most of these drugs are utilized to increase the oxygen supply and decrease the oxygen demand through a decrease in the work of breathing. Antibiotics are used to combat infection. These drugs can affect exercise tolerance by slowing metabolism which leads to early fatigue.

Osteoporosis

Osteoporosis in the elderly population must be considered when prescribing cardiovascular reconditioning exercise programs. The risk of stress fracture is one component of this concern. The unavailability of calcium, an element crucial in the strength of myocardial muscle contracture, is another important concern. The estimated loss of bone from its peak in young adulthood to age 80 is comparable to the reported 35% to 45% decline in muscle strength during the life span.[108] Since a clear relationship between muscle strength and bone mass has been established,[109–112] physical activity has gained attention as a method for improving bone mass, maximizing muscle strength, and facilitating the absorption and utilization of calcium. The mechanisms by which the skeleton responds to activity are discussed in Chapter 11. The evidence suggests that bone mass increases in response to application of mechanical stress.[113–115] Bone density appears to be higher in physically active people and the literature suggests that exercise significantly reduces the rate of age-related bone loss.[116,117,118]

Currently it is known that the type of exercise best for improving bone mass involve aerobic, weight-bearing activities, such as walking and jogging, in addition to weight lifting and extension exercises to promote the piezoelectric effects. All of these exercise forms directly impact the cardiopulmonary system. It is important to evaluate the elderly patient with osteoporosis for cardiovascular and cardiopulmonary involvement, and likewise to determine if the individual with cardiac, pulmonary, and/or vascular problems is at a higher risk for stress fractures as a result of osteoporosis.

Congestive Heart Failure/Cardiomyopathy

There was a time in the not-too-distant past when exercise was contraindicated in an individual with cardiomyopathy and congestive heart failure. However, as the research (to follow) indicates, although precautions need to be taken in relation to the pathophysiological cardiovascular dynamics in these patients, exercise, starting just above rest and gradually progressing to the submaximal ranges, is beneficial for those elders with cardiac failure.

Exercise performance in chronic heart failure is severely impaired, due in part to a peripherally mediated limitation.[119] In addition to impaired maximal exercise capacity, the O_2 uptake (VO_2) response during submaximal exercise may be affected, with a greater reliance on anaerobiosis leading to early fatigue. Therefore, exercise periods need to be shorter and at lower intensities in the initial phases of reconditioning. Hepple and associates[119] studied the relationship between oxygen utilization and peripheral response to exercise in a group of elderly patients with chronic heart failure compared to healthy sedentary elderly individuals at submaximal exercise levels. Heart failure subjects displayed a significantly prolonged VO_2 kinetics response at similar absolute workloads compared to healthy controls. In addition, heart failure subjects demonstrated a lower maximal calf blood flow compared to the controls. These results indicate that patients with heart failure have a prolonged VO_2 kinetics on-response compared with healthy subjects at a similar absolute work rate, but not at a similar relative work rate. Thus, despite a reduced maximal calf blood flow response associated with heart failure, it does not appear that this contributes to an impairment of the submaximal exercise response beyond that explained by a reduced maximal exercise capacity [VO_{2max}].[119]

Peripheral microvascular function plays an important role in congestive heart failure (CHF). Decreased exercise blood flow and microvascular dysfunction have been described in the condition and influences exercise capacity in the CHF patient. Sorensen and associates[120] demonstrated that these factors are related to or can be characterized by clinical severity of CHF. Patients with CHF have reduced exercise skeletal muscle blood flow, which is a limiting factor for the reduced maximal exercise capacity. Moreover, microvascular distensibility in skeletal muscle is reduced and correlates to maximal exercise skeletal muscle blood flow.[120] It was determined that skeletal muscle blood flow correlates to exercise time. This implies that increased skeletal muscle microvascular stiffness may contribute to reduced blood flow during exercise, and skeletal muscle blood flow may partly limit length of exercise performance in CHF patients diagnosed with idiopathic dilated cardiomyopathy.[120]

In normal subjects during exercise, there is vasoconstriction of nonexercise resistance vessels and an increase in blood pressure. It has been found that impairment in the reflex venoconstriction in patients with hypertrophic cardiomyopathy is related to syncope or exercise hypotension.[121] Thomson[122] investigated patients with vasovagal syncope with structurally normal hearts and patients with hypertrophic cardiomyopathy compared with normal controls and found a failure of vasoconstriction in both compared groups with normal subjects. This was evidenced by exercise hypotension. There is an association between exercise hypotension and sudden death. The author of this study speculates that in patients with vasovagal syncope and structurally and electrically normal hearts, exercise hypotension is well tolerated. However, in patients with structurally abnormal hearts, exercise hypotension can have catastrophic consequences.[122]

Another concern in cardiomyopic patients is the low ejection fraction and its relationship to potential arrhythmias. The results of a study by Mager and colleagues,[123] however, suggest that patients with a diminished ejection fraction as low as 16% can safely perform an exercise program. A significant improvement in peak VO_2 and maximal work rate was achieved in this study. Moreover, this study suggests that exercise training might diminish the severity of asymptomatic ventricular arrhythmia.[123]

Peripheral adaptations and ventricular abnormalities influence physical performance in chronic heart failure. However, the role of the heart in determining exercise capacity has not been completely elucidated. To define cardiac determinants of exercise capacity in patients with dilated cardiomyopathy, Pepi and associates[124] measured peak exercise oxygen consumption, left ventricular ejection fraction, left and right atrial and ventricular cavity dimensions, and mitral and tricuspid valvular flows.[124] These researchers concluded that in patients with dilated cardiomyopa-thy, peak VO_2 is related to left and right ventricular dimensions, left and right ventricular filling patterns and ejection fraction. It was determined that both systolic and diastolic dysfunction influence functional capacity in chronic heart failure patients.[124] Other researchers assessed the ventricular-arterial coupling at peak exercise in patients with dilated cardiomyopathy coupled with respiratory gas analysis and concluded that ventricular arterial coupling is further altered at peak exercise in these patients because of a lack of increase in contractility and not due to altered effective arterial elastance response.[125]

The utility of metabolic gas exchange measurements in evaluating the severity and determinants of exercise limitation was studied during upright symptom-limited cardiopulmonary exercise with hypertrophic cardiomyopathy and healthy age- and gender-matched subjects.[126] It was concluded that the peak VO_2 is significantly related to the functional class as defined by the New York Heart Association in patients with hypertrophic cardiomyopathy and that peak VO_2 was a superior measure of cardiovascular performance. The data from this study indicate that mechanical obstruction has an adverse pathophysiologic effect on functional capacity and that VO_2 provides an indicator to support treatments aimed at gradient reduction. Low peak VO_2 characteristics suggests that measurement of VO_2 may aid in differential diagnosis between a cardiomyopic and healthy heart.[126] In chronic heart failure, oxygen delivery during exercise is impaired mainly because of failure of cardiac output to increase normally.[127] Compensatory mechanisms are that hemoglobin concentration increases and there is a rightward shift in the oxyhemoglobin dissociation curve. In addition, as previously mentioned, blood flow redistribution from the non-exercising organs and muscles to the exercising muscles occurs.[127] Changing the exercising muscle group alters the ventilatory response to exercise in chronic heart failure. The recognized muscle abnormalities previously described in CHF may contribute to the ventilatory abnormalities of this condition during increasing levels of activity.[128]

Constant workload exercise at submaximal levels of exercise intensity is frequently used in physical training programs. Faggiano and associates[129] studied the hemodynamic changes induced at a steady workload in CHF patients and found a marked increase in right heart pressure. Cardiac output and heart rate were significantly higher during submaximal exercise at higher workloads, though the systolic pulmonary artery pressure was not statistically different at increasing levels of exercise. Additionally, the hemodynamic profile during submaximal exercise at the anaerobic threshold was similar to that observed during symptom-limited exercise. It was concluded that in patients with heart failure, submaximal exercise performed at a constant workload, even at low exercise intensity, may determine relevant pressure changes in pulmonary circulation thereby influencing the availability of oxygen and affecting endurance.[129]

Mancini and co-researchers[130] investigated the impact of alteration of glycogen stores and metabolism on exercise performance in patients with heart failure. In normal subjects, muscle glycogen depletion results in increased exertional fatigue and reduced endurance. Skeletal muscle biopsies have revealed reduced glycogen content in patients with congestive heart failure (CHF).[130] Whether glycogen depletion contributes to reduced endurance and abnormal ventilation in CHF patient is not entirely known. The Mancini study indicated that glycogen depletion minimally affects maximal exercise performance, endurance or ventilation in CHF patients, whereas slowed glycogen utilization markedly enhances exercise endurance. This demonstrates that low-level therapeutic interventions that speed up or slow down use of glycogen stores may have great clinical significance in the individual with cardiomyopic heart failure.[130]

Webb-Peploe and colleagues[131] examined the benefits and complications of a home-based exercise program in patients with ischemic versus idiopathic dilated cardiomyopathy. Training in both groups resulted in a higher peak oxygen consumption, a higher peak heart rate, and improved sense of well-being. Patients with idiopathic dilated cardiomyopathy showed a significant increase in exercise time and peak oxygen consumption as well as a decrease in left ventricular end-diastolic and end-systolic measures in contrast to those with coronary artery disease, who developed a reduction in septal excursion and shortening following training.[131] Complications of training were more common in those patients with ischemic cardiomyopathy and these individuals experienced greater left ventricular workloads and poorer exercise tolerance with fluid retention and exercise-induced ventricular tachycardia. Conversely, those elders with idiopathic dilated cardiomyopathy, despite poorly functioning left ventricle status, exercised without complications. It was concluded that home-based exercise programs, particularly in those patients with idiopathic origin of the pathology, can proceed safely, with close monitoring for the development of complications.[131]

HORMONE REPLACEMENT THERAPY AS A SECONDARY PREVENTATIVE INTERVENTION

The protective effect of estrogen on the cardiovascular system has been supported by the higher age-specific risk of coronary artery disease in young and middle-aged men compared with women.[132] A woman has a very low risk of coronary artery disease (CAD) before menopause, which normally occurs around age 50 years. The frequency of myocardial infarction in women begins to increase in the perimenopausal period and continues to increase throughout the postmenopausal years. By her seven-

ties, a women's risk for CAD is approximately the same as that of a man.[133–135]

Data clearly indicate an association between estrogen production and the risk of CAD. One analysis of the Nurses' Health Study, a large trial of approximately 120,000 women, examined women who underwent bilateral oophorectomy (removal of the ovaries) and hysterectomy, a menopause equivalent, and compared the occurrence of nonfatal myocardial infarction and CAD death as a composite end point with that of a control group.[136] Subjects who underwent surgical menopause were divided into two groups according to hormone replacement therapy (HRT). The outcomes of these two groups were compared with those of a control group consisting of healthy premenopausal women with intact hormone systems. Women who began HRT after surgical menopause had a relative risk of developing CAD of approximately 0.9, a slight decrease that did not reach statistical significance. Therefore HRT conferred neither benefit nor harm compared with premenopausal women. In contrast, women who did not take HRT after surgical menopause were at increased risk of CAD compared with controls. This increased risk was statistically significant.[136]

An abundance of in vivo and in vitro data indicate beneficial effects of estrogen or estrogen in combination with progestin on particular cardiovascular risk factors. Overall a significant decrease in total cholesterol is seen with estrogen replacement therapy (ERT). A small rise in triglycerides also occurs, but this potential negative is overpowered by the beneficial increase in high-density lipoproteins (HDL) and decrease in low-density lipoproteins (LDL) that is conferred by ERT. In addition, ERT has a significant effect on lipoprotein a [Lp(a)], decreasing it by up to 50%.[132,137,138]

When cyclic HRT regimens containing progestins were added to traditional unopposed estrogen to decrease endometrial hyperplasia, the question of whether the addition of progestin would attenuate the beneficial cholesterol effects of estrogen was raised. The Postmenopausal Estrogen-Progestin Interventions (PEPI) trial indicated that progestins do not appear to have a major impact on lipoprotein benefits conferred by estrogen monotherapy.[139] The combination still results in a rise in HDL.[138,139]

In addition to its effects on cholesterol, estrogen is responsible for many effects that exert a positive influence on coronary artery disease. Both ERT and HRT cause increased insulin sensitivity and decreased glucose levels.[139,140] They also have effects on the vessel wall via several vasoactive proteins. Estrogen decreases renin and angiotensin-converting enzyme, endothelin-1, and angiotensin II receptor expression, and increases nitric acid. These effects, individually and combined, promote vasodilation.[141] Of particular interest in the area of secondary prevention of CAD are actions of the natural vasodilators nitric acid and acetylcholine. Normal, healthy vasculature relaxes in their presence. In diseased tissue, such as arteries with atherosclerotic plaque, the substances induce a paradoxic vasocontriction. Introducing estrogen reverses vasocontriction and restores the normal vasodilating response to these agents.[141,142] This is a key finding that illustrates the positive effect of estrogen on artherosclerotic tissue. Furthermore, after endothelial injury, estrogen inhibits vascular smooth muscle proliferation and promotes growth of healthy endothelial cells. Both actions improve long-term vascular health.[141,143]

Antioxidant activity has also been recognized with estrogen therapy. Alpha-Tocopherol, or vitamin E, and ß-carotene, both antioxidants, are being studied in numerous settings for their ability to prevent or treat disease. In comparison, the antioxidant activity of estrogen is equal or superior to these agents. Estrogen as an antioxidant may decrease the oxidation of LDL, which decreases the amount of oxidized LDL that is incorporated into atherosclerotic plaques.[142,143]

The duration of estrogen replacement therapy is also important. Studies indicate that long-term therapy is more beneficial for primary prevention of CAD than short-term therapy.[132,144] In another analysis, benefit was increased with current estrogen relative to both past and no estrogen therapy for prevention of myocardial infarction.[145] It is important to note that whereas past use did not confer as large a risk reduction compared with current HRT, it was still better than never having taken HRT.

Estrogen, with or without the addition of progestin, is associated with a number of systemic and local effects in addition to those seen in CAD. Substantial data have come from observational studies and small clinical trials on the effects of estrogen replacement in postmenopausal women and cognition. As with CAD, there is biologic plausibility and preliminary evidence for a favorable effect by estrogen on cognition and dementia. Estrogen also reduces the morbidity of osteoporosis by reducing fractures, and it improves the symptoms associated with menopause.

While many benefits are associated with estrogen use, there are also adverse effects. Data from the Heart and Estrogen/Progestin Replacement Study (HERS), the Nurses' Health Study[136] previously mentioned, and other studies have clearly shown an increased incidence of venous thromboembolic events associated with ERT. There is also an increase in endometrial cancer with unopposed estrogen therapy, and though this risk is attenuated with the addition of a progestin, the long-term consequences of estrogen and progesterone on endometrial hyperplasia are uncertain. Breast cancer, however, is perhaps the most well-known, and controversial, potential adverse effect of ERT. In the Nurses' Health Study, despite an overall reduction in mortality, there was a 43% increase in the risk of breast cancer mortality in women taking hormones for more than ten years. This risk increases proportionally with the length of time on hormone replacements.

Current data support an individualized approach to HRT in postmenopausal women. There are subgroups in which estrogen currently offers more risk than benefit. However, for the majority of women, we must explain the risks and benefits as we currently understand them. The decision of whether or not to proceed with HRT should ultimately be left with the patient, with guidance and counseling from her physician.

The preventive aspects of exercise in relationship to CAD and other diseases should not be overlooked. Increased activity and exercise levels have been directly linked to the prevention of heart disease and peripheral vascular pathologies. It has also been found that exercise mobilizes stores of inactive estrogen, using cholesterol to convert the dormant estrogen to the active form, and that women who exercise on a regular basis have higher levels of circulating estrogen without hormone replacement therapy.[146]

COMPLEMENTARY THERAPIES AND CARDIOVASCULAR DISEASE

Many complementary therapies have been implicated as effective modalities in the treatment of cardiovascular and cardiopulmonary disease. The exercise forms of Qi Gong and T'ai Chi, and the use of biofeedback, all of which have a meditative component, are particularly useful for geriatric rehabilitation therapists.

Cardiovascular endurance improves with Qi Gong and T'ai Chi exercises. These movement therapies have been found to increase the resistance to cardiovascular diseases and may actually delay the decline of cardiorespiratory function in older adults.[147,148] Qi Gong improves the ability to maintain activity levels and allows for a high energy return for daily activities. Though Qi Gong exercise does not appear to be an aerobic activity, research has found that it is in fact a low-to-moderate-intensity exercise with a significant aerobic effect.[147,149] It has also been found to be a safe exercise for individuals at high risk for cardiovascular disease.[147,150] Qi Gong may be prescribed as a suitable aerobic exercise for older adults[147,151] and is the most recommended aerobic exercise for coronary artery disease.[152] An additional benefit to Qi Gong and T'ai Chi exercise has been realized by a significant reduction in both systolic and diastolic blood pressure.[147,153] Respiratory function has also been shown to improve with enhanced ventilatory capacity without cardiovascular stress. Research indicates that one of the primary benefits is the efficient use of ventilatory volume and extremely efficient breathing patterns.[147,150]

Studies show that stress hormones (as measured by salivary cortisol levels) significantly drop during and after exercise practice.[154–156] This is not only important in managing stress- and tension-related pathologies, but also in improving the immune system's ability to maintain homeostasis. Sun and coworkers found a significant immune response as measured by a marked increase in blood T-cells during and after T'ai Chi practice.[157,158]

Based on Qi Gong and T'ai Chi exercisers' self-reports, there is a significant effect on mood and anxiety states. The improved sense of well-being has been documented by reported reduction in tension, anxiety, fatigue, depression and confusion. [154–156] Additional benefits included an improved mental attitude toward work, self, and life in general; a greater ability to cope with stress; more regular, restful sleep patterns; healthier eating habits; a greater ability to avoid or control mild depression; and a sense of harmony reported by a better communication pathway among body, mind, and spirit (e.g., a sense of well-being).

The use of biofeedback has also been shown to positively affect cardiovascular and cardiopulmonary status and to reduce stress. The effect of psychological strategies upon cardiorespiratory and muscular activity during aerobic exercise has been widely employed in sports therapy. Hatfield and associates[159] demonstrated that all cardiovascular parameters (e.g., heart rate, respiratory rate, depth of ventilation, blood pressure) could be consciously altered using biofeedback monitoring.[159] Leisman and coworkers[160] investigated the effects of fatigue and task repetition on the relationship between integrated electromyogram and force output of working muscles.[160] This study showed that with fatigue, integrated EMG activity increased strongly and functional force output of the muscle remained stable or decreased. Fatigue results in a less efficient muscle process. Through training using biofeedback, the efficiency of muscle contraction could be improved with volitional control, and the level of fatigue reduced.[160]

The central mechanisms and possibilities of biofeedback of the systemic arterial pressure have been investigated extensively.[159,161,162] McGrady[161] studied a group of patients with essential hypertension for the effects of group relaxation training and thermal biofeedback on blood pressure and on other psychophysiologic measures: heart rate, frontalis muscle tension, finger temperature, depression, anxiety, plasma aldosterone, plasma renin activity, and plasma and urinary cortisol. A significant decline in blood pressure was observed in 49% of the experimental group. Of that group 51% maintained lower blood pressure at a ten-month follow-up examination, suggesting that relaxation training has beneficial effects for short-term and long-term adjunctive therapy of essential hypertension in selected individuals.

Saunders and associates[163] examined the therapeutic effects of thermal biofeedback-assisted autogenic training in a group of diabetic and vascular disease patients with symptoms of intermittent claudication. The individuals received thermal feedback from the hand for five sessions, then from the foot for sixteen sessions, while hand and foot temperatures were monitored simultaneously. Within-session foot temperatures rose specifically in response to

foot temperature biofeedback, and starting foot temperature rose between sessions. Post-treatment blood pressure was reduced to a normal level. Attacks of intermittent claudication were reduced to zero after twelve sessions and walking distance increased by about a mile per day over the course of the treatment. It would appear that thermal biofeedback and autogenic training are potentially promising therapies for persons with diabetes and peripheral vascular disease.

Rice and Schindler[164] investigated the effect of relaxation training/thermal biofeedback on blood circulation in the lower extremities of diabetic subjects. A within-subject experimental design was used. During phase 1, all subjects used a self-selected relaxation method and recorded toe temperatures daily. During phase 2, subjects were taught biofeedback-assisted relaxation techniques designed to elicit sensations of warmth in the lower extremities and increase circulation and temperature. Subjects relaxed at home with the use of a designated relaxation tape. Each phase of the study lasted four weeks. Mean temperature change scores between phases 1 and 2 were 8.73% (phase 1) and 31.88% (phase 2). The greater increase in phase 2 was attributed to the biofeedback-assisted relaxation techniques. The authors concluded that diabetic patients show significant increases in peripheral blood circulation with this technique. This noninvasive method could serve as an adjunct treatment for limited blood flow in some complications of diabetes, such as ulceration.

Respiratory sinus arrhythmia, the peak-to-peak variations in heart rate caused by respiration, can be used as a noninvasive measure of parasympathetic cardiac control. A study by Reyes del Paso and associates[165] showed that subjects could actually alter their respiratory sinus arrhythmia (i.e., decrease or increase the rate) by monitoring respiratory biofeedback apparatus in conjunction with consciously concentrating on their depth and rate of respiration. Shahidi and Salmon[166] also demonstrated that individuals classified as Type A adults were able to modify their heart rates volitionally when instructed in relaxation techniques using EKG biofeedback monitoring.

When we are truly relaxed, very definite and measurable changes take place in the body.[161,167–169] These changes distinguish relaxation from the opposite states of tension or arousal. Some of the most significant changes are triggered by the two branches of the autonomic nervous system. The sympathetic branch of the nervous system controls body temperature, digestion, heart rate, respiratory rate, blood flow and pressure, and muscular tension. The parasympathetic nervous system lowers oxygen consumption and reduces the following bodily functions: carbon dioxide elimination, heart and respiratory rates, blood pressure, blood lactate, and blood cortisol levels.[161,167–171] These bodily changes are collectively referred to as the "relaxation response."

Recent research also suggests that among the biochemical changes triggered by relaxation there is an increase in the body's manufacture of certain mood-altering neurotransmitters.[170,171] In particular, production of serotonin (the naturally expressed biochemical equivalent to Prozac) is increased. Seratonin is associated with feelings of calmness and contentment.

Other complementary therapies have been shown to have beneficial effects on cardiovascular health, such as nutrition, herbal remedies, and acupuncture. However, for the purpose of this chapter, only the modalities that are used in rehabilitation therapies are discussed. Nutrition and herbal intervention for cardiovascular health are discussed in Chapter 7. The topic of acupuncture is clearly beyond the scope of this text.

CONCLUSION

It would be impossible to overlook the great therapeutic potential of physical exercise in the elderly. As Ernst Jokl[172] has noted,

> The theoretical basis for understanding the unimpaired adaptability to exercise with aging was provided more than 100 years ago by the great pathologist, Julius Cohnheim, who pointed out that irrespective of age, physiological challenges of all kinds are reliable in that they invariably result in an enhanced functional status. Training for strength increases strength; training for endurance increases endurance; training for skill increases skill.

Physical exercise and nutrition provide a solid foundation for a sound and healthy old age and can delay the inevitable deterioration of the aging process. The body's adaptability to exercise remains unimpaired with age, although, adaptation to exercise is less reliable when pathologic processes are present. Reports in medical literature and clinical experience provide numerous instances in which physical exercise and activity benefitted patients with coronary artery disease, diabetes mellitus, hypertension, pulmonary disorders, and other chronic illnesses. Physical exercise and training not only improve the physical capacities and skills of older people, they also affect the body's adaptability to physiological stresses.

Several physiologic mechanisms maintain homeostasis during an acute bout of external or internal stress. Age-related changes affect each of these responses limiting exercise performance and VO_2 max. Exercise has been shown to alter and reverse some of these changes and slow the decline in functional aerobic capacity. In doing so, an elderly individual's ability to perform activities of daily living are improved and the quality of life enhanced. Exercise and functional mobility exercises should be considered an integral part of a rehabilitation program for the elderly.

The impact of the growth of the number of older persons in our population on our health care system is emphasized by the rapidity of the increase. The over-85 age group is the fastest growing segment. As age increases, the comorbidity, complexity, and chronicity of health and functional impairments of our cardiopulmonary and cardiovascular patients increase, producing progressive vulnerability to the physical, psychological, and social perturbations confronted by our older patients. Associated with these changes are the economic implications of the rising health care and social welfare costs of advancing age. This presents a challenge to health care providers in terms of assessing quality as well as quantity of life and distinguishing those conditions that are reversible from those that are not. As rehabilitation specialists, we understand the preventive effects of exercise, nutrition, and lifestyle changes. So we must face this challenge of these converging exponents and be prepared for both the opportunities and the economic and social risks and burdens posed by our aging society. Cardiovascular health care professionals have a particular obligation to assume a position of leadership in responding to these challenges: by conducting research to demonstrate the efficacy of preventive as well as treatment interventions; by providing education; and by bringing about improvements in health care delivery.

PEARLS

- Cardiovascular disease is the major cause of death after age 65, accounting for more than 40% of deaths in this population.
- Cardiopulmonary and cardiovascular changes related to aging include decreases in aerobic capacity, vital capacity, minute volume, maximum cardiac output, maximal obtainable heart rate, stroke volume, maximal oxygen consumption, and an increase in blood pressure.
- Prolonged inactivity and bed rest quickly and markedly impairs cardiovascular functional capacity.
- The outcomes of aging on the pulmonary system are an increased mechanical workload for breathing, a decrease in the efficiency of gas exchange, and a compromise in the ability to efficiently supply oxygen to peripheral tissues.
- A decline in cardiac output is absent in physically fit older persons without heart disease.
- The components of a thorough cardiopulmonary and cardiovascular evaluation include assessment of the neuromusculoskeletal system, the sensory system, and cardiopulmonary screening—along with appropriate modifications of stress testing measures.
- Submaximal stress testing can be done safely for older persons. The various types of tests (step test, modified chair-step test, walking test, treadmill

testing, and cycle ergometer testing) are all useful for evaluating cardiovascular status in the elderly.
- An objective means of measuring peripheral circulation is to time the emptying and filling times of the lower extremities. This is best accomplished using the *Buerger-Allen testing protocol* for peripheral circulation.
- Intensity, duration, and frequency—the three major components of exercise prescription—are different for the elderly. Intensity is safe at 60%, duration, which is usually twenty minutes, may need to be cut to four to five minutes initially; frequency should be daily.
- When prescribing exercise for an older person, special considerations and modifications should be made for obese, diabetic, osteoporotic patients; those with pacemakers or on cardiopulmonary medications; and patients with CHF.
- Epidemiologic evidence indicates a beneficial effect of HRT on the development of CAD, improved mortality outcomes in women with existing cardiac and vascular disease, as well as having an impact on other systemic diseases.

REFERENCES

1. National Center for Health Statistics. *Health, United States, 1999 with Health and Aging Chartbook.* 1999; Hyattsville, MD: National Center for Health Statistics, 34–35.
2. National Center for Health Statistics. *Health, United States, 1999 with Health and Aging Chartbook.* 1999; Hyattsville, MD: National Center for Health Statistics, 36–37.
3. Shepard RJ. The cardiovascular benefits of exercise in the elderly. *Top Geriatr Rehabil.* 1985; 1(1):1–10.
4. US Bureau of the Census. *Statistical Abstract of the United States: 1997.* 117 Edition; 1997; US Bureau of the Census: Washington, DC.
5. Centers for Disease Control and Prevention. *Unrealized Prevention Opportunities: Reducing the Health and Economic Burden of Chronic Disease.* 1997; Centers for Disease Control and Prevention, National Center for Chronic Disease Prevention and Health Promotion: Atlanta, GA.
6. Verbrugge L. Recent, present, and future health of American adults. In: Breslow L, Fielding JE, and Lave LB, eds. *Annual Review of Public Health.* 1999; Vol. 20. Annual Reviews Inc., Palo Alto, CA.
7. Cheitlin MD, Gerstenblith G. Management of patients over age 75 with cardiovascular disease. Presented at the American Heart Association 72nd Scientific Sessions, Atlanta, GA: November 7–10, 1000. Plenary Session XIII, November 10, 1999.
8. Palmore EB. Trends in the health of the aged. *Gerontologist.* 1986; 26:298–302.
9. Astrand PO. Exercise physiology and its role in disease prevention and in rehabilitation. *Arch Phys Med Rehabil.* 1987; 68:305–311.
10. Lee IM, Paffenbarger RS, Hennekens CH. Physical activity, physical fitness and longevity. *Aging.* 1997; 9(1–2):2–11.
11. Blair SN, Kohl HW 3rd, Barlow CE, et al. Changes in physical fitness and all-cause mortality. A prospective study of healthy and unhealthy men. *JAMA.* 1995; 273(14):1093–1098.
12. Rowe JW and Besdine RW. *Health and Disease in Old Age.* Boston: Little, Brown & Co.; 1982.
13. Crimmins EM, Saito Y, Ingegneri D. Changes in life expectancy and disability-free life expectancy in the United States. *Population and Development Review.* 1989l 15(2):235–267.
14. Shepard RJ. *Physical Activity and Aging,* 2nd edition. Gaithersburg, MD: Aspen; 1987.
15. Bruce RA. Functional aerobic capacity, exercise and aging. In: Andres R, Bierman EL, and Hazzard WR, eds. *Principles of Geriatric Medicine.* New York: McGraw-Hill; 1985:87–103.
16. Cress ME, Schultz E. Aging muscle: functional, morphologic, biochemical, and regenerative capacity. *Top Geriatric Rehabil.* 1985; 1(1):11–19.
17. Gerstenblith G, Weisfeldt ML, and Lakatta, EG. Disorders of the heart. In: Andres R, Bierman EL, Hazzard WR, eds. *Principles of Geriatric Medicine.* New York: McGraw-Hill; 1985:515–526.
18. Wei JY. Heart disease in the elderly. *Cardiovasc Med.* 1984; 9:971–998.
19. Wei JY. Cardiovascular anatomic and physiologic changes with age. *Topics Geriatr Rehabil.* 1986; 2(1):10–16.
20. Redden WG. Respiratory system and aging. In: Smith EL and Serfass RC, eds: *Exercise and Aging: The Scientific Basis.* Hillside, NJ: Enslow Publishers; 1981:89–108.
21. Irwin SC, Zadai CC. Cardiopulmonary rehabilitation of the geriatric patient. In: Lewis CB, ed: *Aging: The Health Care Challenge.* 2nd edition. Philadelphia, PA: FA Davis; 1990:181–211.
22. Zadai CC. Cardiopulmonary issues in the geriatric population: implications for rehabilitation. *Top Geriatr Rehabil.* 1986; 2:1:1–9.
23. Hurst W. *The Heart, Arteries and Veins.* 9th edition. New York,: McGraw-Hill; 1998.
24. Mann DL, Deneberg BS, Gash AK, et.al. Effects of age on ventricular performance during graded supine exercise. *Am Heart J.* 1986; 111:108–115.
25. Rodeheffer RJ, Gerstenblith G. Effect of age on cardiovascular function. In: Johnson HA, ed. *Relations Between Normal Aging and Disease.* Aging Series. 1985; 28:85–99.
26. Gerstenblith G, Lakatta EG, Weisfeldt ML. Age changes in myocardial function and exercise response. *Progr Cardiovasc Dis.* 1976 19:1–21.
27. Port S, Cobb FR, Coleman RE, et.al. Cardiac ejection fraction in aging. *New Engl J Med.* 1980; 303:1133–1137.
28. Rodeheffer RJ, Gerstenblith G, Becker LC, et al. Exercise cardiac output is maintained with advancing age in healthy human subjects: Cardiac dilatation and increased stroke volume compensate for a

diminished heart rate. *Circulation.* 1984; 69: 203–213.

29. Harris R. *Clinical Geriatric Cardiology: Management of the Elderly Patient.* Philadelphia: JB Lippincott Co; 1986; 29–42.

30. Weisfeldt ML, Gerstenblith ML, and Lakatta EG. Alterations in circulatory function. In: Andres R, Bierman EL, Hazzard WR, eds. *Principles of Geriatric Medicine.* New York: McGraw-Hill;1985; 248–279.

31. Niinimaa V, Shepard RJ. Training and oxygen conductance in the elderly. *J Gerontol.* 1978; 33: 354–367.

32. Horvath SM, Borgia JF. Cardiopulmonary gas transport and aging. *Am Rev Respir Dis.* 1984; 129(suppl):569–571.

33. Aniansson A, Hedberg M, Henning GB, et al. Muscle morphology, enzymatic activity, and muscle strength in elderly men: A follow-up study. *Muscle Nerve.* 1986; 9:585–591.

34. Coggan AR, Spina RJ, King DS, et al. Skeletal muscle adaptations to endurance training in 60–69 year old men and women. *J Appl Physiol.* 1992; 72:1780–1786.

35. Martin WH III, Kohrt WM, Malley MT, et al. Exercise training enhances leg vasodilatory capacity of 65-year-old men and women. *J Appl Physiol.* 1990; 69:1804–1809.

36. Smith EL, Serfass RC, eds. *Exercise and Aging: The Scientific Basis.* Hillside, NJ: Enslow: 1981.

37. Shimada K, Kitazumi T, Sadakne N, et al. Age-related changes of baroreflex function, plasma, norepinephrine, and blood pressure. *Hypertension.* 1985; 7:113–118.

38. Irwin SC. Cardiac rehabilitation for the geriatric patient. *Top Geriatr Rehabil.* 1986; 2:44–54.

39. Turner JM, Mead J, Wohl ME. Elasticity of human lungs in relation to age. *J Appl Physiol.* 1968; 25 (6):664–683.

40. Pump KK. Fenestrae in the alveolar membrane of the human lung. *Chest.* 1965; 65:799–802.

41. Loke J, Mahler DA, Paul-Man SF, et al. Exercise impairment in chronic obstructive pulmonary disease. In: Symposium on Exercise: Physiology and Clinical Applications. *Clin Chest Med.* 1984; 5(1): 121–129.

42. Paffenbarger RS, Wing AL, Hyde RT, Jung DL. Physical activity and incidence of hypertension in college alumni. *Am J Epidemiol.* 1983; 117: 245–256.

43. Paffenbarger RS, Hyde RT, Wing AL, Hsieh CC. Physical activity, all-cause mortality and longevity of college alumni. *New Engl J Med.* 1986; 314: 605–613.

44. Baker PB, Arn AR, Unverferth DV. Hypertrophic and degenerative changes in human hearts with aging. *J Coll Cardiol.* 1985; 5:536A.

45. Krotkiewski M, Lonroth P, Mandroukas K, et al. The effects of physical training on glucose metabolism in obesity and type II (noninsulin-dependent) diabetes mellitus. *Diabetologia.* 1985; 28: 881–890.

46. Sidney KH, Shepard RJ. Frequency and intensity of exercise training for elderly subjects. *Med Sci Sports.* 1978; 10:125–131.

47. Verg JE, Seals DR, Hagberg JM, et al. Effects of endurance exercise training on ventilatory function in older individuals. *J Appl Physiol.* 1985; 58: 791–794.

48. Heath GW, Hagberg JM, Ehsani AA, et al. A physiological comparison of young and older endurance athletes. *J Appl Physiol.* 1981; 51: 634–640.

49. Allen WK, Seals DR, Hurley BF, et al. Lactate threshold and distance running performance in young and older athletes. *J Appl Physiol.* 1985; 58: 1281–1284.

50. Seals DR, Hagberg JM, Hurley BF, et al. Effects of endurance training on glucose tolerance and plasma lipid levels in older men and women. *JAMA.* 1984; 252:645–649.

51. Thomas SG, Cunningham DA, Rechnitzer PA, et al. Determinants of the training response in elderly men. *Med Sci Sports Exerc.* 1985; 17: 667–672.

52. Frontera WR, Evans WJ. Exercise performance and endurance training in the elderly. *Top Geriatr Rehabil.* 1986; 2(1):17–32.

53. Seals DR, Hagberg JM, Hurley BF, et al. Endurance training in older men and women. I. Cardiovascular responses to exercise. *J Appl Physiol.* 1984; 57:1024–1029.

54. Farrar RP, Martin TP, Murray Ardies C. The interaction of aging and endurance exercise upon the mitochondrial function of skeletal muscle. *J Gerontol.* 1981; 36:642–647.

55. Beyer RE, Stames JW, Edington DW, et al. Exercise-induced reversal of age-related declines of oxidative reactions, mitochondrial yield and flavins in skeletal muscle of the rat. *Mech Ageing Dev.* 1983; 24:309–323.

56. Suominen H, Heikkinen E, Liesen H, et al. Effects of 8 weeks' endurance training on skeletal muscle metabolism in 56-70-year-old sedentary men. *Eur J Applied Physiol.* 1977; 37:173–180.

57. McKay DL, Perrone G, Rasmussen H, Dallal G, Blumberg JB. Multivitamin/Mineral supplementation improves plasma B-vitamin status and homocysteine concentration in healthy older adults consuming a folate-fortified diet. *J Nutr.* 2000; 130(12): 3090–3096.

58. Graham IM, Daly LE, Refsum HM, et al. Plasma homocysteine as a risk factor for vascular disease: The European Concerted Action Project. *JAMA.* 1997; 277(22):1775–1781.

59. VonEckardstein A, Assmann G. Plasma homocysteine levels and mortality in patients with coronary artery disease. *N Engl J Med.* 1997; 337(22): 1632–1633.

60. Ebel A, Kim D. Exercise in peripheral vascular disease. In: Basmajian JV, Wolf S, eds. *Therapeutic Exercise.* 4th edition. Baltimore MD: Williams and Wilkins Publishers; 1990: 371–386.

61. Wisham MB, Lawrence H, Abramson MD, Arthur S, Ebel A. Value of exercise in peripheral arterial diseases. *JAMA.* 1953; 153:10–12.

62. Bottomley JM. A comparison of the effects of Buerger-Allen exercises, walking, and high galvanic electrical stimulation on lower extremity blood

flow in elderly patients.(Submitted to circulation-unpublished)

63. Thiele BL, Strandness DE. Disorders of the vascular system: peripheral vascular disease. In: Andres R, Bierman EL, Hazzard WR, eds. *Principles in Geriatric Medicine.* New York: McGraw-Hill; 1985: 527–535.

64. Nagle FJ, Balke B, Naughton JP. Gradual step tests for assessing work capacity. *J Appl Physiol.* 1965; 20:745–752.

65. Smith EL, Gilligan C. Physical activity prescription for the elderly. *Phys Sports Med.* 1983; 11: 91–101.

66. McGavin CR, Cupta SP, McHardy GJR. Twelve-minute walking test for assessing disability in chronic bronchitis. *Br Med J.* 1976; 1:822–826.

67. Enright PL, Sherrill DL. References equations for the six-minute walk in healthy adults. *Am J Respir & Critical Care Med.* 1998; 158:1384–1387.

68. Kline G, Parcari JP, Hintermeister R, et al. Estimated VO$_2$ max from a one-mile track walk, gender, age, and body weight. *Med Sci Sports Exerc.* 1987; 19:253–259.

69. Ellestad NH. *Stress Testing: Principles and Practice.* Philadelphia: FA Davis; 1979.

70. Bruce RA. Exercise, functional aerobic capacity, and aging—another viewpoint. *Med Sci Sports Exerc.* 1984; 16:8–15.

71. Rowbotham JL, Gibbons GW, Kozak GP. Guidelines in examination of the diabetic leg and foot. In: Kozak GP, Hoar CS, Rowbotham JL, et al., eds. *Management of Diabetic Foot Problems.* Philadelphia: WB Saunders Co.; 1984: 9–16.

72. Nawoczenski D, Birke J, Graham S, et al. The neuropathic foot—a management scheme. *Phys Ther.* 1989; 69(4):287–291.

73. Birke JA, Sims DS. Plantar sensory threshold in the ulcerative foot. *Leprosy Review.* 1986; 57: 261–267.

74. Dorairaj A, Reddy R, Jesudasan K. An evaluation of the Semmes-Weinstein 6.10 monofilament as compared with 6 nylon in leprosy patients. *Indian Journal of Leprosy.* 1988; 60(3):413–417.

75. Pollock DL. Breaking the risk of falls: An exercise benefit for the older patients. *Phys & Sportsmed.* 1992; 20(11):146–156.

76. Greco EM, Guardini S, Citelli L. Cardiac rehabilitation in patients with rate responsive pacemakers. *Pacing Clin Electrophysiol.* 1998; 21(3): 568–575.

77. Sharp CT, Busse EF, Burgess JJ, Haennel RG. Exercise prescription for patients with pacemakers. *J Cardiopulm Rehabil.* 1998; 18(6):421–431.

78. Jarret RJ. Is there an ideal body weight? *Br Med J.* 1986; 293:493–495.

79. Stallones R. Epidemiologic studies of obesity. In: Foster WR, Burton BT, eds. Health implications of obesity. *Ann Intern Med.* 1985; 103(6 pt 2): 1003–1005.

80. Kannel WB, Gordon T. *An Epidemiologic Investigation of Cardiovascular Disease.* Section 5. Washington DC: US Public Health Service, US Dept of Health, Education, and Welfare publication; 1968.

81. Ashley FW Jr, Kannel WB. Relation of weight change to changes in atherogenic traits: the Framingham study. *J Chronic Dis.* 1974; 27:103–114.

82. Havlik RJ, Hubert HB, Fabsitz RR, et al. Weight and hypertension. *Ann Intern Med.* 1983; 98(2 pt5): 855–859.

83. Harlan WR, Hull AL, Schmouder RL, et al. High blood pressure in older Americans: the first national health and nutrition examination survey. *Hypertension.* 1984; 6(pt 1):802–809.

84. Jannel WB, Gordon T, Castelli WP. Obesity, lipids, and glucose intolerance: the Framingham study. *Am J Clin Nutr.* 1979; 32:1238–1245.

85. Wilson PWF, Garrison RJ, Abbott RD, et al. Factors associated with lipoprotein cholesterol levels: the Framingham study. *Arteriosclerosis.* 1983; 3: 273–281.

86. McGandy RB. Nutrition and the aging cardiovascular system. In: Hutchinson ML, Munro HN, eds. *Nutrition and Aging.* Orlando, FL: Academic Press, Inc.;1986.

87. Wolf RN, Grundy SM. Influence of weight reduction on plasma lipoproteins in obese patients. *Arteriosclerosis.* 1983; 3:160–169.

88. Zimmerman J, Kaufman NA, Fainaru M, et al. Effective weight loss in moderate obesity on plasma lipoprotein and apolipoprotein levels and on high density lipoprotein composition. *Arteriosclerosis.* 1084; 4:115–123.

89. Drizd T, Dannenberg AL, Engel A. Blood pressure levels in persons 18–74 years of age in 1976–80, and trends in blood pressure from 1960 to 1980 in the United States. *Vital Health Stat.* 1986; 234(11):1–68.

90. Dannenberg A, Drizd T, Horan, et al. Cardiovascular Disease: *Epidemiology Newsletter.* 1985; 68(abstract).

91. Higgins M, Kannel WB, Garrison R, et al. Hazards of obesity: the Framingham experience. *Acta Med Scand.* 1987; 723(suppl):23–26.

92. Chernoff R. *Geriatric Nutrition: The Health Professional's Handbook.* Rockville, MD: Aspen Publishers, Inc.; 1991.

93. Kannel WB. Nutrition and the occurrence and prevention of cardiovascular disease in the elderly. *Nutr Rev.* 1988l 46:68–78.

94. Reaven GM. Pathophysiology of insulin resistance in human disease. *Physiol Rev.* 1995; 75: 473–486.

95. Felber JP. From obesity to diabetes: Pathophysical conditions. *Int J Obes.* 1992; 16:937–952.

96. DiPietro L, Seeman TE, Stachenfeld NS, Katz LD, Nadel ER. Moderate-intensity aerobic training improves glucose tolerance in aging independent of abdominal adiposity. *J Am Geriat Soc.* 1998; 46(7): 875–887.

97. Shimokata H, Muller DC, Eleg JL, et al. Age as an independent determinant of glucose tolerance. *Diabetes.* 1991; 40:44–51.

98. Wang JT, Ho LT, Tang KT, et al. Effect of habitual physical activity on age-related glucose intolerance. *J Am Geriatr Soc.* 1989; 37(2):203–209.

99. Zavaroni I, Dall'Aglio E, Bruschi F, et al. Effect of age and environmental factors on glucose tolerance and

insulin secretion in a worker population. *J Am Geri-atr Soc.* 1986; 34(3): 271–275.

100. Kissebah A, Krakower G. Regional adiposity and morbidity. *Physiol Rev.* 1994; 74:761–811.

101. Kohrt WM, Kirwan JP, Staten MA, et al. Insulin resistance is related to abdominal adiposity. *Diabetes.* 1993; 42:273–281.

102. Rosenthal MJ, Hartnell JM, Morley JE, et al. UCLA geriatric grand rounds: diabetes in the elderly. *J Am Geriatr Soc.* 1987; 35:435–447.

103. Saltin B, Lindgarde F, Houston M, et al. Physical training and glucose tolerance in middle-aged men with chemical diabetes. *Diabetes.* 1979; 28(suppl 1):30–32.

104. Bogardus C, Ravussin E, Robbins DC, et al. Effects of physical training and diet therapy on carbohydrate metabolism in patients with glucose intolerance and noninsulin-dependent diabetes mellitus. *Diabetes.* 1984; 33:311–318.

105. Helmrich SP, Ragland DR, Leung RW, et al. Physical activity and reduced occurrence of non-insulin-dependent diabetes mellitus. *N Eng J Med.* 1991; 325:147–152.

106. Karam JH. Therapeutic dilemmas in type II diabetes mellitus: improving and maintaining B-cell and insulin sensitivity. *West J Med.* 1988; 148: 685–690.

107. Pacini G, Valerio A, Beccaro R, et al. Insulin sensitivity and beta-cell responsivity are not decreased in elderly subjects with normal OGTT. *J Am Geriatr Soc.* 1988; 36:317–323.

108. Johnson T. Age-related differences in isometric and dynamic strength and endurance. *Phys Ther.* 1982; 62:985–989.

109. Doyle F, Brown J, LaChance C. Relation between bone mass and muscle weight. *Lancet.* 1970; 1: 391–393.

110. Aloia JF, Cohn SH, Babu T, et al.. Skeletal mass and body composition in marathon runners. *Metabolism.* 1978; 27:1793–1796.

111. Sinaki M, Offord K. Physical activity in postmenopausal women: effect on back muscle strength and bone mineral density of the spine. *Arch Phys Med Rehabil.* 1988; 69:277–280.

112. Sinaki M, McPhee MC, Hodgson SF. Relation between bone mineral density of spine and strength of back extensors in healthy postmenopausal women. *Mayo Clin Proc.* 1986; 61:116–122.

113. Rubin CT, Lanyon LE. Regulation of bone mass by mechanical strain magnitude. *Calcif Tissue Int.* 1985; 37:411–417.

114. Rubin CT, Lanyon LE. Regulation of bone formation by applied dynamic loads. *J Bone Joint Surg.* 1984; 66:397–402.

115. Carter DR, Fyrie DP, Whalen RT. Trabecular bone density and loading history: regulation of connective tissue biology by mechanical energy. *J Biomech.* 1987; 20:785–794.

116. Talmadge RV, Stinnett SS, Landwehr JT, et al. Age-related loss of bone mineral density in non-athletic and athletic women. *Bone Miner.* 1986; 1:115–125.

117. Brewer V, Meyer BM, Keele MS, et al. Role of exercise in prevention of involutional bone loss. *Med Sci Sports Exer.* 1983; 15:445–449.

118. Smith EL, Redden W, Smith PE. Physical activity and calcium modalities for bone mineral increase in aged women. *Med Sci Sports Exerc.* 1981; 13:60–64.

119. Hepple RT, Liu PP, Plyley MJ, Goodman JM. Oxygen uptake kinetics during exercise in chronic heart failure: influence of peripheral vascular reserve. *Clin Sci.* 1999; 97(5):569–577.

120. Sorensen VB, Wroblewski H, Galatius S, Haunso S, Kastrup J. Exercise skeletal muscle blood flow is related to peripheral microvascular stiffness in idiopathic dilated cardiomyopathy. *Microvasc Res.* 1999; 58(3):268–280.

121. Thomson HL, Morris-Thurgood J, Atherton J, McKenna WJ, Frenneaux MP. Reflex responses of venous capacitance vessels in patients with hypertrophic cardiomyopathy. *Clin Sci.* 1998; 94(4): 339–346.

122. Thomson HL. Exercise vascular responses in health and disease. *Aust N Z J Med.* 1997; 27(4): 459–461.

123. Mager G, Reinhardt C, Kleine M, Rost R, Hopp HW. Patients with dilated cardiomyopathy and less than 20% ejection fraction increase exercise capacity and have less severe arrhythmia after controlled exercise training. *J Cardiopulm Rehabil.* 2000; 20(3):196–198.

124. Pepi M, Agostoni P, Marenzi G, et al. The influence of diastolic and systolic function on exercise performance in heart failure due to dilated cardiomyopathy or ischemic heart disease. *Eur J Heart Fail.* 1999; 1(2):161–167.

125. Cohen-Solal A, Faraggi M, Czitrom D, Le Guludec D, Delahaye N, Gourgon R. *Chest.* 1998; 113(4): 870–877.

126. Sharma S, Elliot P, Whyte G, et al. Utility of cardiopulmonary exercise in assessment of clinical determinants of functional capacity in hypertrophic cardiomyopathy. *Am J Cardiol.* 2000; 86(2):162–168.

127. Agostoni P, Wasserman K, Perego GB, et al. Oxygen transport to muscle during exercise in chronic congestive heart failure secondary to idiopathic dilated cardiomyopathy. *Am J Cardiol.* 1997; 79(8): 1120–1124.

128. Harrington D, Clark AL, Chua TP, Anker SD, Poole-Wilson PA, Coats AJ. Effect of reduced muscle bulk on the ventilatory response to exercise in chronic congestive heart failure secondary to idiopathic dilated and ischemic cardiomyopathy. *Am J Cardiol.* 1997; 80(1):90–93.

129. Faggiano P, D'Aloia A, Gualeni A, Giordano A. Hemodynamic profile of submaximal constant workload exercise in patients with heart failure secondary to ischemic or idiopathic dilated cardiomyopathy. *Am J Cardiol.* 1998; 81(4):437–442.

130. Mancini D, Benaminovitz A, Cordisco ME, Karmally W, Weinberg A. Slowed glycogen utilization enhances exercise endurance in patients with

heart failure. *J Am Coll Cardiol.* 1999; 34(6): 1807–1812.

131. Webb-Peploe KM, Chua TP, Harrington DL, Henein MY, Gibson DB, Coats AJ. Different response of patients with idiopathic and ischaemic dilated cardiomyopathy to exercise training. *Int J Cardiol.* 2000; 74(2–3):215–224.

132. Spencer AP. Hormone replacement therapy should be administered as secondary prevention of coronary artery disease. *Pharmacotherapy.* 2000; 20(9): 1028–1033.

133. Mosca L, Manson J, Sutherland S, Langer R, Manolio R, Barrett-Conner E. Cardiovascular disease in women: a statement for healthcare professionals from the American Heart Association. *Circulation.* 1997; 96:2468–2484.

134. American Heart Association. Cardiovascular diseases, 1999. 2000. Available from: *http://www.americanheart.org/statistics/03cardio.html.*

135. American Heart Association. About women heart disease and stroke, 1999. 2000. Available from: *http://www.americanheart.org/statistics/02about.html.*

136. Colditz G, Willet W, Stampfer M, Rosner B, Hennekens C. Menopause and the risk of coronary heart disease in women. *N Engl J Med.* 1987; 316: 1105–1110.

137. Taskinen M, Puolakka R. Hormone replacement therapy lowers plasma Lp(a) concentrations: comparison of cyclic transdermal and continuous estrogen-progestin regimes. *Arterioscler Thromb Vasc Biol.* 1996; 16:1215–1221.

138. Kim C, Min Y, Ryu W, Kwak J, Ryoo U. Effect of hormone replacement therapy on lipoprotein (a) and lipid levels in postmenopausal women. *Arch Intern Med.* 1996; 156:1693–1700.

139. The writing group for the PEPI trial. Effects of estrogen or estrogen/progestin regimens on heart disease risk factors in postmenopausal women. The Postmenopausal Estrogen Progestin Interventions (PEPI) trial. *JAMA.* 1995; 273:199–208.

140. Barrett-Conner E, Laakso M. Ischemic heart disease risk in postmenopausal women. Effects of estrogen use on glucose and insulin levels. *Arteriosclerosis.* 1990; 10:531–534.

141. Mendelsohn M, Karas R. The protective effects of estrogen on the cardiovascular system. *N Engl J Med.* 1999; 340:1801–1811.

142. Subbiah M. Mechanisms of cardioprotection by estrogens. *Proc Soc Exp Biol Med.* 1998; 217(1): 26–29.

143. Bakir S, Oparil S. Estrogen replacement and heart disease. *Clin Rev Spring.* 2000; 67–72.

144. Henderson B, Paganni-Hill A, Ross R. Decreased mortality in users of estrogen replacement therapy. *Arch Intern Med.* 1991; 151:75–78.

145. Henderson B. Estrogen replacement therapy and protection from acute myocardial infarction. *Am J Obstet Gynecol.* 1988; 159(2):312–317.

146. Timio M, Lippi G, Venanzi S, et al. Blood pressure trend and cardiovascular events in nuns in a secluded order: a 30-year follow-up study. *Blood Press.* 1997; 6(2):81–87.

147. Sancier KM. Medical applications of Qigong. *Alternative Ther Health Med.* 1996; 2(1):40–46.

148. Lai JS, Lan C, Wong MK, Teng SH. Two-year trends in cardiorespiratory function among older T'ai Chi Chuan practitioners and sedentary subjects. *J Am Geriatr Soc.* 1995; 43 (11): 1222–1227.

149. Zhuo D, Shephard RJ, Plyley MJ, Davis GM. Cardiorespiratory and metabolic responses during T'ai Chi Chuan exercise. *Can J Appl Sport Sci.* 1984; 9(1):7–10.

150. Schneider D, Leung R. Metabolic and cardiorespiratory responses to the performance of Wing Chun and T'ai Chi Chuan exercise. *Int J Sports Med.* 1991; 12(3):319–313.

151. Lai JS, Wong MK, Lan C, Chong CK, Lien IN. Cardiorespiratory responses of T'ai Chi Chuan practitioners and sedentary subjects during cycle ergometer. *Journal of the Formosan Medical Association.* Oct 1993; 92 (10): 894–899.

152. Ng RK. Cardiopulmonary exercise: a recently discovered secret of T'ai Chi. *Hawaii Medical Journal.* 1992; 51 (8): 216–217.

153. Channer KS, Barrow D, Barrow R, Osborne M, Ives G. Changes in haemodynamic parameters following T'ai Chi Chuan and aerobic exercise in patients recovering from acute myocardial infarction. *Postgrad Med J.* 1996; 72(848): 349–351.

154. Jin P. Efficacy of T'ai Chi, brisk walking, meditation, and reading in reducing mental and emotional stress. *J Psychosom Res.* 1992; 36 (4): 361–370.

155. Jin P. Changes in heart rate, noradrenaline, cortisol and mood during T'ai Chi. *J Psychosom Res.* 1989; 33:197–206.

156. Jin P. Efficacy of T'ai Chi, brisk walking, meditation, and reading in reducing mental and emotional stress. *J Psychosom Res.* 1992; 36:765–775.

157. Sun XS, Xu Y, Xia YJ. Determination of E-rosette-forming lymphocytes in aged subjects with Tai Chi quan exercise. *International J of Sports Med.* 1989; 10:217–219.

158. Levine DM. Behavioral and psychosocial factors, processes, and strategies. In: Pearson T, Criqui MH, Luepker RV, Overman A, Winston M, eds: *Primer in Preventive Cardiology.* Dallas: American Heart Association; 1994.

159. Hatfield BD, Spalding TW, Mahon AD, Slater BA, Brody EB, Vaccaro P. The effect of psychological strategies upon cardiorespiratory and muscular activity during treadmill running. *Medicine & Science in Sports & Exercise.* 1992; 24(2): 218–225.

160. Leisman G, Zenhausern R, Ferentz A, Tefera T, Zemcov A. Electromyographic effects of fatigue and task repetition on the validity of estimates of strong and weak muscles in applied kinesiological muscle-testing procedures. *Perceptual & Motor Skills.* 1995; 80(3 pt 1):963–977.

161. McGrady A. Effects of group relaxation training and thermal biofeedback on blood pressure and related physiological and psychological variables in

essential hypertension. *Biofeedback & Self Regulation.* 1994; 19(1):51–66..

162. Vasilevskii NN, Sidorov YA, Kiselev IM. Biofeedback control of systemic arterial pressure. *Neuroscience & Behavioral Physiology.* 1992; 22(3): 219–223.

163. Saunders JT, Cox DJ, Teastes CD, Pohl SL. Thermal biofeedback in the treatment of intermittent claudication in diabetes: a case study. *Biofeedback & Self Regulation.* 1994; 19(4):337–345.

164. Rice BI, Schindler JV. Effect of thermal biofeedback-assisted relaxation training on blood circulation in the lower extremities of a population with diabetes. *Diabetes Care.* 1992; 15(7): 853–858.

165. Reyes del Paso GA, Godoy J, Vila J. Self-regulation of respiratory sinus arrhythmia. *Biofeedback & Self Regulation.* 1992; 17(4):261–275.

166. Shahidi S, Salmon P. Contingent and non-contingent biofeedback training for Type A and B healthy adults: can Type A's relax by competing? *Journal of Psychosomatic Research.* 1992; 36(5):477–483.

167. Blumenstein B, Breslav I, Bar-Eli M, Tenenbaum G, Weinstein Y. Regulation of mental states and biofeedback techniques: effects on breathing pattern. *Biofeedback & Self Regulation.* 1995; 20(2): 169–183.

168. Montgomery GT. Slowed respiration training. *Biofeedback & Self Regulation.* 1994; 19(3): 211–225.

169. Lehrer PM, Carr P, Sargunaraj D, Woolfolk RL. Stress management techniques: are they all equivalent, or do they have specific effects? *Biofeedback & Self Regulation.* 1994; 19(4): 353–401.

170. Freedman RR, Keegan D, Rodriguez J, Galloway MP. Plasma catecholamine levels during temperature biofeedback training in normal subjects. *Biofeedback & Self Regulation.* 1993; 18(2):107–114.

171. Van Zak DB: Biofeedback treatments for premenstrual and premenstrual affective syndromes. *International Journal of Psychosomatics.* 1994; 41(1–4):53–60.

172. Jokl E. Abstract: XII International Congress of Gerontology. Hamberg, Germany. July 12–17, 1981.

BUERGER-ALLEN INITIAL EVALUATION

PATIENT_____ AGE_____ SEX_____ RM#_____
DIAGNOSIS_____ PHYSICIAN_____
DATE INITIAL EVAL_____ THERAPIST_____
Signature

	RIGHT LE	LEFT LE
APPEARANCE:	_____	_____
SKIN INTEGRITY:	_____	_____
SKIN TEMP:	_____	_____
EDEMA PRESENT:	0☐ +1☐ +2☐ +3☐	0☐ +1☐ +2☐ +3☐

CIRCUMFERENTIAL:

	RIGHT	LEFT
☐MET HEADS	_____	_____
☐ARCH	_____	_____
☐ANKLE	_____	_____
☐SUPRA MALLEOLAR	_____	_____
☐MID CALF	_____	_____
☐SUB PATELLAR	_____	_____

PULSES:

		RIGHT	LEFT
DORSAL PEDALIS		0☐ +1☐ +2☐ +3☐	0☐ +1☐ +2☐ +3☐
POST TIBIALIS		0☐ +1☐ +2☐ +3☐	0☐ +1☐ +2☐ +3☐
POPLITEAL		0☐ +1☐ +2☐ +3☐	0☐ +1☐ +2☐ +3☐
FEMORAL		0☐ +1☐ +2☐ +3☐	0☐ +1☐ +2☐ +3☐

SENSORY TESTING:

VIBRATORY SENSE:

	RIGHT	LEFT
	☐PRESENT	☐PRESENT
	☐DIMINISHED	☐DIMINISHED
	☐ABSENT	☐ABSENT

PROTECTIVE SENSATION:

1 = 01 gr (4.17 for Normal)
2 = 10 gr (5.07 Protective Sense)
3 = 75 gr (6.10 Loss Protective Sense)
4 = No Protective Sensation

	RIGHT	LEFT
DORSUM:	1☐ 2☐ 3☐ 4☐	1☐ 2☐ 3☐ 4☐
PLANTAR DIGIT 1:	1☐ 2☐ 3☐ 4☐	1☐ 2☐ 3☐ 4☐
PLANTAR DIGIT 3:	1☐ 2☐ 3☐ 4☐	1☐ 2☐ 3☐ 4☐
PLANTAR DIGIT 5:	1☐ 2☐ 3☐ 4☐	1☐ 2☐ 3☐ 4☐
MET HEAD 1:	1☐ 2☐ 3☐ 4☐	1☐ 2☐ 3☐ 4☐
MET HEAD 3:	1☐ 2☐ 3☐ 4☐	1☐ 2☐ 3☐ 4☐
MET HEAD 5:	1☐ 2☐ 3☐ 4☐	1☐ 2☐ 3☐ 4☐
PROXIMAL HEAD 5:	1☐ 2☐ 3☐ 4☐	1☐ 2☐ 3☐ 4☐
ARCH:	1☐ 2☐ 3☐ 4☐	1☐ 2☐ 3☐ 4☐
HEEL:	1☐ 2☐ 3☐ 4☐	1☐ 2☐ 3☐ 4☐

STRENGTH:

RIGHT		LEFT
_____	Anterior Tibialis	_____
_____	Extensor Hallucis Longus	_____
_____	Flexor Hallucis Longus	_____
_____	Posterior Tibialis	_____
_____	Peroneus Longus	_____
_____	Gastroc / Soleus	_____
_____	Intrinsics (S / W / A)	_____

DEFORMITIES:

	RIGHT	LEFT
Hammer/Claw:	_____	_____
Boney Prominence:	_____	_____
Drop Foot:	_____	_____
Charcot Foot:	_____	_____
Hallux Limitus	_____	_____
Rear/ForeFt Varus:	_____	_____
Plantar flexed 1st:	_____	_____
Equinus:	_____	_____
Amputation:	_____	_____

FOOTWEAR: ☐STANDARD ☐SPECIAL DESCRIBE_____
☐ADEQUATE ☐INADEQUATE DESCRIBE_____

BLANCHING/FILLING TIMES: _____ ELEVATED _____ HORIZONTAL _____ DEPENDENT

TREATMENT RECOMMENDATIONS:*
☐BUERGER-ALLEN EXERCISES CYCLES_____ TIMES/DAY_____ MODIFIED Yes / No
☐PATIENT EDUCATION ☐SKIN CARE ☐FOOTWEAR ☐ORTHOTICS

Figure 13A–1. *Buerger-Allen Evaluation Form. Buerger-Allen evaluation form created by: Jennifer M. Bottomley, Ph.D, MS, PT © 1996.*

*Refer to Buerger-Allen Treatment FIlowsheet for intitial blanching/filling times etc.

BUERGER-ALLEN TREATMENT FLOW SHEET

PATIENT _____

INITIALS _____

DIAGNOSIS _____ ☐ PRESENT ☐ NOT PRESENT

WOUND: ☐ PRESENT ☐ NOT PRESENT

AGE _____ SEX _____ RM# _____ THERAPIST _____

☐ DIABETES ☐ PVD ☐ AMPUTEE ☐ CARDIAC ☐ HTN

DESCRIBE _____

BUERGER-ALLEN PROTOCOL: CYCLES _____ TIMES/DAY _____ MODIFIED _____

PARAMETER	INITIAL EVAL	FOLLOW-UP	FOLLOW-UP	FOLLOW-UP	FOLLOW-UP	NOTES
DATE / THERAPIST INITIALS						
RESTING HEART RATE (Supine)						
BLOOD PRESSURE (Supine)						
RESPIRATORY RATE (Supine)						
PLANTAR SKIN TEMPERATURE	L / R	L / R	L / R	L / R	L / R	
DORSAL PEDALIS PULSE LEFT	☐0 ☐+1 ☐+2 ☐+3	☐0 ☐+1 ☐+2 ☐+3	☐0 ☐+1 ☐+2 ☐+3	☐0 ☐+1 ☐+2 ☐+3	☐0 ☐+1 ☐+2 ☐+3	
DORSAL PEDALIS PULSE RIGHT	☐0 ☐+1 ☐+2 ☐+3	☐0 ☐+1 ☐+2 ☐+3	☐0 ☐+1 ☐+2 ☐+3	☐0 ☐+1 ☐+2 ☐+3	☐0 ☐+1 ☐+2 ☐+3	
POST. TIBIALIS PULSE LEFT	☐0 ☐+1 ☐+2 ☐+3	☐0 ☐+1 ☐+2 ☐+3	☐0 ☐+1 ☐+2 ☐+3	☐0 ☐+1 ☐+2 ☐+3	☐0 ☐+1 ☐+2 ☐+3	
POST. TIBIALIS PULSE RIGHT	☐0 ☐+1 ☐+2 ☐+3	☐0 ☐+1 ☐+2 ☐+3	☐0 ☐+1 ☐+2 ☐+3	☐0 ☐+1 ☐+2 ☐+3	☐0 ☐+1 ☐+2 ☐+3	
EDEMA (Supine)	☐0 ☐+1 ☐+2 ☐+3	☐0 ☐+1 ☐+2 ☐+3	☐0 ☐+1 ☐+2 ☐+3	☐0 ☐+1 ☐+2 ☐+3	☐0 ☐+1 ☐+2 ☐+3	
CIRCUMFERENTIAL MEASURES						
MET HEADS	L / R	L / R	L / R	L / R	L / R	
ARCH	L / R	L / R	L / R	L / R	L / R	
ANKLE (figure 8)	L / R	L / R	L / R	L / R	L / R	
SUPRA MALLEOLAR	L / R	L / R	L / R	L / R	L / R	
MID CALF	L / R	L / R	L / R	L / R	L / R	
SUB PATELLAR	L / R	L / R	L / R	L / R	L / R	
BLANCHING TIME ELEVATED						
FILLING TIME HORIZONTAL						
FILLING TIME DEPENDENT						
COMMENTS						

Figure 13A-2. © 1996 Jennifer M. Bottomley, Ph.D, MS, PT.

APPENDIX 13B METABOLIC EQUIVALENT (MET) VALUES FOR ACTIVITY AND EXERCISE

APPROXIMATE METABOLIC COST OF ACTIVITIES a,b

MET Levels	Self-Care Activities	Occupational/Work Activity	Recreational Activity
1.5–2.0 METs[c] 4–7 ml O_2/min/kg 2–2.5 kcal/min (70 kg BW)[d] Very Light/Minimal	Eating Shaving, Grooming Getting in & out of bed Standing Walking (1.6 km or 1 mph)	Desk work Typing, writing Auto driving[e]	Standing Walking (1.6 km or 1 mph) Flying,[e] motorcycling[e] Playing cards[e] Knitting, sewing
2–3 METs 7–11 ml O_2/min/kg 2.25–4 kcal/min (70 kg BW) Light	Showering in warm water Walking (3.25 km or 2 mph)	Ironing Light woodworking Riding lawn mower Auto repair Radio, TV repair Janitorial work Manual typing Bartending	Walking (3.25 km or 2 mph) Level biking (8 km or 5 mph) Billiards, bowling Skeet,[e] shuffleboard Powerboat driving[e] Power golf cart driving Canoeing (4 km or 2.25 mph) Horseback riding (walk) Playing a musical instrument
3–4 METs 11–14 ml O_2/min/kg 4–5 kcal/min (70 kg BW) Moderate	Dressing, undressing Walking (5 km or 3 mph)	Cleaning windows Making beds Mopping floors, vacuuming Bricklaying, plastering Machine assembly Wheelbarrow (100 kg or 220 lb load) Trailer-truck in traffic Welding (moderate load) Pushing light power mower	Walking (5 km or 3 mph) Biking (10 km or 6 mph) Horseshoe pitching Volleyball (noncompetitive) Golf (pulling bag cart) Archery Sailing (handling small boat) Fly fishing (standing in waders) Horseback riding (sitting to trot) Badminton (social doubles) Energetic musician
4–5 METs 14–18 ml O_2/min/kg 5–6 kcal/min (70 kg BW) Heavy	Showering in hot water Walking (5.5 km or 3.5 mph)	Scrubbing floors Hoeing Raking leaves Light carpentry Painting, masonry Wallpaper hanging	Walking (5.5 km or 3.5 mph) Biking (13 km or 8 mph) Table tennis Golf (carrying clubs) Dancing (fox-trot) Badminton (singles) Tennis (doubles) Calisthenics
5–6 METs 18–21 ml O_2/min/kg 6–7 kcal/min (70 kg BW) Very Heavy	Walking (6.5 km or 4 mph)	Digging in garden Shoveling light earth	Walking (6.5 km or 4 mph) Biking (16 km or 10 mph) Canoeing (6.5 km or 4 mph) Horseback ("posting" to trot) Stream fishing Ice/roller skating (15 km or 9 mph)

(continued)

APPENDIX 13B (CONTINUED)

APPROXIMATE METABOLIC COST OF ACTIVITIES a,b

MET Levels	Self-Care Activities	Occupational/Work Activity	Recreational Activity
6–7 METs 21–25 ml O_2/min/kg 7–8 kcal/min (70 kg BW) Very Heavy	Walking (8 km or 5 mph)	Snow shoveling 10/min (10 kg or 22 lb) Splitting wood Hand lawn-mowing	Walking (8 km or 5 mph) Biking (17.5 km or 11 mph) Badminton (competitive) Tennis (singles) Folk (square) dancing Light downhill skiing Ski touring (4 km or 2.5 mph) Water skiing
7–8 METs 25–28 ml O_2/min/kg 8–10 kcal/min (70kg BW)		Digging ditches Carrying 80 kg or 175 lb Sawing hardwood	Jogging (8 km or 5 mph) Biking (19 km or 12 mph) Horseback (gallop) Vigorous downhill skiing Basketball Mountain climbing Ice hockey Canoeing (8 km or 5 mph) Touch football Paddleball
8–9 METs 28–32 ml O_2/min/kg 10–11 kcal/min (70 kg BW)		Shoveling 10/min (14 kg or 31 lb)	Running (9 km or 5.5 mph) Biking (21 km or 13 mph) Ski touring (6.5 km or 4 mph) Squash/Handball (social) Fencing Basketball (vigorous)
10 plus METs 32 plus ml O_2/min/kg 11 plus kcal/min (70 kg BW)		Shoveling 10/min (16 kg or 35 lb)	Running 6 mph = 10 METs 7 mph = 11.5 METs 8 mph = 13.5 METs 9 mph = 15 METs 10 mph = 17 METs Ski touring (8+ km or 5+ mph) Squash/Handball (competitive)

[a]Includes resting metabolic needs.

[b]Source of MET listing: American Heart Association

[c]1 MET is the energy expenditure at rest, equivalent to approximately 3.5 ml O_2/min/kg

dBW = Body Weight

[a]A major increase in metabolic requirements may occur due to excitement, anxiety, or impatience, which are common responses during some activities. The individual's emotional reactivity must be assessed when prescribing or sanctioning certain activities.

Bottomley JM. Metabolic Equivalent (MET values) For activity and exercise In: Bottomley JM. Quick Reference Dictionary Thorofare, NJ: Slack Incorporated; 2000: 474–477.

CHAPTER 14

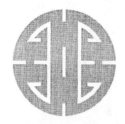

Integumentary Treatment Considerations

It is important to understand the normal aging of the skin and the process and effects of common diseases on skin status and wound healing. It is also important to consider the influence of various interventions in the healing of wounds in the elderly. Although the older adult is often predisposed to wounds because of poor hydration and nutrition, poor circulation, and inactivity, skin breakdown can be prevented through proper seating and positioning. Given the right circumstances, older individuals with wounds also heal well, despite age-related problems and nutritional deficiencies.

This chapter will focus on skin and wound care in the elderly patient. From a geriatric rehabilitation perspective, positioning, seating devices and mattresses, and a focus on the prevention of skin breakdown is an

important component of therapy. Often, in an older population, we encounter wounds that are chronic and slow to heal. The aging of the skin, nutritional status, and hydration, in addition to immobility will impact the integrity of the external integumentary system. Integumentary conditions that therapists treat will be discussed followed by an appraisal of how a wound repairs itself and what complicating factors in the healing process exist in an aged individual. Evaluation, staging of a wound and documentation will be discussed. The importance of nutrition and hydration in maintaining skin health and the importance of its role in healing will be presented. The types of ulcers, venous, arterial, and diabetic will be reviewed as they impact treatment approaches. Other types of wounds seen in the elderly, such as extravasation sites, abrasions and skin tears, dehisced surgical wounds, fistulas, and radiation burns will be discussed. Finally, a review of treatment modalities for wound management, surgical indications, and wound care products will be presented.

This is a new chapter to the second edition of *Geriatric Rehabilitation: A Clinical Approach*. The authors have added this chapter because of the variation in healing and treatment approaches and responses inherent in an aging population. There are natural delays in the healing of wounds of older individuals.[1] Open wounds contract more slowly and incised wounds gain strength more slowly. Experimental studies indicate that cellular proliferation, wound metabolism, and collagen remodeling occur at a delayed rate in older people.[1,2]

DEFINING INTEGUMENTARY CONDITIONS

Integumentary problems involve any covering or lining of the body. Therefore, the topic of integumentary system conditions could potentially cover skin and wound care to gastrointestinal conditions such as diverticulosis, constipation, or gastric ulceration, and respiratory conditions such as tuberculosis. Though the status of these systems will impact the functional status of our elderly patients and may be affected by exercise, positioning, nutrition, and hydration, physical or occupational therapists primarily treat integumentary problems affecting the external covering of the body (e.g., the skin). Despite this, it is important that the therapist not ignore the other integumentary conditions in assessing, evaluating, and treating the whole patient. It is vital that a therapist is cognizant of integumentary conditions that affect the gastrointestinal or respiratory systems and the influence these conditions might have on mobility and functional capabilities. These pathologies, when they exist, should be cared for as a part of an interdisciplinary team approach to patient care.

This chapter deals specifically with the external integument and wound healing. Normal age-related changes that affect wound healing and the conditions necessary for healing need to be understood for successful wound care in older adult populations.

THE SKIN AND THE AGING PROCESS

It is well recognized that the skin of the elderly differs in many ways from that of a younger person.[2] While great variance exists among individuals' physiologic responses to aging, certain characteristics are inherent to the aging process. In order to understand gerontodermatological changes and the effects they have on delayed wound healing, it is important to review what is normal so that the changes that take place can be put into perspective.

On average there is approximately 20 square feet of skin (if laid out flat) and the skin is often called "the body's biggest organ." It is the only organ that is exposed to the external environment. It is an all-purpose covering in that it is water-proof (it keeps the water out and in), and it assists in regulating body temperature.

The skin has three distinct layers. The epidermis, dermis, and subcutaneous layers. Figure 14–1 provides a pictorial representation of the layers of normal skin. The epidermis is the uppermost layer of skin. This is divided into the stratum corneum (top layer), stratum spinosum (middle layer), and stratum germinativum (innermost layer). The stratum corneum, or the horny layer, is somewhat acidic and referred to as the acid mantle. It is the major barrier to the environment and effectively prevents the penetra-

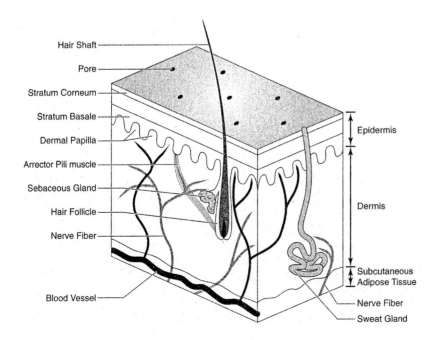

Figure 14–1. *Structure of skin, including accessory structures. Hair with the follicles located deep in the dermis are shown with the associated arrector pili muscles that cause the hairs to become erect and form "goose flesh" in the cold. Sweat glands with their coiled portion deep in the dermis and openings onto the surface of the skin are also depicted. Sebaceous glands are associated with hair follicles and secrete their oily sebum onto the skin to help retain moisture. Also note the relative thickness of the dermis, which is about 10 times thicker than the epidermis, the presence of sensory receptors in the dermis, and blood vessels in the dermis.*

Hair Shaft
Pore
Stratum Corneum
Stratum Basale
Dermal Papilla
Arrector Pili muscle
Sebaceous Gland
Hair Follicle
Nerve Fiber
Blood Vessel

Epidermis
Dermis
Subcutaneous Adipose Tissue
Nerve Fiber
Sweat Gland

tion of most environmental substances. The middle layer, or stratum spinosum is called the prickle-cell layer. This is the thickest of the epidermal layers. The cells in the stratum spinosum are squamous cells, which essentially are basal cells that have matured and migrated upward. The basal layer, the stratum germinativum, continuously reproduces new cells. This layer contains basal cells and elanocytes, in addition to melanocytes, the cells which produce melanin (providing the skin color).[3]

The dermis is the second layor. It contains collagen and elastic fibers, which are complex proteins responsible for the support and elasticity of skin. This layer enables the skin to regain its shape after being stretched or deformed. The circulatory supply is contained in the dermis, as well as the nerve endings, and the oil and sweat glands. Skin nutrition and oxygenation are supplied by numerous arteries, veins, and capillaries coursing upward through the dermis. Incredibly, each square inch of the dermis houses numerous small, nutrient-providing blood vessels. Their constriction and dilation, in response to ambient temperature changes, are responsible for keeping the body temperature constant. These small vessels also keep the skin healthy and viable by providing nutrients and remove metabolic waste materials. (See Figure 14–1.)

The subcutis or subcutaneous is the fatty layer, which gives the skin its smooth appearance. It is loosely connected to itself but adheres to the dermis and the underlying fascia. This allows skin to dissipate both pressure and shear forces. In areas where bony prominences such as the greater trochanter or heel are immediately adjacent to the subcutaneous fat layer without any muscle or other soft tissue protection, the ability of the skin to dissipate pressure is compromised. The disproportionate pressure placed on these areas can occlude blood flow, causing tissue breakdown and leading to tissue death. As well as mechanical protection, the subcutaneous layer also provides thermal insulation. Fat also acts as an energy store. By volume, fat stores approximately 20 times as much energy as the storage form of carbohydrate called glycogen.

As the skin ages, there are certain changes which occur that will ultimately impact the healing process in the event of an injury or wound. These changes are summarized in Table 14–1.

WOUND REPAIR

The body's response to injury of the skin, the repair sequence, is the same regardless of the origin of the wound—whether it is a traumatic injury, a pressure sore, a venous stasis ulcer, or a diabetic ulcer. Wound repair starts the moment the tissue is injured. The healing process involves several predictable stages, which are summarized in Figure 14–2. Wound healing consists of four basic phases: inflammation, proliferation, epithelialization, and remodeling.[4,5] This healing process can easily be remembered by the 3 **Rs** of wound healing: **R**eaction (inflammation), **R**egeneration (proliferation and epithelialization), and **R**emodeling.

The inflammatory response is decreased with age,[6,7] and undoubtedly this bears on some of the alterations in healing that will subsequently be discussed. The proliferative phase traditionally includes cell migration, proliferation, and maturation, all of which are changed with age. Remodeling encompasses the tertiary binding of collagen molecules, whish is also altered with age.[7] Although all of these stages of wound healing differ with age, the changes are qualitative. Events begin later, proceed more slowly, and often do not reach the same level. However, there are neither new events nor an absence of expected events in the healing of wounds in the elderly.

Uninterrupted Wound Repair

After the injury, inflammation allows the destruction of foreign material and microbes. Neutrophils are usually the first cells to the site of injury, and they function to destroy microbes. Macrophages come later, and aid in wound healing by removing debris and attracting and promoting proliferation of fibroblasts. Fibroblasts secrete the molecules that form the ground substance and fibers of the scar tissue that fills the tissue loss. The tissue that is generated forms in small piles, resembling the pebbled surface of a basketball, and because of the formation of leaky, new blood vessels, it is beefy red and shiny. This tissue is called granulation tissue, and from this, fibers are generated in random directions, but provide little of the tensile strength of normal skin (this is scar tissue). During the proliferation phase, myofibroblasts in the wound pull the wound edges toward the middle, producing wound contraction. Concurrent with and continuing after the wound has completed granulation, is the process of epithelialization. As granulation tissue fills in from the sides of the wound, new epithelial cells are regenerated to cover the scar tissue below. Although mature scar tissue has many of the same components of dermis, it lack the accessory structures (sweat glands, sebaceous glands, hair follicles, nails) and blood vessels of natural dermis. The remodeling phase consists of reinforcement of collagen in the direction of stress and removal of collagen bundles that are unstressed so that a mature scar has approximately 80% of the strength of normal skin.[4,5] In fact, during the first two weeks of healing, an acute wound regains one-third to one-half of the skin's original strength. It takes approximately three months for a wound to regain nearly 80% of the tensile strength of the original skin. The maturation or remodeling phase of healing continues for a year or more, thus, care in the older person must be taken to protect healed areas from re-injury, particularly in the first three-month period.

TABLE 14–1. AGING-RELATED CHANGES IN THE SKIN THAT AFFECT THE HEALING PROCESS

Aging Change	Result
Thinning and flattening of epidermis	• Increased vulnerability to trauma • Increased susceptibility to shearing stress leading to blisters and skin tears • Decreased tissue barrier properties • Impairment of barrier functions causing problems by allowing certain drugs and irritants to be more easily absorbed
Decreased epidermal proliferation	• The production on new skin cells slows down and the epidermis cannot replace itself as rapidly • Decreased wound contraction • Delayed cellular migration and proliferation
Cells in horny layer become less elastic	• The skin is unable to return to original position when stretched(i.e., like a worn rubber band)
Atrophy of the dermis	• Underlying tissues are more vulnerable to injury • Increased rate of wound dehiscence • Decreased wound contraction
Decreased vascularity of the dermis	• Easy bruising and susceptibility to injury • Poor temperature regulation (usually making skin cool) • Increased vulnerability to trauma • Decreased wound capillary growth • Increased rate of wound dehiscence
Changes and loss in collagen and elastin fibers	• Underlying tissue more vulnerable to injury • Decreased tensile strength • Delayed collagen remodeling
Decrease in number of oil and sweat glands	• The skin is not as moist or as well lubricated
Vascular response is compromised	• Cutaneous immune and inflammatory response are impaired • Reduced ability to clear foreign materials and fluids • Decreased wound capillary growth • Altered metabolic response
Nerve endings become abnormal	• Altered or reduced sensation
Fragility of the subcuteous layer	• Easy bruising and tearing of the skin • Loss of cushion effect of subcutaneous layer • Skin no longer feels as thick

An acute wound, such as a surgical incision, may be expected to complete this process in a more rapid and orderly manner than a wound dehiscence or a pressure ulcer in an elderly malnourished individual. The stages of chronic wound repair may not follow the sequence of an acute wound.

Certain conditions need to be in place in order for a wound to heal in a timely manner. Appropriate cells need to be present, including macrophages, granulocytes, fibroblasts, platelets, and both red and white blood cells. Circulation needs to be adequate in order to provide oxygen and nutrients essential for wound healing. A proper electrolyte and fluid balance create the ideal healing environment. Sufficient amounts of calories to fuel the very high-energy expenditure needed for healing should be present, as well as appropriate amounts of vitamins, minerals, and proteins. Finally, in order to heal 100%, wounds need to be free from infection.

The Effects of Aging on Wound Healing

There is a potential for problems in wound healing related to the aging process itself, as well as age-associated disease and slower healing as described in Table 14–1. Elderly individuals may have a decrease in sensory input or neurological involvement such as paralysis and peripheral neuropathies that may negatively impact their ability to detect potentially destructive pressures. Older patients may experience decreased cognitive ability, fluctuating mental states, or weakness and debilitation, and chronic illnesses that lead to immobility, which may predispose them to skin breakdown.[6,7]

These factors are not the only ones that will affect wound healing in an older population. Tissue and vascular changes related to decreased activity levels will diminish the nutritional health of tissue and increase their vulnerability to injury.

In an older individual with an impaired inflammatory response, blastema cells may appear within days of injury. This is indicative that the tissue repair process is not starting.[8,9] The inflammatory response may also be prolonged in an older patient, lasting from seven to fourteen days following the initial injury (generally lasts around two to four days). The proliferation period is also extended. Typically this phase of healing lasts for about three weeks. In the elderly, it is more commonly five to six weeks in duration.[10] A delay in wound contraction and cellular migration and proliferation may occur in older patients, and the remodeling phase varies, ranging anywhere from two years to five years (sometimes even more).[11] In an older adult, it is also important to keep in mind

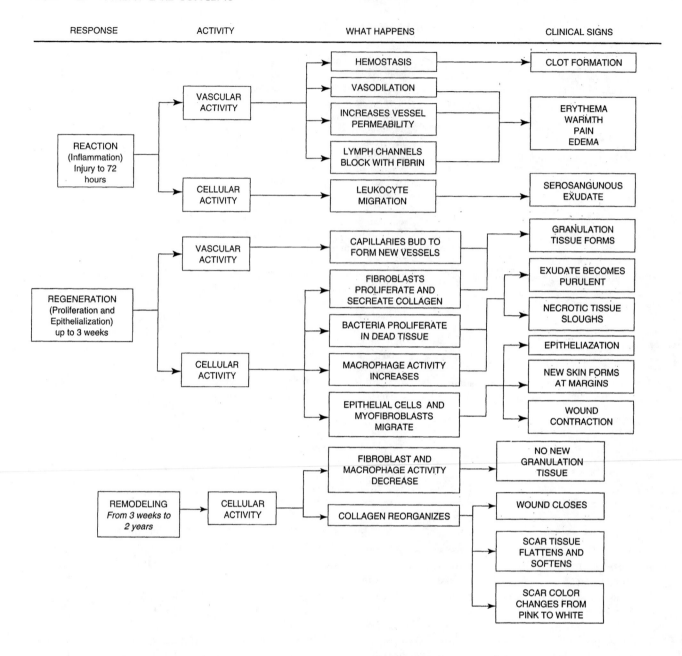

RESPONSE	ACTIVITY	WHAT HAPPENS	CLINICAL SIGNS

Figure 14–2. Reaction • Regeneration • Remodeling • *Wound healing process – The 3Rs.*

that the scar tissue is generally weaker and less elastic than that seen in a younger population.

The aging changes affecting tissue repair as depicted in Table 14–1 influence the rate of healing in older adults. Thinning and flattening of the epidermis results in an increased vulnerability to trauma from shear and frictional forces. The skin is more likely to blister or tear, resulting in a partial thickness injury. Additionally, changes in sensation and perfusion allow the skin to become macerated or overhydrated, which can lead to breakdown. Once the epidermis has been damaged, it takes longer for the older adult to replace these tissue layers.[6;7]

Healing also takes longer in the older adult because the epidermal proliferation or turnover time is slowed. The production of new skin cells decreases and the surface layer simply does not replace itself as readily. The end result is delayed wound contraction and decreased cellular migration and proliferation resulting in an inefficient and slower rate of healing.[7]

Atrophy of the dermis results in less elasticity and a thinning of the tissues. This leaves the underlying tissues more exposed and more vulnerable to breakdown. This circumstance also increases the likelihood of dehiscence and delayed wound contraction.[12]

An older individual's skin also shows a decrease in vascularity, not only compromising sensation because of nutrient deficiency, but altering the ability to regulate body temperature. Capillary growth decreases resulting in a reduction in the amount of blood being delivered to the tissues.[6;7] Consequently, the tissues become more susceptible to injury and breakdown. Due to the poor vascularity and nutrient status, the skin is more likely to bruise. Small insults can result in hemorrhages that are disproportional to the actual injury.

The quality of the tissue is also compromised in the elderly. The loss of collagen and elastic fibers and a delay in collagen remodeling leave the underlying tissue more vulnerable to trauma. The scar tissue of a healed wound is less flexible and much more fragile than the original skin tissue.[6;7]

The number of sebaceous and sweat glands also decreases making the skin less moist, lubricated, and resilient. The skin becomes drier, more easily cracked, and is susceptible to infection and fungal development. Because of the loss of hair follicles and touch/pressure receptors, coupled with dehydration, the sensory system is compromised, increasing the chance of injury.

A diminishment in the responsiveness of the vascular system impairs cutaneous immune and inflammatory responses.[6,7] It also results in delayed wound closure. There is a reduction in the ability to clear foreign materials or fluids, a decrease in wound capillary growth, and an alteration of metabolic responses.

With age, the ability to discriminate touch, temperature, and vibration declines. The skin is more prone to trauma and burns, often without perception.

Last, the subcutaneous tissue, which is a natural padding system, is reduced. This leaves bony prominences directly exposed to external forces without a protective layer for shock absorption. Because of the abundant circulatory network in the subcutaneous layer, the loss of this layer of tissue also impacts the ability to regulate systemic temperature through vasodilation and vasocontriction. The elderly are much less efficient at coping with ambient temperature changes.

In addition to alterations in skin condition related to aging, many disease processes will affect the status of the skin. Peripheral vascular disease, for instance, leads to a poor nutritional state and an increased risk for ulceration. Wounds related to the peripheral neuropathy seen in diabetes mellitus are extremely common in the older population.

Factors Complicating Wound Repair

Elimination of exogenous and endogenous impediments to wound repair and meticulous local care are required for humane and cost-effective patient care and satisfactory treatment outcomes.

This section of the chapter provides an overview of factors which might impair healing in an elderly population. Infection, nutrition, and the aging process are the major factors in overall success of wound healing in an older population. Additionally, the patients complex medical status and potential medical complications may compromise would healing.

The presence of infection increases the metabolic demands for wound healing and normal cellular functioning.[6] The most common complication of wound repair is wound infection. Due to the changing homeostatic mechanism of core body temperature (see Chapter 3) and decreased responsiveness of blood cell production, the body temperature may not be elevated and white blood cell production may not appear to be increased based on laboratory findings. As a result, the presence of infection may go undetected. It is important, therefore, for the clinician to look for indicators of infection, such as wound color, odor, drainage, pain, and edema, or changes in cognition such as lethargy, confusion, or restlessness. Patients with infection may also report dizziness or lightheadedness. In fact, sometimes a fall is the first indicator of an infection. The therapist must be alert to these signs and symptoms, especially when a wound is present.

Many drugs that an older patient may be on compromise wound repair.[12] These include:

- Steroids
- Nonsteroidal anti-inflammatory drugs (NSAIDs)
- Narcotics and sedatives
- Immunosuppressive agents
- Antineoplastic drugs
- Anticoagulants
- Antiprostaglandins

The use of many medications can affect the skin and can lead to an increased risk of breakdown and delay in healing. Steroids and nonsteroidal anti-inflammatory drugs (NSAIDS) are only a few of the many drugs that affect the skin in older adults. In fact, the use of steroids before or shortly after injury can prolong healing by inhibiting epidermal regeneration and collagen synthesis and decreasing the tensile strength of wound tissues. Not only is the function of fibroblasts and collagen synthesis impaired, but the use of steroids may affect the phagocytic and antibacterial elements of wound repair.[7]

The use of NSAIDs can delay the reepithelialization of the stratum corneum. Oral NSAIDs, which have been shown to reduce the inflammatory response, may have a significant effect on wounds during the acute phase, or on those wounds where inflammation is a desired response.

Narcotics and sedatives can increase the risk for skin disruption simply by decreasing the patient's mental alertness, thus leading to decreased mobility and activities.

Chemotherapy (immunosuppressive agents) is associated with an increased risk of infection and alteration of collagen synthesis, metabolism, and fibroblast and myofibroblast function.[11] The use of immunosuppressive agents may decrease the tensile strength of tissues, as well as negatively influence a patient's response to customary wound care.

Other important drug categories that can affect healing are antineoplastic drugs, anticoagulants, and antiprostaglandins. Complications may also occur as a result of other numerous factors and need to be considered:

- Immunosuppressive diseases
- Cytotoxic cleaners, dressings, agents
- Radiation therapy
- Patient's environment
- Lack of attention to primary etiology of the wound (inadequate pressure relief, inappropriate shoegear, inadequate compression with venous disease) and poor patient care
- Patient noncompliance
- Inappropriate wound care
- Nutritional state (including obesity or malnutrition)
- Decreased sensation or paralysis
- Altered mental status
- Urinary incontinence
- Hypovolemia
- Physical disability and chronic illness leading to immobility

Diseases of the immune system result in an increased risk of infection. A decrease in hematocrit (red blood cells as a percentage of blood volume) or diminished hemoglobin (red blood cell volume) will decrease the availability of oxygen to the system. Any disease that reduces red blood cell production will lead to anemia. Too many red blood cells will also affect healing due to the predisposition of blood clot formation. Low platelet counts can increase the risk of bleeding because of the impaired coagulation function.

Diabetes mellitus is not only associated with poor circulation and ischemia from mechanical factors, but this disease is complicated by an impaired immune system. These patients are less resistant to bacteria that can lead to infection. A decrease in perspiration resulting from the autonomic involvement allows the skin to crack and fissure, and increases the vulnerability to infection. Infection can lead to necrosis, gangrene, and amputation.

Chronic venous insufficiency is another problem that increases the risk for infection and is a common medical problem among the elderly. This condition also increases the risk of acute thrombophletitis with potentially life-threatening results. Arterial insufficiency leads to ulceration due to an insufficient blood supply to the lower extremities. Any of these circulatory conditions can be exacerbated by smoking, diabetes, hypertension, or trauma. There is poor perfusion in the lower extremities with arterial insufficiency leading to claudication and self-restricted activity levels (see Chapter 13).

Pulmonary diseases reduce the amount of oxygen introduced into the system thereby affecting peripheral perfusion. Neurological disorders not only reduce mobility, but impair sensation and increase the risk of breakdown.

Obesity is a neglected problem in the older adult population. With obesity, adipose tissue is poorly vascularized, decreasing the nutrients supplies to the various layers of the skin. The increased load places undue stress on the tissues. These patients, though this may not be suspected, are most often malnourished. They consume large amounts of empty calories that do not contain sources of vitamins and minerals.

Converse to obesity is emaciation in the elderly. This clearly will increase vulnerability of tissues, especially over bony prominences, and the likelihood that skin status will be compromised as a result of nutritional deficiencies is great.

Older adults are often plagued with urinary or bowel incontinence. Many elders with incontinence suffer from skin breakdown due to the irritants in excrements and the chronic exposure to moisture. The destruction of the skin's integrity from moisture, combined with bacteria and acidic pH from urine and feces, make the skin more susceptible to infection.

Prolonged hypovolemia can result in reduced venous return and a decrease in cardiac output (see Chapter 13) and can lead to a decrease in leukocyte production and activity and compromise collagen production.[13]

Factors affecting repair of wounds in the older patients include, but are not limited to, delayed cellular activity, decreased wound breaking strength, decreased barrier properties, diminished biosynthetic activity, delayed collagen remodeling and contraction, and decreased vascularity.[12] While caution is suggested in treating the elderly, particularly those with friable skin, not all aged individuals have decreased ability to heal. Variations in medical status and health allow many elderly to heal as well as the younger population. Surgeries are frequently performed on the elderly with no problems with healing. When treating the elderly for healing wounds from any origin:

- Exercise caution when using adhesives and tapes on friable skin
- Avoid frequent scrubs
- Avoid irritating and cytotic agents[12]

Complication of wound repair may occur because of numerous intrinsic and extrinsic factors. It is important for the wound care team to consider the whole of a patient's medical status when dealing with a wound in an elderly person. When a wound shows no response to treatment after two weeks, the patient's medical and wound status should be reevaluated. When there are no new findings regarding medical status, a different wound care approach (product, modality, medication) should be considered.

NUTRITIONAL CONSIDERATIONS IN WOUND CARE

Optimal nutritional status is essential for healing a wound, regardless of the age of a patient.[14] However, protein-calorie, vitamin, and mineral malnutrition, especially in those hospitalized postsurgical elderly patients, occurs in about 50% of older individuals. In fact, it has been determined that nutritional status often deteriorates during a hospital stay.[15] Elderly patients discharged from the hospital with open wounds are likely to have tenuous nutritional status and need careful attention to diet if their wounds are to heal. Nutritionally, the immune system can be bolstered through attention to the diet. See Chapter 7 for further discussion of nutrition and the immune system. Dietary changes specific to wounds and healing will be presented in this chapter.

Pressure ulcers and diabetic ulcers frequently develop in malnourished elderly individuals (regardless of setting). In a 21-day, double-blind study, malnourished elders applied 20 ml of a solution containing either essential fatty acids (linoleic acid extracted from sunflower oil) plus vitamins A and E, or the same solution without the essential fatty acids (control solution) to their skin. Each solution was applied to the skin three times per day. Compared with the control solution, the solution containing essential fatty acids significantly reduced the incidence of pressure ulcers and improved elasticity and hydration of the skin in the malnourished elderly study group.[16]

In another study of twenty-eight malnourished elderly individuals with pressure ulcers, those who were given a diet containing 24% protein showed a significant reduction in the size of the ulcer, whereas those given a diet containing 14% protein had no significant improvement.[17] This study suggests that increasing dietary protein in malnourished elders can improve wound healing.

Assessing elderly patients for signs of malnutrition is discussed comprehensively in Chapter 7. However, as a review specific to wound care, screening for malnutrition becomes extremely important in high-risk patients. Patients at high risk include:

- Patients weighing less than 80% of ideal body weight
- Patients having lost more than 10% of usual body weight in the past 6 months
- Alcoholic patients
- Elderly patients
- Patients with malabsorption conditions such as diverticulosis, irritable bowel syndrome, or Crohn's disease (see Chapter 5)
- Patients on hemodialysis

Factors that might lead to malnutrition during hospitalization may include poor nutritional intake, orders for nothing-by-mouth (NPO) related to surgical or other medical interventions, weight loss, obesity, multiple trauma and burns, elders admitted with gastrointestinal disorders, fistulas, or short bowel syndrome, and draining wounds (increased nutrient losses). It must be noted that obese patients are often erroneously felt to benefit from calorie restriction during an acute illness. The truth is, that given such stressors as trauma or sepsis, obese patients are quite susceptible to protein-calorie malnutrition and resultant poor wound healing despite the excess in adipose tissue.[18] The overall status needs to be evaluated. Regardless of admission weight or physique, recent weight loss (particularly greater than 10% of usual weight), elders weighing less than 80% of their height and weight norms, the presence of edema, excessive hair loss (a reflection of compromised nutritional status), or a low serum albumin (less than 3.5 gm/dl) should be triggers for a more thorough evaluation of nutritional status. Each of these symptoms is indicative of protein-calorie malnutrition.[19]

The edema seen in patients with protein-calorie malnutrition is due to low serum colloid osmotic pressure with resultant accumulation of interstitial fluid.[19,20] Wound edema can impair healing by increasing the distance oxygen and other nutrients must travel to reach the cells, and by inhibiting movement of cellular waste products causing buildup around the wound. Edema also results in weight gain and can cause the clinician to erroneously believe a patient's weight is stable when lean body mass is what is decreasing. While no one of these factors alone is indicative of malnutrition, the more factors present, the higher the suspicion of malnutrition.

Serum proteins have long been used as indicators of visceral protein stores (see Chapter 7).[21] Albumin is the most well studied. An albumin level of less than 3.5 gm/dl indicates that nutritional status should be assessed. Low albumin, less than 3.0 gm/dl, is certainly correlated with poor patient outcomes.[22] Protein-calorie malnutrition has a high mortality rate. If an elderly patient has hypoalbuminemia, edema, and easy hair-pluckability, the patient is in need of urgent and intensive nutritional intervention. It is preferable to implement optimal nutritional intervention upon admission, especially if the admission is for wound care.

Many nutrients are thought to be important in the healing process. Dietary modifications and nutritional and herbal supplements may improve the quality of wound healing by influencing inflammatory or reparative processes.

The results of poor protein ingestion include hypoalbuminemia, edema, lymphopenia, and an impairment in cellular immunity. *Protein* intervention enhances wound repair, facilitates clotting factor production, white blood cell production and migration, and increases cell-mediated bacterial killing. In addition, protein is directly involved in fibroblast proliferation, neovascularization, collagen synthesis, epithelial cell proliferation, and wound remodeling.[18,19,21]

Provision of adequate amounts of *carbohydrates* is a very important component of the diet for wound healing. With an insufficient supply of carbohydrates, the body actually uses its own visceral and muscle tissue to acquire proteins necessary for the production of energy and wound repair. This will result in weight loss, sarcopenia, and overall emaciation. With the resultant catabolism of body protein, protein is no longer used for repair but to provide the needed glucose for the maintenance of normal cellular activities. Carbohydrates added to the diet of an elderly individual with a postsurgical, diabetic, arterial, venous, vasculitic, or pressure ulcer assists in wound repair by supplying cellular energy and sparing the proteins ingested for the work of collagen synthesis and fibroblast proliferation.

Though *fats* are often omitted from an older patient's diet because of cardiovascular pathologies, they become important during wound healing. A lack of fat decreases the conversion of many dormant stores of endocrines (which are stored in fat cells) from being converted to their active form. Deficient fat in the diet will result in poor wound healing. Fats supply cellular energy and are crucial for furnishing the essential fatty acids required for wound repair. Additionally, fat is a major component in the manufacture of cell membranes, thereby an important element in the repair of the dermis and epithelial layers of the skin. The fatty acid arachidonic acid, a precursor of prostaglandins, has an influence on the inflammatory process, thereby affecting the healing process.

Vitamin C participates in wound healing by enhancing the membrane integrity, fibroblast function, the function of leukocytes, angiogenesis, and an increased resistance to infection. A deficiency in vitamin C results in poor wound healing and capillary fragility. Vitamin C also participates in the process of wound healing by promoting the synthesis of collagen. In a study of elderly individuals with oral wounds, supplementation with vitamin C (1 to 2 grams per day) increased the rate of healing.[23] In a double-blind study of older surgical patients with decubitus ulcers, supplementation with 500 mg of vitamin C twice a day accelerated ulcer healing.[24]

The mineral *zinc* plays a role in cell division and cell proliferation, both of which are involved in the process of wound healing. Zinc is also necessary for amino acid metabolism and collagen synthesis. Deficiencies in zinc increase susceptibility to infection by impairing the immune system and also result in epithelial thickening, decreased tensile strength, disruption of granulation formation, and abnormal neutrophil and lymphocyte function. Zinc deficiency is associated with impaired wound healing.[25] The healing time of a surgical wound was reduced by 43% in elderly patients following oral supplementation with zinc sulfate in the amount of 50 mg 3 times per day.[26] Zinc supplementation also improved healing in elderly people suffering from chronic leg ulcers[27] and pressure sores.[28] In another study, intravenous administration of zinc significantly reduced the number of postoperative complications in elderly surgical patients.[29]

Zinc sulfate or other zinc extracts are often used in wound care in topical ointments and dressings. In a study of people deficient in zinc, topically applied *zinc oxide* (as an additive to a gauze bandage) enhanced the regeneration of epithelial tissue on leg ulcers. In addition, inflammation and bacterial growth were reduced.[30] In a study of thirty-seven elderly individuals with leg ulcers, application of zinc oxide compresses promoted ulcer healing.[31] Although zinc oxide produced beneficial effects in these studies, topically applied zinc sulfate was ineffective. This is an important finding as zinc sulfate is effective when ingested as noted above.

Iron is an essential component for hemoglobin synthesis for the transportation of oxygen to the tissues. A reduction in iron can result in bleeding complications, especially following surgical procedures. Deficiency also results in poor oxygenation of the tissue which slows the healing process.

Vitamin A has also been studied in relationship to its wound-healing properties. Subjects fed a vitamin A supplemented diet showed enhanced wound healing, compared with those fed a standard diet.[32] The beneficial effect of vitamin A on wound healing may be due to an increase in collagen synthesis.[33] Supplementation with vitamin A also reversed the impairment of wound healing in diabetics.[34]

Supplementing *vitamin E* can decrease the formation of unwanted adhesions following a surgical wound. In addition, wound healing was more active in subjects fed a vitamin E-rich diet than those fed a standard diet.[35] However, in another study, wound healing was inhibited by supplementation with a massive amount of vitamin E (35,000 IU.) This adverse effect of vitamin E was prevented by supplementation with A. Although these findings require further investigation, physicians of natural medicine recommend supplementing with both vitamins A and E in order to enhance wound healing and prevent adhesion formation.

Vitamin K is essential for proper hemostasis and synthesis of clotting factors. Deficiencies can result in excessive bleeding, as well as the formation of hematomas.

Copper is a required cofactor for the enzyme lysyl oxidase, which plays a role in the cross-linking (and strengthening) of connective tissue.[36] Copper is often a recommended supplement as a part of a comprehensive nutritional program to promote wound healing.

Thiamine (vitamin B_1),[37] *pantothenic acid* (vitamin B_5),[38] and other B vitamins[39,40] have been shown to play a role in wound healing. A vitamin B supplement is often used to promote wound healing, especially in the elderly who tend to have deficiencies in the components of the B complex.

An interesting nutritional element associated with wound healing is *bromelain.* Bromelain is an enzyme derived from pineapple and has been used for decades by trainers to accelerate the healing of soft tissue injuries in boxers.[41] Ingestion of bromelain prior to and following a surgical procedure has been shown to reduce swelling, bruising, healing time, and pain.[42]

Table 8–30 provides a list of herbal remedies commonly used in the treatment of wounds. In addition to those listed, the following herbs have also been shown to enhance wound healing.

Calendula is used by herbalists in a topical dressing to assist in wound healing. Studies indicate a potent anti-inflammatory effect.[43,44] Traditional herbalists frequently recommend a combination of herbs for wound healing in order to achieve the desired effect. The herbs *St. John's wort,* calendula, *chamomile,* and *plantain* have been shown to exert anti-inflammatory effects in combination.[45] It is unknown whether a synergistic effect may be achieved by using the combination of these herbs rather than single herbs. These herbs have shown to have independent beneficial actions; for example, plantain acts as an anti-inflammatory when used externally, and St. John's wort in a topical application demonstrates an anti-inflammatory action.[45]

In addition, *comfrey* is an external anti-inflammatory that may decrease bruising.[45] *Witch hazel* can be used both internally and externally to decrease inflammation and stop bleeding.[45] *Horsetail* can be used both internally and externally to decrease inflammation and promote wound healing.[46] *Aloe vera* has proven beneficial in decreasing inflammation and promotion cellular repair.[47]

Evaluation of the older adult being treated with integumentary problems needs to include vitamin and mineral assays to confirm any suspected deficiencies. As noted above, many naturally occurring nutrients and supplements have been shown to have beneficial effects in promoting wound health and healing. Proper assessment of nutritional status and nutritional interventions to meet the protein, calorie, vitamin, and mineral needs of elderly patients with wounds cannot be overemphasized in wound healing.

PATIENT AND WOUND EVALUATION

Accurate assessment and evaluation of a wound is very important. Identifying causation problems (positioning, diagnoses, functional capabilities) will assist the clinician in treating the current wound and preventing future wounds from occurring.

Thorough knowledge and assessment of the physical and pathological etiologies of wounds are prerequisites to treating lesions successfully. Patient evaluation should include a comprehensive review of systems, review of medications, prior and current treatment modalities, the patient's awareness of the problem, the external environment that may affect wound care and future prevention, and nutritional status. If possible, the date of wound onset should be established in addition to identifying contributing factors. A history of significant medical diagnoses such as diabetes, hypertension, congestive heart failure, renal disease, COPD, peripheral vascular disease, lymphatic insufficiency, recent weight loss, and other problems that may impact the effective treatment of the wound should be established. A history of previous wounds and the types of treatments and results is also an important area of assessment. Medications that may affect wound healing such as steroids or anticoagulant need to be documented. Identifying allergies to topical medications or whirlpool additives should be determined.

Laboratory findings, especially culture reports of the wound if available will assist in establishing the direction of intervention. Any malnourished geriatric patient is not at a greater risk for the development of an ulceration, but will require more healing time. As described above, testing the protein and serum albumin levels is crucial to predicting wound healing. A low protein level will impede collagen synthesis, fibroblast proliferation and wound remodeling. Phagocytosis and the immune response will also be impaired. An elderly patient with a wound will need higher protein sources. Low serum albumin levels respresent late manifestation of protein deficiency. Normal albumin levels are 3.5 to 5.0 gm/dL. A severely compromised albumin level would be less than 2.5 to 3.0 gm/dL.

Laboratory evaluation may also be needed to determine the availability of other nutrients, such as the vitamins and minerals previously discussed, which will expedite wound healing. For example, vitamins A and C assist in collagen synthesis. Vitamin C affects fibroblastic and immune function, while vitamin A promotes re-epithilialization. Minerals such as zinc may increase epithelialization and cell production.

Chapter 13 provides a model for assessing peripheral circulation and central cardiovascular status. Evaluating the presence of pulses, particularly in distal wounds of the lower extremity, will determine the viability of the tissues for healing. Assessing the overall skin integrity including hydration, turgor, and areas of discoloration will provide information on the tissue's nutritional status and the prospect of healing the wound.

Arterial pathologies need to be assessed in an objective manner. It is crucial that the tissue receive oxygen. If blood flow to a wound is impeded, oxygenation and nutrients will be blocked and CO_2 and metabolic by-products will not be removed. Without oxygen, collagen synthesis and fibroblast differentiation will not occur. In the course of the physical exam, beyond assessing dorsal pedis pulse and a posterior tibial pulse, if a portable Doppler is available, this is an objective means of evaluating peripheral circulation. The Buerger-Allen protocol of assessment described in Chapter 13 is also an excellent means of objectifying the status of peripheral circulation.

Venous problems will affect the removal of waste products from the lower extremities and affect the nutritional health of the tissues.[48] Has the patient ever experienced a leg injury? A previous injury often leads to increased venous hypertension, which will progress to lipodermatosclerosis —the visible brown pigmentation and induration of the legs. Edema will keep oxygen and vital nutrients from entering the wound site.

Determine the neurosensory status (e.g., anesthesias, paresthesias, pain, pressure) using the Symmes-Weinstein filaments as described in Chapter 13 to establish the integrity of sensory input. Assessing pain patterns will help to identify symptoms and activities that increase or decrease pain.

Determining mobility status including ADLs, flexibility, strength, locomotion, self positioning will be predictive of rate of healing as well as the potential efficacy of preventive interventions. Assess position needs and equipment to promote wound healing. Immobility is the leading cause of pressure ulceration.[48] A healthy individual capable of feeling noxious stimuli over a bony prominence will alleviate pressure by moving that part. On the other hand, elderly patients who are immobilized secondary to illness with sensory deprivation, friable skin, and poor circulation have no comparable defense. Nor do diabetics, who have a diminished protective sensory threshold. If the individual can not reposition her or himself or move the affected limb, an ulcer sets in via hypoxia. This is a patient that needs pressure-relieving devices and repositioning on a regular schedule.

The presence of incontinence is another risk factor that increases the potential for skin breakdown by creating a moist environment which, if not attended to, leads to maceration and chemical irritation. If incontinent patients move their extremities in a urine or bowel-soaked environment, shear and friction will easily tear the outer layer of soft wet skin, eventually resulting in a breach in integument and paving the way for the possibility of wound infection.

When evaluating a wound, it is important to augment the assessment by appraising risk factors:

■ Is the patient ambulatory?
■ Is the patient oriented and able to understand directives?
■ Is the patient eating independently or receiving nourishment through other sources (supplements, tube feeding)?
■ Does the patient have a sensory deficit, or can pain be felt in the wound area?
■ Does the patient have a significant other or caretaker who can assist with care of the wound?

■ Are there other contributing factors, such as urinary incontinence, poor nutrition, arterial occlusions, venous insufficiency or perhaps diabetes?

DOCUMENTATION AND STAGING OF WOUND STATUS

In the present arena of wound care, accurate documentation is critical for securing reimbursement. While the principle rationale for documentation is to legally record information, equally important is communication with other health care professionals and third-party payors. Over time, documentation can also be used as a database for clinical research, outcomes, peer review and the quality improvement process.

Wound evaluation and documentation includes determination of:

■ Etiology and type of wound
■ Infection versus contamination
■ Size of wound
■ Undermining of sinus tracts
■ Quality and quantity of exudate
■ Underlying structures (muscles, tendons, bones)
■ Stage of healing
■ Chronicity
■ Response to previous treatment

In evaluating the wound, it is important to document the location of the wound and the type of wound (e.g., arterial versus venous insufficiency, vasculitic, pressure ulcer, diabetic ulcer, burn, abrasion, surgical, laceration, shearing, hematoma, stasis). The charting of the size of the wound should include the length, width, depth, presence of undermining and description of the shape of the wound. The status of the wound bed and the surrounding tissue should be described in a clear and concise manner. Color, odor, and exudate are all indications of wound status. The color of the wound is indicative of the stage of repair. Odor is the best way to determine if the wound is infected. It is helpful to evaluate odor after a wound has been cleansed with sterile water or saline. Foul odor may result from accumulation of wound exudate, necrotic tissue and dressing by-products, especially after the use of occlusive dressings. Common examples of appearance of wounds are provided in Table 14–2. Necrotic tissue promotes bacterial growth and when left in a wound will slow the formation of granulation tissue and epithelialization, inhibiting angiogenesis.[48]

The presence of the exudate should be recorded and the description of the drainage would include the amount, color, and viscosity (i.e., serous, serosanguineous, sanguineous or purulent). The condition of the wound tissue includes a description including the presence of granulation, epithelialization, slough, eschar, or hemorrhage. It is also important to note the condition of the surrounding tissue in terms of pain,

TABLE 14–2. COMMON DESCRIPTIONS OF WOUND APPEARANCE IN DOCUMENTATION

DESCRIPTION	IMPLICATION
Red-reepithelializing	Bright red with indications of superficial cell migration. Good wound bed and healing well.
Red-granulating	Bright or true red in appearance associated with islands of granulation tissue and good healing.
Red-chronic	Red appearance but no indication of granulation. Poor or delayed healing
Red-dusky	Dull, gray, or dark red in appearance without signs of granulation, with or without signs of localized ischemia. Poor healing with possibility of infection.
Yellow-granulating	Areas of fibrotic tissue (not usually classified as healthy or unhealthy) present in conjunction with areas of granulating tissue. No necrotic tissue present. Delayed healing.
Yellow-chronic	Areas of fibrotic tissue without areas of granulation. Poor healing.
Yellow-ischemic	Fibrotic tissue in conjunction with signs of ischemia or tissue necrosis. Delayed or poor healing.
Black-dry	Dry, desiccated eschar whether black or brown in appearance. Poor healing with tissue death.
Black-wet	Wet gangrenous appearance. Tissue death with progressive infection.
Black-mixed	Areas of necrotic tissue present with areas of yellow and/or red tissue. Tissue death with areas of infection and sporadic areas of healing.

Formulated with information from: Mulder GC, Fairchild PA, Jeter KF. *Clinician's Pocket Guide to Chronic Wound Repair.* 3rd Edition. Long Beach, CA: Wound Healing Institute Publications; 1995.

swelling, tenderness, erythema, discoloration, maceration, inflammation, skin temperature, skin texture, and hair loss. If edema is significant, baseline girth measurements need to be taken.[48]

It is important that the wound be graded in some fashion so that all health care professionals know the nature of the wound they are dealing with. There are many acceptable staging guidelines. Many clinicians use the Wagner's ulcer grade classification system which is specific to foot ulcerations, others prefer the more general staging system developed by the National Pressure Ulcer Advisory Panel. Both provide a means of objectifying wound status and facilitating consistent communication of the status of the wound.

Wagner's classification[49] was developed to objectively evaluate foot condition and ranks vascular dysfunction in grades of 0 to 5 as follows:

Grade 0: The skin is without ulceration. No open lesions are present, but potentially ulcerating deformities, such as bunions, hammer toes, and Charcot's deformity, may be present. Healed partial foot amputation may also be included in this group.

Grade 1: A full-thickness superficial skin loss is present. The lesion does not extend to bone. No abscess is present.

Grade 2: An open ulceration is noted deeper than grade 1. It may penetrate to tendon or joint capsule.

Grade 3: The lesion penetrates to bone, and osteomyelitis is present. Joint infection or plantar fascial plane abscess may also be noted.

Grade 4: Gangrene is noted in the forefoot.

Grade 5: Gangrene involving the entire foot is noted. This is not salvageable with local procedures.

The National Pressure Ulcer Advisory Board[48] provides a staging scheme for nonfoot ulcers. This staging is as follows:

Stage I: Nonblanchable erythema of intact skin, heralding lesion of skin ulceration. Dangerous if left unprotected. Often progresses quickly to Stage II or greater.

Stage II: Partial-thickness skin loss involving epidermis and/or dermis. Clinically, the lesion presents as a large blister or abrasion. Displayed most commonly under heels of the elderly due to friction and shear from heel movement, and especially in the immobile elderly following hip surgery.

Stage III: Full-thickness skin loss involving damage or necrosis of subcutaneous tissue, which may extend down to, but not through, underlying fascia. It is imperative to check for undermining or sinus tracts.

Stage IV: Full-thickness skin loss with extensive destruction, tissue necrosis or damage to muscle, bone or supporting structures.

These classification systems assist in describing the severity of the wound. In many cases these staging systems have prognostic value and, in some instances, reimbursement value. Complete description and classification are essential components of the diagnostic and therapeutic process in wound care.

Included in the grading or staging of a wound, the following descriptors should be provided in the initial and ongoing documentation of the wound.

- Location of wound
- Surface dimension of wound
- Color of wound base

- Presence of necrotic tissue (amount and color)
- Depth and tissue layers involved
- Exudate (amount, color, odor)
- Condition of the surrounding skin
- Undermining
- Clinical signs of infection (see the subsequent section on microbiology)

There are several methods that can be used to determine the size and shape of a wound. Whichever method is chosen, it is imperative that the therapist continues to use the same method consistently throughout the healing process, as different methods give different results. The therapist may wish to use a combination of methods. For example, measuring length and width as well as volume gives an excellent three-dimensional representation of the wound's actual size. As the wound heals, the length and width may actually become larger, yet the total volume of the wound will decrease. It is imperative to document which methods are being utilized, so the same techniques can be followed by other therapists. Therapists must also coordinate measuring procedures with the nursing staff or wound care team members.

It is helpful to keep the time intervals between measurements consistent. A decline in the rate of healing may be the first indication of a need to change treatment approaches.

In the presence of an ulceration, objective documentation of wound size is best accomplished by tracing the wound on sterilized x-ray film or through photographs on a line-graphed film. This is helpful in monitoring improvement or decline in wound status. Some x-ray type films are available with a bull's eye pattern that provides diameter and metric measures. This sort of industry-prepared measuring tool is use-ful in objectively tracing wound perimeters. Figure 14–3A provides an example of this sort of device.

Tracings, tape measurement guides, volumetric displacement, plain meter and photographic measurement are all excellent ways of documenting wound status. The combination of measurement techniques employed will be dictated by the patient's individualized status and plan of care. Wounds may be measured in a linear fashion and described as an area (e.g., 6 cm by 4 cm) or traced on an acetate measuring guide as presented in Figure 14–3A. Length and width of a wound to obtain size may be accomplished by using a clear ruler and measuring the longest and the widest aspects of the wound. Tracings on acetate can be transferred to a grid as shown in Figure 14–3B. As depicted in this drawing, the wound is represented by the solid line and the measured area of undermining is represented by the dashed line. Periodic tracing can be superimposed on this graph in varying colors and dated to indicate ongoing status of the wound. This gives a wonderful visual representation of the change in wound size and status. By utilizing graph paper, width and length measures are easy to obtain. Area of the wound can be calculated by counting the number of squares contained within the boundaries of the wound.

If acetate film is not available for tracing, placing two layers of plastic wrap over the wound and using a permanent ink marker to trace the outline of the wound is an inexpensive way of tracing the wound. Dispose of the bottom layer of plastic as infectious waste and photocopy the top layer onto the metric graph paper. Approximate the area within the wound by counting the boxes within the wound's borders (see Figure 14–3B).

Tracings enable more accurate comparison of change in wound perimeter over time. These small

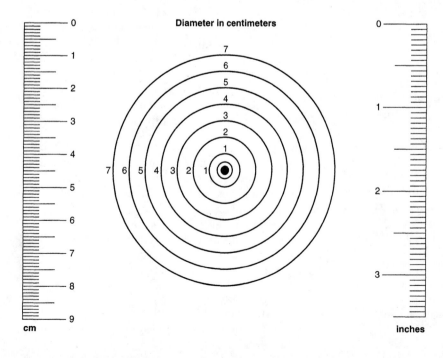

Figure 14–3A. Bull's eye and linear measurement acetate (x-ray) film for tracing and measuring size of wound. Center of bull's eye is placed in center of wound and periphery of wound is traced.

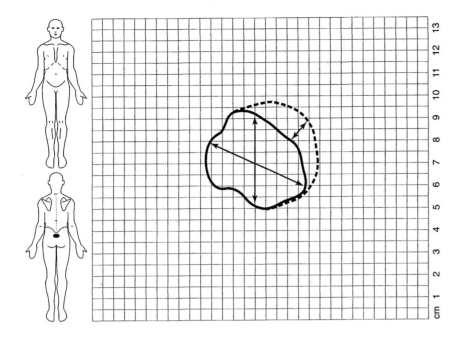

Figure 14–3B. Grid documentation of location and area of a wound.

acetate (x-ray film) measuring sheets are provided at no charge by numerous companies that provide wound care products. Many clinicians add photographic documentation.[50] A series of accurate photos taken over time provides historic data about the wound and its progress and serves as visual support for written documentation. A photograph of the wound is the most reliable documentation. Serial photographs provide objective evaluation of wound healing as demonstrated in Figure 14–4.

Measuring wound depth can be accomplished by putting a cotton-tipped applicator or tongue depressor into the base of the wound and then placing the acetate or ruler across the wound surface and marking the point it encounters the cotton swab or depressor. This measures the distance from the tip of the swab to where the applicator is even with the intact skin and provides a measure of the depth of the wound.

Undermining, which is defined as skin overhanging a dead space, should be measured with a gloved finger or a cotton-tipped applicator. To measure undermining place a cotton-tipped applicator into the wound to the extent of the undermining. Gently lift the applicator towards the skin surface until the skin is raised slightly. Mark this location with a skin pencil. Repeat at close intervals around the perimeter of the wound. On the grid paper the areas of undermining and their depth can be indicated with dashed lines as indicated in Figure 14–3B. This area, as it is probed, can be traced on the plastic wrap or acetate film as described above.

When sinus tracts are suspected, they should be probed gently with a cotton-tipped applicator or a small red rubber catheter to determine their length. A cotton-tipped applicator is placed into the tract and the distance is measured from the tip of the swab to where the tract enters the wound bed. The position of the tract should be noted by using a clock system with 12 o'clock the head of the patient, and 6 o'clock the feet. Measurement techniques for depth, sinus track, and undermining are provided in the drawing in Figure 14–5A.

Volumetric measures are also very helpful. By filling the wound with sterile water or saline just to the point of over flowing and then suctioning the water out of the wound using a needleless syringe, the volume of water it takes to fill the wound can be measured in ccs or mLs by reading the syringe markings. This gives an accurate measure of the volume of the wound. (Note: the wound must be in a position that it can be filled without the water spilling out.) Figure 14–5B provides a pictorial demonstration of this technique.

One technique for measuring volume is to use a substance called Jeltrate. This is a hydrocolloid substance that will not adhere to the wound or damage granulation tissue. A word of caution, however: This gel-like substance should not be used in wounds with very small surface openings or with large areas of undermining or tracking. The Jeltrate technique involves adding water to the Jeltrate powder according to the package instructions. Then pour the liquid into the wound and allow it to solidify (takes around five minutes). Remove the mold from the wound and place it into a graduated cylinder partially filled with a premeasured amount of water. Record the amount of water displaced as demonstrated in Figure 14–5C. This water displacement represents the volume of the wound. This mold is also an excellent teaching tool for patients, family members, or nursing staff.

There are many excellent wound assessment tools available that provide a standardized format for documenting wound status. A helpful tool, because it objectively scores each parameter for accurate monitoring of the patient's condition, was developed

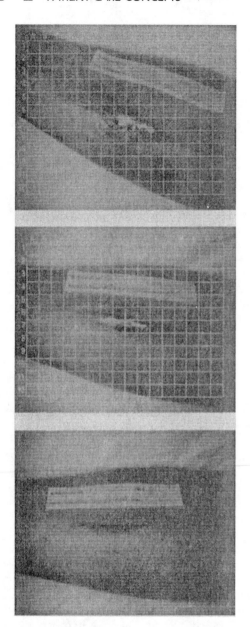

Figure 14–4. Photographic documentation of wound status over time. (*Reprinted with permission from Susan E. Morey. Originally appeared In: Morey SE. Photos supplement written documentation. Physical Therapy Products. Jan/Feb 1998; 66–67.*)

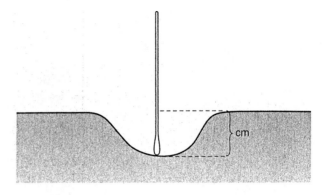

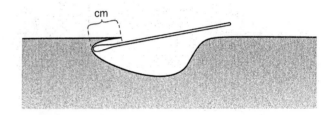

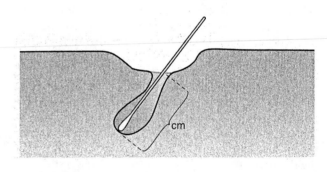

Figure 14–5A. Measuring the depth of a wound using a cotton-tipped swab. Measuring the extent of undermining of a wound. Measurement techniques for determining the depth, extent of undermining and sinus tract of a wound using a cotton swab applicator.

by Barbara Bates-Jensen. A description of the use of this tool and the tool itself is provided in Figures 14–6A and 14–6B, respectively.[51,52]

Accurate documentation enables critical evaluation of the wound-healing process and helps to inform clinicians of the wound status in an objective way. The key to future research in the pathophysiology of chronic wounds and in therapeutic efficacy depends upon precise reporting of incidence and types of chronic wounds and the use of consistent terminology. Documentation can provide the database of healing as well as nonhealing wounds required to establish the need for physical therapy or the database of healing needed to secure reimbursement from intermediaries.

MICROBIOLOGY

Bacteria is often found in chronic wounds. There is a distinction drawn between a contaminated wound and an infected wound. According to Mulder and associates,[12] wound appearance can be misleading. The degree of contamination and the distinction between contamination and infection are difficult to determine; other signs of wound infection may need to be assessed.[12]

Indicators of wound contamination may include periwound erythema, inflammation, nonpurulent drainage, malodorous (foul smelling) wound prior to cleansing, and multiple organisms present on swab culture. The same signs are present with infection,

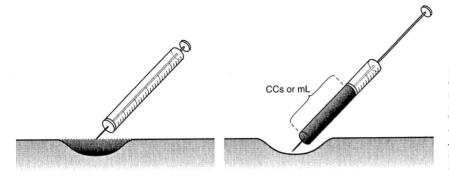

Figure 14–5B. *Measuring area of wound using a volume measurement. Fill wound with sterile watre or saline to level point. Suction fluid from wound to get volume measure in cc's or mLs. Volumetric measurement using Jeltrate mold of wound and determining displacement of water in a premeasured vessel.*

however, other established signs of infection are elevated body temperature, cellulitis, purulent drainage, wet gangrene, increased leukocytosis, persistently malodorous wound (even after cleansing), and greater than 10^5 organisms per gram tissue on culture.[12] Other indications of infection might include pain, swelling, redness, inflammation, and heat.

Swab cultures are of questionable value as multiple bacteria are often present in wound fluid and wound surface, particularly when occlusive dressings have been used. Surface organisms do not correlate well with number and type of organisms present in the tissue. Other clinical signs of infection must be present when determining that organisms present on culture are of clinical significance. For the most accurate results, it is important that the wound be thoroughly cleansed prior to culturing. Organisms found need to be coupled with other clinical indicators of infection.

LOWER EXTREMITY ULCERS

Different wound types exhibit different characteristics depending on their underlying etiology and cannot all be treated identically. Combinations of wound types further complicate the identification and treatment of wounds, especially in the elderly. For example, many diabetic ulcers result from pressure. Likewise, many patients with peripheral vascular disease may also be diabetic or have other chronic disabilities that limit their activity levels, which puts them at greater risk for breakdown as a result of immobility and pressure. The type of pressure causing diabetic ulcers is repetitive,

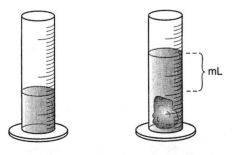

Figure 14–5C. *Volumetric measurement using Jeltrate mold of wound and determining displacement of water in a premeasured vessel.*

callus-forming pressure, whereas pressure ulcers are an ischemic event. Therefore, identification and treatment of a diabetic ulcer is different from that of a pressure ulcer. The fact that current treatment strategies are based on proper wound classification illustrates the need for the clinician to assess and classify wounds properly, even if a particular wound type is not seen in the clinician's practice setting. Table 14–3 provides five different types of wounds that may be encountered in the clinic and describes characteristics that differentiate each one.[53–57]

Arterial Ulcers

Inadequate blood supply can result in poor oxidative and nutritive status in the tissues and lead to an arterial ulcer. Vascular insufficiency can be the consequence of various diseases such as arteriosclerosis obliterans or atheroembolism. They can also occur when blood supply is restricted because of constriction or pressure that impedes blood flow into an area. Typically these ulcers occur in the distal appendages (lower extremities more than upper extremities) and occur over bony prominences. Clinical manifestations include claudication when walking, rest pain, pain in lower extremities when legs are elevated for extended periods of time, poor quality or absent pulses, atrophic changes, and history of wounds with minor trauma.[4]

Characteristically, individuals with arterial ulcerations will complain of very painful lower extremities which are often relieved in the dependent position and aggravated by elevation.[58] Wounds present with minimal drainage, are usually superficial, irregular in shape and borders, are often associated with dry necrotic eschar, and present almost anywhere on the leg, though are most commonly found on the dorsum of the foot or on the toes. The tissues surrounding the wound may be blanched or purpuric in appearance and the peri-wound tissue is often shiny and tight.[12]

Vascular testing is often used to substantiate the presence of hypoperfusion due to arterial insufficiency. The presence of vascular plaques (arteriosclerotic plaques) is associated with a resistance to blood flow and a decrease in "downstream" pressure. The diagnosis of peripheral arterial disease hinges on a thorough history and physical examination. Labora-

NAME: _____

Complete the rating sheet to assess pressure sore status. Evaluate each item by picking the response that best describes the wound and entering the score in the item score column for the appropriate date.

LOCATION: Anatomic site. Circle, identify right (R) or left (L) and use "X" t mark site on body diagrams:
_____ Sacrum & coccyx   _____ Lateral ankly
_____ Trochanter   _____ Medial ankle
_____ Ischial tuberosity   _____ Heal   _____ Other site

SHAPE: Overall wound pattern; assess by observing perimeter and depth. Circle and *date* appropriate description:
_____ Irregular   _____ Linear or elongated
_____ Round/oval   _____ Bow/boat
_____ Square/rectangle   _____ Butterfly   _____ Other shape

Item	Assessment	Date	Date	Date
		Score	Score	Score
1. SIZE	1 = Length × width <4 sq cm 2 = Length × width 4 – 16 sq cm 3 = Length × width 16.1 – 36 sq cm 4 = Length × width 36.1 – 80 sq cm 5 = Length × width <80 sq cm			
2. DEPTH	1 = Nonblanchable erythema on intact skin 2 = Partial-thickness skin loss involving epidermis &/or dermis 3 = Full-thickness skin loss involving damage or necrosis of subcultaneous tissue; may extend down to but not through underlying fascia; &/or mixed partial- &/or full-thickness &/or tissue layers obscured by granulation tissue 4 = Obscure by necrosis 5 = Full-thickness skin loss with extensive destruction, tissue necrosis, or damage to muscle, bone, or supporting structures			
3. EDGES	1 = Indistinct, diffuse, none clearly visible 2 = Distinct, outline clearly visible, attached, even with wound base 3 = Well defined, not attached to wound base 4 = Well defined, not attached to base, rolled under, thickened 5 = Well defined, fibrotic, scarred or hyperkeratotic			
4. UNDERMINING	1 = Undermining <2 cm in any area 2 = Undermining 2 – 4 cm involving <50% wound margins 3 = Undermining 2 – 4 cm involving >50% wound margins 4 = Undermining >4 cm in any area 5 = Tunneling &/or sinus tract formation			
5. NECROTIC TISSUE TYPE	1 = None visible 2 = White/gray nonviable tissue &/or nonadherent yellow slough 3 = Loosely adherent yellow slough 4 = Adherent, soft, black eschar 5 = Firmly adherent, hard, black eschar			
6. NECROTIC TISSUE AMOUNT	1 = None visible 2 = <25% of wound bed covered 3 = 25% to 50% of wound covered 4 = >50% and <75% of wound covered 5 = 75% to 100% of wound covered			
7. EXUDATE TYPE	1 = None or bloody 2 = Serosanguineous: thin, watery, pale red/pink 3 = Serous: thin, watery, clear 4 = Purulent: thin or thick, opaque, tan/yellow 5 = Foul purulent: thick, opaque, yellow/green with odor			

Figure 14–6A.   *Pressure Sore Status Tool. (© 1990 Barbara Bates-Jensen. Used with permission.)*

tory finding are also very important adjuncts in confirmation of arterial insufficiency.[12,58]

Intermittent claudication is a classic symptom of arterial disease. Intermittent claudication is fatigue or pain in the muscles of the lower extremities produced by activity (typically walking) and relieved by rest. Claudication is distinguished from other pain in the extremities because some exertion is always required to produce this symptom and it does not occur at rest.[58] For differential diagnosis, the two conditions that may be confused with claudication are osteoarthritis of the hip or knee and neurospinal compression due to osteophytic narrowing of the lumbar neurospinal canal (spinal stenosis).

When rest pain is present, this is a sign of advanced arterial ischemia which can lead to gangrene if arterial reconstruction or other interventions (e.g., Buerger-Allen exercises—see Chapter 13) are not implemented. In contrast to claudication, rest pain does not occur in a specific muscle group, rather the patient

Item	Assessment	Date	Date	Date
		Score	Score	Score
8. EXUDATE AMOUNT	1 = None 2 = Scant 3 = Small 4 = Moderate 5 = Large			
9. SKIN COLOR SURROUNDING WOUND	1 = Pink or normal for ethnic group 2 = Bright red &/or blanches to touch 3 = White or gray pallor or hypopigmented 4 = Dark red or purple &/or nonblanchable 5 = Black or hyperpigmented			
10. PERIPHERAL TISSUE ENEMA	1 = Minimal swelling around wound 2 = Nonpitting edema extends <4 cm around wound 3 = Nonpitting edema extends ≥4 cm around wound 4 = Pitting edema extends <4 cm around wound 5 = Crepitus &/or pitting edema extends ≥4 cm			
11. PERIPHERAL TISSUE INDURATION	1 = Minimal firmness around wound 2 = Induration <2 cm around wound 3 = Induration 2–4 cm extending <50% around wound 4 = Induration 2–4 cm extending ≥50% around wound 5 = Induration >4 cm in any area			
12. GRANULATION TISSUE	1 = Skin intact or partial thickness wound 2 = Bright, beefy red, 75% to 100% of wound filled &/or tissue overgrowth 3 = Bright, beefy red, <75% & > 25% of wound filled 4 = Pink &/or dull, dusky red &/or fills ≤25% of wound 5 = No granulation tissue present			
13. EPITHELIALIZATION	1 = 100% of wound covered, surface intact 2 = 75% to <100% of wound covered &/or epithelial tissue extends >0.5 cm into wound bed 3 = 50% to <75% of wound covered &/or epithelial tissue extends to <0.5 cm into wound bed 4 = 25% to <50% of wound covered 5 = <25% of wound covered			
TOTAL SCORE				
SIGNATURE				

PRESSURE SORE STATUS CONTINUUM

1   10   13   15   20   25   30   35   40   45   50   55   60   65

Tissue health   Wound regeneration   Wound degeneration

Plot the total score on the Pressure Sore Status Continuum by putting an "X" on the line and date beneath the line. Plot multiple scores with their dates to see at a glance regeneration or degeneration of the wound.

Figure 14–6A. (Continued)

Instruction for use

General guidelines:
Fill out the attached rating sheet to assess a pressure sore's status after reading the definitions and methods of assessment described below. Evaluate once a week and whenever a change occurs in the wound. Rate according to each item by picking the response that best describes the wound and entering that score in the item score column for the appropriate date. When you have rated the pressure sore on all items, determine the total score by adding together the 13 item scores. The higher the total score, the more severe the pressure sore status. Plot total score on the Pressure Sore Status Continuum to determine progress.

Specific instructions:
1. **SIZE:** Use ruler to measure the longest and widest aspect of the wound surface in centimeters; multiply length × width.
2. **DEPTH:** Pick the depth, thickness, most appropriate to the wound using these additional descriptions:
    1 = Tissues damaged but no break in skin surface.
    2 = Superficial, abrasion, blister, or shallow crater. Even with, and/or elevated above, skin surface (e.g., hyperplasia).
    3 = Deep crater with or without undermining of adjacent tissue.
    4 = Visualization of tissue layers not possible due to necrosis.
    5 = Supporting structures include tendon, joint capsule.
3. **EDGES:** Use this guide:

Indistinct, diffuse	= Unable to clearly distinguish wound outline.
Attached	= Even or flush wound base; *no* sides or walls present; flat.
Not attached	= Sides or wall *are* present; floor or base of wound is deeper than edge.
Rolled under, thickened	= Soft to firm and flexible to touch.
Hyperkeratosis	= Callous-like tissue formation around wound and at edges.
Fibrotic, scarred	= Hard, rigid to touch.

4. **UNDERMINING:** Assess by inserting a cotton-tipped applicator under the wound edge; advance it as far as it will go without using undue force; raise the tip of the applicator so it may be seen or felt on the surface of the skin; mark the surface with a pen; measure the distance from the mark on the skin to the edge of the wound. Continue process around the wound. Then use a transparent metric measuring guide with concentric circles divided into four (25%) pie-shaped quadrants to help determine percent of wound involved.
5. **NECROTIC TISSUE TYPE:** Pick the type of necrotic tissue that is predominant in the wound according to color, consistency, and adherence using this guide:

White/gray, nonviable tissue	= May appear prior to wound opening; skin surface is white or gray.
Nonadherent, yellow slough	= Thin, mucinous substance; scattered throughout wound bed; easily separated from wound tissue.
Loosely adherent, yellow slough	= Thick, stringy, clumps of debris; attached to wound tissue.
Adherent, soft, black eschar	= Soggy tissue; strongly attached to tissue in center or base of wound.
Firmly adherent, hard/black eschar	= Firm, crusty tissue; strongly attached to wound base *and* edges (like a hard scab).

6. **NECROTIC TISSUE AMOUNT:** Use a transparent metric measuring guide with concentric circles divided into four (25%) pie-shaped quadrants to help determine percent of wound involved.

Figure 14–6B.   Instructions for use of the Pressure Sore Status Tool. (© 1990 Barbara Bates-Jensen. Used with permission.)

Instructions for use

7. **EXUDATE TYPE:** Some dressings interact with wound drainage to produce a gel or trap liquid. Before assessing exudate type, gently cleanse wound with normal saline or water. Pick the exudate type that is predominant in the wound according to color and consistency, using this guide:

Bloody	=	Thin, bright red.
Serosanguineous	=	Thin, watery, pale red to pink.
Serous	=	Thin, watery, clear.
Purulent	=	Thin or thick, opaque tan to yellow.
Foul purulent	=	Thick, opaque yellow to green with offensive odor.

8. **EXUDATE AMOUNT:** Use a transparent metric measuring guide with concentric circles divided into four (25%) pie-shaped quadrants to determine percent of dressing involved with exudate. Use this guide:

None	=	Wound tissues dry.
Scant	=	Wound tissues moist; no measurable exudate.
Small	=	Wound tissues wet; moisture evenly distribute in wound; drainage involve ≤25% of dressing.
Moderate	=	Wound tissues saturated; drainage may or may not be evenly distributed in wound; drainage involves > 25% to ≤75% of dressing.
Large	=	Wound tissues bathed in fluid; drainage freely expressed; may or may not be evenly distributed in wound; drainage involves >75% of dressing.

9. **SKIN COLOR SURROUNDING WOUND:** Assess tissues within 4 cm of wound edge. Dark-skinned persons show the colors "bright red" and "dark red" as a deepening of normal ethnic skin color or a purple hue. As healing occurs in dark-skinned persons, the new skin is pink and may never darken.

10. **PERIPHERAL TISSUE EDEMA:** Assess tissues within 4 cm of wound edge. Nonpitting edema appears as skin that is shiny and taut. Identify pitting edema by firmly pressing a finger down into the tissues and waiting for 5 seconds; on release of pressure, tissues fail to resume previous position and an indentation appears. Crepitus is accumulation of air or gas in tissues. Use a transparent metric measuring guide to determine how far edema extends beyond wound.

11. **PERIPHERAL TISSUE INDURATION:** Assess tissues within 4 cm of wound edge. Induration is abnormal firmness of tissues with margins. Assess by gently pinching the tissues. Induration results in an inability to pinch the tissues. Use a transparent metric measuring guide with concentric circles divided into four (25%) pie-shaped quadrants to determine percent of wound and area involved.

12. **GRANULATION TISSUE:** Granulation tissue is the growth of small blood vessels and connective tissue to fill in full-thickness wounds. Tissue is healthy when bright, beefy red, shiny and granular with a velvety appearance. Poor vascular supply appears as pale pink or blanched to dull, dusky red color.

13. **EPITHELIALIZATION:** Epithelialization is the process of epidermal resurfacing and appears as pink or red skin. In partial-thickness wounds it occurs throughout the wound bed as well as from the wound edges. In full-thickness wounds it can occur from the edges only. Use a transparent metric measuring guide with concentric circles divided into four (25%) pie-shaped quadrants to help determine percent of wound involved and to measure the distance the epithelial tissue extends into the wound.

Figure 14-6B.   (Continued)

TABLE 14–3. DIFFERENTIATING BETWEEN ULCER TYPES BY CHARACTERISTICS

TYPE OF ULCER:	Arterial Ulcer	Venous Ulcer	Diabetic Ulcer	Pressure Ulcer	Vasculitic Ulcer
Ulcer Characteristic					
Predisposing factors/cause	Peripheral vascular disease, diabetes mellitus, advanced age	Valve incompetence in perforating veins, history of deep vein thrombophlebitis and thrombosis, failed calf pump, history of ulcers, obesity, age	Diabetic patient with peripheral neuropathy and/or peripheral vascular disease	Multiple medical diagnoses, age, impaired mobility, poor nutrition, decreased cognitive satus, incontinence, impaired circulation	Often accompanied by history of recurrence; almost always accompanied by connective tissue disease and systemic inflammatory conditions
Location and depth	Usually distal to impaired arterial supply, between toes or tips of toes, over phalangeal heads, around lateral malleolus, at sites subjected to trauma or rubbing of footwear; usually relatively shallow, but may be deep	On medial lower leg and ankle, on malleolar area, usually shallow	Any sites on the foot and lower limb subjected to pressure, friction, shear or trauma; plantar aspect, metatarsal heads, great toe, heal; shallow to deep; may have sinus tracking or undermining	On heels, sacrum, coccyx, occiput, any bony prominence subjected to pressure, friction or shear, depth ranges from blanchable erythema of intact skin to deep destruction and loss of tissue	Below malleolus on dorsum of foot; shallow in depth
Wound bed and wound appearance	Pale, gray, or yellow, with no evidence of new tissue growth; gangrene, necrosis, or cellulitis may be present; almost always accompanied by wound bed eschar; often accompanied by exposed tendons	Variable appearance frequently ruddy, beefy red, granular tissue; calcification in wound base is common; a superficial fibrinous gelatinous necrosis may occur suddenly with healthy appearing granulation tissue underneath	Granular tissue unless PVD present; often has deep, dry, necrotic area; cellulitis or esteomyelitis may be present, neuropathic ulcers almost always accompanied by eschar and often accompanied by exposed tendon	Extensive necrotic tissue may be present; extensive undermining, sinus tracts, tunneling may be present (tissue necrosis is usually greater than suggested by the external appearance of the epidermal defect)	Typically arise from small reddened areas which continue to increase in size; necrotic with marked vascularity; wound bed contains mixed necrotic and red granulation tissue
Exudate/drainage	Minimal exudate	Frequently moderate to heavy exudate	Low to moderate exudate; an infected ulcer may have purulent drainage	Exudate varies	Exudate varies
Wound shape and margins	Smooth, even; regular; shape will conform to injury if caused by	Tend to be large with irregular margin	Smooth, even; may be small at surface with large subcutaneous	Usually well-defined; shape frequently is round but will conform	Irregular, blistering edge; purple-red, hemorrhagic, "angry

	trauma; punched out appearance		abscess, characterized by callus around the ulcer and undermined edges	form to cause of ulcer and may be irregular if large	"looking", intense surrounding erythema
Surrounding skin	Pale, blanched, gray, cool, thin; no hair on legs/toes; little or no edema; often accompanied by *livedo reticularis*	Pigmented, edematous, macerated; characterized by hyperpigmentation, dermatitis, and lipodermatosclerosis; often accompanied by *livedo reticularis*	Dry, thin, frequently callused	Nonblanchable erythema; clinical infection is indicated by redness, warmth, induration or hardness, swelling	Hyperemic; characterized by *atrophie blanche, livedo reticularis*, and *purpura*; often accompanied by hyperpigmentation
Pain	Often accompanied by severe pain at rest and numbness, parasthesias; pain often increases with leg elevation; sudden onset with acute, gradual onset with chronic; claudication relieved by rest; rest pain relieved by dependency; with total occlusion no position gives complete relief	Varies unpredictably; small but deep ulcers around malleoli are typically the most painful; pain often improves with leg elevation; deep muscle pain with acute deep vein thrombosis; mild pain post-phlebetically	No sensation, or constant or intermittent numbness or burning; neuropathic ulcers are almost always accompanied by numbness and parathesias	Varies	Often accompanied by severe pain at rest, numbness, parasthesias
Healing	Must have increased blood supply to heal	Epithelialization often fails despite good granulation; healing using compression may take 4 to 6 months, depending on degree of lipodermatosclerosis, and presence of cardiovascular disease	Patient must comply with diet, glucose regulation, exercise, and foot care/wear, aggressive revascularization and appropriate antibiotics may be needed for healing	Must eliminate/reduce pressure, shear, and friction and implement appropriate skin care for healing	Must control the inflammatory process and establish adequate circulation to heal

Table compiled from the following references:

Alvarez OM, Gilson G., Auletta MJ. Local aspects of diabetic foot ulcer care: assessment, dressings, and topical agents. In: Levin ME, O'Neal LW, Bowker JH, eds. *The Diabetic Foot*. 5th edition. St. Louis: Mosby Year-Book; 1993:259–281.

Falanga V, Eaglstein WH. *Leg and Foot Ulcers: A Clinician's Guide*. London: Martin Dunitz Limited; 1995.

Hess CT. *Nurse's Clinical Guide to Wound Care*. 2nd edition. Springhouse, PA: Springhouse Corporation; 1997:28–29.

Holloway GA. Arterial ulcers: assessment, classification and management. In: Krasner D, Kane D, eds. *Chronic Wound Care: A Clinical Source Book for Healthcare Professionals*. 2nd edition. Wayne, PA: Health Management Publications, Inc.; 1997:158–164.

Maklebust J, Sieggreen MY. *Pressure Ulcers: Guidelines for Prevention and Nursing Management*. 2nd edition. Springhouse, PA: Springhouse Corporation; 1996:30.

atrophie blanche—a scrinkage and whitening of the skin surrounding the wound

livedo reticularis—a netlike dermatitis

purpura—easy bruising

describes the pain as a burning discomfort most notably confined to the foot. Typically, it is aggravated by elevation of the extremity and relieved by dependency. Rest pain is part of a continuum in arterial vascular disease. It is classically preceded by claudication.

When atherosclerotic disease is present, the distal pulses are usually diminished. If there is an occlusion present the pulse distal to the occluded artery is barely palpable or absent. Bruits may be present and are indicative of turbulent blood flow due to a partially obstructed vessel. It can be heard through a stethoscope and is the loudest during systole.[58]

As described in Chapter 13 in relation to peripheral vascular disease, the pallor of the foot indicates the stage of ischemia. Elevated only slightly, the foot will blanch white and when the foot is dependent it turns a deep red to bluish-purple hue. Rubor is a cyanotic, purple discoloration of the foot on dependency. It appears because, with reduced inflow, blood in the capillary network is relatively stagnant and oxygen extraction is high. Hemoglobin becomes de-oxygenated and the capillary blood has an increasing blue hue. In arterial disease, this peripheral discoloration clears upon elevation. (Note: In venous insufficiency the discoloration does not resolve with positional changes.)

In an individual with chronic ischemia, the temperature of the skin of the lower extremity decreases and the foot is cool to touch.

Ulcerations due to ischemia are usually very painful and accompanied by ischemic rest pain as described above. The margin of the ulcer is sharply demarcated or punched out, and the base is devoid of healthy granulation tissue. The surrounding skin is pale and mottled, and signs of chronic ischemia are invariably present. Tissue necrosis first becomes apparent in the distal extremity or at an ulcer site. It stops at the point where blood supply is sufficient to maintain tissue viability.[58] The first stage of necrosis associated with ischemia is dry gangrene. This becomes wet gangrene if infection sets in.[12]

Moderately severe degrees of chronic ischemia produce muscle atrophy and loss of strength in the ischemic zone.[58] Frequently, there is associated decreased joint mobility; subsequent changes in foot structure and gait increase the likelihood that the individual will develop an ulcer.

Chronic ischemia is accompanied by loss of hair growth in the undernourished areas of the lower extremity. The skin becomes frail and transparent and appears dehydrated. Skin appearance is usually shiny and scaly. Poor circulation also leads to thickening of the nails, which become dense and brittle. Due to poor nutritional status, the lower extremity undergoes a pigment change which presents as a darkening (brownish) of the skin in the poorly nourished areas.[12] Simply looking at the foot will be sufficient for identifying significant arterial insufficiency.

Vascular Testing Screening for vascular insufficiency is accomplished through noninvasive vascular testing which may include segmental extremity pressure measures, toe pressures, Doppler waveform analysis, pulse volume recording (PVR), or transcutaneous measurement of oxygen (TCPO^2).

An easy way to screen for vascular insufficiency is to measure the resting systolic blood pressure at the brachial artery and at the posterior tibial or dorsalis pedis artery. The ankle/brachial index (ABI) is determined by dividing the pressure obtained at the ankle by the brachial arterial pressure. The ratings of the ratios[12] are as follows:

Ratio	Pathological Implication
> 1.2	Suspect vessel wall calcification, stiffness
1.0–1.2	Normal
0.3–0.9	Claudication
0.0–0.3	Ischemic rest pain, non-healing ulcers

The ABI is a helpful tool in substantiating the presence of pathology. A ratio greater than 1.2 indicates that the vessel walls are inelastic and stiff. Blood pressure measures are elevated and often the pulses are visible bounding on the surface without palpation. A ratio of 1.0 to 1.2 is considered normal. The lower ratios indicate poor tissue perfusion. A ratio of 0.3 to 0.9 is associated with claudication, which indicates ischemia on increasing oxygen demands during exercise and activity. Minimal variation between the ankle and the brachial blood pressures result in low ratios (0.0 to 0.3) and would result in ischemic rest pain. The lower the ABI the poorer the rate or possibility of healing.

In addition to the standard ABI, segmental pressures can be obtained at various levels on the leg for localization of occlusive disease. Segmental pressures are performed with the patient in supine and by applying the blood pressure cuff to various levels of the lower extremity (e.g., high thigh, lower thigh, upper calf, ankle). The brachial blood pressure is taken and the highest brachial pressure is used for the denominator. From this, a segmental pressure measurement is obtained. Gradients of more than 20 mmHg between sites are diagnostic of occlusive disease in the intervening segment.

Another helpful means of testing vascular status is toe pressure. Because of the common finding of inaccurately high ABIs in diabetic patients, measurements of toe pressure is particularly useful. In the normal patient, there is a gradient of 20 to 30 mmHg between the ankle and the toe, so a correction must be made when toe pressures are being used. Healing of distal wounds can be expected when toe pressures are greater than 40. Healing rarely, if ever, occurs if toe pressures are less than 20 mmHg, and pressures between 20 and 40 are at risk.

Every clinician has used or at least been exposed to the more commercial form of assessing vascular status, the Doppler waveform analysis. This measurement provides an analog signal that is proportional to the velocity of blood in the vessel being evaluated. The signal is displayed on a screen or recorded for latter analysis. The overall shape of the waveform reflects the status of the vessel proximal to the point studied. In the lower extremity, the normal velocity wave is triphasic, with reverse flow in early diastole. Proximal stenosis first eliminates the reverse flow; and with more severe lesions, there is bunting of the systolic upstroke and increasing flow during diastole.

Another valuable measurement of vascular status is the pulse volume recording (PVR). The blood entering a limb during systole causes an increase in the total volume in the extremity. During diastole, volume returns to normal. This phenomenon results in the pulse pressure oscillation seen with the sphygmomanometer while taking blood pressure. A variety of plethysmograph recorders have been devised using a mercury gauge, water displacement, and impedance. In the 1970s, the pulse volume recorder (PVR) was developed to diagnose peripheral vascular disease.[12] The diagnosis is based on the qualitative evaluation of the PVR waveform. Severe occlusive disease produces a flattened wave with a slow upstroke and downstroke. The absolute amplitude measurements are of limited value from patient-to-patient because substantial changes result from variations in cardiac output and vasomotor tone. Nonetheless, comparison of amplitudes from one side to the other in the same patient may be very useful for assessing unilateral disease. Like toe pressures, the PVR is particularly helpful when ABIs do not seem accurate.

The transcutaneous measurement of oxygen (TCPO^2) can be performed percutaneously using a special instrument. Determination of accurate TCPO^2 is fraught with many difficulties in the elderly, however, and requires an experienced clinician, patience, a warm room, and absence of vasoconstriction from other factors. TCPO^2 should be measured on the dorsum, not the plantar surface of the foot. Ideally, a reference value is obtained at the chest. Analogous to absolute toe pressures, a TCPO^2 value of 40 correlates with good healing. A TCPO^2 below 20 mmHg indicates poor or absent healing, whereas, a measurement between 20 and 40 mmHg places the individual in the at-risk zone.

Venous Ulcers

Venous ulcerations are caused by venous hypertension, valvular incompetence, and generally accompanied by a history of deep vein thrombosis. There are numerous theories that exist regarding the etiology of venous ulcers. The most predominant theories hypothesize that wounds develop because of the failure of the calf and foot muscle pump; that there is damage to the veins secondary to WBC adhesion to capillaries; that poor nutrition and waste removal results from pericapillary fibrin deposition; and the vein damage leading to ulceration is the result of previous trauma.[59] The veins in the lower extremities lose their tone and become distended allowing for the pooling of blood. Figure 14–7 demonstrates the appearance of the veins damaged by venous pathology. The veins can be damaged by gravitational stresses of prolonged standing, obesity, or pregnancy and become distended. Many veins in the lower extremities have semi-lunar valves that prevent back flow of blood during diastole (as demonstrated in the inset of Figure 14–7) and become frail and unable to prevent blood from being directed towards the heart. The blood pools in the lower extremities, resulting in lower extremity stasis, edema, and visible distention of the veins.

This chronic stasis and edema is the reason tissues become vulnerable to breakdown. Stale blood pools in the lower extremities, waste products are not removed, the provision of oxygen is low, and the toxic effects of accumulating metabolites results in breakdown in tissue health. Under the weight of the edematous lower extremities, the stress on the poorly nourished, vulnerable epithelium results in shallow skin breaks and ultimately venous stasis ulcers.

Characteristic of the venous ulceration is that it is not often painful, and that patients are usually comfortable with their legs elevated. If there is pain in the area of the ulcer, this discomfort is relieved by elevation. Acute deep vein thrombosis (DVT) is often accompanied by severe muscle pain and the arterial pulses are normal. Eczema or stasis dermatitis along with edema and dark pigmentation are generally associated with the presence of venous ulcers.[59] The location of these ulcers is usually on the medial aspect of the distal third of the lower extremity and behind the medial malleolus.[12] The so-called gaiter area around the ankle is rich in perforated veins. Venous ulcers occur predominantly in an ambulatory population, though in the elderly, they may be found in nonambulatory patients who spend most of their time in a chair or bed bound.

The appearance of lower extremities in patients with venous ulcers includes a firm (brawny) edema, reddish-brown discoloration with postphlebitic syndrome, evidence of healed ulcers, dilated and tortuous superficial veins, swollen limbs; increased warmth and erythema indicate acute DVT.

Wounds related to venous insufficiency are associated with lipdermatosclerosis. The characteristic appearance of a venous ulcers is that they are superficial wounds with periwound and leg hyperpigmentation, lipodermatosclerosis, and a moderate-to-high exudate. These ulcers usually have uneven edges, ruddy granulation tissue, and though they are superficial, associated with bleeding.

The clinical signs, etiologic classification, anatomic distribution, physiologic dysfunction tool (CEAP) is a helpful wound assessment scale for venous ulcers.[60] This scoring system of chronic venous dysfunction provides a base for comparison of limb condition and evaluation of treatment outcomes. This

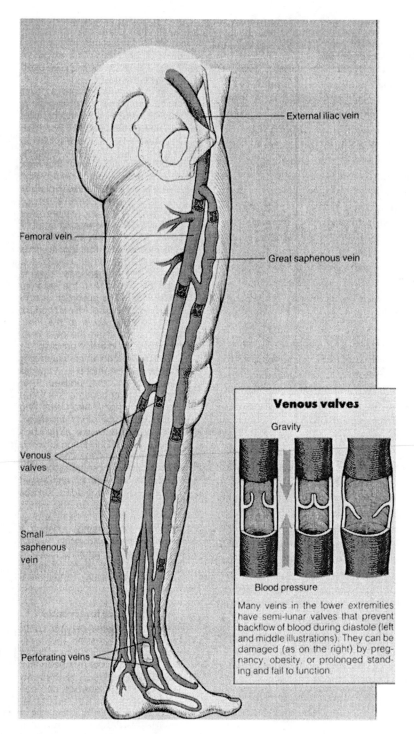

Figure 14–7. Anatomy of a problem: How venous stasis ulcers develop.

tool classifies clinical signs from Class 0 (no visible or palpable signs of venous disease) to Class 6 (skin changes with active ulceration). The remaining three elements each have three categories based on type of venous dysfunction, anatomic extent of the disease, and clinical signs/symptoms of venous dysfunction.[60] Although the grading of symptoms is subjective, the grading of signs is objective.

To rule out arterial disease it is important to carefully assess the patient's vascular status. This can be accomplished by manual palpation of pulses, Dop-

pler examination, and plethysmography.[12] Refer to Table 14–3 for differentiation between arterial and venous ulcers.

Treatment goals in the intervention with venous pathology and ulceration include increasing venous return, decreasing venous stasis and the associated edema, providing compression, and addressing the wound environment. Dressing and pharmacological intervention is dependent on the stage of the ulcer. Generally, in Stage I nonblanchable erythema of the skin with venous ulcers, the use of hydrogels and hydrocolloid dressings or semipermeable foam wafers are used to dress the area. Hydrocolloids and hydrogels are also used for Stage II and III ulcers, however, the dressings are changed more frequently. With the deeper wounds of Stage II and III, the use of calcium alginates is often used to enhance autolysis, especially in a draining wound. Stage IV ulcers are generally treated with hydrogel sheets and hydrogel-amorphous dressings when there is a low level of exudate. In the presence of high exudate wounds, calcium alginates are employed similar to Stage III.

Compression modalities such as stockings, elastic wraps, medicated wraps, and Unna boots are often used to control stasis and edema. Compression modalities vary in the amount of stretch and elasticity, both intrinsically and extrinsically, and in the manner in which they are applied. Correct application is extremely important to product effectiveness. Considerations for the prescription of compression method include the patient's daily activities and her or his tolerance of the chosen modality. Cost, especially in the elderly, is an important variable in choosing the appropriate modality. The presence of a wound and its status will also play a role in the selection of compression intervention.

In the elderly, compression stockings are difficult to apply and often improperly donned, creating constriction and frictional pressures. They may be expensive, especially the custom-fitted stockings. Compression stockings should not be used with arterial disease if there is infection present, weeping dermatitis, or friable tissue. It is also not advisable to use stockings when a wound is present as they are usually non-absorptive of exudates and do not address the skin status.

Elastic wraps are easy to apply, inexpensive, and available at a local pharmacy. Often, these are compression modalities that, if properly applied, accommodate the older person's need for compression in a more user-friendly manner. The same contraindications apply to ace wraps as the stockings. They should not be used with arterial disease, severe infection, weeping dermatitis, or friable tissue. One difficulty encountered is the problem of keeping elastic wraps in place. If improperly applied, they may also result in uneven compression. They tend to lose elasticity quickly and require frequent replacing.

Medicated elastic wraps and Unna boots are often used as they protect and medicate the wound. The cost of these devices is moderate.

Pneumatic compression devices are sometimes applied to decrease lower extremity edema. With sequential cuff filling, these devices address the underlying pathology. Pneumatic pumps do not eliminate the need for compression stockings or elastic wraps and should be avoided in the presence of CHF and severe arterial disease.

Wound dressings provide an optimal environment for wound repair, but do not address the problem of increased venous return. They are used to promote re-epithelialization and granulation when the underlying pathophysiology has been treated. Occlusive compression dressings, bandages, wraps, and pneumatic sequential compression devices should not be used in the presence of clinical signs of infection, cellulitis, or severe arterial disease.

Prevention interventions are extremely important. Venous ulcers may reoccur within days after healing if venous disease is neglected after wound closure. Wound closure does not signify resolution of the patient's primary vascular problem. Continued use of compression therapy, particularly stockings and pneumatic compression devices, is helpful for ulcer prophylaxis.

Diabetic Ulcers

Ulceration in the foot in diabetic patients is the most common location and causes serious disability and considerable consumption of scarce resources. The high morbidity and mortality rates associated with diabetic ulcers is attributed to the pathophysiology of the disease and inadequate knowledge of treatment principles for these ulcers.[12] Accurate identification of those patients at particular risk means that ulcers could be prevented. It is important to understand those factors in the diabetic elder that cause ulceration. Figure 14–8 provides a schematic representation of the probable interaction between major factors responsible for diabetic foot ulcerations.

As Figure 14–8 depicts, the pathology of foot ulceration is a multifaceted combination of contributory factors including neuropathy, abnormal blood flow, mechanical stresses, and a suppressed immune system response to infection.

Vascular disease found in diabetics is significantly different from that in nondiabetic patients. Diabetic vascular disease occurs at a younger age and is more accelerated. Occlusion usually involves the multisegmental small vessels (microvascular). Large vessel occlusion is rare.[61]

The classical symptom of arterial circulation impairment, intermittent claudication, occurs more commonly in diabetics compared with nondiabetic individuals.[62,63] In addition to the effects of diabetes, all the usual risk factors for atheroma such as smoking, hypercholesterolemia, and hypertension are as relevant in diabetics as in nondiabetics, and these factors will add to the risk of developing lower limb ischemia and consequent ulceration.

In addition to large vessel atheroma, degenerative arterial changes are also found more distally in diabetes.[62] In the evaluative process, changes similar to those discussed under the section on arterial ulcers will be observed. Care must be taken not to confuse the nocturnal foot pains of ischemia with pain due to peripheral neuropathy. The former is usually associated with absent peripheral pulses and cold feet, while the latter presents with bounding pulses and a warm foot. Absent peripheral pulses, cold peripheries (especially in a warm environment) and

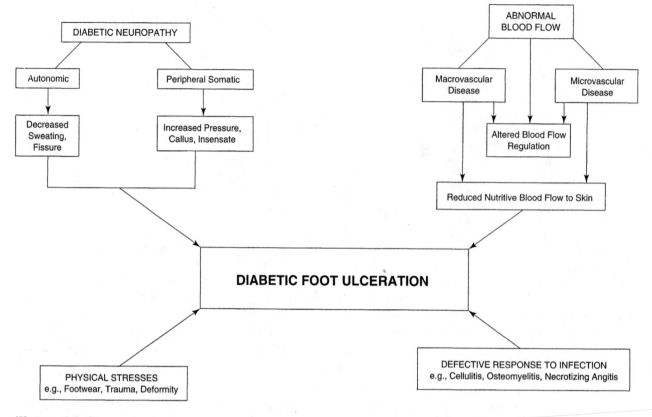

Figure 14–8. Probable interaction between the major risk factors responsible for diabetic foot ulceration.

slow capillary return are all indicative of peripheral vascular disease and susceptibility to ischemic ulceration. Noninvasive measurement of blood pressure in the peripheral arteries using a Doppler ultrasound provides an objective measurement that is more sensitive to peripheral circulatory changes and not masked by edema. The most commonly used measurement in physical therapy is the ratio of ankle to brachial supine systolic blood pressure (Ankle Pressure Index–API), a value of greater than 0.9 being normal. As long as there is not extensive peripheral vascular calcification, which prevents arterial compression by the sphygmomanometer cuff, a reduced API is a reliable guide to impaired circulation.

Macroangiopathy is associated with the arterial/venous involvement associated with poor peripheral circulation. Microangiopathy comprising capillary occlusion and nutrition to the extremities is associated with ulceration in the diabetic. Abnormal autoregulation of skin blood flow results in poor perfusion of the tissue and nutritional breakdown of the sensory tissues creating the classic neuropathy. Calcification of the vascular walls is a well-recognized radiological feature in diabetes. It is thought to be related to sympathetic denervation of the blood vessels. Vascular calcification influences blood pressure recordings.[64]

In diabetic individuals, blood flow velocity is increased, possibly owing to arteriovenous shunting. Reduced peripheral perfusion of distal tissues is pre-

sumed to result. Clinically, microvascular involvement presents with insensate feet that are warm to touch with distension in the dorsal foot and lower calf veins. Generally an elevated venous pressure can be demonstrated by the height to which the leg needs to be elevated before the veins collapse. Peripheral pulses are bounding, ankle pressure index is high, and venous pO_2 in the dorsal foot veins is high.[65,66]

On evaluation, the typical appearance of the lower extremity with circulatory involvement includes shiny skin, digital redness, dependent rubor, loss of hair growth, delayed superficial venous plexus filling time, and subcutaneous fat atrophy. These are important and classic features that require documentation on initial assessment of the elderly diabetic patient.

Neuropathy generally affects the motor, sensory, and autonomic nerves of the leg and often presents as a stocking-like parasthesia of the foot. Loss of sensation in the diabetic foot results in absence of sensitivity to pain, temperature, and pressure. When trauma occurs, the patient is unaware of tissue damage, inflammation, and infection until an ulcer becomes evident. Neurotrophic ulceration in the feet of patients with peripheral neuropathy but no evidence of occlusive peripheral vascular disease is a familiar problem in diabetes. The primary lesion is often complicated by secondary infection.

Early microvascular and nutritional deficits in peripheral somatic neuropathy in diabetic patients presents with complaints of lancinating, stabbing, or burning pains or paresthesia. Such symptoms are very uncommon in patients with neurotrophic foot ulceration due to the sensory loss. On comparative clinical examination stocking-like peripheral sensory loss to pinprick, cold/warm, light touch, and vibration is extensive, and loss of tendon reflexes is greater in patients with neurotrophic ulceration than those with painful early symptoms of neuropathy.[61] Often there is clawing of the toes, indicating motor denervation of the intrinsic foot muscles which releases an unopposed action of the long extensor tendons. On EMG studies in diabetics, evoked nerve action potentials are exceptionally attenuated implying a much greater large fiber axonal loss.[61]

A striking feature of diabetic symmetrical sensory polyneuropathy is the concurrent involvement of autonomic nerves. It has been suggested that autonomic neuropathy may be the principle cause of neurotrophic ulceration.[62,63,64] The diabetic foot rarely sweats suggesting autonomic involvement.

Increased mechanical stresses in the presence of neuropathy places the foot at great risk for breakdown.[67,68] In clinical practice it is often obvious that pressure from inappropriate footwear greatly increases the susceptibility of ulceration. Additionally, the characteristic clawed toe deformity, secondary to motor denervation, exposes the metatarsal heads and toes to increased pressure and trauma.[68] Charcot foot deformity or a high medial plantar arch are important endogenous factors causing areas of increased pressure. Extensive callus formation occurs at sites of increased pressure and intensifies the forces on the subcutaneous tissues.[68] Plantar ulcers frequently result from pressure points, particularly calluses. Predominant areas of occurrence are submetatarsals, distal digits, medial 5th, 2nd metatarsal head, and 1st metatarsophalangeal joint.

Whatever the cause of the initial skin break, infection almost invariably exploits the situation and rapidly becomes an integral component of the clinical lesion. The type (e.g., *Staphylococcus aureus, Streptococcus,* anaerobic organisms) and severity (e.g., superficial cellulitis, osteomyelitis, deep abscess, or necrotizing angiitis) of the associated infection is a major determinant of outcome (e.g., healing, chronicity, gangrene).

There is an increased susceptibility to infection in patients with diabetes. It has been found that there is an impairment in neutrophil function in diabetes which is thought to comprise defective vascular adherence/escape and to defective phagocytosis/killing. Defective lectin receptors on macrophages have also been described.[69] All of these abnormalities are related to the prevailing level of hyperglycemia, so that any diabetic patient with poor glycemic control is at greater risk for infection. Infection is also more probable if foot hygiene is poor.

The characteristic presentation of a diabetic foot ulceration[12] includes:

- Round, punched-out lesion with elevated rim
- Periwound hyperkeratosis
- Surrounding hyperkeratosis and anhydrosis
- Eschar and necrotic debris in ulcer base uncommon (unless accompanied by vascular disease or infection)
- Low to moderate drainage (unless infected)

Evaluation of the diabetic patient with ulceration includes the diabetic status, nutritional status, vascular status of affected extremity, neurological status, ulcer status, and footwear. The ulcer evaluation includes the parameters described above: size, precise anatomical location, stage of ulcer (Wagner's Scale is more commonly used in diabetics as it incorporates the level of infection of a wound),[49] appearance of ulcer base, description of amount and type of exudate, periwound appearance, and documentation of exploration for sinus tracts, fistulas, and bone exposure. In addition to the Wagner Scale,[49] the Diabetic Wound Classification System[70] is a tool that grades wound status. This tool, developed at the University of Texas, is based on wound grade and stage to categorize foot wounds in diabetics. Depth is graded 0 (pre- or postulcerative lesion) through grade III (wound is penetrating to bone or joint). Within each grade there are four stages (A through D) that take into account infection and peripheral vascular disease.[70]

Treatment of the diabetic ulceration includes pressure relief, debridement, attention to the types of dressings used, total contact casting, treatment of infection, and steps taken toward prevention of future skin breakdown once the ulcer is healed.[71]

Ideal pressure relief for a foot ulcer is no weight bearing at all and bedrest. However, in the elderly who are already at greater risk for the complications associated with inactivity (see Chapter 9), it is crucial that ADL and exercise be incorporated into the daily treatment plan.[72,73] In an ambulatory patient, footwear should be modified to relieve pressure on the ulcer and maintain ambulation. Felt or high-density foam inserts, moldable plastazote or other soft insoles, soft-soled healing sandals or shoes or modified shoes may be of benefit. Use of walking aids such as crutches or walkers helps to further decrease trauma to the ulcer during weight-bearing activities. A total contact cast is helpful, not only in providing the best mode of intervention for pressure relief for ambulation, but also in providing an ideal healing environment for the wound.[71] The authors recommend fabrication of a total contact cast and subsequent bifurcation to provide a removable splint.[74] This redistributes the forces and protects the wound during weight-bearing activities and allows the wound to be more closely monitored for stages of healing.

Most diabetic ulcers are surrounded by a thick rim of keratinized tissue. Untreated, this will impede healing.[73] Surgical debridement should extend through the callus and expose underlying pink viable tissue. All necrotic tissue needs to be debrided from the wound. Once the wound is debrided surgically, physical therapy and nursing care should maintain the debridement of the wound as needed. Sharp debridement is usually the most effective and efficient form of debridement, but should be done by an experienced clinician. Eschar and fibrotic debris may be removed by enzymatic debriding agents (when minimal debris is present) or by dressings that will be described subsequently. Hydrotherapy (whirlpool) is used for brief periods to soften and loosen eschar and debris and cleanse the wound, however, in the elderly diabetic patient, it is not recommended.

The majority of diabetic ulcers occur on weight-bearing surfaces making it difficult for dressings such as hydrocolloids, hydrogel sheets, and thin film dressings to stay in place. They may be used on non–weight-bearing wounds with minimal drainage. Silver sulfadizine and gauze have been found to be effective in reducing bacterial colonization on all stages of low exudate diabetic ulcers—on both weight-bearing and non– weight-bearing surfaces.[73]

As mentioned before, total contact casting is a below-the-knee cast that limits excessive foot motion and redistributes the body's weight over the entire foot.[71,74] Patient compliance is improved because ambulation is permitted. Casts are padded over all bony prominences to prevent further tissue injury and total relief of pressure is provided surrounding and over the wound. Casts are changed on a seven- to fourteen-day protocol to assess wound status. Often, while contained in the cast, nature does its own healing so that when the cast and dressings are removed, autolysis has occurred. Despite maintenance in a closed environment, the wound often looks healthier after total contact casting then it did when the casting was originally done. Appropriate training from individuals experienced with this technique is mandatory prior to applying contact casts, as these are very different from standard plaster casts. Casts are generally discontinued when re-epithelialization occurs.[71,74]

One of the most common complications of diabetic ulcers is bacterial infection. The presence of hyperglycemia, as mentioned, greatly increases the risk for infection.[69] Because of this, the assessment and evaluative processes become ever more important. Early diagnosis and treatment will reduce the threat of sepsis and limb loss. However, early detection is difficult. The typical symptoms of infection, pain, erythema, and increased skin temperature may be masked by peripheral vascular disease, microvascular pathology, and neuropathy. In fact, the appearance of the wound and surrounding tissues may not verify the presence of infection at all. Hyperglycemia over a prolonged period may actually be the first indicator of infection.[69] Cultures for polymicrobial organisms will also assist in confirming the presence of bacteria.

Complications, such as progressive cellulitis, unresponsiveness to oral antibiotics, systemic signs of infection, abscess formation and osteomyelitis require aggressive use of IV antibiotics and hospitalization. Osteomyelitis may be difficult to differentiate from diabetic osteopathy and chronic inflammation with either x-ray or bone scan. A bone biopsy is the only definitive diagnostic tool for establishing the presence of osteomyelitis. Surgical debridement of the infected bone followed by IV antibiotics is often required to eradicate the infection.[12] Another complication requiring surgery is an infected diabetic foot ulcer compromised by gangrene.

To summarize, treatment of the diabetic ulcer consists of local wound care and the use of systemic broad-spectrum antibiotics. Nonviable tissue is debrided and the wound and surrounding tissue are protected; once the ulcer is healed, preventive intervention is paramount. Prevention incorporates instruction on daily foot care and appropriate footwear, daily inspection of feet and foot hygiene, regular monitoring of glucose levels and insulin administration, and regularly scheduled checkups with a health care professional.

Pressure Ulcers

The destructive process of epithelial tissue-related ischemia, immobility, inactivity, and poor nutrition can lead to the development of a pressure ulcer. In addition, frictional and shear forces, and moisture damage to the skin contribute to the breakdown of integumentary tissues. An individual's inability to interpret discomfort related to chronic pressure and pathologies that lead to insensate conditions may also add to the risk of developing a pressure ulcer.[75–77]

In an older population prevention is key. Based on the evaluative information already discussed, the risk for developing a pressure ulcer should be determined. The ability to predict the potential for skin breakdown may be the best means of preventing ulceration from occurring. All pressure ulcers are preventable if attention is directed to insensate areas, malnutrition, skin fragility, and the physical or cognitive inability to accomplish pressure relief without guidance or assistance.

Upon first encounter with an elderly patient, whether it be in the home or in a health care setting, screening to determine risk for pressure ulcers should be done. There are several valuable risk assessment tools which have been proved reliable and valid for the prevention of pressure ulcers. The tools utilized with the geriatric patient population are the Braden scale, the Norton tool, the Knoll Assessment Scale, or the Gosnell Scale. The selection of tools is primarily based on the setting of care and the tool that is used by various wound care teams in a given setting.

The Braden scale[78] was developed for an acute-care setting. It is also a useful tool in both the long-term care and home settings. As a result of its versatility, it is the tool this author most frequently utilizes. The Braden scale assesses six risk factor and scores each risk on a scale of 1 to 4 (worst to best scenario). The numerical score provides an objective means of grading risk.

The Norton tool[79] has been found reliable and valid in elderly patients with chronic wounds. This risk assessment tool provides a numerical score based on five areas of risk in patients with a history of long-standing integumentary problems.

Developed in an acute care setting, the Knoll Assessment Scale[80] addresses variables specific to that care environment (e.g., surgical status, medical complexity, hydration, polypharmacy). This tool is valid and reliable and widely used. The scale has been modified by Aronovitch and co-workers[81] to identify the common elements that require the employment of specialized pressure relief surfaces for pressure reduction.

Last, the Gosnell scale[82] was developed specifically for long-term care geriatric patients. The scale assesses five risk factors and scores these on a best to worst rating scale. It goes a step beyond other tools by providing information on vital signs, skin appearance, fluid intake and output, interventions, and medications. Although useful, this scale has not yet been validated.

Wound assessment in pressure wounds is described above. The National Pressure Ulcer Advisory Panel (NPUAP) staging system, which is based on the Shea staging system originally published in 1975,[83] is pressure-ulcer specific. Ulcers are staged by describing the extent of tissue damage, from I (nonblanchable erythema) to IV (extending through the deep fascia into underlying anatomic structures). Another wound assessment tool which is very helpful is the Sessing Scale.[84] This tool is a seven-point observational scale anchored by verbal descriptions of wound healing. This instrument measures an important domain of healing independent of wound size or depth. The Sessing Scale describes granulation tissue, infection, necrosis, and eschar. It is not designed to measure healing but to predict healing.[84]

Early intervention is also key. If the pressure ulcer is detected and treated in early stages (Stages I OR II) it will take less time to heal and creates fewer, if any, systemic problems. Early intervention includes adequate pressure reduction with frequent reposition and specialized pressure relief surfaces as warranted.[12] Attention to nutritional status and hydration, perineal care if the individual is incontinent, and close monitoring for signs of skin pressure (e.g., redness that doesn't immediately blanch with pressure relief) are important care principles.[75,77] If areas of redness are noted, protective devices such as heel lifts or padding at bony prominences will help in preventing skin breaks and resulting in ulceration.[12]

When a pressure ulcer does occur it is important to address the treatment areas of pressure relief, debridement, a moist wound healing environment, and correction of factors that may be contributing to pressure ulcers (e.g., incontinence, malnutrition).

One of the key areas in wound care management is the ability to remove the source of irritation or pressure to allow normal healing to occur. The areas most likely to break down are those parts of the body where there is little fat between the skin and bone, such as the back of the head, rim of the ears, shoulder blades, spine, coccyx, sacrum, greater trochanter, medial and lateral malleolus, and heels.

Treatment principles inherent in pressure relief include the following:

- Determine what may be the cause of breakdown
  - Pressure over a bony prominence
  - Improper fitting shoes, brace
  - Friction, shearing
  - Immobility
- Incorporate pressure-reducing techniques
  - Inspect skin frequently for signs of redness. Redness normally disappears within 15 minutes after removing pressure from uninjured skin
  - Maintain clean skin and attempt to prevent maceration from moist environments
  - Avoid wrinkles in sheets of bed, chair cushion, and clothing (consider seams of socks and clothing)
  - Avoid shearing forces when transferring or moving in bed (using a draw sheet may be recommended)
  - Bedridden patients should be repositioned at least every two hours
  - Wheelchair patients should perform weight shift every thirty minutes (tilt chair back, lateral and forward weight shift, wheelchair push-up)
  - Use positioning and pressure-reducing devices to avoid pressure on wound as warranted
- Patient instruction if appropriate
  - Skin care and self-inspection techniques
  - Weight-shifting techniques
  - Instruction for patients with sensory loss
    - Proper shoe gear
    - Inspect shoes prior to donning (e.g., shake out sand or other debris that may be in shoes)
    - Never walk barefoot
    - Always test bath water temperature before taking bath or shower
    - Check for wrinkles in socks and clothing
- Once wound is healed
  - Begin subjecting healed area to pressure gradually, checking for signs of pressure and with frequent pressure relief periods
  - Maintain functional scar mobility
- Protect healthy tissue to prevent development of wounds
  - Use a screening tool to identify those who are at risk for development of a pressure sore or other type of wound
  - Educate patient and staff
  - Use position and pressure-reducing devices to prevent pressure ulcer development

When a wound has necrotic tissue, this must be debrided in order to provide a better environment for wound healing and contraction. Debridement can be accomplished by (1) sharp debridement down to the level of viable tissue, (2) debridement through the use of transparent adhesive or hydrocolloid water dressings that adhere to the necrotic tissue and promote autolysis in superficial wounds, or (3) calcium alginates, exudate-absorptive dressings and amorphous hydrogels which absorb necrotic tissue and promote autolysis, especially in dry and low exudate wounds.[12]

For cleansing a wound the use of normal saline or a non-ionic surfactant wound cleanser to remove wound debris and dressing material residue is often employed.[12] In the elderly, as in any age patient with a wound, harsh disinfecting agents that are cytotoxic to granulation tissue should not be used in wound care.

Intervention will be dependent on the stage of the wound. Any lesion with black eschar, soft or hard, should not be staged until the eschar has been debrided free from the wound base. Based on the patient's history and risk factors, treatment strategies incorporate debridement as well as the use of modalities and dressings.

In a stage I pressure ulcer, the objective of treatment is to prevent skin breakdown. This can be accomplished by relieving pressure (e.g., elevating heels off the bed, frequent turning, use of pressure-relieving splints or a special support surface). Elderly bedbound patients who are unable to move and roll must have a mattress for off-loading pressure points evenly. At this stage of ulcer development, transparent film dressing is often used as a protective measure to prevent progression of tissue breakdown beyond stage I.[2,6] There are sprays and gels available that protect and cover the skin, and some clinicians use semipermeable foam in the treatment of stage I ulcers.

Stage II ulcers involve the loss of epidermis and dermis due to friction or pressure. Blister development occurs and there is a break in the tissue. The blister requires debridement and the wound needs to be kept moist to promote healing. The objective of treatment in a stage II ulcer is to cover and hydrate and create a moist environment for healing. Either transparent film, hydrogel, antibiotic, absorption-type, or hydrocolloid dressings are used. In addition to covering, hydrating, and protecting the wound, dressing are chosen for absorption of exudates and insulation. High galvanic electrical stimulation may be employed, especially in the presence of infection. Attention to nutrition is important.

The objectives of treatment of a stage III ulcer are the same as in stage I and II. In addition, prevention of infection is paramount with a stage III ulcer. A primary goal in treatment is to promote granulation and contraction of epithelial tissue. This can be accomplished through the use of modalities, such as high galvanic electrical stimulation or ultrasound, and through the use of dressings. Hydrogel, absorption type, antibiotic, or hydrocolloid dressings, if drainage is low to moderate, are most effective to maintain a moist environment and enhance healing.

The primary goals in the treatment of stage IV ulcerations are to promote granulation and obliterate dead pressure ulcer space. Topical antibiotics, hydrogels, and absorptive type dressing are used to decrease and prevent infection and promote autolysis.

Sometimes saline-soaked, fluffed gauze dressings applied in wet to damp fashion are used to pack a wound and keep it moist. This approach is used in stage II to stage IV wounds. In the elderly, gauze impregnated with silver sulfadiazine may be used in stage III and stage IV ulcers to help decrease the presence of bacteria.

Vasculitic Ulcers

Evaluation and treatment of vasculitic ulcers is the same as other types of wounds. The difference is the etiology of the wound. These types of wounds are due to vasculitis, a term that applies to a diverse group of diseases characterized by inflammation in blood vessel walls. Most of these pathologies are autoimmune diseases—rheumatoid arthritis, systemic lupus erythematosus, systemic sclerosis, tuberculosis, sarcoidosis, and multiple organ dysfunction syndrome—which are complicated by inflammatory vascular conditions. Vasculitic lesions are more frequently found in patients with connective tissue disorders and in patients whose immune system is suppressed (HIV and AIDs).[85] Patients whose immune system has been compromised by medical interventions, such as cancer patients undergoing chemotherapy, are also prone to inflammatory vasculitis, compromised nutritional status, and resultant skin ulcerations.[86]

Blood vessels of various sizes in different parts of the body may be affected causing a wide spectrum of clinical manifestations. The inflammation of the vessels often causes narrowing or occlusion of the vessel lumen and produces ischemia of the tissues. The inflammation may weaken the vessel wall, resulting in aneurysm or rupture with subsequent hemorrhage into the tissues which impedes nutrient and oxygen exchange. These two problems are most commonly associated with skin breakdown and vasculitic ulceration.

As a consequence, evaluation requires assessment of the medical condition and patient stability, as well as the determination of systemic involvement of disease manifestations. The presence of an ulceration may be only a small reflection of widespread involvement. Major symptoms of small blood vessel vasculitis are skin lesions that are accompanied by fever, malaise, and myalgia.[86] Intervention strategies must take into consideration that within the context of both wound healing and autoimmunity/immune suppression, molecular mechanisms of age-related changes (described in Chapter 2) affect an organism's ability to repair damaged cells and tissues. This impacts on the rate of healing. Vasculitic ulcers often turn out to be chronic, non-healing ulcers. They are more likely to become infected because of the compromised vascular and immune systems. It is important that vasculitic conditions be identified early so that preventive interventions can be employed to eliminate the need for wound care.

OTHER TYPES OF WOUNDS

Though the most frequently encountered types of wounds encountered in an older population are pressure, arterial and venous, and diabetic ulcers, other types of wounds may occur as well. These wounds include extravasation sites with necrotic tissue, abrasions and skin tears, dehisced surgical wounds, gastrointestinal and gerito-urinary fistulas, and burns from radiation therapy or other causes. This section of the chapter will deal primarily with the treatments approaches utilized in the elderly for care of these wounds.

Extravasation Sites

An extravasation site is a lesion that involves a bleed from a vessel into the surrounding tissues causing a hematoma. An accumulation of blood which becomes dense and stone-like can constrict blood supply to the area and cause breakdown of the tissues surrounding it, often resulting in death of the tissue.[12] The goal of treatment is the removal of the necrotic tissue and steps to facilitate healing. Autolysis, the spontaneous disintegration of necrotic tissue by the action of the patient's own enzymes, is encouraged through the application of transparent nonadhesive dressings or thin transparent hydrocolloid wafer until the necrotic tissue has been eliminated or the wound fluid leaks out. This approach decreases the trauma typically caused by debridement of the necrotic tissues with a sharp instrument. Once the dead tissue has dissipated, the wound can be cleansed and monitored for granulation and re-epithelialization.

Abrasions And Skin Tears

Abrasions and skin tears are very common in an older population. Due to the tissue-like texture of the skin, dehydration, and poor nutritional condition, even a seemingly minor trauma can result in an abrasion or skin tear.[12] The primary goal of treatment is to protect the area from further damage. Transparent nonadhesive dressings, thin transparent hydrocolloid, or semipermeable foam dressings are helpful in facilitating the drainage of fluids from the wounds and for re-epithelialization.

It is important that ADLs be evaluated and that situations that may place an elderly individual at risk for skin tears or abrasions be minimized.

Dehisced Surgical Wounds

Older patients, due to the fragility of the integumentary tissues, may experience the separation of all the layers of an incision or wound.[12] Treatment goals will include the repair, debridement, and healing of the dehisced lesion. For exuding wounds, calcium alginate dressing are often recommended as these products facilitate wound drainage. Once the surgical wound has stopped draining, a hydrocolloid or hydrogel wafer dressing (preferably transparent) or an amorphous hydrogel dressing is recommended for application to the affected area.

The biomechanical components of ADL need to be evaluated in order to prevent the surgical wound from splitting again. Assistive devices such as reaching tools may be helpful in reducing stress to the surgical site.

GI and GU Fistulas

Fistulas may occur from weakening of the gastrointestinal tract, which may result in communication with the external environment creating a wound, or they may be the result of a surgical procedure, such as the implantation of a feeding tube or a colostomy. The importance of maintaining a clean wound bed is very important in a gastrointestinal (GI) or genito-urinary (GU) fistula.[12] Daily evacuation and collecting of wound drainage is usually accomplished through suctioning. Saline or a non ionic surfactant wound cleanser is used to remove debris in the affected area. The most commonly used dressing is the application of a sealant over all intact skin, which is then covered by a transparent adhesive dressing, and finally, gauze is applied to the immediate fistulated area.

Radiation Burns

Burns resulting from radiation therapy need to be treated to prevent infection and extensive tissue damage.[12] Pain control is accomplished by keeping the wound moist. The application of amorphous hydrogels to exuding wounds covered by nonadherent dressings is most frequently used. It is important not to use dressings that adhere to the wound or surrounding radiation-damaged skin as this may result in further tissue trauma. Activated charcoal dressings or gauze soaked with chlorophyllin copper complex solution are also used to control odor as well as promote healing. For lightly draining wounds, hydrocolloid or hydrogel wafer dressings, semipermeable foam dressings or nonadherent dressings are used. For a large wound with profuse drainage, an ostomy-type pouch with a drainage collector may be employed.[87,88,89]

Burns

Due to a loss in sensation resulting from many pathologies, poor visual acuity, diminished temperature sensation, and decreased cognitive capabilities, elders are at a much higher risk of burns due to accidents (e.g., touching a hot surface, scalding from bath water that is too hot). The principle of classifying a wound in order to treat it properly extends to understanding the mechanics of burn care and different types of burns. The goals of acute burn wound management are the same as those of managing any wound.[87] All wounds heal differently depending on the depth of the injury. Wounds that extend only into the epidermis or dermis can heal by tissue regeneration. Wounds that extend more deeply through the dermis heal by scar formation and contraction, because structures such as subcutaneous tissue, glands, and hair follicles are unable to regenerate.[88,89]

Burns also heal by different mechanisms depending on depth. Partial-thickness burns (which may involve the entire epidermis but still have intact hair follicles and sweat glands) will experience revascularization within a short period of time following the burn (one to two weeks).[88] However, full-thickness burns (which extend through the entire thickness of the skin with possible involvement of connective tissue, muscle, or bone) experience occlusion of the arterial vascular supply, with revascularization delayed for several weeks, and are incapable of healing by self-regeneration (requiring grafting). Table 14–4 provides a summarization of the characteristics of wounds causes by burns and the variations in healing expected from each type of wound.[87–89]

With burns in the elderly, like with any burn victim, emphasis needs to be placed on hydration, nutrition, and the maintenance of mobility. Pain is often a limiting factor in accomplishing activities of daily living. Occupational therapy often will provide splinting to maintain proper joint and extremity alignment, as well as determining the assistive devices that may facilitate independence while allowing for a decrease in pain experienced during those activities.

WOUND MANAGEMENT

Because advanced age is associated with delayed wound healing and repair, prevention remains the cornerstone of wound care in the older population. Healing is complicated by the increased prevalence in older patients of conditions that predispose them to pressure ulcers, such as malnutrition, immobility, and systemic disease. If preventive measures fail, there are treatments available to minimize surface contact at pressure points and therapeutic agents to promote wound healing.[2] These treatment approaches include physical modalities, debridement, incontinence care, topical dressings that create an optimal healing environment, specially designed support surfaces, growth factor topicals, and nutritional interventions that can increase the proliferation, migration, and protein biosynthesis of cells in the wound bed.

Electrical Stimulation

Numerous research articles are available on the effects and benefits of electrical stimulation on healing. Electrical stimulation used as an adjunct to other interventions has been found to be effective.[90,91,9293] The use of electrical stimulation, particularly high galvanic, is the modality of choice in elderly with chronic wounds.[90,91,93]

Electrical stimulation works by enhancing the body's bioelectric system on a cellular level. When the skin is wounded, it conducts a current generated between the surface skin (a negative current) and the inner tissues (a positive current) in an attempt to attract healing cells, which are responsible for releasing growth factors that are involved in the process of collagen synthesis.[92] This process is referred to as the "current of injury," and continues until the injury has healed.

A moist environment is required for the body's bioelectrical system to function properly. There must be a medium to conduct "natural" current. If the wound is dry then that medium is lost. Lack of current, or current disruption, is suspected to be one of the reasons why chronic wounds do not heal without outside stimulus to jump-start the healing process. The rationale for applying electrical stimulation is that it mimics the natural current and initiates or accelerates the wound-healing process.[90,91,92]

The wound-healing process, which includes the inflammation, proliferation, epithelialization, and remodeling phases, is enhanced with electrical stimulation. Electrical stimulation facilitates these steps via an electrical current which transfers energy to a wound through the electrodes.[90,91,92] One electrode is placed on the external skin a distance away from the wound and the other in the wound bed to assist the flow of current for healing.

Although there are many waveforms available for electrotherapy, high voltage (galvanic) electrical stimulation, the most commonly used current for wound healing, is a monophasic twin-peaked high voltage pulsed current that gives the cells an interrupted type of stimulus at a high frequency, and causes the body to respond to the stimulation by laying down collagen.[93] High galvanic stimulation also allows for the control of the polarity and variation in pulse rates, which are both important to the healing process.[90,91]

As uninjured skin has a negative potential which shifts to positive when the skin is injured, the use of polarization (e.g. placing the negative lead over the wound) increases the rate of epithelialization.[93] There is strong evidence that a negative polarity increases protein, DNA, and collagen synthesis and fibroblast proliferation. A theoretical effect of high voltage current is that it accelerates soft tissue healing by elevating tissue temperature and stimulating cellular metabolism.[90,91,92] It also increases cutaneous circulation, which promotes wound healing and improves the oxygen and nutritional exchange. It cannot be assumed that high galvanic electrical stimulation causes similar wound reactions as continuous low voltage direct current. Low volt current has bactericidal and sclerosing effects at the cathode (negative

TABLE 14-4.   CHARACTERISTICS OF WOUNDS CAUSES BY BURNS AND THE VARIATIONS IN HEALING.

Type of Burn:	Superficial	Superficial Partial-Thickness	Deep Partial-Thickness	Full-Thickness	Subdermal
Characteristics					
Predisposing Factors/ Cause	Sunburn, ultraviolet exposure, minor flash	Brief exposure to flash flame, liquid spills; brief exposure to dilute chemicals	Hot liquids or solids; flash flame, direct flame; intense radiant energy, chemicals	Prolonged contact with flames, hot liquids, steam, chemicals, high voltage electrical current	Electrical injury
Location and depth	Only minimal epithelial (epidermis) damage	Damage to epidermis, with minimal to dermis	Entire epidermis and more dermal involvement than superficial partial-thickness burn (epidermis, papillary dermis, and reticular dermis); intact hair follicles and sweat glands	Entire thickness of skin through reticular dermis (epidermis, dermis, epidermal appendages, portion of subcutaneous fat; possible involvement of connective tissue, muscle, or bone)	Damage extends beneath dermis to subcutaneous tissue
Wound bed and Wound appearance	Red or pink	Moist, bright pink or red color; large, intact blisters; brisk capillary refill when skin is blanched	Mix of red and waxy white; sluggish capillary return when skin is blanched	Mosaic of colors, including black, tan, red, white, pale yellow, brown; reddened area stays red when pressure is applied	Mummified and devitalized appearance
Exudate/drainage	Dry or with small blisters	Large amounts of exudate when blisters rupture or are removed	May have large amounts of exudate	Tissue is leathery, rigid, and dry	Dry
Swelling and Capillary refilling	Some swelling, particularly if eyes are involved	Brisk capillary refill when skin is blanched	Massive swelling can cause problems with range of motion; slow, sluggish capillary return when skin is blanched	Swelling below eschar but not in area of eschar; reddened areas stay red when pressure is applied; poor circulation to distal area of full-thickness injury	Little swelling; thrombosed blood vessels
Pain	Delayed pain	Extremely painful	Generally dull pain; decreased pinprick sensation, but pressure sensation intact	Insensate areas from nerve destruction	Insensate areas
Healing	Spontaneous healing in 3 to 5 days; generally no scar	Spontaneous healing in less than 21 days, usually 7 to 10 days; minimal scarring	Spontaneous healing in 2 to 3 weeks, possible conversion to full-thickness injury; hypertrophic scarring and scar contracture likely	Incapable of self-regeneration; requires skin graft to heal; scarring around periphery of wound between skin grafts	Incapable of self-regeneration; requires skin graft or flap to heal neurologic involvement possible; muscle paralysis possible; scarring around periphery of wound or between skin grafts

Table compiled from information in the following references:
Greenfield E, Jordan B. Advances in burn wound care. *Critical Care Nurs Clin North Amer.* 1996; 8(2):203–215.
Staley M, Richard R. Management of the acute burn wound: an overview. *Adv Wound Care.* 1996; 10(2):39–44.
Yarbrough DR. Pathophysiology of the burn wound. In: Wagner MM, ed. *Care of the Burn-Injured Patient. Multidisciplinary Involvement.* Littleton, MA: PSG Publishing Company, Inc.; 1981:19–3.

electrode) and anode (positive electrode) respectively. High galvanic current does not deliver enough charge on the skin to alter skin pH or cause electrochemical reactions, compared with low voltage direct current.[90,91]

Contraindications to the use of high voltage pulse current include osteomyelitis, malignancy, pacemakers, and electrical current should not be used over topical agents with metal ions (e.g., zinc-containing substances and the like). The recommended pulse rate/voltage is 100 pps/high voltage (100V) or above. Daily frequency of intervention is recommended with a length of therapy ranging from 30 to 60 minutes. The coupling agent is usually a lead (sterilized product lead or aluminum foil with an alligator clip) over a sterile saline-soaked gauze placed directly in the wound.

Polarity will vary based on the intent of the therapy. The positive electrode will enhance autolysis and epithelialization, The negative lead promotes granulation and is used for infection or inflammation.

Generally, high galvanic current is utilized with the deeper stage II, III and IV wounds. Although the specific means by which electrical stimulation may promote healing is still being explored, more and more evidence exists to support the hypothesis that electrical current creates the proliferation of connective tissue and decreases the inflammatory response. There is a modification of endogenous electrical potentials of tissue; stimulation of cellular biosynthesis and replication occurs; there are antibacteriacidal effects, enhanced circulation, and the generation of a cellular electrophyiological effect.[90,91,92,93] Electrochemical effects at electrode sites, such as increased cell temperature, changes in pH, or release of ions from the electrodes, may possibly occur during low voltage electrical stimulation, though these reactions have not been substantiated in high voltage current interventions.[90-93] Nonetheless, the rate of healing is decreased when high galvanic current is employed as a wound-healing agent.[90,93] Ulcers treated with high galvanic pulsed current demonstrate a significantly greater rate of wound contraction (measured by a decrease in wound size)[90] and ultimately the healing time is reduced.[90,93]

Ultrasound

Ultrasound is used as a physical therapy modality for the treatment of soft tissue trauma, hematosis and inflammation, and induration. Therapeutic benefits are well documented.[94,95,96,97] Ultrasound has been purported to benefit healing by increasing O_2 transport, decreasing pain, expediting tissue repair and wound closure, increasing angiogenesis, and decreasing edema.[94]

Ultrasound works in two ways, dependent on the variable of continuous versus pulsed delivery. Continuous ultrasound is primarily utilized to heat the tissues, whereas, pulsed ultrasound produces a non-thermal effect.[97] It is the nonthermal effect that stimulates wound healing by causing changes in cell membrane, which in turn stimulate tissue repair. However, the heating effects of continuous ultrasound is also beneficial as circulation to the wound is improved, which enhances oxygen and nutrient availability to the healing tissues.

Dyson[97] has demonstrated that when soft connective tissues are injured, platelets and mast cells become activated and release chemotactic agents, which attract leucocytes and monocytes to the site of injury. Ultrasound can stimulate the release of histamine and enhance calcium transport thereby stimulating metabolic activity and furthering the production of these chemotactic agents.[97] The primary role of leucocytes is to remove debris and pathogens from the wound, while monocytes develop into phagocytic macrophages, which release growth factors essential for the development of new connective tissue. Therefore, it is proposed that this is one of the mechanisms by which ultrasound promotes wound healing.[94-97]

Not only does ultrasound appear to have an impact on cellular activity during the inflammatory phase of healing, during the proliferation phase it has been demonstrated that fibroblasts exposed to therapeutic levels of ultrasound can be stimulated to synthesize collagen. The entry of calcium ions is also increased and facilitates reparative responses.[97] When ultrasound is applied to a wound, the rate of contraction can be accelerated, presumably because of direct or indirect effects on the myofibroblasts during the proliferative stage.[97]

The increase in collagen formation has also been determined to increase the strength of scar tissue in addition to normalizing the cross-linking fiber pattern of repair, so that scar tissue following ultrasound is more elastic and stronger.[97]

Contraindications to the use of ultrasound include acutely infected wounds, malignancies, pacemakers, deep vein thrombosis or emboli, and osteomyelitis. The chosen frequencies are 3 Mhz for superficial wounds and 1 Mhz for deep wounds with an intensity of 0.5 to 1.0 w/cm. Treatment frequency will depend on setting, however, it is recommended daily for acute wounds and a minimum of three times per week for chronic wounds. Coupling agents might include hydrogel dressings, degassed water, and ultrasound gel pads.

Whirlpool

The use of whirlpool, in the elderly, to immerse an extremity should be used sparingly. Long periods of time spent with the extremity soaking in water will result in emaciation and sloughing of healthy tissues. If the whirlpool is used, it should be used for brief periods of time (less than 10 minutes) to soften necrotic tissue for debridement, remove exudate, and provide a way of vigorously cleansing and rinsing the wound. Short periods of immersion in a warm whirlpool bath with the turbulent and agitated water massaging the extremity will increase cutaneous vasodilatation and oxygen transport, ease discomfort associated with the wound, and decrease muscle spasm.[98] The use of whirlpool prior for debridement is particularly helpful when there is necrotic tissue present or when preparing burn patients for wound debridement. Whirlpool intervention should be discontinued as a mode for cleansing the wound once the ulcer no longer requires debridement.[99]

Whirlpool intervention is contraindicated in elders with moderate to severe cardiac or pulmonary dysfunction, recent skin grafts, acute febrile conditions, advanced arterial disease, tendency for hemorrhaging, gangrene, venous insufficiency, and in the presence of a comatose or persistent vegetative state. If total or half-body immersion is employed, urinary incontinence or incontinence of bowel are also considerations.

If the goal of treatment is to keep the wound hydrated (which in most cases it is), soaking in water may actually result in dehydration.[53] Additionally, good granulation tissue may be damaged with agitation of the water. Temperature of the water should not exceed 115° to avoid skin burns; in a hypertensive patient, the temperature should not exceed 104° as this may cause a sustained elevated blood pressure.

Debridement

Sharp debridement is the removal of necrotic tissue utilizing scissors, tweezers, forceps, and scalpels. Blunt debridement is mechanically removing necrotic tissue by gently cleansing the wound surface with gauze, Q-tips, or other blunt materials.

Debridement of the wound is typically done by medical personnel, including physical therapists, that have been specifically trained in the skill of debridement. The goal of debridement is to provide a clean wound bed to enhance healing. The frequency and duration of debridement is based on the amount and pace of necrotic tissue formation. While debridement of the entire eschar down to viable tissue is the most efficient means of gaining healthy tissue, it may not be a reasonable alternative for some chronic wounds.

Great caution needs to be employed when debridement is performed in a patient with diabetes, sensory loss, or exposed tendons, ligaments, or bone. If there is excessive bleeding at the wound site, debridement should be curtailed until bleeding is controlled. Sharp debridement must be avoided in patients who have low platelet counts or in those taking anticoagulants.

Hyperbaric Oxygen Therapy

Hyperbaric oxygen therapy (HBO) has been advocated for selected nonhealing wounds and anaerobic wound infections. Patients are treated in chambers that provide O_2 to an isolated spot or to an entire extremity. In fact, treatment of ischemia in elderly subjects has been found to significantly enhance wound healing.[100]

There are topical oxygen bandages and plastic chambers for extremities that deliver oxygen to the wound, however, these are not considered hyperbaric. Their value in treating chronic wounds is questionable and the cost of treatment is expensive.[12]

Incontinence Care

Elderly patients who are incontinent and immobile are at a greater risk for skin breakdown and the development of pressure ulcers. Both fecal and urinary incontinence have been positively associated with the development of ulcers.[99] Skin care, focusing on maintaining a dry environment, thorough cleaning following an accident, moisturizers, barrier creams, ointments, and films are often recommended to prevent ulceration.

Frequent toileting is important in the older patient who requires assistance with bed mobility, ambulation, transfers, and managing clothing. (See Chapter 5). It is also important to provide proper cleaning using perineal washes with surfactants and humectants to decrease bacterial growth. Soaps and cleaning agents with detergents, such as sodium laurel sulfate or alcohol, should be avoided. These substances cause drying and irritation of the skin, which could lead to bacterial infection and breakdown.

Lotions to moisturize the skin assist in maintaining the viability of the skin surface. Moisturizing products should not contain alcohol, which will create excessive drying of the skin and may lead to skin dehydration, cracking, and subsequent ulceration.

Often, water-repellent barrier creams, ointments, or films are used if a patient is continually wet from incontinence or wound drainage. Patients with occasional incontinence may benefit from a perineal wash and moisturizer, however, others with continuous drainage may require a barrier to moisture. Powder may be used to absorb surface moisture followed by the application of a barrier cream or medicated ointment.

If an older individual, exposed to organisms in the urine or feces, develops a fungal infection, a rash will develop. Generally a prescription antifungal agent will be required. These medicinal substances come in powders or creams. There are also OTC antifungal powders which are used preventively for patients on antibiotics and those with mild rashes characterized by redness and itching.[12]

SURGICAL INDICATIONS

Topical treatment that provides a moist healing environment will encourage but not guarantee a successful cascade of wound-healing events. Debridement continues to be important in the healing process. It accelerates healing by removing necrotic debris and can be accomplished autolytically, chemically, mechanically, or surgically. For example, a venous ulcer covered with fibrinous necrotic tissue may heal faster if the fibrinous tissue is debrided to reveal healthy granulation tissue underneath. When necrotic tissue is deep and extensive, debridement is usually a surgical procedure.

The most important goal in wound care is rapid and lasting closure. Surgery is indicated in nonhealing ulcers. Skin grafts are indicated when spontaneous healing is compromised by the size and depth of the wound and when inadequate perfusion of the skin decreases the likelihood of healing.[101] The problem of compromised healing is even greater in diabetic patients if neuropathy and/or vasculopathy is present.[102] Surgical grafting of cultured autologous skin grafts is complemented by rehabilitation involvement inclusive of immobilization of the area with a removable cast or splint, and biostimulation with pulsed electrical fields.[103]

The following acrostic developed by Mulder and associates[12] delineates guidelines warranting surgical evaluation and potential surgical intervention:

N = necrotic tissue
O = osteomyelitis

H = hidden sinus tracts and tunnels
E = eschar (unresponsive to minor sharp debridement or dressing)
A = abscess and arterial insufficiency
L = large defects too big to close by secondary intervention
I = ischemia
N = nonhealing wound after 30 to 45 days treatment
G = graft-ready wound beds and wound beds with tendon and bone exposed

Several different companies have attempted to develop materials that will act as temporary skin coverings. These materials contain any combination of cultured keratinocytes, fibroblasts, collagen, and synthetic materials.[104] The products are used with burns and chronic wounds. Skin replacements may be the wound dressing of the future, replacing current synthetic and semi-synthetic dressings. Skin equivalents with dermal and epidermal layers have been found to be useful on full-thickness wounds when surgically applied.[103,105]

Conservative healing without the need of surgery and anesthesia is preferable in the elderly patient. Combined innovative approaches to wound care that incorporate non-invasive interventions such as growth hormones, biosynthetic dressings, electrical stimulation and other modalities are the preferred methods in the older patient

SUPPORT SURFACES

By controlling the parameters of friction and pressure it is possible to prevent pressure ulcers from forming and to treat stage I and II ulcers successfully with conservative measures. A major consideration in such treatment is the selection and use of effective support surfaces such as wheelchair cushions and mattresses.[106] In this regard, the perfect support surface would have the following characteristics:

- Minimizes the pressures under the bony prominences
- Controls the pressure gradient in the tissue
- Provides stability
- Allows weight shifts
- Allows ease of transfer
- Controls the temperature at the skin interface
- Controls the moisture at the skin interface
- Is lightweight
- Has a low cost
- Is durable and easy to clean
- Meets required infection control standards

Although a number of products have been introduced to the market, the perfect support surface does not exist. Many of the support products fulfill some criteria of the perfect support surface, but none seems to provide maximum protection for all individuals. As a result, provision of support surfaces needs to be an adjunct of intervention.[106]

As an adjunctive intervention special support surfaces play a key role in the prevention and treatment of pressure ulcers. The best support surface, as described above, needs to have properties that include interface pressure, friction and shear characteristics, moisture vapor transmission rate, thermal insulation properties, indentation load deflection, density, ease of use, safety, and patient comfort.

Interface pressure is the most commonly used measure when comparing support surfaces. Interface pressure is a measure of the force the support surface applies to the tissue it is supporting. Interface pressure measures are in millimeters of mercury (mm Hg) and are described as pressure relief and pressure reduction. Pressure relief is defined as pressure below 25 to 32 mm Hg.[12] Pressure reduction is defined as the reduction of interface pressures to 26 to 32 mm Hg.[12] While somewhat useful in objectively evaluating support surfaces, interface pressures are not the precise standard that would be ideal for managing patient care. They should not be used as the sole parameter in evaluating the efficacy of the surface in determining pressure relief and reduction.

The choice of support surfaces will also depend on the following variables:

- Patient's diagnosis
- Number of hours the patient uses the support system
- Types of activities performed

- Usage environment (climate, continence, etc)
- Living arrangements (independent, varying levels of assistance, residential facility)
- Tissue history (history of ulcers, decreased sitting tolerance, surgery to repair ulcers)
- Body build
- Pressure magnitude and distribution

For both mattress and seating products available for support surfaces, Table 14–5 provides the advantages and disadvantages of various pressure reducing materials used in these products.

Though this chapter is not the forum for a thorough review of every available support surface, it is important that the reader explore the many invaluable resources available for determining the best product for individual patients.[5,12,106] The selection of a support surface, whether for the bed, chair, or wheelchair, is a complex multi-factorial process. It is evident that no single device serves all elderly persons with the multiplicity of system involvement seen with advancing age. Furthermore, even the most sophisticated devices will not prevent tissue breakdown. Support surfaces are part of the total pressure management regimen that must be individualized for each older person.

WOUND CARE PRODUCTS

There are numerous wound care products required for appropriate healing beyond support surfaces. These include cleansers and moisturizers, pharmaceutical, agents and various types of dressings. Mulder and associates provide a comprehensive list of these products in the *Clinicians' Pocket Guide to Chronic Wound Repair*.[12] Wound products include:

- Wound cleansers
- Skin moisturizers
- Ointments
- Skin sealants
- Lubricating sprays, ointments, and dressings
- Enzymatic debriding agents
- Transparent adhesive dressings

- Hydrocolloid wafer dressings
- Hydrocolloid paste, granules, and powder dressings
- Exudate absorptive dressings
- Exudate absorptive dressings with antimicrobial activity
- Calcium alginates
- Semipermeable foam dressings
- Hydrogels
- Impregnated gauzes
- Nonadherent dressings
- Composites (island dressings)
- Contact layers
- Specialty absorptive dressings
- Activated charcoal dressings
- Wound pouches

Pharmaceutical Agents[12]

Wound cleansers are applied directly into the wound for purification. Moisturizers add moisture to the epidermis and assist in maintaining the intact skin. Ointments provide a petrolatum-based barrier or water-resistant cream against bodily secretions or chemical injury.[107]

Skin sealants provide some degree of protection from mechanical and chemical injury by providing a copolymer film on the skin. These sealants usually contain alcohol and need to be a cautiously used in the treatment of the elderly. Due to the problem with dehydration in older adults, the alcohol may exacerbate this condition. Extra emphasis on adequate hydration and moisturization of the wound bed is important in conjunction with the use of skin sealants.

Lubricating sprays, ointments, and dressings provide a protective dressing and add moisture to the epidermis.[107]

Enzymatic debriding agents are pharmaceutical agents, which assist in obliterating necrotic tissue, exudates, and denatured collagen.[107] The destructive process is accomplished through proteolytic enzyme action. Some enzymatic debriding agents are provided in dressing products.[12]

TABLE 14–5. ADVANTAGES AND DISADVANTAGES OF PRESSURE-RELIEVING PRODUCTS

PRODUCT	ADVANTAGES	DISADVANTAGES
Air-Filled Products	Light weight Easy to clean Effective with many patients	Subject to puncture Not easily repaired Inflation must be checked frequently User instability
Liquid-Filled Flotation Devices	Easy to clean Effectiveness	Subject to puncture Heavy
Gel-Filled Devices	Adjusts to body movement Easy to clean	Heavy
Foam Products	Availability Many variations/densities Inexpensive Light weight Can be easily modified	Wears out quickly Not easily cleaned Properties change with time Can support combustion

Dressings[12,107]

Historically, wound dressings were used in order to protect the wound from the external environment. It is now understood that dressings play an active, not passive, role in wound management. Dressings create an environment that will optimize the wound-healing process. Key to this is maintaining moisture in the wound. Extensive research has demonstrated that healing of normal wounds is significantly enhanced in a moist environment compared to those allowed to dry.[1,2,8,99]

Dressing choice will be influenced by the wound's stage in its healing process. A wound in the inflammation stage must be treated differently from one with significant epithelialization. Since a wound is constantly in a state of change, dressing choices must periodically be re-evaluated.[107]

Transparent adhesive dressings provide a semipermeable, sterile, thin film that creates a moist environment. This type of dressings is nonabsorptive and enables autolysis of devitalized tissue. Transparent adhesive dressings protect the skin and wound against friction and are referred to as "second skin."

Dressings that interact with the wound environment and contain pharmaceutical agents are helpful in enhancing healing.[107] These include calcium alginates, as well as certain hydrocolloid and hydrogel wafer dressings that can deliver substances to the wound to stimulate healing.[12]

Hydrocolloid wafer dressing and hydrocolloid paste, granules, and powder dressings are commonly used in the treatment of wounds in the elderly.[12] Wafers contain hydroactive, absorptive particles that interact with the wound exudate to form a gelatinous mass which then can be debrided with dressing removal. They provide minimal to moderate absorption (depending on the product) and enable autolysis of devitalized tissue. These dressings are contraindicated where anaerobic infection is suspected.[12] In the elderly, the hydrocolloid dressings are preferred for use in the coccyx area as they require no secondary dressing (which could add to frictional stresses and moisture) and cover and protect the area similar to the transparent adhesive second skin dressings.

Exudate absorptive dressings absorb draining exudate and fill dead space.[107] They conform to the wound surface and keep the wound surface clean and moist. Exudate absorptive dressings enable autolysis of devitalized tissue.[12] These dressing often come with pharmaceutical agents with antimicrobial activity. These dressings absorb exudate, conform to the wound surface, keep the wound clean, and reduce bacterial load in the wound.[107] The disadvantage of use of the antimicrobial absorptive dressings is that they require a secondary dressing.

Calcium alginates are highly absorbent and provide an interactive pharmaceutical dressing. These dressings convert into a viscous hydrophilic gel after contact with exudate. Trapped fibers in the wound are biodegradable and the meshing of the dressing with the wound makes possible the autolysis of devitalized tissue.[12]

Semipermeable foam dressings absorb exudate while maintaining a moist wound surface. The outer layer of the foam dressings is hydrophobic, which helps to maintain moisture in the wound. These dressings also permit autolysis of devitalized tissue.[107]

Hydrogel dressings maintain a clean and moist wound surface. They are oxygen-permeable, allowing for oxygenation of the wound. The hydrogels cool the surface and are often refrigerated to enhance the cryotherapeutic effects of reducing pain and inflammation.[107] The hydrogel dressings absorb minimal exudate. Some products require a secondary dressing. These dressings enable the autolysis of devitalized tissue upon removal.[12]

Impregnated gauzes are nonadherent fine or open mesh gauze that enable autolysis of devitalized tissue.[12] Nonadherent dressings, or more appropriately termed low-adherent, are used on dry or lightly exudating wounds to provide absorptive and autolytic properties in the treatment of a healing wound. Composite dressings, also called island dressings, are nonadherent absorbent dressings with a pad located in the center. They provide absorption of minimal exudate and are bacteria- and moisture-resistant adhesive dressings. Contact layers are also classed as nonadherent dressings and are used on wounds under absorbent cover dressings.[12] Specialty absorptive dressings are low-adherent dressings used on dry or lightly exudating wounds and often used as a secondary dressing.[107]

Activated charcoal dressings absorb exudate and reduce the concentration of wound odor. They are frequently used with high exudate wounds. Enzymatic debriding agents embedded in gauze dressings are designed to destroy necrotic tissue, exudate, or denatured collagen through proteolytic enzyme action.[12]

Wound pouches, which look like ostomy pouches, have attached skin barriers and can be cut to fit the wound shape and size. Hinged caps allow for treatment or inspection and can be adapted for continuous drainage.[12]

Living skin equivalents (synthetic approximations) are also used as temporary skin coverings. These materials contain any combination of a number of substances including cultured keratinocytes, fibroblasts, collagen, and synthetic materials.[12] Substances such as hyaluronic acid, which is a naturally occurring lubricant and a component in the synthesis of connective tissues, has been found to be effective in enhancing healing of chronic wounds.[105,107]

Growth Factors

Several growth factors that stimulate wound healing have been isolated. Autologous growth factors can be harvested from a patient's blood and applied to the patient's nonhealing wound.[108] Genetic recombinant growth factors are being researched in many centers with promising results.

During coagulation and inflammation, platelets, neutrophils, macrophages, and lymphocytes are the predominant cell types as they function to kill bacteria and clear the wound site of cellular debris and foreign material prior to the reparative phases. This type of cells, especially platelets, also acts to initiate and sustain the proliferative and remodeling stages of wound repair by synthesizing and releasing growth factors that serve to regulate healing.[108]

Besides serving as an important source of several growth factors, fibroblasts serve other vital functions—making them the most important cell type during this phase of healing. They produce matrix proteins, of which collagen is the most important, providing strength and integrity to the healed wound. Also, fibroblasts convert into myofibroblasts within the granulation tissue of the open wound, leading to contraction and healing. Other cells, such as keratinocytes and vascular endothelial cells, are active in producing granulation tissue and restoring the epithelium and vascular integrity.

Continuous synthesis and degradation of collagen characterize the remodeling phase, which relies on a balance between factors that promote synthesis of extracellular matrix components and enzymes that degrade these components. Growth factors, which are synthesized and released locally at the wound site, regulate the functions of each of the cell types. The growth factors include platelet-derived growth factor, transforming growth factor-beta (TGF-β), epidermal growth factors.[108]

At the molecular level, chronic wounds may result ultimately from a deficiency in growth factors or inhibition of their function. This deficiency may be partly the result of elevated levels of proteinases that act to degrade growth factors and extracellular matrix components at the wound site. It has been demonstrated that the healing response can be induced in chronic wounds by either adding exogenous growth factors or inhibiting proteinase activity at the wound site.[108] Recently developed pharmaceutical dressings containing growth factors are being utilized with successful results in elderly populations.

Nutritional Agents'

Scientists have discovered that a multipurpose protein found in several bodily fluids has another important function, it can promote the healing of abnormal skin wounds, which are a significant problem in the elderly. Researchers demonstrated that the protein, called secretory leukocyte protease inhibitor (SLPI), plays a critical role in normal wound healing and enhances healing in wounds that are slow to heal.[109,110] SLPI is found in fluids that bathe mucosal surfaces such as bronchial fluids, cervical fluids, and saliva,

and is a remarkably versatile substance. It has anti-inflammatory, antiviral, antifungal, and antibacterial properties. In recent years, investigators demonstrated that SLPI found in saliva blocks HIV-1 infection.[110,111]

Many elderly patients that have delayed healing processes lack the SLPI gene and this is demonstrated markedly by impaired wound healing with an increase in inflammation and the activity of the enzyme elastase, which destroys tissue.[109,111] Without the presence of SLPI to act as a molecular brake, a cascade of events occurs that results in the destruction of tissue and impaired wound healing. However, the topical application of SLPI actually reverses the abnormal response and enhances the rate of healing.[109] Researchers believe that SLPI has three major functions in wound healing. It inhibits elastase, controls the activation of leukocytes, and reduces TGF-β activation. SLPI appears to be a component of innate or natural host defense mechanisms that maintain a balance between protective inflammation responses and overzealous or uncontrolled inflammation that can lead to tissue destruction and failure to heal.[109,110,111] Interestingly, the fact that animals tend to lick their wounds may be nature's way of delivering SLPI to the wound site via saliva.

With aging, the skin is thinner, more fragile, and more susceptible to injury. Progressive normal and pathological aging changes increase the risk for chronic health problems that may lead to open wounds and delayed healing. Optimum care of chronic wounds supports the older person's specific health and care needs, progresses to cleansing and debridement of the wound, then uses appropriate nutrition, modalities, coverings, and protective interventions to promote healing.

ALTERNATIVE MEDICINE AND WOUND HEALING

Alternative and complementary medicine includes a vast array of wound care modalities which requires at least mention in this chapter. Many elderly individuals, disenchanted with the outcomes of allopathic care, seek these forms of treatment for chronic wounds. In addition to nutritional (see Chapter 7) and herbal (see Chapter 8) approaches to wound healing, some alternative and complementary therapies may offer benefits for patients with wounds and wound pain. These therapies include acupuncture, energy healing, guided imagery, hypnosis, prayer, and relaxation techniques.[112] Although we will not go into wound healing and each alternative intervention, it is important that the therapist be aware of the complement of state-of-the-art wound care practices in wound care clinics. In some studies these interventions have been shown to effectively heal wounds and provide relief of wound pain during the healing process.[112]

CONCLUSION

Each year, more than four million older people suffer from chronic, nonhealing wounds such as diabetic ulcers, pressure sores, vasculitic, arterial, and venous ulcers. Inflammation and bacterial infection are two of the major complications that contribute to delayed healing in the elderly. This chapter has addressed the need for preventive approaches to wound care, in addition to early intervention. Even acute wounds are at risk for becoming chronic, nonhealing wounds as a result of poor nutrition, dehydration, and diminished circulation. This chapter has addressed the causes and prevention of problems in the integumentary system, reviewed the stages of wound repair and skin changes affecting the elderly, and provided a discussion regarding the importance of thorough evaluation and documentation of wound status. The staging and grading of wounds and the differentiation between the various types of ulcers has been considered in the management of wounds. Other integumentary considerations were presented with regard to their occurrence in elderly patients including wounds created by extravasation sites, abrasions and skin tears, dehisced surgical wounds, GI and GU fistulas, oral or gastrointestinal ulcers, radiation, and thermal burns. Treatment adjuncts using surface support systems, pharmaceutical agents, dressings, and nutritional approaches were also presented as a part of comprehensive intervention program for the elimination of undue pressure, provision of movement, and enhancement of circulation, nutrition and healing.

The way in which the body responds to wounding depends on many factors including debridement to establish a healthy wound base, tissue oxygenation, age, underlying pathologies, nutritional status, continence, wound dehydration, and whether or not the patient smokes. Assessing tissue blood supply to the wound site and treating/preventing infection are crucial to the process of healing wounds and burns of all types in the elderly.

PEARLS

- The *skin has three distinct layers: the epidermis, dermis, and subcutaneous layers.*
- The healing process can easily be remembered by the 3 **Rs** of wound healing: **R**eaction (inflammation), **R**egeneration (proliferation and epithelialization), and **R**emodeling.
- The effects of aging and age-associated diseases slow the wound healing process.
- Thinning and flattening of the epidermis results in an increased vulnerability to trauma from shear and fricitonal forces in the older adult.
- Nutritional status will directly impact the rate of healing. Many nutrients aid the healing process, such as protein, carbohydrates, fats, vitamin C, zinc, iron, vitamins A, E, and K, copper, thiamine, pantothenic acid, and other B vitamins.
- *Wagner's classification is used to objectively evaluate and stage (rank) vascular dysfunction in grades of 0 to 5.*
- Inadequate blood supply can result in poor oxidative and nutritive status in the tissues and lead to an arterial ulcer.
- Venous ulcerations are caused by venous hypertension, valvular incompetence, and generally accompanied by a history of deep vein thrombosis.
- *Diabetic neuropathy affects the motor, sensory, and autonomic nerves of the leg and often presents as a stocking-like paresthesia of the foot.*
- All pressure ulcers are preventable if attention is directed to insensate areas, malnutrition, skin fragility, and the physical or cognitive inability to accomplish pressure relief without guidance or assistance.
- Inflammation of blood vessel walls can lead to vasculitic ulcers.
- Treatment approaches for wound healing in the elderly population include physical modalities, debridement, incontinence care, topical dressings, and nutritional interventions.

REFERENCES

1. Goodson WH, Hunt TK. Wound healing and aging. *J Invest Dermatol.* 1979; 73(1):88–91.
2. Reed MJ. Wound repair in older patients: preventing problems and managing healing. *Geriatrics.* 1998; 53(5):88–94.
3. Irion G. *Physiology: The Basis of Clinical Practice.* Thorofare, NJ: Slack, Inc; 2000:181–189.
4. McCulloch JM, Kloth LC, Feedar JA. *Wound Healing: Alternatives in Management.* 2nd edition. Philadelphia, PA: F.A. Davis Company; 1995.
5. Sussman C, Bates-Jensen BM. *Wound Care: A Collaborative Practice Manual for Physical Therapists and Nurses.* Gaithersburg, MD: Aspen Publishers, Inc.; 1998.
6. Boynton PR, Jaworski D, Paustian C. Meeting the challenges of healing chronic wounds in older adults. *Nurs Clin North Am.* 1999; 34(4): 921–932.
7. Eaglstein WH. Wound healing and aging. *Dermatol Clin.* 1986; 4(3):481–484.
8. Van Rijswijk L. General principles of wound management. In: Gogia PP, ed. *Clinical Wound Management.* Thorofare, NJ: Slack, Inc.; 1995.
9. Wong RA. Chronic dermal wounds in older adults. In: Guccione A, ed. *Geriatric Physical Therapy.* St Louis, MO: Mosby Publishers; 2000: 376–398.
10. Myer AH. The effects of aging on wound healing. *Top Geriatr Rehabil.* 2000; 16(2):1–10.
11. Stotts N, Wipke-Tevis D. Co-factors in impaired wound healing. In: Grasner D, Kane D, eds. *Chronic Wound Care: A Clinical Source Book for Healthcare Professionals.* Wayne, PA: Health Management Publications, Inc; 1997.

12. Mulder GC, Fairchild PA, Jeter KF. *Clinicias' Pocket Guide to Chronic Wound Repair*. 3rd edition. Long Beach, CA: Wound Healing Institute Publications; 1995.

13. Jones P, Millman A. Wound healing and the aged patient. *Nurs Clin North Am.* 1990; 25(1): 263–277.

14. Campbell S. *Pressure Ulcer Prevention and Intervention: A Role for Nutrition*. Westerville, OH: Ross Products; 2001

15. Nicolle LE, Huchcroft SA, Cruse PJ. Risk factors for surgical wound infection among the elderly. *J Clin Epidemiol.* 1992; 45(4):357–364.

16. Declair V. The usefulness of topical application of essential fatty acids (EFA) to prevent pressure ulcers. *Ostomy Wound Manage.* 1997; 43(5): 48–54.

17. Breslow RA. Hallfrisch J, Guy DG. The importance of dietary protein in healing pressure ulcers. *J Am Beriatr Soc.* 1993; 41(4):357–362.

18. Munro HN, Suter PM, Russell RM. Nutritional requirements of the elderly. *Am Rev Nutr.* 1987; 7: 23–49.

19. Lemon P. Is increased dietary protein necessary or beneficial for individuals with a physically active life? *Nutr Rev.* 1996; 54(1):S169–S175.

20. Cahill GF. Starvation in man. *N Engl J Med.* 1970; 282:668–675.

21. Young VR, Pellett PL. Plant proteins in relation to human protein and amino acid nutrition. *Am J Clin Nutr.* 1994; 59(suppl):1203S–1212S.

22. Greenblatt DJ. Reduced albumin concentration in the elderly: a report from the Boston collaborative drug surveillance program. *J Am Geriatr Soc.* 1979; 27:20–23.

23. Ringsdorf WM, Cheraskin E. Vitamin C and human wound healing. *Oral Surg Oral Med Oral Pathol.* 1982; 53(3):231–236.

24. Taylor TV, Rimmer S, Day B, Butcher J, Dymock IW. Ascorbic acid supplementation in the treatment of pressure sores. *Lancet.* 1974; 2:544–546.

25. Weismann K. What is the use of zinc for wound healing? *Int J Dermatol.* 1978; 17:568–570.

26. Pories WJ, Henzel JH, Rob CG, Strain WH. Acceleration of healing with zinc sulfate. *Ann Surg.* 1997; 201:432–436.

27. Carruthers R. Oral zinc sulphate in leg ulcers. *Lancet.* 1969; 1:1264–1266.

28. Cohen C. Zinc sulphate and bedsores. 1968; 2: 561–563.

29. Faure H, Peyrin JC, Richard MJ, Favier A. Parenteral supplementation with zinc in elderly surgical patients corrects postoperative serum-zinc drop. *Biol Trace Elem Res.* 1991; 30(1): 37–45.

30. Agren MS. Studies on zinc in wound healing. *Acta Derm Venereol Supll* (Stockholm). 1990; 154(1): 1–36.

31. Stromberg HE, Agren MS. Topical zinc oxide treatment improves arterial and venous leg ulcers. *Br J Dermatol.* 1984; 111(4):461–468.

32. Seifter E, Crowley LV, Rettura G. Influence of vitamin A on wound healing. *Ann Surg.* 1975; 181(6): 836–841.

33. Demetriou AA, Levenson SM, Rettura G, Seifter E. Vitamin A and retinoic acid: induced fibroblast differentiation in vitro. *Surgery.* 1985; 98(11): 931–934.

34. Bartolomucci E. Action of vitamin E on healing of experimental wounds on parenchymatous organs. *JAMA.* 1939; 113:1079 [abstract].

35. Ehrlich HP, Tarver H, Hunt TK. Inhibitory effects of vitamin E on collagen synthesis and wound repair. *Ann Surg.* 1972; 175:235–240.

36. Rucker RB, Kosonen T, Clegg MS. Copper lysyl oxidase, and extracellular matrix protein cross-linking. *Am J Clin Nutr.* 1998; 67(5 suppl): 996s–1002s.

37. Alvarez OM, Gilbreath RL. Effect of dietary thiamine on intermolecular collagen cross-linking during wound repair: a mechanical and biochemical assessment. *J Trauma.* 1982; 22(1):20–24.

38. Aprahamian M, Dentinger A, Stock-Damge C. Effects of supplemental pantothenic acid on wound healing. *Am J Clin Nutr.* 1985; 41(3):578–589.

39. Bosse MD, Axelrod AE. Wound healing with biotin pyridoxin, or riboflavin deficiencies. *Proc Soc Exp Biol Med.* 1948; 67:418–421.

40. Tassman G, Zafran J, Zayon G. A double-blind crossover study of a plant proteolytic enzyme in oral surgery. *J Dent Med.* 1965; 20:51–54.

41. Blonstein J. Control of swelling in boxing injuries. *Practitioner.* 1960; 203:206–207.

42. Della Loggia R, Tubaro A, Sosa S. The role of triterpenoids in the topical anti-inflammatory activity of *Calendula officinalis* flowers. *Planta Med.* 1994; 60(6):516–520.

43. Zitterl-Eglseer K, Sosa S, Jurenitsch J. Anti-oedematous activities of the main triterpendiol esters of marigold (*Calendul officinalis L.*). *J Ethnopharmacol.* 1997; 57(2):139–144.

44. Shipochliev T, Dimitrov A, Aleksandrova E. Anti-inflammatory action of a group of plant extracts. *Vet Med.* 1981; 18(6):87–94.

45. Blumenthal M, Busse WR, Goldgerg A. *The Complete German Commission E Monographs. Therapeutic Guide to Herbal Medicines*. Austin, TX: American Botanical Council, 1998.

46. Davis RH, Stewart GH, Bregman PJ. Aloe vera and the inflamed synovial pouch model. *J Am Podiatr Med Assoc.* 1992; 82(3):140–148.

47. Davis RH, Leitner MG, Russo JM, Byrne ME. Wound healing. Oral and topical activity of aloe vera. *J Am Podiatr Med Assoc.* 1989; 79(11): 559–562.

48. Grossman MR. Treating pressure ulcers in the geriatric patient. *Podiatry Today.* July/August 1996; 66–73.

49. Wagner FW. The dysvascular foot: a system for diagnosis and treatment. *Foot Ankle.* 1981; 2(1): 64–69.

50. Morey SE. Photos supplement written documentation. *Physical Therapy Products.* Jan/Feb 1998; 66–67.

51. Bates-Jensen BM, Vredevoe DL, Brecht ML. Validity and reliability of the Pressure Sore Status Tool. *Decubitus.* 1992; 5(6):20–28.

52. Bates-Jensen BM, McNees P. Toward an intelligent wound assessment system. *Osteotomy Wound Manage.* 1995; 41(7A):80–87.

53. Alvarez OM, Gilson G, Auletta MJ. Local aspects of diabetic foot ulcer care: assessment, dressings, and topical agents. In: Levin ME, O'Neal LW, Bowker JH, eds. *The Diabetic Foot.* 5th edition. St Louis: Mosby Year-Book; 1993:259–281.

54. Falanga V, Eaglstein WH. *Leg and Foot Ulcers: A Clinician's Guide.* London: Martin Dunitz Limited; 1995.

55. Hess CT. *Nurse's Clinical Guide to Wound Care.* 2nd edition. Springhouse, PA: Springhouse Corporation; 1997:28–29.

56. Holloway GA. Arterial ulcers: assessment, classification and management. In: Krasner D, Kane D, eds. *Chronic Wound Care: A Clinical Source Book for Healthcare Professionals.* 2nd edition. Wayne, PA: Health Management Publications, Inc.; 1997: 158–164.

57. Maklebust J, Sieggreen MY. *Pressure Ulcers: Guidelines for Prevention and Nursing Management.* 2nd edition. Springhouse, PA: Springhouse Corporation; 1996:30.

58. McCulloch J, Hovde J. Treatment of wounds due to vascular problems. In: Kloth L, McCulloch J, Feedar J, eds. *Wound Healing: Alternatives in Management.* Philadelphia: Davis; 1990:177–195.

59. Phillips T, Machado F, Trout R, Porter J, Olin J, Falanga V. Prognostic indicators in venous ulcers. *J Am Acad Dermatol.* 2000; 43(4):627–630.

60. Beebe HG, Bergan JJ, Bergqvist D. Classification and grading of chronic venous disease in the lower limbs: a consensus statement. *VASA.* 1995; 24(4):313–318.

61. Young RJ, Zhou YQ, Rodriguez E, Prescott RJ, Ewing DJ, Clarke BF. Variable relationship between peripheral somatic and autonomic neuropathy in patients with different syndromes of diabetic polyneuropathy. *Diabetes.* 1986; 35(2): 192–197.

62. Levin M. Diabetic foot wounds: pathogenesis and management. *Adv Wound Care.* 1996; 10(2): 24–30.

63. Steed DL. Diabetic wounds: assessment, classification and management. In: Krasner D, Kane D, eds. *Chronic Wound Care: A Clinical Source Book for Healthcare Professionals.* 2nd ed. Wayne, PA: Health Management Publications, Inc.; 1997: 72–177.

64. Edmonds ME, Morrison M, Law JW, Watkins PJ. Medial arterial calcification and diabetic neuropathy. *Br Med J.* 1982; 284:928–930.

65. Boulton AJM, Hardisty CA, Betts RC, et al. Dynamic foot pressure and other studies as diagnostic and management aids in diabetic neuropathy. *Diabetes Care.* 1983; 6:26–33.

66. Corbin DOC, Morrison DC, Young RJ, et al. Blood flow in the diabetic foot: analysis of doppler ultrasound waveforms by the Laplace transform damping method. *Diabetes Res Clinical Practice.* 1985; 9:S109–110.

67. Edmonds ME, Nicolaides KH, Watkins PJ. Autonomic neuropathy and diabetic foot ulceration. *Diabetic Med.* 1986; 3(4):344–349.

68. Nawoczenski DA, Birke JA. Management of the neuropathic foot in the elderly. *Top Geriatr Rehabil.* 1992; 7(3):36–48.

69. Matthews DM, Glass EJ, Stewart J, Collier DA, Clarke BF, Weir DM. Impairment of human monocyte 'lectin-like' receptor activity in insulin dependent diabetics. *Diabetic Med.* 1986; 3(4): 358–366.

70. Lavery LA, Armstrong DG, Harkless LB. Classification of diabetic foot wounds. *J Foot Ankle Surgery.* 1996; 35(6):528–531.

71. Birke JA, Patout CA. The contact cast: an update and case study report. *Wounds* 2000; 12(2): 26–31.

72. American Diabetes Association: Position statement: Office guide to diagnosis and classification of diabetes mellitus and other categories of glucose intolerance. *Diabetes Care* 1992; 15 (suppl.2): 4.

73. Gambert SR: *Diabetes Mellitus in the Elderly: A Practical Guide.* New York: Raven Press; 1999.

74. Bottomley, JM. A conservative approach in the treatment of a foot ulceration in a homeless diabetic patient: A case report. *PT Magazine.* Publication pending 2002.

75. Allman R. Epidemiology of pressure sores in different populations. *Decubitus.*1989 2(2):30–33.

76. Bennett L, Lee B. Pressure versus shear in pressure sore causation. In: Lee B, ed. *Chronic Ulcers of the Skin.* New York: McGraw-Hill; 1985:39–56.

77. Kosiak M. Prevention and rehabilitation of ischemic ulcers. In: Kottke F, Stillwell G, Lehman J, eds. *Krusen's Handbook of Physical Medicine and Rehabilitation.* 3rd ed. Philadelphia: Saunders; 1982:881–888.

78. Bergstrom N, Braden BJ, Laguzza A, Holman A. The Braden Scale for predicting pressure sore risk. *Nursing Research.* 1987; 36:205–210.

79. Norton D, McLaren R, Exton-Smith AN. An investigation of geriatric nursing problems in hospitals. London: Churchill-Livingston; 1975.

80. Rubin CF, Dietz RR, Abruzzese RS. Auditing the decubitus ulcer problem. *Am J Nurs.* 1974; 74(10): 1820–1821.

81. Aronovitch S, Millenbach L, Kelman GB, Wing P. Investigation of the Knoll Assessment Scale in a tertiary care facility. *Decubitus.* 1992; 5(3):70–76.

82. Gosnell DI. An assessment tool to identify pressure sores. *Nursing Research.* 1973; 22(1):55.

83. Shea JD. Pressure sores: classification and management. *Clin Orthop Relat Res.* 1975; 112:89–100.

84. Ferrell BA, Artinian BM, Sessing D. The Sessing Scale for assessment of pressure ulcer healing. *J Amer Geriatr Soc.* 1995; 43(1):37–40.

85. Hunder GG. Vasculitic syndromes: An update on diagnosis and management. *J Musculoskel Med.* 1993; 10(1):50–60.

86. Kudravi SA, Reed MJ. Aging, cancer, and wound healing. *In Vivo.* 2000; 14(1):83–92.

87. Greenfield E, Jordan B. Advances in burn wound care. *Critical Care Nurs Clin North Amer.* 1996; 8(2):203–215.

88. Staley M, Richard R. Management of the acute burn wound: an overview. *Adv Wound Care.* 1996; 10(2):39–44.

89. Yarbrough DR. Pathophysiology of the burn wound. In: Wagner MM, ed. *Care of the Burn-Injured Patient. Multidisciplinary Involvement.* Littleton, MA: PSG Publishing Company, Inc.; 1981: 19–31.

90. Griffin JW, Tooms RE, Mendius RA, Clifft JK, Zwaag RV, El-Zeky F. Efficacy of high voltage pulsed current for healing of pressure ulcers in patients with spinal cord injury. *Phys Ther.* 1991; 71(6):433–444.

91. Jaskoviak PA, Schafer RC. High voltage therapy. *Amer Chiropractor.* 1986; 12:68–84

92. Sussman C. Electrical stimulation. In: Sussman C, Bates-Jensen BM, eds. *Wound Care: A Collaborative Practice Manual for Physical Therapists and Nurses.* 2nd Edition. Gaithersburg, MD: Aspen Pubs.; 2001.

93. Feedar JA, Kloth LC, Gentzkow GD. Chronic dermal ulcer healing enhanced with monophasic pulsed electrical stimulation. *Phys Ther.* 1991; 71 (9):639–649.

94. Sussman C. Ultrasound. In: Sussman C, Bates-Jensen BM, eds. *Wound Care: A Collaborative Practice Manual for Physical Therapists and Nurses.* 2nd Edition. Gaithersburg, MD: Aspen Pubs; 2001.

95. Nussbaum EL, Biemann I, Mustard B. Comparison of ultrasound/ultraviolet-C and laser for treatment of pressure ulcers in patients with spinal cord injury. *Phys Ther.* 1994; 74(9): 812–823.

96. Byl NN, McKenzie A, Wong T, West J, Hunt TK. Incisional wound healing: A controlled study of low and high does ultrasound. *JOSPT.* 1993; 18(5):619–628.

97. Dyson M. Mechanics involved in therapeutic ultrasound. *Physiotherapy.* 1987; 73(3):116–120.

98. Sussman C. Whirlpool. In: Sussman C, Bates-Jensen BM, eds. *Wound Care: A Collaborative Practice Manual for Physical Therapists and Nurses.* 2nd Edition. Gaithersburg, MD: Aspen Pubs; 2001.

99. Feedar JA, Kloth LC. Conservative management of chronic wounds. In: Kloth LC, McCulloch JM, Feddar JA, eds. *Wound Healing: Alternatives in Management.* Philadelphia, PA: F.A. Davis; 1990.

100. Quirinia A, Viidik A. The impact of ischemia on wound healing is increased in old age but can be countered by hyperbaric oxygen therapy. *Mech Ageing Dev.* 1996; 91(2):131–144.

101. Leung PC, Hung LK, Leung KS. Use of the medial plantar flap in soft tissue replacement around the heel region. *Foot Ankle.* 1988; 8(3):327–330.

102. Cevera JJ, Bolton LL, Kerstein MD. Options for diabetic patients with chronic heel ulcers. *J Diab Complic.* 1997; 11(3):358–366

103. Faglia E, Manuela M, Gino M, Quarantiello A, Signorini M. A combined conservative approach in the treatment of a severe Achilles tendon region ulcer in a diabetic patient: A case report. *Wounds.* 11(5):105–109.

104. Campoccia D, Doherty P, Radice M. Semisynthetic resorbable materials from hyaluronan esterification. *Biomaterials.* 1998; 19:2101–2127.

105. Harris PA, Di Francesco F, Barisoni D, Leigh IM, Navsaria HA. Use of hyaluronic acid and cultured autologous keratinocytes and fibroblast in extensive burns. *Lancet.* 1999; 353(1):35–36.

106. Krouskop TA, Garber SL, Cullen BB. Factors to consider in selecting a support surface. In: Krasner D, ed. *Chronic Wound Care: A Clinical Source Book for Healthcare Professionals.* King of Prussia, PA: Health Management Publications, Inc.; 1990:142–151.

107. Ovington LG. Dressings and Adjunctive Therapies. AHCPR Guidelines revisited. *Ostomy Wound Management.* 1999; 45(suppl 1A):94S–106S.

108. Perricone N, Kerstein MD, Kirsner RS, Norman RA, Phillips TJ. How to approach acute and chronic wound healing in the elderly. *Wounds.* 1999; 11(6):145–151.

109. Wahl SM, Arend WP, Ross R. The effect of complement depletion on wound healing. *Am J Pathol.* 1974; 75(1):73–89.

110. Schmidtchen A. Degradation of antiproteinases, complement and fibronectin in chronic leg ulcers. *Acta Derm Venerol.* 2000; 80(3):179–184.

111. Barron LG, Meyer KB, Szoka FC. Effects of complement depletion on the pharmacokinetics and gene delivery mediated by cationic lipid-DNA complexes. *Hum Gene Ther.* 1998; 9(3):315–323.

112. Papantonio C. Alternative medicine and wound healing. *Ostomy Wound Manage.* 1998; 44(4):44–50.

CHAPTER 15

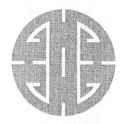

Establishing Community Based Screening Programs

The prevention of disease or mitigation of disability can improve a person's quality of life at any age. Anyone can benefit from gains in function, fewer periods of acute illness, more days free of disability, and less need for long-term care.[1] Prevention strategies can also conserve health resources. In 1988, those over age 65 years represented 12% of the population, but they accounted for more than 30% ($175 billion) of public health care costs.[2] Health care expenditures by older people totaled $73 billion, an average of $2394 per person.[2,3] Expenditures for health care grew from 13% in 1977 to an average of more than 18% of an elderly individual's 1988 personal income. Since the older age group is the fastest growing segment of the population, these health care cost estimates signal the need to examine strategies that might lower expenditures, such as health promotion and disease prevention, for those over age 65 years. In the next 25 years, the number of people over the age of 60 years will double; and those over 85 years are projected to increase more than any other age group.[5]

Nearly $1 of every $4 spent on health care each year can be attributed to behavioral factors, including crime, drug abuse, and the use of alcohol and to-bacco; therefore behavior accounts for $171 billion of the $666 billion Americans spend on health care.[2] The health care crisis cannot be successfully resolved unless damaging patterns of behavior are altered. Twenty-two billion dollars in annual health care costs are attributable to cigarette smoking and other forms of tobacco use, and alcohol abuse may add another $85 billion a year. Other behavioral cost factors include failure to use technology like seat belts and smoke detectors, failure to have routine medical check-ups that could expose cancer and other treatable conditions, and participating in dangerous recreational activities.

There are many factors that contribute to the concept of "successful aging,"[6] the most important of which is optimal health. The human being's resiliency is incredible. It allows many elderly individuals to function adequately with considerable degrees of disability because of their inconceivably large amount of reserve. A person's ability to function independently is closely associated with optimum health status because it impacts the ability of the elderly person to successfully reside in the community at the highest possible level of independence rather than being institutionalized. Other factors that directly impact an individual's ability to maintain independence in the community are adequate financing and the individual's support system (e.g., significant others such as family, kin, friends, or church).[7] In a report published by the Department of Health and Human Services, this conclusion was reached:

> Many analysts of the Medicaid program argue that one of the major problems of both Medicare and Medicaid is the total reliance on institutional care, acute hospital care, and long-term nursing home care. Presently under Medicaid, approximately 70 percent of total program dollars are spent on institutional care: 33 percent in hospitals, 37 percent in long-term care facilities. According to these analysts, both forms of institutional care are some of the more expensive available options. The critics of Medicaid's heavy reliance on institutional care argue that Medicaid incorrectly emphasizes curing the ills of the elderly as opposed to preserving the health of the elderly. They state that in order to increase the preventive aspects of Medicaid, both the federal and state government should encourage the growth of community-based alternatives to institutional care. They argue that in many cases people who could live on their own with very little help with shopping, cooking, or medical care are inappropriately placed in nursing homes.[8]

The allocation of resources focuses on long-term care in an institutional setting like nursing homes rather than on preventative care, a costly alternative. There is a gap in the system between the income support provided to the "well" elderly and the intense health care provided to the "sick" elderly. There is nothing in between. Physical and Occupational therapists have a unique opportunity to demonstrate innovation and leadership in the development of community screening programs that combine health care, personal care, and social maintenance; maximize effective preventive approaches; use the special knowledge of physical rehabilitation potentials to reduce unnecessary institutionalization; and ensure proper use of limited resources. This chapter focuses on screening programs that are community based and enhance the elderly individual's ability to maintain the highest level of physical functioning and independence.

Physical problems affecting the older adult are often undetected until they cause a debilitating loss in the person's capability to independently maintain activities of daily living (ADLs) and functional ambulation. The complications of many chronic diseases can be minimized or prevented by early detection through community based screening programs, regular medical care, environmental adaptations to facilitate function, and fitness programs that promote independence and the overall well being of the elderly. Few elders have annual physical checkups, and rarely, if ever, are functional limitations directly ad-

dressed. In light of this, preventive screening programs have the triple benefit of identifying high-risk individuals, detecting medical and physical problems, and preventing them from progressing into a loss of functional independence.

PREVENTION/HEALTH PROMOTION

Every day clinical experiences in working with the elderly reveal that prevention is probably the single most effective strategy for any significant gains in their functional and health status. Even the policymakers and third-party payers, in their efforts at cost containment, are showing particular interest and greater acceptance of the role that prevention and health promotion can play in decreasing the overall costs of medical care for the aged[9] and improving the quality of life by the avoidance of institutionalization. Many chronic illnesses that affect health and functional status are not merely part of the aging process. The elderly understand and appreciate the impact that life-style, behavior, and environment have on the development of some possibly preventable diseases, such as heart disease, cancer, and lung disease.[10] Interventions, such as exercise, diet, stress reduction, and smoking cessation, have been shown to positively affect the musculoskeletal, cardiovascular, cardiopulmonary, sensory, and neuromuscular systems (see Chapters 11, 12, and 13). These preventive modalities can lead to corrective and ameliorative changes that have the potential of delaying the onset of pathologies, as well as preventing the disabling effects of existing chronic disease(s).[11] Even in the oldest old population, those 85 years of age and older, research reveals that improvements can be made in every system of the body through exercise.[12] Proper attention to diet significantly modifies the onset of certain disease processes,[13] and the implementation of dietary control in combination with exercise has the potential of reversing, if not avoiding, some pathological manifestations, such as diabetes[14,15] and coronary artery disease.[16] Stress reduction and exercise also have positive effects on hypertension.[17] It is never too late to stop smoking. For example, a study by Rogers and associates[18] showed a significant improvement in cerebral blood flow in elderly subjects who stopped smoking and this improvement happened in a matter of 3 to 5 days. In a relatively short period of time, the abstinence from cigarettes also significantly improves cardiovascular and cardiopulmonary circulation and perfusion.[19] In terms of the quality of life for the elderly, preventive interventions can have a substantial impact on health care needs and days free of disability.

Types of Prevention

There are three levels in preventive health care: primary, secondary, and tertiary. Primary aging is the maturation of an organism exclusively attributable to the passage of time. Primary prevention is the prevention of any ill effects that may occur as a result of microtrauma during that maturation process. The goal of primary prevention is to avoid or delay the onset of debilitating pathologies and functional disabilities. An example would be a fitness program for the well elderly that included aerobic as well as stretching and strengthening exercises to enhance the cardiovascular, musculoskeletal, and neuromuscular systems. Primary prevention is synonymous with health promotion and seeks to prevent disease in susceptible individuals by reducing the exposure to risk factors. The basic interventions include better diet, more exercise, smoking cessation, better sanitation, and accident prevention. Primary prevention uses education to encourage individuals to modify behaviors.

Secondary aging relates to systemic or organ-specific changes associated with either acute or chronic disease. Secondary prevention is the implementation of therapeutic interventions at the earliest possible time within the acute phase of an illness. For instance, with pneumonia, the early intervention with chest physical therapy and the early resumption of ambulation and exercise avoids the debilitating effects of bed rest and increases the individual's ability to ward off the infection.[20] Secondary prevention in chronic illness deals with the earliest possible intervention to reverse or maintain existing impairments and prevent further deficits from impeding maximal functional capabilities of the elderly individual. Screening programs are the hallmark of secondary prevention at the community level.

Tertiary aging refers to functional impairments that have already progressed to the level of disability (see Chapter 9) and impede ADLs. Tertiary prevention attempts to minimize the ill effects of diseases once they have occurred and to rehabilitate the elderly individual's residual capacities. Functional activities and therapeutic interventions, such as proprioceptive neuromuscular facilitation (PNF) and Bobath techniques, in addition to strength and endurance training, are all important elements in restoring function and preventing further decline in chronic illnesses.

Webster[21] states, "It is increasingly clear that what was previously accepted as normal primary aging actually relates much more to unappreciated secondary or tertiary influences." Preventive measures that address the most prevalent diseases, such as heart disease, cancer, and cerebral vascular accidents, are particularly applicable in the elderly population. There is a correlation between healthful interventions like diet and exercise and the development of disease, and there is compelling evidence that suggests that the control of risks, such as smoking, an unhealthy diet, high blood pressure, physical inactivity, and exposure to toxic substances in the environment, could significantly diminish the prevalence of the three leading causes of death in the United States.[10]

HEALTH PROBLEMS IN THE ELDERLY/ SYMPTOM PREVALENCE

Studies estimate that of the US population who are 65 years of age and older, 86% have at least one chronic disease that limits their functional activities and decreases the number of "disability-free" days progressively with advancing age.[22] Chronic diseases that affect older adults are sometimes misidentified as normal age changes and can go untreated for years.

Heart disease, cancer, and cerebral vascular disease cause almost 70% of deaths in the United States.[10] According to the National Center for Health Statistics, the elderly population is afflicted (in decreasing order of frequency) by arthritis (48%), heart disease (40%), hypertension (39%), cataracts (36%), diabetes (28%), cancer (26%), osteoporosis/hip fracture (16%), and stroke (9%). Comorbidites are common, and the frequency of these disorders increases with advancing age.[23]

The major causes of fraility and disability in the elderly relate to the broad functional problems of immobility and instability. Intellectual impairment is also a major component of functional decline. Confounding factors with the elderly include depression and transient dementias, isolation, urinary and bowel incontinence, sexual dysfunction, immune deficiency and infections, malnutrition, sleep disorders, impairment of sensory abilities, and iatrogenesis. Many of the health problems of the elderly are especially well suited for preventive efforts. For instance, impaired mobility, injuries, sensory loss, adverse drug reactions, deconditioning due to lack of exercise, depression, malnutrition, alcohol abuse, hypertension and cardiovascular disease, cancers, osteoporosis, urinary incontinence, and abuse and neglect are all preventable or can be postponed as a result of screening programs that identify these problems and follow-up intervention to address each individual's risk factors.

SCREENING CONCERNS IN THE ELDERLY

Planning preventive care packages and counseling approaches for older people requires special considerations. Most older people suffer from one or more chronic diseases or syndromes and total risk increases as a function of the number of individual risk factors.[24]

Screening tests and lab standards have not been developed or adapted specifically for the elderly.[25] "Aging, even without disease, changes physiology, which can alter lab test results."[26] Most of the normal lab values are based on 20- 40-year-old subjects. This makes it difficult to determine what is abnormal in terms of a test result in the elderly. Aside from lab values, normal physiological changes of aging and the use of medications to treat chronic diseases may mask the symptoms of other physical problems.

Some diseases and conditions, such as coronary heart disease, may manifest themselves differently in older patients than in younger.[27] For example, an elevated serum cholesterol level becomes less predictive of heart related morbidity in an older individual. In fact, a low serum cholesterol level is a predictor of mortality in people of advanced age,[28] because they are associated with an increased risk of cancer and hemorrhagic stroke.

Some chronic conditions common in old age have competing risk factors. For example, obesity is a major risk factor for heart disease, diabetes, and other chronic diseases, but modest obesity is protective for osteoporosis.[29] Conversely, low body weight is a significant risk factor for hip fracture.[30]

In older individuals, functional disabilities associated with chronic diseases become as important as preventing the onset of disease.[31] Of the population aged 65 years who live independently, 24% have some degree of functional impairment, 15% are unable to perform major activities, and 11% are less impaired. Of those who are dependent on others for daily care, 6% are in nursing homes and 14% are homebound.[22]

What to Screen for

Many diseases can be prevented or forestalled by identifying and avoiding high-risk behaviors, while others can be treated in the early stages, thereby reducing the risk of disability or death. Yearly physical assessments are the preferred method for identifying problems, however, the majority of people 65 years of age and over do not seek medical attention on an annual basis. As a result of initiatives implemented by the surgeon general in the early 1980s, many agencies now offer preventive health programs, including screening for high-risk behaviors and the presence of disease. The costs associated with the treatment of chronic disease are clearly not desirable in today's malnourished economy. Health screening and early detection of disease processes can reduce costs substantially.

Screening programs for the elderly need to address behavior patterns, such as smoking, level of activity, dietary habits, living environment, health care needs such as dental and foot care, and immunization history. These programs aim to determine what the problems are, and how to address them from an educational perspective. Ideally, screening programs should have a follow-up mechanism or referral sources for evaluating and treating physical or medical problems identified during the screening. Screening programs for the elderly can be holistic, and screen all systems of the body, or they can be system or disease specific (e.g., blood pressure screening, diabetes screening, cholesterol screening, or dental screening).

Primary prevention screening programs include immunizations, accident prevention, exercise programs, posture and flexibility assessment, nutritional modifications, and smoking and alcohol cessation. Secondary prevention screening focuses on early detection and treatment and is particularly applicable in disorders such as hypertension, vision and hearing impairments, musculoskeletal problems, neuromuscular involvement, depression, and iatrogenic adverse drug affects. Tertiary preventive screening focuses on functional assessment and maximizing physical potential and environmental efficiency to prevent the progression of functional decline.

The United States Preventive Services Task Force[32,33] has identified screening interventions that successfully alter the outcomes of various diseases, and emphasizes the importance of educating the elderly population in high-risk behavior modification. For instance, the Task Force advised that elderly individuals be provided with educational material regarding the benefits of physical activity in disease prevention and that guidance in establishing appropriate exercise levels and selected modes of exercise be provided on an individual basis to each person screened. Other components in the Task Forces recommendations include smoking cessation programs; dietary modification to prevent diseases associated with dietary excesses or imbalances (e.g., osteoporosis, heart disease, some cancers, cerebral vascular accidents, or dental diseases); alcohol cessation programs when abuse is identified; home modification screening to reduce the potential for accidental injuries; vaccination programs for pneumococcal, influenza, and tetanus immunization; and screening for preventive "chemoprophylaxis" programs, such as low-dose aspirin therapy (325 mg every other day) for those at risk for cardiovascular diseases and estrogen replacement therapy for women who are at increased risk of developing osteoporosis.

Prescreening for High-Risk Populations

Before a comprehensive community based screening program is initiated, it is valuable to prescreen the community served to identify groups within the older population that would benefit from specific health screening procedures. Health questionnaires or interviews are helpful tools in identifying subgroups within the elderly population that may require special attention (e.g., diabetes mellitus, cardiovascular or pulmonary problems, a decrease in functional ADLs, or foot problems). There are some particularly valuable prescreening tools available. For instance, the Self-Evaluation of Life Function questionnaire developed by Linn and Linn[34] includes questions about health behaviors, existing diseases, symptoms, level of basic and instrumental ADLs, medication use, cognitive status, and socioeconomic well-being.

Another useful tool for prescreening the community elderly is the Health Hazard Appraisal (HHA), which is used in many preventive health care programs in both the United States and Canada[35] to determine high-risk populations for screening in community based settings. Safer[35] demonstrated that through the use of the HHA prescreening tool, Milwaukee residents reduced their health risk by 32% as a result of the health screening, follow-up counseling, and interventions that were employed to address the health care needs determined by the prescreening. The HHA prescreening is based on the assumption that "an individual's response to health threats depends on how he or she feels physically rather than on a rational calculation of health benefits and risks." The HHA is a valuable educational tool. By questioning elderly individuals and generating a "health hazard score," it informs people about how their health habits and life-styles affect their probability of dying within 10 years from potentially preventable causes. The HHA also helps to target the population that are most likely to benefit from health screening and follow-up counseling and intervention programs.

Secondary Prevention Screening Tests

Screening and assessments necessary for health promotion in the elderly should include the evaluation of the presence of chronic diseases; symptoms that may suggest the presence of disease; health habits including nutrition, exercise and activity levels, smoking, medication use, and substance abuse; the evaluation of musculoskeletal, neuromuscular, and sensory deficits; safety; and mental status.

Cardiovascular Disease

Routine monitoring of blood pressure is an important component in controlling and reducing high blood pressure. Individuals with diagnosed high blood pressure need to be counseled regarding appropriate exercise levels, weight reduction, dietary sodium reduction and alcohol consumption. Periodic screening with the finding of persistent high blood pressure (e.g., greater than 140/90 mm Hg) may direct the health care professional to refer the individual for possible drug therapy to control excessively high blood pressure. Routine monitoring of the ECG is recommended in individuals who are symptomatic (e.g., had a previously positive ECG, angina, or dyspnea on exertion), but it is not recommended for those elderly who as asymptomatic. Though somewhat controversial, total serum cholesterol measurements are often employed to determine the presence of elevated blood cholesterol levels that have also been shown to place an individual at a higher risk for the development of cardiovascular diseases.

Cardiovascular screening should also include weight monitoring, and in those individuals who are 20% overweight by the height/weight standards, appropriate dietary and exercise counseling should be implemented as a preventive measure. Additionally, information on transient ischemic attacks, the presence of diabetes mellitus, cardiac arrhythmias, clau-

dication, and any musculoskeletal limitations that place the individual at a high risk of developing problems associated with inactivity should be recorded and monitored. Peripheral vascular status and skin condition are important to evaluate, especially in the diabetic or someone with known peripheral vascular disease.

Cancer

There is little agreement as to the efficacy of screening for cancer in the elderly, and there is conflicting data regarding the accuracy and efficiency of the screening strategies in all ages (e.g., breast exams, mammography, and Papanicolaou [Pap] testing). Because certain cancers are more easily treated if diagnosed early, the consensus is that regular screening for cancer is recommended until more substantial evidence is presented that negates the value of the screening strategies in question. *Summary of Current Guidelines for the Cancer-Related Checkup: Recommendations,*[36] the recommendations for cancer screening are:

■ Annual Pap smears and pelvic examinations for all women who are sexually active or are 18 years of age or older. After three consecutive normal annual examinations, Pap tests may be performed less frequently or at the discretion of the physician.
■ Endometrial tissue samples at menopause for women who are at high risk.
■ Baseline mammogram between 35 and 39 years of age. Repeat every two years from age 40 to 49 and annually thereafter.
■ Breast physical examination every three years for women between 20 and 40 years of age and yearly thereafter.
■ Breast self-examination monthly for all women 20 years and older.
■ Stool guaiac slide test every year for men and women over 50.
■ A sigmoidoscopic examination every three to five years for men and women over age 50.
■ Yearly digital/rectal examination for men and women over age 40 to screen for prostate and rectal cancer.
■ Cancer examination and health counseling every three years after age 20 and yearly after age 40.

The second most common neoplasm in the United States is colorectal cancer, and it also has the second highest mortality rate.[36] Sigmoidoscopy and fecal occult blood testing are important in the early detection of this disease, especially in a known high-risk population (e.g., family or personal history of cancer, colonic polyps, or inflammatory bowel disease). High-risk patients include those with ulcerative colitis involving the entire colon with a duration of seven or more years, a past history of an adenoma of the colon, or a past history of colon cancer or female genital cancer.[37] Early detection is particularly important in colorectal cancer as the survival rate in asymptomatic patients is 90% compared to 43% in those with more advanced disease.[37] Once symptoms of colorectal cancer occur, the disease is usually in an advanced and nonlocalized stage, which decreases the likelihood of successful surgical removal. There are home screening tests for occult blood that are reliable and available through a pharmacist, however, the tests require several stool smears over a 3 day period with dietary restrictions and are difficult to accurately accomplish when elders have physical or cognitive deficits. Cost effectiveness studies clearly indicate that the early detection of colorectal cancer significantly reduces the overall medical costs and improves survival.[38]

Breast cancer is the second leading cause of cancer deaths in women, and of those deaths, 50% occur in women over the age of 65 years[39] and 75% of all breast cancers occur in women over the age of 50 years.[40] There is some controversy regarding the accuracy of both self-breast exams and mammography, however, it is recommended that breast examination be taught to all women, especially to those over the age of 50, and that a breast self-examination be done monthly. After the age of 40, the American Cancer Society recommends that women have a breast examination by a physician and a mammogram annually.[36]

Cervical cancer is accurately detected by a Pap test, however, many older women do not have Pap smears on a regular basis. For the most part, women diagnosed with cervical cancer after the age of 65 years are usually in the advanced stages of the disease, and 41% of all deaths from cervical cancer occur in women over the age of 65 years. Yearly screening using the Pap smear for three consecutive years is recommended by the American Cancer Society.[36] If the test is negative for three years it is recommended that Pap tests be done at the discretion of the physician or at least once every five years thereafter.

Digital rectal examination is the best way to screen for prostate cancer in men. The American Cancer Society recommends that men receive a yearly screening for prostate cancer after the age of 40, and every three to five years after the age of 50 as the greatest incidence of this form of cancer occurs in the age range of 40 to 50 years.

A total skin examination is an important part of the routine physical examination. Inspection of the mouth is also recommended for those who are known smokers and for those who use excessive amounts of alcohol. Seventy-five percent of deaths from oral cancers occur in individuals 55 years of age and older.[41] Screening for oral cancer can be done routinely during periodic dental care, however, many elderly individuals do not go to the dentist on a regular basis, and it is recommended that oral screening be done by the physician or other health care personnel at community based screening clinics and health fairs since it is a noninvasive assessment.

Diabetes Mellitus

Over 4.5 million people in the United States over the age of 65 have diabetes mellitus.[41a] Diabetes has been found to contribute to cardiovascular diseases, end-stage renal failure, amputations, blindness, and peripheral neuropathies.[42] The American Diabetes Association[42] recommends that periodic serum glucose measurements be taken in the elderly population as the incidence of diabetes mellitus increases exponentially with increasing age. In known diabetics, the recommendations include periodic testing for asymptomatic bacteriuria, hematuria, and proteinuria by urinalysis screening.

Osteoporosis

The elderly population, particularly white females over the age of 60, have the highest risk for developing osteoporosis. Subtle changes in posture related to the breakdown of vertebral body height directly affect the individual's flexibility and strength. The person may report that he or she is "shrinking," or that he or she has pain in the cervical, thoracic, or lumbar region(s) of the back. Because height changes are frequently the first clinical indication of osteoporosis, regular screening should include height measurement. Reed and Birge[43] found that 75% of the elderly that they screened who had a 2 inch loss in height had osteoporotic changes on x-ray. Measuring height is a reliable, inexpensive, and noninvasive screening tool for osteoporosis.

Other valuable screening information for the evaluation for osteoporosis include nutritional information and dietary habits (e.g., calcium intake, excessive caffeine or soda consumption, or excessive protein intake), level of activity or inactivity, family history of osteoporosis, and alcohol and tobacco consumption. All of these factors have been found to have a contributory effect toward the development of osteoporosis. Low estrogen levels in women have also been found to influence the integrity of bone.[44] It is particularly important in postmenopausal women that height measurements be taken periodically to screen for osteoporotic changes. Since osteoporosis contributes to more than 1 million fractures in people over the age of 65 years annually,[44] screening becomes a vital component in the identification of risk factors and the prevention of accidental injury.

Health Habits

Nutrition, exercise levels, smoking, substance abuse, and medication use need to be considered when screening the elderly. Optimal health is the key factor in maintaining an independent and productive life. Health promotion and disease prevention activities have the potential of interrupting or slowing the progression of aging and disease before pathological changes become irreversible. The expected outcome of health promotion must reach beyond longevity toward an acceptable quality of life without debilitating physical or mental disabilities.[23,45] Preventive measures seek to detect the precursors that allow for early intervention and risk factors for disease that can be modified,[45a] because modification of personal health habits could have a potential impact on disease outcomes. For instance, smoking cessation improves physical stamina and lessens susceptibility to infections, while it reduces the risk of lung cancer and heart disease.[10]

To meet the needs of the elderly population, health care practitioners involved in screening strategies should educate individuals on ways to promote good health by adopting better life-style habits and a safer local environment; assist people to identify their own genetic/familial predispositions and risk factors for specific diseases; and promote public awareness of the myths, as well as the realities, pertaining to good health.[29]

One of the most significant advances in the past decade has been the convergence of opinion on what constitutes a "proper diet." Two documents, the 1988 *Surgeon General's Report on Nutrition and Health*[46] and the 1989 National Research Council's *Report on Diet and Health,*[47] summarize the consensus of the scientific community and make dietary and health recommendations for the general public,[48] including reducing dietary fats and cholesterol; limiting salt intakes; limiting the use of alcohol; maintaining adequate but not excessive protein intakes; eating more fruits, vegetables, and complex carbohydrates; balancing caloric intake with expenditure to maintain a healthy weight; and avoiding the use of dietary supplements in excess of the NRC's recommended dietary allowances (RDAs). Both documents caution against unsafe dietary practices, health fads, and outright health fraud, much of which is directed at older persons.[46] Screening for nutritional problems is best accomplished by a registered dietitian, however, if this is not feasible, the collection of information on socioeconomic status, food supply, eating patterns, and self-perceived nutritional and dietary status is valuable in establishing the need for further counseling and education.

The effects of inactivity mimic the effects of aging.[49] Almost 50% of the functional decline attributed to aging may, in fact, be related to inactivity.[50] Increasing energy expenditure through exercise appears to influence mortality and morbidity through a number of complex physiological mechanisms (see Chapter 13).

Despite these benefits, there has been some reluctance in recommending fitness programs for elderly because exercising too intensely may injure muscles or joints, provoke heart attacks and irregular heart rhythms, increase blood pressure, and increase fall-related fractures.[51] Regular exercise training can increase protein turnover (37% higher muscle catabolism) in the elderly. As a result, elderly individuals prescribed an exercise program should be advised to increase their protein intake.[52] Some elderly are unable to maintain high-intensity training programs because of the weight reductions association with the loss of lean muscle mass.[53] Therefore special attention to the dietary needs of the exercising elder need to be considered when prescribing a fitness program. It is important to determine the intensity, duration, and frequency of physical training to delay declines in functional capacity. These variables vary from one elderly individual to the next.

Combined with a calorie-appropriate diet, regular physical activity maintains a reasonable body weight, delays loss of lean muscle mass, and promotes good physical performance. A high activity level can predict survival for both institutionalized and people living in the community aged 60 to 80.[54,55] High-intensity training appears to decrease fat cell hypertension, increase insulin resistance, and slow the rate of decline of VO_2 max in older persons.[56–58]

Exercise programs designed for the elderly can reduce bone loss and strengthen skeletal muscle in both men and women of very advanced age,[56–59] thus decreasing the risk of falls and fractures.[60,61] For example, a group of sedentary men and women aged 86 to 96 years, including those with a past history of falling, increased the strength in the knee extensors by as much as 167% to 180% after an 8 week course in weight-lifting exercise.

It is never too late to quit smoking. At any age, cigarette smoking imposes higher risks of coronary heart disease, lung and mouth cancers, stroke, and osteoporosis.[62] Smoking cessation results in a decline of body nicotine within 6 months, a reduced risk of sudden heart attack in 1 to 2 years, and a lowered risk of cancer in about 15 years. Smoking combined with low calorie intakes can also compromise vitamin C status, which is essential in wound healing, infection, and maintenance of the connective tissue health. Smokers take two to three times longer to heal wounds, require longer to recover from acute illnesses such as pneumonia, and are twice as likely to die prematurely of coronary artery disease.[62]

The use of medications is another risk factor to look for when screening an elderly population. The 1991 National Disease and Therapeutic Index indicates that 42.7% of all prescription drugs are doled out to people 60 years of age and older in the United States. The average number of prescriptions per elderly American is 15.7, and there are over 9 million adverse drug reactions in people over the age of 65 years each year.[63] Normal aging results in changes in the way older adults absorb, metabolize, distribute, and excrete medications. The half-life of drugs is longer in the elderly and the cumulative effects of drugs last longer. Because the elderly are often existing on polypharmacy, they are more likely to overdose and experience adverse effects when medication combinations are inappropriate. Falls and fractures can be related to drug effects, for instance, β-blockers often induce an orthostatic hypotensive response on standing. Certain drugs actually induce neurological symptoms, such as tardive dyskinesia and parkinsonism, and many drugs create mental impairment. These drugs are discussed more thoroughly in Chapter 8. Additionally, noncompliance has been found to be a problem in close to 50% of the elderly.[63] Wolf and co-workers[63] found that the factors related to older persons not taking their medications were financial difficulties, language barriers, sensory deficits, accidental overdoses, and cognitive impairments.

Pharmacists often evaluate and monitor medication problems that may occur, but the elderly do not always go to the same pharmacy. Over 13% of all expenditures for medications by the elderly are for over-the-counter medications, which makes monitoring that much more difficult.[64] Screening and education for medication use often takes the form of health education programs combined with a review of current medications by a pharmacist or nurse in a community screening program.

According to Maddox[65] over 5% of the elderly population abuse, alcohol. Late-onset alcohol related problems occur in less than 1% of the elderly, however, because most were abusers before reaching the age of 65 years.[65] In addition, as an individual ages the alcohol tolerance diminishes: Less alcohol is required to produce intoxication in the elderly, so dependency may develop at a level of drinking that would not cause addiction in a younger individual. Willenbrig and Spring[66] have developed a screening tool that contains four questions and is accurate for identifying alcohol abuse 95% of the time. One question is designed to elicit subtle defensiveness while the other three directly ask about drinking habits and patterns. While individual screening by health care professionals is recommended, mass screening is not because of the low incidence of late-onset alcoholism and the fact that the screening has not been shown to lead to a decrease in morbidity or mortality.[28]

Drug abuse is not an issue in the elderly population. It can be expected, however, that as those individuals who use substances, such as cocaine, heroin, marijuana, and so forth, age, drug abuse may become a significant problem.

Sensory Deficits

Visual acuity testing in asymptomatic older adults should be done routinely. Although many older persons maintain nearly normal vision, their eyesight is subject to various changes and disabilities as discussed in Chapters 3 and 5. Yearly eye exams are recommended to detect the presence or progression of presbyopia, as well as the presence of disease. Three disorders—cataracts, glaucoma, and senile macular degeneration—are commonly found through screening.[28]

Anyone with impaired hearing should receive an otoscopic examination and audiometric testing. Between 30% and 60% of people over age 65 and up to 90% of nursing home residents in that age group are estimated to suffer from some degree of hearing loss.[67] Screening for hearing loss can range from a thorough history and interview of family members to testing by a clinical audiologist. A tuning fork is a wonderful screening tool. According to Alpert,[68] if the health care provider can hear the fork's hum when the client can no longer hear it and visual inspection of the ear shows no gross pathology (e.g., cerumen, serous otitis), then there is a hearing deficit. With a suspected hearing deficit, a more definitive audiometric screening by a trained individual can be easily employed in a community setting.

Psychological Problems

Elderly individuals should be specifically screened for depression and the potential for suicide. This screening needs to include a family history of depression/suicide, the presence of a chronic illness, recent loss (real or perceived), problems with sleep disorders, the presence of multiple somatic complaints, recent divorce or separation, unemployment, alcohol abuse, living alone, and the presence of prolonged bereavement. Depression is more prevalent in the older population than any other age group. White men, in particular, are at the highest risk for suicide. Alpert[68] recommended the Beck Depression Inventory as a reliable test in elderly populations.

Dementia

The Mental Status Questionnaire, Fact-Hand Test, and Dementia Rating Scale are frequently used along with screening for other mental, neurological, and physical deficits to determine if patients are suffering from dementia. In the early stages, however, it is difficult to distinguish true dementia from depression, the adverse effects of medication, and other mental and physical illnesses. Screening can only determine whether or not a problem exists, not what the underlying cause is. Magaziner and associates[69] were able to show that a shortened version of the Mini-mental Status Examination could be used as a reliable predictor of scores on the longer version of the test. The shortened version makes screening easier and more cost effective.

Urinary Incontinence

Urinary incontinence affects a significant number of elderly persons. In fact, urinary incontinence contributes to nursing home admission in nearly half of the elderly admitted to long-term care facilities. Women have a weakening of the muscles of the pelvic floor and abdomen following pregnancy, which can be treated with Kegal exercises. In addition, birth injuries, hormonal changes, infections, tumors, or side effects of medications may cause urinary incontinence. Men develop urinary incontinence most often because of bladder or prostate disease. Causes of urinary incontinence need to be determined to prevent the need for institutionalization.

Safety

Elderly individuals account for almost 30% of all accidental deaths and about 15% of all hospitalized accident victims. Baker and Harvey[70] report that for every fall that results in a hip fracture, the incidence of mortality is higher. Decreased mobility, reduced independence, and a higher incidence of illness are common after a hip fracture. Impaired hearing and eyesight, slower physical reactions, poor balance and coordination, circulatory changes, orthostatic hypotension, and decreased physical stamina are among the reasons for the high accident rate in elders. For these reasons it is important to assess the older adult's risk for falls as well as the presence of fall hazards in the home. The US Consumer Product Safety Commission has developed a "Home Safety Checklist for Older Consumers" to help spot possible safety problems in the home. These were distributed through Area Agencies on Aging (AAAs) to senior centers, public health departments, and other community groups. Copies may be obtained from the US Consumer Safety Commission, Washington, DC, 20207.

PRIMARY PREVENTION

Advancing primary prevent for those over the age of 65 requires a change in attitude that accepts the growing proof that individuals of any age may benefit from adopting health-promoting behaviors.[27] The attitude that diseases of old age are irreversible and inevitable needs to be dismissed. Life expectancy has been extended, accounting for the growth in population of those over the age of 85. In fact, those who are presently age 65 years can expect to live an average additional 17 years (19 years for women and 14.5 years for men).[22]

Primary preventive efforts directed at personal health practices are among the most effective interventions available to health care practitioners caring for older adults. Traditional clinical activities, such as routine unfocused testing, are generally of less value in preventing disease than counseling. Although demonstrated advantages of preventive services for older people are limited, emerging research is quite convincing. For instance, research on cancer etiology suggests that a 10- to 20-year latent period exists between events that may induce some cancers and the clinical expression of disease. Based on an average 15-year latency period, cancer detected after age 70 could have begun between ages 55 and 60 years. Therefore, many of the quarter of a million cancers induced in people after age 60 might have been prevented by primary prevention measures,

such as smoking cessation and dietary changes.[71] Comprehensive screening strategies should be tailored to the individual risk profile of each elderly person.

Older individuals are more susceptible to acute diseases and episodes, such as infections, pneumonia, food poisoning, and orthostatic hypotension with resulting falls and injury.[72] Most of these conditions are preventable with proper intervention to maintain optimum health, thereby warding off these acute episodes. The growth of community "wellness" services or activities for older people signals a growing commitment to postponing disease and disabilities in older persons. Using Title IIIB grants from the federal government in response to Surgeon General Koop's efforts, 37 states had initiated community wellness programs for the elderly by 1985.[72]

Over the past 20 years, some of the major causes of morbidity and mortality in old age have declined, although the extent to which health promotion efforts are responsible has not been determined. Over these two decades, stroke deaths declined 55%, heart attacks decreased by 40%, and substantial progress had been made in hypertension control.[1] Evidence indicates that those who reach old age in good health tend to stay healthy until shortly before death, often well into the seventh or eighth decade of life.[73]

A COMMUNITY BASED SCREENING PROGRAM/MODEL PROJECT

Screening for Foot Problems

Many systemic diseases manifest themselves in the lower extremity, including diabetes, peripheral vascular disease, heart and kidney disease, arthritis, and nutritional deficiencies.[74–76] Many orthopedic conditions, arising from long-standing biomechanical imbalances, ill-fitting shoes, or both, plague the elderly patient and interfere with functional mobility. The most common foot disorders in individuals over the age of 65 years include pes planus (flat feet), excessive calluses, hallux abducto valgus, painful bunions, and toe deformities.[76,77] With advancing age the plantar fat pads atrophy,[78] resulting in increased stress on and microtrauma to the underlying soft tissue and osseous structures. Degenerative joint diseases compromise the articular surfaces of the joints of the foot, interfering with weight bearing and leading to decreased mobility. Circulatory changes further compromise the integrity of the tissues of the foot. Elders may not even be aware of losses in sensation to pain, pressure, and temperature. The loss of "protective sensation" to shoe pressures, wrinkles in the socks, or foreign objects in the shoe may be the beginning of a pressure point that may quickly become a callus or an open sore, which, if let untreated, may develop ulceration, infection, or gangrene, and lead to eventual amputation.[77–80] Routine foot screenings can help eliminate small problems and keep them from becoming larger.

Foot problems are the fourth leading cause of complaint in institutionalized elderly individuals.[75] Lack of ambulation and the ability to independently get to the bathroom are often reasons for admission to nursing homes. Individuals who are mobile and ambulatory in their own homes and community retain their dignity and generally live longer than those who are immobilized or institutionalized.[74,79]

Low-income elders are particularly at risk for poor foot care, because podiatric services are not covered by insurance companies. Elders who are on a fixed pension or receive a small social security check cannot afford out-of-pocket visits to have toe nails cut. Medicare will not cover the cost of protective shoe gear for the diabetic person at risk for amputation, but it will cover the cost of shoes following an amputation (as part of the prosthetic costs). Complications from foot problems are the cause of 20% of all diabetic admissions to hospitals, and 50% of all non-traumatic amputations is enormous. Inpatient hospitalization, surgical procedures, and rehabilitation programs including prostheses, result in costs of $10,000 to $30,000. Both the personal and financial impacts of foot problems in diabetic patients are of serious magnitude. Findings from the Medicare Shoe Demonstration Project strongly supports the cost benefits of providing protective foot gear to diabetic patients.[80,82]

Low-income elders often wear shoes that are inadequate, ill-fitting, and therefore, dangerous. Ill-fitting shoes may create excessive pressure to the foot or repetitive pressures leading to foot lesions that are difficult to heal in the diabetic. Ill-fitting shoes increase the likelihood of falling and hip fractures are a major factor in the morbidity of elders.[83]

Medicare's lack of reimbursement for routine foot care forces elders to attempt self-care of the feet. Limited limb mobility, decreased eyesight, diminished sensation, and unsteady hands may lead to wounds that fail to heal and result in eventual amputation.

Foot care is a unique medical specialty that contributes to the physical, psychological, and social health of the elderly individual. Delivery of a comprehensive foot care program reduces the problems associated with foot pain and discomfort, lower extremity fatigue, and the secondary problems associated with lack of ambulation.

The "Community Foot Care Project" servicing low income elders in 14 communities in Central Massachusetts was inspired by the nonambulatory status of patients that were being admitted to hospitals and nursing homes. In one nursing home, 72% (based on an unpublished clinical data collection at Cushing Hospital in Framingham, Massachusetts) of the patients returned to an ambulatory status after receiving foot care, shoes, and orthotics. Preventing foot problems was key to keeping the community elders from becoming institutionalized elders. The foot care program was developed to screen low-income elders in the community for foot and medical problems, provide education on foot care, and dispense orthotics and free shoes.

The Foot Care Project uses an interdisciplinary team of a community coordinator, social worker, podiatrist, and physical therapist who work together to provide 18 community clinics held yearly in 14 different communities. The community coordinator schedules the clinics at community senior centers, and the social worker takes a detailed medical history on the 18 to 20 patients seen at each clinic. A podiatrist renders free nail cutting and debridement of excessive calluses, and the physical therapist evaluates the elder person for lower extremity problems and specific foot dysfunction using the screening tool shown in Figure 15–1. After the initial evaluation in the community setting, if the screening reveals foot dysfunction or biomechanical problems leading to functional losses, the patient is scheduled for an outpatient clinic visit for orthotic fabrication and shoe distribution by the physical therapist and physical therapy intervention as needed for musculoskeletal/biomechanical problems. Patients return to the outpatient clinic for 2- and 6-month reassessments. Foot care is taught to family members when patients are unable to care for themselves. Knowledge of foot care (Figure 15–2) is assessed by a questionnaire before and after treatment. Guidelines for foot care by the patient and family are provided and explained at the first visit (Figure 15–3). This project is funded by a Federal III B grant from the Massachusetts Baypath Area Agency on Aging. Over 100 letters were drafted and sent to area stores and manufacturers of shoes asking for donations, which yielded 1500 pairs of shoes. Research projects were also established, with area shoe manufacturers donating 36 to 50 pairs of shoes for each of these projects. Shoe drives among hospital employees also yield numerous pairs of adequate shoes.

Goals for any community foot care program should be to promote pain-free ambulation, restore maximum function, maximize foot care knowledge and safety awareness and decrease hospitalizations related to foot problems.

To meet these goals the following methods are proposed

1. Offer foot care at community centers close to home for the greatest possible participation. (Greater participation was seen when the foot care team went to the patients rather than having them attend a hospital or outpatient-based clinic. For many, lack of transportation was a major deterrent to seeking help and needed foot care.)
2. Establish an easy screening tool that is reliable and highly reproducible.

Foot Screening Tool

Date _____

Name _____

Address _____

Phone (   ) _____

Sex _____ DOB _____

Language or Communication problems: ☐ No
    ☐ Yes   (describe) _____

Primary Doctor/Podiatrist _____

Address _____

Phone (   ) _____

SUBJECTIVE DATA

Medical History: _____
_____

1. Do you have:
    - ☐ Arthritis _____
    - ☐ Circulatory Problems_____
    - ☐ Heart Disease _____
    - ☐ Diabetes Mellitus _____
    - ☐ Kidney Problems _____
    - ☐ High Blood Pressure _____
    - ☐ Foot Problems _____
    - ☐ Eye Problems _____
    - ☐ Thyroid Problems _____
    - ☐ Hearing Problems _____
    - ☐ Vertigo _____
    - ☐ Dizziness _____
    - ☐ Fx hip _____

2. Did you have an injury in the:

		Left Leg		Right Leg	
		Sprain	Fx	Sprain	Fx
No					
Yes	hip				
	knee				
	ankle				
	foot				
	back				

3. Are you experiencing any leg pain?

	Left Leg	Right Leg
No		
Yes Hip		
Knee		

If yes, describe:

Night cramps		
Claudications		
Radiating		

— Continued —

Continued from previous page

4. Are you experiencing any foot pain?

	Left Leg	Right Leg
No		
Yes Aching		
Burning		
Stabbing		
Nail pain		
Shoe pain		
Met heads		
Toes		

Pain increased:	Left Leg	Right Leg
When standing		
When walking		
When wearing shoes		
In the morning		
In the afternoon		
At other times (describe)		

OBJECTIVE DATA

1. Ambulates without assistance?   ☐ No   ☐ Yes

2. Ambulates with assistive devices?   ☐ No   ☐ Yes

cane	
walker	
crutches	
other	

3. Falls? ☐ No ☐ Yes   describe _____

4. Distance ambulated?   ☐ Home   ☐ 1 block   ☐ 2 blocks   ☐ 5 blocks
                             ☐ 1 mile   ☐ Unlimited

5. Regular exercise?   ☐ No   ☐ Yes

Continued

Continued from previous page

6. Examination of Feet (Removing shoes and stockings)

	Left Foot		Right Foot	
	Unacceptable	Acceptable	Unacceptable	Acceptable
Cleanliness of foot?				
Socks/stockings a good fit?				
Proper fitting shoes?	☐ Short		☐ Short	
	☐ Long		☐ Long	
	☐ Narrow		☐ Narrow	
	☐ Worn down		☐ Worn down	
Shoe Wear: Heel				
Sole				
Lateral Counter				

7. Problems

☐ Bunions

	Left Foot	Right Foot
HAV		
Taylor		

		Left Foot					Right Foot				
		I	II	III	IV	V	I	II	III	IV	V
☐ Calluses	Spin										
	Pinch										
	IPK										
	Sub										
	Shear										
☐ Corns	Met Heads										
	Heloma Molle										
	Heloma Durum										
☐ Involuted Nails											
☐ Ingrown Toenails											
☐ Nail Trophic Changes											

Continued

Continued from previous page

	Left Foot					Right Foot				
	I	II	III	IV	V	I	II	III	IV	V
☐ Circulatory Problems										

	DPP: ☐ 0 PTP: ☐ 0	DPP: ☐ 0 PTP: ☐ 0
	☐ 1+ ☐ 1+	☐ 1+ ☐ 1+
	☐ 2+ ☐ 2+	☐ 2+ ☐ 2+
	☐ 3+ ☐ 3+	☐ 3+ ☐ 3+

		Left Foot					Right Foot				
☐ Toe Clubbing											
☐ Toe Deformities	Hammer										
	Claw										
	Mallet										
	Crossing										
	Hallux										
		I	II	III	IV	V	I	II	III	IV	V

	Left Leg	Right Leg
☐ Foot/Ankle Deformities		
☐ Dermatitis/[PI]Fungus Infection		
☐ Dry, Scaly Skin		
☐ Edema Foot		
Ankle		
Extremity		

☐ Infection (Describe) _____

☐ Other _____

ASSESSMENT

_____
_____
_____
_____
_____
_____
_____
_____

Continued

——————— Continued from previous page ———————

Recommend: ☐ None
            ☐ Refer to orthotics clinic   Date: _____ Time: _____
            ☐ Refer for shoes _____
            ☐ Refer to pediatrist
            ☐ Refer to podiatrist
            ☐ Educated in _____
            ☐ Orthotics fabricated   Date: _____ Time: _____

_____

_____

            2-month follow-up: Date: _____ Time: _____
            6-month follow-up: Date: _____ Time: _____

Comments:

Figure 15–1.

Foot Care Knowledge Questionnaire

Name: _____

Date: _____

1. Do you inspect your feet
   A. Once a month
   B. Once a week
   C. Once a day

2. Do you wash your feet
   A. Daily
   B. Two times a week
   C. Weekly

3. When you wash your feet do you use
   A. Cool water
   B. Lukewarm water
   C. Hot water

4. At night do you walk around barefoot
   A. Never
   B. Sometimes
   C. Always

5. Daytime, do you walk around barefoot
   A. Never
   B. Sometimes
   C. Always

6. How often do you change your socks
   A. Every day
   B. Twice a day
   C. Less than three times a week

7. Do you buy shoes that
   A. Are tight and need to be broken in
   B. Just fit
   C. Are a little big

8. Do you
   A. Trim your toenails straight across
   B. Trim your toenails in a curve
   C. Never trim your toenails

9. Do you treat your own corns/calluses
   A. With a razor blade
   B. With medicine to dissolve them
   C. Wait for the podiatrist or other doctor

10. If you have a blister, do you
    A. Open it up
    B. Keep it covered so it does not pop open
    C. Ignore it

Figure 15–2.

Self-Care Guidelines: Recommended Foot Care

1. Inspect feet daily for swelling, sores, cracks, reddened areas or cuts. Observation of bottom of feet can be done with a mirror.

2. Wash feet daily. Use mild soap and lukewarm water. Rinse thoroughly. Dry carefully and gently with clean, soft towel, especially between the toes.

3. If skin is dry, apply lanolin or other lubricating lotions or creams. Do not put lanoline or other preparations between toes or around the toenails. Avoid excess of lanolin or other preparations. Polysorb Hydrate, Carmol, or Nivea can be used.

4. Powder or cornstarch can be used when feet tend to perspire.

5. Do not go barefoot. Always protect feet, especially when on the beach or in swimming. Sharp stones, glass, cans, ringworm, ticks, chiggers, staples, pins are hazardous for feet.

6. Wear clean stockings or socks at all times. Avoid socks or elastics that constrict legs (i.e., knee socks with tight tops).

7. Break in new shoes gradually (wear for a few hours each day). Recommended heel height: 1/2″ for men, 3/4″ for women. No tapered or pointed shoes.

8. Check shoes before putting them on. Shake them to make sure nothing is in them.

9. Do not use hot water bottles or heating pads on feet.

10. Do not soak feet.

11. Never perform bathroom surgery. Go to your doctor or podiatrist about corns, calluses, ingrown toenails, bacterial and fungal infections, abscess, and lacerations.

12. Trim your toenails frequently. Cut them straight across and not too short.

13. Care of your feet should include doing exercise several minutes a day to speed up blood flow. Bend feet up and down and side to side, and move feet in circles at the ankle. When sitting, place your feet as high as your chair and NEVER CROSS YOUR LEGS!

14. When buying shoes you should have 1/2″ space in front of your longest toe and shoe shape should fit the contour of your foot. The best shoe is a tie shoe with a wide and deep toe box and strong heel counter.

15. Smoking constricts the blood vessels. Smoking is discouraged.

Figure 15–3. *(Courtesy of Jennifer M. Bottomley, PhD, M.S., P.T. and Holis Herman, M.S., P.T. Department of Physical Therapy, Cushing Hospital.)*

3. Determine whether the foot dysfunctions are complications associated with tissue changes, biomechanical abnormalities, or chronic disease processes.

4. Provide easy to read literature and offer corrective treatment so that the elders can participate in community and personal activities.

5. Arrange the details for getting the patient to the outpatient clinic for orthotic fabrication and treatment.

6. Have local radio or newspaper spots explaining the service.

7. Team up with agencies conducting screening clinics (i.e., the American Diabetic Association) so that patients can be identified and treated within the same clinic appointment.

Resources for meeting these objectives are provided in Figure 15–4. It is evident from the remarkable response to the program that a desire for foot

Patient Educational Resources

Krames Communications
312 90TH Street
Daly City, CA 94015-1898

Pamphlets:
1. The Foot Book (#1078)
2. Foot Owner's Manual (#1005)
3. Ankle Owner's Manual (#1073)
4. Foot Surgery (#1119)
5. Laser Foot Surgery (#1321)
6. Walking For Fitness (#1263)
7. Running (#1117)
8. Diabetes and Your Feet (#1372)

Thermal-Moldable Shoes, Inc
100 DeVille
Williamsville, NY 14221-4408

Pamphlet:
1. For Diabetics On the Go
2. For Arthritics On the Go
Thermold Shoes

P.W. Minor and Son, Inc
3 Treadeasy Avenue
P.O. Box 678
Batavia, NY 14021-0678

Extra Depth Shoes

The Langer Foundation
1011 Grand Blvd
Deer Park, NY 11729

Pamphlets:
1. Walking As an Exercise
2. "Facts for Runners and Other Athletes"
3. When Your Feet Hurt You Hurt All Over

Channing L. Bete Co., Inc
Scriptographic Booklet
South Deerfield, MA 01373

Pamphlet:
1. About Foot Care
2. Fun, Fitness and Your Feet

The Arthritis Foundation
Massachusetts Chapter
Parker Building
124 Watertown, MA 02172

Pamphlet:
1. Arthritis Surgery Information to Consider
2. Arthritis Basic Facts
3. Arthritis—Exercise and Your Arthritis
4. Arthritis—A Serious Look At the facts

Fund for Podiatry Education and Research
9312 Old Georgetown Road
Bethesda, MD 20814

Newsletter
"Foot News"

US Department of Health, Education, and Welfare
US Government Printing Office
Washington, DC 20402

Pamphlet:
Feet First—A Booklet About Foot Care

PAL Health Technologies, Inc
293 Herman Street
Perkin, IL 61554

Pamphlets:
1. Maybe You Need Orthotics
2. What Is Pronation?
3. Oh My Aching Feet!
4. Foot Surgery
5. Walking—Make It Easy On Yourself
6. Running . . . and Jogging
7. Skiing—Your Feet . . .
8. Ice Skating/Roller Skating

Department of Public Health
Center for Health Promotion
150 Tremont Street
Boston, MA 02111

Pamphlet:
Walking—A Lifetime Activity

Figure 15–4.

care and a willingness to participate in order to remain an active and useful member of the community was enhanced.

SPECIAL CONSIDERATIONS IN SCREENING PROGRAMS

The majority of elderly adults are highly motivated to seek out strategies for improving their health. Annual physical examinations provide screening for problems in the older adult, however, screening procedures are often not paid for by third-party payers, and regular check-ups become an out-of-pocket expense for the elderly. In many cases they are abandoned. Older adults seek acute care much more frequently than younger people.[22] This may be the result of insidious symptoms left unchecked by the lack of annual physical examinations. Additionally, many older adults, especially the groups at highest risk, such as minorities (who make up 10% of the total elderly population) and those living at or below the poverty level (who make up 20% of the elderly population),[84] do not have their own physicians and are treated only on an acute-care basis through clinics and emergency rooms.

These problems need to be addressed through an interdisciplinary approach using a variety of community service settings. Groups, such as public health and social services departments, senior centers, and area agencies of aging (AAAs), need to come together to identify potential barriers to the provision of health promotion, screening, and assessment programs. The collaborated effort will enable health care practitioners to pool information and resources and provide the most successful and well-attended programs for screening in the elderly.

CONCLUSION

Much emphasis has been placed on prevention. "We must protect what we can't replace," as some wise old gentleman once said. Helfand states, "Ambulation is many times the key or the catalyst between an individual remaining in a community living environment or being institutionalized."[79] The remarkable response to screening programs in the community setting demonstrates that elderly individuals desire preventive care and wish to remain active and useful members of the community.

PEARLS

- Prevention strategies can improve the quality of life and conserve health resources.
- "Successful aging" is a combination of good lifestyle and behavioral habits, including exercise, diet, and socioeconomic well-being.
- Resiliency of the human being is incredible.
- There is a need to change the health care approach from curative to preventive interventions. It is important to convince third-party payers through research efforts of the efficacy of preventive approaches.
- Primary, secondary, and tertiary prevention are the three levels of health intervention.
- Eighty-six percent of those aged 65 and older have at least one chronic disease.
- "We must protect what we can't replace."

REFERENCE

1. McGinnis JM. Year 2000 health objectives for the nation. In: *Surgeon General's Workshop on Health Promotion and Aging.* Washington, DC: US Dept of Health and Human Services, 1988:20–25.
2. Roybal ER. Elderly health care cost likely to rise to one-fifth of income. *Congressional Record.* March 23, 1989; E978–E980.
3. NCHS Health Statistics on Older Persons. United States, 1986: *Analytical and Epidemiological Studies.* Series 3. NCHS: Washington, DC: US Dept of Health and Human Services; Publication No. 25 (PHS): 87–1409.
4. Sundwall D. Health promotion and Surgeon General's workshop. *Surgeon General's Workshop on Health Promotion and Aging.* Washington, DC: US Dept of Health and Human Services; 1988.
5. Fisk CF. *Address, Opening Plenary Session.* Surgeon General's workshop. Surgeon General's Workshop on Health Promotion and Aging. Washington, DC: US Dept of Health and Human Services; 1988.
6. Rowe JW, Kahn RL. Human aging—usual and successful. *Science.* 1987; 237:143–149.
7. Shore H. Therapeutic strategies and institutional care. In: Lesnoff-Caravaglia G, ed. *Handbook of Applied Gerontology.* New York: Human Sciences Press, Inc.; 1987; 447–452
8. Department of Health and Human Services. *Recent Medicaid Cutbacks: Shocking Impacts on the Elderly.* HHS Pub. 148; 1992.
9. Wallack SS, Tompkins CP, Gruenberg L. A plan for rewarding efficient HMOs. *Health Affairs.* Summer, 1988; 80–96.
10. Havas S. Prevention of heart disease, cancer and stoke: the scientific basis. *World Health Forum.* 1987; 8:344–351.
11. Frame PS. Clinical prevention in primary care: the time is now! *J Fam Pract.* 1989; 29:150–156.
12. Liarson EG, Bruce RA. Exercise and aging. Ann Intern Med. 1986; 105:783–785.
13. Chernoff R. *Geriatric Nutrition: The Health Professional's Handbook.* Rockville, MD: Aspen Publishers; 1991.
14. Bogardus C, Ravussin E, Robbins DC, et al. Effects of physical training and diet therapy on carbohydrate metabolism in patients with glucose intolerance

and non-insulin-dependent diabetes mellitus. *Diabetes*. 1984; 33:311–318.

15. Helmrich SP, Ragland Dr, Leung RW, et al. Physical activity and reduced occurrence of non-insulin-dependent diabetes mellitus. *N Engl J Med.* 1991; 325:147–152.

16. Astrand, PO. Exercise physiology and its role in disease prevention and in rehabilitation. *Arch Phys Med Rehabil.* 1987: 68:305–311.

17. Paffenbarger RS, Hyde RT, Wing AL, Hsieh CC. Physical activity, all-cause mortality and longevity of college alumni. *New Engl J Med.* 1985; 314: 605–613.

18. Rogers R, Meyer J, Judd B, et al. Abstention from cigarette smoking improves cerebral perfusion among elderly chronic smokers. *JAMA.* 1985; 253 (20):2:970–974.

19. McGinnis JM, Nestle N. The Surgeon General's report on nutrition and health: policy implications and implementation strategies. *AM J Clin Nutr.* 1989; 49(1):23–28.

20. Gladman JRF, Barer D, Venkatesan P, et al. The outcome of pneumonia in the elderly: a hospital survey. *Clin Rehab.* 1991; 5:201–205.

21. Webster JR, Prevention, technology, and aging in the decade ahead. *Top Ger Rehab.* 1992; 7(4):1–8.

22. Crimmins EM, Saito Y, Ingegneri D. Changes in life expectancy and disability-free life expectancy in the United States. *Pop Develop Rev.* June, 1989; 15(2):235–267.

23. Center for Disease Control. Comorbidity of chronic conditions and disabilities among older persons—United States, 1984. *MMWR.* 1989; 38:788–791.

24. Tinetti ME, Speechley M, Ginter SF. Risk factors for falls among elderly persons living in the community. *N Engl J Med.* 1988; 319(26):1701–1707

25. Celentano D, Klassen A, Weisman C, et al. Cervical cancer screening practices among older women; results from the Maryland Cervical Cancer Case-Control Study. *Clin Epidemiology* 1988; 41(6): 531–541.

26. Garner B. Guide to changing lab values in elders. *Ger Nurs.* 1989; 10(3):144145.

27. Ory MG. Considerations in the development of age-sensitive indicators for assessing health promotion. *Health Promotion.* 1988; 3(2):139–149.

28. Frame PS. A critical review of adult health maintenance: part 4. Prevention of metabolic behavioral and miscellaneous conditions. *J Fam Pract.* 1985; 23(1):2939.

29. Koop CE. *Keynote Address, March 2023, 1988: Surgeon General's Workshop on Health Promotion and Aging.* Washington, DC: US Dept of Health and Human Services; 1–4, 1988.

30. Pruzansky ME, Turano M, Luckey M, et al. Low body weight as a risk factor for fracture in both black and white women. *J Orthop Res.* 1989; 7(2): 192–197.

31. Fried LP, Bush TL. Morbidity as a focus of preventive health care in the elderly. *Epidemiol Rev.* 1988; 10:4864.

32. Woolf SH, Kamerow DB, Lawrence RS, et al. The periodic health examination of older adults: the

recommendations of the US Preventive Service Task Force. *J Am Ger Soc.* 1990; 38:871823.

33. Woolf SH, Kamerow DB, Lawrence RS, et al. The periodic health examination of older adults: the recommendations of the US Preventive Service Task Force. *J Am Ger Soc.* 1990; 38(part II):933942.

34. Linn M, Linn B. Self-Evaluation of Life Function (SELF) scale: a short, comprehensive self-report of health for elderly adults. *J Gerontol.* 1984; 39(5): 603–612.

35. Safer M. An evaluation of the Health Hazard Appraisal based on survey data from a randomly selected population. *Pub Health Rep.* 1982; 97(1): 3137.

36. American Cancer Society. *Summary of Current Guidelines for the Cancer-related Checkup: Recommendations.* Atlanta, Ga: American Cancer Society; 1988. Pamphlet No. 334701PE.

37. Winawer S. Screening for colorectal cancer: an overview. *Cancer.* 1980; 45(5 suppl):1093–1098.

38. Allison J, Feldman R. Cost benefits of hemocult screening for colorectal carcinoma. *Dig Dis Sci.* 1985; 30(9):860–865.

39. Verbrugge LM. Long life but worsening health? Trends in health and morbidity of middle-aged and older persons. *Milbank Memorial Fund Quarterly/Health and Society.* 1989; 82:475–519.

40. Hayward R, Shapiro M, Freemen A, et al. Who gets screened for cervical and breast cancer? Results from a new national survey. *Arch Intern Med.* 1988; 148(5):1, 177–181.

41. American Cancer Society. *Cancer Facts and Figures.* New York: American Cancer Society; 1985.

41a. National Center for Health Statistics. Advance report of final mortality statistics. *Monthly Vital Statistics Report.* Hyattsville, Md: US Public Health Service; 1988. US Dept of Health and Human Services, publication PHS 88-1120;37: 6 (suppl).

42. American Diabetes Association. Position statement: office guide to diagnosis and classification of diabetes mellitus and other categories of glucose intolerance. *Diabetes Care.* 1992;15(suppl 2):4.

43. Reed A, Birge S. Screening for osteoporosis. *J Gerontol.* 1988; 14(7):18–20.

44. Dowd T. The female climacteric. *Nat OB-GYN Group.* 1990; 6:1:32–54.

45. Walker SN. Health promotion for older adults: direction for research. *Am J Health Promotion.* Spring 1989; 3(4):47–52.

45a. National Institutes of Health. Nutrition Coordination Committee, Program in Biomedical and Behavioral Research and Training, 11th Annual Report of the National Institutes of Health. Washington, DC: US Dept of Health and Human Services; 1987: 111.

46. Surgeon General's Report on Nutrition and Health. *Dietary Fads and Frauds.* US Public Health Service. Washington DC: US Government Printing Office; 1988. US Dept of Health and Human Services publication No. 88-50210; Stock No. 017-001-00465-1.

47. Commission on Life Sciences, National Research Council. *Report on Diet and Health.* Washington, DC: National Academy Press; 1989.

48. McGinnis JM. *Promoting Health-Preventing Disease: Year 2000 Objectives for the Nation.* Office of the Assistant Secretary for Health, Office of Disease Prevention and Health Promotion. Washington DC: US Government Printing Office; 1989.

49. Drinkwater BL. *The Role of Nutrition and Exercise in Health. Continuing Dental Education.* Seattle, Wash: University of Washington; 1985.

50. Nieman DC. *The Sports Medicine Fitness Course.* Palo Alto, Calif: Bull Publishing, Co.; 1986.

51. Peck WA, Avioli LV. Physical exercise and bone health. In: *Osteoporosis the Silent Thief.* Washington, DC; American Association of Retired Persons; 1988.

52. Suominen H, Heikkinen E, Liesen H. Effect of 8 weeks endurance training on skeletal muscle metabolism in 56–70 year old men. *Eur J Appl Physiol.* 1987; 37:173–180.

53. Shepard RJ. *Physical Activity and Aging.* 2nd ed. Rockville, Md: Aspen Publishers, Inc.; 1987.

54. Kaplin GA, Seeman TE, Cohen RD, et al. Mortality among the elderly in the Alameda County study: behavioral and demographic risk factors. *Am J Pub Health.* 1987; 77(3):307–312.

55. Stones MJ, Dornan B, Kozma A. The prediction of mortality in elderly institution residents. *J Ger Psychol Sci.* 1989; 44(3):72–79.

56. Evans W. Exercise and muscle metabolism in the elderly. In: Hutchinson ML, Munro HN, eds. *Nutrition and Aging.* Orlando, Fl: Academic Press; 1986.

57. Craig BW, Garthwaite SM, Holloszy JO. Adipocyte insulin resistance: effects of aging, obesity, exercise, and food restriction. *Am Physiol Soc.* 1987; 62(1):95.

58. Wang JT, Ho LT, Tang KT, et al. Effect of habitual physical activity on age-related glucose tolerance. *J Am Ger Soc.* 1989; 37(3):203–209.

59. Smith EL, Gilligan C, Smith PE, et al. Calcium supplementation and bone loss in middle-aged women. *Am J Clin Nutr.* 1989; 50:833–842.

60. Tinette ME, Speechley M. Prevention of falls among the elderly. *N Engl J Med.* 1989; 320(16): 1055–1059.

61. Blake AJ, Morgan K, Bendall MJ, et al. Falls by elderly people at home: prevalence and associated factors. *Age Ageing.* 1988; 17(6):365–372.

62. Hemenway D, Coldtz GA, Willet WC, et al. Fractures and lifestyle: effects of cigarette smoking, alcohol intake and weight on risk of hip fracture in middle-aged women. *Am J Pub Health.* 1988; 78: 1554–1558.

63. Wolf S, Fugate L, Halstrand E, et al. *Worst Pills Best Pills.* Washington, DC: Public Citizen Health Research Group; 1988.

64. Gibson R, Waldo D. National health expenditures. *1980 Health Care Financing Rev.* 1981; 3:1–54.

65. Maddox G. Aging, drinking, and alcohol abuse. *Generations.* 1988; 12(4):14–16.

66. Willenbrig M, Spring W. Evaluating alcohol use in elders. *Generations.* 1988; 12(4):27–31.

67. Kart C, Metress E, Metress S. *Aging, Health and Society.* Boston: Jones & Bartlett; 1988.

68. Alpert M. Health screening to promote health for the elderly. *Nurse Pract.* 1987; 12(5):42–44, 48–51, 54–58.

69. Magaziner J, Bassett S, Hebel J. Predicting performance on the Mini-Mental Status Exam: use of age and education specific equations. *J Am Ger Soc.* 1987; 35(11):996–1000.

70. Baker S, Harvey A. Fall injuries in the elderly. *Clin Ger Med.* 1985;1(3):501–512.

71. Sorenson AW, Seltser R, Sundwall D. Primary cancer prevention as an attainable objective for the elderly. In: Yancik R, ed. *Perspectives on Prevention and Treatment of Cancer in the Elderly.* New York: Raven Press; Raven Press Aging Series: 1983:24.

72. Maloney S. Healthy older people. In: *Surgeon General's Workshop on Health Promotion and Aging.* Washington, DC: US Dept of Health and Human Services; March, 1988.

73. Munro HN. Aging and nutrition: a multifaceted problem. In: Hutchinson ML, Munro HN, eds. *Nutrition and Aging.* Orlando, Fl: Academic Press; 1986.

74. Collet BS. Podiatry and public health: a systematic approach. *Cur Podiatry.* 1979; 28:32–37.

75. Collet BS, Katzew AB, Helfand AE. Podiatry for the geriatric patient, *Annual Review of Gerontology/ Geriatrics.* 1984; 4:221–234.

76. Evanski PM. The geriatric foot. In: Jahss M, ed. *Disorders of the Foot.* Philadelphia: WB Saunders; 1982:964–978.

77. Gould N, Schneider W, Ashikaga T. Epidemiological survey of foot problems in the continental United States: 1978–1979. *Foot Ankle.* 1980; 1:8–10.

78. Helfand AE. *Clinical Podogeriatrics.* Baltimore: Williams and Wilkins; 1981.

79. Helfand AE. Common foot problems in the aged and rehabilitative management. In: Williams TF, ed. *Rehabilitation in the Aging.* New York: Raven Press; 1984:291–303.

80. Soulier SM. The use of running shoes in the prevention of plantar diabetic ulcers. *J of Am Podiatric Med Assoc.* 1986;76(7):395–400.

81. Bessman AN. Foot problems in the diabetic. *Comprehensive Ther.* 1991; 8(1):32–38.

82. Mathmatica. *The Medicare Shoe Demonstration Project: Preliminary Findings.* Summary for HCFA, Unpublished document; October, 1990.

83. Jette AM, Harris BA, Cleary PD. Functional recovery after hip fracture. *Arch Phys Med Rehab.* 1987; 68:735–740.

84. American Association of Retired Persons (AARP). *A Profile of Older Americans.* Washington, DC; 1988. AARP pamphlet No. PF3049 (1228)-D996.

CHAPTER 16

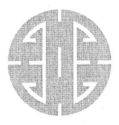

Communication

Normal Changes with Age Affecting Communication	The Team
Hearing	Writing
Vision and the Other Senses	Compliance and Motivation
Voice Changes with Age	Conclusion
Ethnicity	

A patient gets better, a child graduates from college, a pain is felt, a new idea comes to mind, and yet this information is unable to be communicated. Why? Is it old age? Is it because the recipients of the information do not understand? Is there some pathological process that is going on that is impairing the communication process?

This chapter will attempt to answer some of these questions. The first section will explore the older individual in terms of normal and pathological changes with age that impact communication. A special section discusses the ethnic influences on aging and communication. Impediments and enhancements to communication with the health professional will also be examined. The final sections of this chapter will explore writing skills and the important topic of compliance and motivation.

NORMAL CHANGES WITH AGE AFFECTING COMMUNICATION

Hearing

Normal Changes with Age Affecting Hearing   Hearing loss is second only to arthritis as the most common physical complaint of the aged.[1] Statistics show that approximately 24 million persons over the age of 65 suffer from hearing loss.[1] In addition, with each consecutive decade after 70, the prevalence of those affected increases dramatically.[1]

Changes in the major structures of the ear establish the three main types of hearing loss: conductive, sensorineural, and mixed. Conductive hearing loss is a result of changes in the outer or middle ear that

blocks the acoustic energy. The changes in the external and middle ear follow.

Changes in the external ear

1. Decreased sensation that causes the patient to be unaware of a build-up of wax.
2. Excess hair growth in the outer ear, especially in men, that can aid in the accumulation of wax.
3. A decrease in the wax-producing glands and a subsequent tendency for the wax to become drier.

Changes in the middle ear

1. The tympanic membrane becomes more rigid and translucent with age.
2. Negative pressure in the middle ear as a result of a decrease in the elasticity and displacement of tissue in the nasopharynx causes the eustachian tube to resist opening.[2]

Sensorineural hearing loss occurs because of changes in the inner ear. These changes follow.

Changes in the inner ear

1. Death of hair cells in the cochlea.
2. Damage to the basilar membrane within the cochlea.[2]

Mixed disorders are a combination of sensorineural and conductive. In general, conductive hearing disorders may be reversed, sensorineural disorders cannot, and mixed disorders can be partially reversed.

A common term used to describe the hearing loss of old age is presbycusis. This general type of hearing

549

loss is sensorineural and, therefore, not reversible. The characteristics of presbycusis are

1. A reduced sensitivity to high-pitched sounds, such as sh, s, t, z, v, f, ch, and g.
2. Bilaterally the hearing loss is equal.
3. Men are more affected than women.
4. A decreased hearing of pure tones.

The hearing loss often associated with old age is usually insidious. It gradually appears, and often patients do not realize that they are misinterpreting communications. For example, when an older person with presbycusis is asked, "How old are you?" The answer may be "fine." This inappropriate response may lead to frustration on the part of the patient, family, and health professional. In addition, the older person with hearing loss may feel depressed, isolated, and angry.[4]

Pathological Changes with Age Affecting Hearing
The classification, manifestation, and approach to the pathological changes with age affecting hearing are similar to the normal changes already listed. In conductive hearing loss, some of the common causes might be infection and osteosclerosis.[2] In the area of sensorineural changes, some causes may be drug toxicity, brain tumor, or Meniere's disease.[2] Finally, in mixed disorders, a foreign body or an infection can cause the problem.

Evaluation For both normal and pathological changes in hearing with aging, thorough screening is imperative to delineate the cause and type of hearing loss. Table 16–1 lists several signs of hearing impairment.

In addition, once a person is suspected of having a hearing loss, the "Hearing Handicap Inventory" can be administered. This test evaluates the person's response to the hearing loss emotionally and socially. Figure 16–1 is a sample hearing handicap test.

After the hearing-impaired person completes this test, the care giver totals the numerical value of the responses for a total score and two subscores delineating values for the emotional and social/situational areas. Patients who avoid social encounters and are becoming emotionally isolated are identified by a high "S" score value. Persons whose emotional supports are weak would score high points in the "E" category.

A rough estimate of total scores is as follows[2]:

- 0–16   The individual does not have a perceived handicap due to hearing loss. These persons either have little objective hearing loss or enjoy adequate coping skills.
- 17–42   The person has a mild-to-moderate self-perceived handicap. This person requires evaluation for other stressors and may need help with realistic goal setting, defining needs, and following through with care.
- 43+   The person's coping skills are extremely limited. This person requires concrete direction in terms of self-care and seeking proper assistance for the hearing loss.

Interventions Interventions for hearing loss range from specific rehabilitation programs to appropriate assistive devices (i.e., hearing aides). In addition, the health team can keep in mind measures and aides to communication (Tables 16–2 and 16–3).

Vision and the Other Senses

Hearing obviously impacts communication. Nevertheless, changes in the other senses also impact communication. The major, but normal, change with age in vision, called presbyopia, begins as early as the fourth decade. (For specific information on presbyopia and vision changes, see Chapter 3.) Most vision deficits normally caused by aging can be managed by changes in lenses.[5] In addition, environmental modifications can enhance communication as well as ensure safety.[6]

The literature also notes a decline in the senses of touch, taste, and smell.[7] Lack of information in

TABLE 16–1. CLUES TO DETECTING HEARING IMPAIRMENT

The person states that words are difficult to understand.
The person is unable to hear high-pitched sounds (a faucet dripping, high notes of a violin).
The person may complain of a continuous hissing or ringing background noise.
The person ceases to enjoy concerts, TV programs, and social get-togethers because he or she is unable to understand much of what is being said.
The person understands a conversation that takes place in a quiet room, but misunderstands most of the conversation when the room is noisy.
The person can participate in a conversation with one other person but has difficulty if two or more conversations are going on.
You may need to get the person's attention before speaking to him or her.
The person understands you when you are speaking face to face but is confused when your back is turned or your mouth isn't clearly visible. This person may be "speech-reading" (watching lips, facial expressions, and gestures) to understand the message.
The person becomes angry and frustrated when he or she misunderstands something.
The person may attempt to blame hearing loss on outside factors. He or she may accuse you of talking too fast or of mumbling or they may say, "It's too noisy in here."
The person becomes irritable and tires easily during conversation, because listening is hard work.
The person may become annoyed when spoken to loudly (recruitment). This occurs commonly with presbycusis.

Reprinted with permission from Dwyer B. Detecting hearing loss and improving communication in elderly persons. In: *Focus on Geriatric Care & Rehabilitation*. Rockville, Md: Aspen Publishers; 1987; 1(16)3–4.

The Hearing Handicap Inventory for the Elderly

The purpose of this scale is to identify the problems your hearing loss may be causing you. Answer YES, SOMETIMES, or NO for each question. *Do not skip a question if you avoid a situation because of your hearing problem.* If you use a hearing aid, please answer the way you hear *without* the aid.

		YES (4)	SOME-TIMES (2)	NO (0)			YES (4)	SOME-TIMES (2)	NO (0)
S-1.	Does a hearing problem cause you to use the phone less often than you would like?	☐	☐	☐	E-14.	Does a hearing problem cause you to have arguments with family members?	☐	☐	☐
E-2.	Does a hearing problem cause you to feel embarrassed when meeting new people?	☐	☐	☐	S-15.	Does a hearing problem cause you difficulty when listening to TV or radio?	☐	☐	☐
S-3.	Does a hearing problem cause you to avoid groups of people?	☐	☐	☐	S-16.	Does a hearing problem cause you to go shopping less often than you would like?	☐	☐	☐
E-4.	Does a hearing problem make you irritable?	☐	☐	☐	E-17.	Does any problem or difficulty with your hearing upset you at all?	☐	☐	☐
E-5.	Does a hearing problem cause you to feel frustrated when talking to members of your family?	☐	☐	☐	E-18.	Does a hearing problem cause you to want to be by yourself?	☐	☐	☐
S-6.	Does a hearing problem cause you difficulty when attending a party?	☐	☐	☐	S-19.	Does a hearing problem cause you to talk to family members less often than you would like?	☐	☐	☐
E-7.	Does a hearing problem cause you to feel "stupid" or "dumb"?	☐	☐	☐	E-20.	Do you feel that any difficulty with your hearing limits or hampers your personal or social life?	☐	☐	☐
S-8.	Do you have difficulty hearing when someone speaks in a whisper?	☐	☐	☐	S-21.	Does a hearing problem cause you difficulty when in a restaurant with relatives of friends?	☐	☐	☐
E-9.	Do you feel handicapped by a hearing problem?	☐	☐	☐	E-22.	Does a hearing problem cause you to feel depressed?	☐	☐	☐
S-10.	Does a hearing problem cause you difficulty when visiting friends, relatives, or neighbors?	☐	☐	☐	S-23.	Does a hearing problem cause you to listen to TV or radio less often than you would like?	☐	☐	☐
S-11.	Does a hearing problem cause you to attend religious services less often than you would like?	☐	☐	☐	E-24.	Does a hearing problem cause you to feel uncomfortable when talking to friends?	☐	☐	☐
E-12.	Does a hearing problem cause you to be nervous?	☐	☐	☐	E-25.	Does a hearing problem cause you to feel left out when you are with a group of people?	☐	☐	☐
S-13.	Does a hearing problem cause you to visit friends, relatives, or neighbors less often than you would like?	☐	☐	☐					

FOR CLINICIAN'S USE ONLY: Total Score: _____
Subtotal E: _____
Subtotal S: _____

Figure 16–1. *(Reprinted with permission from Ventry I, Weinstein B. The hearing handicap inventory for the elderly: a new tool. In: Ear Hear. Baltimore: Williams & Wilkins; 1982; 128–134.)*

TABLE 16–2. COMMUNICATING WITH THE HEARING IMPAIRED

Keep the following measures in mind

Get the person's attention by calling his or her name but do not shout or touch the person first, since this may startle him or her.

Keep your conversation focused and introduce the topic (for example, "Mr A, I'd like to talk with you about your family"). The person then can focus on ideas and key words. Let the person know when you are going to change topics.

If the person does not understand you, phrase your thought differently rather than repeating the same statement over and over. Repetition only leads to frustration.

Face the person directly during conversations. A distance of 3 to 6 feet is ideal. In group situations, no speaker and listener should be more than 6 feet apart.

Your face should be visible to the listener. Do not eat, chew gum, or smoke while talking to hearing-impaired persons.

Do not speak to hearing-impaired persons from another room or while they are concentrating on an activity, such as reading or watching television.

Speak at a slightly greater than normal loudness and at a normal rate.

Do not overarticulate. This distorts the sounds of speech and the speaker's face, thus limiting the use of cues from facial expression.

Reduce the amount of background noise when carrying on conversations. Turn off the radio or TV. If there are other conversation nearby, move to a quieter area.

Be certain that hearing-impaired persons wear their eyeglasses and hearing aids, if they have these devices.

Use body language, facial expressions, and gestures to help convey what you have to say.

Never speak directly into the person's ear. Although this amplifies the sound of your voice, it decreases clarity, and the listener is unable to make use of visual cues.

Provide a public address system for group situations or meetings. Many elderly persons complain that they enjoy meetings, but for various reasons the speaker avoids using a microphone.

Reprinted with permission from Dwyer B. Detecting Hearing Loss and Improving Communication in Elderly Persons. *In: Focus on Geriatric Care & Rehabilitation.* Rockville, Md: Aspen Publishers, 1987; 1(6):6.

TABLE 16–3. AIDS TO COMMUNICATION

The following tips are hearing-impaired individuals, who by definition experience difficulty communicating.

Do not strain to hear or to read lips. A combination of hearing and seeing enables you to understand most speakers better.

Watch the speaker carefully so that you can observe the lips, as well as other body language.

Look for ideas rather than isolated words. As you become familiar with the rhythm of a person's speech, you will pick up key words that will help you put together what the speaker is trying to communicate.

Position yourself directly across from the speaker. Avoid facing a bright light.

Try to determine the subject under discussion as quickly as possible. Ask your friends to give you a lead, such as, "We are talking about the housing situation."

Remember that conversation is a two-way affair. Do not monopolize it in an attempt to control it. Listening takes more energy, but you learn more.

Don't be afraid that people will think you are staring at them while you are trying to understand what they are saying. It is always polite to look at the person who is talking to you.

Tell the speaker what part of what he or she said that you don't understand. Merely saying, "I didn't understand," does not provide the necessary information to correct your problem. Let speakers know that they are talking too softly, that their hand is in front of their mouth, and so on.

If you don't understand something, ask the speaker to rephrase the statement. If you have understood some part of what has been said, use those words in your question, asking the speaker to supply the words you have missed.

Don't get into the habit of allowing anyone else, such as your spouse of friends, to speak or listen for you.

Everyone needs time to relax. At such times, a person simply does not listen. Allow yourself the luxury of withdrawing at times, but do not confuse this with your hearing loss.

Reprinted with permission from Dwyer B. Detecting hearing loss and improving communication in elderly persons. In: *Focus on Geriatric Care & Rehabilitation.* Rockville, Md: Aspen Publishers, 1987; 1(6):6.

these areas can alter normal communication. Suggestions for health professionals in this area are

1. Try to use touch as much as possible to enhance communications.
2. Bring in the other senses as much as possible. For example, describe the smell of the bread the patient is making or the roses they just received.
3. Instruct the family or staff in methods of seasoning food to enhance the sense of taste (i.e., different healthy seasonings).
4. Make a mental checklist to include the other senses in a treatment session (for example, show the patient the menu for the day, and discuss the taste and smell of the food).

Voice Changes with Age

A person's ability to vocalize is another important variable in communication. Studies on voice cues alone have shown that older speakers tend to be negatively rated as compared to younger speakers.[89] There are normal changes that occur with age in the voices of men and women, however, they do not cause significant problems with communication. Men, according to Honjo and Isshiki,[30] experience a higher fundamental frequency due to "vocal fold atrophy." Women, on the other hand, experience a lower frequency due to a slight hoarseness and vocal fold edema.[10]

Normal aging changes can affect voice production. A list of the changes with age in the human body that can affect speech follows.

1. Reduced respiratory efficiency caused by
   a. Degeneration of vertebral discs (senile kyphosis).[11]
   b. Decreased elasticity of the rib cartilages, as well as ossification, and calcification of these cartilages.[12]
   c. Reduced recoil and elasticity of the lungs[13] resulting in lower frequencies, decreased loud-

TABLE 16–4. PATHOLOGICAL CAUSES OF IMPAIRED COMMUNICATION

Name	Characterized By	Disease Associated	Speech Muscles	Communications
Flaccid dysarthria	Damage to the peripheral nervous system Cranial nerve Motor muscle Spinal or cranial nerve axons Myoneural junctions	Bulbar palsy Myasthenia gravis Muscular dystrophy Polymyositis	Weak Hypotonic	Slurred Slow Breathy Weak Hypernasality
Spastic dysarthria	Damage to central nervous system Bilateral upper motor neuron lesions	Multiple cerebrovascular accidents (CVA) Multiple sclerosis (MS) Traumatic brain injury	Hypertonicity Disintegration of movement	Slow Labored Low pitch Imprecise consonants Monopitch Hypernasality
Ataxic dysarthria	Damage to cerebellum or its tracts	CVAs Tumors MS Toxic or metabolic disorders Encephalitis	Uncoordination of force, speed, timing, range, and direction	Imprecise consonants Inconsistent nasality Scanning speech Vocal tremor Loudness variation
Dyskinetic dysarthria	Damage to extrapyramidal motor system Hypokinetic Hyperkinetic	Parkinson's disease Epilepsy Tics Chorea Ballism Encephalitis	Rigidity Reduced range of force Tremor at rest Abnormal Interrupted	Monopitch loudness Breathy or hoarse Short rushes of speech Difficulty initiating speech Erratic changes in pitch and loudness Intermittent hypernasality Harshness
Mixed dysarthria	Damage to multiple lesions in the central nervous system	Multiple strokes Tumors Head trauma Degenerative disease—ALS or MS	Combination of hypokinetic and hyperkinetic depending on motor system affected	Combination of hypokinetic and hyperkinetic depending on motor system affected
Wernicke's aphasia	Damage to the left cerebral hemisphere (posterior lesion of temporal lobe)	CVA Brain tumor Cerebral trauma Cerebral infection Intracranial surgical procedures		Impaired auditory comprehension Fluent, flowing verbal output, low in information Word substitution
Broca's aphasia	Damage to the left cerebral hemisphere (anterior lesion of frontal lobe)			Restricted vocabulary and grammar Word retrieval difficulties Slow, labored, halting
Verbal apraxia	Same—coexists with Broca's aphasia			Impairment in motor programming, not muscle function Difficulty initiating speech Inconsistent articulation errors
Right hemisphere	Damage to right hemisphere (nondominant side of brain)	CVA		Attention and perceptual deficits Unable to comprehend emotional and perceptual tone Flat effect, monotone
Dementia	Progressive degeneration to central nervous system	Hydrocephalus Alzheimer's Vitamin deficiency Multi-infarct dementia Endocrine disorders		**Initial stage** Fluent conversation with elaborate detail Reduced attention and memory Disorientation Repetition and blame

(continued)

TABLE 16–4. (CONTINUED)

Name	Characterized By	Disease Associated	Speech Muscles	Communications
		Pick's disease (See Chapter 4 for further listing)		**Mid stages** As above plus word-finding deficits Perseverative responses Self-correction absent **Advanced** Unable to communicate or understand Echolalia
Laryngectomy	Surgical removal of larynx due to cancer	Cancer	No muscles of speech in larynx	No voice—person communicates with facial expression and writing Uses esophageal muscles to speak Restricted loudness and pitch range Chronic hoarseness Difficulty with energy expenditure of talking
COPD	Chronic airflow obstruction with reversible or irreversible components	Emphysema Bronchitis Asthma		

ness, and shortening of the length of utterances per breath.[14]

2. Changes in the oral cavity caused by
   a. Changes in the structure of the lower jaw.
   b. Loss of dentition.
   c. Weakening and loss of sensitivity of the pharyngeal muscles.
   d. Reduced activity of the salivary glands.[15]
   e. Atrophy of the lips and tongue[16] resulting in an alteration in resonance, increased nasality, and reduced articulatory accuracy.
3. Changes in the laryngeal cavity caused by
   a. The laryngeal cartilages undergoing ossification and calcification.
   b. Drying out of the laryngeal mucosa.
   c. Reduced vascular supply to the mucosa.
   d. Progressive thinning and shortening of the vocal folds resulting in vocal tremors, roughness, breathiness, and hoarseness.[17]

As mentioned earlier, the changes listed essentially have minimal effect on communication; however, pathological causes, such as dysarthria, apraxia, aphasia, dementia, laryngectomy, and chronic obstructive pulmonary disease (COPD), can cause significant impairment in communication (Table 16–4).

Evaluation of pathologies of the voice should be done by a trained speech and language professional. The treatment, however, cannot be done solely by these professionals. To maximize the benefits of treatment, the family, staff, and rehabilitation team must become involved. Table 16–5 provides a list of strategies for improving communication for the various pathologies already noted.[3]

Ethnicity

How can a person's origins, rules, and contrasts affect communication between the person, family, and health professional? Is cultural diversity a major concern when looking at the demographics in the United States? In the year 2000, an estimated 30% of the population was Asian, Hispanic, Native American, and African American.[18] Often, people tend to overgeneralize or overemphasize cultural differences and therefore miscommunicate. Table 16–6 provides a list of possible verbal and nonverbal miscommunication sources between cultural groups.[19]

So how does one work most effectively with cultural differences? Like other areas of human intervention, the therapist must make an appropriate evaluation of the situation. Table 16–7 provides examples of assessment categories for ethnic behavior.[20]

The therapist should consider this checklist when working with older adults; however, prior to implementing any intervention the therapist should rank its importance. In a study done by Chee and Kane,[21] the priority of ethnic factors was addressed. They discovered that Japanese-Americans highly rated ethnic factors in a nursing home, such as similar ethnic background of staff, ethnic foods, programming activities, and community involvement.[21] The blacks in this study placed more emphasis on access to family than on the ethnic considerations.[21]

The key to ethnic considerations in communications with older persons is to evaluate effectively the needs of the patient, become more sensitive to their concerns, and to provide modifications in the environment commensurate with the needs identified.

TABLE 16–5. STRATEGIES FOR IMPROVING COMMUNICATION

Aphasia

1. Be familiar with the person's level of comprehension and adjust rate, length, and complexity of language to a level at which the person can respond with success.
2. Use concrete, familiar vocabulary in short, clear sentences.
3. Use gesture and facial expression to augment what is said, or demonstrate the information you are trying to convey.
4. Provide written and visual cues.
5. Phase questions for short responses, multiple choice, or yes/no responses.
6. Rephrase a message if not understood initially.
7. Give the person adequate time to respond.
8. Encourage the aphasic person to use gestures, facial expressions, and writing, if appropriate, to augment what is said.
9. Let the person know that you have understood the message by repeating it back conversationally.
10. Be patient and supportive to reduce any stress associated with communicating.
11. Treat the person as an adult at all times.

Right Hemisphere Dysfunction

1. Minimize external distractions in the environment.
2. Position yourself and any materials within the person's visual field if he or she has a left visual field defect.
3. Establish eye contact to ensure attention to the conversation.
4. Provide orienting materials like clocks and calendars.
5. Provide structured activities.
6. Help the person structure responses by cueing with relevant details; if the person goes off on a tangent, cue him or her back to the topic at hand.
7. Be concrete and direct in language use; avoid figurative language and sarcasm.
8. This person may not understand lengthy, complex directions, so repeat and rephrase to assure understanding of important details.

Dementia

1. Establish eye contact prior to addressing the person to ensure attention.
2. Use short, gramatically simple, and concrete input. Avoid the use of pronouns.
3. Keep to one topic at a time. Be redundant; repeat and rephrase critical information.
4. Provide multisensory input, both visual and tactile, to enhance comprehension. For example, provide illustrations or photographs, write down key words, or use gesture and demonstration.
5. Ask yes/no and either/or questions.
6. Provide external orientation and memory aids, such as name bracelets, reminder signs, and calendars.
7. Share successful communication techniques with the patient's care givers.

Dysarthria

1. Communicate in a quiet, nondistracting environment.
2. Encourage the person to speak at a slower rate.
3. Have the person exaggerate production of consonants and separate syllables within words.
4. Encourage the use of shorter utterances compatible with breath support and meaning.
5. Provide honest feedback about the intelligibility of the message.
6. Provide appropriate feedback about loudness level.
7. Become familiar with the person's alternate or augmentative communication methods, such as language boards and gestures.

Laryngectomy

1. Talk in a quiet environment.
2. Consider facial expressions, gestures, speech-reading cues, and situational and linguistic context, if you have difficulty understanding the person.
4. Provide support and encouragement for the use of the new voice.

Chronic Obstructive Pulmonary Disease

1. Encourage short utterances compatible with breath supply.
2. Encourage a reduced rate of speech.
3. Do not engage in conversation while the person is involved in physical activity.

Reprinted with permission from Cherney L. *Aging and communication.* In: Lewis C, ed. Aging: The Health Care Challenge. Philadelphia: Davis; 1989.

THE TEAM

Why place the team in the middle of a chapter on communication? There are two reasons: First, to explore the method in which the team interacts with itself and its effectiveness in this effort; and second, to examine the team or the individual on the team's ability to communicate with the older patient.

What is the role of the team in geriatric rehabilitation? There is no definitive answer to this question. In the studies to follow, the team is a constantly changing variable. It can simply be a doctor and a nurse, or it can be expanded to include a social worker, dietitian, occupational therapist, speech-language pathologist, physical therapist, leisure services professional, psychologist, or dentist.[22]

Is the team more effective in delivering care to the older person? The results of several studies on this subject follow.

TABLE 16-6. SOME POSSIBLE VERBAL AND NONVERBAL SOURCES OF MISCOMMUNICATION BETWEEN CULTURAL GROUPS

Blacks	Opposing View	Hispanics	Opposing View
• Touching of one's hair by another person is often considered offensive.	• Touching of one's hair by another person is a sign of affection.	• Hissing to gain attention is acceptable.	• Hissing is considered impolite and indicates contempt.
• Preference for indirect eye contact during listening, direct eye contact during speaking as signs of attentiveness and respect.	• Preference for direct eye contact during listening and indirect eye contact during speaking as signs of attentiveness and respect.	• Touching is often observed between two people in conversation.	• Touching is usually unacceptable and usually carries a sexual overtone.
• Public behavior may be emotionally intense, dynamic, and demonstrative.	• Public behavior is expected to be modest and emotionally restrained. Emotional displays are seen as irresponsible or in bad taste.	• Avoidance of direct eye contact is sometimes a sign of attentiveness and respect; sustained direct eye contact may be interpreted as a challenge to authority.	• Direct eye contact is a sign of attentiveness and respect.
• Clear distinction between "argument" and "fight." Verbal abuse is not necessarily a precursor to violence.	• Heated arguments are viewed as suggesting that violence is imminent.	• Relative distance between two speakers in conversation is close.	• Relative distance between two speakers in conversation is farther apart.
• Asking "personal questions" of someone one has met for the first time is seen as improper and intrusive.	• Inquiring about jobs, family, and so forth of someone one has met for the first time is seen as friendly.	• Official or business conversations are preceded by lengthy greetings, pleasantries, and other talk unrelated to the point to business.	• Getting to the point quickly is valued.
• Use of direct questions is sometimes seen as harassment (e.g., asking when something will be finished is seen as rushing that person to finish).	• Use of direct questions for personal information is permissable.		
• Interruption during conversation is usually tolerated. Access to the floor is granted to the person who is most assertive.	• Rules of turn-taking in conversation dictate that one person has the floor at a time until all points are made.	**Asians**	**Opposing View**
		• Touching or hand-holding between members of the same sex is acceptable.	• Touching or hand-holding between members of the same sex is considered as a sign of homosexuality.
• Conversations are regarded as private between the recognized participants. "Butting in" is seen as eavesdropping and is not tolerated.	• Adding points of information or insights to a conversation in which one is not engaged is seen as being helpful.	• Hand-holding/hugging/kissing between men and women in public looks ridiculous.	• Hand-holding/hugging/kissing between men and women in public is acceptable.
• Use of expression "you people" is seen as pejorative and racist.	• Use of expression "you people" tolerated.	• A slap on the back is insulting.	• A slap on the back denotes friendliness.
• Accusations or allegations are general rather than categorical and are not intended to be all-inclusive. Refutation is the responsibility of the accused.	• Stereotypical accusations or allegations are all-inclusive. Refutation or making exception is the responsibility of the person making the accusation.	• It is not customary to shake hands with persons of the opposite sex.	• It is customary to shake hands with persons of the opposite sex.
		• Finger beckoning is only used by adults to call little children and not vice-versa.	• Finger beckoning is often used to call people.
• Silence denotes refutation of accusation. To state that you feel accused is regarded as an admission of guilt.	• Silence denotes acceptance of an accusation. Guilt is verbally denied.	**American Indians**	**Opposing View**
		• Personal questions may be considered prying.	• Personal questions are acceptable particularly when establishing case history information.
		• Gushing over babies may endanger the child.	• Gushing over babies shows admiration of the child.
		• A bowed head is a sign of respect.	• Lack of eye contact is a sign of shyness, guilt, or lying.
		• It is acceptable to ask the same question several times, if you doubt the truth of the person.	• It is a sign of inattention if the same question is asked several times.

Reprinted with permission from Cole L. *E Pluribus Unum: Multicultural Imperatives for the 1990s and Beyond*. Rockville, Md: American Speech-Language—Hearing Association; September 1989: 69.

556

TABLE 16–7. ASSESSMENT CATEGORIES WITH WHICH TO ELICIT RITUALS, BELIEFS, AND SYMBOLS OF CARE ACTIVITIES

Sleep

Condition of room/environment: Occupancy of rooms and bed/sleeping surface, kind of bed/sleeping surface and other furniture, condition of room (temperature, lights, doors and windows open or closed, other artifact/symbols in room).

Kinds of covering, comforting materials: Pillow/head support (height/number of supports used, type, positioning); covering (blanket type, sheet type, other).

Sleepwear: Covering on head, body, legs, feet (type and variation by season or event).

Care of bed linen: Kind of cleaning, frequency, how, by whom.

Bedtime ritual: Time, tasks, others involved, food or liquid consumed, sensory stimulation, symbols/icons used.

Rules for sleeping: When, with whom, how, in what positions, where, beliefs related to rules.

Rules for awakening: By whom/what, how, mechanisms used.

Awakening rituals: Time, tasks, others involved, food or liquid consumed, sensory stimulation, symbols/icons used.

Personal Hygiene

Tending one's body: Rituals for mouth care (tools and substances used, time, who can assist); rituals for body and hair care (how, when, where, how often, substances used, taboos, gender rules, symbols, beliefs associated with aspects of ritual).

Associations with health/illness: Care associated with body fluids/excretions, symbolism, body temperature, activities of tending one's body, substances used in rituals, seasonal/climate taboos, kinds of activities, time of day/year, gender rules, beliefs.

Eating

Kinds of foods: Preferences, dislikes, specific to an event, ritual, specific to time of day/week/month/year, seasonal, rules or taboos for hot foods, cold foods, rules for amount, type, composition, beliefs, and symbolism associated with specific foods.

Schedule of foods: Rules for when/when not to eat; amount related to time of day; healthy/ill status; associated with certain rituals, beliefs, symbols; before/after meal rituals, symbols/icons used/present.

Environment for eating: Place, people, position, taboos/rules, symbols/icons used/present.

Implements/utensils: Kind, number, rules for use of each, taboos, utensils as symbols.

Reprinted with permission from Rempusheski V. The role of ethnicity in elder care. *Nursing Clinics of N Am.* September 1989;24(3).

1. The use of a geriatric consultation team resulted in a comprehensive view of the elderly and reduced early recurrent readmissions.[23]
2. The geriatric consultation service improves awareness of functional problems, and increases use of rehabilitative services, but does not decrease the rate of readmission.[24]
3. The geriatric consultation team was unable to alter the degree of functional decline.[25]
4. The geriatric consultation team in the acute care hospital caused a 21% decline in the census of older patients.[26]

5. The patients who received consultation from the geriatric team fared similarly to the control group.[27]

It appears from these results that the efficacy of the geriatric team is not completely proven in controlled studies. Some of the negative outcomes may be a direct result of poor communication among the team. To improve this communication, Lee, Pappius, and Goldman[28] suggest

1. Direct communication (preferably face-to-face or by phone).
2. Frequent follow-up notes.
3. Agreement on the reason and roles of the team's intervention.
4. Limited suggestions to other team members.[28]

Finally, Blumfield and associates[29] suggest providing a complete educational program prior to implementing the geriatric team in an acute hospital.[29]

The most important member of the team, and one that is classically left out of studies of the type listed, is the patient. Patients desire information. However, they do not engage in information seeking behavior when communicating with doctors.[30] Beisecker and Beisecker's study[30] in this area provides five important points to consider when working with patients (Table 16–8).

In addition, health professionals tend to spend less time with older patients as is evidenced by the startling results of Radecki and co-authors' study[31] on the amount of time physicians spent with older patients. In this study, the authors found that internists and cardiologists spend more time with patients (approximately 18 minutes), as compared to general practitioners (approximately 12 minutes). All types of physicians studied spent less time with the older patient (2 to 3 minutes less).[31]

TABLE 16–8. PATIENT INFORMATION-SEEKING BEHAVIOR WHEN COMMUNICATING WITH DOCTORS

1. Patients express a uniformly strong desire for medical information.
2. Patients are much less willing to assume responsibility for medical decision making, preferring to delegate that responsibility to doctors.
3. Patients, on the average, exhibit relatively low rates of information-seeking behavior when interacting with doctors.
4. Situational variables explain information-seeking communication behavior for all types of patients better than do patient attitudes and sociodemographic characteristics.
5. Patient attitudes toward medical decision making are related to patient information-seeking communication behaviors only for patients with long interactions with physicians.

Reprinted with permission from Beisecker A, Beisecker B. Patient information-seeking behaviors when communicating with doctors. *Medical Care* January 1990;28(1):19–28.

Finally, in communicating with this valuable member of the team, what is an appropriate label to use? According to Barbato and Feezel,[32] the only terms rated positively by both young and old were, retired person, mature American, and senior citizen. All other terms were rated negatively.[32]

The key to communicating effectively with the older patient is best described by Purtillo in *The Allied Health Professional and the Patient: Techniques of Effective Interaction*.[33] Table 16–9 summarizes simple steps to more effective communication.

The success of verbal communications depends on (1) the way material is presented—the vocabulary used, the clarity of voice and the organization; (2) the attitude of the speaker; (3) the tone and volume of his voice; (4) the degree to which both speaker and receiver are able to listen effectively.[33]

WRITING

The topic of writing is adequately covered in numerous books and articles.[34–41] This section will define the different types of writing and give suggestions for the specialist to improve them.

The first major type of writing for communication is clinical documentation, which is composed of initial, progress, daily, and discharge note writing. For both legal and reimbursement purposes, the keys to effective note writing are

1. Accuracy: State exactly what you plan to do and did.
2. Completeness: Provide all necessary information and avoid extraneous comments.
3. Timeliness: Chart as close to the time of interaction as possible.
4. Honesty: Tell exactly what happened, do not assume, appear, or seem.

Appendix A provides samples of initial, discharge, progress, daily, and plan of care notes. (Table 16–10 provides a list of Dos and Don'ts for charting.[42]

Another important area of writing is professional writing. Professional writing includes articles for

TABLE 16–9. SIMPLE STEPS TO MORE EFFECTIVE LISTENING

- Be selective in what you listen to.
- Realize that words are only symbols—we impose our meanings on others' words.
- Concentrate on central themes rather than isolated statements.
- Judge content rather than style or delivery.
- Listen with an open mind—do not focus on emotionally charged words.
- The average person can listen four times faster than he or she can speak—use extra time to summarize.

Reprinted with permission from Walker R. Effective listening. *Am J Med Technol.* 1969;35:8–10.

TABLE 16–10. THE DOS AND DON'TS OF CHARTING

Do
Chart concisely, completely, and accurately.
Be objective and avoid tentative or vogue statements.
Chart promptly.
Be neat and legible.
Make entries in sequence, beginning with the most important data.
Use standard abbreviations and those approved by the agency.
Sign all timed entries with written signature and credentials.
On flow sheets, include as much routine data as possible.
Record problem-focused client information.
Make corrections appropriately.
Omit unnecessary words like "client" when the meaning is clear.
Include refusals of or omissions in care with the reason for the refusal or omission.

Don't
"Block" time on the chart.
Skip lines or leave white space.
Use ditto marks to repeat information.
Erase or use correct fluid over a notation.
Chart before the fact.
Use pencil or colored pens other than black or dark blue.
Make personal comments, argue, or complain on the medical record.

Reprinted with permission from Ignatevicius D. *Documentation.* Focus on Geriatric Care and Rehabilitation. Rockville, Md: Aspen Publishers, 1988;2(4).

publication and business letters. One of the best reference sources for writing business letters is by Piotrowski.[35] One of the best reference sources for the health professional in the area of article writing is by Lynch.[34] Appendix B contains two excellent articles on starting to write, and an outline from a series done by Dr Lynch for the *PT Forum.*

TABLE 16–11. HINTS TO GAINING INSIGHT INTO PATIENTS' INTERNAL MOTIVATING FACTORS

- Read the case history with care.
- Talk with the client about his/her history.
- Ask the client about his/her current and past expectations about performing activities of daily living.
- Ask family members about their performance expectations for the client.

Stay alert for past experiences and value that could affect motivation. Listen and look for
- Successful past motivators
- Cultural factors that could influence behaviors.
- Past experiences of pain.
- Need for approval.
- Need for independence.
- Need for control.
- Fear.
- Depression.

Reprinted with permission from Duchene P. Motivation of older adults. Focus on Geriatric Care and Rehabilitation. Rockville, Md: Aspen Publishers; 1990;3(8):2.

INDIVIDUAL PERCEPTIONS   MODIFYING FACTORS   LIKELIHOOD OF ACTION

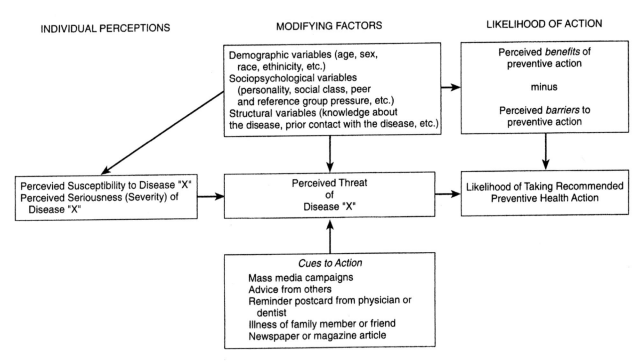

Figure 16–2. Health belief model. *(Reprinted with permission from Becker MH, et al. A new approach to explaining sick-role behavior in low-income populations. AJPH. March 1974;64(3):206.)*

COMPLIANCE AND MOTIVATION

The final areas to be discussed in this chapter are compliance and motivation. Motivation is an inner urge that moves a person to action.[43] Compliance is following orders and doing what is instructed.[44] As important as all the skills used in evaluation and treatment are in the rehabilitation realm, a person's drive and ability to follow through with a program may be just as important as the actual program itself.

Motivation may be broken up into internal and external motivations. Internal motivation is made up of the person's past values and experiences (desire, fear, thirst, and hunger).[43] The therapist can gain insight into a person's internal motivation by learning as much as possible about them. Table 16–11 provides a checklist to assist the therapist in gathering this information.

External motivation is characterized by the factors in the person's physical and social environment. Some of these factors are privacy, rewards, expectations from others, lighting, and temperature.[43] It is obvious that the therapist can influence external factors with a well designed environment and appropriate interaction with the patient.

Additional compliance and motivation factors can be described by various models. One of the most widely accepted models for health behavior is the Health Belief Model by Becker,[45] which is illustrated in Figure 16–2. Its main benefit in understanding patient behavior is isolating factors in individual patient compliance.

Orem's Self-Care Model is a particularly useful model for the rehabilitation of older patients. It differentiates between self-care (a patient's choice to act in a way that promotes health) and compliance (the patient's choice to follow instruction).[46] Figure 16–3 is a visual representation of the Orem model.[47] To use this model, the therapist must assess and contrast the

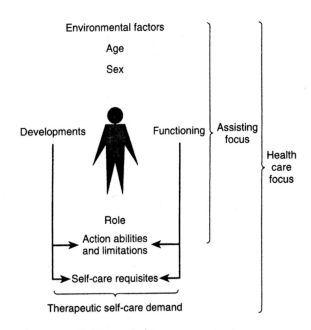

Figure 16–3. *Orem's self-care model. (Reprinted with permission from Orem DE. Nursing: Concepts of Practice. 3rd ed. New York: McGraw-Hill; 1985.)*

TABLE 16–12.   PINKSTON'S BEHAVIORAL INTERVENTIONS INTO SELF-CARE BEHAVIORS

Step	Implementation
1. Defining desired behavior	Select specific behavioral outcome (i.e., client will dress in underwear, slacks, shirt, shoes, and socks; client will wash face 3 times a day; client will use washroom 4 times a day).
2. Setting and using a schedule	Designate a time to begin and end each occurrence of self-care.
3. Providing response opportunity	Arrange or ask client to arrange materials (e.g., clothing, soap, and towel) so that they are usable and within easy reach.
4. Prompting correct behavior	Have the support person prompt the client to go through each step of the task in the correct order. If there is no response, the prompt is repeated once or twice, then 2 minutes later if necessary.
5. Allowing time for behavior to occur	If the client is attempting to complete a self-care task, instruct the care giver to wait until the task is completed. This should occur within 5 minutes.
6. Praise appropriate behavior	If the client is able to complete the task, the care giver offers praise or touching (food, token, or point on the recording form may also be used) and then prompts the client to go on to the next step.
7. Assistance if the behavior does not occur	If the client does not respond to the prompt within 30 seconds, the care giver guides the older person through the various steps required. The care giver provides help with any items the client is unable to complete because of physical impairment or pain.
8. Ignoring inappropriate behavior	If the client engages in inappropriate behavior, such as complaining, arguing, or any behaviors that serve to bring about an unnecessary delay in the process, the care giver should remove his or her attention from the client until the behavior ceases. Care giver then returns to step 4.
9. Recording	Behavior is recorded on recording form.

Reprinted with permission from Pinkston EM, Linsk NL. Behavioral family intervention with the impaired elderly. *Gerontologist.* 1984;24:576–583.

An Example of Pinkston's Behavioral Record

Name: Mr. Green   Date: Wednesday, November 3
Behavior: *Conversation—Communication or talking where Mr. G says at least three words in response to questions or statements by another family member.*
Please note when the behavior occurs and what happens before and after.

TIME		BEFORE	DURING	Describe what others did AFTER the behavior occurred. Check box.					
start	stop	What happened before the behavior occurred?	What happened when the behavior occurred?	Did not notice	Ignored	Criticized	Asked to do something else	Praised or rewarded	Other
9:00	9:03	Sitting at table	Asked for more breakfast	☐	☐	☐	☐	X	Gave more eggs
9:05	9:07	Asked what will do today	Said he would like to go for a walk	☐	☐	☐	☐	X	☐
10:30	10:33	Returned from walk	Complained about cold	☐	☐	☐	X	☐	☐
TOTAL			3				1	2	

Figure 16–4. *(Reprinted with permission from Pinkston EM, Linsk NL.* Care of the Elderly: A Family Approach. *Elmhurst, NJ: Pergamon Press; 1984;30.)*

TABLE 16–13. MOTIVATION LIST

The following is a list suggested by Dr. Raymond Harris to assist a leader (or therapist) to motivate an older individual to participate in the physical exercise program.

1. Recognition that the approach requires mental, emotional, and physical engagement.
2. Individualization of the program to the group or to the person.
3. Satisfaction of some of the participant's basic psychic needs.
4. Provision of choice elements and alternatives.
5. Social support and reinforcement.
6. Continuous productive measurement certifications from the beginning by assessment devices.
7. Incorporation of creative opportunities, such as novelty, change of pace, or improvisations.
8. Engagement of recreational elements, such as play and game qualities.
9. Personal projections of the leader as a concerned, interested, competent, and helpful person.
10. Attention to the aesthetics of the environment and the propitious atmosphere.
11. Counseling to some degree as an adjunct.

Reprinted with permission from Harris R, Frankel L. *A Guide to Fitness After Fifty.* New York: Plenum Press; 1977.

TABLE 16–14. YOUR CLIENT AND MOTIVATION FOR SELF-CARE

- Learn what the client believes is important and identify the client's priorities.
- Set mutual goals together.
- Recognize that your client's goals are more important than the staff's or institution's goals.
- Incorporate the individual's past experiences in the goal determination process.
- Help your client to have realistic expectations by discussing program goals.
- Stress that increasing independence in self-care is often a long, slow process.
- Reinforce positive and independent behaviors by giving concrete feedback on goal attainment.
- Use concrete, visible, and personally significant rewards.
- Involve the family in the goal-setting process whenever possible.

Use contracts as motivators
- Establish a contract with the client emphasizing choices based on realistic short-term goals.
- Include a realistic plan and time frame for goal accomplishment.
- Be certain to include reinforcers for goal attainment.
- Encourage the individual to agree verbally or consent to the contract.
- Have the contract signed by the individual and the health care providers.

Reprinted with permission from FOCUS on your client and motivation for self-care. In: *Focus on Geriatric Care and Rehabilitation.* Rockville, Md: Aspen Publishers; 1990.

person's assets and liabilities along the following dimensions: cognitive, psychological, and physical, and they must design a strategy based on these findings.[46]

The Pinkston Behavioral Model is another useful model for geriatric rehabilitation, especially for patients with cognitive impairments. It requires mutual participation of care giver and patient, the use of behavioral reinforcement, and continued care giver involvement.[46] Table 16–12 lists Pinkston's behavioral interventions for self-care behaviors, and Figure 16–4 provides an example of Pinkston's behavioral record. Besides models, various lists have been generated to help the practitioner in the area of motivation (Tables 16–13 and 16–14).

The final concept in compliance and motivation, and a thoughtful end to this discussion of communication, is an exploration of the Advocacy Model as it relates to compliance and motivation as discussed by Guccione.[48] In this model, the therapist acts on behalf of the patient based on the patient's desires. Getting to this point, however, takes five steps.

1. Provide the patient with all the information, so he or she is able to fully exercise free choice.
2. Assist the patient in determining which information is relevant to the decision.
3. Disclose personal views, so the patient realizes that the clinician may have a personal as well as professional bias.
4. Assist the patient in clarifying his or her own values.
5. Ascertain how patients comprehend their individuality.[48]

CONCLUSION

To truly be an advocate for and with the patient requires open communication. This chapter provides a means of understanding the normal and pathological changes that occur with age that affect communication, the senses, and the voice. This chapter also explored communication across cultures and among the team. In addition, writing as a means of communication was investigated. Finally, compliance and motivation were described as a possible outcome of adequate communication.

PEARLS

- *Changes in the major structures of the ear establish three main types of hearing loss: conductive (which can be reversed), sensorineural (which cannot be reversed) and mixed (which can be partially reversed).*
- *Detecting hearing loss in a physical therapy setting can range from the use of cues to screenings to more formal tests, such as the Hearing Handicap Inventory.*
- *Simple interventions, such as changes in the mode of communication and environment (i.e., speaking*

slowly in a noncompeting environment), will enhance communication.

- *All five major senses tend to decline with old age, and yet they are needed to enhance communication; therefore, physical therapists should bring in the other senses as much as possible.*

- *The voice of an older person changes with age because of reduced respiratory efficiency and changes in the oral and laryngeal cavities. Nevertheless, these changes have little impact on the older person's ability to communicate.*

- *Understanding the effectiveness of all the team members, especially the patient, will help to enhance communication.*

- *Accuracy, completeness, timeliness, and honesty are the keys to effective note writing.*

- *To motivate older persons, the therapist must first assess the person's internal motivation (i.e., values and experience) and then assess and appropriately modify the external factors of motivation (i.e., the physical and social environment).*

REFERENCES

1. Kelly LS. Are we ready for the year 2000? *Hear J.* 1985; 38:15–17.

2. Dwyer B. Detecting hearing loss and improving communication in elderly persons. *Focus Ger Care & Rehab.* Nov/Dec 1987; 1(6).

3. Cherney L. Aging and communication. In: Lewis C, ed. *Aging: The Health Care Challenge.* Philadelphia; Davis; 1989.

4. Heller B, Gaynor E. Hearing loss and aural rehabilitation of the elderly. *Clin Nurs.* 1981;3:1.

5. Boone D, Bayles K, Koopmann C. Communication aspects of aging. *Otolaryngol Clin N Am.* May 1982; 15(2).

6. Cullinan TR, Silver JH, Gould ES, et al. *Lancet.* 1979; 24:1642–1644.

7. Maguire G. The changing realm of the senses. In: Lewis C, ed. *Aging: The Health Care Challenge.* Philadelphia; Davis; 1989.

8. Ryan EB, Capadano HL. Age perceptions and evaluative reactions toward adult speakers. *J Ger.* 1978; 33:98–102.

9. Stewart MA, Ryan EB. Attitudes toward younger and older adult speakers: effects of varying speech rates. *J Language and Social Psych.* 1982; 1:91–109.

10. Honjo I, Isshiki N. Laryngoscopic and voice characteristics of aged persons. *Arch Otolaryngol.* 1980; 106:149–150.

11. Kahane JC. Anatomic and physiologic changes in the aging peripheral speech mechanism. In: Beasley DS, Davis GA, eds. *Aging: Communication Processes and Disorders.* New York; Grune & Stratton; 1981:21–46.

12. Noback GJ. Correlation of stages of ossification of the laryngeal cartilages and morphologic age changes in other tissues and organs. *J Gerontol.* 1949; 4(abstract):329.

13. Lynne-Davies P. Influence of age on the respiratory system. *Geriatrics.* August 1977; 57–60.

14. Meto M. Aging and motor speech production. *Top Geriatr. Rehabil.* July 1986; 1(4).

15. Massler M. Oral aspects of aging. *Postgrad Med.* 1971; 49:179–183.

16. Cohen T, Gitman L. Oral complaints and taste perception in the aged. *J Ger.* 1959; 14:294–298.

17. Mysak E, Hanley T. Aging processes in speech: pitch and duration characteristics. *J Ger.* 1958; 13:309–313.

18. Meadows J. Cultural diversity. *Community Health Section Newsletter.* 1993.

19. Cole L. E Pluribus Unum: multicultural imperatives for the 1990s and beyond. *ASHA.* September 1989; 69.

20. Rempusheski V. The role of ethnicity in elder care. *Nurs Clin N Am.* September 1989; 24(3).

21. Chee P, Kane R. Cultural factors affecting nursing home care for minorities. *J Am Ger Soc.* February 1983; 31(2).

22. Maguire G. *Care of the Elderly: A Health Team Approach.* Boston; Little Brown & Co; 1985.

23. Berkman B, Campion E, Swagerty E. Geriatric consultation team: alternate approach to social work discharge planning. *J Ger Social Work.* Spring 1983; 5(3):77–87.

24. Campion E, Jette A, Berkman B. An interdisciplinary geriatric consultation service: a controlled trial. *J Am Ger Soc.* December 1983; 31(12): 792–796.

25. McVey L, Becker P, Saltz C, et al. Effect of a geriatric consultation team on functional status of elderly hospitalized patients: *An Intern Med.* January 1989; 110(1):79–84.

26. Barker W, Williams F, Zimmer J, et al. Geriatric consultation teams in acute hospitals: impact on back-up of elderly patients. *J Am Ger Soc.* June 1985; 33(6):422–427.

27. Gayton D, Wood-Dauphinee S, deLorimer M, et al. Trial of a geriatric consultation team in an acute care hospital. *J Am Ger Soc.* August 1987; 35(8): 726–736.

28. Lee T, Pappius E, Goldman L. Impact of inter-physician communication on the effectiveness of medical consultation. *Am J Med* January 1983; 74:106–112.

29. Blumenfield S, Morris J, Sherman F. The geriatric team in the acute care hospital. *J Am Ger Soc.* October 1982; 30(10):660–664.

30. Beisecker A, Beisecker B. Patient information-seeking behaviors when communicating with doctors. *Medical Care.* January 1990; 28(1):19–28.

31. Radecki S, Kane R, Solomon D. Do physicians spend less time with older patients? *J Am Ger Soc.* August 1988; 36(8):713–718.

32. Barbato C, Feezel J. The language of aging in different age groups. *Gerontologist.* 1987; 27(4):527–532.

33. Purtillo R. *The Allied Health Professional and the Patient: Techniques of Effective Interaction.* Philadelphia; Saunders; 1973.

34. Lynch B, Chapman C. *Writing for Communication in Science and Medicine.* New York; Van Nostrand Reinhold Co.; 1980.

35. Piotrowski M. *Rewriting Strategies and Suggestions for Improving Your Business Writing.* New York; Harper & Row; 1989.

36. Aslanian M, Manalio G, Taylor C. The joys of paperwork: care plans really can work. *Caring.* October 1986; 92–94.

37. Austin MJ, Skelding AH, Smith PL. Managing information. In: *Delivering Human Services.* New York; Harper & Row; 1977:360–371.

38. Bouchard MM, Shane HC. Use of the problem-oriented medical record in the speech and hearing profession: Special Reports. *ASHA.* March 1977; 157–159.

39. Griffith J, Ignatavicius D. *The Writer's Handbook.* Baltimore; Resources Applications, Inc.; 1986.

40. Lampe S. Focus charting: streamlining documentation. *Nurs Man.* 1985; 16–7,43.

41. Murphy J, Beglinger JE, Johnson B. Charting by exception: meeting the challenge of cost containment. *Nurs Man.* 1988; 19:2,56–72.

42. Ignatavicius D. Documentation. *Focus on Geriatric Care and Rehabilitation.* September 1988; 2(4):1–8.

43. Duchene P. Motivation of older adults. *Focus on Geriatric Care and Rehabilitation.* February 1990; 3(8):1–8.

44. Ransdem E. Compliance and motivation. *Top Geriatr Rehabil.* April 1988; 3(3):1–15.

45. Becker MH, McVey LJ, Saltz CC, et al. A new approach to explaining sick-role behavior in low-income populations. *AJPH.* March 1974; 64(3):206.

46. Thibodaux L, Shewchuk R. Strategies for compliance in the elderly. *Top Geriatr Rehabil.* April 1988; 3(3):21–34.

47. Orem D. *Nursing: Concepts of Practice.* 3rd ed. New York; McGraw-Hill; 1985.

48. Guccione A. Compliance and patient autonomy: ethical and legal limits to professional dominance. *Top Geriatr Rehabil.* April 1988; 3(3):62–74.

Appendix A Sample Notes

Initial Note	Initial Plan of Care
Initial Evaluation	Daily Note
Initial Discharge	

Initial Note

PHYSICAL THERAPY SERVICES OF WASHINGTON, D.C., INC.

1150 18th Street, N.W.
Suite 4
Washington, D.C. 20036

June 19

Dear Dr.

Thank you for referring _____ to Physical Therapy Services for treatment of her left shoulder adhesive capsulitis. She was evaluated on 6/19 and at that time revealed a history of having had a frozen shoulder for approximately one year. Functionally, _____ is unable to perform routine ADLs, such as overhead dressing, lifting objects of more than 2 pounds, and washing her hair, secondary to pain and weakness. The pain is in the deltoid area and at night radiates into the arm and wrist.

On objective evaluation, _____ is extremely limited in range of motion with active shoulder abduction to 68° and flexion to 85° with reports of pain at end range of both movements. Internal rotation is limited to 42°, external rotation to 11°. The patient presents with 3+/5 strength in external rotation, 4/5 strength in internal rotation, 4/5 strength in flexion and abduction. Patient reports extreme pain on resistance to all these movements. Right grip strength is 53 pounds, left grip strength is 42 pounds. On a postural evaluation, _____ presents with 8/10 forward head as well as 8/10 rounded shoulders.

The program we would like to pursue with _____ is one of heat, electrical stimulation, ultrasound, exercise, and ice, and a strong home exercise program. We will continue to see _____ twice a week for 2 months depending on patient's progress with goals being normal range of motion, normal strength, and ability to perform ADLs without pain.

If you have any questions or comments please don't hesitate to contact me. For billing and insurance purposes please sign and return the enclosed treatment plan.

Sincerely,

Carole Lewis, P.T., G.C.S., Ph.D.

Figure 16A–1.

Initial Evaluation

Date: _____

Patient's Name: _____ Phone: _____

Address: _____

Attending Physician's Name: _____

Diagnosis for which treatment has been prescribed: _____

_____

_____

Patient's Program: _____

_____

_____

Goals: _____

_____

History: _____

_____

_____

Function: _____

_____

Pain Where: _____

When: _____

ROM: _____

_____

Strength: _____

_____

Gait: _____

_____

Posture: _____

_____

Sensation: _____

Figure 16A–2.

Initial Discharge

PHYSICAL THERAPY SERVICES OF WASHINGTON, D.C., INC.

1150 18th Street, N.W.
Suite 4
Washington, D.C. 20036

September 19

Dear Dr.

Thank you for referring _____ to Physical Therapy Services. She received her last treatment on 8/19 and at that time had made significant improvements. Her shoulder flexion has increased from 85° to 171°. Her abduction is now 167°, external rotation has improved from 11° to 79°, internal rotation has improved from 42° to 79°. _____ now has presented with 4+/5 strength in all motions, although she still reports pain at end range. She is independent with all her ADLs at this time. She is also independent on a very comprehensive exercise program of strengthening and stretching that she will perform on a daily basis. She will contact us in 1 month as to her status.

If you have any questions or comments please don't hesitate to contact me.

Sincerely,

Carole Lewis, P.T., G.C.S., Ph.D

Figure 16A–3.

Initial Plan of Care

PHYSICAL THERAPY SERVICES

1150 18th Street, N.W.,
Suite No. 4
Washington, D.C. 20036

OF
WASHINGTON, D.C., INC.

Patient _____ Physician _____

Age _____ Diagnosis _____

Treatment received during the total course of therapy:

____ Hot Packs	____ Ultrasound	____ Taping	____ Therapeutic Exercise
____ Cold Packs	____ Electrical Stim.	____ TENS	____ Act. Range of Motion
____ Cervical Traction	____ Phonophoresis	____ Soft Tissue Mob.	____ Act. Assistive ROM
____ Pelvic Traction	____ Joint Mobilization	____ Massage	____ Pas. Range of Motion
____ Back School	____ Myofascial Release	____ Paraffin	____ Spray and Stretch
____ Posture Evaluation	____ Functional Electrical Stim.	____ Iontophoresis	____ Medcosonolator
____ Functional Activities	____ Neuromuscular Reeducation	____ Gait Training	____ Whirlpool
____ Home Visit	____ Office Assessment	____ Other (_____)	

Admission Goals   1. _____

2. _____

3. _____

4. _____

5. _____

Frequency _____ times per week   Duration for _____ weeks

Notes _____

_____

_____

_____

_____

Therapist _____ Date _____ Physician _____ Date _____

Therapist _____ Date _____ Physician _____ Date _____

Therapist _____ Date _____ Physician _____ Date _____

Please sign and return to Physical Therapy Services. Thank you.

Figure 16A–4.

Daily Note

MODALITIES

PHYSICAL THERAPY SERVICES

OF
WASHINGTON, D.C., INC.

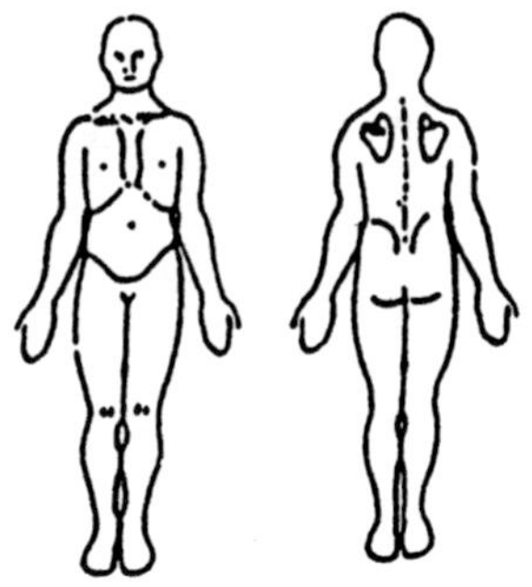

Date: _____

Patient Name: _____

Notes: _____

_____

_____

_____

_____

_____

_____

_____

_____

_____

_____

_____

_____

_____

_____

_____

_____

_____

_____

Figure 16A–5.

Appendix B
Selected Portions of Workshops
by B. Lynch*

SESSION I: WANTED: THE PT WRITER

Do you at moments think that you have an important observation to share with others? Or maybe a helpful hint, a solution to a management problem, a strong opinion, the results of a study? Perhaps you have mentioned your idea to a colleague, who responded with an enthusiastic suggestion to write about it in an article for a professional journal, such as *Physical Therapy Forum* or *Topics in Geriatric Rehabilitation*. Which of the following was your response to the suggestion?

1. Your mouth felt dry and your chest tightened.
2. You scoffed, commenting that your idea was not so important.
3. You reddened, saying that the idea was too personal and not significant to anyone else.
4. You felt satisfied with the praise of your colleague and friend, but feared that anyone else would think, "So what?"
5. You said that you didn't have time to write.
6. You sighed: "I did that once and my article was rejected."
7. You said: "I can't write well, and writing is laborious, even painful."

None of the above? or most of the above? especially Number 7?

The PT: Predisposed to Be a Writer

The responses are common, but they are not logical for the physical therapist. Having seen first hand the remarkable results physical therapists achieve with their patients, and the skills and observations required of the PT in working with patients, I know that PTs not only have important information to communicate to one another, but also have a special predisposition, by virtue of their training and practice, to develop and improve writing skills. The PT is already trained to:

■ Observe each patient critically and note overt and subtle diagnostic signals.
■ Perceive small increments of progress.
■ Expect specific outcomes, not immediately but down the line.
■ Communicate carefully and explain thoroughly.
■ Practice patience.

These are precisely the characteristics a developing writer must have.

How can you best develop professional writing skills? Ordinarily I would recommend participating in an interactive program, such as a workshop or seminar. However, given the above characteristics you have already cultivated as a PT, and given your professional motivation, I believe that you can advance considerably through this series of articles, which will guide you incrementally through the basics of writing well and of identifying the symptoms of faulty writing. This Workshop series offers instruction and programmatic exercises that you may patiently apply in improving your own writing. To get the most benefit from the "therapy," you should participate in *all* the exercises, because they build progressively, each honing some aspect of writing ability necessary for later exercises.

Record each exercise in a singular-to-purpose notebook so that you will have a permanent record of your responses and can review your writing progress. The notebook, henceforth referred to as a *journal*, should be bound (not loose-leaf or spiral). Number and date each exercise as you enter it into your journal.

Although you may do this program alone, consider sharing it with one or two colleagues. In working with others, meet once a week and review the exercises. By interacting with others, you will learn more and will probably have more fun.

*Reproduced with permission from Lynch B, Chapman C. Writing for Communication in Science & Medicine. New York: Van Nostrand Reinhold Company; 1980.

Motivation

The first step in becoming a writer is to think of yourself as a writer and to understand your motives for writing. Writing can be pleasurable, satisfying, and even fulfilling. A writer may have published 1 article or 200 articles; but, as in biomedical research and clinical practice, fulfillment comes as much through the habit of writing as with the product itself. With the habit comes the identity of self as writer. I hope to lead you not only to the habit of but also to an addiction to writing.

Meanwhile, other rewards are possible—fame, for example, or at least professional recognition. In writing a piece, you become the *author;* in having it read, you become an *authority.* Please be encouraged by the knowledge that authority begins with *author.*

Among the great wonders of professional and academic life is a syndrome known as *publish-or-perish.* Lamentations have been voiced about the demand by universities and medical institutions that faculty members and even staff write, submit, and publish research, clinical, and observational information. Health professionals may see themselves as pressured to pursue an artificial goal of publication rather than that of satisfying specific needs, obligations, and services. Nonetheless, an alternative view is that publication overtly proves one's professional competence and fulfills one's responsibility to inform colleagues of new ideas—and even opinions. Furthermore, the number of publications generally seems to correlate directly with professional promotion and institutional reputation. Finally, a reputation built through publications means grant money for more programs, in turn leading to more publications about the results. Publish-or-perish may seem a poor motive for writing, but it is decidedly evolutionary in the survival of the fittest. If this is your stimulus for writing, you are eager, if not anxious, to get articles written and published. With luck, as you struggle for publishing success, you will strive for excellence and satisfaction in writing as well.

I hope that you want not only to be published but also to be *read.* If so, you must write *well.* If all clinical articles were clearly written, imagine how much more would be read and how many more patents and practitioners would benefit.

Standards, Audience, and Opportunity

Coincident with a writer's idealistic or altruistic motive to write well so that his or her message will serve humanity is the countering fear of rejection. Such fear is soundly based. Journals are becoming more and more particular about what they accept. They do not lack materials; to the contrary, most publishers of professional journals are swamped with submissions. And printing costs are much higher today than they were just a few years ago. So publishers can afford to be choosy. While you may be perishing, they are enjoying the benefit of publishing. They must be strict about both the content and the style of writing; after all, the prestige of their journals depends on both.

A frequent occurrence, however, is not out-and-out rejection, but the acceptance of an article "contingent on editing." What do you do then? Chances are that when you wrote and submitted the paper, you thought it was reasonably coherent and lucid. Or, possibly you knew it had problems, but you could not figure out what they were or how to correct them when you did spot them. Could you edit a manuscript that an author returned? Do you know how to spot and correct the problems of syntax, organizational structure, or content? Publication of the paper depends on your editing and rewriting skills—but I expect that as you complete this writing program you will be able to edit and rewrite credibly.

Also, remember that editors and reviewers are human. Besides stacks of work, they have moods. If your writing is confusing, muddled, boring, or abstruse, no matter how important the content, the editor might become annoyed and impatient and, consequently, overly critical of your manuscript; or he or she might ignore it altogether, except, of course, for the brief moment taken to reject it. But, with all these human variables, the challenge of writing becomes that much more intriguing because the writing hypothesis is communication—whether or not you are able to make others comprehend ideas from your own mind as represented in your writing.

The first step toward success in writing is to understand who your audience is and what publications are available to you as a PT writer. The focus in this program is on the physical therapist as the primary audience, and on physicians and other professionals who work with PTs as the secondary audience. The available publications are weekly newspapers, professional journals, research journals, books, and book chapters. Each publication has its range of subjects, types of articles, and standards for writing. The subjects covered in the publications range from announcements and reports of special meetings to accounts of personal professional experiences, helpful tips for the practitioner, case reports, research reports, and suggestions for improving business administration and professional skills (including those involved in writing).

The first program of exercises will help you understand the opportunities and standards for publishing in the PT field, and to perceive yourself as a potential conveyor of information within the profession. Remember to enter every exercise in your writing journal; record all related observations and thoughts.

Program 1

Exercise 1 In the next 2 weeks, look at the available physical therapy journals and newspapers with the points of view of writer/editor, rather than simply as reader. Analyze each publication for:

1. Types of articles.
2. Lengths and numbers of each type of article.
3. Format for each type, that is, the order in which the information is organized.

Exercise 2   List or photocopy pertinent information from the "Instructions for Authors" page of each publication, noting specifically the types of materials called for, the name and address of the publisher, and all particulars relating to manuscript preparation and submission.

Exercise 3   Identify all of your own motives for writing, and record those motives in your journal.

Exercise 4   Think about your own work experiences, case encounters, techniques for client management, and what might be said that is worth saying. Write a list of these ideas. Also, list the publications in which your subject matter would be most appropriate. Note the format that would suit your topics best.

SESSION II—OUTLINING

Many writing courses begin with the teacher expecting the students to write a complete outline of the articles they will write. Unfortunately, and realistically, for the novice writer the very thought of being able to have a complete plan at the start paralyzes minds and fingers. The reaction is similar to focusing on the mountain you intend to climb and thinking that you will never make it. I find it easier to look up the trail a few hundred yards to an agreeable spot that will offer an encouraging view of what I have, in fact, so effortlessly (!) managed to traverse. Soon enough, I am on top of the mountain and have a complete overview.

Composing an article can proceed similarly— idea to idea, section to section. Sometimes when you begin writing, you do not really know where the trail of thoughts will lead you, and it is a good practice to keep your mind open to forks in the trail. An opportunity to explore an unexpected line of thought may lead you to an important discovery.

So, view the overall article as a series of steps. You use individual words to construct phrases, phrases to construct clauses, clauses to construct sentences. Each piece, considered separately, is easy to write. Composing the larger part is just another step—a matter of putting together what you have already written so clearly. Remember, because you have edited each word so carefully, and have made your sentences so logical, constructing paragraphs will be a simple matter of organization. That organization relates to the overall composition (or idea movement) of the entire article; therefore, we will now look at how to conceptualize the article, and in a subsequent session we will look at the internal organization of paragraphs.

Go Back to the Beginning

In the first few sessions of this Workshop, we considered the three steps you should take before beginning your article. You may have now written 12–16 paragraphs of the article, so now is a good time to return to your original intention (you noted this in your journal) and consider whether or not you should revise those steps. Or, perhaps you were not sure at that time and now can complete the steps. The three steps are

1. Decide on the audience you want to read your article: physical therapists; all allied health professionals; specialists; subspecialists; technicians; lay public; students; adults/children, etc.
2. Pick the publication you will submit your article to. Consider the type of publication suitable to your purposes: professional journal; professional newspaper; popular magazine. Consider several that may be appropriate for your article. Carefully review each candidate publication for *content* (Does it seem to match what you have to offer?); *audience appeal* (the same audience as your target audience?); *use of figures and tables; the average length of the articles.*
3. Carefully review the "Information for Authors" page from the journal you have chosen. Note any particular details pertinent to your article: photos, tables, figures, bibliography, etc.

Try an Outline

Although some writers can dictate an entire article without the benefit of a definitive outline, most writers find outlines helpful at some draft stage. In fact, outlines are helpful in many ways—in organizing the writing of the first draft; in preparing the abstract or summary; in preparing spinoff works such as professional lectures, class notes, and even letters to colleagues and friends; and in preparing experimental protocol.

An outline is by no means required before or while you write your article. Indeed, some authors are stymied and stifled by outlines. However, it is a good idea to try working with an outline at least once to find out if the mode suits you.

Outlining the Research Article

If you are doing experimental or clinical research, the outline tends to evolve by itself in your lab notes— with the hypothesis stated at the beginning of the research project, the steps of the method briefly described, and results listed as data are analyzed. When your research is finished, complete the outline, keeping in mind the journal you have selected. The clearest example of an outline is that for an IMRAD article. IMRAD is an acronym for introduction, materials and methods, results, and discussion.

The first marks you should make on paper are rather skeletal and simple: just write the name of each formal section of the IMRAD used by the journal. To leave plenty of space between each heading, write each heading on a separate sheet of paper. Assign a roman numeral to those headings.

I. Introduction
II. Methods and Materials
III. Results
IV. Discussion
V. Summary/Conclusion/Abstract

That was simple, but you are not yet finished with this step. Each of those headings represents a sizable body of words, some more than others, but each sizable enough to warrant the assumption that there is a succinct theme to each, that is, a major idea you are expressing. Everything you will say in a given section should relate to that major idea. Formulate the theme of each section in a single sentence and write it after the appropriate heading in the outline.

I. Introduction: (thematic statement)
II. Method and materials: (name method)
III. . . . etc.

If you have already done some scribbling and scratching in your lab book, the next activity will be easier than if you are thinking about your article for the first time. Take your outline and, section by section, reflect on each thematic statement. On scratch paper, scribble down the main points you think should be made about that theme. Remember, these are only main ideas, not the supporting details or the supporting reasons that prove or illustrate the ideas. These main ideas are the topics of the section's theme and, as such, warrant a full paragraph of explanation in your article. The one-sentence statement of the topic should be assigned a capital letter, beginning the list with "A."

I. Introduction: (thematic statement)
  A. (Topic statement)
  B. (Topic statement)
II. Method: (state method)
  A. (Description of patients or materials)
  B. (Description of method in study)
III. Results:
  A. (Topic sentence—results, category 1)
  B. (Topic sentence—results, category 2)
IV. Discussion
  A. (Conclusion 1)
  B. (Conclusion 2)
  C. (Implications)

If you have done that much, that is, if you have thought through all the main ideas in topic form, you have done a lot. In fact, the crisis is over and what fol-lows is the fun of developing each topic by dissecting it into its various components. Those components may be dissected by logic (inductive or deductive), by cause-and-effect relationships, by physical description, by chronological directions, or by syntheses. (You will learn how to do this in the session on paragraphs.)

Whether or not you develop your outline into components or even into further detail (a, b, c, etc.) is a matter of personal style. Some writers like to item-ize so thoroughly in outline form that they need only supply transitional and connecting phrases to actu-ally write the article. Others prefer to let thoughts flow more randomly on paper at the outline stage. Some find it best not to write full sentence in an out-line and instead use phrases, producing what is called a topic outline.

Whichever, when you have completed the out-line, study it for overall flow of thesis. Does each topic sentence lead in some order, whether logical, chronological, or spatial, to the next topic sentence? If not, you probably have some rearranging to do, or maybe you have left out an important thought-step. If two topic sentences within a single section seem re-dundant, maybe combining them is in order.

You probably remember the rule that if there is an A there must be a B, if a 1, a 2. The reason is that the divisions of an outline *divide* thoughts into com-ponents. With only one component, only one idea is given; thus, there is no division. The component should be represented, therefore, as a single idea. Conceivably, for example, the Introduction might in one, short succinct paragraph stating the central the-sis of the entire article. In that event, the thematic sentence accompanying roman numeral I should suf-fice. However, if the Introduction has at least two components, those should be specified.

Outlining the Essay-Type Article

Now let's outline an article that does not have a pre-determined format. An essay is a short article on one subject usually presenting the personal views of the author. The essay may argue for or against an idea, or present an objective discussion or description of the subject. Physical therapists find the essay a useful form for describing and encouraging the use of a ther-apeutic technique. The essay's structure is not for-malized, but several sections are typical: an introduc-tion, idea development or argument, and conclusion.

The following is an outline of an article by Re-becca A. Davidson that appeared in the *PT Forum*, January 14, 1991. If you have that issue, follow the ar-ticle's developments as you read through the outline. I will use a full-sentence outline.

Outline of "The Art of Listening—The Heart of a Caring Profession"

A. During a physical therapy session, a patient re-veals that his last therapist was not very good because the therapist "didn't listen."

B. Diagnostic and therapy machinery and a lack of time tend to preempt the essential listening skill.

I. PTs should carefully listen to patients for several reasons.

A. To confirm a diagnosis or to discover a different reason for the patient's problem, the therapist must listen to the patient's account of his symptoms and behaviors.

B. To develop appropriate treatment plans and goals, health care providers must take into account the patient's goals and cares.

C. To engender trust and gratitude in the patient relationship, the therapist must show interest—by listening.

D. To demonstrate to the patient that you care about him and his progress you must show that you are open to him—by listening.

II. Here's how you can become a good listener.

A. Make eye contact.

B. Focus your attention exclusively on the patient.

C. Express compassion.

Conclusion: By listening, you can help the patient to restore a sense of self-worth and improve your quality of care.

The above outline is broad, not detailed. It's the sort of outline you might be able to construct from your basic ideas even before beginning to write. As you write, you "flesh out" the subcomponent and begin to discover what you know and think about each topic. As you complete a section or subsection, go back and fill in more details in your outline. For example, Part I.C. might develop with the following details:

I.

A. To engender trust and gratitude in the patient relationship, the therapist must show interest—by listening.

1. People need to be heard.
2. Patients expect you to be interested in hearing about their ailments.
3. A person feels better physically after speaking and feels better emotionally.
4. Refusing to listen will produce resentment and magnify physiological problems.

The actual paragraph is written as follows:

A less practical, but no less important motive for listening is patient gratification. People feel the need to be heard. Patients assume that you are interested in their bodies; they expect you, of all people, to listen to their ailments. We cannot deny psychosomatic realities—when a person feels emotionally relieved after speaking, he/she is likely to feel better physi-

cally as well. Likewise, if a person is denied a listening ear, feelings of hostility, resentment, or disappointment tend to magnify physiological and functional problems. Listen, and make someone's day.

Outlining with a Gimmick

Occasionally, use of a gimmick might be an original and appropriate way to develop an article. For example, in the article "Early Intervention—Bedside PT" in *PT Forum* (March 15, 1991), Mary Russell uses the word "bedside" as the title, the subject, and the sectional development gimmick of her article. To give suggestions on maximizing your bedside care of patients, she instructs: "Think B.E.D.S.I.D.E.!" then develops a topic for each letter of the word. A topic outline of her article would look like the following:

Introduction:	My experience as bedside PT		
	I.	B:	Body Mechanics
	II.	E:	Equipment
	III.	D:	Document!
	IV.	S:	Scheduling
	V.	I:	Initiative
	VI.	D:	Demonstrate
	VII.	E:	Encourage!
Conclusion:	You can make a difference.		

The proper form of the outline is not so important as the flow of development, and you should not let formalities block your writing process early in the article's development. At this stage, just get your thoughts in order and under control. As you write the sections you can refer back to the outline, altering its structure with the flashes of perception that come from the illuminating (!) writing process itself. To make your outline even more useful, you might leave an oversized margin on the left or right, in which you can make notes concerning ideas, figures, tables, and references corresponding to appropriate topics.

Program

Exercise One   Make a broad outline of any three published articles.

Exercise Two   Make a broad outline (roman numerals and capital letters) of the article you are writing. Remember first to review the first three steps.

Exercise Three   Add another level of detail to your outline (1, 2, 3, etc.)

(Dr Lynch, author of the book *Writing for Communication in Science and Medicine,* is a freelance writer in the Washington, DC, area and a former university professor. She welcomes your comments and questions about writing. She may be contacted at: 815 Bowie Road, Rockville, MD 20852.)

PART III

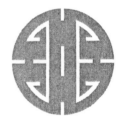

Administration and Management

CHAPTER 17

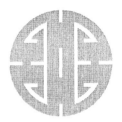

Attitudes and Ethics in Gerontology

HOW MEDICAL CARE IS CHANGING

In today's world, the growing elderly population, advances in technology, and philosophical attitudes are changing the way we think ethically. In the past, the medical treatment of a patient was primarily humanistic due to the paucity of scientific knowledge. Patients were treated spiritually rather than the disease being treated. Given the rapid advances in medical science, there is a great concern that spiritual treatment or meeting the patient's emotional needs will take a back seat to more technologically oriented treatments.[1] As this concern grows, the ability to meet the emotional needs of the elderly has also diminished, which has been a natural consequence of the increased specialization in medical technology.[1] An older person with multiple problems may have several different physicians and therapists to care for his or her different needs. With the demise of the general practitioner, the intimate relationship between clinician and patient likewise ceases.

In addition to technological changes, attitudes are changing and a concern for patients' "rights" is growing. The Miranda decision,[2] which required that people accused of a crime be informed of their rights under the law, has dramatically changed the legal institution. Likewise, an analogous development is occurring in the health care system with more of an emphasis placed on informing patients of their rights. Medicine is shifting away from a paternalistic role to giving the patient more responsibility in decision making, and this may be threatening, especially to the elderly who may be more comfortable with traditional roles.[3] Clinicians in the past have used paternalism to express compassion and minimize the patient's fear and pain, but patients have often taken this role to mean, "They will decide and do what is necessary for me." The shift away from this relationship requires patients, with proper guidance and information, to determine their own medical care.

Ethics and Managed Care and Medicare

Changes in health care in the form of shrinking economic resources, increased patient participation in decision making, and ongoing professional turf battles are dilemmas facing practitioners. Managed competition and care are mechanisms that function to varying degrees to limit access to rehabilitation therapists in choice of treatment and number of visits. Under managed care, there is the potential for therapists to be "double agents" with contractual obligations to the managed care plan and professional fiduciary responsibilities to the patient. These competing needs of differing groups (e.g., consumer, provider, insurer, and purchaser of care) affect therapists' clinical decision making in a managed care environment. Therapists must be able to analyze clinical cases and use moral reasoning and ethical judgement in deciding upon resource allocation and distribution of justice. While every professional educational program in rehabilitation must teach some content in ethics, the degree to which ethics is integrated into clinical practice and part of professional development varies. Under the managed care model of care, practicing the ethics of care becomes increasingly difficult, especially in the area of geriatrics.

The United States has focused attention on the rising costs of health care coincident with the increasing age of the population. Arguments have been made to overtly ration care to older persons; however, general acceptance of the need to ration scarce resources, whether or not such a policy is actually formalized, can lead to covert rationing. Overt rationing under managed care has already occurred. Some of the data put forth to justify that rationing must be challenged, and ethical principles should be applied to provide appropriate and perhaps less costly care.[4] Because the concept of managed care is involved with medicine, a moral enterprise, public and private policy enters the ethical arena.[5,6,7] Health care costs have risen steadily for many years as a result of an inflationary reimbursement system, technological advances, an aging population, and increasing patient expectations. This has accelerated the growth of managed care organizations in an attempt to control costs. Medicare has evolved towards managed care model of health care delivery through the implementation of prospective payment systems and capitation on many services, inclusive of rehabilitation.

PERSONAL ATTITUDES

How the aged are dealt with depends on how they are viewed. When negative stereotypes exist and therapists have a negative view of the elderly, the health care the individual receives is compromised.

Most studies of attitudes toward the elderly have focused on gender, contact, race, and socioeconomic status. Even though labels are an important descriptive tool, attitudes may develop toward a group as a whole that ignores individual differences.[8,9] Increased contact with the elderly allows people to view them on a more personal level rather than generalizing or stereotyping about the meaning of being old. Harris and Fiedler[10] demonstrated that the more contact preadolescents had with the elderly, the more positive their attitude was to that population. Preadolescent attitudes are important to examine since according to Piaget, preadolescence is a transitional stage between concrete and formal operations, as well as the beginning of attitude judgments and stereotyping.[10]

At a very young age, people learn that all old people must be looked after and attribute personality traits to them, such as childishness, irritability, incapability of reasoning or of learning new information, and inability to make important decisions about their lives. If the rehabilitation therapist makes these generalizations regarding the elderly, he or she may fail to notice or investigate personality changes that have recently occurred, such as confusion. It may be assumed that the patient has been confused for a long time because he or she is old, when in reality the onset of confusion was a week prior to contact and due to physiological or pharmaceutical causes.[11]

Society also tends to believe that body image is not important to an older person and does not view the elderly as sexual beings. It is easy, therefore, to overlook the emotional needs of an 85-year-old woman who has just had a mastectomy and fail to explain the prosthetic options that are available.[11]

MEDICAL DECISION MAKING

One of the basic ethical principles that guides health care providers in making decisions is called *beneficence*. This involves providing benefits to the patient, including preserving life. When a clear medical picture is present, the clinician and patient usually agree on the decisions that must be made, however, when it is not present, "defensive medicine," which does not necessarily benefit the patient but instead builds evidence against malpractice, is often practiced.[12]

The paradigm of good decision making is properly informing competent patients of their care options, and the possible outcomes and risks of treatments so they can decide the course of treatment, which should be limited only by the clinician's availability and willingness to provide the treatment.[13] The clinician should not be a neutral party and should take an active role in encouraging acceptance of an appropriate treatment, but the patient must not be coerced or deceived.[14]

An important consideration in medical decision making is the individual's value system. What constitutes quality of life to the patient may be very different from the clinician's philosophical beliefs, and when making decisions, the *self-determination or autonomy* of the patient should always prevail.[12] Decisions in rehabilitation therapy treatment, which have usually been based on scientific knowledge and professional experience, can be deficient since the moral aspect of the treatment may have been ignored. The value system of the patient must be considered, especially with regard to goal setting. What may be considered functional by the therapist may not meet the goals the patient has set.[15]

Decisional capacity must be assessed by the health provider before intervention is implemented and should be based on the individual's mental status, judgment, and short-term memory. The greater the risk of the treatment, the more carefully the decisional capacity must be evaluated. Many elderly people who are not capable of making their own decisions are treated as if they are, because they nod their head and agree with everything the clinician says. Elderly patients are denied the right to choose proper medical care if they are not properly evaluated by the health care team.[14]

If it is determined that an elderly patient is no longer able to make his or her own decisions, the first appeal should be to any specific documents of empowerments executed while the patient was capable. These empowerments or advanced directives, which include power of attorney and living wills, make it possible for health care professionals to determine the wishes and values of the patient and will be covered in depth later.

If the patient is unable to make medical decisions and advanced directives are not present, a surrogate decision maker must be chosen. This surrogate is usually a spouse or, as is often the case with the elderly, a son or daughter. For the elderly who have outlived all family and friends, the only alternative may be a court–appointed guardian. In special cases where the court feels the patient is unable to make medical decisions but the clinician and family feel the patient is capable, both the patient and the court–appointed surrogate must agree on a course of treatments.[14]

Conflicts regarding medical decisions may exist within the elderly patient, such as retaining a normal appearance versus attaining the best cure possible, or deciding whether to spend one's life savings on a costly treatment knowing it will be a financial burden to the rest of the family. In these cases, the patient should be the one to resolve the dilemma with the help and support of the clinician. The responsibility of the clinician is to present the facts regarding the treatment choices, but it may be more helpful to supply information about others who have been through similar experiences.[13]

Professional conflicts may be present that affect decision making by placing the patient's needs in competition with the clinician's interests. For example, a therapist may want a patient to reach a normal, functional status but also hopes the patient will need his or her services for a long period of time to financially support the practice. In this case, the clinician must obviously serve the needs of the patient and disregard his or her own incentives.[13]

Other difficult situations arise when a competent patient has poor judgment regarding his or her ability to function at home or in society (such as driving a car), in which case the clinician is responsible for weighing the risks of performing these activities and must act to preserve the safety of the patient and others. In such cases, the therapist must not act in ways that would be only

moderately beneficial to the patient but would also be detrimental to society or the patient's overall safety.[13]

Insufficient legal focus has been placed on discharge planning, which has become more of an issue with the formation of diagnostic related groups (DRGs). It has been determined, however, that if a patient is capable of making decisions, it is illegal to place that patient in a residential facility against his or her will. The family would have to petition the court for guardianship in order to override the patient's discharge preference.[14]

ALLOCATION OF RESOURCES

The growth of the elderly population, especially of that over the age of 85, poses economic and ethical dilemmas due to the rapid increase in the demand for health care services at a time when resources are scarce. Some important questions are: (1) how should these resources be rationed; (2) who should be responsible for allocating these resources; and (3) how should the scarcity of these resources affect medical policy decisions.[4]

Allocation of resources is commonly based on need and the belief that society should take care of its members. The disproportionate amount of medical care the elderly needs makes this group particularly vulnerable when it comes to rationing resources. Critics of Medicare view the program as "overgenerous and unwarranted" for people who do not have the need for this special help. Some feel that the dispensing of Medicare funds should be based on financial need rather than on medical need. Public opinion on this topic is indicated in a state poll showing moderate support (36%) for age criteria in health care, and the feeling that resources should be given to people who will receive the most long-term benefit from the treatment, which can exclude the elderly.[2,16]

Clinicians have always felt age is an important consideration when making medical decisions, but they are unclear about the ethical and moral implications of their actions. Sometimes it is felt that it is better to allocate resources to the young, who have their whole lives ahead of them rather than the elderly who have already experienced life, since the young are more capable of adjusting to handicaps and will be able to repay the costs with future contributions. Productivity has always been a criteria of need, which is ironic because elderly people are forced out of the workplace due to mandatory retirement and are, therefore, considered less productive. However, one must also consider that the elderly have contributed to society and that society has a responsibility to take care of them.[8,9,16,17]

One difficulty in basing medical decisions on age is the uncertainty of the prognosis in determining how long a person will live, particularly for an older person who is suffering from multiple illnesses. Another important factor that age criteria fails to recognize is that each person's life is important to him or her, and a longer life is not more valuable than a shorter one. Society must be careful not to devalue the life of an older individual, particularly one who is dependent, since this may lead to abusive discrimination of the elderly. Each person has an equal right to life no matter how old the individual is, and the quality of life should be evaluated by the patient only and not the clinician.[14,16]

When limited resources exist obviously not everyone will be entitled to every possible medical benefit, but the question remains of how rationing should be implemented. Should health care be distributed according to ability to pay or is it a social obligation to supply care regardless of financial ability? Ideally, everyone should have the right to proper health care, which should not be considered a luxury but a basic need. Conflicts arise when people use resources without replenishing them by either paying personally or having insurance that will pay. When this occurs, society is harmed because other people, in addition to not receiving the services, will have to replenish the funds.[18,19]

Who should be responsible for distributing these scarce resources? If the therapist is given the chore of making funding decisions the trust between the patient and the practitioner may be jeopardized. Patients trust that the physical therapist will provide the treatment needed regardless of financial concerns. Controlling expenditures are counterbalanced by the ethical obligations of the practitioner and negligence laws that demand that maximum effort should be made to cure the patient.[14]

With the growth of the health maintenance organization (HMO) industry, clinicians are given the new role of "gatekeeper" and, given the limited resources, must face the situation where resources spent on one patient will mean fewer resources for another. When a patient's health provider or insurance policy does not provide payment for health care services, the clinician should respect the right of the patient to limit treatment he or she does not value if it involves using personal funds. Conflicts for the clinician arise when the patient wants the treatment more than the provider and will pay for the care with personal funds. In this scenario, the clinician must consider that even though financial resources will not be compromised, access to resources (space and equipment) may hinder other patients from receiving care who need it more.[3]

In the past, the patient had to be cautious because reimbursement policies encouraged clinicians to provide unnecessary treatment. Today with the change in public policy and the addition of DRGs, the patient's rights are in danger of being violated due to incentives to limit treatment, decreasing the role of the clinician as the patient's advocate. The presence of these DRGs will affect the elderly the most since treatment will be discontinued prematurely for individuals with long-term illnesses. When economic incentives provided to clinicians lead them to deny beneficial care, there is a direct threat to the requirement that clinical decisions be competent and respect the patient's decision-making autonomy. For example, one cost–control method is rewarding an institution for offering a treatment at a lower cost. Hospitals that deliver treatment for less than the DRG rate can keep the difference. As a result, hospital administrators are examining the decisions of the clinicians to use resources and are applying pressure to physicians to deny beneficial treatment and the patient's right to choose that treatment.[9,18]

Another new medical policy that creates a conflict of interest is the addition of case managers to insurance companies because the managers' dominant measure of success is keeping costs low even though they want the patients to be satisfied with their care. If the patient's interests were always served, obviously the cost-saving goal would not be achieved. Therefore, formal ethics do not provide the answer. One suggestion is to give the balancing responsibility to the direct-care provider who is given incentives to conserve costs, but also possesses the moral and professional desire to meet the needs of the patient. This, however, creates a conflict of interest for the clinician, who is left with a situation in which the balance between the benefit for the patient and the cost to the system is unclear: to deny the patient the resource without informing him or her about the denial is ethically wrong. Providers have an obligation to inform patients regarding care options, even though they are denied these options by the system.[13]

Because of all these conflicts regarding allocation of resources, one can see that health care professionals will become frustrated with not being able to supply quality treatment unless they become more directly involved with health care policy formation and evaluation. The true challenge for the medical care system in the future will be learning how to balance the increasing medical needs of the elderly with the financial limitations of the system.[8,13]

CAREGIVER STRESS

Contrary to what many people believe, a majority of elderly people are being cared for at home by family members. It was estimated that by the year 2000 1 million people suffering from dementia would reside in nursing homes, while 1.5 to 2.5 million people would be living at home.[4] Studies show that family members who provide care to disabled relatives experience emotional, physical, and social strain. They also suffer from higher rates of depression, perceived burden, social isolation, family discord, and poor physical health than people who do not have this responsibility. A study done by Rabins and associates[20] of a small sample of elderly chronically ill individuals revealed family care givers underwent some adaptations over a two-year period. It was found that anger and anxiety toward their situation decreased but guilt and depression persisted.[20]

Two reasons physical or occupational therapists would naturally involve the family of an elderly patient is that they are a valuable source of information and they will provide care for the patient. However, the practitioner should be aware that the plan of care worked out by the patient and the clinician may be a burden on family members, and there are limits to the burdens of care that should be placed on the family. This creates a conflict of interest between the patient and the family.[3]

If the care of the elderly patient places a financial burden on the family, there is an ethical obligation to allow the family to participate in decision making. Conflicts arise when the decisions of the family and the patient differ, putting pressure on the two parties and possibly compromising the autonomy of the patient. Problems also occur when the family underestimates the difficulty or cost to them of the proposed patient care, which may lead to harm to all parties. Caring for an elderly relative at home impairs the freedom, independence, and satisfaction of others in the home, and responsibilities fall more on the functional family members, which causes resentment. In this case, it is the moral obligation of the clinician as well to help the family evaluate the responsibility they are undertaking.[3]

ELDER ABUSE

Identification and the subsequent reporting of elder abuse is an unfortunate circumstance to which many health care providers are exposed to in geriatrics. As the practice of rehabilitation involves the development of an ongoing relationship with patients during the course of treatment, and may also include frequent contact with the patients' families, it is critical that physical and occupational therapists know how to identify and effectively intervene in situations of suspected abuse.

Elder abuse occurs most commonly in residential rather than institutional settings, and the most likely perpetrators are known by the victim.[21,22] Although a defined set of risk factors has not yet been developed, careful questioning and assessment can help determine whether a patient is at increased risk. Some potential risk factors for mistreatment of older people include age, race, low income, functional or cognitive impairment, a history of violence, and recent stressful events.[21,23] Both depression and dementia have been identified as particularly strong risk factors associated with abuse of the elderly.[24,25] There is little information in the literature concerning the clinical profile of mistreated older people.

The common types of elder maltreatment include caregiver and self-neglect, emotional and psychological abuse, fiduciary exploitation, and physical abuse.[23] Assessment consists of comprehensive physical examination, including scrutiny of the musculoskeletal system, neurologic and cognitive testing, and detailed social and sexual histories.[26] Clues that cannot be explained medically may signal elder abuse. To properly intervene, clinicians should be familiar with state laws governing reporting procedures and patient privacy.[27,28]

Though as clinicians we are less likely to explore abuse beyond the physical, psychological, and cognitive realms, there is a dearth of literature on financial exploitation of elderly persons.[29] In fact, financial abuse accounts for up to one-half of all types of elder abuse in the United States, accounting for over 500,000 victims. Psychological abuse, including deception, intimidation, and threats, always accompanies financial exploitation.[29] Despite the devastating emotional and financial losses incurred, rehabilitation professionals are reluctant to recognize, diagnose, and assist impaired elderly victims of financial exploitation. This type of abuse, if suspected, should provoke a referral to a social worker or legal consultant by the rehabilitation professional.

PATIENT DIGNITY

Elderly people should be able to live out their lives with dignity, security, and independence. The tendency in American society is to place the elderly in nursing homes where they lose their identity, self-esteem, and individuality instead of encouraging and helping them to spend their remaining years in the dignity of their own homes. The readiness to place the elderly in these institutions stems from a negative basic attitude toward the elderly in this country. In Scandinavia, there is a system called "open care" where the elderly are not dependent on the charity and patience of relatives: Older people in this system retain their independence through programs that allow them to live in their own homes safely with outside help. The cost of this expensive program is paid for by the Scandinavian people through extremely high taxes. This basic attitude, that it is the responsibility of society to take care of its elderly, differs from the United States, which tends to be motivated by politics and would not consider advocating the costly care the Scandinavians have chosen.[30]

Principle I of the American Physical Therapy Association (APTA) Code of Ethics states that physical therapists must respect the rights and dignity of all individuals.[31] Likewise, Principle 2 of the American Occupational Therapy Association (AOTA) states that occupational therapy personnel shall respect the rights of the recipients of their services (autonomy, privacy, confidentiality).[32] This must be considered when implementing medical intervention because to ignore this principle is to treat the individual as less than human. When the therapist is not able to see the older person as an individual, treating the patient with dignity is compromised.[8]

One way the clinician can maintain the dignity of patients is to respect their autonomy and right to make decisions regarding their care. The health care professional must remember that even though elderly persons may be in a dependent state, the individuals have had a whole lifetime of self-determination that should not cease because they are temporarily or permanently disabled. This includes their right of confidentiality with respect to family members at the onset of treatment. This does not preclude the clinician from exploring the reasons the patient desires this confidentiality, especially when bad feelings are present, but ultimately the desires of the patient should prevail.[3]

There is also a tendency for health care professionals to treat the elderly, given their dependent state, like children, which is an assault on the individual's self-esteem and dignity. Because of this view, the clinician may assume that sons and daughters of the elderly should assume a parenting role, and important decisions will be discussed with the patient's children rather than with the patient. The health care provider may treat the older patient like a child on a smaller scale, such as assume the patient may be addressed by his or her first name, placing bows in an elderly woman's hair, or referring to an elderly man or woman as "cute," all of which compromise a patient's dignity.[11]

The main way to promote self-esteem and dignity in the elderly population is to change the attitude that society has toward growing old. Given the difficulty of changing this global problem, it may be a start to at least change the way rehabilitation therapists feel toward the elderly.[11]

PATIENTS' RIGHTS

The rehabilitation therapist is responsible for the maintenance of the basic rights of human beings during their illnesses, such as independence of expression, decision, and action. The APTA House of Delegates has adopted rights* for the individual referred or admitted to the physical therapy service that include but are not necessarily limited to:

1. The selection of a physical therapist of one's own choosing to the extent that it is reasonable and possible.
2. Access to information regarding practice policies and charges for services.
3. Knowledge of the identity of the physical therapist and other personnel providing or participating in the program of care.
4. Expectation that the referral source has no financial involvement in the service. If this is not the case, knowledge of the extent of any financial involvement in the service by the referring source must be explained.
5. Awareness of the physical therapy goals, desired outcomes, and procedures that are being rendered.
6. Receipt of information necessary to give informed consent prior to the initiation of services.
7. Participation in decisions involving the physical therapy plan of care to the extent reasonable and possible.
8. Access to information concerning his or her condition.
9. Expectation that any discussion or consultation involving the case will be conducted discreetly and that all communications and other records pertaining to the care, including the source of payment for treatment, will be treated as confidential.
10. Expectation of safety in the provision of services and safety in regard to the equipment and the physical environment.
11. Timely information about impending discharge and continuing care requirements.
12. Refusal of physical therapy services.
13. Information regarding the practice's mechanism for the initiation, review, and resolution of patient complaints.[33]

The AOTA† has established a similar set of statements regarding the rights of patients when referred for occupational therapy:

1. Occupational therapy personnel shall collaborate with service recipients or their surrogate(s) in determining goals and priorities throughout the intervention process
2. Occupational therapy personnel shall fully inform the service recipients of the nature, risks, and potential outcomes of any intervention.
3. Occupational therapy personnel shall obtain informed consent for subjects involved in research activities indicating they have been fully advised of the potential risks and outcomes.
4. Occupational therapy personnel shall respect the individual's right to refuse professional services or involvement in practice, research or educational activities.
5. Occupational therapy personnel shall protect the confidential nature or information gained from educational, practice, research, and investigational activities.[34]

There is a particular need to safeguard the rights of elderly individuals in nursing homes. Ombudsmen funded by Medicare are available to provide informa-

---

* Patients' Rights reprinted with permission of the American Physical Therapy Association.

†Patients' Rights reprinted with permission of the American Occupational Therapy Association.

tion regarding patient rights and protection in long-term care facilities.[14] Task forces have also been formed consisting of nursing home staff members and administrators, government officials, and medical, legal, and social service professionals to help protect the rights of elderly people in long-term care facilities. One accomplishment of the task force was to determine when it is appropriate for a patient to receive "supportive care" in a facility by setting up recommendations and guidelines. In the past, nursing homes abused patients by placing them on supportive care orders regardless of their health status.[35] Sometimes supportive care is taken to mean "no care necessary," leading to neglect of the elderly patient's basic needs. The task force defines supportive care as "care that is intended not to prolong life but to promote the dignity of the patient, minimize pain, preserve hygiene, and support the psychological, social, emotional, and spiritual needs of the patient and family."[36,37]

The Right to Refuse

One right that has the interest of lawyers and ethicists but has not been focused on by health professionals is the right to refuse. One may wonder if a refusal is due to the patient's denial of his or her illness or even to suicidal desires, or if it is a result of a well-thought out balancing of the risks and benefits of a particular treatment. The courts have distinguished between a suicide and refusal of care that may or may not prolong life and protects the rights of the individual to refuse treatment. When dealing with the elderly where chronic irreversible and debilitating conditions are present for which there is often no cure, limited treatment may be desired by the patient. One reason for this is that although the care is meant to prolong life, it is actually prolonging death. The American Medical Association's (AMA) Council on Ethical and Judicial Affairs states that competent patients have the moral and legal right to refuse treatment whether it is life sustaining or not. This may be overridden in the case where the refusal of treatment affects another person, particularly minor children.[14,37]

One important fact the clinician must remember is a refusal does not mean the patient is incompetent or crazy, and it has been suggested that for some groups of chronically ill patients, refusal should be offered as an option before treatment is initiated.[35] The single greatest reason for refusal of care is misunderstanding or miscommunication of the treatment involved.

A study by Applebaum and Roth[37] concluded many patients refuse treatment as a way to find out more information regarding their care. When psychological factors were implicated in reasons for refusal it was usually due to the distinctive way that individual deals with stress; the denial of illness was not commonly a direct cause.[14,37]

Often the clinician did not investigate the reason why the patient was refusing and, therefore, did not respond accordingly. For example, if a patient refused because he or she misunderstood the treatment plan, the response of the clinician would not be to offer clearer information since the reason for the refusal was not sought. Forced treatment by health professionals as a response to refusal was not uncommon but was usually limited to patients who were incompetent and unable to make their own decisions. Substitute consent was not usually obtained in these cases before treatment was started. When dealing with competent patients, there were responses of what was termed "forceful persuasion," where patients were told they had no choice if the treatment was considered essential by the chnician.[37]

In rehabilitation therapy, refusal of care can be as obvious as refusing treatment or as subtle as not performing the prescribed home exercise program. These patients are typically labeled noncompliant, and it is usually assumed that this problem exclusively lies with the patient, and the only solution is the person's compliance. The patient's right to autonomy over his or her body is not recognized, and the right of the patient not to comply with the advise of the physical therapist is not acknowledged. In a long-term care facility, noncompliance is often the only way a patient can exert control over his or her life, particularly in a rehabilitation setting. Reasons for the patient's noncompliance should be sought with the intention of understanding the rationale for nonparticipation. When a clinician places the problem of noncompliance totally on the patient, it is easy for therapists to avoid examining their own behavior or the influence of the health care setting on the patient's nonparticipation. The therapist can enhance compliance by taking the time to explain routine procedures, listening to the patient's concerns and fears, and involving the patient in goal setting. Although persuading the patient with clear and accurate information is encouraged, the autonomy of the patient must always be respected, even when the patient chooses to continue noncompliance.[38]

The rehabilitation therapist must also be wary of patients who unquestioningly follow every directive of the clinician and should not assume these patients understand the treatment being implemented. Often, this behavior is motivated out of fear of the health professional or fear of a bad medical outcome. The need to evaluate the decision-making capacity of a compliant patient is easy to miss because it is patients who refuse care who are usually having their competency challenged. From a moral point of view, therefore, unquestioned compliance may be as much of a problem as noncompliance.[38]

Rights of Demented Patients

In order to respect the rights of demented patients, their wishes regarding medical intervention must be documented when they are still in a competent state.

Often family understanding of the patient's wishes or prior values without specific documentation is not sufficient to make decisions about life-sustaining treatment. Given the difficulty of determining what best serves the interests of a severely demented patient, the court system recommends that the individual state specific preferences before the onset of disability. Discontinuing treatment that would prolong severe pain in the patient is clearly permissible according to the courts, because it is universally accepted that death is preferable to living with unrelenting pain. The clinician must also consider the pain and suffering that is present when treatment is forced on the incompetent patient against his or her wishes. An incompetent patient often can have strong preferences regarding treatment even though these preferences are not based in reality, and forcing unwanted treatment may cause the patient to experience a painful and humiliating violation.[39,40]

As previously mentioned, when it has been determined by careful evaluation that a patient is unable to make his or her own decisions regarding medical care, a surrogate decision maker must be chosen. It is believed that to the extent possible the rights of the incompetent patient should be an extension of the rights of the competent, and respect, self-determination, and promotion of well-being should be observed.[17]

For the clinician, it is clear that one must yield to the wishes of a competent patient, but dealing with a surrogate who may be acting in bad faith or have conflicts of interest is more complicated. For example, if the surrogate demands treatment that the clinician deems unnecessary, the clinician must make it clear that treatment is not indicated. If the family member still insists on the treatment, a court order must be obtained. This is an expensive and time-consuming process and tends to discourage a family member acting out of guilt or self-serving motives. Only the court can authorize a plan of care that is opposed by an incompetent patient's next of kin. If the health care professional has concerns regarding the decision made by the surrogate, the surrogate appointment should be reviewed by an ethics committee or consultant but can be legally changed only by the court system. Even though the surrogate should be more limited in his or her decision-making power than a competent patient, the family members should have some range of discretion so that they are not just carrying out the desires of the clinician.[13]

When considering the ability of the mentally impaired to make medical decisions, a precise mental evaluation is critical since the legal system has customarily taken an all–or–nothing approach to this decision. Either an individual is capable of making all decisions or he or she is declared incompetent and denied the right to make any decisions at all.[41,42,43] Elderly patients with fluctuating mental abilities need to be carefully evaluated before they are judged incapable of making medical decisions. "Windows of lucidity" may exist in patients where, in their more lucid mo-

ments, they are able to understand information that is given to them and consequently make clear decisions. An elderly person may experience what is called "sundowning" in which he or she experiences increased confusion at night and may need to be evaluated at different times of day in order to evaluate his or her ability to understand information.[14,42]

General mental status exams may be a good assessment for impairments when cognition is already severely compromised, but they are not adequate in assessing gradations of decision-making capacity.[44] In assessing competence, the most important part of the formal evaluation should be testing of the patient's ability to understand his or her medical situation. For example, the patient may not know what day it is but appears to understand the benefits of physical therapy and, therefore, is capable of making decisions even though disorientation is present.[12]

It is often assumed that preconceived beliefs about the elderly, as well as the paternalistic patterns of medical practice, may lead clinicians to underestimate the decisive capabilities of the older patient. However, in a study done by Fitten and associates[44] it was found that when clinicians rely on brief medical evaluations, test of recall, and their own judgment, they are most likely to assume incorrectly that the decision-making capacity of the patient is intact. The outcome of this research stresses the importance of a systematic evaluation that directly probes the patient's understanding of the issues involved and the reasoning underlying his or her treatment decisions.[44]

Future scenarios for the prevention and delay of Alzheimer's disease (AD) draw attention to a variety of ethical issues that need to be considered. The determination through genetic susceptibility testing in asymptomatic persons at high risk for AD, may eventually prove accurate enough to be of use in identifying at-risk individuals decades before probable onset (see Chapter 2). The ethical dilemmas created by both genetic testing and the genome projects in altering genetic make-up present a number of value-based issues for many clinicians, public policy makers, and insurers. Early identification of genetic susceptibility could lead to the application of pharmacologic and lifestyle interventions that delay onset of the disease and maximize preventive efforts.[45] By delaying or preventing the onset of AD, the patient may ultimately die of unrelated ailments of old age before they lose their capacity to communicate and to recognize loved ones. The other side of the coin is that the early identification of the possibility of developing AD could bias insurers in coverage for such benefits as long-term care insurance or rehabilitation.

INFORMED CONSENT

The legal and ethical foundation of informed consent is self-determination and autonomy, or, in other words, the right to decide what is done to one's body. Medical professionals are obligated to provide information regarding the risks and benefits of the recommended treatment plan in a language and style that the patient can understand, as well as to inform the patient about alternate treatment options. By giving the patient proper and clear information the health professional is allowing the patient to execute his or her right to choose.[14]

All states have a combination of statutes, common laws, and regulations that require that the informed consent of a competent patient must be obtained before treatment is started. Some states do recognize *therapeutic privilege,* which is an exception to the informed consent process and allows a physician to withhold information if, in the opinion of the physician, the patient would suffer direct harm as a result of the knowledge. This doctrine is not usually appropriate.[14]

The perception of the elderly as being too old to learn new information can compromise their right to be informed. The health professional must remember that learning is a lifelong process, even though age–related changes can affect learning and comprehension. Some variables that may affect learning in the older patient are alterations in sensory perception, motivation, response time, memory, and sleep-wake cycles, all of which require modified teaching strategies in order to enhance the comprehension of information (see Chapter 18). One of the major factors in the learning process is sensory perception, such as sight and hearing, and because this is often compromised in the elderly, it should be evaluated and compensated for, if needed, before the clinician begins to present information. One can compensate for the increased response time that may be present in an older person by decreasing the rate and amount of information presented. Creating a relaxed, private atmosphere may be necessary to decrease anxiety and increase the client's capacity to comprehend.[46] The clinician must take responsibility to implement these strategies in order to ensure that elderly patients can understand what medical treatments are being considered and can exercise their right to be informed.

Informed consent is generally recognized as necessary when providing potentially dangerous treatment, such as chemotherapy, blood transfusions, and surgery. However, in treatments like physical therapy, which is considered noninvasive, the necessity of consent is often overlooked. From a moral point of view obtaining consent to perform "harmless" treatment is just as important as hazardous treatment. Physical or occupational therapy may be considered routine, however, rehabilitation can be considered extremely invasive considering the amount of time patients need to dedicate to it and the impact it has on their lives.[38,42]

It is felt that it is the therapist's responsibility to ensure that information presented to the patient is understood and to be sensitive to cues regarding the patient's level of understanding. Purtilo feels it is better to give the patient too much rather than too little information.[8] Those who do not believe informed consent is appropriate feel patients cannot possibly understand the complexity of the medical situation and are, therefore, incapable of making decisions. However, what these individuals fail to recognize is that it is not necessary for the patient to understand every detail but only the major issues.[47]

Therapists are also in a special situation regarding informed consent since their main focus is management of disability and pain control. Patients who are experiencing pain, changes in lifestyle, and anxiety may agree to anything that could possibly make their situation better. The clinician should not take this eagerness for granted and should always properly explain what is being implemented.[47] Informed consent should not simply be obtained for legal or malpractice reasons but to protect the patient's right to know and preserve patient autonomy.

DEATH ISSUES

Advances in medical technology that tend to prolong the dying process have created a new group of ethical issues regarding patient autonomy and death.[48] Dying at home has become rare; it now occurs most frequently in hospitals and long-term care settings that are dominated by professionals and their use of technology. Medical management is usually geared toward promoting life at all costs, which often can overlook the value systems and desires of the individuals involved.

Advanced directives, which are documented desires of medical management, can be used to ward off unwarranted care and promote death with dignity. Specificity is important in order for advanced directives to be as effective as possible. The documents should include a statement that the person has presence of mind and is able to make decisions regarding specific possible medical events of the future. A list of interventions that is undesired in the event of certain illnesses should also be included. A competent individual can delegate decision rights to someone else by giving that person power of attorney. Legally, in order for that power to continue after the onset of incompetence, a durable power of attorney must be obtained.[42]

Living Wills

A living will is one example of an advanced directive in which a competent adult expresses his or her wishes regarding medical management in the event of incapacitation. In November 1990, President Bush signed the *Patient Self-Determination Act,* which was created to increase patient involvement regarding decisions involving life-sustaining equipment and encourage more patients to prepare documents, such as living wills, in advance by providing them with the proper information. The *Patient Self-Determination Act* requires hospitals and skilled nursing facilities to develop written policies regarding advanced directives as a condition of Medicare and Medicaid payment. These facilities are required to ask all new patients whether or not they have prepared these documents, as well as to provide written information regarding facility policy and patient rights under the law. In December 1991, requirements went into effect that provide immunity to physicians and other health professionals when they are carrying out the wishes of the patient.[49]

The importance of clear, advanced directives was demonstrated in the US Supreme Court decision of *Cruzan v. Director of Missouri Department of Health*, the first case in which a high court considered termination of life-prolonging measures for an incompetent patient. The court upheld the Missouri decision not to remove the feeding tube of Nancy Cruzan, who was in a vegetative state, at the request of her parents since there was no "clear and convincing" evidence that the patient, if competent, would want it removed.[50]

There are many shortcomings regarding living wills that can make the document ineffective. For example, a living will is only applicable for the terminally ill, and there are limitations on the types of treatments that can be refused by the patient. There is also no penalty for the health provider who refuses to honor the document and there is a tendency for physicians to make medical decisions based on their interpretation of the living will. For this reason it is important to accompany the document with a durable power of attorney to make it mandatory for the clinician to discuss treatment options with an individual selected by the patient.[51]

Durable power of attorney is present in every state and was primarily developed in order to manage financial matters of incapacitated individuals. Additional proxy laws are being developed state to state that specifically deal with health care. These laws would give an agent named by the patient the same authority for decision making as the patient would have if competent. The decision of the agent prevails when disagreements among family members are present regarding medical management. Since the physician may have difficulty honoring a living will over the objections of the family, the presence of this agent is essential to ensure that the wishes of the patient are respected.[43,51]

Euthanasia

According to *Webster's Dictionary*, euthanasia is defined as the action of inducing the painless death of a person for reasons assumed to be merciful. A moral distinction is made, which is accepted by most physicians, between passive and active euthanasia in which it is considered acceptable to remove life-sustaining treatment but it is unacceptable to actively terminate another person's life. A statement adopted by the House of Delegates of the AMA in 1973 considered "mercy killing" to be contrary to the medical profession's ethical position. On the other hand, the opinion of the AMA was that ceasing extraordinary treatment that prolongs the life of a body when death is imminent is the decision of the patient, family, or both, with the aiding advice of the physician.[52]

Controversy is centered around active voluntary euthanasia that, for instance, would allow the physician at the request of the patient to administer a lethal medication. The concept that killing someone is morally worse than letting them die is one reason why people believe there is a moral difference between active and passive euthanasia. However, this belief does not account for the patient who is in severe unrelieved pain with days to live and who desires to terminate his or her own life. According to the AMA doctrine, the physician is permitted to stop treatment that prolongs the pain thereby causing the patient to suffer more than if direct action were taken.[52,53]

The American Geriatric Society (AGS) opposes active euthanasia and feels that while lethal injections may be appropriate for the few patients suffering from unrelenting pain, there is too much of a risk for abuse of frail, disabled, and economically disadvantaged members of society. The AGS is also concerned that legalized active euthanasia would weaken the motivation of society to develop solutions for proper care of the dying, such as hospice programs and that, given our fiscally obsessed society, active euthanasia may be viewed as a way to contain medical costs.[53]

The mental anguish caused by having to face another day waiting to die may be a growing reason for requests for voluntary active euthanasia. The presence of intractable pain is no longer as widely used as a justification for active euthanasia given the presence of anesthetic levels of pain-relieving medications. The psychological suffering of the patient would be minimized if the individual were able to legally choose the time and place of their death.[54] It has also been argued that making these choices regarding death is fundamental and honors the autonomy of the patient.[55]

If patients were legally given the choice of active euthanasia, the question is how many patients would pursue it. Hospice physicians report that although the topic of active euthanasia frequently arises in passing conversation, only a few patients seriously and persistently pursue its implementation.[55,56,57]

The debate regarding legalizing voluntary active euthanasia is far from over, and the degree to which supportive services for the dying should be made available must be addressed. Society must develop policies for the dying that will benefit the patient and enhance autonomy but not lead to potential abuses of the weaker members of society.

Cardiopulmonary Resuscitation

In the health care setting cardiopulmonary resuscitation (CPR) is considered a routine procedure administered to patients suffering cardiopulmonary arrest. It has always been assumed that consent to perform CPR is present since the patient is incapacitated and inaction will lead to death. The practice of performing CPR on any patient experiencing cardiac arrest regardless of the state of their illness and chances for survival is a cause of concern.[42,58] The right of the patient to refuse treatment also applies to the use of resuscitation, and a patient may express in advance that this procedure be withheld.[59]

The right of the patient to have do not resuscitate (DNR) orders placed in his or her medical chart is established, but the question is how involved is the patient in the decision making? One study revealed that 95% of a group of physicians believed that patients should be involved in resuscitation decisions, but only 10% discussed this issue with their patients. Another study showed that only 20% of the patients with DNR orders in their chart discussed their preferences with their physician prior to the initiation of the orders.[59] Even though decreased mental capacity may be one reason preferences were not discussed, the difficulty both physicians and patients have with discussing death may be another reason for inadequate patient participation. However, the need for this discussion is essential in order for the patient to participate in the decision-making process. In order to assist physicians in managing patients who are not appropriate for CPR, guidelines have been established by the Council on Ethical and judicial Affairs.[59]

Another concern is that the presence of DNR orders will affect other therapeutic care given to the patient. A study done by Zimmerman and co-authors[60] showed that within 1.7 days of placement of a DNR order in the chart the patient either died or was discharged from the ICU. These results suggest that even though DNR orders only specify withholding of CPR, other therapeutic limits may accompany the order.[60]

A difficult situation arises when the patient, family, or both insists on CPR orders even when the procedure would clearly be futile. Inappropriate resuscitation may even cause harm by producing a chronic vegetative state. Patients and their families may insist on resuscitation out of guilt or fear, as well as out of unrealistic hopes for a cure. In this situation patient autonomy cannot be the only guide and does not allow a patient to demand treatment that is nonbeneficial and potentially harmful.

However, in this scenario, the question arises as to what is the point of offering the patient the choice in an attempt to preserve his or her rights of autonomy if these wishes are later denied. For this reason some physicians believe CPR should not be offered to this type of patient since the choice represents a potential for benefit when there is none.[58]

The issue of CPR in the nursing home setting is a complex one. The benefits are difficult to assess given the degree of debilitation in individuals present in a skilled nursing facility. Furthermore, the violence of the procedure and its small likelihood of success argue against it. However, to withhold lifesaving therapy from a certain population just because they are dependent can be construed as discriminatory. A limited study done by Finucane and coworkers[61] demonstrated that there is an implicit policy by most nursing homes to withhold CPR from their residents.

The debate on proper policies regarding performing CPR in nursing homes continues and, like other treatments that tend to prolong the life of an already debilitated individual, it is difficult for the clinician to balance patient autonomy with supplying a treatment that is considered nonbeneficial.[62]

Terminal Care

Terminal care is geared toward providing a protective, nurturing, and homelike environment in which there is a large involvement of the health care team in decision making for the patient.[62] Since the elderly resident is dependent on the staff for personal hygiene, meals, and medication, the resident assumes a subservient role by trading his or her autonomy and dignity for the attentive care received.[3]

The older person's own home has a certain therapeutic value that is often not recognized. Home health care is, therefore, receiving new recognition. In this setting, individuals will be more likely to exercise their right to make decisions. There is, however, a danger of a patient becoming overconfident and having unrealistic views regarding his or her capacity to care for him- or herself, which the home care provider must be careful in assessing.[3]

Unlike an acute care setting, the treatment in a long-term care facility is routine and repetitive, making violations of the individual's autonomy more probable. Older people often may have the power to decide but are unable to carry out their personal decisions without the aid of the staff. Without this assistance their freedom to decide is useless and their autonomy infringed upon.[63]

Value systems are important to examine when considering the long-term care setting. An individual may be placed in a facility that does not share his or her values and goals or the patient's status may change while in the facility, making the setting no longer appropriate. It is important for the primary care physician to manage this and prevent or resolve ethical mismatches.[3] For example, the elderly resident in a nursing home may not share the enthusiasm of the rehabilitation therapist to participate in an exercise program.

Although nursing home residents vary in age, degree of function, and levels of cognition and interests, a common denominator is the difficulty in exercising choice. In order to enhance patient autonomy in long-term care facilities, increased staff, space, and resources are needed. Society is responsible for making the decision whether or not this should be a priority.

The changes that do not require extra funds should of course be investigated first, and efforts should be made to find out the preferences of nursing home residents themselves.[64,65]

Hospice

The question of how society should deal with their dying population has always represented a void in the health care system that, in the past two decades, has been filled with the fast growth of the hospice. The growth of the hospice setting has received widespread support in the United States, sparking the interest of the health professional specializing in geriatrics, since approximately 66% of the patients in hospices are over 65.[66]

In the hospice, health care and service is provided for the patient and the family and is available at all times. Care is planned and provided by a medical interdisciplinary team, as well as by using family and volunteers to provide physical, emotional, and spiritual care to the patient with an emphasis on palliative care. The hospice is sensitive to needs of the family who obviously experience stress with the patient's terminal illness and also provides follow–up care after the patient dies.[66]

The focus of the hospice is to help the dying patient live the remaining time as fully as possible instead of concentrating on the disease process itself. The care is directed primarily at symptom and pain control to improve quality of life rather than disease control. There are major philosophical differences between hospices and the traditional health care setting, with hospice rules and regulations being extremely flexible to enhance the life of the dying patient.[67]

The rehabilitation therapist does play a palliative role in the hospice setting, using pain control modalities but more importantly, he or she functions as an educator for both the patient and the family. As in a home care setting, the physical or occupational therapist teaches the patient functional and safe tasks, and the family is present to learn as well. Each member of the hospice health care team, including the physical therapist, assumes the role of counselor, which demands good listening and communication skills. The involvement of the therapist is dependent on the resources available as well as the desires of the patient and family.[67]

Suicide

The suicide rate of older people is double that of any other age group. These rates are most likely underestimated, given that the probability of not reporting suicides is highest in the elderly population. Older people are also more likely to complete the task of suicide, use a more violent means, and have a greater male to female ratio than any other age group. Conwell and co-authors[68] found that older suicide victims had a lower incidence of psychopathy and were responding to physical illness and loss.

Ethical debate regarding suicide and the elderly leaves health care providers confused about what their response should be. One question is whether suicide in the elderly should be treated like suicide in any other age group with an attempt to prevent it or to respect the right of the older person to choose to die. Health professionals desiring to prevent suicide rarely view it as a rational act well-thought out by the individual but as a symptom of depression and mental dysfunction. It is equally important to discuss whether or not killing oneself for reasons of old age alone without the presence of terminal illness is ethically justified.[11]

Arguments against the concept of a justifiable suicide are dominated by the belief that killing one's self is a terrible act regardless of the circumstances. Clinicians concerned with suicide prevention may argue that the state of mind of the older person may be temporary and, though circumstances may be bad, they may get better in the future. However, elderly individuals who have deliberated about suicide over a long period of time are not experiencing a passing mental state and, unlike their younger counterparts, the future of an older person is more predictable and less bright.[11]

There is a great desire to promote both "death with dignity" and the right to choose one's own destiny; however, there is a concern that society, as well as the elderly, will view suicide as a solution to problems associated with aging. Taking this a step further, elderly people who do not choose suicide may be viewed as selfish for not committing the act in order to remove their presence as a burden to society.[11]

The issue of suicide and the elderly is complicated by desires to preserve patient autonomy, as well as the fear that making suicide acceptable in the elderly will contribute overall to the reprehensible attitude that the older person is a burden and should be removed. Perhaps these ethical issues will become clearer when the young and old are able to come to terms with their own aging process and mortality.

RESTRAINTS

Restraint issues arise frequently in the practice of rehabilitation therapy in geriatric settings and create many ethical, as well as legal, ramifications. In 1987, Congress passed the *Omnibus Reconciliation Act* (OBRA) to reform the use of physical and chemical restraints in nursing homes in the United States. OBRA prohibits nursing homes from inappropriately using physical and chemical restraints on nursing home residents for nonmedical purposes. Before OBRA, many nursing homes used restraints for the convenience of nursing home staff. For example, if an individual wandered, the staff did not have to watch that individual if they simply tied the resident to a chair. OBRA sought to stop this kind of abuse.

Nursing homes may not use "as needed" or PRN orders for nursing home residents' restraint use under OBRA. OBRA only allows the use of restraints as a last resort after the facility completes a comprehensive assessment of the resident and determines that less restrictive alternatives have failed. Even if the nursing home facility proves that alternatives have failed, numerous other rules apply to protect residents from being restrained indefinitely. On-going assessment and attempts to remove restraints are required.

According to OBRA, that assessment should include input from the therapists involved in care of the residents in the facility. The "Interpretive Guidelines on Physical Restraints," which was implemented in October 1990, states that "a facility must have evidence of consultation with appropriate health professionals, such as occupational or physical therapists in the use of less restrictive supportive devices, *prior to* using physical restraints as defined in this guideline for such purposes."

The four major types of patients that are candidates for physical restraints according to OBRA are:

■ The cognitively impaired wanderer;
■ The aggressive patient;
■ Patients who interfere with medical treatment; and
■ The unsteady patient.

The physical and occupational therapist are the most qualified health professionals in effectively assessing the necessity for restraining devices, especially in the fourth group. There are clear benefits associated with improving function and stability with the goal of aiding these patients in maintaining their quality of life. Assessing the risk of falls or decline in function if physical restraints are applied are primary parameters in the evaluation of restraints for elderly patients (see Chapter 6 for assessment tools).

From an ethical perspective, to tie or not to tie the elderly is a difficult question. Understaffed nursing homes are fearful of guidelines that may cause an increase in the responsibilities of overburdened and underpaid staff. In addition, the possibility of increased legal pressure has been a source of apprehension regarding nonadherence to the guidelines. The proponents of untying the elderly, however, are advocating unassailable issues in the area of quality of life that must be considered in a comparison of risks and benefits.

The issues of freedom, dignity, self-choice, and enhanced function and mobility are very important ethical issues that arise regarding the choice not to use restraining devices. The physical and occupational therapists are extremely important players in allaying the fears of nursing home staff, improving functional capacity and stability, as well as helping to ensure that the least restrictive and most freedom enhancing environment for older persons is established.

MINORITY ISSUES AND ETHICS

Demographically, the number of different ethnic groups in the United States has grown considerably in the past decade.[69,70] Inherent in a discussion of attitudes and ethics, it is important to introduce the cross-cultural and diversity phenomena affecting health care. Individuals from different ethnic groups will have grown up and been socialized in accordance with their various cultures. As a result, their health beliefs and practices may be considerably different from the traditional beliefs regarding health care in our western civilization.[71,72] Minorities often assume a subgroup within society and maintain their own "neighborhoods." Assimilation into the common culture may not occur and it is important that the health care professional respect ethnic diversity by identifying, acknowledging, and accepting cultural beliefs and tendencies.

Cultural expectations are important to consider. The stronger the ties to the old-country practices, language, and rituals, the more likely it is that the individual will not share the beliefs and values of contemporary US health care. It is worthwhile to discuss with each elderly patient and their families their perspectives on aging, health and wellness, and what it is they perceive to be the proper practice for care in their condition (a herb, a ritual?).[73]

"Cultural pluralism emphasizes mutual respect between various groups that allows minorities to express their own culture without suffering prejudice or hostility."[74]

The rehabilitation professional has been culturalized through whatever professional educational program they have experienced. Yet, what they have been taught may not be the way an elderly individual from a different ethnic background sees things. Perhaps their thought is that they are old, they've served their community, and now it is time from them to be served — so, 'why is it important to do these exercises?' We as clinicians need to respect that view. In order to practice effectively, cognizant of the ethics of care,[31,32] it is also important that ethnic considerations and respect for the different beliefs and values be the centerpiece in the care of our elderly patients with diverse cultural backgrounds.

CONCLUSION

The ethical treatment of patients is an important but underemphasized aspect of medical care. Given the current trend away from high cost, high technology health care, today's health professional must reevaluate the role ethical issues play in their attitudes toward providing the best care, especially for older patients. This chapter has addressed the therapist's attitude toward the older patient, and how these attitudes impact decision making in rehabilitation. In addition, the more controversial areas of medical ethics,

CASE STUDIES: ETHICAL DILEMMAS

CASE STUDY 1
A childless, 78-year-old woman was admitted to the hospital on July 14, 2001, because of weight loss and fever. Her husband died in 1999 and after his death she become depressed, refused to eat, and lost weight. An ileostomy tube was inserted for feeding purposes. It was successful, and the patient gained weight. Psychological interviews revealed her to be well oriented but possibly slightly demented because of her simple answers, and she did not show interest or awareness of events happening around her. She lost the ability to ambulate and developed multiple contractures. She also developed anemia secondary to poor nutrition. On November 30, 2001, when she was transferred to another facility, she still had the ileostomy, which had not been used for feeding for some time. The patient often complained about the tube and stated she would like it removed. On or around April 27, 2002, the end of the "J tube" broke off and the remaining portion appeared to be "flush" with the surface of the skin. On April 28, 2002, the tube slipped inside, causing the physicians to maintain a close observation of her status. The physician believed the tube would pass through the rectum in the feces, which it did several days later. The patient then stated she thought she was going to die and appeared quite depressed. The ethical question in this case is: Should the tube have been removed at the request of the patient given her presumed competence?

CASE STUDY 2
A 95-year-old woman living at home independently with diabetes and congestive heart failure was hospitalized after developing gangrene of one foot. While hospitalized she refused amputation but consented to continue management of her other medical problems, including medication and localized treatment for her foot. She became unpopular with the hospital staff and other patients because of the foot's odor and the related infection control hazards. The house staff on her case expressed that she must be crazy since she refused life-sustaining treatment. The physician and a psychologist experienced in competency assessment evaluated the patient and determined that the patient's cognitive abilities were intact. The evaluation also concluded that the patient refused the surgery due to personal values of not wanting to continue life at her age without her foot even if death without intervention was imminent. Presentation of positive examples of life as an amputee did not change her position. In order to pacify the concern of the staff regarding infection and odor, the ward was visited frequently by in infection control specialist and the patient received whirlpool treatments of the foot. The patient died several weeks later with her wishes respected.[12] The ethical question here: Should surgery have been performed to prolong life?

CASE STUDY 3
An 83-year-old woman whose status postoperatively included a right cerebral vascular accident, was admitted to a nursing home directly from the hospital. At the time of admission, the patient was extremely dependent and could only ambulate short distances with the maximum assistance of two people. She refused to use an assistive device. A mental evaluation performed by the nursing home staff physician revealed the patient was not oriented to time or place but was aware of her medical condition and recognized her daughter who visited her frequently. The physician and the patient's daughter agreed it was important to continue the physical therapy that was initiated in the hospital in order to promote restoration of function as well as independence. When the transporter arrived to take the patient to her first physical therapy session, the patient verbally refused, but she was placed in the wheelchair by the transporter under the direction of the nurse in charge on the floor. In the physical therapy department, the patient expressed the desire to return to her room repetitively and reluctantly cooperated during the evaluation performed by the therapist. Even after a great deal of coaxing and encouragement the physical therapist was unable to convince the patient to ambulate with a walker or a quad cone. In spite of the patient's verbal refusals, she was brought to physical therapy daily where she ambulated short distances with the assistance of two people but refused to perform any other exercises. The ethical question: Should this individual's refusal to participate in therapy have been respected given her cognitive status?

such as allocation of resources, care giver stress, elder abuse, patient dignity and patient rights, informed consent, and death and dying issues were discussed. The topic of restraints was presented with the ethical implications inherent in preventing an individual freedom to move around their environment. The ethical issues related to the increased cultural diversity and the need to see things from each individual's perspective was discussed. Finally, the chapter stressed that these issues not only play a critical role in the day-to-day care of patients, but have a long-term impact on the ethical practice of rehabilitation.

PEARLS

- The shift in modern medicine from a paternalistic role toward giving the patient more responsibility in decision making may be threatening to the aged who are more comfortable with traditional roles.
- Rehabilitation therapists should practice beneficence in medical decision making and not be a neutral party. They should encourage acceptance of an appropriate treatment, being careful not to coerce or deceive the patient.
- Ombudsmen funded by Medicare are available to provide information regarding patient rights and protection in long-term care facilities.
- In informed consent, therapists are obliged to provide information in language a patient can understand regarding risks, benefits, and alternate treatment options, except when the therapist exercises therapeutic privilege (e.g., withdrawing information that the therapist feels will cause the patient direct harm as a result of knowledge).
- The common types of elder maltreatment include caregiver and self-neglect, emotional and psychological abuse, fiduciary exploitation, and physical abuse.
- Advanced directives, such as a living will, are documented desires of medical management used to ward off unwarranted care and promote death with dignity.
- The American Geriatric Society opposes active euthanasia and feels that while lethal injections may be appropriate for a few patients suffering from unrelenting pain, there is too much at risk for abuse for frail, disabled, and economically disadvantaged elderly.
- Older people have double the suicide rate of any other age group.
- OBRA prohibits nursing homes from inappropriately using physical and chemical restraints on nursing home residents for nonmedical purposes.
- The stronger the ties to the old-country practices, language, and rituals, the more likely it is that the individual will not share the beliefs and values of contemporary US health care.

REFERENCES

1. Spencer FC. The vital role in medicine of commitment to the patient. *Am Coll Surg Bull.* 1990; 75:7–19.
2. *Miranda v. Arizona,* 384 U.S. 436 (1966).
3. Talar GA, Waymack MH. Ethics and the elderly. *Primary Care.* 1989; 16;529–541.
4. Blanchette PL. Age-based rationing of health care. *Hawaii Med J.* 1995; 54(4):507–509.
5. Gonsoulin TP. Ethical issues raised by managed care. *Laryngoscope.* 1997; 107(11 Pt 1):1425–1428.
6. Rodwin MA. Conflicts of interest and accountability in managed care: the aging of medical ethics. *J Am Geriatr Soc.* 1998; 46(3):338–341.
7. Evans JG. Economic, political and ethical implications of aging. *Aging.* 1998; 10(2):141–142.
8. Purtilo RB. Ethical considerations. In: Jackson OL, eds. Therapeutic Considerations for the Elderly. New York: Churchill Livingstone; 1987:173.
9. Purtilo RB. *Ethical Dimensions in the Health Professions.* 3rd edition. Philadelphia, PA: WB Saunders Co.; 1999.
10. Harris J, Fiedler CM. Preadolescent attitudes toward the elderly: an analysis of race, gender, and contact variables. *Adolescence.* 1988; 23:335–340.
11. Lesnoff-Caravaglia G. *Values, Ethics and Aging.* New York: Human Sciences Press; 1985.
12. Goldstein NIK. Ethical care of the elderly: pitfalls and principles. *Geriatrics.* 1989; 44:101–106.
13. Lynn J. Conflicts of interest in medical decision-making. *J Am Geriatr Soc.* 1988; 36:945-950.
14. Dubler NN. Legal issues. *Merck Manual.* Rahway, NJ: Merck, Sharp, and Dohme Research Laboratories; 1990:1142–1161.
15. Coates R. Ethics and physiotherapy. *Aust Physiotherapy.* 1990; 36:84–87.
16. Kilner JF. Age criteria in medicine. *Arch Intern Med.* 1989; 149:2343–2346.
17. Barondess JA, Kalb P, Weil WB, et al. Clinical decision-making in catastrophic situations: The relevance of age. *J Am Ger Soc.* 1988; 36:919–937.
18. Daniels N. Why saying no to patients in the United States is so hard. *N Engl J Med.* 1986; 314:1380–1383.
19. Eddy DM. The individual vs. society: is there a conflict? *JAMA.* 1991; 265:1446–1450.
20. Rabins PV, Fitting MD, Eastham J, et al. Emotional adaptation over time in care-givers for chronically ill elderly people. *Age and Ageing.* 1990; 19:185–190.
21. Marshall CE, Benton D, Brazier JM. Elder abuse. Using clinical tools to identify clues of mistreatment. *Geriatrics.* 2000; 55(2):42–44, 47–50, 53
22. Jogerst GJ, Dawson JD, Hartz AJ, Ely JW, Schweitzer LA. Community characteristics associated with elder abuse. *J Am Geriatr Soc.* 2000; 48(5):513–518.
23. Collins KA, Bennett AT, Hanzlick R. Elder abuse and neglect. Autopsy Committee of the College of American Pathologists. *Arch Intern Med.* 2000; 160(11):1567–1568.

24. Dyer CB, Pavlik VN, Murphy KP, Hyman DJ. The high prevalence of depression and dementia in elder abuse or neglect. *J Am Geriatr Soc.* 2000; 48(2):205–208.

25. Anetzberger GJ, Palmisano BR, Sanders M, et al. A model of intervention for elder abuse and dementia. *Gerontologist.* 2000; 40(4):492–497.

26. Gray-Vickery P. Recognizing elder abuse. *Nursing.* 1999; 29(9):52–53.

27. Ciolek DE, Ciolek CH. *Guidelines for Recognizing and Providing Care for Victims of Elder Abuse and Neglect.* Alexandria, VA: Section on Geriatrics—American Physical Therapy Association. 1999.

28. Wolf RS, Li D. Factors affecting the rate of elder abuse reporting to state protective services program. *Gerontologist.* 1999; 39(2):222–228.

29. Tueth MJ. Exposing financial exploitation of impaired elderly persons. *Am J Geriatr Psychiatry.* 2000; 8(2):104–111.

30. Szulc T. How we can help ourselves age with dignity. *Parade.* May 29 1988;4–7.

31. Bottomley JM, ed. *Quick Reference Dictionary for Physical Therapy.* Thorofare, NJ: Slack, Incorporated; 2000: 237.

32. Jacobs K, ed. *Quick Reference Dictionary for Occupational Therapy.* 2nd Edition. Thorofare, NJ: Slack, Incorporated; 1999; 229.

33. American Physical Therapy Association. *Code of Ethics.* Alexandria, VA: American Physical Therapy Association.

34. American Occupational Therapy Association. *Code of Ethics.* Bethesda, MD: American Occupational Therapy Association.

35. Marcus EL, Berry EM. Refusal to eat in the elderly. *Nutr Rev.* 1998; 56(6):163–171.

36. Moon MA. Task force to protect rights of nursing home patients. *Intern Med News. 1983;* 16:23.

37. Appelbaum PS, Roth LH. Patients who refuse treatment in medical hospitals. JAMA. 1983; 215: 1296–1301.

38. Coy JA. Autonomy-based informed consent: ethical implications for patient noncompliance. *Phys Ther.* 1989; 69:826–833.

39. Arras JD. The severely demented, minimally functional patient: an ethical analysis. *J Am Ger Soc.* 1988; 36:938–944.

40. Jones DG. Aging, dementia and care: setting limits on the allocation of health care resources to the aged. *N Z Med J.* 1997; 110(1057):466–468.

41. Gunn AE. Mental impairment in the elderly: medical-legal assessment. *J Am Ger Soc.* 1977; 25:193–198.

42. Scott RW. *Professional Ethics: A Guide for Rehabilitation Professionals.* St. Louis, MO: Mosby Year-book, Inc.; 1998.

43. Scott RW. *Promoting Legal Awareness in Physical and Occupational Therapy.* St. Louis, MO: Mosby Year-book, Inc., 1997.

44. Fitten LJ, Lusky RL, Hamann C. Assessing treatment decision-making capacity in elderly nursing home residents. *J Am Ger Soc.* 1990; 38:1097–1104.

45. Post SG. Future scenarios for the prevention and delay of Alzheimer disease onset in high-risk groups. An ethical perspective. *Am J Prev Med.* 1999; 16(2):105–110.

46. Rendon DC. The right to know, the right to be taught. *J Gerontol Nurs.* 1986; 12: 33–37.

47. Simm J. Informed consent: ethical implications for physiotherapy. *Physiotherapy.* 1986; 72:584–587.

48. Gadow S. Aging as death rehearsal: the oppressiveness of reason. *J Clin Ethics.* 1996; 7(1):35–40.

49. Greco PJ, Schulman KA, Lavizzo-Mourey R, et al. The patient self-determination act and the future of advance directives. *Ann Intern Med.* 1991; 115:639-643.

50. Malloy DW, Clametle RM, Braun EA, et al. Decision making in the incompetent elderly: "the daughter from California syndrome." *J Am Ger Soc.* 1991; 39:396–399.

51. Annas GJ. The health care proxy and the living will. *N Engl J Med.* 1991; 324:1210–1213.

52. Rachels J. Active and passive euthanasia. *N Engl J Med.* 1975; 292:78–80.

53. AGS Public Policy Committee. Voluntary active euthanasia. *J Am Geriatr Soc.* 1991; 39:826.

54. Kane RS. The defeat of aging versus the importance of death. *J Am Geriatr Soc.* 1996; 44(3):321–325.

55. Teno J, Lynn J. Voluntary active euthanasia: the individual case and public policy. *J Am Ger Soc.* 1991; 39:827–830.

56. Loewy EH. Living well and dying not too badly: integrating a whole life into a tolerable death. *Wien Klin Wochenschr.* 2000; 112(9):381–385.

57. Muller MT, Kimsma GK, van der Wal G. Euthanasia and assisted suicide: facts, figures and fancies with special regard to old age. *Drugs Aging.* 1998; 13(3): 185–191.

58. Blackhall LJ. Must we always use CPR? *N Eng J Med.* 1987; 317:1281–1285.

59. Council on Ethical and Judicial Affairs, American Medical Association. Guidelines for the appropriate use of do-not-resuscitate orders. *JAMA.* 1991; 265: 1868–1871.

60. Zimmerman JE, Knaus WA, Sharpe SM, et al. The use and implications of do not resuscitate orders in intensive care units. *JAMA.* 1986; 255:351–356.

61. Finucane TE, Boyer JT, Bulmash J, et al. The incidence of attempted CPR in nursing homes. *J Am Ger Soc.* 1991; 39:624–626.

62. Iris MA. The ethics of decision making for the critically ill elderly. *Camb Q Healthcare Ethics.* 1995; 4(2):135–141.

63. Collopy BJ. Ethical dimensions of autonomy in long-term care. *Generations.* 1990 XIV:9–12.

64. Kane RL, Kane RA. Long-term-care financing on personal autonomy. *Generations.* 1990; XIV:86–94.

65. Hoehner PJ. Ethical decisions in perioperative elder care. *Anesthesiol Clin North America.* 2000; 18(1): 159–181, vii-viii.

66. Greer DS. Hospice: Lessons for geriatricians. *J Am Ger Soc.* 1983; 31:67–70.

67. Toot J. Physical therapy and hospice, concept and practice. *Phys Ther.* 1984; 64:665–671.

68. Conwell Y, Rotenber M, Caine ED. Completed suicide at age 50 and over. *J Am Ger Soc.* 1990; 38:640–644.

69. Leavitt RL. Introduction. In: Leavitt RL, ed. *Cross-Cultural Rehabilitation: An International Perspective.* Philadelphia, PA: WB Saunders; 1999:1–7.

70. Luckman J. *Transcultural Communications.* Canada: Delmar Thomson Publications; 2000.

71. Spector R. *Cultural Diversity in Health & Illness.* Stamford, Conn: Appleton & Lange; 1996.

72. Mouton CP, Johnson MS, Cole DR. Ethical considerations with African-American elders. *Clin Geriatr Med.* 1995; 11(1):113–129.

73. Fadiman A. *The Spirit Catches You and You Fall Down. A Hmong Child, Her American Doctors, and the Collision of Two Cultures.* New York, NY: Farrar, Strauss and Giroux; 1997.

74. McDonald H, Galgopal P. Conflicts of American immigrants: assimilate or retain ethnic identity. *Migration World Mag.* 1998; 127(4):14–19.

C H A P T E R   1 8

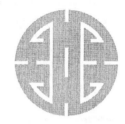

Education and the Older Adult: Learning, Memory, and Intelligence

Elders of the tribe were once considered teachers, the founts of wisdom. Today, little respect is given to the experiences of a lifetime, and myths perpetuate the notion that learning abilities and memory capabilities decline with age. On the contrary, in our society, elderly individuals must learn new skills as new technology alters basic systems of communication, transportation, finance and recreation on nearly a daily basis. As values change, societal rewards change, and new learning is required.

Learning means the acquisition of information or skills, and it is usually measured by looking for improvements in task performance. When someone improves their performance at a given intellectual or physical task, we say that they have learned. Studies of performance in elderly individuals indicate a decline with age. Clearly, there are a number of factors other than learning ability that affect performance. Some of these include physiological responses, physical health status, pathology, depression and motivation. In practice, it is extremely difficult to separate the components of performance in order to examine the influence of learning ability, although a number of studies have attempted to do so. Despite evidence that other factors contribute to the decline in task performance, most researchers still attribute part of

this decline to a diminished ability to learn new tasks or acquire new information with age.[1-6]

All age groups can learn. Older individuals just require more time. Tasks that involve manipulation of distinct and familiar symbols or objects, unambiguous responses, and low interference from prior learning are particularly conducive to good performance by older individuals.[7-9]

At various points in time, different approaches to the study of learning and memory have been dominant. In the 1960s, the associative view of learning was most popular. In the 1970s, theories on information processing or conceptual learning were established as the mode for learning and memory. Now, a growing emphasis in learning theories concerns a contextual approach.[10] Thus, it is important to briefly review research on learning and memory from each of these approaches.

Learning and memory are closely related concepts. People must learn before they can remember, and learning without memory has limited utility. Learning is often assessed by memory tasks. "How much have you learned?" is translated to "How much do you remember?" Learning is defined as the acquisition of a new skill or information through practice and experience. Remembering is defined as the retrieval of information that has been stored in memory.[10]

The general learning/memory system involves three processes: acquisition, storage, and retrieval. Memory is often discussed in terms of information: How you put information into the system, how you store it and how you retrieve it. This is the approach of modern information processing theories, and in this view, learning is part of memory; that is, the acquisition, registration, or encoding phase.

When adding the dimension of age, there are many questions that arise. How do learning abilities change? How does memory change? Does it fade? Do old people forget new things and remember the past? How do societal demands affect learning and memory?

ASSOCIATIVE LEARNING

Based on the assumption that learning and memory involve the association of ideas or events that occur together in time, the associative learning theory involves a stimulus-response bond, and paired association is the most commonly employed mode for testing memory using this theory. The task is to learn an association between two commonly unrelated items, such as basket—therefore, or orange—until. The subject is first presented with two unrelated words, and the subsequent task is to give a correct response to each stimulus word as it appears alone. The ability to recall a paired stimulus represents the contents of memory. There are several factors that appear to influence the amount of information that can be processed with increasing age, including the pace of learning and the environment in which learning occurs, which may be influenced by cautiousness, anxiety, and interference from previously learned information.

The pace of learning is the speed with which a task is performed and is one variable known to affect older learners more than young ones. The pace of learning can be manipulated in two ways. The anticipation interval is the time allotted for a response. Older subjects perform poorly when this interval is short and do much better when they are given more time to respond.[3,11] Younger subjects also improve as the anticipation interval increases but less than older subjects. If a method called "self-pacing" is permitted, (i.e., if learners are allowed as much time as they want), older subjects improve in the number of correct responses they are capable of giving. The second element of pacing in paired associative learning is the time the pair of items is presented for study. This period is referred to as the study time or inspection interval. Increasing the study time also improves performance by older learners, although old and young subjects have been shown to benefit equally from more time.[2,12] Again, if "self-pacing" is allowed, older subjects benefit more than younger subjects.[13]

The ability to perform associative learning tasks may be affected by variables such as cautiousness, anxiety, and interference. These factors are often associated with errors of omission (not responding) or errors of commission (responding incorrectly). Errors of omission occur most often in fast-paced associative learning situations (rather than errors of commission). Errors of omission are reflective of cautiousness or a reluctance to venture a response unless one is absolutely certain of its accuracy. It has been suggested by researchers that the poorer performance of older adults, as reflected in omission errors, is a function of their being more cautious.[10,13]

To overcome cautiousness, or test this hypothesis, experimenters have requested or demanded responses be made, even if they are wrong. This failed to improve the learning rate of older subjects or to reduce the number of errors of omission.[14] However, in another test of the cautiousness hypothesis, a small monetary reward was given for each correct response and each incorrect response was also rewarded at a slightly lower value, and the absence of a response received no reward. In this situation older learners significantly reduced the number of errors of omission,[15] which suggests that older learners could do better if they took a few more chances.

Another hypothesis regarding the poorer performance of the elderly on paired associative learning suggests that anxiety affects performance. Eisdorfer and associates[16] tested this theory by introducing a drug that blocked physiological arousal. This resulted in significantly fewer errors in older subjects on associative learning tasks compared to elders given a placebo.

A final hypothesis suggests that in some instances of associative learning, older adults are more susceptible to the effects of interference from prior learning. When one word is frequently associated with another word in everyday situations, such as dark-light and water-ocean, the pair is said to have high associative strength. When one word is infrequently associated with another, such as dark-fast and water-book, the pair has low associative strength. If the associative habits of older individuals are more established through a greater number of years of experience, it follows that the age-related difference should be least for high associative pairs.[13] This appears to be the case. In a comprehensive study, Botwinick and Storandt[17] found no age-related differences in performance on an easy list but marked age-related differences in performance on moderate to high difficulty lists. The older adults appear to be more handicapped when learning and recall involves forming associations that are contrary, or in competition with, previously learned verbal associations.

Salthouse[13] conducted studies to determine the mechanisms by which processing speed contributes to the relations between adult age and associative learning. The results of these studies indicated that increased age was related to poorer associative learning largely because of a failure to retain information about previously correct responses. This in turn was related to the effectiveness of encoding briefly presented information in an associative memory task, which was related to measures of processing speed. It was suggested that age-related decreases in speed of processing lead to less effective encoding or elaboration, which results in a fragile representation that is easily disrupted by subsequent processing.[13]

Judging from studies of associative learning, the rate of learning slows gradually through the adult years. Only after the age of 65 does one's learning become demonstrably poorer than that of young adults. The nature of the age deficit remains unclear. Older subjects profit from a slower pace of learning much more than do young adults. Moreover, the older learner may get too anxious or cautious, or may encounter interference from previously learned associations.

INFORMATION PROCESSING

How information is processed has to do an the older adult's learning style, which is unique to each learner. Information processing has to do with the typical manner in which an individual receives, retains, and retrieves information, as well as how the individual responds emotionally in a learning experience. The term "information processing" as a means of learning grew from analogies with computer operations and has become a prominent theory in discussions of memory and perception. It involves associative, conceptual, and contextual learning. Information processing is the mechanism through which an individual processes, stores, and remembers events, tasks, lists, and the like. It involves the wiring of the human hard drive, the brain.

In an interesting study by Spitzer and associates,[18] functional magnetic resonance imaging (MRI), in conjunction with carefully designed, psychometrically optimized stimulation procedures (e.g., word-pairs, lists of words, color discrimination tasks), were used to investigate the relationship between brain activation and the processing of word associations. A semantic discrimination task of word-pair similarity selectively activated the left frontal and left frontotemporal areas. Cortical activation was decreased during language activities but highly active when an individual was performing a color similarity task. A similar study[19] used functional MRI to identify cortical areas involved in category learning by prototype abstraction. Elderly participants studied forty dot patterns that were distortions of an underlying prototype and were asked to make yes or no category judgments regarding the objects depicted by the dot patterns. Activity in four cortical areas correlated with the category judgment task. A sizeable posterior occipital cortical area exhibited significantly less activity during processing of the categorical patterns than during

processing of noncategorical patterns. Significant increases in activity during processing the categorical patterns were observed in left and right anterior frontal cortex and right inferior lateral frontal cortex. Decreases in activation of the visual cortex when categorical patterns were being studied suggest that these patterns could be processed in a more rapid or less effortful manner after the prototype had been learned. The researchers suggest that increases in prefrontal activity associated with processing categorical patterns could be related to any of several processes involved in retrieving information about the learned exemplars.[19]

Performance of complex motor tasks, such as rapid sequences of finger movements or lower extremity sequencing activities, can be improved in terms of speed and accuracy over several weeks by daily practice sessions.[5] This improvement does not generalize to a matched sequence of identical component movements, nor to the contralateral extremity. In a study by Karni and colleagues,[5] the underlying neural changes of learning of complex motor tasks was studied using functional magnetic resonance imaging of local blood oxygenation level-dependent signals evoked in the primary motor cortex (M1). Before training, a comparable extent of M1 was activated by both upper and lower extremity sequences. However, two ordering effects were observed: repeating a sequence within a brief time window initially resulted in a smaller area of activation (habituation), but later in a larger area of activation (enhancement), suggesting a switch in M1 processing mode within a fast learning session. By week 4 of training, concurrent with asymptotic performance, the extent of cortex activated by the practiced sequence enlarged compared with the unpracticed sequence, irrespective of order (slow learning). These changes persisted for several months. The results suggest a slowly evolving, long-term, experience-dependent reorganization of the older adult M1, which may underlie the acquisition and retention of the new motor skill.[5]

Cortical functions concerned with the execution of skilled movements can also be studied through complex interactive tasks. The learning of skilled performance tasks (SPT) offers the greatest amount of information about the electrophysiological components reflecting preprogramming, execution of the movement and control of the results. Overall, these components are indicated as movement-related brain macropotentials (MRBMs). Among them, Bereitschaftspotential (BP) reflects cerebral processes related to the preparation of movement, and skilled performance positivity (SPP) reflects control processes on the result of performance. There is some evidence supporting a training effect on MRBMs, but less clear is whether long-term practice of a skilled activity could modify learning strategies of a new skilled task.[20] Fattapposta and associates[20] recorded MRBMs in elderly subjects trained for a long time to perform a highly skillful activity (i.e., sequencing dancing steps) and compared electrophysiological brain activity to a group of elderly control subjects without any former experience in these skilled motor activities. Their findings demonstrated the existence of a relationship between pre-programming and performance control, as suggested by decrease in the BP amplitude and an increase of the SPP amplitude in the presence of high levels of performance. Long-term practice seems to develop better control models on performance that reduce the need of a high mental effort in preprogramming a skilled action.[20]

CONTEXTUAL LEARNING

Associative learning is often supported by the individual placing some contextual meaning to lists of words, activities, or other learning endeavors. For example, if an important piece of information is presented in **bold** type, it is more likely to be perceived as important because its importance has been stressed through visual intonation. In other words, learning occurs because the information has been presented in context.

In a study by Naveh-Benjamin and Craik,[21] memory for words and the font in which they appeared (or the voice speaking them) was compared in younger and older persons to explore whether age-related differences in episodic word memory are due to age-related differences in memory for perceptual-contextual information. In each of the experimental sessions, young and old participants were presented with words to learn. The words were presented in either one of two font types, or in one of two male voices, and participants paid attention either to the fonts or voices or to the meaning of the words. Subjects were tested on both work and font or voice memory. The results showed that younger participants had better explicit memory for font and voice memory and for the words themselves but that older participants benefited at least as much as younger people when perceptual characteristics of the words (e.g., *italics*, **bold,** tone of voice) were utilized. This study concluded that there was no evidence of an age-related impairment in the encoding of perceptual-conceptual information.[21] This is an important finding for geriatric rehabilitation professionals. Much of the printed or spoken information we provide for our elderly patients/clients could conceivably be learned better if it were presented in a perceptual-contextual format.

In a study by Spencer and Raz,[22] age-related differences in memory for facts, source, and contextual details were examined in healthy young (18 to 35 year olds) and old (65 to 80 year olds) volunteers. In all tested memory functions, decline over time was greater in the elderly than in the young. A time-dependent increase in the prevalence of source amnesia errors was clearly associated with old age. Contrary to other studies, measures of frontal lobe functions did not predict source memory.[22] Nevertheless, some of these putative frontal function measures were related to memory for contextual details. The number of perseverative responses on testing was inversely related to performance on both factual and contextual memory tests, but the association with contextual memory was stronger. Difficulties with response selection predicted poor contextual memory in young but not in old adults.[22]

In a subsequent study, Spencer and Raz[23] reviewed the evidence of age differences in episodic memory for content of a message and the context associated with it. Specifically, the authors tested a hypothesis that memory for context is more vulnerable to aging than memory for content. In addition, the authors inquired as to whether effort at encoding and retrieval and type of stimulus material moderate the magnitude of age differences in both memory domains. The results confirmed the main hypothesis: Age differences in context memory are reliably greater than those in memory for content. Tasks that required greater effort during retrieval yielded larger age differences in content but not in context memory. The greatest magnitude of age differences in context memory was observed for those contextual features that were more likely to have been encoded independently from content.[23] The possible mechanisms that may underlie age differences in context memory, as suggested by these researchers, are attentional deficits, reduced working memory capacity, and/or a failure of inhibitory processing. The findings of the Spencer and Raz studies[22,23] are substantiated by numerous other studies.[24–27] The major clinical implication of these findings is that elderly humans overwhelmingly seek, create, or imagine context in order to provide meaning when presented with information. The importance of this will be discussed further in a subsequent section of this chapter in relationship to teaching strategies for the elderly.

HUMAN MEMORY

There are many myths about the effects of aging on memory. For example, people are supposed to forget things they've recently learned, but memories from the distant past are supposed to be clear and vivid, sometimes startlingly so. Early learning also appears to have a significant impact on an elderly individual's resourcefulness for both verbal and physical skills in later life. [1,8,9]

Memory is closely related to both intelligence and learning, since remembering is part of the evidence of learning and learning is part of the measurement of intelligence. For example, if a person does not learn, that person has nothing to remember. Conversely, if the individual cannot remember, there is no sign of their having learned.[28]

There are essentially four types of memory. Short-term or immediate memory involves recall after very little delay (as little as five seconds up to thirty seconds). Recent memory involves recall after a brief period (from one hour to several days). Remote memory refers to recall of events which took place a long time ago but which have been referred to frequently throughout the course of a lifetime. Old memory refers to recall of events that occurred a long time in the past and which have not been thought of or rehearsed since.[9]

Regardless of type, there are three stages of memory: registration (encoding), retention (storage), and recall (retrieval). Registration refers to the recording of learning or perceptions, and is more commonly referred to as encoding. In concept, it is analogous to the recording of sound on a tape recorder. Retention refers to the ability to sustain registration over time. Recall is retrieval of material that has been registered and retained. Obviously in any type of memory, a failure at any one of these stages will result in no measurable memory.

It is commonly believed that all kinds of memory show a decline with advancing age; however, studies do not consistently support this idea. While it is true that there is an age-related deficit in recall of various types, it is not clear whether this deficit results from declining memory or declining ability to learn in the first place. If one is interested only in whether or not there is a decline in the ability to reproduce previously exposed material with age regardless of what the basis for the decline may be, the evidence seems to point to an age deficit in the performance of both immediate and delayed recall.[29]

There appears to be a greater loss with age in short-term and recent memory than in remote or old memory. Also, the decline with age in memory function is less for rote memory (i.e., material that has been deliberately memorized) than for logical memory (i.e., material requiring problem solving from past learning).[8-10]

People with higher intelligence are less susceptible to memory loss with increasing age than are their less intelligent counterparts, and some older people escape memory loss altogether.[30] This pattern suggests that the memory loss that is associated with age may not in fact be due to processes of senescence. It suggests that perhaps memory losses are associated with disuse. In fact, people who exercise their memories tend to maintain both remote and recent memory.[10]

Any attempt to try to reverse or compensate for a decline in memory functions must obviously depend on some notion of why people forget. There are a number of theories of forgetting, and each has implications for various treatment solutions.

One biological theory proposed that memory is located in RNA (ribonucleic acid). This theory states that loss of memory is the result of loss of RNA with age due to the influence of certain enzymes. Studies of subjects with severe memory decline suggest that memory is improved by administering RNA either orally or by intravenous injection.[31] Cameron[31] has asserted that this procedure (RNA therapy) is the only method that has reversed memory deterioration in cases of organic brain syndromes, but scant follow-up research does not substantiate this claim.

Another theory proposed has to do with previously learned material interfering with new learning.[10] If the interference theory is accurate, then all that could be done to ward off memory decline would be periodic rehearsal. Faulty encoding could be at least partly countered by allowing plenty of time for learning, perception, or both to take place. Not much could be done, according to this theory, about a decline in ability to retain material that has been registered.

The information processing theory deals with the acquisition of learned material. According to this approach, learning is viewed as part of memory and is based in the acquisition phase.[32] Studies of memory encoding often overlap with studies of perception, for both involve initial processing. Memory psychologists distinguish three phases of memory: encoding, storage, and retrieval.

Learning is often called encoding. Just as information must be translated into the proper code (or language) for a computer to process it further, information from the environment must be encoded for the human processing system to store, use, and later retrieve.

Encoding is the learning or acquisition phase of memory, but storage is perhaps the phase most people think of as memory. It is the laying away of encoded information in "storehouses" for later use. The sensory store is conceptualized as a very brief way station for essentially unprocessed information from the environment.[33] In order for information to be recalled, it must be processed and transferred to later stores (short-term and long-term). Short-term store is presumed to hold relatively small amounts of information for a slightly longer time than the sensory store (a phone number from directory assistance), commonly on the order of a few seconds, whereas, the long-term store is seen as having a very large capacity for storing information which can be retained over long periods of time. Figure 18–1 provides a schematic representation of the memory system.[34]

The final phase of memory is retrieval, which is the finding of the information when it is needed. The major age differences in memory performance are related to short-term and long-term store.[35] There do not appear to be significant age differences in sensory store, but there is evidence that some of the age difference in memory lies specifically in the retrieval phase. Older people may have the necessary information in storage, but they can't get to it as easily as younger people.[36] One way to show that retrieval is the problem, rather than learning or storage difficulties, is to compare two common methods of retrieval: recall and recognition. Recall is the remembrance of what has been learned or experienced, while recognition is the perception that an object or person has

ENCODING ————————→ STORAGE ————————→ RETRIEVAL

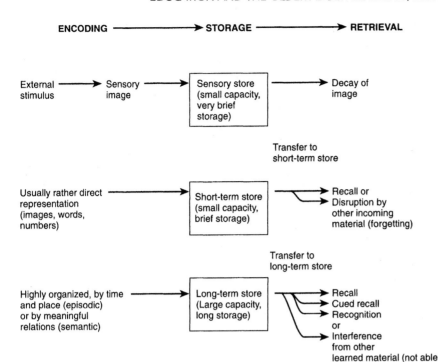

FIGURE 18–1. The memory system is a rough approximation of memory theories. This chart's primary purpose is to illustrate (1) the three phases of memory (encoding, storage, and retrieval) and (2) the three storage systems (sensory, short-term, and long-term) The additional material shows the differences in encoding, storage, and retrieval for the three stores. (*Reproduced with permission from* Atkinson JW, Shiffrin RM. Human memory: a proposed system and its control processes. In: Spence KW, Spence JT, eds. *The Psychology of Learning and Motivation.* New York: Academic Press; 1968;2)

been encountered and learned before. What does it mean, then, that one can recognize material that one cannot recall? It means that the information was learned and stored, because it can be recognized as correct, but it also means that the individual could not retrieve it when asked for simple recall, though she or he can if presented with multiple choices. It means that the failure of recall was a failure in retrieval; that the search for the desired information in the storehouses of memory failed, even though the information was there.

Research suggests that encoding and retrieval problems are the cause of the memory difficulites of older adults.[36] Some of these difficulties occur because older adults do not spontaneously use effective encoding and retrieval strategies. When instructed in these strategies, their performance improves.

The relationship of age to encoding has been cross-sectionally studied, and the findings indicate only a slight decline in encoding ability until age 65.[35] Are there age differences in encoding? Encoding, when viewed from the information processing theory, is the learning or acquisition phase. The earlier discussion suggests that encoding will be found to be less efficient in older subjects. In particular, a slower pace of learning leads to a more efficient encoding of the information.[37] If initial learning between young and old groups is compared, memory will be essentially the same, although elderly individuals need more repetition. The implication of this is that older subjects are less efficient in encoding the material and they require more repetitions or better organization of the material to build an adequate code.

One of the best ways to encode information for later retrieval is to organize it.[38] Evidence suggests that many older subjects do not spontaneously organize information for later recall.[36] In one investigation, lists of words with "clusters" based on similarity in meaning (ocean/sea) or relatedness (piano/music) were used to test age-related differences.[39] These natural ways to organize and encode the list of words were used by younger learners but rarely used by older learners. If older subjects were instructed in memory-enhancing advantages of organization, they improved their position relative to younger subjects.[40] This was true of subjects who were old and measured as low intelligence on verbal ability.[41] An example of this type of study is one in which subjects were first given experience in sorting words into categories, which trains them in organizing words.[42] Later, given a similar list to learn, older subjects did better relative to younger subjects who did not have the prior training in sorting words into categories (Figure 18–2).

Another way to encode information for later retrieval is to use what are commonly called mnemonic devices.[43] These techniques use verbal or visual associations to link pieces together that might not by themselves have clear relationships. A common verbal mnemonic: "i before e, except after c." An example of visual mneumonics might be "picturing" a shopping list (milk, mushrooms, and sun lotion) by visually imagining a cow sunning on a mushroom.

In a study of the effectiveness of various types of encoding instructions,[44] younger and older adults were given pairs of unassociated words to learn. Three different groups were instructed to simply learn the pairs as best they could; or to think of some

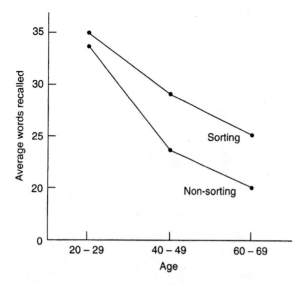

FIGURE 18–2. *Average number of words learned as a function of age. Prior to learning, about half of the subjects carried out a sorting task designed to aid in organizing word lists; the rest of the subjects performed a task that did not involve sorting. (Reproduced with permission from Hutsch D. Adult age differences in free classification and free recall. Dev Psych. 1971; 4:338–342. " 1971 American Psychological Association.)*

property or characteristic common to both words; or to form a visual image of an interaction. To test retention, one word of a pair was given and the subject was asked to recall the second word. Both age groups who were instructed to use imagery did better. Encoding was facilitated by the use of imagery and retrieval was facilitated by using cues to stimulate recall.

In another investigation,[45] individuals in their 60s and 70s were instructed in a venerable memory trick called the "method of loci." This method involves imagining items to be remembered in various familiar locations. The older subjects who learned this trick remembered significantly more than those not instructed in this method.

Another way to examine age differences in the encoding phase of memory is to consider the "depth" at which information from the environment is processed. The depth-of-processing approach was first proposed in 1972 to explain why some tasks involve greater memory demands than others.[46] In general, deeper levels of processing involve reviewing or evaluating words at a semantic level; that is, they involve examining the meaning of the word rather than superficial characteristics of the stimuli. The deeper the level, the more remembered. As with their apparent difficulties with organization and mediation, older subjects do not seem to process information as deeply as younger subjects. The data suggests that without direct and detailed instructions, older subjects process words in a list simply by thinking about their sounds (acoustic encoding), whereas younger subjects process them by thinking about their meaning (semantic encoding).[36,47]

Age differences in memory can be reduced or eliminated altogether if older adults are instructed in the use of encoding strategies and given additional time to complete memory tasks.[33] Age differences in encoding and the use of organizational strategies are most evident in "effortful" tasks; those that require constant attention or are novel or unfamiliar (for example, following a new recipe, driving an unfamiliar car, or driving to a familiar place by a different route). Automatized tasks require little attention or conscious awareness (such as routine household chore, playing a familiar tune on piano).[48]

Several lines of evidence suggest that part of the age difference typically observed in studies of memory lies in the encoding phase of memory.[12,41] Older subjects do not spontaneously organize information as quickly or as effectively as younger ones. It appears that it is harder for older learners to form associations, and it takes them longer to do so. They use less effective verbal mediators when they mediate at all. Also, older adults do not seem to process information as deeply as younger adults; therefore, they store less information and consequently can retrieve less. This has been explained by researchers as a problem in motivation or anxiety, because elderly persons are either unwilling or unable to explore the lists at a deeper level. Another factor could be less education and a different learning mode. In the early 1900s, rote learning (memorization) was the emphasized mode for learning.

THE STORAGE PHASE OF MEMORY RELATED TO AGE

The second phase of memory, storage, involves retention or loss of information. Traditionally, studies of memory storage deal with capacity or how much information an individual can store. Another important consideration in the study of memory storage in addition to capacity is duration, or how long the information can remain in storage before it is lost or displaced and forgotten. The three storage systems defined earlier guide studies of retention and storage.[34] Sensory and short-term stores are viewed as limited-capacity structures in that they ordinarily retain information for only brief periods of time. The long-term store is considered to have an almost unlimited capacity and information is rarely lost from it.

Sensory memory is considered to be sense-specific, that is, the information is stored according to the sensory modality that receives it. Two types of sensory modalities are defined within this context of memory. The visual memory store is called iconic memory. This is considered to be a fleeting memory based on visual information. Facsimiles of auditory stimuli are termed echoic memory. Many psychologists consider these brief facsimiles to be an initial stage of information processing. There is almost no information available on the effects of aging on echoic memory.[49] Iconic memory is often studied by briefly presenting a stimulus (for example, a letter or letters) to a subject and then presenting a second stimulus that interferes with or "masks" the first one. Iconic memory is assessed as the extent to which the initial stimulus is recalled after the mask.[50] Since visual abilities decline with age, it might be expected that the declines in the sensory store would be larger than they are. It is possible that age differences in sensory store make some stimuli more difficult for older people to attend to and remember. Speech comprehension is one likely candidate, but the minor deficits in sensory store that do occur probably do not contribute significantly to the more severe memory problems in long-term store experienced in the elderly.[35] This is because age differences in short-term memory, the next stage in the information-processing system, appear to be small, and it is in short-term memory that information is prepared for long-term memory.

The short-term store is considered to be temporary memory with a limited capacity (e.g., six to nine items with acoustic encoding). The purpose of the short-term store is to work on organizing the information so that it is in proper form for storing in the more permanent long-term store. As a result, the short-term memory store is sometimes called "working memory." The short-term store uses the encoding processes of organization, mediation, and depth of processing, which helps prepare or encode information for permanent storage. There are age differences in the facility with which adults use these encoding processes, as previously discussed. If information is bumped out of short-term store before it is properly encoded, it probably will be lost forever.

While there are age differences in encoding in the short-term store, there do not appear to be age differences in the capacity of short-term store.[35,51,52] Studies of memory span (the ability to recall the longest string of items, such as numbers, letters, words, that can be repeated after a single, brief presentation) show few age differences. An example would be hearing a phone number from directory assistance with no pen in hand. Lack of age differences in short-term storage is provided by a second line of evidence called the recency effect. Subjects typically do best on the first (primary effect) and the last few words given (recency effect). The only age difference found is the pace with which the lists are presented. Older learners need more time.[52] Old and young people do not differ in the capacity of the short-term store, but when encoding information into long-term store, the problems experienced by older adults may be a result of the tendency to use repetition rather than a more appropriate encoding strategy.

The long-term store is what people generally think of as memory. There may be large age differences in long-term memory, particularly when the material to be remembered exceeds the capacity of short-term

store.[10] Since the probability of diseases that can affect brain tissue (e.g., cardiovascular)[53] or brain functions (e.g., neurological)[54–57] or psychological problems like depression[58] is much greater in old people, this sort of loss may be a factor in age differences in memory. Most of the discussion of age differences in long-term storage focuses not on capacity or loss of information but rather on the ease or difficulty people have when trying to locate information in this vast repository of facts and ideas. This is the issue of retrieval, the third phase of memory.

RETRIEVAL RELATED TO AGE

As with encoding, older adults also have more difficulty retrieving the information they have stored, because older people have more trouble getting the information into their long-term stores and more trouble getting it out. Difficulties in encoding and retrieval account for most of the overall age differences observed in memory experiments.[35]

The distinction between recall and recognition is key to studying the retrieval process of memory. Often elderly subjects can recognize words but they cannot recall them. An example of this is that older subjects might not be able to recall BASKET, but can recognize it when asked: "Was BASKET on the list?" Studies show that age differences on recognition tests are small or nonexistent, whereas age differences found for recall of factual information are significant.[35,59] Recall and recognition may be affected by different encoding strategies,[60] and the use of efficient encoding strategies may be especially important for recall. In a comprehensive twenty one-year longitudinal study,[61] word recognition showed modest gains until age sixty and only moderate decline thereafter. In contrast, the word recall test showed marked age changes beginning in young adulthood and accelerating in old age.[61] The conclusion of this study was that older subjects have a lot of information in memory storage that they cannot get to in difficult retrieval tasks that involve recall. Older subjects benefit more than younger subjects when retrieval cues are improved; recognition tests provide more and better cues than recall tests. Cued recall (e.g., starts with . . . , or categories: animals, names, professions, vegetables, etc.) aided elderly individuals in better recall.[62]

The magnitude of age differences in recall and recognition may also be affected by the subjects' verbal ability.[4] Several studies showed no differences between younger and older groups who had high verbal ability, but age differences were found between young and old groups with low verbal ability.[63,64]

Recall of ancient memories is an interesting area in the study of memory and aging. Another of the myths of aging is that old people cannot remember recent events but can recall, with great clarity, events in the distant past.[8,9,65] In the nineteenth century, one theorist went so far as to formulate what has come to be known as Ribot's Law,[8,44] which states that information is forgotten in a sequence that is the reverse of the order in which it was acquired. As a general rule, memory for an event is greatest immediately following the event and then declines systematically; recognition memory declines less rapidly than recall. The literature on age differences in remote memory suggests that such differences are minimal. Even though remote memory holds up well in older adults, it is not superior to the recall of recent events.[65]

Remote memory is commonly evaluated by recall and recognition of public events (e.g., World War II, Kennedy's assassination). No age-related difference in recall of recent events as compared to remote events has been found.[66] What is probably happening when people feel that ancient events are clearer in their mind is that a particularly sharp memory from the past is being compared with some vaguely encoded events of the last day or two.[65] Strong memory, called a "flashbulb memory," is evident when a remote event was of such personal significance that it has strong emotions associated with it or was thought about (rehearsed) many times.[67]

Young and middle-age adults experience this strange reversal of memory strengths where remote memories are stronger than recent memories.[67] Old people encode recent events less well than younger adults, and it is possible that they rehearse ancient memories more often (reminiscing), but the reversal of memory strengths is a natural phenomenon that occurs at all ages and is incorrectly viewed as a sign of aging.[8] The truth is that memory is a notoriously leaky repository in humans of all ages. The myth that old memories are set in mental concrete that has hardened to the extent that it will not accept new inputs is pure nonsense!

Atypical difficulties in encoding new events often result from temporary or permanent changes in brain function or changes in brain chemistry.[68] In humans, such changes can be induced in adults of all ages by prescription drugs or voluntary use of alcohol or drugs. These effects are usually transient. In elderly adults, and sometimes in younger adults, brain disease that results in biochemical imbalance is often reflected in the inability to remember recent events (because they are not encoded and stored), although memory for less recent events is unimpaired.[69]

Everyday memories have been studied as a more relevant area of memory testing in older subjects.[70] The older subjects may have more difficulty in encoding word lists into memory and later retrieving them. They do not seem to have difficulties remembering the time and place of the experiment, and they retrieve with ease information about income, education, or number of grandchildren, and they have no difficulty encoding the instructions for the experiment.[70] Elders may not spontaneously organize word lists for effective recall, but ask an 80-year-old fan of soap operas to recount the last two weeks of "The Young and the Restless" or "Days of Our Lives" and you are likely to observe a confident, highly organized, and accurate response.

Some memory researchers distinguish episodic memories, which concern specific events (episodes) that occurred at a specific time and place, and semantic memories, which concern general context-free facts about the world, such as the meaning of words, rules of grammar and arithmetic, personal beliefs. Episodic memory studies investigate recall of activities which have already occurred. In contrast, prospective memory involves remembering something in the future (i.e., a dental appointment or turning off the oven when the cake is done). Though elders reported problems with forgetting prospective memory, most studies indicate they performed as well or better than younger subjects.[71] Time monitoring strategies, such as a calendar or a kitchen timer, were found to be important modalities for enhancing prospective memory for both young and older adults.

The contextual approach to learning and memory takes into account the subject's prior knowledge, level of verbal ability, motivation, and other factors. Contextual approach studies involve the interaction between the characteristics of the subject, the type of material used in the task, and memory performance.[72] These studies investigate the processing of information from prose passages which are common in everyday experience (e.g., from newspapers, magazines). Age differences are not as common in text (prose) memory performance as they are in recall of lists. The presence or absence of age differences is a function of the contextual factors that mediate the subject's processing of text materials. Age differences have been found to be smaller when text is well organized, when there is prior knowledge and when the subject has above-average verbal ability. Recalling the gist of a well-organized text passage proved to be strong in the older subjects as well as young adults.[72] The old may focus on the main idea, whereas the young may be more observant of detail. What appears to be inefficient processing in older people may actually reflect adaptive changes. As a result of life experiences or lower levels of energy, the old may focus on higher levels of meaning devoting less attention to detail.[73]

Self-reports of memory are included in the contextual approach to investigating learning and memory in older adults. It was found that all age learners may present a distorted picture of what actually occurred. When questioned however, older adults report more memory failures and are more likely to be upset when memory failure occurs.[74] Older adults reported that they forget names, routines, and objects more often than younger adults. This self-reporting of memory problems was more common in unfamiliar situations or when required to recall information they have not recently used.[70,71] External aids, such as visual cues, proved to be very helpful tools in assisting with recall, particularly with regard to prospective memory.

Distortion of long-term memory has been found to occur in all age groups.[75] Theorists suggest that information is permanently stored once it has been placed in long-term memory; that information is not lost even when it cannot be retrieved. Research in which subjects witnessed a complex event (e.g., a crime or accident) and were subsequently given misleading information confirmed distortion of memory consistent in all age groups. Provided with the initial event and a confounding piece of information, both young and older subjects later recalled the event incorrectly. Distortions in memory are more likely when the interval between the event and the misinformation is long. Memories of violent events are more likely to be distorted and postevent information is more likely to be accepted if it is presented in an auxiliary clause than if it appears in a main clause of a sentence. Memory distortion is minimized if subjects are warned that the postevent message contains misinformation.[76]

Memory complaints, depression, and drug use are important variables to consider when assessing memory loss. The extent of memory problems is probably exaggerated with age, especially when posited against depression, drug use, or both.[77] Complaints of memory problems do not correlate with scores on objective tests of memory performance.[78–80] But significant correlations between depression and complaints of poor memory have been found.[70,77] There is a tendency for depressed persons to underestimate their abilities.

Drug side effects may also affect cognitive function in general and memory in particular. Drugs, such as tranquilizers, antidepressants, and sedatives reinforce some cognitive-slowing tendencies. Inappropriate dosages or the interaction of drugs (multiple drug use) can result in mental confusion and memory loss.[69]

There is also the potential for drugs to improve cognitive functioning and memory by improving neurotransmitter and neuroendocrine functioning.[35,68] But, no drug, to date, has been found that significantly improves memory function. To find a drug that improves memory function, the researcher must first target a specific cognitive process that a drug is supposed to influence. Also, problems resulting from metabolic variations often mask any significant changes in study groups of elderly.

PROBLEM SOLVING

Many of the learning and memory tasks described in previous sections involved relatively simple problems. Another type of cognitive activity, problem solving, is more complex and may involve aspects of learning and memory not previously discussed. Problem solving requires that a person assess the present state of a situation, define the desired state (or goal), and find a way to transform the present state to the desired state.[81]

The process of solving a problem has been broken down into four steps.[82] The first step is to understand the problem, which involves gathering information on the problem and identifying its important elements. The second step is to devise a plan, using past experience for guidance. The use of a relevant strategy would ensure that one devises an efficient plan. The third step is to carry out the plan, and the final step is to review what has been done (i.e., was the problem solved?).

There are many types of studies that address problem solving from a "laboratory" perspective (using prefabricated laboratory situations that do not necessarily duplicate problems encountered in real life). One such mode of testing is termed concept attainment. In concept attainment tasks, items in a set are divided into two subsets in accordance with some characteristics or rule. The subject demonstrates mastery of the rule by distinguishing the items that reflect the rule from those that do not. An example of this would be "choose the red circle; do not choose the green circle." Another example is presenting meal content lists with the rule that certain food types may induce illness and having the subjects identify those meals that would make them ill following consumption. A number of studies of this type, in which performance of younger and older adults were compared, found that the old solved fewer problems than the young.[83–85] Some of the difficulties encountered were that older subjects failed to ignore irrelevant information and tended to fixate on useless hunches.[85] Although the elderly people do not spontaneously employ effective strategies, several training studies have found that their performance could be improved with brief training procedures.[86,87]

"Twenty questions" is another means of testing problem-solving abilities. In this type of task, the subject is presented with an array of pictures or words, only one of which is the correct choice. The task is to determine the correct choice by asking less than twenty questions that can be answered with a "yes" or "no." The most efficient strategy is to ask questions that are constraint-seeking (e.g., "Is it a vegetable?"), each of which eliminates a set of possible answers. Asking questions that refer to only one item is inefficient. Again, the elderly tend to do less well on these tasks than younger groups,[88] but their performance improved significantly after training in the use of constraint-seeking questions.

Piagetian theory has been applied to problem-solving measurement as well. Piagetian theory assumes that concrete operational abilities (the ability to think logically about concrete or tangible problems), such as classification and conservation (the recognition that the amount of matter does not change when it is rearranged), develop during middle childhood and that formal operational abilities (the ability to think logically about hypothetical situations or problems) are achieved in adolescence. Do these abilities decline in old age? One hypothesis suggests that operational abilities decline in reverse of the order in which they develop.[9,89,90] In other words, formal operational thought would decline before conservation. Studies of performance by elderly persons on various Piagetian tasks have yielded mixed results. Some show that the elderly do less well than younger people;[91] others find no age differences in formal operational tasks.[92] Success is positively correlated with higher levels of education and higher intelligence scores. Training has been shown to improve performance by the elderly as well.

In summary, these studies suggest that there are age differences in problem-solving abilities and the elderly do less well on a number of types of tasks. Several explanations have been offered. It may be that problem-solving ability is a function of educational level, fluid intelligence, or both, rather than aging per se. These factors, in turn, may reflect cohort differences. Additionally, brief educational training has been shown to improve all types of problem solving discussed.[93] This suggests that the elderly possess the competence to perform the tasks but do not spontaneously employ the necessary strategies. Even after training, the elderly may not transfer the use of these strategies to the problems encountered in real life.

INTELLIGENCE

When considering intelligence, a potential and actual ability are implied. In practice, however, measured ability is always dealt with. Thus, intelligence, as it is studied conceptually by psychologists, has three aspects: potential intelligence; actual intelligence; and measured intelligence. This discussion will center around age changes in measured intelligence.

Measured intelligence is actual mental ability (i.e., measured performance of basic cognitive abilities) defined in terms of responses to items on a test. Yet no matter how extensive or well-prepared a test is, there is always a margin of error in its measurement of actual mental ability. The most frequently used test in studies of adult intelligence and age-related changes is the Wechsler Adult Intelligence Scale (WAIS).

Intelligence quotient (IQ) is a test score that is compared with the normal or average score of 100. When the WAIS is used for adults aged 20 to 75 and older, there is an age factor built into the determination of what is normal. In Figure 18–3, the heavy black line indicates the mean raw scores on the WAIS by age. Note that measured performance peaks about age 25 and declines thereafter, particularly after age 65. In scoring measured performance, a handicap or advantage is built into the WAIS IQ score to control for age. There could be a 40-point difference between the score at age 25 and the score at age 75, and yet the IQ score would be the same. The importance of this is that the most frequently used test of mental ability incorporates an assumption that a 40-point drop in score from age 25 to age 75 is normal.

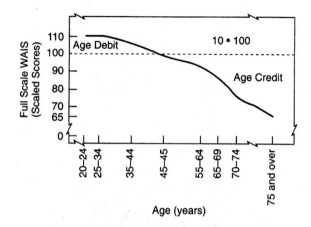

FIGURE 18–3. *Full scale WAIS scores as a function of age. (Reproduced with permission from Botwinick J. Cognitive Processes in Maturity and Old Age. New York: Springer; 1967:3.)*

In practical terms, however, the average decline with age in WAIS scores masks a large amount of individual variation. Any given older person might have an extremely high IQ even when compared to the young. In fact, the correlation between age and IQ is not particularly high, only around –0.40. This means that if the odds against predicting the IQ score were 10 to 1, then knowledge of age would reduce these odds to 6 to 1, not a particularly stunning reduction.

Intelligence testing does not measure a single ability, but rather a set of abilities. Broadly, the WAIS yields separate scores for verbal and performance IQ. The WAIS includes subtests measuring information, vocabulary, comprehension, arithmetic, similarities, digit span, picture completion, object assembly, block design, picture arrangement, and digit symbol tasks.[41] Elderly subjects do best on the information subtest and worst on the digit symbol subtest. The subtests can be broken into two sets; one set dealing with verbal ability and the other dealing with performance ability. Older people consistently do better on the verbal tests than they do on the performance tests. Subtest patterns on the WAIS indicate that stored information and verbal abilities are sustained in old age at a much higher level than are psychomotor-perceptual-integrative skills.[41,94] Of relevance here is that most of the performance subtests are timed while many of the verbal subtests are not. Timed tests may be influenced by reaction time which shows an age-related decline (see Chapter 3).

There are a number of factors which influence age changes in IQ. Perhaps the most important is the individual's initial level of function. People with scores in the 95th percentile (i.e., with scores high enough that 95 percent of all scores fall below theirs), show a leveling off in vocabulary scores between the ages of 20 and 30. Thereafter, these individuals scores show a plateau or a slight rise with advancing age.[95] On the other hand, people in the 25th percentile show a marked decline in vocabulary scores after the age of 30. This suggests that those with a stronger verbal base to begin with continue to acquire verbal intelligence as the years progress, and those with a weaker verbal foundation initially show a progressive decline in ability as the years go by.

Performance on an intelligence test is closely related to such factors as motivation, anxiety, and cooperation. An environment producing anxiety, or a poorly motivated or uncooperative individual will prevent accurate measurement of what that individual is actually capable of accomplishing intellectually.

Another factor that has great influence on performance on an intelligence test is the level of education: the higher the educational level, the higher the test scores. It is difficult to determine whether intelligence or education comes first, but they are highly correlated.

IQ is also affected by the health status of the individual being tested. Suboptimal levels of health have been shown to have a negative influence on performance on IQ tests. In fact, it has been hypothesized that rapid declines in IQ after the age of 65 could very likely be the result of poor health. Arteriosclerosis has been correlated to markedly decreased scores.

Most studies of intelligence and age compare test scores of people of different ages using a cross-sectional study model and assume that the only variable is age. This assumption is obviously difficult to defend. Older people have lived through a different era and developed a different body of "symbols" than younger people. Life experience is likely to be a strong influencing variable. The studies discussed measured age differences as opposed to age changes in intelligence. The most accurate study design in the examination of age changes in intelligence would be a longitudinal study following the individual through life with periodic measures of intelligence. Such studies have been conducted and have shown the same patterns of changes noted above except that the declines observed in overall scores were much smaller. This would suggest that at least part of what appears to be the decline in intelligence of older people is actually a change in skills that are being emphasized by the culture.

Memory is also a factor influencing an older individual's performance on intelligence tests. Studies have shown that short-term memory tends to lose efficiency with advancing age, as previously discussed. Since perceptive and integrative skills depend heavily on short-term memory, and vocabulary and information skills depend mainly on long-term memory, these findings may account for much of the observed difference in IQ test performances between older and younger individuals.

MOTOR LEARNING

Beyond the cognitive components of learning (e.g., memory, intelligence), motor learning is a very important part of therapeutic interventions with the el-

derly. Considerable age-related changes in the neuromuscular and sensory systems, as described in Chapter 3, paint a picture of progressive decline, however, practicing movement patterns has been found to be very effective in re-establishing ease of movement patterns and postural control.[96–98] Motor learning can occur at any age. Many of the declines in functional capabilities are the result of compensation for muscle imbalances, postural changes, and pain. Rehabilitation efforts that address these compensatory problems will result in relearning of sequential movements.

Recent studies of the improvement of perceptual performance as a function of activity training (i.e., perceptual learning) have provided new insights into the neuronal substrates of this type of skill learning in the adult brain. Issues such as where in the brain, when, and under what conditions practice-related changes occur have been investigated.[99] Karni and Bertini[99] suggest that a behaviorally relevant degree of plasticity is retained in the older adult cortex, even within early, low-level representations in sensory and motor-processing streams. The acquisition and retention of skills may share many characteristics with the functional plasticity subserving early-life learning and development. While the specificity of learning provides localization constraints, an important clue to the nature of the underlying neuronal changes is the time course of learning or relearning activity in a healthy older adult.[99] If, however, a neuromuscular pathology exists, learning is often impaired.

Prior studies have shown that procedural learning is severely impaired in patients with diffuse cerebellar damage (cortical degeneration) as measured by the serial reaction time task (SRTT). Gomez-Beldarrain and associates[53] hypothesized that focal cerebellar lesions can also have lateralized effects on procedural learning. They studied elderly patients with single, unilateral vascular lesions in the territory of the posterior-inferior or superior cerebellar artery, and compared the study group to age- and sex-matched controls. The results of their intervention showed that the study group did not acquire procedural knowledge when performing a task with the hand ipsilateral to the lesion, but showed normal learning with the contralateral hand. This suggests a critical role for the cerebellum and crossed cerebellar-prefrontal connections, or both, in this type of motor learning.[53]

Evidence suggests that patients suffering from Parkinson's disease (PD) demonstrate less sequence learning in the SRTT. One of the problems with this task is that it is motor-intensive and, given the motor difficulties which characterize Parkinson's disease (e.g., tremor, impaired facility of movement, rigidity, and loss of postural reflexes), there is the possibility that patients with PD are capable of sequence learning but are simply unable to demonstrate this because of a decrease in reaction time. Westwater and colleagues[54] examined the performance of patients with PD and healthy controls matched for verbal fluency, on a verbal version of the SRTT where the standard button-pressing response was replaced by a spoken response. The PD group demonstrated less sequence learning than the controls and this was independent of age and severity of illness. These results add support to other studies that have found impaired sequence learning in PD patients.[54]

Individuals with PD have difficulty initiating and performing complex, sequential movements. Practice generally leads to faster initiation and execution of movements in healthy adults, however, whether practice similarly improves motor performance in patients with PD remains controversial. To assess the effects of practice on motor performance, Behrman and associates[55] compared patients with PD to control subjects doing rapid arm-reaching tasks with different levels of movement complexity for 120 trials over two days. Response programming was studied by analyzing the overall reaction time latency of each movement and its fractionated subcomponents, premotor, and motor time. Practice effects were investigated by comparing pretest performance to immediate and delayed retention test performances (ten minutes and 48 hours rest intervals, respectively). Both patients with PD and control subjects improved speeded performance of sequential targeting tasks by practice and retained the improvement across both retention test intervals. Finding a learning effect for persons with Parkinson's disease supports practice as an effective rehabilitation strategy to improve motor performance of specific tasks.

Huntington's disease (HD) is another neuromuscular disease where learning, both cognitive and motor learning, can be compromised. Skill learning in early-stage HD patients was compared with that of normal controls on two perceptual-motor task, rotary pursuit and mirror tracing, in a study by Gabrieli and associates.[56] HD patients demonstrated a dissociation between impaired rotary pursuit and intact mirror tracing skill learning. These results suggest that different forms of perceptual-motor skill learning are mediated by separable neural circuits. A striatal memory system may be essential for sequence or open-loop skill learning but not for skills that involve the closed-loop learning, of novel visual response mappings. It is hypothesized by these researchers that working memory deficits in HD result from frontostriatal damage and account broadly for intact and impaired long-term learning and memory in HD patients.[56]

TEACHING STRATEGIES FOR THE ELDERLY

Life is an educational process. Some education occurs in formal settings, such as schools, but most learning occurs informally through everyday experiences. It has been shown that adults of all ages benefit from education and that formal educational experiences can assist the older adult to prepare for career changes and retirement. Learning environments are also useful in compensating for deficits in sensory input, memory, and physical changes that may occur with aging.

Though the research previously reviewed indicates that older adults may have more difficulty in the acquisition or encoding of information and in retrieving stored information, these age differences have been found to be quite minimal. Clearly, adults of all ages, in the absence of pathology, have no difficulty in learning.[100] Most of the studies on memory training involve encoding of information into long-term store and focus on training older learners in encoding strategies. Older adult learners do not automatically employ encoding strategies,[101] although when instructed in their use, elderly learners utilize these techniques effectively.

Face-name recall (i.e., remembering people's names) is one of the most common memory problems. Yesavage,[102] in a series of studies, examined the effectiveness of imagery in name-face recall. Elderly subjects were taught to form associations using visual imagery,[102,103] and those subjects who learned this technique were found to have significantly improved face-name recall. In a subsequent study, pretraining in muscle relaxation techniques reduced performance anxiety and significantly improved learning in the same subjects using imagery.[103] These imagery studies used elderly subjects living in the community, which raises the question, "Can similar procedures in memory training be used to improve functioning of elderly individuals with dementia?" So far, the evidence is not very encouraging. In a study examining the effectiveness of visual imagery training among subjects with cognitive declines, subjects improved somewhat in tests given immediately following the training, however, there was no latency or long-term retention and these improvements were not maintained.[104] However, with intensive memory training in subjects with retrograde and anterograde amnesia and head injury patients, Wilson and Moffat[105] found some improvement in both immediate and latent recall.

It appears that memory performance of healthy elderly people can be improved through memory training.[62] Whether this improvement is maintained over time has not been well documented. It is also not evident that elderly spontaneously employ these training strategies in everyday situations. Rehearsal of encoding strategies is effective in keeping information in short-term memory, but for encoding information into long-term memory, organizational strategies, mnemonics, and imagery are more useful. Likewise, in prospective memory (i.e., remembering an appointment), using of time monitoring strategies, like calendars or timing devices, have been shown to be particularly effective. Most of the research on memory focuses on the use of internal memory aids (encoding strategies). As most people, young or old, generally use external aids, such as making lists, it would be helpful for future research to examine external strategies for improving memory in the elderly.[106–109]

The elderly do just as well as younger people on recognition tasks but have more difficulty with verbatim recall.[61] They are adept at retaining the gist of a text but have difficulty remembering the details. These findings are important when developing a means of assessing learning in the elderly. For example, multiple-choice or true/false items may be more effective procedures, since both involve recognition memory. Short answer or fill-in-the-blank questions, on the other hand, would be difficult because they require recall of specific information. Providing sufficient time for recall is also important.[108]

When teaching the elderly, it must be kept in mind that there may be some loss of vision or hearing. Compensation for these losses could facilitate processing of the information. Aids, such as larger print, avoidance of rapid speaking, seating the hearing impaired near the speaker to facilitate lip reading, and repetition of the main points, are helpful in assisting the elderly in learning tasks and retaining information. The capacity to pay attention may decline with age,[108] and repetition ensures the learners can grasp a point even if they were inattentive when it was first presented.

Many principles of learning amplify the information-processing model of learning: people learn best in pleasant surroundings; they are most likely to repeat activities which they experience as pleasant; overlearning allows task performance to be accomplished automatically; and people are most likely to remember those tasks in which they have been actively involved (i.e., "doing" influences the depth of encoding and storage). In addition, if an individual "forgets" something they once knew, they relearn it faster than if they'd never learned it before.[10]

TEACHING IN THE THERAPEUTIC SETTING

In the process of implementing treatment, allied health professionals consistently function in the role of "teacher." It is important for them to be knowledgeable not only about the content of the information they are conveying, but even more importantly, about the capability of the elderly individual for learning. Therapists must understand the developmental changes that occur in older persons that ultimately affect their learning capabilities, and adapt instructional sessions to enhance the learning process.

Documented changes in sensory function can limit or distort reception, perception, monitoring, feedback, and transmission of incoming stimuli. A general slowing of neural processes seems to occur with age as demonstrated by decreased conduction over multisynaptic pathways.[110] There is also progressive age-related changes in response to cutaneous, proprioceptive, vestibular and other stimuli.[110] There are reported visual declines in acuity, accommodation, field luminance factors, color sensitivity, perception of ambiguous figures and illusions, figural aftereffects, serial learning, figure ground organization, closure, spatial abilities, and visual memory.[111] Some of these variables have been considered in the IQ and memory research reviewed, though not comprehensibly in any one study. If all of these factors are not considered, then these sensory variables may be confounding with cognitive variables.

Aging changes also occur in the outer ear, the inner ear, and central auditory processing that are reflected in a decreased ability to inhibit background noise and other irrelevant signals, and which decrease auditory acuity and perception of high-frequency sounds. The older person's ability to hear and understand speech in less than ideal listening environments is particularly affected.[112] Attentional deficits further compromise the accuracy of input and registration of stimuli. Inaccuracies in the first stage of learning (input and registration) affect the subsequent stages of information processing. Stimuli which is not adequately registered cannot be effectively encoded (stored) or retrieved.

A marked slowing in learning ability in the elderly is reported whether a simple motor movement or a complex cognitive process is involved. Older adults benefit from having longer periods of time for inspection and response. Self-paced learning leads to the best performance.[113] The elderly tend to make more errors of omission than errors of commission.[114] Concrete information is learned more accurately and efficiently than abstract information,[115] and concept learning is also better when information is conveyed in concrete (as opposed to abstract) language.[114] When the opportunity to practice psychomotor tasks is given, learning and performance improve, regardless of the difficulty of the task.[116] When unlimited numbers of trials are given for the mastery of a task, the elderly can recall information as effectively as younger persons; however, more trials are required by elderly, to attain this goal.[114] Elderly who are given verbal feedback concerning their performance improve significantly on subsequent related problems. As a general rule, they perform best when instructions are given in a supportive manner.[114] These factors that influence older adult information aquisition should be considered if learning is to be accomplished in the therapeutic setting.

In considering age-related changes in learning, it becomes clear that health care professionals who interact with the elderly must be particularly sensitive to learner needs and diligent in structuring teaching settings to maximize and individualize learning. For example, some people are auditory learners, and some are visual learners, while others need kinesthetic input and learn by doing. Some tasks are better taught by demonstration and some by verbal instruction.

The learning environment determines and influences the educational experience. An environment that is conducive to learning promotes the process, and as a general rule, an environment that is familiar to the learner is the preferred environment for learning new skills. Familiar settings induce a sense of security in which pertinent new information can be attended to. Learning in the natural environment (i.e., the home or work environment) eliminates the need for the client to transfer or generalize information to a home or work setting. In unfamiliar settings, the learner is more likely to be attracted by, and responsive to, novel environmental stimuli. When unfamiliar treatment environments must be used, they should be structured to simulate the natural environment whenever possible and to diminish the number of competing stimuli. Once a new skill is learned, practice in a variety of environments will assist in generalizing its use.

Environments and procedures that are orderly and organized enhance the learner's ability to process information in an orderly and organized fashion. A cluttered or busy environment creates irrelevant, distracting stimuli in the learning environment and impedes the learning process.

Physical and psychological comfort are also important to consider in the treatment setting. Noise levels, color schemes, adequate lighting, ventilation, and comfortable room temperature should all be considered. Glossy, highly waxed floors and work surfaces that distort and reflect light should be avoided. Comfortable chairs and proper table heights are also recommended. Background noises (e.g., computers, air conditioners, running water, and other appliances) should be eliminated so they don't interfere with foreground sound perception. Most kitchen and bathroom settings compromise hearing; the lack of carpeting, drapes, and padded furniture impose additional noise and reverberating sounds.

The persona of the therapist is also an important source of psychological comfort for the elderly learner. A calm, patient, unhurried, interested, knowledgeable and assured health care provider can decrease situational stress and promote a climate of acceptance and reassurance. Conveying verbally and nonverbally that the elderly individual is a valued person with valuable ideas to contribute and that experimentation and failure are important processes in learning new skills enhances the environment. Positive reinforcement for good efforts, as well as good performance, is crucial in facilitating the learning process in an elderly person.

Teaching methods and techniques in the therapeutic setting include all those behaviors employed by instructors to communicate particular pieces of information to the learners.[114] Variables that influence learning include: the organization of material, the rate of presentation, the choice of task, the mode of presentation and covert strategies.[108]

Organization of Information

New information needs to be presented in a highly organized fashion. Visual displays should be simple configurations that explicitly demonstrate a few salient points. Verbal instructions and directions must emphasize the most important information in a simple manner. Written instructions need to be clearly written in large print with section headings and with emphasis on the major points. Only information relevant to the task at hand should be presented. Differences and similarities between new and old tasks need to be identified. Whole-part-whole learning is a recommended strategy with the elderly. With this technique the entire task and anticipated goal are introduced, then the parts are identified, and each is related to the preceding steps and to the whole. For instance, the person whose end goal is independent meal preparation has to accomplish many component steps in the process of reaching that goal. The individual will have to understand the importance of each step (e.g., mobilizing joints and strengthening particular muscle groups or increasing fine motor coordination and endurance) and how each step relates to the end objective.

Rate of Presentation

Information should be presented at a rate compatible with the learner's ability to comprehend and respond. Generally, this rate will correspond with the complexity of concepts and tasks being taught. Simple, concrete tasks require less time to learn. When instructing the elderly, directions should be presented slowly and ample time for practice provided. If fatigue or confusion occur, the instructional sessions should be kept shorter.

Task Choice

It is important that the choice of task be directed toward attainment of a pre-established, desirable goal. The task should allow the learner to express and fulfill their own personal needs (e.g., creativity, socialization, mastery). Tasks that interest the learner should be selected, if possible. A preliminary development of an interest inventory will identify what is important to the individual learner. In other words, activities chosen need to be relevant and meaningful to the learner, and the purpose for learning each task needs to be clear. Self-care tasks seem to have the greatest relevance for most elderly individuals. Goals, such as transfer training, eating, and dressing, are concrete and usually experienced as meaningful. Practice of self-care tasks in a familiar environment is best for obtaining follow through of the learned tasks. Activities, such as mat exercises or fine hand coordination exercises may not seem relevant to the older learner. In these cases, it is important to relate the activities to the established treatment goals. Explain and demonstrate the mobility and strengthening components of mat activities as they relate to functional goals. This will help in making the activities more concrete and necessary for accomplishing the end goal.

Tasks should be sufficiently challenging but easy enough to assure successful experiences. Building on past successes will promote advancing toward the treatment goals. A knowledgeable, enthusiastic therapist can help to motivate learners to engage in the necessary tasks to be learned.

Presentation of Information

Instructions for the older learner should to be concrete, simple, clear, and one step at a time. The learner should be given the opportunity to practice each step before subsequent steps are introduced. Demonstrations, which are carefully planned, are also helpful modes of education. With a good demonstration, the learner is given the opportunity to initiate the exact movement until each step has been completed. It is also advised that demonstrations be done in the same position as the learner will be doing the task. For demonstration to be effective in influencing the learner, it requires skillful observation and visual memorization of the teacher's movements, followed by a transfer of the complex visual information to an opposite orientation. This can be frustrating for the older learner.

To accommodate for hearing loss, the instructor needs to be within ten feet of the listener, use a low pitched speaking voice with a moderate volume (shouting distorts sound in the presence of hearing losses), and find a position so that the listener can see the speaker's mouth. Since much information is communicated by facial expression, gestures, and body language, these should be acknowledged as important facilitators for conveying information. Verbal and nonverbal language needs to be congruent, because understanding is enhanced when nonconfusing visual stimuli accompany auditory information.

To compensate for some of the aging changes in vision with aging use a large, bold print on a solid background for printed material. The use of a visual aid, such as a magnifying glass, may be used when large print is not available. Lighting is also important. Too much light can create glare, and too little light will diminish the older learner's ability to see anything.

Motor learning may be enhanced by physically guiding the learner's extremities through the desired patterns of movement. It is preferable for the teacher to stand behind the learner so that the learner can concentrate on the sensation of movement. Movements should be repeated several times without any alteration in the motion. The learner is eventually weaned from guided patterning and asked to perform the movement without the teacher's tactile, proprioceptive, and motoric assistance.

Covert Strategies

Older adults tend not to spontaneously use organized methods or ploys to enhance learning and memory, as previously discussed. They do, however, benefit from instructions in memory strategies. The use of memory strategies is a means of compensating for real or anticipated deficits in memory.

It is important to optimize overall health status by implementing the concept of independence. The more one can do for oneself, the more one is capable of doing independently. The more that is done for an aged individual, the less capable they become of functioning on an optimal independent level and the more likely the progression of a disability. The advancing stages of disabilities increase an individual's vulnerability to illness, emotional stress, and injury. Aged persons' subjective appraisal of their health status influences how they react to their symptoms, how vulnerable they consider themselves, and when they decide they can or cannot accomplish an activity. Often an aged person's self-appraisal of health is a good predictor of the rehabilitation clinician's evaluation of the individual's health and functional status, but such assessments may also differ in many ways. In older persons, perceptions of their health may be determined in large part by their level of psychological well-being and by whether or not they continue in rewarding roles and activities.[117]

As older persons' perception of their health status is an important motivator for their compliance with a rehabilitation program, it is important to discuss this further. One notable study showed that even when age, sex, and health status (as evaluated by physicians) were controlled for, perceived health and mortality from heart disease were strongly related.[118] Those who rated their health as poor were two to three times as likely to die as those who rated their health as excellent. A Canadian longitudinal study of persons over 65 produced similar results.[119] Over three years, the mortality of those who described their health as poor at the beginning of the study was about three times the mortality of those who initially described their health as good, regardless of their actual (or measured) health status.

Despite this awareness among older persons of their actual state of health, the aged are known to fail to report serious symptoms and wait longer than younger persons to seek help. It is with this in mind that rehabilitation professionals need to listen carefully to their aged clients. It appears that, contrary to the popular view that older individuals are somewhat hypochondriacal, the aged generally deserve serious attention when they bring complaints to their caregivers. Their perceived level of health will greatly impact the outcomes of functional goals in the geriatric rehabilitation setting whether it be acute, rehabilitative, home, or chronic care.

Rosillo and Fagel[120] found that improvement in rehabilitation tasks correlated well with patients, own appraisal of their potential for recovery but not very well with others' appraisal. Stoedefalke[121] reports that positive reinforcement (frequent positive feedback) for older persons in rehabilitation greatly improved their performance and feelings of success. This indicates that aged persons can improve in their physical functioning when modifications in therapeutic interventions provide more frequent feedback. Some research indicates that older persons with chronic illness have low initial aspirations with regard to their abilities to perform various tasks.[122] As situations in which they succeeded or failed occurred, their aspirations changed to more closely reflect their abilities. Older persons may have different beliefs about their abilities compared to younger persons.[123] When subjects were given an unsolvable problem, younger subjects ascribed their failure to not trying hard enough, while older subjects ascribed their failure to inability. On subsequent tests, younger individuals tried harder and older subjects gave up. These age differences indicate a variation in the perceived locus-of-control. This holds extreme importance in the rehabilitation potential of an aged person. If the cause of failure is seen as an immutable characteristic by the person, then little effort in the future can be expected.

Aged individuals may have a higher anxiety level in rehabilitation situations because they fear failure or are afraid of looking bad to their family or therapist.[124] Eisdorfer[124] found that if anxiety is high enough, then the behavior is redirected toward reducing the anxiety rather than accomplishing the task. Weinberg[125] found that subjects set their own goals for task achievement even if they are directed to adopt the therapist's goals. In another study, Mento, Steel, and Karren[126] reported that the best performance at difficult tasks (as many rehabilitation tasks are) occurs when the aged person sets a very specific goal, such as walking ten feet with a walker. If the person simply tries to do better, then performance is not improved as much.

Depression also plays a big role in learning and memory. King and associates[58] compared the verbal learning and memory of elderly patients with major depression and nondepressed control participants. Except for verbal retention, the depressive group had deficits in most aspects of performance, including cued and uncued recall and delayed recognition memory. As well, there were interactions between depression effects and age effects on some measures such that depressives' performance declined more rapidly with age than did the performance of controls. The results indicate that the integrity of learning and memory are compromised in the presence of late-life depression. Depression of an elderly individual in a rehabilitation setting needs to be addressed as a part of a comprehensive therapeutic intervention. Failure to do so will result in poor learning capabilities for new activities, and failure at a task could further exacerbate the depression.

These are important motivational components to keep in mind when working with an aged client, because the therapeutic approach of the clinician may have the greatest impact on the successful functional outcomes in a geriatric rehabilitation setting.

CONCLUSION

The process of aging may inexorably bring with it changes that interfere with learning, especially in the presence of pathology. An elderly individual's competence may decline, and environmental influences may also be a prominent impediment to learning. Therefore, if the elderly are to gain maximum benefit from therapeutic interactions which are educational in nature, therapists must give much thought and attention to learning style, sensory changes, the environments in which they teach older adults, as well as to the methods they rely upon to convey information.

PEARLS

- Learning is defined as the acquisition of a new skill or information through practice and experience, whereas remembering is the retrieval of information that has been stored in memory.
- Encoding and retrieval problems are the cause of memory difficulties in older adults, and instruction in organizing, slower pacing, and verbal and visual associations can improve performance.
- Sensory and short-term stores of memory are limited in capacity, whereas long-term stores have unlimited storage capacity.
- Problem-solving ability appears to decline with age and may be due to education level and fluid intelligence. Training can improve older patients, problem-solving abilities, however, they may not transfer these strategies to problems encountered in real life.
- Memory performance of healthy elderly can be improved through memory training.
- Orderly environments enhance an older person's ability to process information, whereas, a cluttered, busy environment creates distracting stimuli and impedes learning.
- Variables that positively influence learning for the older person are:
    - A supportive approach by the therapist with much positive reinforcement.
    - Highly organized presentation of material. Simple, concrete, step-by-step information presentation.
    - Appropriate rate of presentation of information.
    - Choosing meaningful tasks.
    - Use of memory strategies.
    - Ample time for repetition and practice.
- An elderly person's perception of their health status will impact the progress they make in rehabilitation.

- Depression, anxiety, and motivation will influence learning and memory abilities.
- One is never too old to learn.

REFERENCES

1. Zauszniewski JA, Martin MH. Developmental task achievement and learned resourcefulness in healthy older adults. *Arch Psychiatr Nurs.* 1999; 13(1): 41–47.
2. Vakil E, Agmon-Ashkenazi D. Baseline performance and learning rate of procedural and declarative memory tasks: younger versus older adults. *J Gerontol B Psychol Sci Soc Sci.* 1997; 52(5): P229–234.
3. Norman GR. The adult learner: a mythical species. *Acad Med.* 1999; 74(8):886–889.
4. Woodruff-Pak DS, Finkbiner RG. Larger nondeclarative than declarative deficits in learning and memory in human aging. *Psychol Aging.* 1995; 10(3):416–426.
5. Karni A, Meyer G, Jezzard P, Adams MM, Turner R, Ungerleider LG. Functional MRI evidence for adult motor cortex plasticity during motor skill learning. *Nature.* 1995; 377(6545):155–158.
6. D'Eredita MA, Hoyer WJ. An examination of the effects of adult age on explicit and implicit learning of figural sequences. *Mem Cognit.* 1999; 27(5): 890–895.
7. Gardner DL, Greenwell SC, Costich JF. Effective teaching of the older adult. *Top Geriatric Rehabil.* 1991; 6(3):1–14.
8. Hodgson C, Ellis AW. Last in, first to go: age acquisition and naming in the elderly. *Brain Lang.* 1998; 64(1):146–163.
9. Rubin DC, Rahhal TA, Poon LW. Things learned in early adulthood are remembered best. *Mem Cognit.* 1998; 26(1):3–19.
10. Merriam SB, Cafferella RS. *Learning in Adulthood.* San Francisco, CA: Jossey-Bass; 1991.
11. Arenberg D and Robertson-Tchabo EA. Learning and aging. In: Birren JE, Schaie KW, eds. *Handbook of the Psychology of Aging.* New York, NY: Van Nostrand Reinhold; 1977.
12. Canestrari RE. Age changes in acquisition. In: Talland, GA, ed. *Human Aging and Behavior.* New York, NY: Academic Press; 1968.
13. Salthouse TA. Aging associations: influence of speed on adult age differences in associative learning. *J Exp Psychol Learn Mem Cogn.* 1994; 20(6): 1486–1503.
14. Taub HA. Paired associates learning as a function of age, rate and instructions. *J of Genetic Psych.* 1967; 111:41–46.
15. Leech S and Witte KL. Paired-associate learning in elderly adults as related to pacing and incentive conditions. *Dev Psych.* 1971; 5:174–180.
16. Eisendorfer D, Nowlin J, Wilkie F. Improvement of learning in the aged by modification of autonomic nervous system activity. *Science.* 1970; 170: 1327–1329.
17. Botwinick J and Storandt M. *Memory, Related Functions and Age.* Springfield, IL: Charles C. Thomas; 1974.
18. Spitzer M, Bellemann ME, Kammer T, et al. Functional MR imaging of semantic information processing and learning-related effects using psychometrically controlled stimulation paradigms. *Brain Res Cogn Brain Res.* 1996; 4(3):149–161.
19. Reber PJ, Stark CE, Squire LR. Cortical areas supporting category learning identified using functional MRI. *Proc Natl Acad Sci USA.* 1998; 95(2): 747–750.
20. Fattapposta F, Amabile G, Cordischi MV, et al. Long-term practice effects on a new skilled motor learning: an electro physiological study. *Electroencephalogr Clin Neurophysiol.* 1996; 99(6): 495–507.
21. Naveh-Benjamin M, Craik FI. Memory for context and its use in item memory: comparisons of younger and older persons. *Psychol Aging.* 1995; 10(2):284–293.
22. Spencer WD, Raz N. Memory for facts, source, and context: can frontal lobe dysfunction explain age-related differences? *Psychol Aging.* 1994; 9(1): 149–159.
23. Spencer WD, Raz N. Differential effects of aging on memory for content and context: a meta-analysis. *Psychol Aging.* 1995; 10(4):527–539.
24. Sekiya H, Magill RA, Sidaway B, Anderson DI. The contextual interference effect for skill variations from the same and different generalized motor programs. *Res Q Exerc Sport.* 1994; 65(4):330–338.
25. Lee YS. Effects of learning contexts on implicit and explicit learning. *Mem Cognit.* 1995; 23(6): 723–734.
26. Bernasconi J, Gustafson K. Contextual quick-learning and generalization by humans and machines. *Network.* 1998; 9(1):85–106.
27. Koutstaal W, Schacter DL, Johnson MK, Gallucio L. Facilitation and impairment of event memory produced by photographic review in younger and older adults. *Mem Cognit.* 1999; 27(3):478–493.
28. Fisher J and Pierce RC. Dimensions of intellectual functioning in the aged. *J Gerontol.* 1967; 22: 166–173.
29. Botwinick J. *Cognitive Processes in Maturity and Old Age.* New York: Springer; 1967.
30. Ryan EB. Beliefs about memory changes across the adult life span. *J Gerontol.* 1992; 47:1:41–47.
31. Cameron DE. Ribonucleic acid in psychiatric therapy. In: Masserman JH, ed. *Current Psychiatric Therapies.* New York: Grune and Stratton; 1964.
32. Craik FIM, Byrd, M. Aging and cognitive deficits: The role of attentional resources. In: Craik FIM and Trehub S, eds. *Aging and Cognitive Processes.* New York: Plenum; 1982.
33. Hoyer WJ, Plude DJ. Attentional and perceptual processes in the study of cognitive aging. In: Poon L, ed. *Aging in the 1980's.* Washington, DC: American Psychological Association; 1980.
34. Atkinson JW, Shiffen RM. Human memory: A proposed system and its control processes. In: Spence

KW, Spence JT, eds. *The Psychology of Learning and Motivation.* Vol. 2. New York: Academic Press; 1968:2.

35. Poon L. Differences in human memory with aging: Nature, causes, and clinical implications. In: Birren JE, Schaie KW, eds. *Handbook of the Psychology of Aging.* 2nd ed. New York: Van Nostrand Reinhold; 1985.

36. Craik FIM, Rabinowitz JC. Age differences in the acquisition and use of verbal information. In: Long J, Baddeley A, eds. *Attention and Performance.* Hillsdale, NJ: Erlbaum. 1984.

37. Bryan J, Luszcz MA. Speed of information processing as a mediator between age and free-recall performance. *Psychol Aging.* 1996; 11(1)3–9.

38. Kausler DH. *Experimental Psychology and Human Aging.* New York: Wiley; 1982.

39. Denney NW. Classification abilities of the elderly. *J Gerontol.* 1974a; 29:309–314.

40. Schmitt FA, Murphy MD, Sanders RE. Training older adult free recall rehearsal strategies. *J Gerontol.* 1981; 36:329–337.

41. Ackerman PL, Rolfhus EF. The locus of adult intelligence: knowledge, abilities, and nonability traits. *Psychol Aging.* 1999; 14(2):314–330.

42. Hultsch D. Adult age differences in free classification and free recall. *Dev Psych.* 1971; 4:338–342.

43. Hartley JT, Harker JO, Walsh DA. Contemporary issues and new directions in adult development of learning and memory. In: Poon L, ed. *Aging in the 1980's.* Washington, DC: American Psychological Association; 1980.

44. Rabinowitz JC, Craik FIM, Ackerman BP. A processing resource account of age differences in recall. *Canadian J Psych.* 1982; 36:325–344.

45. Robertson-Tchabo EA, Hausman CP, Arenberg DA. A classic mnemonic for old learners: A trip that works. *Ed Gerontol.* 1976; 1:215–226.

46. Craik FIM, Lockhart RS. Levels of processing: A framework for memory research. *J Verbal Learning and Verbal Behavior.* 1972; 11:671–684.

47. Treat N, Reese H. Age, imagery, and pacing in paired associate learning. *Dev Psych.* 1976; 12: 119–124.

48. Shiffrin RM, Schneider W. Controlled and automatic human information processing: II. Perceptual learning, automatic attending and a general theory. *Psych Rev.* 1977; 84:127–190.

49. Crowder RG. Echoic memory and the study of aging memory systems. In: Poon LW, Fozard JL, Cermak LS, Arenberg D, Thompson LW, eds. *New Directions in Memory and Aging: Proceedings of the George A Talland Memorial Conference.* Hillsdale, NJ: Erlbaum; 1980.

50. Cerella J, Poon L, Fozard J. Age and iconic readout. *J Gerontol.* 1982; 37:197–202.

51. Fozard JL. A time for remembering. In: Poon L, ed. *Aging in the 1980's.* Washington, DC: American Psychological Association; 1980.

52. Poon L, Fozard J. Speed of retrieval from long-term memory in relation to age, familiarity and datedness of information. *J Gerontol.* 1980; 5:711–717.

53. Gomez-Beldarrain M, Garcia-Monco JC, Rubio B, Pascual-Leone A. Effect of focal cerebellar lesions on procedural learning in the serial reaction time task. *Exp Brain Res.* 1998; 120(1):25–30.

54. Westwater H, McDowall J, Siegert R, Mossman S, Abernethy D. Implicit learning in Parkinson's disease: evidence from a verbal version of the serial reaction time task. *J Clin Exp Neuropsychol.* 1998; 20(3):413–418.

55. Behrman AL, Cauraugh JH, Light KE. Practice as an intervention to improve speeded motor performance and motor learning in Parkinson's disease. *J Neurol Sci.* 2000; 174(2):127–136.

56. Gabrieli JD, Stebbins GT, Singh J, Willingham DB, Goetz CG. Intact mirror-tracing and impaired rotary-pursuit skill learning in patients with Huntington's disease: evidence for dissociable memory systems in skill learning. *Neuropsychology.* 1997; 11(2):272–281.

57. Oscar-Berman M, Pulaski JL. Association learning and recognition memory in alcoholic Korsakoff patients. *Neuropsychology.* 1997; 11(2): 182–189.

58. King DA, Cox C, Lyness JM, Conwell Y, Caine ED. Quantitative and qualitative differences in verbal learning performance of elderly depressives and healthy controls. *J Int Neuropsychol Soc.* 1998; 4(2):115–126.

59. Schonfield D, Robertson EA. Memory storage and aging. *Canadian J Psych.* 1966; 20:228–236.

60. Smith A. Age differences in encoding, storage, and retrieval. In: Poon LW, Fozard JL, Cermak LS, Arenberg D, Thompson LW, eds. *New Directions in Memory and Aging: Proceedings of the George A Talland Memorial Conference.* Hillsdale, NJ: Erlbaum; 1980.

61. Schaie KW. Cognitive development in aging. In: Obler LK, Alpert M, eds. *Language and Communication in the Elderly.* Lexington, MA: Heath; 1980.

62. McKitrick LA, Friedman LF, Brooks JO 3rd, Pearman A, Kraemer HC, Yesavage JA. Predicting response of older adults to mnemonic training: who will benefit? *Int Psychogeriatr.* 1999; 11(3): 289–300.

63. Bowles NE, Poon, L. An analysis of the effect of aging on memory. *J Gerontol.* 1982; 37:212–219.

64. Cavanaugh J. Effects of presentation format on adult's retention of television programs. *Exp Aging Res.* 1984; 10:51–54.

65. Erber JT. Remote memory and age: A review. *Exp Aging Res.* 1981; 1:189–199.

66. Poon L, Fozard J, Paulshock D, Thomas J. A questionnaire assessment of age differences in retention of recent and remote events. *Exp Aging Res.* 1979; 5:401–411.

67. Brown R, Kulick J. Flashbulb memories. *Cognition.* 1977; 5:73–99.

68. Marsh GR. Introduction to psychopharmacological issues. In: Poon L, ed. *Aging in the 1980's.* Washington, DC: American Psychological Association; 1980.

69. Butler RN, Lewis MI. *Aging and Mental Health.* 3rd ed. St Louis, MO: Mosby; 1982.

70. West RL. Practical memory mnemonics for the aged: Preliminary thoughts. In: Poon L, Rubin D,

Wilson B, eds. *Everyday Cognition and Memory.* Hillsdale, NJ: Erlbaum; 1986.

71. Poon L, Schaffer G. Prospective memory in young and elderly adults. Paper presented at the meeting of the American Psychological Association, Washington, DC; August, 1982.

72. Hultsch D, Dixon R. Memory for text materials in adulthood. In: Baltes PB, Brim OG, eds. *Life-Span Development and Behavior.* New York: Academic Press; 1984;6.

73. Labouvie-Vief G, Schnell D. Learning and memory in later life. In: Wolman BB, ed. *Handbook of Developmental Psychology.* Englewood Cliffs, NJ: Prentice-Hall; 1982.

74. Cavanaugh J, Grady J, Permutter M. Forgetting and use of memory aids in 20 to 70 year olds' everyday life. *Int J Aging Hum Dev.* 1983; 17:113–122.

75. Loftus E. Misfortunes of memory. *Philosophical Trans Royal Society London.* 1983; 302:413–421.

76. Loftus E, Fienberg S, Tanur J. Cognitive psychology meets the national survey. *Am Psych.* 1985; 40:175–180.

77. Zarit SH. *Aging and Mental Disorders.* New York: Free Press; 1980.

78. Kahn RL. The mental health system and the future aged. *Gerontologist.* 1975; 15: 24–31.

79. Perlmutter M. What is memory aging the aging of? *Dev Psych.* 1978; 14:330–345.

80. Thompson L. Testing and mnemonic strategies. In: Poon LW, Fozard JL, Cermak LS, Arenberg D, Thompson LW, eds. *New Directions in Memory and Aging: Proceedings of the George A Talland Memorial Conference.* Hillsdale, NJ: Erlbaum; 1980.

81. Reese HW, Rodeheaver D. Problem solving and complex decision making. In: Birren JE, Schaie KW, eds. *Handbook of the Psychology of Aging.* 2nd ed. New York: Van Nostrand Reinhold; 1985.

82. Polya G. *How to Solve It: A New Aspect of Mathematical Method.* 2nd ed. Princeton: Princeton University Press; 1971.

83. Crovitz E. Reversing a learning deficit in the aged. *J Gerontol.* 1966; 21:236–238.

84. Offenbach SI. A developmental study of hypothesis testing and cue selection strategies. *Dev Psych.* 1974; 10:484–490.

85. Hartley AA. Adult age differences in deductive reasoning processes. *J Gerontol.* 1981; 36:700–706.

86. Sanders JA, Sterns HL, Smith M, Sanders RE. Modification of concept identification performance in older adults. *Dev Psych.* 1975; 11:824–829.

87. Sanders RE, Sanders JA, Mayes GJ, and Sielski KA. Enhancement of conjunctive concept attainment in older adults. *Dev Psych.* 1976; 12:485–486.

88. Denney NW. Task demands and problem-solving strategies in middle-age and older adults. *J Gerontol.* 1980; 35:559–564.

89. Papalia D, Bielby D. Cognitive functioning in middle and old age adults: A review of research based on Piaget's theory. *Hum Dev.* 1974; 17:424–443.

90. Muhs PJ, Hooper FH, Papalia-Finlay DE. An initial analysis of cognitive functioning across the life-span. *Int J Aging Hum Dev.*1980; 10:311–333.

91. Rubin KH. Decentration skills in institutionalized and noninstitutionalized elderly. Proceedings of 81st Annual Convention, American Psychological Association; 1973; 8(Part 2):759–760.

92. Papalia-Finley DE, Blackburn J, Davis E. Training cognitive functioning in the elderly—Inability to replicate previous findings. *Int J Aging Hum Dev.* 1980; 12:111–117.

93. Willis SL. Towards an educational psychology of the older adult learner: intellectual and cognitive bases. In: Birren JE, Schaie KW, eds. *Handbook of the Psychology of Aging.* 2nd ed. New York: Van Nostrand Reinhold; 1985.

94. Hulicka IM. Age changes and age differences in memory functioning. *Gerontologist.* 1967; 7(2, partII):46–54.

95. Jones HE. Intelligence and problem-solving. In Birren JE, ed. *Handbook of Aging and the Individual.* Chicago: University of Chicago Press; 1959: 700–738.

96. Wolf SL, Barnhart HX, Ellison GL, Coogler CE. The effect of Tai Chi Quan and computerized balance training on postural stability in older subjects. *Phys Ther.* 1997; 77(4):371–384.

97. Wolf SL, Coogler C, Xu T. Exploring the basis for Tai Chi Chuan as a therapeutic exercise approach. *Arch Phys Med Rehabil.* 1997; 79:886–892.

98. Bottomley JM. The use of Tai Chi as a movement modality in orthopaedics. *Ortho Phys Ther Clin No Amer.* 2000; 9(3):361–373.

99. Karni A, Bertini G. Learning perceptual skills: behavioral probes into adult cortical plasticity. *Curr Opin Neurobiol.* 1997; 7(4):530–535.

100. Poon L, Rubin D, Wilson B. *Everyday Cognition and Memory.* Hillsdale, NJ: Erlbaum; 1986.

101. Poon L, Walsh-Sweeney L, Fozard J: Memory skill training for the elderly: Salient issues on the use of imagery mnemonics. In: Poon L, ed. *New Directions in Memory and Aging: Proceedings of the George A Talland Memorial Conference.* Hillsdale, NJ: Erlbaum; 1980.

102. Yesavage JA. Imagery pretraining and memory training in the elderly. *Gerontology.* 1983; 29: 271–275.

103. Yesavage JA, Rose T. The effects of a face-name mnemonic in young, middle aged, and elderly adults. *Exp Aging Res.* 1984; 10:55–57.

104. Zarit SH, Zarit J, Reever K. Memory training or severe memory loss: Effects of senile dementia. *Gerontologist.* 1982; 22:373–377.

105. Wilson B, Moffat N. *Clinical Management of Memory Problems.* Rockville, MD: Aspen. 1984.

106. Chasseigne G, Mullet E, Stewart TR. Aging and multiple cue probability learning: the case of inverse relationships. *Acta Psychol (Amst).* 1997; 97(3):235–252.

107. McGeorge P, Crawford JR, Kelly SW. The relationship between psychometric intelligence and learning in an explicit and an implicit task. *J Exp Psychol Learn Mem Cogn.* 1997; 23(1):239–245.

108. Whitman N. Learning and teaching styles: implications for teachers of family medicine. *Fam Med.* 1996; 28(5):321–325.

109. Wilkniss SM, Jones MG, Korol DL, Gold PE, Manning CA. Age-related differences in an ecologically based study of route learning. *Psychol Aging.* 1997; 12(2):372–375.

110. Kenney RA. *Physiology of Aging.* Chicago: Year Book Medical Publishers, Inc.; 1982.

111. Cristarella MC. Visual functions of the elderly. *Am J Occup Ther.* 1987; 31:432–440.

112. Gladstone VS. Hearing loss in the elderly. *Phys & Occup Ther Geriatr.* 1992; 2:5–20.

113. Feldman HS, Lopez MA. *Developmental Psychology for the Health Care Professions: Adulthood and Aging.* Boulder CO: Westview Press; 1982;2.

114. Okun MA. Implications of geropsychological research for the instruction of older adults. *Adult Education.* 1987; 27:139–155.

115. Rabbitt P. Changes in problem solving ability in old age. In: Birren JE, Schaie KW, eds. *Handbook of the Psychology of Aging.* New York: Van Nostrand Reinhold Co.; 1987; 606–625.

116. Botwinick J. *Aging and Behavior.* 3rd ed. New York: Springer; 1983.

117. Siegler IC, Costa PT Jr. Health behavior relationships. In: Birren JE, Schaie KW, eds. *Handbook of the Psychology of Aging.* 2nd ed. Van Nostrand Reinhold, New York; 1985.

118. Kaplan E. Psychological factors and ischemic heart disease mortality: a focal role for perceived health. Paper presented at the annual meeting of the American Psychological Association, Washington, D.C.; 1982.

119. Mossey JM, Shapiro E. Self-rated health: A predictor of mortality among the elderly. *Am J Pub Health.* 1982; 72:800–808.

120. Rosillo RA, Fagel ML. Correlation of psychologic variables and progress in physical therapy: I. Degree of disability and denial of illness. *Arch Phys Med Rehabil.* 1970; 51:227–232.

121. Stoedefalke KG. Motivating and sustaining the older adult in an exercise program. *Top Geriatr Rehab.* 1985; 1:78–83.

122. Nader IM. Level of aspiration and performance of chronic psychiatric patients on a simple motor task. *Percept Mot Skills.* 1985; 60:767–771.

123. Prohaska T, Pontiam IA, Teitleman J. Age differences in attributions to causality: Implications for intellection assessment. *Exp Aging Res.* 1984; 10:111–117.

124. Eisdorfer L. Arousal and performance: experiments in verbal learning and a tentative theory. In: Talland GA, ed. *Human Aging and Behavior.* Academic Press, New York; 1968.

125. Weinberg R, Bruya L, Jackson A. The effects of goal proximity and goal specificity on endurance performance. *J Soc Psychol.* 1985; 7:296–301.

126. Mento A, Steele RP, Karren RJ. A metaanalytic study of the effects of goal setting on task performance: 1966–1984. *Organ Behav Hum Decis Process.* 1987; 39:52–58.

CHAPTER 19

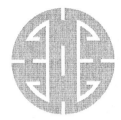

Administration of Geriatric Services

As the role of the geriatric rehabilitation therapist continues to evolve, the development of excellent clinical skills and the ability to interpret research in the literature has become more important to the geriatric therapist. In addition, as the nation's health care system is revised, nursing homes, hospitals, rehabilitation centers, outpatient clinics, and home health agencies will be looking for therapists with good administrative skills to provide administrative advisement and supervision for professional, as well as adjunct staff.

It is imperative, therefore, that rehabilitation therapists become aware of all aspects of administration. A greater understanding of administrative services will facilitate communication not only within the discipline but also with other disciplines.

This chapter has two goals: first, to familiarize therapists with administrative terms and concepts, and second, to serve as a reference for therapists working in a rehabilitation facility or a physical or occupational therapy department.

DESCRIPTION OF ADMINISTRATION

Administration is an extremely complex term. It involves not only paperwork for developing a policy and procedure manual, finance, and budgeting, but also developing guidelines for effectively managing and motivating people. For the purposes of this chapter, administration will be divided into five areas:

1. Finance and budgeting;
2. Policies and procedures;
3. Legal concerns;
4. Employee relations;
5. Marketing.

The needs of administration vary by position. For example, if the therapist is a staff therapist, his or her administrative needs may be minimal. This therapist may be asked to fill out documentation forms, send in billing slips, and play a very limited role in managing employees. On the other hand, if a therapist is in charge of an entire department, he or she may need to develop personnel information, such as employee handbooks, billing procedures, documentation procedures, or finance and budget procedures, as well as equipment use forms and marketing strategies. Therefore, the best approach to acquiring an understanding of administrative needs is to gain an understanding of the information in each of the five major areas listed.

FINANCING AND BUDGETING

Financing and budgeting can be defined as a monetary sketch of the needs and plans of a department in any setting. If a therapist works in an outpatient facility, for example, items that must be budgeted are rental of space, equipment, staff time, and ancillary personnel (such as receptionists or aides), as well as laundry and other line items. Based on the number of patients that will be seen, the income, and the costs, the therapist must establish a workable formula for the amount of money dispersed versus the amount of incoming money.

A realistic budget is essential to the financial well-being of a physical or occupational therapy business. No matter how effective the treatment and how dedicated the staff, the hard reality is that if income does not exceed expenditures, the business will fail. Descriptions of the nuances of finance and budget can be gleaned from any elementary course in business, but the difficult part is applying the practices to an actual business.

Figure 19–1 is a notational example of a budget for a medium-sized (gross annual income between $500,000 and $1,000,000), physical therapy business, adapting data from an actual practice in a large metropolitan area. While the specifics are dependent on a wide range of variables, the rough order of magnitude of the percentages spent on various services should be a useful guide.

Figure 19–1 illustrates several points. First and foremost, a profit *must* be made to ensure the long-term viability of the practice. Next, the income comes from services delivered, and expenses should only be made for those items that contribute to earning that income. Finally, there are controllable and noncontrollable expenses. Time and effort should be spent on the controllable expenses, such as salary, postage, and so on, without agonizing over those expenses that cannot be controlled (i.e., taxes or repairs).

Budgets should also be living documents. No matter how well planned a budget is, actual income and expenses will vary, and the budget should be modified accordingly during the year.

The financial health of the business should be checked at least once a month. This is a useful time period, since it coincides with the normal cycle of bank statements, as well as payments by insurers and other health care agencies.

In a nursing home setting, therapists who are planning and working in a department will use a similar type of budget and have similar types of concerns. Figures 19–2A and 19–2B give examples of a financial report and budget for a nursing home.

ORGANIZING AND PLANNING FOR PERSONNEL, EQUIPMENT, AND SUPPLIES

Equipment and supplies can be broken up into the equipment and supplies needed by the department versus the equipment and supplies needed for the patient. With respect to departmental equipment, therapists specializing in geriatrics must assess whether or not their equipment will provide a return on investment.

For example, if one were to purchase an expensive piece of exercise equipment, would this in fact provide enough revenue to justify the expense? If for

example, the piece of equipment is $10,000, the therapist must assess in what way this $10,000 will be returned to the facility. If a therapist could put a patient on this piece of equipment for ten minutes, this would free the therapist up to work with another patient. Doing this approximately eight times during the day would free up eighty minutes. Over the course of the year, this amounts to approximately three hundred fifty hours. A piece of equipment that supplies this magnitude of additonal time for a therapist, plus the effects of the machine (i.e., strengthening, motivation, and endurance training) will recoup its cost in one year (an excellent pay back rate).

When writing requests for equipment or in looking for equipment for self-purchase, the therapist should keep in mind these variables: need, advantages, disadvantages, and cost. Therapists, for example, can purchase parallel bars, and these bars provide needed standing support for gait, balance, and posture work. The advantage of parallel bars is that there is a well-documented history of use in the clinical setting. The main disadvantages are that they are expensive and space-consuming. Access to a sturdy railing might be an alternative. In this type of setting, the railing also can be used for gait training.

A department can be sparse, with hooks on the wall for attachment of exercise bands to be used in progressive resistance exercises, or it can be more high technology, with isokinetic equipment and high-tech balance machines. However, this level of sophistication is not always necessary. Table 19–1 presents a listing of the minimum equipment necessary for a nursing home, as well as a more comprehensive listing for a high-tech facility.

Another important category of equipment and supplies is durable medical equipment. To administer efficiently what a facility needs of this type of equipment, therapists must develop policies and procedures to monitor rental, purchase, and resale of the equipment. Therapists in the administrative capacity must develop procedures for purchase or rental of equipment for patient use based on the type of equipment that the patient needs.

Table 19–2 provides a sample of procedural record dispersement of medical supplies in a nursing home facility. This policy and procedure can be modified slightly to be used in an outpatient and hospital setting as well.

DEVELOPING GOALS, PHILOSOPHY, AND ORGANIZATIONAL PLANS

Before developing an outpatient or nursing home department, therapists should carefully review their expected goals and plan accordingly. What is the mission statement of the department? In other words, what are the goals and what kind of plan is one going to use to attain these goals in this setting? In an existing setting, the organizational goals and plans should

Sample Budget for a Medium Sized
Outpatient Physical Therapy Practice.

INCOME

Fees & Services	$745,000
Sales - Equipment	5,000
Total Income	$750,000

EXPENSES

Direct Expenses

Salaries: Owners/officers	$200,000
Salaries: Other employees	230,000
Medical supplies	30,000
Payroll taxes	30,000
Total Direct Expenses	490,000
Gross Profit (Loss)	260,000

Operating Expenses

Accounting	9,000
Advertising	2,000
Annual Report	100
Bank service charges	100
Business meals	4,000
Cleaning	1,000
Contributions	2,000
Data processing	1,000
State income tax (@10%)	5,000
Credit card discount	4,000
Delivery expenses	400
Depreciation	15,000
Dues and subscriptions	1,000
Entertainment	3,000
Education and seminars	2,000
Gifts	2,000
Insurance	24,000
Interest expenses	1,000
Legal fees	4,000
Licenses and permits	500
Miscellaneous expenses	1,200
Office expenses	3,000
Office supplies	6,000
Parking	2,000
Postage	3,000
Printing and stationery	5,000
Publications and books	1,000
Rent	84,000
Repairs and maintenance	2,000
Taxes, personal property	1,500
Tax, sales	200
Telephone	7,000
Travel	5,000
Temporary Help	5,000
Utilities	3,000
Total Operating Expenses	210,000
Income before taxes	50,000
Federal income tax	7,500
NET INCOME	**$42,500**

Figure 19–1. Sample Budget for Medium Sized Outpatient Practice.

Sample SNF Rehab Budget: Small Unit

	Physical Therapy	Occupational Therapy	Speech Therapy	Total Therapy
Charges	157,000	154,000	28,000	339,000
Expenses	84,000	88,000	14,000	186,000
Overhead	71,000	52,000	8,000	131,000
Gross Margin	2,000	14,000	6,000	22,000
Nonbillable	3,000	2,000	2,000	7,000
Adjust to Cost	2,000	14,000	6,000	22,000
Net Loss	(3,000)	(2,000)	(2,000)	(7,000)

ASSUMPTIONS/NOTES

1. 134 bed facility

2. Medicare average daily census = 7.5 beds or 5.7% of total census

3. Therapy unit staffing

	FTEs
Physical therapist	1.00
Physical therapy aide	1.00
Occupational therapist	1.00
Certified occupational therapy assistant	1.00
Speech language pathologist	0.25
Director of rehab (MD)	0.05

4. Square footage

	SQ. FEET
Physical therapy	644
Occupational therapy	50
Speech therapy	0
Total facility	23,677

5. Facility general & administrative expenses = $490,000/year

6. Rehab services payor mix:

	Mix (%)
Medicare - Part A	60
Medicare - Part B	37
Private/other	2
Welfare	1

7. Loss is due to nonbillable services to welfare patients and services under all-inclusive insurance contracts (where services are covered in the per-diem rate).

Figure 19–2A. Sample SNF Rehabilitation Budget: Small Unit. (*Reprinted with permission from Kurtz H. Medical and Rehabilitation Specialists.*)

Sample SNF Rehab Budget: Large Unit

	Physical Therapy	Occupational Therapy	Speech Therapy	Total Therapy
Charges	802,000	268,000	258,000	1,328,000
Expenses	490,000	102,000	66,000	658,000
Overhead	254,000	58,000	32,000	344,000
Gross Margin	58,000	108,000	160,000	326,000
Nonbillable	45,000	50,000	46,000	141,000
Adjust to Cost	55,000	87,000	181,000	273,000
Net Loss	(42,000)	(29,000)	(17,000)	(88,000)

ASSUMPTIONS/NOTES

1. 118 bed facility

2. Medicare average daily census = 15.5 beds or 14% of total census

3. Therapy unit staffing

	FTEs
Physical therapist	5.75
Physical therapist assistant	4.00
Physical therapy aide	1.16
Occupational therapist	2.16
Certified occupational therapy assistant	1.00
Occupational therapy assistant	1.00
Speech language pathologist	1.58
Director of rehab (MD)	0.25

4. Square footage

	SQ. FEET
Physical therapy	2,071
Occupational therapy	496
Speech therapy	134
Total facility	32,584

5. Facility general & administrative expenses = $480,000/year

6. Rehab services payor mix:

	Mix (%)
Medicare - Part A	81
Medicare - Part B	8
Private/other	11
Welfare	0

7. Loss is due to nonbillable services to welfare patients and services under all-inclusive insurance contracts (where services are covered in the per-diem rate).

Figure 19–2B. Sample SNF Rehabilitation Budget: Large Unit. (*Reprinted with permission from Kurtz H, Medical and Rehabilitation Specialists.*)

TABLE 19–1. MINIMUM AND MAXIMUM EQUIPMENT LISTS FOR PT DEPARTMENTS

Basic Equipment Needs	Maximum Equipment Needs
Exercise mat	List A plus
Treatment table (plinth)	Cybex
Mirror(s)	Kinetron
Stairs	UBE
Complete set cuff weights: 1/2 to 10 lbs	Fitron
Parallel bars or sturdy railings	Balance Master
Restorator or bike	KAT
Hot pack (Hydrocollator)	Tekdyne
Wall pulleys	Pro-Stretch
Assortment of ambulation aids: Walkers, pick-up, 2 wheel, 4 wheel canes, single point, quad, hemicrutches	Complete Theraband Line Zelex
Swiss ball	Hip Machine Fitter

Additional Recommended Equipment
Multi-mode electrical stimulator
Ultrasound
Tilt table
Whirlpool

be reviewed periodically to see that they correspond to the current structure of the practice.

Organizational Goals

Reviewing an organization's goals and objectives will provide the therapist with an idea of the direction in which the practice is or should be moving. Is the practice providing standard care to a small community, moving toward high-quality care in the current area, or expanding into a larger area, or both? Therapists must determine if these goals agree with their own goals for the future. Does the therapist want to stay in a small practice, working a regular schedule, and doing the best possible job with available re-

TABLE 19–2. SAMPLE POLICY AND PROCEDURE FOR EQUIPMENT PURCHASE/RENTAL

Short-term rental may be appropriate if there is an occasional need for equipment. If the facility routinely uses the equipment on patients, it would be considered part of the departmental costs and would not be billable as medical supply. All equipment must be ordered by the patient's physician and billed under Part A Medicare Claims.

Examples of billable rental equipment:
1. CPM (constant passive motion machines: Used for total joint replacements.
2. Reclining wheelchairs: Used for patients allowed only minimal hip flexion.
3. Transcutaneous Electrical Neuro Stimulation units.
4. Bucks traction unit for lower extremity fractures.

sources? Or is the therapist trying to expand the practice, get involved in a larger company, or both? In trying to focus on these issues, it is important to clarify the individual therapist's goals as they relate to the organizational goals of the practice.

Table 19–3 provides a sample mission statement and philosophy statement. Therapists in a supervisory role should use the type of guidelines suggested in Table 19–3 to develop their own personal philosophy, taking into consideration not only current goals but expected goals for the next five to ten years.

Organizational Plan

The organizational plan is a visual chart of the administrative hierarchy of the department, facility, or entire company. It is a charting of the various employees' positions in relation to others (Fig. 19–3). This can be done on a small scale (e.g., a one-to-two person department) or on a larger scale (e.g., a company of 1,000).

This can be very useful for getting an idea of how a company's hierarchy operates, how a person fits into the practice, or how a setting will change if a new person is hired. For example, an administrator can simply add the new employee to the chart in various places to see how it affects the chain of command.

TABLE 19–3. SAMPLE MISSION STATEMENT AND PHILOSOPHY STATEMENT

Mission Statement

Our mission is to provide the highest quality rehabilitation services that:
• Meet and maximize each resident's individual needs.
• Promote the quality of life of each resident entrusted to our care.
• Use highly trained rehabilitation professionals.
• Integrate an interdisciplinary approach toward the rehabilitative potential of each resident.

Philosophy of Resident Care
• Our goal in rehabilitation services is to provide the highest quality of service to each individual resident who needs assistance in returning to his or her maximal functional abilities.
• The rehabilitation therapist at the facility plays a vital role in the operation of the skilled nursing facility, not only by being involved with the residents currently receiving therapy, but also by providing input for all residents in the facility through staff education and consultation, attendance at key meetings within the facility, routine therapy programs, and involvement in RNA programs.
• Each resident has some potential for rehabilitation, however small. It is the responsibility of the health care team to evaluate the medical, physical, and psychosocial needs of each resident. From this assessment, a health care plan is designed that encourages maximum functional independence and above all promotes the well-being and quality of life of each resident.

Reprinted with permission for Therapy Management Innovations, Inc.

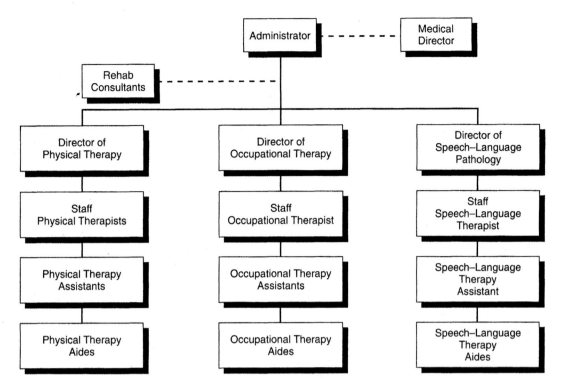

Figure 19–3. Sample Organizational Chart. *(Reprinted with permission from Therapy Management Innovations, Inc.)*

LEGAL CONSTRAINTS

Legal ramifications are extremely important for therapists in both administrative and practicing capacities. Therapists must be certain that they have taken adequate measures to provide an optimal and legally safe environment for their patients.

A major concern of therapists is being sued for malpractice or negligence. The remainder of this section provides information to assist in understanding the legal climate and prepares the geriatric therapist for some common scenarios that may occur.

The malpractice scenario is as follows: the plaintiff, who is the person suing, tries to provide evidence that, through a failure to meet accepted standards, a patient has been injured. The defendant, or the person being sued, tries to show that quality care was given. Therefore, it is imperative that the therapist constantly complies with regulations and safety practices. The safety practices of the clinic should be outlined in the policy and procedure manual, and the therapist must constantly document that safety measures are in place. Legal documentation, separate from the documentation used for the purposes of reimbursement, is therefore essential.

When sued, a health professional must be able to show that they provided care equal to or exceeded by the national, as well as the local, standard. If called to appear in court, local practitioners who can attest to local practices, or national experts who can testify on the differences between local and national standards, may be useful.

If a patient receives minimal or nonspecific harm because of treatment, a suit would be improper. Therapists can only be sued because actual harm resulted from treatment. For example, if a patient states that the therapist did not diagnose a particular problem, but the therapist did not prevent the patient from obtaining an adequate diagnosis, there is no fault. However, if, because of an inadequately maintained piece of equipment, a patient is injured, the therapist is at fault.

Additionally, liability for injury must be based on proximate cause. That is, the therapist's wrongful conduct must have actually caused the problem. For example, if the therapist walks the patient through a puddle of water, and the patient slips and falls, injuring the coccyx, that is considered proximate cause and the therapist may be sued for unsafe practice and negligence.

For the therapist in a supervisory capacity, as well as in a clinical capacity, it is advisable to use a systematic approach in writing notes, to ensure the therapist is legally covered.[1,2] The best system for this is the FACT System,[3] which stands for factual, accurate, complete, and timely. The FACT System states that therapists should write down factual comments, what they see, hear, smell, and feel, not what they suppose or assume. They should be accurate: Never document for someone else and never ask other therapists to document for you. Be complete. Do not leave any blank spaces, because the attorney will allude to the possibility that space was left to be filled in at a later date.

Finally, be timely. Try to write your notes on time. If a late entry is necessary, do not write it in the margins; note that it was a late entry. If a late entry follows other entries and it is dated, it will look as though it was filled in after the fact in a methodical fashion. This reflects a better organized chart compared to squeezing notes in the margins. Do not erase errors, run a line through them and initial the correction. Table 19–4 provides additional dos and don'ts to help in legal documentation.

Finally, from an administrative advisory standpoint, therapists should keep in mind a risk management program to avoid legal complications. To develop an effective risk management program, take the following five steps: (1) identify the potential risks; (2) measure potential risks; (3) select the best technique to control the risks; (4) implement the best technique chosen; and (5) evaluate the technique chosen.

For example, if a potential risk is water spilling from a Hubbard tank, the therapist needs to assess if it is just a minimal amount of water leaking out. If it stays in the Hubbard tank area and does not move to a patient traffic area, there may not be a significant risk. If, however, the drip results in a large puddle, and the patients walk in it, then some measure needs to be taken to keep the environment safe. To drain the excess water, a pump may need to be installed in the floor, or a therapist or aide should be assigned the task of water control and clean up in the hydrotherapy unit. If either measure is used, it should be monitored to see if it is, in fact, solving the problem. If it is, it should be continued; if not, the risk assessment/management should be repeated until the situation is rectified. Some additional red flags that may indicate the liabilities of a law suit and of which therapists should be aware are listed in Table 19–5.[4]

Another area of legal concern for rehabilitation therapists is the malfunction or misuse of equipment. Unlike other specialties in medicine, equipment can play a large role in the legal ramifications of the physical therapy department. Therefore, therapists should be particularly aware of the following areas.

All equipment should be checked and calibrated annually or more periodically, if deemed necessary. The current certification should be clearly displayed on each piece of equipment as well as the last time that the equipment was checked. Finally, the procedure for the checking of equipment should be listed

TABLE 19–4. DOS AND DON'TS FOR LEGAL DOCUMENTATION

- Do put in patient's behavior.
- Don't get personal.
- Do use quotes.
- Don't advertise incident reports.
- Don't use charts to settle disputes.
- Do be neat and legible.
- Don't try to keep secrets.

TABLE 19–5. RED FLAGS FOR POSSIBLE LITIGATION

- A patient refuses or leaves treatment.
- Patient has cardiac arrest during treatment.
- Patient sees doctor at completion of treatment.
- Patient goes to hospital within 72 hours.
- Patient burned during treatment.
- Patient isn't properly prepared or equipment fails.
- Patient falls during visit.
- Patient not informed of his or her condition or complications.
- Postoperative pain is greater than expected.
- Patient not encouraged to call doctor if they have a problem.
- Patient wait longer than 15 minutes.
- Patient uncomfortable about sexual questions.
- Patient given unclear instructions.
- Therapist unfriendly or discourteous.
- Patient feels therapist didn't spend enough time with him or her.

in the policy and procedure manual (see Appendix 19A).

Even simple equipment may pose a problem. For example, thermometers used in hot pack warmers, paraffin machines, and whirlpools may become dysfunctional. Temperature in these pieces of equipment should be checked monthly with a second thermometer to see if, in fact, they are correct. Hot pack covers showing bald spots and other warning signs should be replaced immediately.

Safety regulations should be posted on all pieces of equipment that require sophisticated techniques (e.g., Cybex equipment or balance machines). All timers and call bells should be checked daily, and foot stools should be eliminated if they have worn pads. Wheelchairs and stretchers should be checked to make certain that locks, straps, and belts are in proper working order.

The best idea for assessing safety is to have someone examine the department weekly, as though he or she were an insurance or safety inspector or a skeptical patient, keeping an eye out for hazards.

The final step of any legal administrative program is being prepared to go to court or to be deposed. Table 19–6 presents some useful hints for being an outstanding expert witness, being deposed, or being cross-examined.

The following is a list of the most frequent reasons why therapists are sued, according to the APTA Risk Management Manual:[4]

1. Failure to perform a physical therapy diagnosis;
2. Failure to refer;
3. Failure to properly treat;
4. Failure to monitor the patient;
5. Failure to maintain equipment or equipment failure;
6. Failure to follow doctor's orders.

TABLE 19-6. HINTS FOR EXPERT WITNESS

- Be sure you understand the question.
- Answer directly and simply.
- Don't volunteer information.
- Do not guess.
- Don't be too proud to admit the limits of your expertise.
- Take time to think before you answer.
- Do your homework.
- Speak clearly.
- Say yes or no, don't just shake your head.
- Always complete your answer.
- Don't let the opposing counsel cut you off.
- Be polite but firm, not cocky.
- Stop instantly when the judge interrupts you.
- Never lose your temper or argue with the attorney.
- When in court, talk directly to the members of the jury.
- Explain your answers in layperson's terms for the jury.
- Dress professionally and conservatively.

Improper practice by the therapist may lead to patient injury. Some common causes for patient injury are[5-8]

1. Being improperly treated with heat or electric equipment;
2. Incorrectly performing exercises with various types of equipment;
3. Improper manipulation;
4. A slip and fall accident;
5. Improper range of motion testing.

PERSONNEL MANAGEMENT: EMPLOYEE RELATIONS

Personnel management encompasses policies and procedures for employee orientation, benefits, and other programs. Providing proper supervision is another important part of personnel management. Many books have been written on how to successfully supervise employees. One of the easiest and most succinct books on supervision is *The One Minute Manager*.[9] The text, which takes about one minute to read, states that it takes one minute to acknowledge an employee's positive attributes and only one minute to reprimand them when necessary.

A good supervisor is one that is aware of employee needs and acknowledges good as well as inadequate performances. In addition, a good supervisor gives immediate feedback to the employee frequently.[10]

Employee orientation, quality assurance, in-services, and meeting attendance and orientations for aides are all areas that will require policy development as well as managerial expertise. Providing detailed information on this subject is beyond the scope of this text, but some guidelines for supervisors are provided in Appendix 19A. These guidelines can be used by supervisors to assist in hiring, training, and managing employees.

MARKETING

The final area to be covered in this chapter is marketing. Marketing is often a foreign concept for rehabilitation professionals. Frequently, marketing is thought of as selling, which it is not. Marketing is the process of identifying services to be offered and then, promoting, pricing, and distributing these services to the patients.[10,11]

For example, before opening a rehabilitation therapy department that will provide geriatric care in the Los Angeles suburbs, it is imperative to research the composition of the population in the area to see if it will support the practice. This background information can be developed by reviewing Chamber of Commerce data, performing interviews with citizens, conducting random sampling by telephone or a mail survey, and general information gathering. Once a need has been identified, decisions can be made on pricing and promoting the service.

It is not easy to open a practice. Studies of demographics, compensation, and other factors must be thoroughly examined before a new practice can be opened. It is essential to develop a fair scheme for charging, to prepare a schedule that meets the needs of the community, to establish the most centrally located site for the services, and to make sure that the site is accessible to all clients.

The next step is to promote the service. Let people know that the service is available, show how it differs from other services in the area, and try to expose people to information about the clinic. This can be done in a number of ways, ranging from sending out letters or making telephone calls to preparing seminars or just advertising by word of mouth.

Targeting marketing efforts is very important. In many areas, therapists are dependent on physicians for referrals. Thus, marketing may need to be targeted at physicians. In other areas, targeting patients who may want physical therapy but cannot get physician orders may be the best approach.

Marketing can be divided into two categories: external and internal. External marketing has already been described and it involves letting people from the outside know about the practice's services. Internal marketing focuses on the inner workings of the facility and how the efficiency and high quality of the services provided encourages patients to return or refer others to the clinic. Good questions to assess internal marketing efforts are: (1) Is the staff courteous? (2) Is a visit to the clinic a pleasant experience? (3) Are patients provided with information about the facility? (4) Does the staff know what the goals of the clinic are and act with these in mind?

Internal marketing strategies are discussed widely in the literature and although providing more detail is beyond the scope of this section, additional references are available.[11-16] Table 19-7 provides a simple and succinct marketing strategy handout for therapists, discusses professional level marketing and

TABLE 19–7. MARKETING STRATEGY

Rehabilitation departments frequently succeed or fail due to their ability to plan and implement ongoing marketing programs to showcase rehabilitation services. Marketing concepts must be kept in mind at all times and not only during low volume periods. The following is an example of marketing techniques that each therapist is encouraged to develop relative to their facility and specialized programs.

COMMUNITY LEVEL

- Volunteer to an organization, such as Spinal Cord Club, Multiple Sclerosis, Muscular Dystrophy, Breast Cancer, homeless shelter.
- Advertise facility based community service programs, such as "Caring for the Stroke Patient at Home." Could be for families in the facility as well as on a local community level.
  - Organize a posture screening in a mall or senior center
  - Teach a special exercise class at a retirement center.
  - Develop educational activities for osteoporosis month (May).
- Presentations to Special Interest Groups.
  - Service clubs.
  - Elderly groups.
  - Community business groups.

PROFESSIONAL LEVEL

- Doctor visits
  - Initial introduction to new physicians.
  - Introduce new programs or equipment in the rehabilitation department
  - Discuss continuing education courses.
  - When getting started, you may want to discuss postoperative protocols (i.e., for THR, TKR to determine general approach to weight bearing, exercise).
  - Accompany patients on follow-up physician visits.
  - Send typed discharge summaries frequently.
- Acute Care Rehabilitation Visits
  - Introduce yourself to all staff.
  - If new to area, may ask for information on local APTA chapter, TENS distributors, recommendations on good medical supply companies.
  - Tour the facility.
  - Ask for input on skilled nursing facility (SNF), rehabilitation needs in the community
- Discharge planners
  - Administrator, director of nursing, and rehabilitation professional make a good team to visit hospital discharge planners.
  - Leave brochures and business cards when available.
  - Send discharge planners typed discharge summaries on those patients they referred to you as soon as possible.
- Attend local continuing educational courses, especially those sponsored by your referring hospitals.
- Attend local professional meetings (e.g., APTA, AOTA state chapters).

FACILITY LEVEL

- Admission meetings: attendance by the rehabilitation therapist is mandatory.
- Inservices to Nursing Staff and other disciplines for staff development, body mechanics, range of motion, positions, and teach rehabilitation approach.
- Form teams (e.g., wound care team, fall screening and prevention, etc.)
- Rehabilitation Conferences: used to teach rehabilitation approach to other disciplines.
- Consult with activities director to help coordinate an exercise class.

community level marketing, and gives examples of how to implement these strategies.

CONCLUSION

As stated previously, it is imperative that therapists not only understand the clinical aspects of geriatric rehabilitation but the administrative aspects as well. Most of the information on administration is not directly available in rehabilitation texts, and the therapist may need to consult other sources to find some information. The best sources are business publications and seminars. A mixture of good clinical and administrative skills can provide therapists with a very rewarding practice.

PEARLS

- The components of administration are finance and budgeting, policies and procedures, legal concerns, employee relations, and marketing.
- Budgeting is defined as providing a monetary sketch of the department or clinic, and a realistic budget is essential to the financial well-being of the business.
- Need, advantages, disadvantages, and cost are all important considerations when purchasing equipment.
- An organizational plan is a visual chart of the administrative hierarchy.
- The plaintiff has a case if they can show actual harm resulted from an action, or if the therapist practiced below local or national standards.
- Equipment should be calibrated annually, and more sophisticated equipment should have precautions and directions posted.
- Marketing is identifying services to be offered and promoting, pricing, and distributing these services to the patients.

REFERENCES

1. American Physical Therapy Association. Guide to Physical Therapist Practice: Guidelines for Physical Therapy Documentation. *Phys Ther.* 1997; 77(11): 1634–1636.
2. Bottomley JM. American Physical Association Guideline for Documentation. In: Bottomley JM, ed. *Quick Reference Dictionary for Physical Therapy.* Thorofare, NJ: Slack Incorporated; 2000: 265–271.
3. Bergeson S. More about charting with a jury in mind. *Nursing.* April 1988; 50–58.
4. American Physical Therapy Association. *Risk Management.* Alexandria, VA: APTA; 1990.
5. Morgan MG, Florig HK, DeKay ML, et al. Categorizing risks for risk ranking. *Risk Anal.* February 2000; 20(1):49–58.

6. Schraeder C, Britt T, Shelton P. Integrated risk assessment and feedback reporting for clinical decision making in a Medicare risk plan. *J Ambulatory Care Manag.* October 2000; 23(4):40–47.

7. Raven J, Rix P. Managing the unmanageable: risk assessment and risk management in contemporary professional practice. *J Nurs Manag.* July 1999; 7(4): 201–206.

8. Michael JE, Summers CH. Establishing or enhancing your risk management program. Part II: The key elements of an effective risk management program. *Home Care Manag.* November-December 1997; 1(2): 10–13.

9. Blanchard K, Spencer J. *The One Minute Manager.* New York, NY: Berkley Books; 1982.

10. Solomon R. *Clinical Practice Management.* Gaithersburg, MD: Aspen Publishers; 1991.

11. MacCracken L. *Market-Driven Strategy: An Executive's Guide to Health Care's Integrated Environment.* American Hospital Publishing, Inc.; 1997.

12. Kotler P, Clarke R. *Marketing for Health Care Organizations.* Englewood Cliffs, NJ: Prentice-Hall; 1987: 244.

13. Husted S, Varble D, Lowry J. *Principles of Modern Marketing.* Needham Heights, MA: Allyn and Bacon Publishers, Inc. 1997: 237.

14. Scott J, Warshaw M, Taylor J. *Introduction to Marketing Management.* 5th Ed. Homewood, IL: Irwin Publishers; 1985: 11–12.

15. *Journal of Health Care Marketing.* American Marketing Association. 250 S. Wacker Drive, Chicago, IL 60606.

16. *Journal of Medical Practice Management.* Williams and Wilkins, 428 E. Preston St., Baltimore, MD 21202.

Appendices

- 19A-1. Orientation of Therapy Aides.
- 19A-2. Orientation and Training Checklist: PT Aide
- 19A-3. Physical Therapy Aide Work Performance Evaluation Checklist
- 19A-4. Committee Meetings
- 19A-5. Daily Stand-Up Meeting
- 19A-6. Rehabilitation Meeting
- 19A-7. Resident Care Planning Conference
- 19A-8. Utilization Review
- 19A-9. Department Head Meeting
- 19A-10. Resident Care Policy Review
- 19A-11. Quality Assurance and Assessment

Orientation of Therapy Aides

Policy

All new OT, PT, SLP aides will be oriented in a timely manner by the director of physical therapy or a designee (i.e., other staff therapists). Upon satisfactory completion of orientation and skills assessment, the aide will be assessed at 3 months, 1 year, and yearly thereafter.

Purpose

To assure competent skills in both direct and indirect patient care activities.

Scope

Orientation procedure must be followed on all new therapy aides.

Guidelines

1. Orientation process will vary depending on employee's prior work experience and will be at the discretion of the supervising therapist.
2. The therapy aide will be trained in the use of selective therapy modalities and procedures as deemed appropriate by the supervising therapist. All modalities that may be performed by the aide will be documented on work performance evaluation checklist by the trainer.
3. When responsibilities are added to the tasks performed by therapy aides, these are documented on the work performance evaluation checklist to indicate training has been done.
4. Orientation checklists will be completed on each new therapy aide.
5. Work performance evaluation checklists are updated on an ongoing basis and maintained, and a copy is kept in the aide's personnel file.

Figure 19A–1. Orientation of Therapy Aides. *(Reprinted with permission from Therapy Management Innovations, Inc.)*

Orientation and Training Checklist: PT Aide

General Orientation to Facility

- ☐ Mission/Philosophy Statements
- ☐ Introductions
    Facility Staff
    Rehab Staff
- ☐ Tour
- ☐ Supplies & Equipment
    List supplies or equipment issued (i.e., dept. key, gait belt, etc.)
- ☐ Body Mechanics Instruction

Roles

- ☐ PT Aide Job Description
- ☐ Supervision Requirements
- ☐ Interdisciplinary Team Approach (common goals, communication, etc.)
- ☐ PT Role
- ☐ Other Rehab Roles
- ☐ Other Facility Staff
- ☐ Consultants
- ☐ Nursing/Rehab Integration of Services

Clinical Information

- ☐ Effects of Aging (i.e., systems, multiple dx., myths v. facts, etc.)
- ☐ Common Diagnoses/Problems/Precautions
- ☐ CVA
- ☐ Upper extremity fracture
- ☐ Hip fracture
- ☐ Hip replacement
- ☐ Knee replacement
- ☐ Fracture of spine
- ☐ Arthritis
- ☐ Progressive neurological conditions
- ☐ Head injury
- ☐ Cardiac
- ☐ COPD
- ☐ Amputation
- ☐ Wounds
- ☐ Medical conditions
- ☐ Functional Levels Defined
- ☐ Identifying Change of Condition (functional)
- ☐ Reporting Patient Information what, to whom, when, written, verbal
- ☐ Family Interactions

Treatment Modalities/Procedures

- ☐ Bed Mobility Training (Consider: hemiplegia, UE or LE fracture, hip, replacement, fracture of spine)

- ☐ Transfer Training/Use of Gait Belt (Consider: hemiplegia, LE fracture or joint replacement, amputee)
- ☐ Ambulation Activities/Use of Gait Belt (Consider: hemiplegia, LE fracture, or joint replacement)
    - ■ Types of gait
    - ■ Precautions
    - ■ Safely assisting
    - ■ Equipment—types, adjustments
- ☐ Balance Activities
    - ■ Sitting
    - ■ Standing
- ☐ Positioning (Consider: hemiplegia, UE or LE fracture, UE or LE fracture, LE joint replacement, wounds)
    - ■ Bed
    - ■ Wheelchair
- ☐ Wheelchair Mobility Training
    - ■ Safe transport of patients
    - ■ W/C adjustments
    - ■ Brakes, footpedals, leg rests
    - ■ Propulsion

Therapeutic Exercise

- ☐ Passive ROM
- ☐ Self ROM
- ☐ Active/assisted
- ☐ Active
- ☐ Resistive use of equipment (i.e., pulleys, weights, rickshaw, thera-band, etc.)
- ☐ Group

Other Procedures

- ☐ Whirlpool (Incl. routine use, cleaning, culturing per procedure)
- ☐ Hot Packs
- ☐ Cold Packs
- ☐ Contrast Bath
- ☐ Paraffin

Physiological Monitoring

- ☐ Pulse, Rate, and Rhythm
- ☐ Respirations, Rate, SOB

Use of Specialized Equipment

- ☐ Tilt Table
- ☐ Mechanical Lift
- ☐ CPM

Continued

——— *Continued from previous page* ———

☐ Parallel Bars
☐ Specialized Exercise Equipment

Documentation (if applicable)

☐ Medical Record Format
☐ Patient Subjective & Objective Information
(pt. comments & treatment given)
☐ Acceptable Abbreviations
☐ Functional Levels
☐ Co-signature by PT

Clerical Support

☐ Telephone Protocol

☐ Copying
☐ Faxing
☐ Ordering Supplies/Equipment (therapeutic and office needs)
☐ Scheduling
☐ Therapy Logs (for billing)
☐ Cleaning and Maintenance of Treatment Area

Other

☐ Reporting Incidents/Unusual Occurrences
☐ CPR
☐ Fire Safety Procedures
☐ Infection Control
☐ Disaster Procedures

Figure 19A–2. Orientation and Training Checklist: PT Aide. (*Reprinted with permission from Therapy Management Innovations, Inc.*)

PHYSICAL THERAPY AIDE WORK PERFORMANCE EVALUATION CHECKLIST

Procedure/Modality	INITIAL ASSESSMENT			3-MONTH			YEARLY		
	Date	PT Initials	AIDE Initials	Date	PT Initials	AIDE Initials	Date	PT Initials	AIDE Initials

Figure 19A–3. Physical Therapy Aide Work Performance Evaluation Checklist. (*Reprinted with permission from Therapy Management Innovations, Inc.*)

Committee Meetings

Policy

To improve communication between Rehabilitation Services and the facility, each therapy service is requested to share information at specific committee meetings. This information should be given to the committee coordinator prior to its commencement if the therapist is unable to attend.
The following committee meetings are required, as appropriate, in your facility:

- Admissions.
- Rehabilitation.
- Resident Care Planning Conference.
- Quality Assurance.
- Use Review.
- Department Head Meeting.
- Patient Care Policy Review.
- Corporate/Regional Rehab Meeting.
- Quality Assurance and Assessment.

Procedure

1. Obtain the dates and times of these meetings from your administrator.
2. Schedule meetings accordingly.

Figure 19A–4.   Committee Meetings. *(Reprinted with permission from Therapy Management Innovations, Inc.)*

Daily Stand-Up Meeting

Meeting name: This meeting may be known by different names in different facilities; it may be called the Admissions or Stand-up or Census Meeting.
Purpose: To provide coordinated interdisciplinary communication regarding patient inquiries, admissions, discharges, and room transfers.
Frequency: Every day, for approximately 15 minutes.
Members: Administrator, director of nursing, admissions coordinator, physical therapist, occupational therapist, speech-language pathologist, medical records, bookkeeper and appropriate department heads.
Items Discussed:

- Inquiries pending, level of care/payor status.
- New admissions.
- Discharges.
- Room transfers.
- Patient's change of condition.
- Special programs/activities for the day.

Figure 19A–5.   Daily Stand-up Meeting. *(Reprinted with permission from Therapy Management Innovations, Inc.)*

Rehabilitation Meeting

Purpose: To provide an opportunity for interdisciplinary team members to discuss a patient's plan of treatment.

Frequency: Weekly.

Members: Administrator of nursing, charge nurse, RNA, physical therapist, occupational therapist, speech-language pathologist, social services, and discharge planner. Dietary services and CNA should attend as appropriate.

Items Discussed:

- Interdisciplinary goals.
- Patient's progress.
- Equipment needs.
- Discharge planning.
- Family teaching.

Documentation: Minutes of each meeting should be kept. These should include date of the meeting, members present, patients reviewed, and necessary follow-up. A notebook containing rehabilitation meeting minutes can be kept in the rehabilitation department and used as a reference for each minute.

Figure 19A–6. Rehabilitation Meeting. *(Reprinted with permission from Therapy Management Innovations, Inc.)*

Resident Care Planning Conference

Purpose: To provide the highest quality of care planning through use of a coordinated interdisciplinary approach.

Frequency: Twice weekly or as needed per facility census.

Members: Director of nursing, dietary, social services, activities, physical therapist, occupational therapist, and speech-language pathologist, RNA and CNA staff as needed.

Items Discussed:

- Interdisciplinary problems, goals, and treatment approaches are discussed and listed on the patient care plan.
- New admissions are discussed within 7 days of admit.
- Residents are discussed with updates and deletions recorded at least quarterly.
- Appropriateness of care plan entries.
- Changes in condition.

Figure 19A–7. Resident Care Planning Conference. *(Reprinted with permission from Therapy Management Innovations, Inc.)*

Utilization Review

Purpose: To maintain a medical committee to determine Medicare coverage and to appropriately use facility services.

Members: Two or more physicians, including medical director, administrator, director of nursing, medical records, social services, physical therapist, occupational therapist, and speech-language pathologist.

Committee Functions: In order to promote the highest quality of resident care, the committee is responsible for conducting medical care evaluation studies, extended duration reviews, and consideration of any other cases brought to its attention. The committee will also review discharge plans for individual residents.

Rehabilitation Involvement: The rehabilitation team has an important role to play in the decision made by the utilization review committee. A list of patients should be reviewed prior to the meeting in order for the therapist to give an accurate update on the patient's therapy progress and expected duration of treatment. If a therapist is unable to attend, their patients should be discussed with the director of nursing to ensure their treatment plans are taken into consideration by the committee.

Figure 19A–8. Utilization Review. (*Reprinted with permission from Therapy Management Innovations, Inc.*)

Department Head Meeting

Purpose: To facilitate open communication and sharing of information between key personnel. Each department head is responsible to share appropriate information with his or her staff.

Frequency: Scheduled as needed by the administrator; may be weekly or daily.

Members: Administrator, director of nursing, rehabilitation services, dietary, social services, activities, housekeeping/laundry, maintenance.

Items Discussed:

- Department update.
- Changes in policies and procedures.
- Corporate updates.
- Facility activities.
- Department head and consultant schedules.
- Community education.

Figure 19A–9. Department Head Meeting. (*Reprinted with permission from Therapy Management Innovations, Inc.*)

Resident Care Policy Review

Purpose: To review and revise the Resident Care Policy Manual.

Frequency: At least yearly, usually prior to survey. It may be scheduled more frequently, as needed.

Members: Administrator, director of nursing, rehabilitation services, social services activities, dietary, housekeeping/laundry, maintenance.

Items Discussed:

- Review policies and procedures for accuracy.
- Delete nonexistent policies.
- Update and revise appropriate policies.
- Include new policies and procedures, as appropriate.

The Rehabilitation Policy and Procedure Manual should be reviewed and revised yearly. This may be completed during this meeting. Once completed, the manual is signed and dated.

Figure 19A–10. Resident Care Policy Review. *(Reprinted with permission from Therapy Management Innovations, Inc.)*

Quality Assurance and Assessment

Purpose: To provide a systematic and ongoing self-evaluation process geared toward identifying and re-solving problems, targeting areas for program improvement and development, and enhancement of overall resident care and quality of life.

Frequency: Monthly.

Members: Administrator, medical director, director of nurses, and at least three other staff members from various departments, such as social service, activities, dietary, rehabilitation, or housekeeping.

Items Discussed:

- Identification of areas to be studied.
- Format for data collection and communication of finding.
- Establishment of CQI studies, including time frames, responsibilities, data collection, tools, and re-porting mechanism.

Figure 19A–11. Quality Assurance Assessment. *(Reprinted with permission from Therapy Management Innovations, Inc.)*

CHAPTER 20

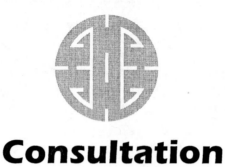

Consultation

Identifying the Rehabilitation Professional's Consultant Role	The Consultant Process
	Conclusion
Settings for Consulting	Appendices
Identifying Consultation Activities	

The consultant role is not new to physical or occupational therapy, because rehabilitation professionals serve as consultants to other health care team members in daily treatment delivery. The therapist's role as a consultant is, however, new in the realm of geriatrics. Most literature on the subject of the consultant in geriatrics has only been published in the last twenty years.

The general literature on geriatric consultation states several reasons for its development. These reasons include patient care, professional education, public relations screening, and quality assurance. In an early article on the topic in the medical literature, the major reasons for requesting geriatric consultation were medical management (25%), discharge planning (18%), evaluation and management of dementia (17%), and failure to thrive (15%).[1] According to another early study, the major reasons for requesting consultation were geriatric evaluation (28%), assessing rehabilitation potential (27%), and mental status evaluation (3%).[2]

Several benefits of geriatric consultation have been enumerated in the literature. These benefits are

1. Decreased length of hospitalization;[3]
2. Increased use of rehabilitation services;[3]
3. Improved patient care;[4]
4. Decreased use of expensive health care resources;[5]
5. Increased identification of new diagnoses;[6]
6. Provides a source of education.[7]

The negative aspects of geriatric consultation are

1. Conflicts may arise among the disciplines when there is a "turf" battle over the overall management of the patient.

2. Geriatric consultation can be time consuming.
3. This type of consultation can also be costly.[7]

The final introductory point on geriatric consultation is efficacy. The general literature reveals no definitive conclusions as to the efficacy of consultation. The literature is fraught with complications about the type of patient classically referred to a medical geriatric consultant. The frailer patients are more frequently referred and are more difficult to manage. Secondly, the recommendations of the consultant are often only partially followed.[8,9] Even with the controversy in geriatric consultation, the potential benefit to the older person in different treatment settings outweighs the negative aspects cited.

IDENTIFYING THE REHABILITATION PROFESSIONAL'S CONSULTANT ROLE

SETTINGS FOR CONSULTING

Nursing Homes

The variety of settings available to the rehabilitation consultant in geriatrics is only limited by the therapist's imagination, but the major areas of consultation are nursing homes, home care, community senior centers, hospitals, rehabilitation centers, outpatient clinics, and industrial settings.

In the nursing home, a therapist can work as a staff therapist and receive a regular salary with all the benefits, or he or she can contract. Contract basis in the nursing home can take many forms, the most common of which are the hourly, per patient, or direct bill. In the hourly arrangement, the therapist charges the nursing home for any hours spent in the facility with the majority of time being spent in direct patient care. In addition, the therapist may set up restorative programs, provide in-service education, conduct screenings, and assist in quality assurance. The therapist is simply reimbursed on a time-spent basis.

The per patient arrangement reimburses the therapist based on how many patients are seen. This can be a flat figure per patient or based on a percentage of charges. The percentage method can be further broken down into the percentage of charges billed and the percentage of charges received. It is obvious that it is more advantageous to the therapist to contract on a percentage-billed basis, while the nursing home would prefer to use the percentage received. The pros of the first situation are that the therapist does not have to wait for the money and is not dependent on the nursing home's filing ability. In addition, the therapist does not risk a denied claim. The therapist who contracts on a percentage basis has several options in providing non-patient care services: They can be included as part of the package on a gratis basis; the therapist can be reimbursed on a hourly basis for any time spent in presentation and preparation; or a flat fee can be assessed on a weekly, monthly, or yearly basis for these extra services.

The final, most common method of consulting in a nursing home with direct patient care as the major emphasis is direct billing of the patient. In this situation the therapist offers to treat any appropriate patients and to bill the respective insurance company. This form of consultation is riskier and more inundated with paperwork than the previously mentioned methods; however, it can prove to be the most lucrative. (For specific information on inpatient and outpatient contracting see Appendix D.)

Home Care

Consultation in home care is identical to the situation already described when the consultant subcontracts with an agency. In this situation the therapist can be salaried, hourly, or per patient. In an even more independent situation, a therapist can hang up a shingle and treat patients in the home. The therapist will direct bill the patient and the insurance company. To treat Medicare home patients, the independent therapist must have a certified office. (See Appendix A for Criteria for a Certified Office.)

Senior Centers

Senior centers and retirement homes provide a creative way of consulting in the geriatric realm, and therapists can serve in several capacities. For example, they can conduct environmental assessments, develop and teach exercise classes, or provide screening programs. The financial arrangements for these types of programs can be quite varied. The consultant can offer the facility a menu of these activities with a cost-per-activity charge. Another alternative is an hourly arrangement to provide whatever services are needed. The consultant can also directly charge the participants. For example, a consultant may charge each exercise class participant $5 per session, or $20 for four sessions. The consultant may want to provide some of the services for free as a public relations effort for future programs.

Hospitals, Rehabilitation Centers, and Outpatient Clinics

Hospital consulting is a new area of physical and occupational therapy; therefore, the therapist seeking hospital privileges is a relatively new and controversial topic. (See Appendix A for practice privileges from the state of California and criteria for a certified office, as well as for information on performance standards for independent practitioners.)

The consultant in the hospital, rehabilitation center, and outpatient clinic can always contract to provide direct patient care on an hourly, per patient, or direct bill basis. He or she can also act to provide special assessment for older patients, which may take the form of a screening, such as an osteoporosis, balance, or foot evaluation. The consultant may also be called in to provide expert advice on how to improve the outcomes of therapy or to perform specific functional assessment specific for older persons (see Chapter 6 for functional assessment tools). In addition to providing these services in the hospital, rehabilitation and outpatient settings, the consultant can provide continuing education and screening programs to the public, as well as quality assurance expertise. The financial arrangement for this could take the form of an hourly contract, fee for service, or flat fee contract.

Industrial Settings

With increasing life expectancy, many elderly individuals choose to remain active in employment settings. In fact, many industrial entities actively recruit the older worker. As a result, industrial rehabilitation for an older population is an excellent platform for the consulting therapist. The consultant in a work-related setting can contract to do screening, functional capacity testing, ergonomic assessments and modifications, conditioning programs, and educational programs on health and wellness related topics for the older worker. Instruction in proper body mechanics for lifting and other repetitive activities can be implemented to prevent injury.

In all of these settings, the geriatric consultant may be asked to design a program where none has existed previously. This will require the consultant to create policy and procedure manuals, employee handbooks, and billing procedures and forms. In the opinion of the authors of this book, the best approach to this type of arrangement is to develop an hourly contract. A flat fee contract can also be used; however, this does not give the consultant the freedom to spend time on unforeseen complications that may arise in the process of designing a program.

IDENTIFYING CONSULTANT ACTIVITIES

Screening Programs

Screening programs are one of the major activities of the geriatric consultant. They can be conducted in any of the settings listed as well as in a public setting (e.g., shopping malls). (Appendix B has examples of screening programs for the community.)

Direct Patient Care

Therapists can provide part-time or full-time direct patient care as another type of activity, and it can be very creative. In many situations the rehabilitation therapist conducts the evaluations and discharges, and the therapist assistant provides the hands-on treatment under the supervision of the physical therapist. Some therapists set up classes for providing care to similar patients in the hospital, nursing home, or community setting. The options for care in this setting are limitless. Nevertheless, the important components of this type of consulting are appropriate evaluation, progressive treatment strategies, and comprehensive discharge. Throughout this process, the therapist must provide appropriate documentation.

Consulting on OBRA

In the nursing home setting, additional consultative roles are constantly developing. In 1989 and 1990, for example, the US government took action on some previous legislation that directly impacted the rehabilitation therapist. The scenario with a consultative view of an approach to the problem follows.

The Omnibus Reconciliation Act (OBRA) and the Federal Nursing Home Amendment are two of the most influential pieces of legislation affecting long-term care. Even though OBRA was published in 1987, the guidelines for the implementation of this legislation are still being written. One portion of these guidelines that will affect physical and occupational therapy dramatically is the "Interpretive Guidelines on Physical Restraints: Implemented October 1, 1990."

A quote from these guidelines illustrates the importance of physical and occupational therapists with regard to interpreting the legislation and administering the guidelines: "A facility must have evidence of consultation with appropriate health professionals, such as occupational or physical therapists in the use of less restrictive supportive devices, *prior to* using physical restraints as defined in this guideline for such purposes."

The four major types of patients who are candidates for physical restraints are

■ The cognitively impaired wanderer;
■ The aggressive patient;
■ Patients who interfere with medical treatment;
■ The unsteady patient.

The physical and occupational therapist will be most effective in assessing the necessity for restraining devices for the fourth group because of the clear benefits associated with aiding these patients to maintain their quality of life. For this group, the guidelines call for several major areas of assessment. The first major area of assessment is the risk of falls or a decline in functional status if physical restraints are not applied. The next area of assessment is the risk of falls or decline in function if physical restraints are applied. The third and fourth areas of concern are to use less restrictive measures and the application of restraints. The final area to be assessed is the facility's ability to provide the least restrictive environment.

To tie or not to tie is a difficult question. Understaffed nursing homes are fearful of guidelines that may cause an increase in the responsibilities of overburdened and underpaid staff. In addition, the possibility of increased legal pressure has been a source of apprehension regarding nonadherence to the guidelines. The proponents of untying the elderly, however, are advocating unassailable issues in the area of quality of life that must be considered in a comparison of risks and benefits.

Physical and occupational therapists can be extremely important players in allaying the fears of staff in this area, as well as in helping to ensure that the least restrictive and most freedom-enhancing environment for older persons is established. Figure 20–1 is a Physical Restraint Consultation (PRC) Form,[10] which is self-explanatory. Questions 1–16 on the PRC Form address the area of risk of falls both intrinsic and extrinsically. The next areas of concern, possible less restrictive measures and application of restraints, respectively, are addressed by the questions under #17 on the PRC form. The third area of the assessment form is the risk of falls or decline in function if physical restraints are applied. The same tools already noted will answer this concern, as well as question #18 on the PRC form. The final area of assessment is the facility's ability to provide the least restrictive environment. This is addressed in question #19.[10]

Quality Assurance and Chart Review

Rehabilitation therapists can also act in a consultative capacity to provide quality assurance and chart review assistance. To provide this type of service the

Physical Restraint Consultation Form

1. Name _____ Date _____
2. Current medical problems _____
3. Medications _____
4. History of falls _____
   Frequency _____
   Time of day _____
   Position _____
   Activity _____
5. Balance with eyes open _____
6. Balance with eyes closed _____
7. Get up and go _____
8. Vertebral artery syndrome _____
9. Blood pressure change with position change _____
10. Flexibility _____
11. Strength _____
12. Posture _____
13. Gait (eyes open) _____ (eyes closed) _____
14. Tandem walk _____
15. Psychological _____
16. Environment
    Noise level _____
    Chairs _____ Stable _____ Locked _____
    Beds _____ Low _____ Locked _____
    Lighting _____ Adequate _____ Glare _____
    Toilet _____ Raised _____ Handrails _____
    Colors _____ Raised _____ Safe _____
17. Recommendations
   A. Physical Restraints Y _____ N _____ (If yes, state time, placement, precautions, and suggestions) _____
   B. Does the resident need devices for alignment, proper body position, or prevention of contractures? Y _____ N _____ (If yes, specify) _____
   C. Does resident need to be in nonrestrained area of constant observation? _____
   D. Other suggestions (P.T., O.T., exercise class, or assistive devices). Specify _____
18. Has the use or will the use of physical restraints cause:
   A. Chronic constipation or incontinence _____
   B. Pressure sores _____
   C. Loss of muscle tone _____
   D. Loss of independent mobility _____
   E. Increased agitation _____
   F. Loss of balance _____
   G. Symptoms of withdrawal or depression _____
   H. Reduced social contact _____
19. Is the least restrictive restraint being used? Y _____ N _____ If no, why not _____
20. When should the resident be reevaluated for use of physical restraints? _____

Figure 20-1. Physical Restraint Consultation Form (*Reprinted with permission from Lewis CB. How to handle upcoming guidelines. PT Bull. June 27, 1990; 18–19.*)

therapist should consult several references in this area. References 11–18 are particularly useful for information on quality assurance. Several groups exist across the country that provide this type of service. However, if it can be done in-house or locally for less money and inconvenience, then the therapist is providing a worthwhile consultant service.

THE CONSULTATION PROCESS

To execute a successful consultation program a methodical and reproducible process should be followed. The steps in this process are

1. Needs assessment;
2. Query;
3. Proposal;
4. Negotiation;
5. Implementation;
6. Evaluation.

A needs assessment can be conducted simply or through a very sophisticated process. In its simplest form, a needs assessment is conducted either by asking people if they think a program would be beneficial or by observing the site. Increasing in sophistication, a needs assessment would be a random phone survey, a written survey to a specific audience, or tapping the data from a community or facility survey.

The query portion of the process entails asking detailed questions to assist in the design of the program. For example, if a posture screening program is to be developed, questions about the time of day, acceptable waiting time, price, expectations, and people and facilities available would be useful (Fig. 20–2).

A proposal can be simple or sophisticated. A simple proposal would be a telephone call to the general manager of a community mall, with a discussion that included information on the therapist's background. If space is available, the therapist should ask what the appropriate times are, about the available manpower, and about additional expense requirements. A letter restating the terms can follow this up. A formal proposal is given in Appendix C.

The negotiation step of the consultation process entails discussing the therapist's needs with the facility. In this process, the therapist must come into the meeting with both an optimal situation and the minimal acceptable situation. Begin the negotiation by describing the optimal situation, and then ask the representative(s) from the facility about their optimal scenario. If the two match, both will be very happy. If the responses are completely opposite, then ask what their minimal acceptable situation is. If this situation is vastly different than the minimal criteria the therapist has established prior to this meeting, then he or she should graciously leave.

The implementation of the consulting process can be divided into four phases: long-term planning, short-term planning, execution, and continuation. Long-term planning begins from the moment the negotiation ends and the contract is signed and lasts until the day before the project begins. Activities to be accomplished during this phase are the design or completion of any administrative forms. For example, if a therapist consults to provide an exercise class, in the long-term phase he or she will need to develop medical releases and get them filled out before the class begins (Figures 20–3A & 20B). Participant evaluation forms will be needed as well as handouts and contracts, and the class will need to be advertised (see Appendix C). The final aspect of the long-term implementation is preparing the exercise class. In preparing for the first class, an introduction must be designed for the therapist and a way of meeting the class's participants must also be designed. Then a format for the class must be developed. Finally, the class should be practiced several times so the therapist is comfortable teaching it.

In the short-term phase of implementation (one to two days before the class) areas to plan for are environmental and advertising. Environmentally, check the room one more time before the class. Is there enough room? Is the temperature correct? Is the music system appropriate and do the tapes work on the equipment? Do you have tapes and do you feel comfortable working the equipment? The therapist is also part of the environment. What are you going to wear? There are several considerations here. First,

---

Sample Query

Your group has expressed an interest in a low back exercise class. To design the class to meet your needs, please take a few moments to fill out the questions below.

1. What time of day is good for you?
2. Is five dollars per class acceptable?
3. What do you expect from this class?
4. How often would you like to come to the class?

Figure 20–2. *Sample query for design of a program.*

Implementation Phase

	EXERCISE CLASSES	SETTING UP	PHYSICAL THERAPY DEPT.
Long-term	Medical releases Evaluation forms Contracts with individual Handouts Sign-in sheet Advertise		
Short-term	Check space Get equipment Get music Appropriate clothes Advertise		
Execution	Check water Check temperature Check music Check handouts Check lights		
Continuation	New handouts Reevalulate forms New equipment/music Advertise		

Figure 20–3A. Implementation of the consulting process divided into long-term planning, short-term planning, execution, and continuation phases.

Implementation Phases—Long-Term

	NURSING HOME	HOSPITAL
Long-term		
Short-term		
Execution		
Continuation		

Figure 20–3B. Long-term program planning during implementation phases by a consultant.

Patient Satisfaction Survey

The following is a survey that Crescent City Physical Therapy sends to patients within 30 days of their discharge date. What we hope to accomplish is to determine if we are meeting your needs and expectations. Crescent City Physical Therapy cares about what you think. We want to offer you the highest quality of patient care. So, please take a brief moment and complete this short survey, and return it in the stamped, self-addressed envelope. Thank You!!

1. The treatment you received from your physical therapist was?

   ☐ Excellent   ☐ Average   ☐ Poor   ☐ No response

2. The treatment you received from your physical therapy aid was?

   ☐ Excellent   ☐ Average   ☐ Poor   ☐ No response

3. The service you received from the front desk when you first set up an appointment was?

   ☐ Excellent   ☐ Average   ☐ Poor   ☐ No response

4. The service you received at the front desk when checking in for your appointment was?

   ☐ Excellent   ☐ Average   ☐ Poor   ☐ No response

5. The service you received at the front desk when setting up a return appointment was?

   ☐ Excellent   ☐ Average   ☐ Poor   ☐ No response

6. The manner or promptness in which billing the responsible party (insurance company, attorney, workman's compensation, or private pay) was?

   ☐ Excellent   ☐ Average   ☐ Poor   ☐ No response

7. Was the manner in which statements were sent easily understood?

   ☐ Excellent   ☐ Average   ☐ Poor   ☐ No response

8. The manner in which the Crescent City Physical Therapy office handled your telephone calls was?
   ☐ Excellent   ☐ Average   ☐ Poor   ☐ No response

Figure 20–4.   Patient Satisfaction Survey. (*Reprinted with permission from Cresent City Physical Therapy & Sports Rehabilitation Services, Inc.*)

you need to look professional, and yet you need to move around to teach an exercise class. Tailored slacks and a professional blouse will work. Second, the colors should be in the optimal appreciation range for the older person, that is the reds, oranges, and golds. See Chapter 9 for more information on colors.

The final aspect of the short-term implementation phase is intense advertising. In the last 24 to 48 hours, advertisements can be repeated for one more time. Flyers can be used to attract potential participants.

The execution phase is teaching the class. Do a last-minute check of the environment. Check to be sure the temperature and lighting are correct and that water is close by. Check to be sure the handouts are ready and that the music is working. At the very last minute, check to be sure that you are relaxed and comfortable.

The continuation phase is composed of what it takes to continue the consulting activity. In the preceding example, the continuation phase is relatively simple, but in a contracted physical therapy department, it can be much more difficult. For example, in the department setting the consultant is frequently confronted with patient load fluctuations and staff shortages. These types of problems constantly plague these settings and should be planned for in the continuation. Returning to the example of the continuation phase in the exercise classes, activities to enhance this phase are developing new handouts, programs, equipment usage, musical background, and continuing advertisement. In addition, frequent re-evaluations of the class participants, using the initial evaluation to show progress, can help to motivate individuals to continue in an exercise program.

The final phase of the consultant process is the evaluation phase, which can be accomplished simply or in a more sophisticated fashion. In the simplest form, evaluation can be done by asking the recipients if they like the services. This can be done by spontaneous feedback or by a formal questionnaire (Fig. 20–4).

In the hospital or nursing home setting, the recipients of the service are not the only consumers. Nurses and referring doctors should also receive questionnaires on the services. Evaluations can be done periodically or at set intervals (e.g., every six months), and they can also be used to assess outcomes.

Outcomes can be broken down into two broad categories. The first is patient or recipient outcomes. In the example of the exercise class, comparing initial and follow-up data can easily assess the participant outcome. The same is true for direct service consulting. Patient initial evaluation and subsequent evaluation comparison can show outcomes. (See Chapter 21 for statistical analysis.) The second outcome variable of overall institutional benefits is much more elusive and difficult to assess. The simplest way of assessing this variable is to choose one outcome. For example, in the direct service area, you may want to compare the number of falls prior to implementation of your rehabilitation program and after.

CONCLUSION

The possibilities of consulting in the realm of geriatrics are limitless, because the consultant has the luxury of designing unique programs in a variety of settings. Through this, the therapist can contribute worthwhile information to the rehabilitation process.

PEARLS

- The primary reasons for consultation services in geriatrics are patient care, professional education, public relations, screening, and quality assurance.
- The benefits of geriatric consultation are:
  1. Decreased length of hospitalization and responsible use of expensive health care resources.
  2. Increased use of rehabilitative services and identification of new diagnoses.
  3. Improved patient care.
  4. Greater access to educational resources.
- Rehabilitation therapists may serve as consultants in nursing homes, senior centers, hospitals, rehabilitation centers, fitness centers, industrial settings, as well as home care. The consultant's role will change in each setting.
- The four major types of patients that are candidates for restraints are:
  1. Cognitively impaired wanderers;
  2. Aggressive patients;
  3. Patients who interfere with medical treatment;
  4. Unsteady patients.
- The steps in a successful consultation process are needs assessment, query, proposal, negotiation, implementation, and evaluation.
- The most important phase of the consultation process is the evaluation or outcome phase. The step can be as simple as checking patient satisfaction or as sophisticated as statistical analysis of post-program scores.

REFERENCES

1. Duthie EH, Gambert SR. Geriatrics consultation implication for teaching and clinical care. *Gerontol Geriatric Education*. 1983; 4:59.
2. Burley L Currie C, Smith R, et al. Contribution from geriatric medicine within acute medical wards. *Br Med J*. 1979; 2:90.
3. Hogan DB, Fox RA, Badley BWD, et al. Effects of a geriatric consultation service on management of pa-

tients in an acute care hospital. *Can Med Assoc J.* 1987; 136:713.

4. Allen C, Becker P, McVey L, et al. A randomized controlled clinical trial of a geriatric consultation team. *JAMA.* 1986; 255:2617.

5. Barker WH, Williams TF, Zimmer JG, et al. Geriatric consultation team. *J Am Ger Soc.* 1985; 33:422.

6. Lichtenstein H, Winograd CH. Geriatric consultation: a functional approach. *J Am Ger Soc.* 1984; 32:356.

7. Lee T, Pappus EM, Goldman L. Impact of interphysician communication on the effectiveness of medical consultation. *Am J Med.* 1983; 74:105.

8. Katz P, Dube D, Calkins E, et a1. Use of a structured functional assessment format in a geriatric consultation service. *J Am Ger Soc.* 1985; 33:681.

9. Campion EW, Jette AM, Beckman B. An interdisciplinary geriatric consultation service: a controlled trial. *J Am Ger Soc.* 1983; 31:792.

10. Lewis C. How to handle upcoming guidelines. *PT Bull.* June 27,1990; 18–19.

11. Borden LP. Patient education and the quality assurance process. *QRB.* 1985; 11(4):123–127.

12. Chauhan L, Hutchings D, LePoer K. Quality assurance manual in PT services. *Clin Manage in Phys Ther.* 1986; 6(5):28–31.

13. Filingliim CT, Deschler MJ. Quality control circles. *Clin Manage in Phys Ther.* 1985; 5(5):42–43.

14. Gaynor L. Quality assurance quarterly screening review. *Clin Manage in Phys Ther.* 1985; 5(5): 38–41.

15. Glendinning M. Quality assurance in physiotherapy. *Austin Clin Rev.* November 1981; 1(3):22.

16. Goocle DH, Jamieson HD, Warrington DM. Quality assurance in physiotherapy. *Laser NZ J Physiother.* April 1984; 12(l):27–28.

17. Quality Assurance. *Hosp Peer Rev.* March 1980; 5(3):29–40.

18. Lewis C, Campanelli L. *Health Promotion and Exercise for Older Persons.* Rockville, MD: Aspen Publishers; 1990.

Appendices

Performance Standards for Registered Physical Therapists in Long-Term Care Facilities

The purpose of these standards shall be to ensure that Physical Therapy services rendered in Long-Term Care facilities shall subscribe to Standards of Practice as established by the American Physical Therapy Association.

I. Admissions

The Registered Physical Therapist shall advise and/or participate in the Admissions Process to ensure:

A. That sufficient information is available at the time of admission review including a comprehensive summary of previous physical therapy received by the patient;

B. That restorative services and equipment available in the facility are appropriate to meet the needs of patients being considered for admission;

C. That a record review of every patient admitted to the facility is accomplished to determine the need for physical therapy evaluation services, or maintenance care.

II. Direct Services

A. The Registered Physical Therapist shall provide direct service to any patient upon referral by the physician.

B. The therapist shall conduct a:

1. physical therapy evaluation and in consultation with the patient, the physician and other members of the patient care team develop a goal and treatment plan or recommend to the physician that no treatment or maintenance care only is indicated;

2. provide skilled physical therapy services directly or direct the services performed by the qualified PT assistant;

3. maintain progress notes at designated intervals in the clinical record indicating:

a. progress toward goals;

b. changes in status or new problems;

c. re-evaluations.

C. The RPT will periodically reassess goals and review and revise the patient care plan accordingly.

D. Contact the patients physician as required or indicated.

E. Maintenance programs may be planned by the RPT and carried out by the patient, nursing staff or family members.

1. The therapist should ensure that the maintenance program is clearly understood by the personnel designated to carry out the plan.

2. The therapist should re-evaluate patients on maintenance routines periodically but not less than every 60 days.

F. Discharge Planning:

1. The RPT shall assist in implementing an appropriate discharge plan for those individuals transferring to another facility or returning home.

2. Activities of the therapist may include but not be limited to:

a. developing PT discharge summary;

b. discharge home;

1. home visit to assess architectural barriers and recommend modifications

2. establish home physical therapy program (copy in chart) that is understood by patient and family

c. discharge to another facility;

1. provide a physical therapy summary (including treatment given and patient status on discharge).

III. Indirect Services

A. The Registered Physical Therapist shall provide consultation regarding the rehabilitation needs of patients in the facility by any of the following:

1. Participation in Multi-Disciplinary Patient Care meetings or conferences to:

a. assist in identifying patient problems;

b. state short and long term goals and recommend how these objectives can be reached;

c. review patient's progress and reassess appropriateness of the direct services or maintenance program as part of the total patient care plan.

B. The Registered Physical Therapist shall participate in formal and informal in-service training.

1. provide in-service training to other long term care facility staff;

Continued

Continued from previous page

    2. attend relevant in-service training programs provided in the facility.

  C. Attends UR committee meetings or other conferences at the request of administration.

  D. Submit a written summary of indirect services provided in accordance with facility policy.

IV. Physical Therapy Audit

The Registered Physical Therapist should be encouraged to participate in and/or develop peer review activities as recommended by the Massachusetts Chapter APTA; these activities may include: Physical Therapy Audit, Department structure review, process review, outside review by persons designated by Massachusetts Chapter APTA.

V. Policies and Procedures

The RPT shall have appropriate input into development of parts of policy and procedure manual pertaining to Physical Therapy.

Figure 20A–1. Performance Standards in Long-Term Care Facilities (*Reprinted with permission from Massachusetts Chapter of the APTA Newsletter. June 15, 1979; 4(5):4.*)

Practice Privileges for Physical Therapists: Model Policy and Procedure

Application: Physical Therapists seeking full or limited practice privileges, physical therapy department director, medical staff committee on interdisciplinary practice.

Policy: A physical therapist holding a current license as required by California law to practice physical therapy is eligible for practice privileges in this hospital only if he or she meets the following qualifications:

1. Is a registered physical therapist licensed by the Board of Medical Quality Assurance to practice in the State of California.
2. Adequately documents experience, background, training, demonstrated ability, experience, judgment, and physical and mental health status to demonstrate qualification to exercise practice privileges within the hospital, and that any patient treated will receive that professional level of quality and efficiency of care established by the hospital.
3. Is determined, on the basis of documented references, to adhere strictly to the accepted ethics of the physical therapy profession; to work cooperatively with others in the hospital setting; and to assist the hospital in fulfilling its obligations related to patient care, within the areas of his or her professional competence and credentials.

Purpose: This policy establishes a mechanism for reviewing credentials and granting practice privileges to physical therapists who practice outside the employment of the hospital.

Definitions

1. *Physical Therapists with Practice Privileges:* A physical therapist, eligible for practice privileges by meeting the qualifications set forth under this policy, who chooses to practice outside the employment of the hospital. He or she shall meet the eligibility requirements for employment by the hospital should both parties wish to pursue this arrangement.
2. *Full Practice Privileges:* Includes all areas of practice as defined by the Physical Therapy Practice Act, State of California, as they pertain to the scope of physical therapy services provided in the hospital and defined in hospital department policies and procedures.
3. *Limited Practice Privileges:* Limited to specified areas of practice or patient population, such as but not restricted to, electromyography, cardiac rehabilitation, or neonatal intensive care.

Procedures

1. Granting of Practice Privileges: A physical therapist seeking practice privileges at this hospital must apply and qualify for such privileges. Applications for initial granting of practice privileges and subsequent renewal there of shall be submitted and processed in a parallel manner to that provided in the Medical Staff Bylaws for other practitioners.

   a. A completed Allied Health Professional application with pertinent support documentation is to be submitted to the Medical Staff Office.

   b. Upon written verification of required information, the application is forwarded to the Director of Physical Therapy for review and recommendations. Input from the physical therapy department's Medical Director is obtained as needed. The Application is then forwarded to the medical Staff Committee on Interdisciplinary Practice (CIP), or similar appropriate committee.

   c. While considering applications for practice privileges in physical therapy, the Director of Physical Therapy, or his or her designee, shall be present at CIP meetings. The CIP shall review and recommend approval or denial of the application, then forward it to the Medical Executive Committee.

   d. The Medical Executive Committee's recommendation is then presented to the Board of Trustees for final approval.

   e. The applicant shall be notified in writing as to the approval or denial of his or her request for practice privileges. Individuals whose applications have been denied may have the decision reconsidered by requesting a personal appearance at a regularly scheduled meeting of the CIP.

   f. The CIP reviews the status of all physical therapists with practice privileges biannually and recommends reappointment or denial of continued privileges.

   g. The President of the Medical Staff may grant temporary practice privileges for individual physical therapists.

   h. Assignment: Each physical therapist who is qualified for initial granting of practice privileges shall be assigned to a clinical department appropriate to his or her professional training, and shall be subject to the policies and procedures of that department.

   i. Monitoring requirement: Except as otherwise recommended by the Medical Executive Committee and approved by the Board of Trustees, each physical therapist initially granted practice privileges shall complete a period of monitoring. Monitoring may include direct observation of the therapist's performance and chart review. Each initial appointee shall be assigned a monitor(s) for evaluation of his or her performance. The purpose of the monitoring requirement

——— *Continued* ———

Continued from previous page

is to determine the appointee's eligibility to exercise the practice privileges initially recommended. An initial appointee shall remain subject to monitoring until a favorable recommendation for his or her removal from monitoring is received in writing from his or her Monitor and approved by the CIP, the Medical Executive Committee, and the Board of Trustees.

Term of Monitoring Period: The term of monitoring for initial appointment or modification of privileges shall extend for a minimum period of 6 months and for a minimum number of cases determined by the CIP with input from various Clinical Service Committees as requested.

2. Prerogatives: the prerogatives that may be extended to a physical therapist with practice privileges shall be defined in hospital/departmental policies and procedures. Such prerogatives may include

   a. Provision of specified patient care services consistent with Physical Therapy Department/Hospital policies and procedures; consistent with the practice privileges granted, being full or limited; and within the scope of the physical therapist's licensure or specialized certification, if applicable.

   b. Service on medical staff, department, and hospital committees.

   c. Attendance at the meetings of the department where assigned, and attendance at hospital education programs in his or her special area of practice or at those programs deemed mandatory by the Hospital.

3. Responsibilities: Each physical therapist with practice privileges shall

   a. Meet those responsibilities required by Medical Staff Rules and Regulations, and if not so specified, meet those responsibilities specified in the Medical Staff Bylaws, Section on Membership as generally applicable to the practice of physical therapy.

   b. Retain appropriate responsibility within his or her area of professional competence for the care and supervision of each patient in the Hospital for whom he or she is providing services.

   c. Participate as appropriate in patient care quality review, evaluation, and monitoring activities required of physical therapists; in supervising initial appointees of his or her profession, and in discharging such other functions as may be required from time to time.

   d. Maintain his or her professional competence by pursuing professional development opportunities, which would include, but are not limited to, formal education, seminars, conferences, workshops, self-study, and advanced clinical residencies.

   e. Abide by the Medical Staff Bylaws and Rules and Regulations as they pertain to physical therapists, and all other physical therapy practice standards, departmental policies, and procedures.

   f. Prepare and complete in a timely fashion, the medical and other required records for all patients for which he or she provides services in the hospital.

   g. Abide by the lawful ethical principles of the profession of physical therapy.

   h. Abide by the laws of the State of California, including the California Physical Therapy Act, and the California Business and Professional Code, Section 654.2 (disclosure of ownership interest in a service to which referrals are made).

   i. Work cooperatively with other physical therapists, both institutionally based and those with practice privileges, as well as medical staff members, nurses, and other hospital personnel.

   j. Assist in providing continuing education programs for the physical therapy staff, physicians, nurses, and other hospital personnel.

Figure 20A–2. Practice Privileges for Physical Therapists. (*Reprinted with permission from California Chapter APTA.*)

Medicare Regulations—Conditions for Coverage: Outpatient Physical Therapy Services Furnished By Physical Therapists in Independent Practice

[¶20,698A]

§ 405.1730. Conditions for Coverage—Services Furnished by Physical Therapists in Independent Practice—General.

(a) In order to be covered under the program of health insurance for the aged and disabled as a supplier of outpatient physical therapy services, a physical therapist in independent practice must meet State licensure and requirements set forth in section 1861(p)(4) of the Act, 42 U.S.C. 1395x(p)(4), and other requirements established pursuant to this provision. This section of the law states specific requirements which must be met by such suppliers and authorizes the Secretary of Health, Education, and Welfare to prescribe by regulation other requirements relating to the health and safety of beneficiaries as may be found necessary.

(b) Section 1861(p) provides in pertinent part as follows:

"(p) The term 'outpatient physical therapy services' means physical therapy services furnished by a provider of services, a clinic, rehabilitation agency, or a public health agency, or by others under an arrangement with, and under the supervision of, such provider, clinic, rehabilitation agency, or public health agency to an individual as an outpatient—

* * *

"The term 'outpatient physical therapy services' also includes physical therapy services furnished an individual by a physical therapist (in his office or in such individual's home) who meets licensing and other standards prescribed by the Secretary in regulations, otherwise than under an arrangement with and under the supervision of a provider of services, clinic, rehabilitation agency, or public health agency, if the furnishing of such services meets such conditions relating to health and safety as the Secretary may find necessary"

¶ 20,698A   Reg. § 405.1730

(c) The requirements included in the statute and the additional health and safety requirements prescribed by the Secretary are set forth in the Conditions for Coverage for Outpatient Physical Therapy Services Furnished by Physical Therapists in Independent Practice (see § § 405.1732–405.1737).

.01 Source

As adopted 41 F.R. 20863 (May 21, 1976, effective June 21, 1976); recodified from 20 CFR 405.1730 at 42 F.R. 52826 (Sept. 30, 1977).

[¶20,698B]

§ 405.1731. Definitions Relating to Physical Therapists in Independent Practice

As used in § § 405.1731–405.1737, the following definitions apply:

(a) *Physical therapist.* A person who is licensed as a physical therapist by the State in which he is practicing if the State licenses physical therapists, and—

(1) Has graduated from a physical therapy curriculum approved by the American Physical Therapy Association, or by the Council on Medical Education and Hospitals of the American Medical Association, or jointly by the Council on Medical Education of the American Medical Association and the American Physical Therapy Association, or

(2) prior to January 1, 1966:

(i) Was admitted to membership by the American Physical Therapy Association: or

(ii) Was admitted to registration by the American Registry of Physical Therapists; or

——— *Continued* ———

Continued from previous page

(iii) Has graduated from a physical therapy curriculum in a 4-year college or university approved by a State department of education; or

(3) Has 2 years of appropriate experience as a physical therapist and has achieved a satisfactory grade on a proficiency examination approved by the Secretary except that such determinations of proficiency shall not apply with respect to persons initially licensed by a State after December 31, 1977, or seeking qualifications as a physical therapist after such date; or

(4)(i) Was licensed or registered prior to January 1, 1966; and

(ii) Prior to January 1, 1970, had 15 years of full-time experience in the treatment of illness or injury through the practice of physical therapy in which services were rendered under the order and direction of attending and referring doctors of medicine or osteopathy; or

(5) If trained outside the United States:

(i) Was graduated since 1928 from a physical therapy curriculum approved in the country in which the curriculum was located and in which there is a member organization of the World Confederation for Physical Therapy;

(ii) Meets the requirements for membership in a member organization of the World Confederation for Physical Therapy;

(iii) Has 1 year of experience under the supervision of an active member of the American Physical Therapy Association: and

(iv) Has successfully completed a qualifying examination as prescribed by the American Physical Therapy Association.

(b) *Physical therapist in independent practice:* A person who is licensed as a physical therapist by the State in which he is practicing, meets one of the qualification requirements in paragraph (a) of this section, and furnishes services under the circumstances described in § 405.232(e)(2)(ii).

(c) *Supervision:* The presence, at all times, of a qualified physical therapist when physical therapy services are rendered in the physical therapist's office or in the patient's place of residence.

(d) *Physician.* A person who is—

(1) A doctor of medicine or osteopathy legally authorized to practice medicine and surgery by the State in which he or she performs these functions or actions; or

(2) A doctor of podiatric medicine, but only with respect to the functions which he or she is legally authorized to perform by the State in which he or she performs them.

.01 Source

As adopted, 41 F.R. 20863 (May 21, 1976, effective June 21, 1976); recodified from 20 CFR 405.1731 at 42 F.R. 52826 (Sept. 30, 1977); amended at 53 F.R. 12010 (Apr. 12, 1988, effective May 12, 1988).

[¶ 20,698C]

§ 405.1732. Condition for Coverage—Compliance with Federal, State, and Local Laws

The physical therapist in independent practice and staff, if any, are in compliance with all applicable Federal, State, and local laws and regulations.

(a) *Standard: Licensure of facility.* If any State in which State or applicable local law provides for the licensing of the facility of a physical therapist, such facility is:

(1) Licensed pursuant to such law; or.

(2) If not subject to licensure, is approved (by the agency of such State or locality responsible for licensing) as meeting the standards established for such licensing.

Medicare and Medicaid Guide

(b) *Standard: Licensure or registration of personnel.* The physical therapist in independent practice and staff, if any, are licensed or registered in accordance with applicable laws.

Continued

Continued from previous page

.01 Source:

As adopted, 41 F.R. 20863 (May 21, 1976, effective June 21, 1976); recodified from 20 CFR 405.1732 at 42 F.R. 52826 (Sept. 30, 1977).

[¶ 20,698D]

§ 405.1733. Condition for Coverage—Physician's Direction and Plan of Care

Patients in need of outpatient physical therapy services are accepted for treatment by the physical therapist in independent practice only on the order of a physician who indicates anticipated goals and is responsible for the general medical direction of such services as part of the total care of the patient. For each patient, there is a written plan of care established and periodically reviewed by the physician.

(a) *Standard: Medical findings and physician's orders.* The following is made available to the physical therapist, prior to or at the time of initiation of treatment:

(1) The patient's significant past history,

(2) Diagnosis(es),

(3) Physician's orders,

(4) Rehabilitation goals and potential for their achievement,

(5) Contraindications, if any,

(6) The extent to which the patient is aware of the diagnosis(es) and prognosis, and

(7) Where appropriate, the summary of treatment provided and results achieved during previous periods of physical therapy services or institutionalization.

(b) *Standard: Plan of care.* For each patient there is a written plan of care established by the physician or by the physical therapist who furnishes the services, which indicates anticipated goals and specifies the type, amount, frequency, and duration of physical therapy services. The plan of care and results of treatment are reviewed at least once every 30 days by the attending or other physician and the indicated action is taken.

(c) *Standard: General medical direction.* Patients are seen by a physician at least once every 30 days. General medical direction at appropriate intervals is evident from the clinical record.

(d) *Standard: Notification of physician.* The attending physician is promptly notified of any changes in the patient's condition. If changes are required in the plan of care, such changes are approved by such physician and noted in the clinical record.

Reg. § 405.1733   ¶ 20,698D

(e) *Standard: Indexes.* Clinical records are indexed at least according to name of patient to facilitate acquisition of statistical clinical information and retrieval of records for administrative action.

.01 Source

As adopted, 41 F.R. 20863 (May 21, 1976, effective June 21, 1976); recodified from 20 CFR 405.1736 at 42 F.R. 52826 (Sept. 30, 1977).

[¶ 20,698H]

§ 405.1737. Condition for Coverage—Physical Environment

The physical environment of the office and/or facility of the physical therapist in independent practice affords a functional, sanitary, safe, and comfortable surrounding for patients, personnel, and the public.

(a) *Standard: Building construction.* The construction of the building housing the physical therapy office meets all applicable State and local building, fire, and safety codes.

(b) *Standard: Maintenance of the physical therapy office and equipment.* There is established a written preventive-maintenance program to ensure that equipment is operative and that the physical therapy

Continued

office is clean and orderly. All essential mechanical, electrical, and patient-care equipment is maintained in safe operating condition, and is properly calibrated.

(c) *Standard: Other environmental considerations.* The building housing the physical therapy office is accessible to, and functional for, patients, personnel, and the public. Written effective procedures in aseptic techniques are followed by all personnel and such procedures are reviewed annually, and when necessary, revised.

(d) *Standard: Emergency procedures.* The physical therapist is aware of the possibility of the occurrence of fire and other non-medical emergencies and has documented: (1) A means of providing for safe patient egress from the physical therapy office and the building housing the office, such means being demonstrated by fire exit signs, etc., and (2) Other such provisions necessary to ensure the safety of patients.

.01 Source

As adopted, 41 F.R. 20863 (May 21, 1976, effective June 21, 1976); recodified from 20 CFR 405.1737 at 42 F.R. 52826 (Sept. 30, 1977).

.01 Source

As adopted, 41 F.R. 20863 (May 21, 1976, effective June 21, 1976); recodified from 20 CFR 405.1733 at 42 F.R. 52826 (Sept. 30, 1977); amended at 53 F.R. 12010 (Apr. 12, 1988, effective May 12, 1988).

[¶ 20,698E]

§ 405.1734. Condition for Coverage—Physical Therapy Services

The physical therapist in independent practice provides an adequate program of physical therapy services and has the facilities and equipment necessary to carry out the services offered.

(a) *Standard: Adequate program.* The physical therapist will be considered to have an adequate physical therapy program when services can be provided, utilizing therapeutic exercise and the modalities of heat, cold, water, and electricity; patient evaluations are conducted; and tests and measurements of strength, balance, endurance, range of motion, and activities of daily living are administered.

(b) *Standard: Supervision of physical therapy services.* Physical therapy services are provided by, or under supervision of, a qualified physical therapist.

.01 Source

As adopted, 41 F.R. 20863 (May 21, 1976, effective June 21, 1976); recodified from 20 CFR 405.1734 at 42 F.R. 52826 (Sept. 30, 1977).

[¶ 20,698F]

§ 405.1735. Condition for Coverage—Coordination of Services with Other Organizations, Agencies, or Individuals

The physical therapy services provided by the physical therapist in independent practice are coordinated with the health and medical services provided to the patient by organizations, agencies, or individuals.

(a) *Standard: Exchange of clinical records and reports.* When a patient is receiving or has recently received health and medical services from providers, organizations, physicians, or others that are related to and that may involve the physical therapy program, the physical therapist shall, on a regular basis, exchange with such providers, organizations, physicians, or others in accordance with § 405.1736(a) documented information which has a bearing on the patient's health and welfare so as to ensure that services effectively complement one another.

.01 Source

As adopted, 41 F.R. 20863 (May 21, 1976, effective June 21, 1976); recodified from 20 CFR 405.1735 at 42 F.R. 52826 (Sept. 30, 1977).

——— *Continued* ———

Continued from previous page

¶ 20,698E   Reg. § 405.1734

[¶ 20,698G]

§ 405.1736. Condition for Coverage—Clinical Records

The physical therapist in independent practice maintains clinical records on all patients in accordance with accepted professional standards and practices. The clinical records are completely and accurately documented, readily accessible, and systematically organized to facilitate retrieving and compiling information.

(a) *Standard: Protection of clinical record information.* Clinical record information is recognized as confidential and is safeguarded against loss, destruction, or unauthorized use. Written procedures govern use and removal of records and include conditions for release of information. A patient's written consent is required for release of information not authorized by law.

(b) *Standard: Content.* The clinical *record information.* Clinical record in-record contains sufficient information to identify the patient clearly, to justify the diagnosis(es) and treatment, and to document the results accurately. All clinical records contain the following general categories of data:

(1) Documented evidence of the assessment of the needs of the patient, of an appropriate plan of care, and of the care and services provided,

(2) Identification data and consent forms,

(3) Medical history,

(4) Report of physical examination(s), if any,

(5) Observations and progress notes,

(6) Reports of treatments and clinical findings, and

(7) Discharge summary including final diagnosis(es) and prognosis.

(c) *Standard: Completion of records and centralization of reports.* Current clinical records and those of discharged patients are completed promptly. All clinical information pertaining to a patient is centralized in the patient's clinical record.

(d) *Standard: Retention and preservation.* Clinical records are retained for a period of time not less than:

(1) That determined by the respective State statute or the statute of limitations in the State, or

(2) In the absence of a State statute: (i) 5 years after the date of discharge or, (ii) in the case of a minor, 3 years after the patient becomes of age under State law, or 5 years after the date of discharge, whichever is longer.

Figure 20A–3.   Medicare Regulations. Conditions for Coverage: Outpatient Physical Therapy Services Furnished by Physical Therapists in Independent Practice. (*Reprinted with permission from Commerce Clearing House, Inc., 1998.*)

Foot Care Demonstration Project for Frail, Low-Income Elderly

This project is designed to demonstrate the development, use, and efficacy of a foot care program for low income, frail elders. The focus of the program is several-fold:

1. Preventative education.
2. Screening for identification and treatment of foot disorders before disabling complications occur.
3. Remediation of foot disorders through appropriate home care, education, orthotics, shoes, exercise, or both.
4. Follow-up care for individuals who receive orthoses, shoes, podiatric care, exercise programs, or educational instruction.

The objectives of this program are to improve mobility, function, and quality of life for elders through:

1. Improving foot function.
2. Reducing the incidence of painful feet.
3. Preventing foot dysfunction from producing loss of mobility and independence.

The hypotheses of this demonstration project are that:

1. There is a correlation between foot pain and level of function.
2. There is a significant difference in function with those clients with foot pain/deformity and those without.
3. Specific interventions will result in a decrease of soft tissue abnormalities and pain and an increase in function.

The Foot Care Demonstration Project is carried out by a team, including a physical therapist, podiatrist, orthotist/podiatrist, and social worker. Foot screening, preventive education, intervention and follow-up care is provided to approximately 400 low income, frail elderly individuals in 14 communities located within central Massachusetts.

A data base has been developed describing foot dysfunction, pain, functional ability, and socioeconomic characteristics within the population served. Success of the education and intervention programs will be determined by comparing pain, function, and foot deformity prior to and following 1 year in the Foot Care Program for each client.

This Foot Care Demonstration Project is an outgrowth of a foot care clinic that had been started through Cushing Hospital in January 1986. The Demonstration Project serves to measure the short-term (1 to 2 years) efficacy of this type of intervention in reducing disability, loss of mobility, or hospitalization of elders as a consequence of foot disorders. It will also serve as a basis for a longitudinal study of foot deformities among low income elderly.

Figure 20B–1. Foot Care Demonstration Project for Frail, Low-Income Elderly. (*Reprinted with permission of Jennifer M. Bottomley.*)

A Screening Mechanism to Identify Potential Physical Therapy Geriatric Clients in Institutional Settings

Frequently, for a variety of reasons, patients are not referred to physical therapy. In many instances, there is an inadequate understanding of the physical therapy services available as well as a lack of appreciation for the benefits available to the patient and institution through physical therapy programs.

Informational programs and materials identifying physical therapy services and the skills of physical therapy practitioners are frequently presented to health care practitioners and the community. However, frequently physical therapists do not identify the improved quality of life and cost effectiveness of their services, such as reducing the amount of care and services needed by clients and the prevention of complications as well as further disability.

No formal follow-up was conducted following the program. However, surveys reported using the suggested criteria during survey sessions and found them to be helpful. In Mississippi, state certifying licensure groups were aware of many individuals perceived to need additional service but were unaware of the specific types of patient problems that physical therapists could offer assistance with in the nursing home setting. Furthermore, many of the surveyors felt that more residents should be receiving physical therapy but without guidelines to follow it was difficult to make recommendations with any certainty. However, surveyors had no guidelines for effectively identifying potential patients. So, agency personnel approached a physical therapist requesting an inservice for surveyors. The topic for the meeting was to be "identifying nursing home residents who might benefit from physical therapy services."

The therapist planning the workshop developed the following objectives for the session: (a) describe the professional qualifications and skills of physical therapists; (b) identify quality of life and cost effective outcomes produced through physical therapy; (c) describe problems and diagnoses that frequently require a physical therapy referral and (d) develop an easy mechanism to identify potential physical therapy patients.

To summarize the 2 hour program and provide the participants with a practical, easy to use mechanism for patient identification, a short check list was developed. The surveyors were told that if a patient needed assistance with two or more of the problems listed, had a condition in the diagnostic category, and met onset criteria, a referral for physical therapy evaluation was probably indicated. In addition, they were alerted to check for information on any previous rehabilitation services.

1. Diagnostic Categories: The individual has one or more of the conditions listed:
   a. cerebral vascular accident (i.e., stroke)
   b. fractures
   c. impaired cognitive function or organic brain syndrome (i.e., Alzheimer's)
   d. arthritis
   e. amputation
   f. chronic lung disease
   g. Parkinson's disease
   h. general dehabilitation
   i. cardiovascular problems
   j. postsurgery
   k. cardiovascular disease
2. Onset Criteria: The patient has physical problems:
   a. a recent decrease in mobility skills or activities of daily living
   b. the onset of disease or disability occurred less than 6 months ago
3. Physical Problems: The patient has problems, such as:
   a. muscle weakness in one or both upper and lower extremitiesm
   b. very limited physical endurance

Continued

─── *Continued from previous page* ───

   c. range of motion limitations

   d. diminished sensory function

   e. coordination/balance difficulties

   f. posture

4. Equipment problems: The patient needs assistance with:

   a. self-care activities or using adaptive equipment

   b. learning skills (e.g., one handed skills, wheelchair mobility, ambulation)

   c. adaptive equipment procurement and maintenance

5. Activities of Daily Living Problems: The patient needs to develop and/or practice:

   a. self-care skills

   b. daily living activities

   c. ambulation activities

   d. mobility skills

6. Mental Status Problems: The patient has had a change in:

   a. mental alertness since admission

   b. socialization is limited

7. Previous Rehabilitation Services

   a. what, when, where, response, and discharge status

No formal follow-up was conducted following the program. However, surveys reported using the suggested criteria during survey sessions and found them to be helpful.

Figure 20B–2. Screening Mechanisms in Institutional Settings. (*Reprinted with permission from Greenwald NF. A screening mechanism to identify potential physical therapy geriatric clients in institutional settings. GeriTopics. Winter 1991; 14(1):26.*)

Introductory Letter

Ms. Ann Jones
Mill Vill Retirement Home
South Pond, WY 12345

Dear Ms. Jones:

My name is Carole Smith, and I am interested in talking to you about setting up some very special exercise classes. My background is in physical therapy, and I have worked for more than 10 years with older people. I would like to share some of my expertise with the members of Mill Vill Retirement Home before they need the individualized services of a physical therapist.

My classes are special because they are on different subjects, such as arthritis, back pain, and neck stiffness, to name just a few.

I have enclosed my resumé as well as a list of topics for the exercise group. Please review the information at your leisure. In the meantime, if you have any questions, I can be reached at 555–1212.

I plan to call you to set up a meeting in a week. Thank you for your time.

Sincerely,

Carole Smith, PT

Figure 20C–1. Introduction Letter. (*Reprinted with permission from Carole B. Lewis. Health Promotion and Exercise for Older Adults. Gaithersburg, MD: Aspen Publishers, Inc; 1990.*)

Introductory Phone Call

Hello, Ms. Jones. My name is Carole Smith. I wrote to you about a week ago about the possibility of my conducting an exercise class. I was wondering if you would like to get together and discuss this. What is a good time for you? Good, I look forward to seeing you then.

Figure 20C–2. Introductory Phone Call. *(Reprinted with permission from Carole B. Lewis.* Health Promotion and Exercise for Older Adults. *Gaithersburg, MD: Aspen Publishers, Inc; 1990.)*

Sample Visit

Hi, Ms. Jones. I'm Carole Smith. [Make small talk here; discuss the weather, how nice the facility is.] Did you have a chance to look over the material I sent you? [If not, have an extra copy to give her, and discuss the topics.] Do you think this program would be a welcome addition at Mill Vill? Are you interested? I would like to start doing the class on a weekly basis and see how well it is received. My fee is $100 per class. Is that agreeable to you? Good. I have a contract that I brought to protect both of us. If you will sign it, I can begin in 3 weeks. In the meantime, I have a letter to your residents to introduce me and get their ideas. If you could pass these out, I will be back in a week to get the responses. Then, 1 week before class, I will come around with flyers announcing the class.

Figure 20C–3. Sample Visit. *(Reprinted with permission from Carole B. Lewis.* Health Promotion and Exercise for Older Adults. *Gaithersburg, MD: Aspen Publishers, Inc; 1990.)*

Topic List for Classes

- Fancy footwork
- Lavish legs
- Knowledgeable knees
- Happy hips
- Better backs
- Nice necks
- Supple shoulders
- Agile arms
- Wonderful wrists
- Hardy hands and flexible fingers
- Improving balance
- Realizing relaxation
- Abatable arthritis
- Preventing Parkinson's problems

- Opposing osteoporosis
- Perfect posture
- Getting stronger
- Better breathing
- Stopping stroke
- Ways to walk
- Facts on flexibility
- Correcting coordination
- Understanding aerobics
- All about Alzheimer's disease
- Achieving perfect body weight
- Exercising facial muscles
- Hidden exercises

Figure 20C–4. Topic List for Classes. *(Reprinted with permission from Carole B. Lewis.* Health Promotion and Exercise for Older Adults. *Gaithersburg, MD: Aspen Publishers, Inc; 1990.)*

Sample Contract

I, _____ contract with _____

_____ to provide a _____ exercise/discussion
(frequency)
class on various topics.

I agree to bring handouts and cassette tapes. _____ agrees to provide <u>chairs, stereo,</u>

<u>and batons</u> as well as <u>$100.00</u> (one hundred dollars) per class to be paid within 2 weeks of the class.

This contract can be terminated with 30 days' notice by either party.

_____   _____
Date   Signature

_____   _____
Date   Signature

Note: An attorney can suggest additions and variations of this sample agreement and should be consulted regarding the full implications of any contractual commitments.

Figure 20C–5.   Sample Contract. *(Reprinted with permission from Carole B. Lewis.* Health Promotion and Exercise for Older Adults. *Gaithersburg, MD: Aspen Publishers, Inc; 1990.)*

Sample Letter to Potential Class Members

Dear Mill Vill Residents:

Allow me to introduce myself. My name is Carole Smith and I am a physical therapist with 10 years' experience. My specialty is the bone and muscle problems of older people.

On Monday, June 18, from 11:00 to 12:00, I will be leading an exercise class and a brief discussion of osteoporosis. I will be returning to conduct other discussions as well and would like you to help me determine which ones would be of interest to you. Please check those of interest and add any others. Thank you in advance for your help.

See you in exercise class soon!

Sincerely,

Carole Smith, PT

Please fill out and return to the front desk.

TOPICS

☐ Arthritis   ☐ Increasing Flexibility

☐ Posture   ☐ Getting Stronger

☐ Neck Pain   ☐ Aerobics—Pros and Cons

☐ Relieving Back Pain   ☐ Stress Management

☐ Fixing Shoulder Problems   ☐ Walking Programs

☐ All about Knees   ☐ Exercises for You

☐ Feet Work   ☐ Helping Hands

☐ Improving Balance   ☐ Better Breathing

☐ Correct Coordination   ☐ Hidden Exercises

☐ Walking Better   ☐ _____

Figure 20C–6.   Sample Letter to Potential Class Members. (*Reprinted with permission from Carole B. Lewis.* Health Promotion and Exercise for Older Adults. *Gaithersburg, MD: Aspen Publishers, Inc; 1990.*)

Sample Flyer

OSTEOPOROSIS CLASS

11:00–12:00

Monday, June 18th
in the
Dining Room

MEET

Carole Smith, Physical Therapist

LISTEN, LEARN, & EXERCISE

for Osteoporosis

and

HAVE FUN DOING IT!

Figure 20C–7. Sample Flyer. *(Reprinted with permission from Carole B. Lewis.* Health Promotion and Exercise for Older Adults. *Gaithersburg, MD: Aspen Publishers, Inc; 1990.)*

Participant Consent Form

I understand that the purpose of this (project or program) is to enhance my health-fitness status.

I verify that my participation is fully voluntary, and no coercion of any sort has been used to obtain my participation.

I understand that I may withdraw from the (project or program) without prejudice or malice at any time during the involved period or session.

I have been informed of the procedures and methods that will be used in the (project or program) and understand what will be necessary for me as a participant.

I understand that my participation will remain anonymous unless expressed name permission is given by me.

Signed: _____

Date: _____

Figure 20C–8. Participant Consent Form. *(Reprinted with permission from Carole B. Lewis.* Health Promotion and Exercise for Older Adults. *Gaithersburg, MD: Aspen Publishers, Inc; 1990.)*

Medical Release Form

_____ has my permission to participate in a physical exercise program to be given at _____ . I understand that this course consists of gentle stretching and strengthening programs of a mild exercise performance level. I have listed below any problems that the health professional leading this class should be aware of and that may affect this patient's performance in the class.

Name of Physician _____

Diagnosis _____

Limitation _____

Areas To Emphasize _____

Medications _____
_____

Figure 20C–9. Medical Release Form. (_Reprinted with permission from Carole B. Lewis._ Health Promotion and Exercise for Older Adults. _Gaithersburg, MD: Aspen Publishers, Inc; 1990._)

Physical Activity Profile

Name: _____

Date: _____

We would like to know more about you in order to improve our fitness program and meet your individual needs. Please fill in the following:

1. What was/is the nature of your employment (e.g., manufacturing, sales, teacher)? _____

Year of retirement, if applicable: _____

2. How would you rate the physical activity you perform/performed at work? (Check one)

_____ little (sitting, typing, driving, talking)
_____ moderate (standing, walking, bending, reaching)
_____ active (light physical work, climbing stairs)
_____ very active (moderate and physical work, lifting)

3. My physical activity during the "working hours" of the day has:
_____ stayed the same   _____ decreased   _____ increased

4. What physical and recreational activities are you presently involved in (e.g., dancing, swimming, walking, bowling)? _____
_____ How often? _____

5. My goal(s) for joining a fitness program is:

_____ to lose body fat
_____ because my doctor advised me to

_____ to stay active
_____ because I am concerned
       about my health (e.g.,
       blood pressure, arthritis,
       bad back)

6. Check the activity you participate in and place the appropriate category next to the activity:

1 if total time spent is less than 15 minutes (3 times/day)

2 if total time spent is at least 20 minutes (3 times/week)

3 if activity is sustained for more than 20 minutes (3 times/week)

_____ walking   _____ swimming   _____ golf
_____ jogging   _____ dancing   _____ other _____

Figure 20C–10.   Physical Activity Profile. (*Reprinted with permission from Carole B. Lewis.* Health Promotion and Exercise for Older Adults. *Gaithersburg, MD: Aspen Publishers, Inc; 1990.*)

Medical History Form

Name: _____ Date: _____

1. Have you any medical complaints at present (i.e., lower back pain, arthritis, neck pain, hypertension, diabetes, cardiovascular problems, etc.)? _____
_____

2. What major illnesses required hospitalization (give dates)? _____
_____

3. Smoking status (circle one):
   a. never smoked   b. smoke now   c. smoked in past, not now

4. History of cardiovascular disease:
   NO   YES   Personal, if so, what _____
   _____
   NO   YES   Family history, if so, what _____
   _____
   NO   YES   Other _____
   NO   YES   Other _____

5. (Muscular history) Present or previous injury?
   a. NO   b. YES
   c. If yes, specify: _____

6. (Bone-joint history) present or previous bone or joint disease?
   a. NO   b. YES
   c. If yes, specify: _____

7. Check off each of the following ailments that apply to you:
   _____ Frequent dizziness   Hernia _____   Diabetes _____
   _____ Physical impairments, if any, specify: _____
   _____

8. On the average, how many times do you visit your physician each year?
   _____

9. How many times do you take medication each day? What types of medications are they? _____
   _____

10. Do you have any limitations not mentioned previously that will place limitations on complete participation in the fitness program? _____
   _____

Figure 20C–11.   Medical History Form. *(Reprinted with permission from Carole B. Lewis.* Health Promotion and Exercise for Older Adults. *Gaithersburg, MD: Aspen Publishers, Inc; 1990.)*

Sample Class Invitation

Posture tells people a lot about you. Good posture also helps your body function better.

Posture exercises are easy to learn so join us to find out about . . .

PERFECT POSTURE

at:

_____

on:

_____

in:

_____

Taught by: _____

LISTEN, LEARN, AND EXERCISE!

PERFECT POSTURE

Figure 20C–12. Sample Class Invitation. *(Reprinted with permission from Carole B. Lewis. Health Promotion and Exercise for Older Adults. Gaithersburg, MD: Aspen Publishers, Inc; 1990.)*

Sample Class Outline

PERFECT POSTURE

Lecture/Discussion

Posture tells people a lot about you. Posture affects how you look, obviously; standing with your head in a very forward position makes you look sort of unhappy and depressed, while standing in a very chin-tucked, upright position makes you much more attractive. Good posture can also enhance your musculoskeletal and your cardiopulmonary functioning. For example, try this: stick your head way forward as far as you can (*demonstrate*), take a deep breath, and blow it out. Now, sit back in your chair, pull your head up as high as you can, and take a nice deep breath. Notice that you can take a much bigger breath when you head is back in the chin-tuck position. So, posture is extremely important not only for physical attractiveness, but also for physical functioning.

Good posture can be looked at from either the side or the front. From the side, if you have good posture, you can draw a straight line from your ear, through your shoulder, knee, and ankle. Take a look at my posture. Then stand up, and take a quick look at the posture of the other members of the class (*go around to all the participants, giving quick little hints to people if they have a forward head, rounded shoulders, or bend in their knees; try to be positive, but try to give good useful feedback*).

You can assess posture from the front or the back, too. People often have asymmetries. One shoulder may be higher; one hip may be higher. Such as asymmetry may cause problems. There may be a tightness or soreness in the higher shoulder. A higher hip may cause tightness in the back area as well. So again, stand up, and let me take a look at your posture (*again, go around the room and give individual feedback*).

Good posture is also needed when you are sitting down. For this, you need to support yourself with the back of a chair, behind your low back, and behind your upper back area. So let's all sit back with good posture (*watch the participants, and give feedback to them*).

Try and become aware of your posture, and know when your posture is good. Do not take posture for granted. You really need to work on posture all the time. Put dots around your house or apartment, and every time you see a dot think to yourself that you need to tuck your chin in or pull your shoulders back. I will give you a hand-out before you leave today with some other reminders (*Figure 19C–14; read aloud and discuss, if desired.*) Now we are going to go on to posture exercises.

Exercises

1. Deep breaths. Do three times.
2. Turtle. Push head forward in an exaggerated motion, then pull back. Do three times.
3. Chin tucks. Do three times.
4. Head motions. Do three times each.
   (a) Forward
   (b) Backward
   (c) Side to side
   (d) Over each shoulder
5. Shoulder shrugs. Do three times.
6. Shoulder circles. Do three times.
7. Shoulder backs. Pull your shoulder blades back. Do three times.
8. Arm reaches up. Reach as high as you can to the sky. Do three times.
9. Arm reaches back. Reach as far backward as possible. Do three times.
10. Side tilts. Do three times.
11. Pelvic tucks. Do three times.
12. Gluteal sets. Tighten your buttock muscles as tight as you can. Do three times.
13. Knee ups. Bend your knees up to the ceiling. Alternate knees. Do three times.
14. Knee outs. Let your knees flop outward. Do three times.
15. Knee twists. Turn your knees inward. Do three times.
16. Ankle bends. Do three times.
17. Ankle circles. Do three times.
18. Toe curls. Do five times.
19. Spine lengtheners. As you take a deep breath, imagine your spine extending from your hips to the top of your head. Do three times.
20. Body extenders. Gently pull your spine into extension. Do three times.

Figure 20C–13. Sample Class Outline. (*Reprinted with permission from Carole B. Lewis.* Health Promotion and Exercise for Older Adults. *Gaithersburg, MD: Aspen Publishers, Inc; 1990.*)

Perfect Posture Handout

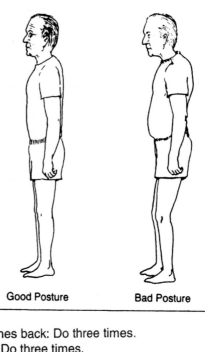

Good Posture   Bad Posture

Dos

1. Tuck in your chin.
2. Pull your shoulders back as much as you can.
3. Try to keep your ear over your shoulders, over your hips, over your ankles.
4. When sitting, support your back and legs as much as possible.
5. Think lengthening.
6. Try to sleep in a position that optimizes good posture and flexibility of muscles.
7. Be aware of your posture as much as possible.

Don'ts

1. Do not sit in one position too long.
2. Do not stand in one position too long.

Exercises

1. Deep breaths: Do three times.
2. Turtle: Do three times.
3. Chin tucks: Do three times.
4. Head motions: Do three times each.
   a. Forward
   b. Backward
   c. Side to side
   d. Over each shoulder
5. Shoulder shrugs: Do three times.
6. Shoulder circles: Do three times.
7. Shoulder backs: Do three times.
8. Arm reaches up: Do three times.
9. Arm reaches back: Do three times.
10. Side tilts: Do three times.
11. Pelvic tucks: Do three times.
12. Gluteal sets: Do three times.
13. Knee ups: Do three times.
14. Knee outs: Do three times.
15. Knee twists: Do three times.
16. Ankle bends: Do three times.
17. Ankle circles: Do three times.
18. Toe curls: Do five times.
19. Spine lengtheners: Do three times.
20. Body extenders: Do three times.

Figure 20C–14.   Perfect Posture Handout. *(Reprinted with permission from Carole B. Lewis. Health Promotion and Exercise for Older Adults. Gaithersburg, MD: Aspen Publishers, Inc; 1990.)*

HOSPITALS' RFP GUIDE: CONTRACTING OUT INPATIENT AND OUTPATIENT PHYSICAL THERAPY

by Jerome B. Connolly, PT

Member of the Executive Committee of the American Physical Therapy Association & Past Chairman of the Montana Board of Physical Therapy Examiners

SCORING SCALE: Rank each proposal on the criteria below and total section scores on the heavy line in front of the section heading.
0 = Not Available
1 = Would Try
2 = Limited Experience
3 = Experienced
4 = Expert

Introduction

With physical therapists and other health professionals in short supply, more hospitals are turning to experienced physical therapists with entrepreneurial skills to manage, market, and maintain high quality, productive departments. Included here are the key factors to consider when contracting for physical therapy services.

1. CONTROL

1.1 The contract stipulates that ultimate control remain with the hospital. The physical therapy services must comply with existing hospital policy.

1.2 The physical therapy department policy and procedure manual development and maintenance is the responsibility of the physical therapy (PT) contractor, but is subject to the approval of the hospital governing board and administrator.

2. INCOME

2.1 The hospital should be able to derive attractive income from the PT services

2.2 while simultaneously divesting itself of the profit-eating expenses of personnel recruitment, retention, benefits, turnover, sick leave, vacation coverage,

2.3 equipment acquisition, and

2.4 continuing professional education Moreover, a long-term commitment to a contract PT service develops a more consistent service, greater market share,

Developed by First Physical Therapy, PC, Billings, MT.

more respect and recognition in the community and a more satisfied medical staff

3. EXPERIENCE

3.1 Experience in PT evaluation and treatment,

3.2 practice management,

3.3 marketing, and promotion are at the top of the list when it comes to selecting the contractor. Experienced PTs with proven track records who can develop programs based on need and drawing from their own experience in such programs are essential for success of this kind of arrangement. The physical therapy contractor must be able to relate professionally to referring physicians, earn respect, and develop rapport.

4. QUALITY

Physical therapy patient care should be of the highest quality with an emphasis placed on

4.1 comprehensive, objective patient evaluation,

4.2 thorough treatment planning and implementation,

4.3 demonstration of progress through reevaluation measures, and

4.4 prompt, complete documentation from intake to discharge. Cooperative interdisciplinary approaches are to be used as appropriate and

4.5 timely communication with all necessary parties is essential.

5. INFORMATION NETWORKS

5.1 Physical therapists who are active in their state and national professional association matters (*The American Physical Therapy Association*) have at their disposal the most recent information in the field.

5.2 They also develop nationwide networks that prove valuable. Physical therapists who have a high profile in the APTA can more easily attract and recruit qualified and dedicated professionals.

5.3 Experience on a State Board of Physical Therapy Examiners is highly desirable.

— **Continued** —

Continued from previous page

_____ **6. Personnel**
_____ 6.1 Recruitment and retention of qualified dedicated, professional, and support staff
_____ 6.2 Payroll, benefits,
_____ 6.3 performance evaluations,
_____ 6.4 staff motivation, communication, and
_____ 6.5 professional development (continuing education).
_____ 6.6 Scheduling of staff including providing adequate relief for vacation, sick, and professional development leave.

_____ **7. Equipment**
_____ 7.1 While maintenance of the hospital's existing equipment in optimal functional condition should remain the responsibility of the hospital,
_____ 7.2 any new equipment acquired should be acquired and maintained by the contractor.
_____ 7.3 New equipment should be acquired promptly as needed to remain competitive and progressive.

_____ **8. Contract Development**
_____ 8.1 Development of the contract language should be accomplished by the PT contractor and be subject to approval of the hospital administrator, governing board, and attorneys. This puts the bulk of the legal expenses in drafting the contract on the contractor rather than the hospital.

_____ **9. Administration**
_____ 9.1 Recruitment and retention of qualified staff.
_____ 9.2 Staffing department for existing and developing need.
_____ 9.3 Scheduling patients on a prompt and timely basis.
_____ 9.3 Fiscal analysis and reporting to hospital administrator.
_____ 9.4 Submission of complete month-end reports to hospital administration.
_____ 9.5 Oversight of complete, timely, and accurate PT documentation.
_____ 9.6 Arrange and comply with fiscal relationship established with hospital (*rent, fee for service, percentage of revenue, etc.*).

_____ **10. Marketing**
_____ 10.1 Determination of existing, emerging, and future needs.
_____ 10.2 Planning to meet identified needs.

_____ 10.3 Assessing satisfaction of referral source.
_____ 10.4 Development of a market-driven service.
_____ 10.5 Program and protocol development. Secure necessary approval of programs and protocols developed.

_____ **11. Strategic Planning**
_____ 11.1 Creation of a mission statement for the service consistent with that of the hospital.
_____ 11.2 Development of an environmental statement as it affects the provision of physical therapy in the area.
_____ 11.3 Development of 1 year specific objectives supplemented by an action plan to accomplish the objectives.
_____ 11.4 Development of a 3 to 5 year long-range plan to include new market niches.
_____ 11.5 Development of an ongoing action plan, regular activities essential to the ongoing operation of a progressive physical therapy service.

_____ **12. Physician Relations**
The contractor should be able to successfully establish and maintain a strong rapport with the medical staff.
_____ 12.1 Evidence of this capability should be demonstrable.
_____ 12.2 Physician references should be provided.

_____ **13. Quality Assurance**
_____ 13.1 Through chart and program review and
_____ 13.2 in-house professional development sessions, high quality standards are promoted and achieved. Cooperation with other hospital departments is essential to this.

_____ **14. Risk Management and Professional Liability**
_____ 14.1 Through an organized and concerted awareness program the professional and support staff should be sensitized to the latest malpractice trends and risks confronting physical therapy. This is the responsibility of the PT contractor in addition to
_____ 14.2 providing proof of insurance at $1 million/$3 million levels and naming the hospital as an additional insured.

Continued

———————— *Continued from previous page* ————————

15. Community Involvement
The physical therapist contractor and staff should have a commitment to the community.
_____ 15.1 Periodic talks, presentations,
_____ 15.2 events,
_____ 15.3 articles, and the like are all part of the quality service that demonstrates the hospital's commitment to the community in terms of prevention and wellness as well as treatment. This is also an effective component of marketing the hospital's PT services and programs.

16. Injury Prevention Programs
The PT contractor should be willing to participate in the hospital's employee orientation program as well as showing a commitment to employee health and
_____ 16.1 well-being by providing back and sports injury prevention programs.
_____ 16.2 Similar programs should be offered to the community and to local and regional business and industry.

17. Program Development
Through frequent and close interaction with the medical staff and consumers the PT contractor should develop
_____ 17.1 programs and services to meet the needs as identified, and
_____ 17.2 should demonstrate the ability to successfully sell and implement these programs.

18. Professional Development and Continuing Education
A significant emphasis should be placed on the continuing professional development of the staff. This should be demonstrated by the contractor through
_____ 18.1 in-house as well as
_____ 18.2 external, formal programs that keep the professionals current in the field.
_____ 18.3 The emphasis must be provided by the PT contractor by whom the cost is borne and the example set.

TOTAL

For more information about contracting for physical therapy services, call Jerry Connolly at First Physical Therapy.

Figure 20D–1A. A Guide for Contracting Out Inpatient and Outpatient Physical Therapy.

SCORING GUIDE

Interpreting the scores and comparing them must of course take into account the size and type of your facility.

After assigning a point rating of 0–4 to each factor (i.e., factor 2.2 received a "3"), add all of the factors up for each section to give an overall score for that area (i.e., Risk Management scored a "7"). Then add all the section scores together for an overall ranking of the proposal. If you use all of the sections, which we recommend, there are 236 points possible on the 59 questions. A minimum threshold score should be no lower than 130. If the potential contractor scores in that range, proceed with caution as their inadequacies and inexperience could well negate most of the benefits of contracting physical therapy services outside the staff. A "C+" score or 2.5 avg. would be 150 points. If some of these sections are deemed by you to be areas already handled elsewhere in the hospital or infeasible for your operation, eliminate the section(s) from the scoring.

If you would like further assistance in this area, First Physical Therapy can develop your facilities' RFP, distribute it, screen and score applicants, and even develop and negotiate the contract for the selected Physical Therapy provider. Simply call us to discuss the possibilities.

Figure 20D–1B. A Guide for Contracting Out Inpatient and Outpatient Physical Therapy: Scoring The Proposals Guide.

Consulting Services Offered by First Physical Therapy for Hospital & Nursing Home Physical Therapy Departments

Whether you are starting, upgrading, fine-tuning, or just evaluating your physical therapy service, First Physical Therapy's wealth of experience in a variety of physical therapy settings and arrangements can assist you in identifying and achieving your goals for your physical therapy services.

Do You Face These Now Common Problems in Physical Therapy Departments?

1. High Staff Turnover
   - Continuous recruiting efforts that result in uneven compensation packages that sap morale.
   - Recent graduates forced into management roles.
   - Difficulty in maintaining the high quality standards that the hospital or nursing home stands for.
   - Staffing unresponsive to physicians' demands and needs.
   - The high cost of traveling PTs/locum tenems (*avg. $320/day*, $83–91,500/yr).
2. Loss of faith in the department by physicians.
3. Underperforming profit center.
4. Inability of the department to contribute fully to the hospital's overall mission.
5. Inattentiveness to equipment maintenance.
6. Loss of continuity and an inability to develop a proactive, market-driven department.
7. A department that is not as responsive as desired to physician demand.

Our Professional Experience

The principals of First Physical Therapy have cumulative experience in excess of 50 years. This has been earned in a multitude of settings, including hospitals, long-term care facilities, home care, outpatient centers, school systems, industry, work-hardening, wellness programs, health clubs, and others. Moreover, the firm currently operates three outpatient clinics and provides physical therapy as a contractor to five nursing homes and hospitals in Montana.

How can First Physical Therapy directly help your hospital or nursing home?

1. Assessment and planning of your physical plant.
2. Identification of local market needs.
3. Determination of local market size for supporting PT services.
4. Competitor analysis.
5. Differentiation of your services from competitors.
6. Other market research.
7. Analysis of current operations' practices and effectiveness.
8. Staff performance assessment.
9. Environmental statement development.
10. Strategic planning.
11. Professional development of current staff.
12. Recruitment strategies.
13. Contract review or development.
14. Equipment needs and use assessment.
15. Physician relations enhancement.
16. Risk management and professional liability analysis.
17. Injury prevention and wellness consulting.
18. Productivity analysis
19. Environmental analysis and forecasting.
20. Marketing and public relations assistance.
21. Department oversight or management.
22. Reimbursement analysis-cash flow.

Continued

Continued from previous page

Examples of Program and Protocol Development of Particular Interest to Hospitals

- Industrial physical therapy.
- Temporomandibular joint (TMJ) protocols
- Sports physical therapy.
- Injury prevention programs.
- Risk management.
- Quality assurance.
- Documentation for optimal reimbursement.
- Customer service practices.
- Dealing with managed care/PT-managed care.
- Work-hardening programs.

Nonbillable time
PHASE I:
Information Gathering
Preliminary Assessment
Scope of Services Defined
Time/Expense Estimate

Billable time
PHASE II:
Assignment Definition
Methodology Selection
Goal & Results Targeted

PHASE III:
Work Plan & Timeline
Implementation
Analyze Findings
Draw Conclusions

PHASE IV:
Report of Findings & Documentation
Formal Presentation

PHASE V:
Oversee Implementation of Recommendations
Conduct Training
Evaluate Outcome
Followup as Appropriate

WHY USE A CONSULTANT WITH YOUR CURRENT PHYSICAL THERAPY DEPARTMENT?

Experience: With over half a century in cumulative PT experience there is little we haven't seen. We offer specialized service management from the perspective of these many years of experience.

Efficiency: Because we are specialized and extensively involved in the profession of physical therapy we have resources at our disposal that allow us to perform an assignment better, faster, and more thoroughly than clients can on their own.

Concentration: We can focus on accomplishing a critical assignment quickly, our clients are free to operate the ongoing services without diversions.

Continued

───── *Continued from previous page* ─────

Confidentiality: We are an independent physical therapist-owned private firm. We do not reveal the identity or purpose of our clients except when permitted to do so. We will not reveal critical information without prior approval.

Objectivity: We can offer a fresh viewpoint, unencumbered by hierarchical pressure, traditions, bias, or conflict of interest. If we are unable to help, we will refer the client to other appropriate resources.

Client Relationships and Billing

Work is carried out in a manner that best satisfies the client. This can be accomplished on an hourly basis or on a retainer for a stipulated period or even as a single project assignment. Itemized billing of time, materials, and expenses will be provided on a monthly basis. Invoices are due payable within 10 days of receipt.

There is no charge for Phase I consulting services. The plan developed is converted to contractual language by FPT and is subject to the approval of the hospital administrator or governing board before implementation.

To discuss your specific needs, contact Lorin Wright or Jerry Connolly at First Physical Therapy.

Figure 20D–2. Consulting Services Offered by First Physical Therapy for Hospital & Nursing Home Physical Therapy Departments.

CHAPTER 21

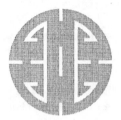

Scientific Inquiry
and Research in Geriatric Therapy

Competency in the area of geriatric physical and occupational therapy would not be complete without
an understanding of research. Evidence-based practice is critical in providing the highest quality of rehabilitative care. The necessity of evaluating current
treatment methods to document efficacy and effectiveness is important not only from a reimbursement
perspective, but assists us in looking to the future for
the most successful means of providing therapy interventions and care.

This chapter will discuss methods of evaluating
research in general and will examine problems with
rehabilitation and aging research in particular. It will
also discuss measurement issues often encountered
in qualitative and quantitative research, and will address research design and outcome measurement in
the clinical setting. The final section of this chapter is
intended to show how to do research and how to
apply research findings in the daily clinical practice
of physical therapy.

CRITICAL INQUIRY

Critical inquiry is something that therapists do routinely at each step of patient/client management.
Daily, the therapist considers possible outcomes such
as the remediation of functional limitations and disability, optimization of patient/ client satisfaction, and
primary or secondary prevention. Critical inquiry is research. The therapist working in geriatric settings en-
gages in outcomes data collection and analysis, the
systematic review of outcomes of care in relation to selected variables (e.g., age, gender, diagnosis, interventions performed, etc), and develops statistical reports
for internal or external use. So, whether the therapist
realizes it or not, they are collecting data, they are making observations, on a small-scale basis—they are
doing research. "Critical inquiry is the process of applying the principles of scientific methods to read and
interpret professional literature; participate in, plan,
and conduct research, evaluate outcomes; and assess

new concepts and technologies."[1] Examples of critical inquiry activities in which therapists engage include:

- Analyzing and applying research finding to therapy practice and education;
- Disseminating the results of research;
- Evaluating the efficacy and effectiveness of both new and established interventions and technologies;
- Participating in, planning, and conduction of clinical, basic, or applied research.[1]

HOW TO ANALYZE RESEARCH ARTICLES

Research articles contain several general elements.[2-4] Most articles start with an abstract, which is a concise paragraph summarizing the primary purpose of the study, methods used in the research project, results, and conclusions drawn from the investigation.[5] The abstract should also state the relevance of the article to clinical practice. Frequently, an abstract can be read to save time and to note results. If the clinician is interested in delving deeper into the topic and wants to more critically evaluate the conclusions reached by the researcher, the entire article should be examined.

The next part of the research article is the introduction, which contains several elements:

1. The problem statement
2. The literature review
3. The purpose of the study
4. The type of study
5. The expected results
6. The research question (null hypothesis)[2-5]

The most important aspect of the introduction is clarity. Did the author clearly state the purpose, type of study, expected results, and research question? The literature reviewed must be complete and exhaustive, and it should note any gaps in the literature that have been idenitified.[5]

The method section provides the reader with specifics as to how the study was conducted. This section should describe the subjects in detail as to their characteristics in regard to age, sex, and diagnosis, and it should describe sample size and the method of selection of the sample. Any instrument used in the study should be described in terms of validity and reliability, and the procedures used should be described in detail so that the reader could replicate the study.

The next section of the article is results and data analysis, which should provide in detail the method of statistical data analysis and applicability to the particular study. In the description of data analysis p-values must be presented. The results section should clearly describe the results generated from the study and define their practical and statistical significance.

The discussion section provides more interpretive information as compared to the results to the results and methods sections. In this part, the author is

defining in greater detail accepted or rejected results of the hypothesis and any weakness in the experimental design. Here the author can further discuss any relevant literature that may apply to the study results. The authors' opinions on how these relate to the research finding can be stated. The conclusion section briefly states the results that should flow logically from the remainder of the article. Table 21–1 outlines these guidelines for assessment of research articles and can assist a clinician by providing more information on evaluating research.

HOW TO SELECT RESEARCH ARTICLES

The volume of research published monthly is often overwhelming. How do you assess research articles for their importance in providing the information that

TABLE 21–1. GUIDELINES FOR EVALUATING A RESEARCH ARTICLE

Introduction
Is problem clearly stated?
Is literature review complete?
Do authors identify a gap in the literature?
Is purpose clearly stated?
Is expectation or hypothesis identified, if indicated?

Methods
Are subjects well described?
How was sample selected?
How large is the sample?
Is a control group used?
Is the instrumentation well described?
Are measuring instruments valid and reliable?
Is the procedure well described?
Could you replicate the study?
Does the design have internal validity?
Is data analysis well described?
What questions are addressed by each test?
Is the analysis appropriate to the question and to the data?
What p-value was used, if indicated?

Results
Are results presented clearly?
Are results statistically significant?
Are results practically significant?

Discussion
Clarifies if hypothesis was accepted or rejected?
Clarifies if results were as expected?
Do authors identify weaknesses in the experimental design?
Is further literature cited to expand on unexpected findings?
Are results applied to clinical practice?
Are suggestions for further study presented?

Conclusions
Are results restated briefly?
Do conclusions follow logically from the results?

Reprinted with permission from Domholdt E, Malone T. Evaluating research literature: the educated clinician. *Phys Ther.* 1965; 65(4): 487–491.

you need related to advances in clinical practice, new assessment tools, new insights into critical clinical pathways and prognosis, breakthroughs in understanding the etiology of disease, and therapeutic improvements? Thompson[6] provides some straightforward strategies for determining whether or not reading a research article is worth your investment of time. She identifies five steps for assessing whether an article is worth reading.

1. Look at the title. Is it potentially interesting or possibly useful in your clinical practice?
2. Review the authors' credentials. What is their track record for careful, thoughtful work? Has their research stood the test of time?
3. Read the abstract. Does the research design and results of the study draw your interest? Would reading this article be important to your clinical practice?
4. Consider the site or clinic that the research was done in. Is the site sufficiently similar to your own so that the research results would be applicable in your setting?
5. Ask the question: does the study focus on what therapists actually do?[6]

If you've answered yes to these questions, you'll probably want to delve deeper into the article. In critically evaluating the research for efficacy, reliability, and validity as you read the article in its entirety, determine the following:[6]

1. Was the assignment of patients/clients to treatment randomized?
2. Were all clinically relevant outcomes reported?
3. Were the patients/clients in the study recognizably similar to the patients/clients in your own clinical setting?
4. Were both clinical and statistical significance considered?
5. Is the therapeutic treatment feasible in your practice?
6. Were all patients/clients who entered the study accounted for at its conclusion?

By following these simple suggestions it will help the busy therapist afford time for the proper evaluation of a subset of clinical literature most likely to yield valid, useful new knowledge that is applicable to your clinical practice.[6]

PROBLEMS WITH REHABILITATION RESEARCH

Before discussing the problems of aging research, it is imperative to look at the difficulties that might be encountered in the area of rehabilitation research. Cicely Partridge[7] did an excellent job of describing research guidelines for physical therapists, and her text developed stages of the research project.[7] Figure 21–1 provides an example of her checklist for following the various stages of research. This can be very

helpful to the therapist in getting started on a research project. In addition, she cites many obstacles that may occur in the rehabilitation setting, making it more difficult for physical therapist to achieve research in this environment:[7]

1. Finding an appropriate question in the research environment;
2. Finding a population that can tolerate research in various rehabilitation techniques;
3. Finding literature to support the research hypothesis;
4. The physical therapists' knowledge of the research process;
5. Availability of funding, and financing facilities;
6. Time to conduct research;
7. Cost of research;
8. Cooperation of the patients/clients to undergo the rigors of the rehabilitation process as well as the study;
9. Availability of subjects that meet specific criteria for the research project;
10. Familiarity with coding and statistically analyzing data;
11. Ethics:
    - Is it ethical to withhold treatment from various subjects for the sake of research?
    - Is it ethical to go through patients'/clients' records?
    - What are the ethical limits of informing patients/clients of the results of the research?
    - Is it ethical to withhold the new therapy from the control group and cause the possible loss of therapeutic benefit?
    - Is it ethical to withhold the standard therapy from the experimental group, again with possible loss of therapeutic benefit?
    - Is it ethical to ask the experimental group to receive a new, unproven therapy, which may have side effects as yet unknown?[8]

PROBLEMS WITH AGING RESEARCH

The problems with aging research are quite numerous, ranging from sampling and subject recruitment to cross-sectional design. In the area of sampling, the article by Wayne et al.[9] showed that people in cross-sectional samples tended to have longer nursing home stays, as well as less social support and more behavioral and functional problems than persons in the admissions sample, who tended to have shorter stays and more acute medical problems. Therefore, looking at a cross-sectional sample could skew the results of research findings. When conducting research in a nursing home, it is imperative to look at the samples chosen to control for the particular and cultural problems already listed.[9]

Research guidelines: A handbook for therapists

	Yes	No	Not applicable

1. Asking questions, developing ideas
   Reading the literature
   Defining the research question
   Statement of objectives for the study, or producing a
   hypothesis for testing			

2. Deciding on appropriate research design
   Organization and approaches to field work
   Writing the research proposal
   Applying to grant-awarding bodies
   Ethical committees or other bodies concerned with the use
   of human subjects			

3. Considering methods of collecting information
   Preparing forms and questionnaires
   Considering analysis of data
   Consulting a statistician			

4. Collection of information
   Pilot work
   Main study			

5. Analysis of results
   Writing the report
   Presentation of oral and written papers			

Figure 21–1. *Research guidelines: A handbook for therapists. (Reprinted with permission from Partridge C, Barnitt R. Research Guidelines: A Handbook for Therapists. Rockville, MD: Aspen; 1986.)*

In the area of subject recruitment, several variables must be considered for the elderly. For example, older persons experience decreased mobility. Therefore, a study requiring mobility, such as the ability to drive a car or use public transportation to get to the test site, may eliminate participants from the study. To generalize the abilities of the subject's recruited is also difficult. For example, the majority of the elderly do not live in nursing homes. Therefore, to assume that they are a representative sample of all older people would be erroneous. In addition, when recruiting subjects from various settings, you may disrupt the normal functioning of the person's day, and therefore, make it difficult to generalize the results of the study.[10]

Gerontological researcher have been painfully aware of the effects of variability in subjects of aging research. Nelson and Dannifer,[11] however, present compelling information to the geriatric researcher to attend to the diversity and analyze the homogeneity of variance on control for aging research methodology. Their work showed an increase in variability with age up to 65%, which was more pronounced in longitudinal versus cross-sectional studies.[11]

Andrews[12] makes a very strong point for controlling cultural variables in aging research and points out that attitudinal, religious, social, and behavioral influences can affect many outcome measures commonly explored by rehabilitation researchers and cites numerous examples, one of which is nutrition.[12] A person's religious background, for example, can strongly influence a person's nutritional intake. This may affect rehabilitation variables, such as the ability to walk, independence, or need for assistance from others. These attitudinal, religious, and social variables should be controlled for when doing rehabilitation research to be sure to check for the effects of the study.[12]

In aging research, methodology can significantly impact research outcomes. Research designs can vary from cross-sectional to longitudinal. In cross-sectional research, all variables are measured at one point in time. Longitudinal research looks at an extended period of time and variables are measured over years. The benefits of cross-sectional studies are the short-term commitment and minimal financial implications. However, the ability to attribute differences between groups to variables of age is very difficult, and this particular study design does not take into consideration other confounding variables. For example, cohort differences can influence demographic variables. People who lived during the Depression developed a specific sense for understanding how to function in the economy when the availability of money was lowered. Therefore, as a group they have a different understanding of functioning. This shared experience is a cohort effect, which is difficult to figure out when using cross-sectional studies.[13]

Longitudinal studies, on the other hand, take a much longer amount of time and can be impractical in terms of time and money involved. In a longitudinal study, for example, a therapist may choose to examine patients/clients at age twenty to check for arthritis of the knee and follow them until they reach ninty years of age. This requires seventy years of study and is, therefore, impractical. Another problem with longitudinal studies in the area of aging research is the discrimination of socialization. How, for example, can a therapist determine if the variables are actually age-related or activity-related? Has a patient's/client's medication or periods of rest or nutrition or depression affected the outcomes of the study or can the findings truly be associated with the aging process?[13]

Dr. Schale[14] proposes a cross-sectional and time-sequential analysis to differentiate the presence of cohort and age differences. He also suggests that this type of research can minimize problems of longitudinal methodologies. His method is called the cohort sequential method[14] and controls for historical events by following two or more cohorts over different age and time ranges. For example, a 20-year-old group, a 50-year-old group, and a 70-year-old group may be followed for ten years to look at the effects of arthritis of the knee. Schale believes this method decreases the time involved in doing aging research and controls for the cohort differences. It does, however, give some longitudinal perspective to the research as to the aging process.[14]

Another problem with aging research can result from the use of the survey used. It is well known that some older persons have problems with vision, hearing, and mentation that may affect the extent to which they are able to respond to the survey instrument. The older person may also be more fearful of test-taking, and, therefore, it may be more difficult to obtain informed consent from older populations.[15] Finally, the degree to which physical or cognitive impairments affect the older population may require special explanations and modifications of methods employed for research participation.[15]

MEASUREMENT ISSUES

Reliability

In reviewing and conducting research, it is imperative that therapists are aware of measurement issues in research. The first area is *interrater reliability*, which is essentially the internal consistency of a measurement tool. For example, if quadriceps strength is measured by one therapist and then another therapist measures quadriceps strength of an 80-year-old person, are the two measures similar? For instance, if the first therapist rates the quadriceps as 3/5 or fair (subjectively comparing strength in an 80-year-old to younger cohorts) and the other therapist rates the quadriceps as 5/5 (subjectively assessing that this is "normal" strength for an 80-year-old), there is no interrater reliability. This means there is a discrepancy between the two therapists' measures. Interrater reliability is, therefore, consistency between examiners. *Intrarater reliability* means that if a therapist rates the quadriceps as 3/5 at one point in time, two months later, assuming that there was no change in quadriceps strength, that same therapist should again rate the quadriceps as 3/5 in the same older person. Intrarater reliability is consistency within an individual therapist's measurements over time. These priniciples must be met or the measures themselves will be inaccurate and inconsistent. Although reliability is essential, it is not the only measurement issue to consider when evaluating measurement tools. Validity of the measurement tools is also very important.

Validity

Validity assesses whether or not the scale measures what it is designed to measure. There are six different types of validity:[16]

1. *Concurrent validity* correlates the test with other test variables. For example, manual muscle testing may be correlated with functional tests. A balance assessment tool should correlate with standard and accepted balance assessment tools.
2. *Content validity* examines the components of a measurement tool. Content validity examines each item of a test as to its representation of the entire sample. For example, if you want to look at balance and you have ten different questions related to balance, it looks at each one to see if, in fact, they individually relate to the final outcome of the variable you are trying to measure.
3. *Predictive validity* looks at the test's ability to predict outcomes. For example, on the Barthel Functional Assessment Test, which has a predictive validity, a score of 50 would predict that a person is not independent, not ready for discharge, and needs excessive help in personal care. Whereas if a person scores a 90, they could probably go home with a minimal amount of assistance.
4. *Internal validity* shows if the independent variable really caused the dependent variable. Internal validity is basically cause and effect. For instance, measurement of quadriceps strength (independent

variable) affects the ability of the individual to get from sit-to-stand (dependent variable).

5. *External validity* determines the extent to which findings can be generalized to other settings in the real world. For example, the results of a study testing muscle strengths on aging rats has external validity to a rat population but lacks external validity in humans.

6. *Face validity* is the easiest form of validity. It states that if you think the measurement tool is measuring what it is supposed to measure, than it is. For example, if you are looking for the components of gait and you are doing a gait analysis, face value would validate the belief that you are measuring gait. Face validity is usually measured through professional judgement as to whether or not it is face valid.

Independent and Dependent Variables

The next major measurement issue is variables identified in the research project. Differentiating between *independent* and *dependent variables* is critical to understanding research design. Independent variables are those that the experimenter manipulates. Dependent variables are what the experimenter assesses as a result of the independent variable. For example, exercise classes to improve balance would be the independent variable, and balance outcomes as a result of the classes would be the dependent variable.

Variability

The concept of variability is under the category of descriptive statistics. Variability has three types of measures:

1. *Range*, essentially describes the highest to the lowest score. This can be very important if you are trying to talk about the person's response to an exercise program. For the data set 1,2,4,6,8,8,10, the range is 9 (e.g., from 1 to 10).

2. *Standard deviation* is another measure of variability that looks at the distribution from the highest to lowest scores by calculating the square root of the variance. *Standard deviation* is the mathematically determined value used to derive standard scores and compare raw scores to a unit normal distribution. It is a univariate measure of variability or dispersion that indicates the average "spread" of observations about the mean. For example, if the mean age of a study sample is 75 years of age with a standard deviation of 10.5, this means that the range of ages of study participant is 64.5–86.0 years of age and would be noted as 75 ± 10.5.

3. *Standard error* is the possible range in the variability of a person's "true" score in a test. This number recognizes the amount by which a score might vary from the norm. The standard error is a statistical measure of the "average" sampling error

for a particular sampling distribution; it is the standard deviation of the sampling distribution and thus a measure of how much results vary from sample to sample.

A normal distribution curve, or bell curve, has a line representing the mean at its center (Fig. 21–2). To either side of the line, up to the dotted line, is the standard deviation. One standard deviation above or below the mean represents 34% of the sample. If it is on both sides it is 68%. To go two standard deviations would encompass almost the entire population or 95%.[16]

Data Analysis

The final area of research is *data analysis*. Therapists need an understanding of when and why certain statistical tests are used, not only when conducting research, but also when reviewing research articles. The first step in selecting a statistical test or evaluating the appropriateness of a statistical test used in a study is to identify the purpose of the study, outcome variable(s), and study design. Next, determine the purpose of statistical analysis. Is data analysis done to (1) determine the significance of the difference among group means? (2) evaluate the degree of relationship between 2 variables? Or (3) predict one variable based on another? Then determine the type of measurement used in data acquisition. Did the study use *nominal, ordinal, interval,* or *ratio* measurement scales?[17]

The major components of descriptive statistical analyses are parametric and nonparametric statistics. Parametric assumptions include random sample selection, normally distributed population, and homogeneity of variance.[16,17] Parametric statistical analysis is based on the evaluation of parameters, which are quantities or constants whose value varies with the circumstances. For example, the mean age of a study population is a parameter which will remain a constant based on the cross-sectional composition of a study population. Measures of central tendency and variance are parametric statistics. Measures of central tendencies can be subdivided into three catagories:[16]

1. *Mean or the average.* To calculate the mean, the sum of all of the scores are added and then di-

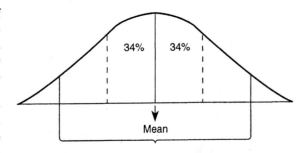

FIGURE 21–2. *Normal distribution curve.*

vided by the number of scores to produce the mean. For example, for the scores 1,2,4,6,8,8, and 10, the mean is 5.57.

2. *Median* is the middle ranked score, the one that occurs exactly in the middle. For example, if the listed scores are 1,2,4,6,8,8, and 10, the median would be 6.
3. *Mode* is the most frequently observed value in the data set. For example, with the above scores, 8 would be the mode or most frequently observed value.

Statistical analysis used for these parametric statistics can be at the nominal or ordinal or interval or ratio level. When looking at numbers and measurements, they can be placed into a hierarchy, which ranges from nominal to ratio.

Nominal numbers essentially describe categories. Something is nominal if it is naming something, such as the months of the year. Strong, weak; male, female; young and old are examples of nominal level data. Nominal level information provides the reader with some descriptive information, but it has no hierarchical value.

Ordinal information has a hierarchical value and uses numbers to order objects with respect to some characteristics. For example, scales of stronger to weaker or faster to slower or intense pain to no pain provide ordinal information. The numbers all represent values relative to each other and are assigned to give qualitative descriptive data some sense of order.

The next level is *interval*. Interval data can be thought of as integers; it describes, provides a hierarchy, and ascribes a numerical difference. Examples of interval level measures are manual muscle tests, number of feet ambulated, a period of time between two events, and number of repetitions.

Finally, the highest level of measurement is *ratio* level data. Ratio level information has all three characteristics, as previously noted, with 0 as a reference point. It is a fixed relation in degree, number, etc. between two similar things and describes a proportion. Examples of ratio data are fractions, goniometric measurements, and timed scores.

Table 21–2 is a chart of statistical procedures commonly used in geriatric therapy research that's shows their use and application.[17,18,19]

To use parametric statistics appropriately you need nominal, ordinal, interval or ratio level data in order to establish the distribution of the study population. To use parametric statistics, you need to make statistical assumptions about the data (e.g., normality or homogeneity of variance), whereas in nonparametric statistics, fewer assumptions need to be made.

Nonparametric statistics, also termed *inferential statistics*, make no assumptions about the form of the underlying distribution except that it be continuous. Nonparametric tests are used when parametric assumptions are not met. Namely, sample selection is not random, the population is not normally distrib-

uted, and/or inhomogeneity of variance occurs. Nonparametric tests are also used when ordinal data cannot be evaluated with comparable parametric tests.[17] Chi-square is an example of a nonparametric statistical analysis. In nonparametric statistics we are looking at the nature of relationships between variables. Chi-square is based on the *null hypothesis:* the assumption that there is no relationship between two variables. Given the observed distribution of values (parametric data) on two separate variables, for instance, the conjoint distribution is computed and the result is a set of *expected frequencies*. Another example is the Mann-Whitney U Test. This is a relatively powerful nonparametric test used to determine the significance of the difference between two group means of independent (unpaired) scores. This test can be applied to ordinal, ratio, or interval measurements and is an alternative to the independent (unpaired) *t*-test.[16–19]

Though space in this chapter does not allow for a thorough review of all parametric and nonparametric statistical tests, the authors of this book have compiled a list of data analysis tests commonly used in geriatric research with indications of their general requirements for use, purpose, and most appropriate application. [See Table 21–2.] When reviewing and conducting geriatric research, it is imperative to examine the most appropriate use of statistical measures employed to analyze the data.

CONDUCTING CLINICAL RESEARCH IN AGING[20–22]

Once a therapist understands how to analyze the problems with aging research and rehabilitation, he or she can begin to evaluate the various forms of clinical research. One of the most interesting approaches was developed by Rothstein and Ecternach and is called the Hypothesis Oriented for Clinicians Algorithm (HOAC model).[23] This method is presented as a means to assist rehabilitation therapists in clinical decision making and patient/client management. Figure 21–3 illustrates the process by which the therapist can collect information and assess the efficacy of their efforts. The stages are:

1. Initial data collection: The therapist, through interview, chart review, or subject information, gathers information from the patient/client.
2. Problem statement: The therapist generates a question to explore.
3. Examination and collection of the data: The therapist conducts the study (e.g., collects data).
4. Working hypothesis: The therapist generates a working hypothesis about why the goals were met or not met and reassesses whether or not the goals were appropriate.
5. Reevaluation: The therapist then does a reevaluation of the methodology.

TABLE 21–2. STATISTICAL TESTS COMMONLY USED IN GERIATRIC RESEARCH

Parametric Test	Use/Purpose	Requirements for Application
t-Test	Compares two independent groups. Determines significance of difference between group means.	– Ratio/interval measurements – Parametric assumptions met – Comparison between two group means – Paired or unpaired data
Paired t-Test	Compares two groups of data where each value in group A is linked in some way to a value in group B.	– Parametric assumptions met – Comparison between two group means – Paired data
ANOVA	Compares multiple groups or treatments. Determines significance of difference among group means.	– Ratio/interval measurements – Parametric assumptions met – Comparison among >3 group means – Paired or unpaired data
ANCOVA	Used to control initial differences when comparing various groups.	– Ratio/interval measurements – Parametric assumptions met – Controls for pre- and postdata differences – Paired or unpaired data
Factorial ANOVA	Compares effects of two or more independent variables.	– Ratio/interval measurement – Parametric assumptions met – Compares differences related to two or more variables
Repeated ANOVA	Compares measurements taken under different conditions or on different occasions in a particular group or groups.	– Ratio/interval measurement – Parametric assumptions met – Determines differences among group means
Bonferroni Test	Determines where differences occur among group means.	– Following ANOVA (preplanned) – Within-subjects or between-subjects or mixed design
Scheffe Test	Determines where differences occur among group means.	– Following ANOVA (post hoc) – Within- or between-subject design – Comparison between group means of all
Tukey Test	Determines where differences occur among group means.	– Following ANOVA (post hoc) – Within- or between-subject design – Pair-wise comparison between group means
Dunnett Test	Determines where differences occur among group means.	– Following ANOVA (post hoc) – Within- or between-subject design – Comparison only to one (control) group mean
Pearson Correlation	Evaluates degree of relations between two variables.	– Ratio/interval measurements – Parametric assumptions met – Linear relationship between variables
Interclass Correlation Coefficient	Evaluates the degree of correspondence and agreement among ratings.	– Ratio/interval measurement – Parametric assumptions met – Reliability testing
Linear Regression	Predicts one variable based on another.	– Ratio/interval measurements – Normal distribution of residuals present – Homogenous variance between variables – Linear relationship between variables

Nonparametric Test	Use/Purpose	Requirements for Application
Chi Square	Determines if distribution of observed frequencies differs from the expected frequencies.	– Nominal/ordinal measurements – Parametric assumptions not required – Comparison among more than two group means – Evaluation of 1 independent variable

(continued)

TABLE 21–2. **(Continued)**

Nonparametric Test	Use/Purpose	Requirements for Application
Mann-Whitney U Test	Determines significance of difference between group means.	– Ratio/interval/ordinal measures – Parametric assumptions not met – Comparison between two group means – Unpaired data – Sample size >30
Wilcoxon Rank Test	Determines significance of difference between group means.	– Ratio/interval/ordinal measures – Parametric assumptions not met – Comparison between two group means – Unpaired data – Sample size >30
Kruskal-Wallis One-Way ANOVA	Determines significance of difference among group means.	– Ratio/interval/ordinal measures – Parametric assumptions not met – Comparison among more than 3 group means – Paired or unpaired data
Spearman Rank Correlation	Evaluates degree of relationship between two variables	– Ratio/interval/ordinal measures – Parametric assumptions not met – Linear relationship between variables

Adapted from Ciccone C. Lecture notes from Geriatrics, An Advanced Tutorial, San Francisco: February 1992 and Kinney LaPier TL, Donovan C. Statistical Case Scenarios in Geriatric Physical Therapy Research. *GeriNotes;* January 2000; 7(1):12.

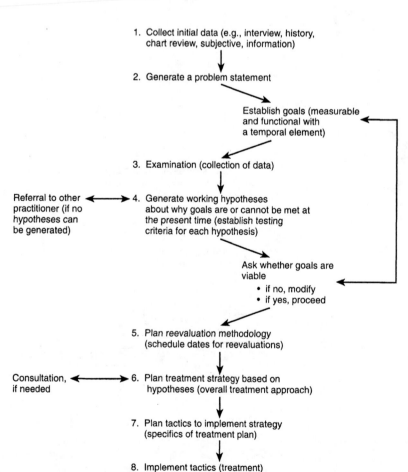

1. Collect initial data (e.g., interview, history, chart review, subjective, information)

2. Generate a problem statement

   Establish goals (measurable and functional with a temporal element)

3. Examination (collection of data)

Referral to other practitioner (if no hypotheses can be generated) ◄──► 4. Generate working hypotheses about why goals are or cannot be met at the present time (establish testing criteria for each hypothesis)

   Ask whether goals are viable
   • if no, modify
   • if yes, proceed

5. Plan reevaluation methodology (schedule dates for reevaluations)

Consultation, if needed ◄──► 6. Plan treatment strategy based on hypotheses (overall treatment approach)

7. Plan tactics to implement strategy (specifics of treatment plan)

8. Implement tactics (treatment)

FIGURE 21–3. Hypothesis-oriented algorithm for clinicians. *(Reprinted with permission from Rothstein J, Echternack J. Hypothesis-oriented algorithm for clinicians—a method for evaluation & treatment planning. Phys Ther. 1986; 66(9):1388–1394.)*

6. Future strategies: The therapist plans future treatment strategies based on the overall hypothesis.
7. Tactic for implementation: The therapist develops a tactic to implement the strategies.
8. Final implementation: The therapist finally implements this specific treatment protocol.

This is an initial way of using a research design for the evaluation and treatment of an individual patient/client or a group of patients/clients.

Single Subject Design

Another interesting research methodology that can easily be used in the geriatric rehabilitation setting is the single subject design. This particular type of design is defined as a detailed documentation summary of the characteristics, diagnosis, problem, treatment, and response of one patient/client. In this study design, the patient/client will be viewed prior to any intervention, then the intervention will be introduced and then withdrawn. When intervention is applied, any changes in patient/client status will be noted and carryover from this particular status will also be noted after termination of the intervention.

This is an easy way of making an analysis of a particular treatment intervention. For example, let's take one Parkinson's patient/client who has a difficult time getting out of a chair. The therapist initially records the difficulties that the patient/client has getting out of a chair and the time spent by the patient/client sitting in the chair. The therapist then applies education and the use of strengthening and flexibility activities to facilitate the patient's/client's ability to get out of the chair. The therapist then records what happens when the patient/client, throughout the day, tries to get up out of the chair independently (e.g., a noted increase in the number of times the patient/client gets up and walks around is documented). The intervention of the strengthening and flexibility activities is withdrawn, and an effect is observed (e.g., number of times the patient/client gets out of the chair independently). This type of study has some difficulties for generalization in that there is only one patient/client being observed.[24,25] However, single case design is helpful in determining effectiveness of intervention in one patient/client, with the potential of that treatment protocol being applied in other patients/clients.

Woolery[25] describes several ways of interpreting the data from single subject research design. Woolery discusses visual analysis of the graph data that relies on visual interpretation of the changes and another strategy of the use of statistical procedures, such as trend estimation (used to looks at changes in data over time), Rn statistic (provides a statement of statistical significance), and time series analysis (an inferential statistic used to analyze data collected at different points in time on the same patient/client), all of which can provide valuable information in the single subject design.[25]

Quantitative Research[2,3]

In *quantitative research* there is numerical representation and manipulation of observations for the purpose of describing and explaining the phenomena that those observations reflect. The logic of data analysis is applied to *quantify* observations and measurements collected during research assessments. A variable is quantitative if its values or categories consist of numbers and if differences between its categories can be expressed numerically. For example, the variable of "joint range-of-motion," measured in degrees over time, represents a quantitative difference. For instance, knee range from $-20°$ to $60°$ measured prior to intervention, and remeasured following treatment at $-15°$ to $68°$ is a quantifiable difference. Often, researchers will assign a numerical value to a typically non-numerical variable, such as in rating pain on a scale from 0 to 10. This is an attempt to quantify this variable for statistical analysis. Another good example of this, especially in geriatric research, is assigning a numerical value to functional levels of activity so that we can quantify clinical findings related to interventions. Many measurement tools utilize numerical scales to quantify subjective, qualitative variables.[26]

Qualitative Research[27]

The more characteristically utilized and often more "clinically friendly" area of research is *qualitative research*. This involves the non-numerical examination and interpretation of observations, for the purpose of discovering underlying meanings and patterns of relationships. A variable is qualitative when it fits into discrete categories, usually designated by words or labels, and there are non-numerical differences between categories. A simple example would be gender. For the most part, the variable "gender" consists of the discrete categories of male and female, and we can make categorical, but not numerical, distinctions between people of different genders. However, often for statistical analysis, you'll see the assignment of a number such as 0 = male; 1 = female. The same sort of numerical assignment is used in functional assessment measures in elderly populations where 0 = independence in activities of daily living—progressing to 4 = totally dependent in activities of daily living.

The basis for data collection in qualitative research is that of making observations. In social research this is termed *field research*. The premise is: If you want to know about something, just go to the place where it's happening and observe what happens. Qualitative research includes *participant observation* (questionnaires, ratings of perceptions, self-assessments of function, etc.), *direct observation*, and *case studies*. Qualitative research differs from other models of observation in that it is not only a data-collecting activity; frequently, it is a theory-generating activity as well. By making initial observations, and developing tentative general conclusions that suggest particular trends, often new hypotheses emerge.

Shepard provides an excellent description of qualitative research in the *Journal of the American Physical Therapy Association*,[28] where she discusses case studies, descriptive research, and quasi-experimental research as examples of both qualitative and quantitative methods for looking at the effects of rehabilitation. The case study method presents one case study and describes a patient/client, and it may have both quantitative and qualitative research methods. However, the qualitative aspect tends to be highlighted. In the area of descriptive research, she describes this as a way the clinician describes a certain patient/client population and the discusses relevant physical therapy clinical problems and how the current literature addresses those problems. It is a description of what actually occurs in the clinical setting.

All experiments involve at least a treatment, an outcome measure, units of assignment, and some comparison from which change can be inferred and hopefully attributed to the treatment. *Randomized experiments* are characterized by the use of initial random assignment for inferring treatment-caused change. It is difficult to assign individuals or larger social groups to treatments at random. It is also more difficult to assign individuals to treatments at random in field settings than in laboratory settings. Such considerations imply that random assignment will be less frequent with humans in community or field settings. *Quasi-experiments* have treatments, outcome measures, and experimental units, but do not use random assignment to create the comparisons from which treatment-caused change is inferred. In-

stead, the comparisons depend on nonequivalent groups that differ from each other in many ways other than the presence of a treatment whose effects are being tested.

In the *quasi-experimental research*, the therapist conducts the actual research. The treatment techniques do not have to be as controlled as the level of laboratory studies, because it would be almost impossible to do this in the clinical or community setting. Variables, such as nutrition, depression, motivation, etc., are common in human research and are not an issue in rat sample studies. Therefore, the majority of research done in the clinical setting is of a qualitative nature and termed *quasi-experimental*. The task confronting researchers who try to interpret the results from quasi-experiments is basically one of separating the effects of a treatment from those due to the initial noncomparability between the average units in each treatment group; only the effects of the treatment are of research interest. To achieve this separation of effects, the researcher has to explicate the specific threats to valid causal inference that random assignment rules out and then in some way deal with these threats.

Jensen[29] presents an outline guide designed for conceptual framework and qualitative research (Table 21–3) that provides an excellent framework for the therapist to understand qualitative research and to implement it in the clinical setting.

Finally, Table 21–4 examines ways to address potential threats to internal validity in qualitative research, which is the biggest threat to conducting qualitative studies. Frequently, the therapist will be questioned as to the scientific basis for this research and will have to face these various problems.

TABLE 21–3. GUIDELINES FOR CONDUCTING QUALITATIVE RESEARCH

Questions	Suggestions
1. Is the description rich?	Provide sufficient detail so the account of observations comes to life. The goal is to capture what you observed. Avoid using abstract or passive words. For example, instead of stating the patient appeared to be in pain, describe what you saw so someone could infer the patient was in pain.
2. Is there concrete detail that portrays what actually happened?	Reconstruction of dialogue is important. Strive to record the subject's own words when possible. Nonverbal expressions should also be noted.
3. Is confidentiality maintained?	Usually, the researcher is dealing with a small number of subjects, and confidentiality is a critical factor. The researcher also relies on building trust and rapport with subjects to collect valid information.
4. Is the material presented pertinent to the research topic?	Once immersed in the research setting, it is easy to get off track and gather data that are not relevant. An initial, yet dynamic, conceptual framework can help guide your data collection.
5. Are multiple perspectives presented?	The researcher must continually look for data that might disconfirm preliminary insights. Field notes should reflect collection of supporting and disconfirming evidence. This evidence can in turn be used to revise the conceptual framework.
6. Has the researcher kept an account of his/her behaviors during data collection?	Because the researcher is the data-collection instrument, it is important to keep track of behaviors, assumptions, or whatever else might affect the construction of field notes.

Reprinted with permission from Jensen G. Qualitative methods in physical therapy research: A form of disciplined inquiry. *Phys Ther.* 1989; 69(6):492–500.

TABLE 21–4. WAYS TO ADDRESS POTENTIAL THREATS TO INTERNAL VALIDITY IN QUALITATIVE RESEARCH

Threat	Recommendation
History	Qualitative researchers assume that history affects the nature of data, because phenomena rarely remain constant. When process and change are the focus of the research, then the researcher must establish which baseline data remain stable over time and which data change. This process can be accomplished through the use of replication and time-sampling strategies.
Observer Effects	Sufficient residence in the field and corroboration from multiple informants can reduce these effects. Participant reaction and confirmation, documented throughout the research process, will also help guard against observer effects.
Selection-Regression	Qualitative researchers do not usually try to control selection and regression effects to isolate a treatment, but distortions in the data may occur by selection of participants. In complex field situations, an adequate inventory of groups, subgroups, events, or social scenes must be completed to ensure the findings are representative.
Mortality	Qualitative researchers assume that growth and attrition are normal processes in a natural setting and that what is important is the identification of their effects.
Spurious Conclusions	Elimination of rival explanation in qualitative research requires effective and efficient data-collection systems and the use of corroborating sources of data. Negative confirming or disconfirming evidence is sought throughout the research process.

Reprinted with permission from Shepard K. Qualitative & quantitative research in clinical practice. *Phys Ther.* 1987; 67(12):1891–1894.

Ethnography

Another method of research that may be employed by therapists in a geriatric setting is ethnography. Ethnography is a branch of anthropology that deals descriptively with whole cultures or groups of people. This is a qualitative form of scientific inquiry and is used to discover and describe human behavior through the perspective of the person studied and through researcher observation. Table 21–5 lists the steps in the ethnography methodology.[30]

Table 21–6 lists the unique aspects of ethnography.[30] Ethnography has both pros and cons. The positive side of ethnography is that it is a very flexible process for data collection. It's a good tool for measuring behavior, which is frequently evaluated in clinical research, and enables the therapist to develop theories about behaviors in the clinical setting. The limitations of ethnography are that it is restricted to human interpretation and interactions that impact human behavior, and the lack of control variables and statistical analysis make the data inappropriate for quantitative statistical hypothesis testing. Nevertheless, because of the role that behavior plays in the success or failure of recovering of function after an illness, it is an appropriate research modality in the rehabilitation environment.

ENCOURAGING THE USE OF RESEARCH[31,32]

The final component of this chapter is how to use research and how to encourage the use of research for evidence-based practice. According to Bohannon and LeVeau[33] the literature suggests that research information is not routinely used by human service professionals. What are some of the major factors that

TABLE 21–5. STEPS IN ETHNOGRAPHIC METHODOLOGY

The steps used in ethnographic methodology are presented in a sequential format, but in practice many of these steps occur simultaneously or concurrently, rather than in a fixed, sequential manner.

1. Identify a topic to study.
2. Pose research questions related to the topic of study.
3. Identify initial methods and sources for data collection based on questions posed (e.g., persons to interview or observe).
4. Develop operational definitions initially or as the need arises during the study.
5. Collect initial data by observations or interviews. Begin analysis of data as they are collected from initial observations or interviews. Preliminary concepts should emerge from the data.
6. Analyze data as they are collected and form tentative concepts that explain them.
7. Collect more data. For example, conduct additional observations, interview persons previously observed, or observe persons initially interviewed.
8. Continue to analyze all accumulated data and refine tentative concepts that explain the data.
9. Continue to collect and analyze data concurrently until the concepts established can explain all of the data collected. If tentative concepts do not explain (fit) the data, they should be modified until they do fit the data.
10. Analyze concepts to establish explanations of the interrelationships of two or more concepts. This analysis results in forming tentative hypotheses or propositions.
11. Formulate hypotheses into substantive theory that describes and explains phenomena that occur. The hypotheses also may serve as the basis for subsequent experimental or quasi-experimental design research.

Although the phases of ethnographic inquiry differ from those of quantitative scientific inquiry, the process for collecting and analyzing data is systematic and rigorous.

Reprinted with permission from Schmoll BJ. Ethnographic inquiry in clinical settings. *Phys Ther.* 1987; 67(12):1895–1897.

TABLE 21–6. UNIQUE ASPECTS OF ETHNOGRAPHY

Ethnography is distinguished from quantitative research by the following characteristics:

1. The study is guided by general questions related to a topic rather than by preestablished hypotheses.
2. A review of the literature is treated as a data source that may be subjected to constant comparative analysis rather than serving as a basis for the generation of hypotheses.
3. The direct contact with the groups under study by observations or interviews, or both, is essential. Other forms of data, such as progress reports, surveys, medical records, quality assurance reports, and a review of the literature, may be used in combination with observations and interviews.
4. Variables are regarded as data.
5. Multiple phases of the inquiry occur simultaneously rather than in a fixed, sequential manner.
6. Ethnography begins with a broad general area for study that increasingly becomes focused more narrowly as the study proceeds.

Reprinted with permission from Schmoll BJ. Ethnographic inquiry in clinical settings. *Phys Ther.* 1987; 67(12):1895–1897.

keep health care professionals from using research as the basis for interventions?

1. Frequently, clinicians view researchers as "different" from themselves, and they question the type of research that is being conducted.
2. The communication of research findings is so overwhelming it may discourage its use by the professional.
3. The use of jargon in research that is not commonly used in the clinic may preclude its use.
4. The results may be too tentative, inconclusive, and not studied thoroughly enough.
5. The research may be delayed in its publication and of interest to only a few of the clinicians available.
6. Frequently, people who are active clinically do not have the time to read new information or they may not be using this type of information in their practice.
7. Clinicians tend to prefer practice articles over research articles because of the vast amount of information available and, when faced with time constraints, may frequently choose to read the clinical versus the research article.
8. Frequently clinicians, even if they do understand the research report, may not be able to implement the findings, and they may resist implementing the various findings because they may go against what they have been taught.[33]

These strategies could be used to increase the use of research information in the clinic:

1. Prepare students to be consumers of research. Teachers, clinicians, and clinical affiliates should use research when talking to students and make it available so they can frequently refer to various articles. Encourage students to do research projects and to work with mentors on research projects. Role models in the area of research are necessary in the various academic and clinical institutions and facilities.
2. Prepare therapists to be consumers of research by exposing them to research articles versus clinical tracts that may extrapolate the research information. Have therapists go to the library and investigate original research. In addition, make research information available by providing annotated bibliographies, notebooks of current research, and highlight clinicians who have done and/or used research. Have a research member assigned on a clinical staff.[33]

Ethical Issues

Special mention must be made about ethical considerations in research. Prior to conducting any study using human subjects, therapists must have potential participants in the study sign a consent form. Figure 21–4 is a sample of a consent form for research and can be modified as needed for various studies. Within the consent form it should be noted that at any time a subject has the right to withdraw from a study and that this must be clearly identified in the consent form.

Funding Research

Refer to Chapter 22 in this text for a more comprehensive listing of grant-giving agencies of the federal government and electronic and printed publications with information related to ongoing grant announcements and availability. For the purposes of this section of the chapter on research, only a few funding resources for research will be presented.

The Foundation for Physical Therapy has research funding available for geriatric-related research projects due to the annual contribution of funds by the Section on Geriatrics of the American Physical Therapy Association. Requests for proposals (RFPs) are available annually for projects that evaluate the effectiveness of physical therapy interventions for elderly patients/clients and for the evaluation of the effectiveness of physical therapist practice in general. The deadline for submitting proposals for research grants is August 15 each year. If the RFP is accepted and the grant awarded, funding begins January 1 of the subsequent year. To be eligible for a research grant, the principle investigator must be a licensed physical therapist. For applications and guidelines, or if you have questions, contact the Foundation for Physical Therapy at 800–875–1378, or e-mail: foundation@apta.org.

The National Institute on Aging (NIA) is another excellent source of funding for research in geriatrics. This agency of the federal government also focuses on grants to support doctoral dissertation research for

Consent Form for Human Subjects

Description

Subject's Name (Please print): _____

Project Title: _____

_____

Project Director/Researcher's Name: _____

_____

Describe the nature of the research project and what will be required of the participants:

Certification

I fully understand the program or activity in which I am being asked to participate and the procedures that will be performed. I have had an adequate chance to ask questions and understand that I may ask additional questions any time while the study is in progress.

I understand that I am participating in this activity of my own free will, and I am free to withdraw my consent and discontinue my participation at any time while the study is in progress.

This is to certify that I agree to participate in this program or activity under the direction of the researcher named above.

_____   _____
Date   Signature of Subject (or other
                                 authorized person, such as a
                                 child's parent or guardian)

                                 _____
                                 Witness (if necessary)

FIGURE 21–4. Consent Form for Human Subjects.

underrepresented minority doctoral candidates. There are four areas of concentration for grants in the area of geriatrics:

- Biology of Aging Program—This program supports research that focuses on the molecular mechanisms involved in the aging process, and how these are affected by genetic and environmental factors
- Behavioral and Social Research Program— This program supports research on social and psychological aging processes and the place of older people in society and its social institutions.
- Neuroscience and Neuropsychology of Aging Program—Research supported by this program focuses on the structure and function of the aging nervous system and the behavioral manifestations of the aging brain.
- Geriatrics Program—Research supported by this program focuses on clinical issues and problems that occur predominantly among middle-aged and older persons or that are associated with increased morbidity and mortality in older people.

Application kits (PHS 398) may be obtained from the Division of Extramural Outreach and Information Resources, National Institutes of Health, 6701 Rockledge Drive, MSC 7910, Bethesda, MD 20892–7910; telephone: 301 435 0714; e-mail: GrantsInfo@nih.gov or from the NIH web site at: http://grants.nih.gov/grants/funding/phs 398/phs398.html.

Last, the Agency for Health Care Policy and Research (AHCPR) Health Services Research has a broad priority of interests for extramural grants for research, demonstration, dissemination, and evaluation projects. Research needs to: (1) support improvements in health outcomes; (2) strengthen quality measurement and improvement, including the use of evidence-based practice information and tools; and (3) identify strategies to improve access and foster appropriate use and reduce unnecessary expenditures, including research on the organization, financing and delivery of health care and the characteristics of primary care practice. The AHCPR has also identified two additional areas of emerging research interest that are becoming increasingly important in today's market-driven health care delivery system. These are research on methodologic advances in health services research, especially cost-effectiveness analysis, and research on ethical issues across the spectrum of health care delivery. For application materials contact: AHCPR contractor: Equals Three Communications, Inc., 7910 Woodmont Avenue, Suite 200, Bethesda, MD 20814–3015; telephone: 301–656–3100; fax: 301–652–5264.

Though it takes a little time and effort to apply for grant funding of research projects, the process is well worth your while and actually assists in your own clarification of the research process.

CONCLUSION

Geriatric research is similar to research in the entire rehabilitation realm with a few exceptions. This chapter points out that the older population is slightly more difficult to study for a variety of reasons. Certain study methodologies might be better for obtaining information, and suggestions for different types of research tools that could be used in the rehabilitation environment were briefly discussed. The future of geriatric rehabilitation truly is in the area of research. As third party payers scrutinize evaluative and intervention procedures for efficacy and cost, we as clinicians need to be prepared to defend and justify the value of the skills we provide. Anecdotal information and casual observations will not have a strong impact on legislative and policy initiatives that dictate what is skilled therapy practice. We need research to quantify and qualify the treatments we purport to be effective. We need evidence-based, outcome-oriented practice. Understanding the differences in aging research, and the various ways of conducting aging research, applying research in our daily practice, and knowing how to use available research information, will clearly improve our future in geriatric rehabilitation.

PEARLS

- A research article is composed of an abstract, introduction, methods, data analysis, results, discussion, and conclusion sections.
- The introduction of a research article should contain: (1) the statement of the problem, (2) the literature reviewed, (3) the purpose of the study, (4) the type of study, (5) the expected results, and (6) the research question.
- The major problems in aging research are sampling, subject recruitment, and design constraints.
- Understanding measurement issues, such as reliability, validity, variability, and data analysis, are essential for therapists to properly interpret aging research reports.
- The major components of descriptive statistical analyses are *parametric* and *nonparametric or inferential* statistics.
- A method suggested to clinicians to assist therapists in clinical decision making related to research findings is the *Hypothesis Oriented Algorithm for Clinicians (HOAC)*.
- A *single subject research* design is defined as a detailed documentation summary of the characteristics, diagnosis, problem, treatment, and response of one patient/client.
- In *quantitative research* there is numerical representation and manipulation of observations for the purpose of describing and explaining the phenomena that those observations reflect.

- *Qualitative research* involves the non-numerical examination and interpretation of observations, for the purpose of discovering underlying meanings and patterns of relationships.
- Ethnography is a qualitative form of research used to describe and discover human behavior from the perspective of the person studied and through the eyes of the research observer of characteristics.

REFERENCES

1. American Physical Therapy Association. Guide to Physical Therapy Practice. *Phys Ther.* November 1997; 77(11):1184–1185.

2. Currier DP. *Elements of Research in Physical Therapy.* Philadelphia, PA: Lippincott, Williams & Wilkins; 1990.

3. Domholdt E. *Physical Therapy Research: Principles and Applications.* Philadelphia, PA: W.B. Saunders; 2000.

4. Cutler SK, Stein F. *Clinical Research in Occupational Therapy,* 4th Edition. Florence, KY: Singular Pub Group; 2000.

5. Domholdt E, Malone T. Evaluating research literature: the educated clinician. *Phys Ther.* April 1965; 65(4):487–491.

6. Thompson LV. Steps to indentify the research article that is beneficial to you. *GeriNotes.* 2000; 7(1): 8–10.

7. Partridge C, Barnitt R. *Research Guidelines: A Handbook for Therapists.* Rockville, MD: Aspen Publishers, Inc.; 1986.

8. Sim J. Methodology and morality in physiotherapy research. *Physiotherapy.* 1989; 75(4):237–243.

9. Wayne S, Rhyne RL, Thompson RF, et al. Sampling issues in nursing home research. *J Am Ger Soc.* 1991; 39(3):308–311.

10. Kelly P, Kroemer K. Anthropometry of the elderly: status and recommendations. *Human Factors.* October 1990; 32(5):571–595.

11. Nelson E, Dannefer D. Aged heterogeneity: fact or fiction? The fate of diversity in gerontological research. *Gerontologist.* 1992; 32(1):17–23.

12. Andrews G. Cross-cultural studies—an important development in aging research. *J Am Ger Soc.* 1989; 37(5):483–485.

13. Schunk C. Research and the elderly. In: Lewis: CB, ed. *Aging: The Health Care Challenge.* Philadelphia: F.A. Davis; 1985:311–320.

14. Schale KW. Quasi-experimental research designs in the psychology of aging. In: Britton SE, Schale KW, eds. *Handbook of the Psychology of Aging.* New York: Van Norstrand Reheinhold; 1985:39.

15. Rayman I, Bloom S. Survey research as a tool for studying problems in the elderly. In: Kent B, Butler RN, eds. *Aging: Human Aging Research—Concepts & Techniques,* Vol. 34. New York: Raven Press; 1988:51–76.

16. Mattson D. *Statistics Difficult Concepts; Understandable Explanations.* Oak Park, Ill: Bolzchazy-Carducco Publishers, Inc.; 1986.

17. Kinney LaPier TL, Donovan C. Statistical case scenarios in geriatric physical therapy research. *GeriNotes.* 2000; 7(1):11–17.

18. Ciccione C. Lecture notes from *Geriatrics: An Advanced Tutorial.* San Francisco, CA: February 1992.

19. Kinney LaPier TL. The when and why of statistical tests. *Cardiopulm Phys Ther.* 1999; 10(1):19–22.

20. Payton OD, Sullivan MS. *Research: The Validation of Clinical Practice.* Philadelphia, PA: FA Davis Co.; 2000.

21. Hicks CM. *Research Methods of Clinical Therapists: Applied Project Design and Analysis.* Philadelphia, PA: Churchill Livingstone; 1999.

22. Seale J, Barnard S. *Therapy Research: Processes and Practicalities.* Newton, MA: Butterworth-Heinemann Medical; 1998.

23. Rothstein J, Echternach J. Hypothesis-oriented algorithm for clinicians—a method for evaluation and treatment planning. *Phys Ther.* 1986; 66(9): 1388–1394.

24. Connolly BH, Criak RL, Krebs DE. Single-case research: when is it valid? *Phys Ther.* 1983; 63(11): 1767–1768.

25. Woolery M, Harris S. Interpreting results of single-subject research designs. *Phys Ther.* 1982; 62(4): 445–452.

26. American Physical Therapy Association. Guide to physical therapy practice. *Phys Ther.* 1997; 77(11): 1184–1185.

27. Hammell KW, Carpenter C, Dyck I. *Using Qualitative Research: A Practical Introduction for Occupational and Physical Therapists.* Philadelphia, PA: Churchill Livingstone; 2000.

28. Shepard K. Qualitative & quantitative research in clinical practice. *Phys Ther.* 1987; 67(12):1891–1894.

29. Jensen G. Qualitative methods in physical therapy research: a form of disciplines inquiry. *Phys Ther.* June 1989; 69(6):492–500.

30. Schmoll B. Ethnographic inquiry in clinical settings. *Phys Ther.* 1987; 67(12):1895–1897.

31. Fuhrer MJ. *Assessing Medical Rehabilitation Practices: The Promise of Outcomes Research.* Baltimore, MD: Paul H. Brookes Pub Co.; 1997.

32. Bury TJ, Mead JM. *Evidence-Based Healthcare: A Practical Guide for Therapists.* Newton, MA: Butterworth-Heinemann Medical; 1998.

33. Bohannon R, LeVeau B. Clinicians' use of research findings. *Phys Ther.* 1986; 66(1):45–50.

CHAPTER 22

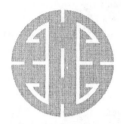

Aging Network Resources

The goal of this chapter is to give the reader a meaningful sampling of available resources for the elderly so that you can create your own network. A definitive list of resources would itself fill a large book and would encompass organizations and services that operate locally as well as nationally. The wonderful thing about the resources selected for this chapter is that they are bound to lead you to others.

HELPFUL ORGANIZATIONS

GENERAL INFORMATION

Diseases and disabilities that afflict enough people have their own organizations. For instance, the American Lung Association, the American Cancer Society, the American Heart Association . . . just for starters.

There are more than 1,000 of these types of disease- or disability-specific, user-friendly repositories of general information. Most of the organizations will send free educational booklets about specific diseases, current treatments available, and newsletters. These organizations are excellent sources of professional as well as patient educational materials.

Some national organizations are listed in the local yellow pages, or you can order a printed listing of private and public sources for $17.25 postpaid by writing to: **Resource Information Guide,** PO Box 990297, Redding, CA 96099, http://www.aoa.dhhs. gov/.

The **National Institutes of Health (NIH)** is the official web site of the NIH, one of the world's foremost research centers. This site is an excellent resource for information for patients and professionals in all areas of health care. The web site is: www.nih.gov/.

The **National Aging Information Center** http://www.202.dhhs.gov/naic is a service of the Department of Health and Human Services Administration on Aging and provides information on aging programs and the needs of the elderly.

The **National Health Information Center** can also refer you to the appropriate organizations. Just call: 800-336-4797. Don't be shy—the center gets calls for every disease imaginable, and its staff is armed with 1,100 phone numbers. The National Health Information Center also has a web site: http://nhicnt. health.org/ This site offers links to publications and several databases with health care information. For less well-known illnesses, the **National Organization for Rare Disorders (NORD),** created by Abbey Meyers after she discovered how hard it was to get information on Tourette's syndrome, which her three children have, is another excellent source for information. This organization supplies the public with the kind of information she wishes she'd had easier access to. There is information available on 950 diseases. The pamphlets and informational materials cover symptoms and therapies for patients with rare diseases, education on the disease, as well as current research reviews for the clinician. The first request is free; subsequent reports cost $3.25 each. Call: 203-746-6518.

The National Institutes of Health (NIH) launched ClinicalTrials.gov, a new web site of clinical trials for serious illnesses. The purpose of this registry, which was mandated by Congress as part of the 1997 FDA Modernization Act, is to provide patients, family members, and members of the public with current information about clinical research studies. The registry can be accessed at http://www.clinicaltrials.gov.

General health information can be obtained via a wonderful internet site called **Healthfinder** at: http://www.healthfinder.gov/. General health information and resources for available services in agency areas is also available from the **National Association of Area Agencies on Aging** at 1112 Sixteenth Street NW, Suite 100, Washington, DC 20036; 202-296-8130.

HOTLINES

Hotlines have been created and are another excellent source of information. The **Medicare Hotline:** 1-800-MEDICARE (800-633-4227; for TTY or TDD service, call 877-486-2048) offers general information about Medicare and detailed comparisons of all Medicare health plans in your community, including quality of care and member satisfaction in Medicare private health plans, such as Medicare HMOs.

ElderCare Locator provides access to information on an extensive network of organizations that serve seniors at state and local levels: 800-677-1116.

A **Prostate hotline,** for instance, offers advice on treatments: 800-543-9632. The **Y-ME National Organization for Breast Cancer** offers information and support to women with breast cancer: 800-221-2141 or 708-799-8228. The **Centers for Disease Control and Prevention** offers information on risk factors for just about any disease and operates an **AIDS hotline:** 800-432-AIDS. For a list of some 100 hot lines call the National Health Information Center (800-336-4797). For $1.00 they will send a roster of toll-free health information numbers. Some operate from nine to five, others are on call 24 hours. The **National Health Information Clearinghouse:** PO Box 1133, Washington, DC 20013; 800-336-4797 or 703-522-2590, will help locate resources pertaining to health information; specific questions about health are referred to appropriate experts or Federal agencies. The **American Dietetic Association's National Center for Nutrition and Dietetics** has a hotline for questions about nutrition and diet and for a referral to a registered dietitian in your area. Call the **Consumer Nutrition Hotline:** 800-366-1655.

SUPPORT GROUPS

Support groups are another excellent source of information. While most people think of such groups merely as sources of emotional support, they also provide the powerful function of information exchange. An example is a patient of the author's. She developed a problem with such frequent urination that she couldn't leave the house. Her doctor told her there was no treatment for urinary incontinence, but, he referred her to a self-help group for people who shared this affliction. From the group, she learned about a drug that offered relief, not yet approved in the United States, but available in Europe and Mexico. Armed with this information, she returned to her doctor, who obtained the drug for her through an experimental program. The drug was effective in resolving her urinary incontinence and her functional level of activity has returned to a desirable balance. The **American Self-Help Clearinghouse** at St Clare's Riverside Medical Center in Denville, New Jersey or http://mentalhelp.net/selfhelp/clrnghse/clrnhse.htm, tracks more than 700 groups and publishes the Self-Help Source-book, available for $10. Call 201-625-7101. They'll also provide numbers for clearing-houses in 19 states: Calif., Conn., Ill., Iowa, Kan., Mass., Mich., Mo., Neb., N.J., N.Y., N.C., Ohio, Ore., Penn., S.C., Tenn., Tex., and the District of Columbia. The regional clearing houses can direct you to specific local support groups. The **National Self-Help Clearinghouse:** http://www.selfhelpweb.org, will also send a list of support group information. Just send a self-addressed, stamped envelope (SASE) to: 25 West 43rd St., New York, NY 10036, 212-840-7606.

For patient and professional educational materials on just about any disease, disability, or social problem afflicting the elderly the **U.S. Department of Health and Human Services** and the **National Institute on Aging:** http://www.nia.nih.gov/ which is a division of this agency are excellent sources. To obtain a comprehensive listing of all available publications from these two institutions write: **Department of Health and Human Services, Public Health Service, Agency for Health Care Policy and Research,** Executive Office Center, 2101 East Jefferson Street, Suite 501, Rockville, MD 20852 and **NIA Information Center,** 2209 Distribution Circle, Silver Spring, MD 20910 or http://www.rwjf.org. In addition, the **Robert Wood Johnson Foundation,** Consumer Information Center, Pueblo, CO 81009 and the **American Association of Retired Persons,** 1909 K Street, NW, Washington, DC 20049, 202-872-4700, http://www.aarp.org will provide numerous materials on issues related to aging and disease/disability.

WOMEN'S HEALTH ISSUES

One of the best sources of information on women's health issues is the **Section on Women's Health** of the American Physical Therapy Association: 1111 North Fairfax Street, Alexandria, VA 22314-3492; telephone: 703-706-8516, Fax: 703-706-8578, e-mail: lacey-toney@apta.org. Information is available on every conceivable topic via fax-on-demand or brochure, in addition to numerous course offerings related to women's health issues. Check this resource prior to exploring elsewhere for information on women's health and related topics.

For women's illnesses, the **National Women's Health Network** provides information and referrals on 75 topics and is an organization that serves as a clearinghouse for information on women's health issues: 202-347-1140 or 202-223-6886 or http://www.womenshealthnetwork.org, 224 Seventh Street, SE, Washington, DC 20024. It also publishes a newsletter on health and lobbying efforts. This is a public interest advocacy organization that works for women's health issues in the United States. The **National Institute on Aging** has a wonderful publication called

Health Resources for Older Women: http://www.nia.nih.gov. It is free of charge and can be obtained by writing: NIA Information Center, 2209 Distribution Circle, Silver Spring, MD 20910 and asking for NIH Publication No. 87-2899. This publication provides resources on age changes and health promotion such as menopause, nutrition and physical fitness, skin changes, use of medicines, and accident prevention. In addition, common disorders such as osteoporosis, osteoarthritis, breast cancer, urinary incontinence, and cognitive changes are discussed and resources available presented. Educational material is available on housing options, financial planning, caregiving, and widowhood as well. The NIA also has an excellent and comprehensive booklet entitled, *Who? What? Where?: Resources for Women's Health and Aging,* which includes resource information of all of the above mentioned areas in women's health in addition to materials and resources on Alzheimer's disease and other cognitive changes, depression, heart disease and current research related to women and aging (NIH Publication No. 91-323, 1999).

The **National Women's Health Information Center (NWHIC)** is the official site of the U.S. Public Health Service's **Office of Women's Health (OWH).** This site answers frequently asked questions, allows access to databases of federal publications and organizations related to women's health: http://www.4woman.org. 800-994-9662.

The **Center for Climacteric Studies,** University of Florida, 901 NW 8th Avenue, Suite B1, Gainesville, FL 32601; 904-392-3184, was established to promote research, public education, and clinical service in areas related to women's health issues. **Hysterectomy Education Resources (HERS),** 422 Bryn Mawr Avenue, Bala Cynwyd, PA 19004; 215-667-7757 is also an excellent source of educational materials on menopause and OB-GYN surgical procedures. This organization publishes a quarterly newsletter that is a valuable update mechanism for research oriented toward women's health problems related to menopause. The **American College of Obstetricians and Gynecologists (ACOG):** 600 Maryland Avenue, SW, Suite 300 East, Washington, DC 20024; 202-638-4680 offers patient education pamphlets entitled *The Menopause Years, Estrogen Use, and Preventing Osteoporosis.*

Other excellent sources of information on health-related topics for women are the **American Association of Clinical Endocrinologists (AACE):** 1000 Riverside Avenue, Suite 205, Jacksonville, FL 32204; 800-393-2223; http://www.aace.com, and the **ACOG's Resource Center:** P.O Box 96920, Washington, DC 20092-6920; http://www.acog.com (No calls: send SASE or visit their Web site).

The **North American Menopause Society (NAMS)** offers ten easy-to-read booklets offering accurate, unbiased health information needed by all women as they approach midlife and beyond. The entire set of booklets can be purchased for $10.00

(plus shipping and handling): PO Box 94527, Cleveland, OH 44101; telephone: 216-844-8748; fax: 216-844-8708; e-mail: nams@apk.net or at their web site: http://www.menopause.org. This organization also provides a list of menopause clinicians and discussion groups by geographical area.

PHYSICAL FITNESS

The best resource for information on physical fitness for all age groups is the **American Physical Therapy Association (APTA):** 1111 North Fairfax, Alexandria, VA 22314; 703-684-2782 or 800-999-2782; http://www.apta.org. Numerous materials on physical fitness and specific conditions are available through the resource center catalogue on the APTA's web site.

Patient education is an important part of the services physical therapists deliver. The **National Exercise for Life Institute (NEFLI),** an organization established by NordicTrack, offers free information brochures entitled: *Exercise and Aging* and *Exercise and Back Pain.* These brochures give easy-to-understand explanations of the effects of aging and the effects of back problems, and provide practical tips and suggestions for starting and maintaining a successful exercise program. For copies of the brochures contact: NEFLI Brochures, PO Box 2000, Excelsior, MN 55331-9967; 800-358-3636.

Melpomene Institute for Women's Health Research is a wonderful source of reliable information on the relationship between women's health and physical fitness. This organization is involved in research, publication, and education. 1010 University Avenue, St. Paul, MN 55104; telephone: 612-642-1951; fax: 612-642-1871; e-mail: melpomen@skypoint.com; Web site: http://www.melpomene.org. Informational packets are available in all areas of women's health. Check out their web site for the numerous publications, research, and speaker availability.

The **American Physical Therapy Association,** 1111 North Fairfax Street, Alexandria, VA 22314-9902; 800-999-2782, http://www.apta. org, can provide valuable information on exercise specific to the aging population. In addition, the **President's Council on Physical Fitness and Sports,** 450 5th Street, NW, Suite 7103, Washington, DC 20001; 202-272-3421, is mandated by an executive order signed by the president for the purpose of explaining to the public the importance of physical fitness. The Council trains professionals to run health and fitness demonstration programs for the elderly and provides brochures, films, and speakers.

NUTRITION

Guidelines on specific nutritional requirements of older people are scarce. Current RDAs divide the adult population into only two age groups—those aged 23 to 50 and those over age 50. Relatively little research has been done to define the impact of age-related physiological changes on human nutritional requirements. However, the few studies that have been done indicate that aging may affect the need for certain nutrients, vitamins, and minerals. For example, the ability of the body to absorb calcium and vitamin D declines substantially with age, possibly increasing older people's susceptibility to osteoporosis and risk of bone fractures.

With age, the need for calories declines while the requirements for protein, minerals, and vitamins remains the same. Also, many people decrease their physical activity somewhat as they grow older, and this also reduces the need for calories. Good health depends on staying physically active. Current evidence from research shows exercise strengthens the heart and lungs, lowers blood pressure, reduces the risk of diabetes, reduces the level of certain fats in the blood, and strengthens bone. Thus, maintaining a regular fitness program is important. Exercise can safeguard health, help control weight, and contribute to a better mental outlook.

The **U.S. FDA/Center for Food Safety and Applied Nutrition (CFSAN):** http:// cfsan.fda.gov/ or 200 C Street SW Washington, DC 20204, provides an overview of every imaginable nutrient and product on the market. This site has links to research based findings on a variety of food products and their relationship to health issues.

The **American Dietetic Association (ADA),** 430 North Michigan Avenue, Chicago, IL 60611; 312-280-5000, http://www.eatright.org, is interested in improving dietary habits of all people and works to advance the science of dietetics and nutrition, as well as to promote education in these areas.

The **National Meals on Wheels Foundation;** telephone: 800-999-6262 is also an excellent resource for determining available nutritional programs in specific geographical locations.

MEDICATIONS

Drugs often affect the body differently as an individual increases in age, probably because of normal changes in body metabolism. Such changes can affect the length of time a drug remains in the body and the amount of the drug absorbed by body tissues. There are precautions that can be taken to reduce the risks associated with drug use. For example, taking the exact dosage prescribed and having a pharmacist or physician monitor the use of multiple drugs to avoid adverse reactions. The **AARP Pharmacy Service,** PO Box NIA, 1 Prince Street, Alexandria, VA 22314; 703-684-9244, http://www.aarppharmacy.com/ provides information on common prescription drugs, side effects, and cost differences between brand name and generic drugs. It has published a series of leaflets called Medication Information Leaflets for Seniors (MILS), which discuss 350 prescription drugs. For copies write to the Pharmacy Service and specify the drugs you are interested in. The service also operates twelve pharmacies throughout the country for members of AARP. Another excellent source of information on drugs, the **American Pharmaceutical Association (APhA),** 2215 Constitution Avenue, NW, Washington, DC 20037; 202-628-4410, http://www.aphanet.org, comprised of practicing pharmacists, manufacturers, researchers, and publishers of pharmaceutical literature, promotes public health by establishing satisfactory drug standards. For answers to questions regarding drug approval, drug reactions, and other issues concerning new or approved medications the **Food and Drug Administration,** Division of Regulatory Affairs, Center for Drugs and Biologics, 5600 Fisher Lane, Rockville, MD 20857; 301-295-8012, http://www.fda.gov/ is a good resource for information.

ALTERNATIVE AND COMPLEMENTARY MEDICINE

The National Institutes of Health (NIH), **National Center for Complementary and Alternative Medicine (NCCAM)** conducts and supports basic and applied research and training and disseminates information on complementary and alternative medicine to practitioners and the public. It provides a list of programs, news and events, and information resources. NCCAM Clearinghouse, PO Box 8218, Silver Spring, MD, 20907-8218; telephone: 888-644-6226; fax: 301-495-4957; http://nccam.nih.gov/. Another wonderful resource for information on alternative medicine and complementary therapies is an internet site entitled: **Alternative Health News Online:** http://www.altmedicine.com.

HEALTH PROMOTION AND WELLNESS

The **National Wellness Institute (NWI)** helps individuals lead better lives by serving an international network of health promotion and wellness professionals and organizations. This organization provides professional education, furnishes information and resources, develops and distributes wellness-related products and services, and provides a list of speakers on health promotion and wellness topics.http://www.national-wellness.org/ or 800-243-8694. The **National Wellness Association (NWA)** is the membership division of NWI. This organization has many services for professionals working in all areas of wellness and health promotion. 1300 College Court, PO Box 827, Stevens Point, WI 54481-0827; telephone: 715-342-2969; fax: 715-342-2979.

ACCIDENT PREVENTION

Accidental injuries become more frequent and serious in later life. Several factors make people in this age group prone to accidents: poorer eyesight and hearing can decrease awareness of hazards; arthritis, neurological diseases, and impaired coordination and balance can affect steadiness; illness, use of medicines or alcohol, and preoccupation with personal problems can cause drowsiness or distraction. Falling is the most common cause of fatal injury in the aged. Each year it causes hip fractures in about 210,000 older persons, 20% of whom die within the first year after an injury. In addition, a fall can result in months of pain and confinement or the fear of falling again. For some older persons it leads to institutionalization. Older women also have a greater chance of developing osteoporosis and in combination with a greater risk of falls this increases the chances of fracture. Automobile accidents are the second most common cause of accidents among older persons. Many of these accidents could be prevented, however, by limiting the distance traveled and number of hours on the road, by using extra caution driving in evening rush hour and in winter weather, and by staying on familiar roads. The **American Association of Retired Persons (AARP),** 55 Alive/Mature Driving Program, Traffic and Driver Safety Program, 601 E Street, NW, Washington, DC; 202-434-2277 or 800-434-2277, http://www.aarp.org/, offers an 8-hour classroom, driver-education refresher course for persons aged 50 or older, taught by instructors who are 50 or older. In some states, a certificate of completion entitles the driver to a discount on automobile insurance. In addition, the **American Automobile Association (AAA),** http://www.aaa.com/, offers the Mature Operator Program, an 8-hour classroom course for persons aged 55 and over to enhance driving knowledge and awareness of new techniques and information about safe driving.

It's also especially important for older people to avoid prolonged exposure to extreme heat or cold. Accidental hypothermia (an abnormally low body temperature) can be avoided by wearing several layers of clothing and keeping the head covered. When older people live alone, they should arrange to have someone check on them daily when temperatures are very low. Overexposure to heat or to the sun can result in hyperthermia (heat stroke), a serious and potentially fatal condition. Older people, especially those with chronic diseases, can avoid hyperthermia by remaining in shady areas outside or in cool rooms during hot weather.

The **National Safety Council,** 444 North Michigan Avenue, Chicago, Il 60611; 312-527-4800, http://www.nsc.org/, is a nonprofit public service organization whose goal is to prevent accidents and improve the health of all Americans. The **National Institute on Aging:** http://www.nia.nih.gov/ has some excellent materials on home safety, accidental hypothermia, and prevention of injury to older adults.

DISEASE-SPECIFIC ORGANIZATIONS

Osteoporosis

Osteoporosis is sometimes called the "silent disease" because it has no symptoms during its early stages. Unfortunately the condition is usually not recognized until it reaches an advanced stage when fractures occur, most often in the spine, wrists, and hips. Current recommendations to prevent osteoporosis involve engaging regularly in weight-bearing exercise, and consuming adequate amounts of calcium and vitamin D throughout life. The **American Academy of Orthopaedic Surgeons,** 222 South Prospect Avenue, Park Ridge, IL 60068; 312-823-7186, http://www.aaos.org/, is a professional association whose members are orthopaedic surgeons. The staff offers an educational brochure entitled: Osteoporosis. The **National Institute of Arthritis and Musculoskeletal and Skin Diseases (NIAMS),** Public Information Office, Building 31, Room B2B15, Bethesda, MD 20892; 301-496-8188, http://nih.gov/niams/healthinfo/, one of the National Institutes of Health, supports clinical research on such chronic disabling diseases as osteoporosis, arthritis, and other musculoskeletal and skin diseases. The **National Institute on Aging,** Public Information Office, Building 31, Room 5C35, Bethesda, MD 20892; 301-496-2947, http://www.nia.nih.gov/, supports biomedical, social and behavioral research on the aging process and special problems common to older people. The National Osteoporosis Foundation, 1625 Eye Street, NW, Suite 1011, Washington, DC 20006; 202-223-2226, http://www.nof.org/, offers programs nationwide to educate professionals and the public about osteoporosis and related research.

Arthritis

Osteoarthritis (OA), one of the most common forms of arthritis, is a degenerative joint disease that develops in a large number of people by the age of 65 years. Only half of those affected experience pain and loss of mobility as a result of OA. It is important to reduce symptoms and prevent disability and handicap resulting from inactivity. The form of treatment recommended depends on how severe the disease is and the joints affected. General approaches to treatment are to control pain with drugs, and to protect the joints from stress through rest and by exercising regularly to strengthen muscles supporting the joints. Surgery for joint replacement is often indicated in the more severe cases of OA. The **Arthritis Foundation,** PO Box 7669, NW, Atlanta, GA 30357-0669; 404-872-7100 or 800-283-7800, http://www.arthritis.org/, is a nationwide program committed to examining the cause and cure for arthritis and to improving treatments for arthritic patients. Services offered include public information and education about arthritis, a variety of publications for patient education, referrals to specialists, and community activities such as arthritis clinics and rehabilitation and home care programs. The **National Institute of Arthritis and Musculoskeletal and Skin Diseases,** as mentioned in the previous section, is also an excellent source of patient and professional informational materials and research.

No matter what your role is on the treatment team for rheumatoid arthritis patients, on of the best resources for professional information is the **Association of Rheumatology Health Professions (AHRP).** The AHRP is affiliated with the **American College of Rheumatologists** and is based on the premise that collaboration among the many health care professionals involved in the care of patients should strengthen care. The organization promotes education, research, and quality care in rheumatic diseases and includes physicians, nurses, physical therapists, occupational therapists, social workers, psychologists, nutritionists, and alternative practitioners. 1800 Century Place, Suite 250, Atlanta, GA 30345; 404-633-3777; e-mail: acr@rheumatology.org.

Urinary Incontinence

Urinary incontinence is especially common in women over the age of 65 years. Because those affected often isolate themselves, incontinence can be both a medical and a social problem. Two common types of incontinence are urge incontinence, in which the individual is unable to hold urine long enough to make it to the bathroom due to bladder irritation or hyperactivity, and stress incontinence, in which leakage occurs during physical exertion or when sneezing, coughing, or laughing. Stress incontinence is also found in younger women as a result of pelvic floor weakening following pregnancy. The treatment methods most often used to relieve incontinence include: exercises (Kegel exercises to strengthen the pelvic floor muscles), medications, and surgery. The **Help for Incontinent People Organization (HIP),** PO Box 544, Union, SC 29379; 803-585-8789, http://www.incontinent.com/, is a self-help and patient advocacy group that offers encouragement, information, and resource listings for incontinent individuals. It also publishes the Resource Guide for Continence Aids and Services and the quarterly newsletter: The HIP Report. The **Simon Foundation,** PO Box 835X, Wilmette, Il 60091; 800-237-4666, http://www.simonfoundation.org/html/, is a nonprofit educational group and serves as a clearinghouse for information on incontinence. It also publishes a newsletter entitled The Informer. **Continence Restored,** 785 Park Avenue, New York, NY 10021; 212-879-3131 or 407 Strawberry Hill Avenue, Stamford, CT 06902; 203-348-0601, is a newly developed self-help organization that provides a wealth of information and support through the assistance of medically trained leaders. The **U.S. Department of Health and Human Services** through the **Department of Health Resources and Service Administration,** http://www.hrsa.dhhs.gov/, has an excellent set of publications that serve as a quick reference for clinicians (AHCPR 92-0041), a more extensive booklet on clinical practice guidelines (AHCPR 92-0038), and a patient's guide (AHCPR 92-0040), all of which are very comprehensive and valuable as educational tools in treating urinary incontinence in both men and women.

Cognitive Changes

Mental decline is not a normal part of growing older. Symptoms of cognitive decline, such as memory loss, bizarre behavior or personality changes, confusion, and extreme combativeness, in an older person may indicate the presence of any number of conditions, some of which are reversible. Two forms of incurable mental impairments that occur in old age are Alzheimer's disease and multi-infarct dementia. What may appear to be profound mental impairment often is a reversible condition that can be easily corrected. Common causes of reversible impairment are poor nutrition, adverse drug reactions, high fever, and minor head injuries. Emotional problems frequently cause a reversible condition as well. Anxiety, boredom, loneliness, and depression can all appear as mental impairment. Depression, in particular, is the most common cause of pseudodementia. The **Alzheimer's Disease and Related Disorders Association,** 70 East Lake Street, Chicago, IL 60601; 800-621-0379, http://www.alzhi.org/, serves as a clearinghouse for all aspects of Alzheimer's disease including medical, psychosocial, research, legal, political, fundraising, and family services and support. The **National Institute of Neurological Disorders and Stroke (NINDS),** Public Information Office, Building 31, Room 8A06, Bethesda, MD 20892; 301-496-5751, http://www.ninds.nih.gov/, one of the National Institutes of Health, supports research on neurological and communicative disorders and on stroke. It offers an excellent booklet entitled: *The Dementias.* Nursing home resources are listed in the "Housing Options" section of this chapter. The **Alzheimer's Disease Education and Referral Center (ADEAR),** PO Box 8250, Silver Spring, MD 20907-8250; 301-495-3311 or 800-438-4380, http://www.alzheimers.org/adear, established by NIA, distributes information to health professionals, patients and their families, and the general public on Alzheimer's disease, current research activities, and available services. There is information on diagnosis, treatment, drugs, clinical trials, and federal programs and resources. The NIA supports an Alzheimer's disease clinical trials database through the ADEAR. The web site is http://www.alzheimers.org/trials/index.html. The **Alzheimer's Association** is also an excellent source

of information related to the diagnosis and treatment of Alzheimer's disease. It is a national voluntary health organization which provides information and services to people with Alzheimer's, caregivers, researchers, physicians, and health care professionals: 919 Michigan Avenue, Suite 1000, Chicago, IL 60611-1676; 800-272-3900; http://www.alz.org.

Depression

The **National Depressive and Manic-Depressive Association (NDMDA)** 730 N. Franklin Street, Suite 501, Chicago, IL 60610-3526; telephone: 800-826-3632 or 312-642-0049; fax: 312-642-7243; web site: http://www.ndmda.org/ is a nonprofit organization that provides educational materials for patients, families and the public concerning the nature and management of depressive and manic-depressive illness as treatable medical diseases. They have a referral service for access to care regionally and provide information on research related to depression. The NDMDA publishes a quarterly newsletter entitled, *Outreach,* and produces and distributes educational materials that are available upon request. Another very helpful organization for the acquisition of resource materials is the **National Foundation for Depressive Illness (NAFDI)** PO Box 2257, New York, NY 10116; telephone: 800-239-1264 or 800-248-4344 (voice), fax: 212-268-4434; e-mail: NAFDI@pipeline.com; web site: http://www. depression.org./ This is a nonprofit corporation that provides educational materials to educate the public about depressive illness, its consequences, and its treatability. Information is available for physicians and other health care professionals. They provide educational materials, information, and referrals upon request. Ongoing research reports are available through the web site or by request through correspondence at the above contact numbers.

Diabetes

The best source for information on diabetes is the **American Diabetes Association (ADA),** Two Park Avenue, New York, NY 10016; 212-683-7444, http://www.diabetes.org. Members of ADA include physicians, research scientists, and dietitians, as well as diabetics and their families. The Association sponsors educational lectures, film presentations, and diabetes screening clinics. A comprehensive prevention program developed at the Bureau of Primary Health Care to reduce lower extremity amputation in individuals with diabetes mellitus, Hansen's disease, or any condition that results in loss of protective sensation in the feet is the **Lower Extremity Amputation Prevention Program (LEAP Program).** They provide protocol for annual foot screening and patient education including daily self inspection and selection of appropriate footwear. Bureau of Primary Health Care, Division of Programs for Special Populations, 4350 East West Highway, 9th Floor, Bethesda, MD 20814; 888-275-

4772; http://www.bphc.hrsa.gov/leap. You can obtain free Symmes-Weinstein filaments with cardboard mountings in quantities of up to 50/order through this web site.

Wound Care

Several wound care organizations and societies that have been formed over the past decade offer specialized information for management of wounds to health care providers. Physical therapists either serve in vital management roles or as key advisors in many of these groups. Education materials and information on current research related to wound care is available from the following wound care organizations: The **American Academy of Wound Management** 1720 Kennedy Causeway, Suite 109, North Bay Village, FL 33141; telephone: 305-866-9592; fax: 305-868-0905; e-mail: woundnet@aol.com, Web site: http://www.members@ aol.com/woundnet/. The **Association for Advancement of Wound Care** c/o Health Management Publications, 950 West Valley Road, Suite 2800, Wayne, PA 19087; telephone: 800-237-7285; e-mail: aawcline @aol.com, Web site: http://members@aol. com/aawcline. Lastly, a particularly good resource for pharmaceutical information is the **Wound Healing Society** 9650 Rockville Pike, Bethesda, MD 20814-3398; telephone: 800-433-2732 x 7120; fax: 301-530-7049; web site: http://www.woundhealsoc.org.

Cancer

The **Cancer Information Service of the National Cancer Institute,** 9000 Rockville Pike, Building 31, Room 10A18, Bethesda, MD 20892; 800-4-CANCER; http:// cis.nci.nih.gov/. This service is provided by the National Cancer Institute (NCI) under the National Institutes of Health (NIH). In this program, trained NCI staff answer questions and offer publications about various aspects of cancer prevention, detection, causes, and treatments. A very comprehensive NCI web site for information on current drug and treatment trials for cancer and other cancer-related research is **CancerNet** at http://cancernet.nci.nih.gov/. The **American Cancer Society** is the nationwide community-based voluntary health organization dedicated to eliminating cancer as a major health problem by preventing cancer through screening, providing referrals for cancer care, and through research, education, advocacy, and service. 800-ACS-2345; http://www.cancer.org.

Ensuring Quality Cancer Care, is a comprehensive and informative report from the National Cancer Policy Board of the Institute of Medicine and the National Research Council. It contains information on the financial costs of cancer care, ensuring access to cancer care, defining quality of care, and the status of cancer-related health services research. This report also includes recommendations for overcoming barriers of access to quality cancer care. Contact the National Academy Press, 2101 Constitution Avenue,

NW, Washington, DC 20418; 202-334-2138 or see the web site at: http://www.nap.edu.

High Blood Pressure

The **High Blood Pressure Information Center,** 120/80 National Institutes of Health, Bethesda, MD 20892, is operated by the National Heart, Lung, and Blood Institute (listed above) and provides information relating to research on the causes, prevention, methods of diagnosis, and treatment of heart, blood vessel, and blood diseases. http://www.nhlbi.nih.gov/ or http:// rover.nhlbi.nih.gov/health/prof/heart/. The **Hypertension Network, Inc.** is an invaluable resource of information regarding medications currently being tested, educational information on exercise and diet, and referral sources in regional areas for clinics focusing on hypertension and related disorders: http://www. bloodpressure.com.

Heart Disease

The **American Heart Association (AHA),** 7320 Greenville Avenue, Dallas, TX 75231; 214-373-6300, http://www.americanheart.org/, supports research, education, and community service programs with the objective of reducing premature death and disability from cardiovascular disease and stroke. Local chapters are found in many communities. In addition, the Mended Hearts, a subgroup of the AHA provides information, encouragement, and services to heart disease patient and their families. The **National Heart, Lung, and Blood Institute (NHLBI),** 9000 Rockville Pike, Bethesda, MD 20892; 301-496-4236, http://www. nhlbi.nih.gov/, one of the National Institutes of Health, provides leadership for a national program of research and education on causes, prevention, diagnosis, and treatment of diseases of the heart, blood vessels, blood, and lungs, and on the use of blood and the management of blood resources. The **American Heart Association National Center** provides many links to information of treatment, research, drugs, and patient educational materials on disease, peripheral vascular disease, and stroke on it's web site: http://www.americanheart.org/.

Cerebral Vascular Accident

The resources listed under heart disease and high blood pressure above are also excellent sources for information on cerebral vascular accidents. Additional organizations that have publications for professionals and the public pertaining to stroke, provide current research and support services to rehabilitation specialists are: The **National Stroke Association** 96 Inverness Drive E, Suite 1, Engelwood CO 80112; telephone: 800-787-6537; fax: 303-771-1886; web site: http://www.stroke.org, and the **National Aphasia Association (NAA)** which can be reached by phone: 800-922-4622 or e-mail: naa@aphasia.org. The NAA in a nonprofit organization that promotes public education, research, rehabilitation, and support services to assist people with aphasia and their families.

Parkinson's Disease

The **National Parkinson Foundation, Inc. (NPF)** Bob Hope Parkinson Research Center, 1501 NW 9th Avenue, Bob Hope Road, Miami, FL 33136-1494; telephone: 305-547-6666 or 800-327-4545; fax: 305-243-4403; e-mail: mailbox@npf.med.miami.edu, web site: http://www.parkinson.org, supports researchers, physicians, physical, occupational, and speech therapists, and psychologists. The NPF has a wealth of educational and medical information for Parkinson's patients, their families, and medical practitioners. There are numerous patient and caregiver resources in addition to on-line publications, free brochures, research reports, and a very comprehensive annotated reading list. One very helpful service provided by the NPF is the caregivers' web site: http://www.parkinsonscare.com which provides referrals to local agencies to assist in the care of Parkinson's patients and lists organizations that can assist with the acquisition of or donation of equipment for managing activities of daily living and mobility.

The **American Parkinson Disease Association, Inc. (APDA)** 1250 Hylan Boulevard, Suite 4B, Staten Island, NY 10305-1946; telephone: 718-981-8001 or 800-223-2732; fax: 718-981-4399; web site: http://www.apdaparkinson.com offers a variety of free services and information. One very helpful resource is *The Parkinson's Handbook: A Guide for Patients and Families;* as well as booklets on diet, exercise, nutrition and a variety of other topics and issues relevant to the Parkinson patient. The *Parkinson's Newsletter* is published three times a year and highlights current research and legislative issues. The APDA also provides referrals to physicians and services throughout the United States. There is a network of APDA information & referral centers across the United States. Other resources include financial consulting, social work, medical research trials and more. Additionally, you can borrow books and videotapes from the APDA for educational purposes free of charge (see web site).

Pulmonary Disease

The **American Lung Association (ALA)** is an organization that provides educational materials and information on every imaginable pulmonary disease. It also provides a listings of smoking cessation programs across the country, and consumer information on pollutants that lead to respiratory pathologies. To contact the ALA for a regional office call 800 LUNG USA (582-4872) or to reach the National Association of the ALA: 1740 Broadway, New York, NY 10019; 212-315-8700; http://www.lungusa.org/. Another source of consumer and professional information and educational materials is the **American Tho-**racic Society, which is an organization that helps to prevent and fight respiratory disease through research, education, patient care, and advocacy. The contact information for the American Thoracic Society is: 1740 Broadway, New York, NY 10019; telephone: 212-315-8700; fax: 212-315-6498; http://www.thoracic.org/.

Asthma and Allergy

Allergy, Asthma & Immunology Online is an excellent resource of information on treatment, seasonal changes in respiratory diseases and allergies, and updates on medications and dietary approaches for the management of restrictive respiratory diseases. http://www.allergy.mcg.edu.

Thyroid Disease

The **American Foundation of Thyroid Patients** is a wonderful resource for patient education and support. It was established to assist persons with a thyroid condition and their family members, health care providers, and other interested parties by providing support groups, a medical advisory board, and a quarterly newsletter. They provide regional referrals to medical practitioners dealing with thyroid problems and have up-to-date information on current treatment modes inclusive of diet. 18534 N Lyford, Katy, TX 77449; 888-996-4460 or 281-855-6608; http://www.thyroid.org. Another excellent source of information on questions about thyroid disease is the **Thyroid Foundation of America, Inc.** This is a nonprofit charitable organization of thyroid specialists that provides education and information for thyroid patients and health professionals. They work to increase public awareness of screening and detection of thyroid pathologies and fund research. Ruth Sleeper Hall 350, 40 Parkman Street, Boston, MA 02114; telephone: 800-832-8321 or 617-726-8500; fax: 617-726-4136; e-mail: info@tsh.org; website: http://www.tsh.org. A professional society of physicians and scientists dedicated to research and treatment of thyroid pathologies is the **American Thyroid Association** Townhouse Office Park 55 Old Nyack Turnpike, Suite 611, Nanuet, NY 10954; fax: 914-623-3736; http://www.thyroid.org. This association is involved in education, research, dissemination of new knowledge for prevention, diagnosis, and treatment. It was established to guide public policies related to thyroid disease and publishes an excellent journal entitled, *Thyroid,* which you can read at their web site.

Visual Problems

The **American Academy of Ophthalmology (AAO)** PO Box 7424, San Francisco, CA 94120-7424; telephone: 515-561-8500; fax: 515-561-8533; website: http://www.aao.org/; e-mail: comm@aao.org is an excellent resource for educational materials on visual problems in the elderly. The AAO offers an on-line education center as well as a variety of public service programs aimed at achieving accessible, appropriate and affordable eye care for the public by serving the educational and professional needs of the ophthalmologist. Another excellent resource for educational pamphlets and other materials is the **American Society of Cataract and Refractive Surgery (ASCRS)**. Their primary mission is to provide clinical and practice management education for eye surgeons and to work with patients, government and the medical community to promote delivery of quality eye care. Educational materials can be obtained by contacting ASCRS at: 4000 Legato Road, Suite 850, Fairfax, VA 22033; telephone: 703-591-2220; fax: 703-591-0614; web site: http://www.ascrs.org. Lastly, the **Glaucoma Foundation** is a nonprofit organization dedicated to research and public education regard screening for, preventing, detecting, and treating glaucoma. Their web site offers many programs and resources: http://www.glaucoma-foundation.org. There is a patient guide on-line which can also be obtained in book form: 116 John Street, Suite 1605, New York, NY 10038; telephone: 212-285-0080 or 800-452-8266; fax: 212-651-1888. This organization publishes a monthly newsletter entitled, *Eye to Eye*.

Hearing Problems

The **American Speech-Language-Hearing Association (ASHA)** 10801 Rockville Pike, Rockville, MD 20852; telephone: 800-498-2071; TTY: 301-897-5700; fax: 301-571-0457; web site: http://www.asha.org/ is the best resource of educational materials and information regarding hearing loss and other auditory problems. Their mission is to promote the interests of and provide the highest quality of services for professionals and advocate for people with communication disabilities. The **American Academy of Audiology (AAA)** 8300 Greensboro Drive, Suite 750, McLean, VA 22102; telephone: 800-AAA-2336 or 703-790-8466, fax: 703-790-8631; web site: http://www.audiology.org is a professional organization dedicated to providing quality hearing care to the public. They provide a wealth of professional and consumer resources in addition to education materials for the health care professional and the patient. The **AAA** has a referral service in addition to access to the latest research on hearing problems linked to their web site.

Alcoholism

The best source of information on alcoholism in the elderly is the **National Council on Alcoholism and Drug Dependence, Inc. (NCADD)**, 12 West 21st Street, New York, NY 10010; 212-206-6770; fax: 212-645-1690; http://www.ncadd.org/. This is a voluntary organization whose purpose is to educate the public about the disease of alcoholism and to promote programs for prevention.

LONG-TERM CARE ISSUES

Housing Options

In later years, changing circumstances often create the need for a new living arrangement. Costly maintenance and utility bills, the desire to relocate closer to family or live in a smaller home, or a need for regular nursing attention are just a few of the considerations older persons have regarding housing. Today, a wide variety of housing options are available, some of which include new types of living arrangements that have evolved only in recent years. Some people arrange for "in-home" services for special needs. These might include homemaker or home health aide services, home-delivered meals, and escort or transportation services. Others consider renting out a portion of their home. Additional options include moving to a smaller home, moving in with family members, moving to a group home where older people share one residence, or moving to a community designed especially for older people. Many types of housing offer support services, as in a continuing care community or a nursing home. The **American Association of Homes for the Aging (AAHA)**, 901 E Street, NW, Suite 500, Washington, DC 20040-2011; telephone: 202-783-2242; fax: 202-783-2255; http://www.aahsa.org/, is a national organization whose members include nonprofit nursing homes, independent housing facilities, continuing care facilities, and homes for the aging. They provide an excellent brochure entitled The Continuing Care Retirement Community: A Guidebook for Consumers. The **National Association of Home Care**, 228 Seventh Street, SE, Washington, DC 20003; telephone: 202-547-7424; fax: 202-547-3540; http://www.nahc.org/, monitors federal and state activities affecting home care and focuses on issues relating to home health care. They publish a magazine bimonthly called the Caring Magazine. The **National Citizen's Coalition for Nursing Home Reform**, 1424 16th Street, NW, Suite 202, Washington, DC 20036-2211; telephone: 202-332-2275; fax: 202-332-2949; http://www.nccnhr.org/, serves as a voice enabling consumers to be heard on issues concerning the development of long-term care systems. The Nursing Home Information Service of the **National Council of Senior Citizens, National Senior Citizens Education and Research Center**, 8403 Colesville Road, Suite 1200, Silver Spring, MD 20910-3314; telephone: 301-578-8800; fax: 301-578-8999; http://www.ncscinc. org/, is a referral center for consumers of long-term care services. They offer information on nursing homes and alternative community and health services, and information on how to select a nursing home.

The **National Center for Assisted Living (NCAL)** is the assisted living voice of the American Health Care Association, the nation's largest organization representing Long Term Care providers. This organization provides professionals and consumers with information and educational resources and seminars on long-term care. 1201 L Street, NW, Washington, DC; 202-842-4444; http://www.ncal.org/. The **National Association for the Support of Long Term Care (NASL)** represents Medicare reimbursed ancillaries providing medical services and products to long term care facilities. Additionally, this association provides numerous services including lobbying, information dissemination and accessibility to health policy makers. 1321 Duke Street, Suite 304, Alexandria, VA 22314; telephone: 703-549-8500; fax: 703-549-8342; http://www.nasl.org/.

Homelessness

The **National Coalition for the Homeless (NCH)** 1012 Fourteenth Street, NW, Suite 600, Washington, DC 20005-3410; telephone: 202-737-6444; fax: 202-737-6445; e-mail: info@nationalhomeless.org; web site: http://www.nationalhomeless.org is a national advocacy network of homeless persons, activists, service providers, and others committed to ending homelessness through public education, policy advocacy, grassroots organizing, and technical assistance. The NCH Online Library is a searchable bibliographic database with references to research on homelessness, housing, and poverty. Also available on the web site are six directories listing contact people, e-mail addresses, and web pages for hundreds of local, statewide and national organization. NCH publishes a very informative bimonthly newsletter entitled *Safety Network* which deals with the many issues of homelessness with focus often on the issues created by homelessness of an elderly population. The **Committee to End Elder Homelessness (CEEH)** 1640 Washington Street, Boston, MA 02118; telephone: 617-369-1555 is a nonprofit organization dedicated to the prevention and elimination of elder homelessness in our communities. They've created and implemented a wide range of strategies and initiatives to guide the access to, and effectiveness of, resources for homeless or "at risk" older adults. Their web site is http://www.ceeh.org.

Financial Planning

Many older people are able to enjoy their retirement years with enough money to meet their basic needs and enjoy some leisure activities. Others face poverty for the first time in old age. Retirement savings often must be used for expensive medical treatment, fixed incomes or savings that many older persons depend on can erode through high inflation rates, and with a longer life expectancy many older people simply outlive their assets.

Women are at a particularly high risk for becoming impoverished. Women generally earn lower salaries than men, and this further limits retirement benefits. Benefits are calculated on average lifetime earnings, so time spent at home to rear children reduces both pension and Social Security income in later life. Women are also more likely to work part-time and to work for employers who do not offer pension benefits, such as in service businesses. Moreover, Social Security is intended to supplement other forms of retirement income, but for 60% of women over age 65 it is the only source of support. Another problem is that a large group of older women do not even receive benefits because they do not know about them or how to get them, or because they are too proud to accept this assistance. Others, especially those for whom English is a second language, may not understand complicated paperwork necessary to initiate payments. Thus, only half of elderly persons eligible for Supplemental Security Income actually receive benefits.

The **Social Security Administration (SSA),** Office of Public Inquiries, 6401 Security Boulevard, Baltimore, MD 21235-6401; 301-594-1234 or 800-772-1213; http://www.ssa.gov/, is a Federal agency that provides information about Social Security coverage, earnings records, claims eligibility, and adjustments. They also have information about Medicare and Medicaid programs. The Supplemental Security Income program is also administered by SSA and provides supplemental payments to older persons who already receive public assistance. Social Security branch offices are located throughout the country and are listed in local telephone directories. The **Women's Equity Action League,** 1250 Eye Street, NW, Suite 305, Washington, DC 20005; 202-898-1588, is a national organization whose members are dedicated to securing legal and economic rights for women by monitoring the implementation and enforcement of equal opportunity laws, conducting research, publishing reports, lobbying, and supporting lawsuits.

Retirement

The SSA (listed above) is an excellent resource for information related to planning for retirement. In addition http://www.quicken.com/retirement has a retirement planning section with forms you can download and fill out. This is a very helpful tool.

Caregiving

Caregiving is the job of helping a relative or friend with meals, shopping, and other daily activities. A recent survey of caregivers for elderly persons showed this role is most often taken on by women, usually wives or daughters. Caregiving is also a policy issue growing in importance today since the number of people over age 85 (those in greatest need of daily help) is increasing rapidly and is expected to more than double within the next 15 years. With this rapid growth in the frail elderly population, a declining birth rate, and more women participating in the labor force, a wider diversity of groups are taking on responsibility for shouldering the tasks of caregiving. Many groups are developing new ways of enabling families to share in partnership with other types of support systems, although the nature of such partnerships and the proper division of responsibility remain complex issues and are subject to much debate. The **Administration on Aging (AoA)**, Office of Human Development DHHS, 330 Independence Avenue, S.W., Washington, DC 20201; 202-245-0724 (general information); 202-245-0641 (publications), is a federal agency and provides information about social services, nutrition, education, senior centers, and other programs for older Americans. It also offers a *Directory of State and Regional Agencies on Aging*, which lists local area agencies on aging. Through the AoA you can also get in touch with the Office of the Assistant Secretary of Aging at 202-401-4541. For congressional and media inquiries, fax requests, questions, or information to 202-260-1012. The AoA web site also links you to all of the above information: http://www.aoa.gov. The **Eldercare Locator** is also managed through the National Aging Information Center of the AoA: 112 16th Street, NW, Suite 100, Washington, DC 20036; 800-677-1116. This agency is helpful in finding local services to answer a specific need and referral to local agencies that can assist in the care of an elder parent or relative. An organization called the **Children of Aging Parents (CAPS)**, 1609 Woodbourne Road, Suite 302A, Levittown, PA 19057; 215-945-6900 or 800-227-7294; http://www. CAPS4caregivers.org, is a cooperative effort of the NIA and the AoA and provides a variety of services, including starter packages for those interested in becoming caregivers, a "matching" service for people starting a support group, workshops for the general community, and printed material. This nonprofit organization has a national mission of assisting caregivers of the elderly by providing information, referrals, and support. They also distribute a monthly newsletter.

The **National Family Caregivers Association (NFCA)** 10400 Connecticut Avenue, Suite 500, Kensington, MD 20895-3944; telephone: 800-896-3650; fax 301-942-2302; e-mail: info@nfcacares.org, web site: http://www.nfcacares.org espouses a philosophy of self-advocacy and self-care that is predicated on the belief that caregivers who choose to take charge of their lives, and see caregiving as but one of its facets, are in a position to be happier and healthier individuals. The NFCA has much to offer through its services in the areas of education and information, support and validation, public awareness and advocacy. There are numerous services available for family caregivers (see web site for a listing).

The **American Association for Continuity of Care (AACC)** PO Box 7073, North Brunswick, NJ 08902, 800-816-1575 (voice), 301-352-7686 (fax); web site: http://www.continuityofcare.com/ is a networking and planning organization of health care professionals concerned with discharge planning and continuity of patient care. The Association provides a forum to exchange information, a network to identify resources, and a support organization for local groups. AACC also tracks pertinent legislation and regulation. It is comprised of a multidisciplinary membership committed to providing leadership and supporting excellence in practice among those involved in continuity of care through education and patient-focused advocacy.

The **National Association of State Units on Aging (NASUA)** 1225 I Street, NW, Suite 725, Washington, DC 20005; 202-898-2578, is a national, nonprofit, public interest organization which operates a National Resource Center on Long-Term Care and the National Information and Referral Support Center. Both are funded by the Administration on Aging (AoA), and operates AGE-NET, an electronic bulletin board.

The **National Association of Area Agencies on Aging, Inc.,** 1112 16th Street, NW, Suite 100, Washington, DC 20036-4823; 202-296-8130, represents a majority of the more than 660 area agencies on aging. Its mission is to assist older Americans, allowing them to stay in their own homes and communities with dignity and independence for as long as possible. This organization publishes a resource entitled, *National Directory for Eldercare Information and Referral.*

The **National Alliance for Caregiving (NAC),** 4720 Montgomery Lane, Suite 642, Bethesda, MD 20814; 301-718-8444 is a nonprofit joint venture of several national aging organizations that focus attention on the issue of family caregiving of the elderly. NAC publishes a free brochure, *LINKAGES, Resources for People Care for Older Relatives,* which is an invaluable source of information. NAC also has sent information on caregiving books and videos to help caregivers find local community services, Internet resources, and resource organizations to libraries across the country, so a quick trip to your local library may yield a wealth of information for the caregiver.

The **AARP** (as listed under "General Information" in this chapter) is also an excellent resource for information to assist the caregiver in identifying agencies for support and referral to available means of care provision. They have an excellent video, *Survival Tips for New Caregivers,* which is available for $4.50 plus postage, and also publish a booklet, *Before You Buy: A Guide to Long-Term Care Insurance* (D12893), which is free and a very concise and comprehensive review of what to look for in insurance policies for the provision of long-term care.

Widowhood

The average age of widowhood for women in the United States is 56, which results in half of all women over age 65 living as widows. The average age of widowhood for men is 72. This high rate of widowhood occurs because women tend to marry men older than themselves and because life expectancy from birth is seven years longer for women than for men. Widowhood is often the end of a relationship that lasted most of a lifetime; it can cause profound grief. Thus recovery is often painful and takes time. The period of most intense grief can last from a few months to a year or more. During this time it is normal for the widowed person to feel despair or depression, irritability, and even anger toward the person who died. After this grieving process, the individual is usually able to increase her/his range of independence and find new friends and activities to enrich life, although most people need special help with the social and psychological problems associated with being widowed.

Loneliness also commonly arises during this period. It sometimes takes an extra effort to find social activities and friends, but many resources are available to draw on. Also, by offering their skills, many elderly individuals make new friendships through a variety of affiliations: with religious or civic organizations, voluntary activities, and other commitments. Women who find themselves alone as a result of widowhood may need to develop new skills for a changing role. For example, some must learn to manage financial matters for the first time, such as paying bills, balancing a checkbook, and handling insurance benefits. To help both widows and widowers, a growing number of national and local organizations provide social and other types of support. **ACTION,** 806 Connecticut Avenue, NW, Washington, DC 20525; 800-424-8580, is a federal agency which administers domestic and international volunteer programs including the Peace Corps, Retired Senior Volunteer Program, Foster Grandparent Program, Senior Companion Project, and others. The **Displaced Homemaker Network,** 1411 K Street, NW, Washington, DC 20005; 202-628-6767, is an agency that fosters the development of programs across the United States with services to help displaced homemakers; these include individual counseling, support groups, employment/training seminars, vocational testing, and a "job club." The **Widowed Persons Service** is a part of American Association of Retired Persons, 1909 K Street, NW, Washington, DC 20049; 202-872-4700 or 800-253-2017 x 4841; http://www.aarp.org/griefprograms/wps.html. This is an outreach program for newly widowed persons. A service of the AARP, it provides group sessions, publication about legal matters, volunteer opportunities, and other services.

POLITICAL ISSUES

The **Gray Panthers** founded by the late Maggie Kuhn is an intergenerational advocacy group comprised of a coalition of activists who work to promote the concerns of the aged through newsletters and publications aimed at fighting various types of abuse and age discrimination. 733 15th Street NW, Suite 437, Washington, DC 20005; telephone: 800-280-5362 or 202-

737-6637; fax: 202-737-1160; website: http://www.graypanthers.org e-mail info@graypanthers.org (e-mail). The **National Coalition on Older Women's Issues (NCOWI),** 2401 Virginia Avenue, NW, Washington, DC 20037; 202-466-7837, is a nationwide network made up of member organizations and individuals concerned with improving the status of older women. Its focus is on the areas of employment, retirement income, and health and well-being of women. NCOWI offers a list of organizations called *Midlife and Older Women: A Resource Directory.* The cost is $4.

The **National Council on the Aging (NCOA),** 409 Third Street, SW, Washington, DC 20024; telephone: 202-479-1200; fax: 202-479-0735; http://www.ncoa.org, in conjunction with other organizations, helps to promote concerns of interest to older persons. NCOA is an advocacy group that conducts seminars on wellness, offers a range of publications on public policy, advocacy, education, and career training, and functions as a resource for public education.

The **National Organization for Women (NOW),** 733 15th Street, NW, 2nd Floor, Washington, DC 20005; telephone: 202-628-8669; fax: 202-785-8576; http://www.now.org/, is an advocacy group that monitors local and national legislation affecting American women. Members participate in activities concerned with women's rights issues, such as economic protections for older women, participation in politics, recognition of the economic value of homemaking, and freedom from racial and educational discrimination. The **Older Women's League (OWL),** 666 11th Street, NW, Suite 700, Washington, DC 20001; 202-783-6686; http://www.owl-national.org, a cooperative effort of NIA and the AoA has a national membership who are committed to helping meet various special needs of middle-aged and older women, especially in the areas of Social Security, pension rights, health insurance, and caregiver support services. OWL uses volunteers to help with mailings, to maintain a referral resource file, and to answer letters from women writing in from across the country with questions.

LEGAL ISSUES

The **Commission on Legal Problems of the Elderly** is an organization managed by the American Bar Association. 740 15th Street, NW, Washington, DC 20005-1022; telephone: 202-662-8640; fax: 202-662-8698; http://www. abanet.org,elderly This is a commission that works to improve the quality and quantity of legal services for older citizens. It refers requests for services to appropriate agencies or groups. The **National Senior Citizens Law Center,** 1101 14th Street, NW, Suite 400, Washington, DC 20005; telephone: 202-289-6976, fax: 202-289-7224; http://www.nsclc. org, is a public interest law firm with attorneys who specialize in areas of federal law having the greatest impact on the elderly poor. This organization advocates, litigates, and publishes on low-income elderly and disability issues including Medicare, Medicaid, SSI, nursing homes, age discrimination, and pensions.

The **National Academy of Elder Law Attorneys (NAELA)** 1604 N. Country Club Road, Tucson, AZ 85716; telephone: 520-881-4005; fax: 520-325-7925; web site: http://www.naela.com/ is an organization comprised of attorneys in the private and public sectors who deal with legal issues affecting the elderly and disabled. Members include judges, professors of law, lawyers, and students. Some of the issues NAELA assists their clients with include, but are not limited to: public benefits, probate and estate planning, guardianship/conservatorship, and health and long-term care planning. This organization is also a wealth of information on printed materials pertaining to topics such as living wills, power-of-attorney, patient rights, elder abuse, and the areas identified above. A very helpful pamphlet entitled: *Questions and Answers When Looking for an Elder Law Attorney* is free and an excellent guide to choosing a lawyer knowledgeable in legal issues pertaining to the elderly.

ELDER ABUSE

The **National Center on Elder Abuse (NCEA)** 1225 I Street, NW, Suite 725, Washington, DC 20005; telephone: 202-898-2586; fax: 202-898-2583; web site: http://www.elderabusecenter.org/ is funded through a grant by the US AoA, and consists of a consortium of six partners: National Association of State Units on Aging (NASUA), the lead agency; Commission on Legal Problems of the Elderly of the American Bar Association (ABA); the Clearinghouse on Abuse and Neglect of the Elderly of the University of Delaware (CANE); the San Francisco Consortium for Elder Abuse Prevention of the Goldman Institute on Aging (GIOA); the National Association of Adult Protective Services Administrators (NAAPSA); and the National Committee to Prevent Elder Abuse (NCPEA). NCEA exists to provide elder abuse information to professionals and the public; offer technical assistance and training to elder abuse agencies and related professionals; conduct short-term elder abuse research; and assist with elder abuse program and policy development. NCEA's web site contains many resources and publications to help achieve these goals. It's absolutely the best resource for comprehensive information on elder abuse. Their web site provides links to every conceivable organization or service addressing elder abuse in the United States, and therefore, once you've connected with NCEA, you've connected with all agencies that deal with elder abuse in this country.

ADVOCACY

Developments in Aging contains reports of activities by federal departments and agencies on behalf of older Americans, including information about ac-

tions taken by the Congress, the administration, and the Special Committee on Aging. Single copies can be obtained from the Senate Committee on Aging, G-31 Dirksen SOB, Washington, DC 20510-6400, e-mail: mailbox@aging.senate.gov. The **National Council of Senior Citizens (NCSC)** 8403 Colesville Road, Suite 1200, Silver Spring, MD 20910; telephone: 301-578-8800; fax: 301-578-8999; web site: http://www.nscerc.org is one of the largest nonprofit organization for senior citizens in the United States with more than 500,000 members in 2,000 affiliated clubs and councils nationwide. Their primary objective is to closely follow the concerns of older Americans and translate those concerns into political muscle. They also sponsor senior housing with nearly 4,000 units in 38 buildings in 17 states across the country. NCSC's affiliate, **National Senior Citizens Education and Research Center (NSCERC)** operates more than 145 Senior AIDS projects with the help of the US Department of Labor grant. The program employs more than 10,500 low-income senior citizens nationwide in jobs ranging from Meals-on-Wheels workers and after-school program staff to library aides and literacy tutors.

The **National Association of Senior Friends (NASF)** 800-348-4886; web site: http://www.senior-friends.com provides advocacy and healthy living programs and healthcare discounts throughout the US. NASF offers a strong national network (220 chapters) which provide exceptional benefits and services for middle aged and older, employed and retired senior citizens. Materials are available from their web site on health screenings, educational health programs, social activities, exercise programs, and senior volunteer programs. [see also "Political Issues" and "Legal Issues" in this chapter].

EDUCATIONAL/CAREER ISSUES

The **American Association of University Women (AAUW)**, 1111 16th Street, NW, Washington, DC 20036; telephone: 800-326-AAUW or 202-785-7700; fax: 202-872-1425; http://www.aauw.org is the largest national organization promoting the advancement of women in education and lifelong learning. For its members the AAUW holds monthly lectures and for the public offers a variety of publications relating to education and career reentry. **Elderhostel,** 75 Federal Street, Suite 400, Boston, MA 02110-1941; 877-426-8056; http://www.elderhostel.org, is a nonprofit educational program for adults age 60 and over. The program consists of one-week courses taught in residence at various college campuses. The courses offer a range of liberal arts subjects presented at an introductory level. It provides liberal arts educational adventure programs for retirement age individuals. Free catalogues are available upon request.

The **National Commission on Working Women,** 1211 Connecticut Avenue, NW, Suite 400, Washington, DC 20036; 202-332-1405, is a private organization that focuses on the concerns of women working in service industries, clerical occupations, retail stores, and factories.

COMPUTER TRAINING AND RESOURCES FOR SENIORS

Many older adults are interested and yet intimidated by computers and the use of the Internet. As an educational tool the Internet is invaluable. Additionally, the use of the Internet can provide product information, health and wellness information, updates on Medicare and other insurance-related information, materials on legislative and policy initiatives and changes, and it can also provide a means of communication with relatives and friends. There are several web sites that offer a wealth of information for seniors.

The **American Association of Retired Persons (AARP)** site, http://www.aarp.org, offers purchasing advice, discounts for gear and Internet access, as well as discussion groups and educational materials.

The **AgeLight Institute,** http://www.agelight.org/ provides assistance in locating a computer site for instructionals in how to use a computer and how to maneuver on the Internet. **Computers for Seniors,** http://www.computersforseniors.org, aims to help seniors overcome their fear of computers and gain confidence in using them. The Web site offers information about classes and has links to other sites of interest. **Senior Tips,** http://www.seniortips.com has computer tips, product reviews, chat and links to sites offering free stuff. **SeniorNet,** http://www.seniornet.org, is a site that helps to locate computer training programs, provides information on current computer technology and coupons for discounts on computer products for seniors. **ThirdAge,** http:// www.thirdage.com, has free on-line classes, e-mail, chat rooms, and a variety of other resources for seniors.

ASSISTIVE TECHNOLOGY

Project LINK is a nationwide information service that mails catalogues and brochures from assistive device companies to consumers and service providers who need such devices. To request a copy of its *Media and Publications Catalogue on Assistive Technology,* which features videos, workshops, and printed materials on assistive technology, call 800-628-2281 or see the catalogue on their web site: http://www.buffalo. edu/dissemination.htm. Of course the **American Occupational Therapy Association (AOTA)** is a vital source on information assistive devices and technology for enhancing independence in activities of daily living.

Lifease Stony Lake Office Park, 2451 15th Street, NW, Suite D, New Brighton, MN 55112; telephone: 651-636-6869; fax: 651-636-7075; e-mail: MCLifease @aol.com, web page: http://www.lifease.com. is a software resource that assesses the physical living environment for safety and makes recommendations for assistive technologies and vendors for obtaining these needed items.

ADMINISTRATION

There are many resources related to administration of health care services. The most comprehensive web site on administrative issues is the **National Information Center for Health Services Administration:** http://www.nichsa.org. There is a collaborative initiative established by health organizations to collect, manage, and provide information on topics related to administration of hospitals, health systems and networks, and health services. This site provides links to numerous other administration-related web pages.

MEDICARE

America's Seniors and Medicare: Challenges for Today and Tomorrow provides a state-by-state snapshot of the unprecedented demographic and health care challenges confronting Medicare. It documents the success of the current program and provides new information about its impact on women, Americans over the age 85, and rural beneficiaries. To view this publication and many other links to vital information, explore the web site: http://www.whitehouse. gov/.

The **Medicare Web site** http://www.medicare.gov provides general information about Medicare as well as up-to-date information about private health plans, such as Medicare HMOs, and the implications of leaving Medicare. The "Medicare Compare" section of this site provides information on the costs and benefits of the Medicare health plans in your community and the quality of care and member satisfaction in Medicare private health plans. In the "Important Contacts" section, you can find the Medicare contacts for your state and local community.

The **National Committee for Quality Assurance (NCQA)** can tell you if it has accredited the HMO you're in or considering. Call 888-275-7585 or search NCQA's web site a http://www.ncqa.org/

Talking With Your Parents About Medicare Coverage is an excellent publication that answers questions about the Medicare program, supplemental insurance, Medicare HMOs and long-term care. This guide also includes a list of agencies in your state to call with specific questions. You can order this guide from the **Kaiser Family Foundation (KFF),** c/o Information Management International, 2548 Zanker Road, San Jose, CA 95131-1127, or find the guide on the KFF Web site at http://www.kff.org.

The **American Association of Retired Persons** also provides the latest information from AARP on

Medicare, managed care, health insurance options, health legislation, and more at *"Explore Health"* on the AARP web place: http://www.aarp.org.

HELPFUL ORGANIZATIONS

The **Section on Geriatrics (SOG),** a component of the American Physical Therapy Association, supports those therapists, assistants, and students that work with an aging population in roles of advocacy, direct patient care, consultation, supervision, and education. This organization is an excellent resource for information in all areas of concern related to geriatric rehabilitation. The Section represents and serves over 7,000 members with a wide array of services and benefits. They provide continuing education, specialist certification in geriatrics, and work closely with the governance department of the APTA in lobbying for legislative and reimbursement policies that meet the needs of older adults. The SOG plays a very strong role as advocates for the senior citizens they serve. Their web site is superb with links to numerous resources including state and federal policy links, health promotion, prevention, wellness materials, research related to the older adult and geriatric rehabilitation, and access to vendors and equipment suppliers. Additionally, a wide range of educational materials is available inclusive of patient education and current bibliographies of research related to specific areas of geriatric rehabilitation. 1111 North Fairfax Street, PO Box 327, Alexandria, VA 22313; telephone: 800-999-2782 x3238; fax: 703-706-8578; web site: http://www.geriatricspt.org.

The **American Physical Therapy Association (APTA)** is a national professional organization representing nearly 70,000 members. Its goal is to foster advancement in physical therapy practice, research, and education. The mission of the APTA, the principle membership organization representing and promoting the profession of physical therapy, is to further the profession's role in the prevention, diagnosis, and treatment of movement dysfunctions and the enhancement of the physical health and functional abilities of members of the public. 1111 North Fairfax Street, Alexandria, VA 22314-1488, 703-684-APTA (2782), 800-999-APTA (2782), TDD: 703-683-7343, fax on demand: 800-399-APTA (2782); http://www.apta.org.

The **American Occupational Therapy Association (AOTA)** is the nationally recognized professional association for over 60,0000 occupational therapists and occupational therapist assistants. The mission of the association is to support a professional community of members and to develop and preserve the viability and relevance of the profession. The organization serves the interests of the members, represents the profession to the public, and promotes access to occupational therapy. They offer fax on demand services with the provision of educational and informa-tional materials related to the practice of occupational therapy, as well as a web site that has numerous links to available resources for the professional and patients. 4720 Montgomery Lane, PO Box 31220, Bethesda, MD 20824-1220, 301-652-2682 or TDD: 800-377-8555; fax: 301-652-7711; http://www.aota.org.

The **Gerontological Society of America (GSA)** 1030 15th Street, NW, Suite 250, Washington, DC 20005-1503; telephone: 202-842-1275; fax: 202-842-1150; web site: http://www.geron.org. This multidisciplinary organization promotes the scientific study of aging, encourages exchanges among researchers and practitioners from various disciplines related to gerontology, and fosters the use of gerontological research in forming public policy. The primary purpose of this society is to provide researchers, educators, practitioners, and policy makers with expanded opportunities to understand, advance, integrate and use basic and applied research on aging to improve the quality of life during processes of aging. Their major methods for accomplishing this include: disseminating information on aging research, policy, education and practice, providing networks for researchers, policy makers, educators and practitioners, linking research with policy, practice and education, advocating for increased public and private funding for research on aging, and promoting career development and advancement of members.

The **National Academy on an Aging Society** 1030 15th Street, NW, Suite 250, Washington, DC 20005-1503; telephone: 202-408-3376; fax: 202-842-1150; web site: http://www.agingsociety.org. This nationally based, nonpartisan Academy is a policy institute that fosters critical thinking about the implications of an aging society. The Academy studies the impact of demographic changes on public and private institutions and families of all ages. The Academy conducts and synthesizes research on a broad range of topics related to income and health security and conveys the findings to policy makers. Thus, the Academy serves as an information broker on issues often associated with Social Security, Medicare, and Medicaid programs. Materials are also available on their web site on topics that include: changes in the labor market, employer-provided health and pension benefits, the health care market, and access to health and long-term care. They sponsor many geriatric-related conferences, publish and disseminate reports and fact sheets, and provide the newsletter on current legislative initiatives entitled: *The Public Policy and Aging Report.*

Recently, the **Association for Gerontology in Higher Education (AGHE)** merged with the GSA to promote the scientific study of aging and to foster growth and diffusion of knowledge relating to problems of aging and of the sciences contributing to their understanding. AGHE is the only national membership organization devoted primarily to gerontological and geriatrics education. Its membership consists of over 300 colleges, universities, and other organizations interested in gerontological education and research and providing aging-related instructional and research programs. A visit to the GSA web site (listed above) will be beneficial in discovery of the many materials and resources this organization has to offer.

The **American Society on Aging (ASA)** 833 Market Street, Suite 511, San Francisco, CA 94103-1834, 800-537-9728 or 415-974-9643; web site: http://www. asaging.org is a national organization comprised of every imaginable discipline related to gerontology. This organization is a wealth of information through educational programming, outstanding publications and state-of-the-art information and training resources, all developed through the knowledge and experience of a large network of professionals working in the field of geriatrics. This unique society brings together researchers, practitioners, educators, business people, and policy makers concerned with the physical, emotional, social, economic, and spiritual aspects of aging. ASA was founded on the premise that the complexity of aging in our society can only be addressed as a multidisciplinary whole. Additionally, ASA advances the new standard of professionalism in aging, with diversity and cultural competence at its core. A visit to their web site is an experience you don't want to miss.

The **American Geriatrics Society (AGS)** The Empire State Building, 350 Fifth Avenue, Suite 801, New York, NY 10118l telephone: 212-308-1414; fax: 212-832-8646; web site: http://www.americangeriatrics.org is a professional organization of health care providers dedicated to improving the health and well-being of all older adults. With an active membership of over 6,000 health care professionals, the AGS has a long history of effecting change in the provision of health care for older adults. The organization provides leadership to health care professionals, policy makers and the public by developing, implementing and advocating programs in patient care, research, professional and public education and public policy. An excellent resource for educational materials related to all areas of patient care, prevention and health promotion, as well as legislative and reimbursement updates and information.

RESEARCH GRANTS

Contact information on the federal government grant-giving agencies, in terms of address and phone numbers, etc., is referenced previously in this chapter. So, for research grant information, the agency and their web site will only be listed here.

Agency for HealthCare (AH) (now known as Agency for Healthcare Research and Quality) (AHRQ)
http://www.ahrq.gov
Centers for Disease Control and Prevention (CDC)
http://www.cdc.gov

Health Resources and Services Administration (HRSA)
http://www.hrsa.dhhs.gov
National Center for Medical Rehabilitation Research (NCMRR)
http://nichd.nih.gov/about/ncmrr
National Institute of Arthritis and Musculoskeletal and Skin Diseases (NIAMS)
http://www.nih.gov/niams
National Institutes of Health
http://www.nih.gov

Several publications are also available that provide either electronic or printed newsletters with grant announcements as they become available. The **Commerce Business Daily** is a publication of notices of proposed government procurement actions, contract awards, sales of government property, and other procurement information. Each issue has about 500 to 1,000 notices, and each notice appears only once. See their web site for additional information: http://cbdnet.access.gpo.gov/index.html. Grant funding opportunities are announced in the **Federal Register.** On this web page you can search current and past issues of the *Federal Register* for announcements of grants: http://www.access.gpo.gov/su_docs/aces/aces140.html. **NIHTOC-L** is also a sign-up to receive the Table of Contents for the NIH Guide for Grants and Contracts via e-mail each week. The Table of Contents includes the web site addresses for the full text of each Guide announcement or article. For instructions on how to subscribe to this mailing list see the NIH Guide web page: http://grants.nih.gov/grants/guide/index.html.

DATABASE RESOURCES

More than any other tool, the computer has diminished the gap between health care providers and patients. There are hundreds of databases, computerized indexes of information. The most important index, and the one on which most searches are based is **Medline,** (www.ncbi.nlm.nih.gov/entrez/query.fcgi) a data base of 3,600 medical journals. With a personal computer, a modem, and a $30 software package (e.g., **Grateful Med**), you can conduct your own search for in-depth articles on any medical subject. For the Grateful Med software: 800-638-8480; for a free demo disk and brochure: 301-496-6308.

A guide to other databases, Directory of Online Healthcare Databases, is available for $38 at 503-471-1627. This is a far-reaching directory with databases on specific diseases and specific treatments. Most major medical libraries subscribe to Medline, and a reference librarian is an excellent source of information and guidance in how to use the system. In addition, some libraries, hospitals, and HMOs have desktop terminals which provide information for the "nonscientific public". For the center nearest you, call: 800-227-8431 and ask for marketing. **MDX Health Digest** contains 200 health-oriented publications: 503-471-1627. Both of these services rely mainly on secondary sources and will link you to more specific informational centers, and both information and materials are usually free.

If you're already into computer technology, or eager to learn, you can scan all kinds of exchanges between people delving into various medical subjects, via numerous Internet sites. You can also send out a message and await the serendipity of a reply. For a list of health-oriented computer sites, send $5 and a SASE to Black Bag BBS, 1 Ball Farm Way, Wilmington, DE 19808, or with a modem, dial: 302-994-3772.

An extension of the computer web sites is the on-line conference, a sort of electronic self-help group accessible from your own living room. The American Self-Help Clearinghouse organized the first on-line conference for agoraphobics (people who are afraid of open or public places). They linked up without having to leave the house, chatting via keyboards. This could also be a boon for elderly people in rural areas.

CompuServe, an on-line information service, hosts several groups (for a membership fee of around $40, plus a small monthly charge). There is, for instance, a diabetes forum. For general information call: 800-848-8199. For cancer patients, there are numerous data bases. Designed both for medical practitioners and the public, they're among the most complete and easy to use. Medline, for instance, offers a separate cancer data base called **CANCERLIT.**

CRISP (Computer Retrieval of Information of Information on Scientific Projects) is a searchable database of federally funded biomedical research projects conducted at universities, hospitals, and other research institutions. The database is maintained by the Office of Extramural Research at the National Institutes of Health. The address is http://www-commons.cit.nih.gov/crisp/.

A list of treatment centers, plus some 1,500 experimental programs, is available through the National Cancer Institute's data base called **Physician Data Query (PDQ).** PDQ also has a directory of physicians and organizations that provide cancer care. It's designed for doctors, however, you can tap into PDQ by using the Grateful Med software. You can also call 800-4-CANCER and request a free PDQ search and they will mail it to you free of charge. If you have a fax, try Cancer-Fax at 301-402-5874 and an automated voice will tell you how to obtain detailed prognosis and treatment summaries on 80 kinds of cancers. The information is updated every month and you can request a version intended for either medical professionals or for the general public.

Database resources are also available through data brokers to meet the needs of health care professionals. The four listed below rely heavily on Medline, tend to be consumer oriented, and are staffed by professionals. The **Health Resource Inc.,** a commercial enterprise, will provide Medline searches, article summaries, book excerpts, medical journal articles, as well as lists of self-help groups. They cover alternative and holistic interventions along with the more mainstream sources of help. A report of 50 to 150 pages costs from $175 up, a mini-report (20 to 25 pages) runs $85. There's a 30-day money-back guarantee if you're not satisfied: 933 Faulkner, Conway, AR 72032; telephone: 501-329-5272 or 800-949-0090; fax: 501-329-9489; http://www.thehealthresource.com/. The nonprofit **Planetree Health Resource Center** provides an in-depth packet on a particular illness for $100; 2040 Webster Street, San Francisco, CA 94115; 415-923-3680 or 408-977-4549; http://www.ihr.com/planetre.html. Planetree will also do a PDQ search for $25 per topic or a Medline search for $35 per topic. Medline searches are included in the comprehensive package, as are book excerpts and magazine articles. The **Medical Information Service of the Palo Alto Medical Foundation** was founded as a nonprofit service for medical professionals. They also provide information for the general public. A standard search, including Medline costs $89: 800-999-1999 or 650-321-4121; 795 El Camino Road, Palo Alto, CA 94301; http://www.pamf.org/. The **Medical Data Exchange** offers a search on its own consumer health data base, MDX Health Digest, at a cost of $25. A Medline search is $48. If you need a more exhaustive, customized search, it's $60 an hour. This company also began as a data source for health professionals, but recently launched into searches for lay people. 503-471-1627 or http://www.medicalexchange.com/.

The **National Center for Health Statistics:** http://www.cdc.gov/nchs is a web site that provides information on mortality data that includes life expectancy and infant mortality rates. It also includes news releases and fact sheets of a variety of health related and demographic topics.

The **U.S. National Library of Medicine (NLM):** http://www.nlm.nih.gov/, is the worlds largest medical library. It collects materials in all major areas of health sciences..

The **Combined Health Information Database (CHID)** is a database produced by health-related agencies of the Federal Government. This database provides titles, abstracts, and availability information for health information and health education resources. It includes thousands of books, journal articles, audio/video tapes, and other patient education materials on a wide variety of health topics. CHID is user friendly and free. Contact the National Institute on Aging web site: http://chid.nih.gov/ or call: 800-438-4380.

Health, United States, 1999 with Health and Aging Chartbook is a comprehensive analysis of the current data on aging, covering population characteristics, health status and health care utilization. Available from the Center of Disease Control, National

Center for Health Statistics, it can be ordered through the web site: http://www.cdc.gov/nchs/agingact.htm.

HELPFUL 'LISTSERVS'

A listserv is an electronic mailing list, much like a broadcast fax. It is used with e-mail and is a great way to share ideas among peers and contemporaries. Access to these listservs is free. The following is a short list of some listservs you may wish to subscribe to. To join any or all of these listservs, send an e-mail to the address indicated, use no subject in the subject line and on the first line in the body of the message type: Subscribe *listname your name* and send it. Voilà!

- Listserv@nihlist.bitnet—DS-H-PI—discussion on independence and handicap issues in ICIDH.
- Listserv@ubvm.bitnet—GERINET—geriatric health issues.
- Listserv@ukcc.uky.edu—HEALTHRE—health care reform.
- Listserv@mizzoul.missouri.edu—MHCARE-L—managed health care.
- Listserv@vm.utcc.utoronto.edu—PARKINSN—Parkinson's disease information exchange.
- Listserv@uky.edu—STROKE-L—CVA discussion list.

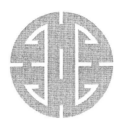

Index